Medical Radiology

Diagnostic Imaging

Series editors
Hans-Ulrich Kauczor
Paul M. Parizel
Wilfred C. G. Peh

For further volumes:
http://www.springer.com/series/4354

Michael Riccabona
Editor

Pediatric Urogenital Radiology

Third Edition

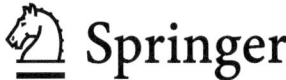

Editor
Michael Riccabona
Division of Pediatric Radiology
University Hospital, LKH Graz
Graz
Austria

ISSN 0942-5373　　　　　　ISSN 2197-4187　(electronic)
Medical Radiology
ISBN 978-3-030-13248-4　　ISBN 978-3-319-39202-8　(eBook)
https://doi.org/10.1007/978-3-319-39202-8

© Springer International Publishing AG, part of Springer Nature 2001, 2008, 2018
Softcover re-print of the Hardcover 3rd edition 2018
This work is subject to copyright. All rights are reserved by the Publisher, whether the whole or part of the material is concerned, specifically the rights of translation, reprinting, reuse of illustrations, recitation, broadcasting, reproduction on microfilms or in any other physical way, and transmission or information storage and retrieval, electronic adaptation, computer software, or by similar or dissimilar methodology now known or hereafter developed.
The use of general descriptive names, registered names, trademarks, service marks, etc. in this publication does not imply, even in the absence of a specific statement, that such names are exempt from the relevant protective laws and regulations and therefore free for general use.
The publisher, the authors and the editors are safe to assume that the advice and information in this book are believed to be true and accurate at the date of publication. Neither the publisher nor the authors or the editors give a warranty, express or implied, with respect to the material contained herein or for any errors or omissions that may have been made. The publisher remains neutral with regard to jurisdictional claims in published maps and institutional affiliations.

Printed on acid-free paper

This Springer imprint is published by the registered company Springer International Publishing AG part of Springer Nature
The registered company address is: Gewerbestrasse 11, 6330 Cham, Switzerland

Preface to the Third Revised Edition

It is an honor for me having been entrusted with editing this new third edition of the standard textbook *Pediatric Uroradiology*; however, it took quite some time and effort get everything done.

Looking back over time to the first edition of this textbook more than a decade ago, one realizes that not that much has changed for many queries in spite of ongoing discussions on varying concepts, experts' opinions and recommendations, new insights into pathophysiology, and new imaging options as well as new applications of existing modalities or refinement of existing techniques. And still, there is restricted high-level evidence for deciding on how to best image our pediatric patients for many pediatric urogenital conditions.

Nevertheless, some basic trends can be observed and are also reflected in this new edition. There is a general tendency towards reducing invasiveness and radiation burden to our pediatric patients, and it is widely recommended to more strictly adhere to a "therapeutic thinking efficacy," i.e., imaging must have an impact on patient treatment and management. Thus, the numbers of voiding cystourethrograms have in most centers significantly decreased, antibiotic treatment for uncomplicated vesicoureteric reflux is less often prescribed, or intravenous urography has been mostly outdated and replaced by modern ultrasound or MRI for the common pediatric queries.

Additionally, the growing economic pressure (in the USA with the aim of making money from health care, in Europe for saving money by restricting medical services) has led to a new thinking and concept in pediatric medicine and also pediatric radiology, i.e., only treatment and related diagnostic measures that impact further outcome, prognosis, and development are administered. Thus, imaging modalities that probably do not necessarily effect patient morbidity and mortality are questioned, particularly if they imply invasiveness or burden such as radiation, sedation, or contrast agent application.

Finally, considering the new development towards "personalized medicine" and the growing demand for interdisciplinary diagnostic and therapeutic approaches, additional in-depth knowledge on clinical basics, diagnostic needs, embryology, and pathogenesis, as well as therapeutic options and consequences, is becoming indispensable for the radiologist to enable an understanding of what imaging must provide in terms of diagnosis and management decision information. In the recent years, fetal imaging has become an established part of pediatric uroradiology, too: not only that it detects conditions that have to be addressed after birth by pediatric radiology but increasingly pediatric radiologists are performing fetal body MR imaging themselves.

Taking all these aspects into consideration, this new edition has been restructured into four main sections: the methods, the anatomy and embryology, the clinical information, and the imaging section. As such, it contains some new chapters – e.g., a completely new chapter on fetal imaging has been introduced, and dedicated clinical chapters are provided that shall offer a comprehensive insight into the various conditions and diseases. Furthermore, all old chapters have been revised or updated and some were completely rewritten. New illustrations have been added and recent new knowledge, insights, and changes in imaging approaches (e.g., contrast-enhanced ultrasonography; modern MRI applications and techniques) have been integrated. Hence, this third edition aims to address all these aspects, but without disregarding the valuable and necessary established "old" imaging procedures that may still be indicated for well-defined diseases and conditions.

As with this diversity of approaches and persisting restricted evidence in many of the pediatric uroradiology conditions, a somewhat varying and partially overlapping presentation of the individual contributors to this third edition is intended – in order to allow for an informed reflection of the continuous re-orientation process in pediatric urogenital imaging. To achieve this objective, a broad context and knowledge of all possible options and conditions that are mandatory for understanding are provided clearly to satisfy the needs of practicing pediatric radiologists, pediatricians, pediatric surgeons, urologists, and nephrologists. Furthermore, up-to-date information and reference are provided for researchers.

Only with the help of the distinguished and renowned faculty of international experts in the field of diagnostic and interventional pediatric uroradiology as well as neighboring fields (e.g., pediatric surgeons/urologists/nephrologists and pediatricians) who contributed to this revised new edition, this new edition hopefully a has become comprehensive volume containing all the latest advances thus fulfilling the demands of a textbook covering all aspects at the most modern and newest of the art.

Last but not least, I want to acknowledge the dedication and expertise of each contributor and I thank all authors sincerely for their hard efforts and their excellent contributions as well as their patience. I do hope that – as the first two editions – this new edition will again become a standard working and reference text for pediatric urogenital radiology that helps in improving our service to the pediatric patients, the future generation.

Graz, Austria Michael Riccabona
2018

Preface to the Second Edition

Never before in the history of pediatric uroradiology have concepts, expert opinions and recommendations changed as significantly and as quickly as over the last 5–7 years. Even established scientific concepts which we thought would never be debated again, are now back on the discussion table. This even applies to the treatment and imaging management of very common but serious nephrourological disorders such as urinary tract infection and vesicoureteric reflux, where the benefit of antibiotic prophylaxis and therefore the role of imaging are called in to question. These changes are not only triggered by the latest scientific findings, some of which contradict formerly established scientific concepts, but by the growing awareness of evidence-based medicine and, last but not least, also by new imaging techniques and technologies.

However, many old concepts still remain and many facts established in the last millennium are still true and pertinent today. This leads to some confusion even among experts, who are still searching for consensus-based imaging management recommendations.

Therefore, the invitation to compile a second revised and extended edition of the book *Pediatric Uroradiology* came at the right moment. In many aspects, the first edition could be used as a reliable basis for the development of the second edition. Thus this new book embraces both the new, taking recent advances in knowledge and technology into account, and the old. It is a complete rewrite where necessary, containing new contents with regard to latest developments such as genetics, and it provides the newest recommendations and discussions on clinical and imaging management of common nephrourologic disorders.

Thanks to the contributions of the distinguished and renowned international experts in the field of diagnostic and interventional pediatric uroradiology and of neighbouring fields such as genetics and pediatric nephrourology, a comprehensive volume containing all the latest advances could again be prepared, fulfilling the demands of a textbook covering all aspects of pediatric uroradiology in its broadest context. This book should satisfy the needs of the practising (pediatric) radiologist, pediatrician, pediatric surgeon and urologist; it should also offer up-to-date information and references to the researcher.

In view of the ongoing, rapid and significant changes, it was the intention of the editor to include a number of somewhat varying and overlapping views of the individual contributors for this second edition. Precisely this approach guarantees the requisite comprehensiveness and allows a degree of diversity reflecting the continuous reorientation process in pediatric uroradiology.

Again, it was a great honour and pleasure to work as an editor for this book project. I would like to acknowledge the dedication and expertise of each contributor, and I thank all of them sincerely.

Mrs. Irene Stradner, my secretary, was an indispensable member of our team; she did a marvelous job for this book project and I would like to express my warmest gratitude to her.

I hope that this second revised edition will again become a standard working and reference text for pediatric uroradiology.

Graz, Austria   Richard Fotter

Preface to the First Edition

A substantial change in the diagnostic and therapeutic management of urogenital disorders in children has taken place in recent years. There are two main reasons for this phenomenon: first, the growing integration of (new) imaging modalities such as magnetic resonance imaging and helical computed tomography and of advanced ultrasound techniques into pediatric uroradiologic imaging protocols; second, dramatic advances in our knowledge on the natural history of important urogenital pathologies of childhood as a consequence of maternal–fetal screening ultrasound.

Changing indications and limitations and comprehensive multimodality interpretation should be in the field of the (pediatric) radiologist's expertise. To enhance the role of the radiologist, she/he should have a profound knowledge of urinary symptoms as well as the principles of medical and surgical treatment in children and should also be able to interpret laboratory data.

This growing challenge for the (pediatric) radiologist seems to justify the idea of a book specifically devoted to pediatric uroradiology. Therefore, we were delighted to be invited by the series editor, Prof. Baert, to write such a book. Thanks to the contributions of the well-known international experts in the field of diagnostic and interventional pediatric genitourinary radiology who wrote the different chapters, a comprehensive volume could be prepared fulfilling the demands on a textbook covering all aspects of pediatric uroradiology in its broadest context. The book is written to satisfy the needs of the practicing radiologist and pediatrician but also to offer up-to-date information and references to the researcher.

In view of the above-mentioned changes in the field, one central goal was to discuss the reorientation of diagnostic and interventional radiological approaches to problems of the pediatric genitourinary tract and to elucidate the contributions made by different diagnostic and interventional uroradiologic techniques.

The focus of this book is primarily the point of view of the (pediatric) radiologist, but it offers all the necessary information for the pediatrician, pediatric surgeon and urologist as well putting decisions on imaging management on a reasonable basis. To meet the demands on a (pediatric) radiologist today, pertinent clinical observations, important pathophysiologic concepts, operative options, postoperative complications and clinical as well as radiological normal values have been included.

Dedicated chapters are devoted to specific problems of the newborn and infant, such as imaging and interpretation of upper urinary tract dilatation, postnatal imaging of fetal uropathies, associated urinary problems with imperforate anus, epispadias–exstrophy complex and lower urinary tract anomalies of urogenital sinus and female genital anomalies.

Detailed discussions focus on the management of common problems in pediatric uroradiology such as urinary tract infection, vesicoureteric reflux and functional disorders of the lower urinary tract including enuresis and incontinence.

In dedicated contributions, embryology and the changing anatomy and physiology and pathophysiology of the growing organism are discussed to facilitate understanding of the disease processes and anticipated complications and form the rationale for interventions.

Specific chapters deal with agenesis, dysplasia, parenchymal diseases, neoplastic diseases, stone disease, vascular hypertension, renal failure and renal transplantation and genitourinary trauma in children. Specific problems of childhood neurogenic bladder are discussed.

Interventional uroradiologic procedures in children are discussed in full detail not only to show their value in treatment and diagnosis of a given problem, but also to serve as a source guiding the performance of these interventions.

It was the intention of the editor to respect the views of the individual contributors as far as possible. This is reflected in a diverse writing style and some degree of overlap and repetition. In the opinion of the editor, just this approach guarantees the necessary comprehensiveness.

After an always enjoyable time as editor I would like to acknowledge the dedication and expertise of each contributor; I thank all of them sincerely. Mrs. Renate Pammer, my secretary, was an important member of our team and I would like to express my warmest gratitude to her for the excellent job she did for this book project.

We all hope that this book will be accepted as the standard working and reference text for pediatric uroradiology. Moreover, we hope that it will prove useful to physicians in training and specialists alike as a reference source during preparation for examinations and conferences. The bibliography should readily satisfy the needs of all kinds of readers.

Graz, Austria   Richard Fotter

Contents

Part I   Diagnostic Procedures

Diagnostic Procedures: Excluding MRI, Nuclear Medicine and Video Urodynamics 3
Aikaterini Ntoulia, Jean-Nicolas Dacher, and Michael Riccabona

MR of the Urogenital Tract in Children 33
J. Damien Grattan-Smith and Richard A. Jones

Nuclear Medicine 93
Marina Easty and Isky Gordon

Video Urodynamics 113
Erich Sorantin, Katrin Braun, and Richard Fotter

Nomenclature and Reporting 117
Pierre-Hugues Vivier and Freddy Avni

Contrast Agents in Childhood: Application and Safety Considerations 123
Michael Riccabona and Hans-Joachim Mentzel

Part II   Fetal Findings, Embryology, Anatomy, Normal Variants

Urinary Tract Embryology, Anatomy, and Anatomical Variants .. 135
Aikaterini Ntoulia, Frederica Papadopoulou, and Gabriele Benz-Bohm

Urogenital Fetal Imaging: US and MRI 151
Marie Cassart

Anomalies of Kidney Rotation, Position, and Fusion 167
Samuel Stafrace and Gabriele Benz-Bohm

Part III   Clinical Statements and Basics: What Every (Pediatric) Uroradiologist Ought to Know

Genetics in Nephrourology 181
Klaus Zerres, Miriam Elbracht, and Sabine Rudnik

**Renal Agenesis, Dysplasia, Hypoplasia, and Cystic Diseases
of the Kidney**... 195
Christoph Mache and Holger Hubmann

Renal Parenchymal Disease.................................. 205
Ekkehard Ring and Birgit Acham-Roschitz

UTI and VUR 219
Rolf Beetz

Congenital Urinary Tract Dilatation and Obstructive Uropathy... 243
Josef Oswald and Bernhard Haid

Surgical Procedures and Indications for Surgery 255
Annette Schröder and Wolfgang H. Rösch

Urolithiasis and Nephrocalcinosis........................... 269
Bernd Hoppe

Renal Failure and Renal Transplantation 283
Ekkehard Ring, Holger Hubmann, and Birgit Acham-Roschitz

Part IV Lower Urinary Tract Anomalies, Malformations and Dysfunctions

Abnormalities of the Lower Urinary Tract and Urachus......... 299
Samuel Stafrace, Marie Brasseur-Daudruy,
and Jean-Nicolas Dacher

Female Genital Anomalies and Important Ovarian Conditions ... 317
Gisela Schweigmann, Theresa E. Geley, and Ingmar Gassner

Imaging in Male Genital Queries 353
Thomas A. Augdal, Lil-Sofie Ording-Müller, and Michael Riccabona

Urinary Problems Associated with Imperforate Anus 373
Erich Sorantin, Michael E. Höllwarth, and Sandra Abou Samaan

Epispadias-Exstrophy Complex............................. 385
Erich Sorantin and Sandra Abou Samaan

**Non-neurogenic Bladder-Sphincter Dysfunction
("Voiding Dysfunction")**.. 397
Michael Riccabona and Richard Fotter

Neurogenic Bladder in Infants and Children................. 423
Erich Sorantin, R. Fotter, and K. Braun

Part V Congenital Malformations, Vesico-Ureteric Reflux, and Postoperative Imaging

Congenital Anomalies of the Renal Pelvis and Ureter........... 433
Freddy Avni, Elisa Amzallag-Bellenger, Marianne Tondeur,
and Pierre-Hugues Vivier

Upper Urinary Tract Dilatation in Newborns and Infants and the Postnatal Work-Up of Congenital Uro-nephropathies 465
Freddy Avni, Marianne Tondeur, and Rene-Hilaire Priso

Imaging in Prune Belly Syndrome and Other Syndromes Affecting the Urogenital Tract 481
Gundula Staatz and Wolfgang Rascher

Vesicoureteric Reflux 491
Freddy Avni, Marianne Tondeur, Frederica Papadopoulou, and Annie Lahoche

Postoperative Imaging and Findings 517
Michael Riccabona, Josef Oswald, and Veronica Donoghue

Part VI Renal Parenchymal and Cystic Disease, Urolithiasis, Renal Failure and Transplantation

Imaging in Urinary Tract Infections 537
Lil-Sofie Ording Muller, Freddy Avni, and Michael Riccabona

Imaging in Renal Agenesis, Dysplasia, Hypoplasia, and Cystic Diseases of the Kidney 553
Michael Riccabona, Ekkehard Ring, and Freddy Avni

Imaging in Renal Parenchymal Disease 579
Michael Riccabona and Ekkehard Ring

Imaging of Urolithiasis and Nephrocalcinosis 603
Michael Francavilla, Kassa Darge, and Gabriele Benz-Bohm

Imaging in Renal Failure, Neonatal Oligoanuria, and Renal Transplantation 615
Maria Beatrice Damasio, Christoph Mache, and Michael Riccabona

Renovascular Hypertension 641
Frederica Papadopoulou and Melanie P. Hiorns

Part VII Urinary Tract Tumors, Trauma and Intervention

Neoplasms of the Genitourinary System 653
Eline Deurloo, Hervé Brisse, and Anne Smets

Urinary Tract Trauma 701
Maria Luisa Lobo and Jean-Nicolas Dacher

Pediatric Genitourinary Intervention 721
Richard Towbin, David Aria, Trevor Davis, Robin Kaye, and Carrie Schaefer

Part VIII   Management, Guidelines, Recommendations and Beyond Including Normal Values

Clinical Management of Common Nephrourologic Disorders (Guidelines and Beyond) 753
Michael Riccabona, Ekkehard Ring, and Hans-Joachim Mentzel

Normal Values 773
Ekkehard Ring, Hans-Joachim Mentzel, and Michael Riccabona

Index 785

Contributors

Sandra Abou Samaan Department of Radiology, Hamad General Hospital, Doha, Qatar

Birgit Acham-Roschitz Department of Pediatrics, Division of General Pediatrics, University Hospital Graz, Graz, Austria

Elisa Amzallag-Bellenger Department of Pediatric Imaging, Jeanne de Flandre Mother and Child Hospital, Lille University Hospitals, Lille, France

David Aria Department of Medical Imaging, Phoenix Children's Hospital, Phoenix, AZ, USA

Thomas A. Augdal Department of Radiology, University Hospital of North Norway, Tromsø, Norway

Freddy Avni Department of Pediatric Radiology, Jeanne de Flandre Hospital, Lille University Hospital, Lille, France

Rolf Beetz Pediatric Nephrology, Center for Paediatrics and Adolescent Medicine, University Medical Clinic, Mainz, Germany

Gabriele Benz-Bohm (Retired) Department of Radiology, Division of Pediatric Radiology, University of Cologne, Cologne, Germany

Marie Brasseur-Daudruy Department of Radiology, University Hospital of Rouen, Rouen, France

Katrin Braun Department of Pediatric and Adolescent Surgery, Medical University Graz, Graz, Austria

Hervé Brisse Department of Radiology, Institut Curie, Paris, France

Marie Cassart Department of Fetal and Pediatric Imaging, Etterbeek-Ixelles Hospital, Brussels, Belgium

Jean-Nicolas Dacher Department of Radiology, University Hospital of Rouen, Rouen, France

Maria Beatrice Damasio Department of Radiology, Division of Radiology, Giannina Gaslini Institute, Genoa, Italy

Kassa Darge Department of Radiology, Children's Hospital of Philadelphia, Philadelphia, PA, USA

Trevor Davis Pediatric Interventional Radiology, Phoenix Children's Hospital, Phoenix, AZ, USA

Eline Deurloo Department of Radiology, Academic Medical Center, Amsterdam, The Netherlands

Veronica Donoghue Departments of Radiology, Temple Street Children's University Hospital, Dublin, Ireland

National Maternity Hospital, Dublin, Ireland

Marina Easty Great Ormond Street Hospital NHS Foundation Trust, London, UK

Miriam Elbracht Institute of Humangenetics, RWTH Aachen University, Aachen, Germany

Richard Fotter (Retired) Department of Radiology, Division of Pediatric Radiology, Medical University Graz, Graz, Austria

Michael Francavilla Department of Radiology, Children's Hospital of Philadelphia, Philadelphia, PA, USA

Ingmar Gassner (Retired) Section of Pediatric Radiology, Medical University of Innsbruck, Innsbruck, Austria

Theresa E. Geley Section of Pediatric Radiology, Medical University of Innsbruck, Innsbruck, Austria

Isky Gordon (Retired) Great Ormond Street Hospital NHS Foundation Trust, London, UK

J. Damien Grattan-Smith Department of Radiology, Children's Healthcare of Atlanta, Atlanta, GA, USA

Bernhard Haid Department of Pediatric Urology, Hospital of the Sisters of Charity, Linz, Austria

Melanie P. Hiorns Great Ormond Street Hospital for Children, London, UK

Michael E. Höllwarth (Retired) Department of Pediatric and Adolescent Surgery, Medical University Graz, Graz, Austria

Bernd Hoppe University of Bonn, Department of Pediatrics, Division of Pediatric Nephrology, Bonn, Germany

Holger Hubmann Department of Paediatrics, Division of General Paediatrics, Medical University Graz, Graz, Austria

Richard A. Jones Department of Radiology, Emory University School of Medicine, Atlanta, GA, USA

Robin Kaye Department of Medical Imaging, Phoenix Children's Hospital, Phoenix, AZ, USA

Annie Lahoche Department of Pediatric Nephrology, Jeanne de Flandre Hospitals, Lille, France

Maria Luisa Lobo Department of Radiology, University Hospital of Santa Maria, HSM-CHLN, Lisboa, Portugal

Christoph Mache Department of Paediatrics, Division of General Paediatrics, Medical University Graz, Graz, Austria

Hans-Joachim Mentzel Section of Paediatric Radiology, Institute of Diagnostic and Interventional Radiology, University Hospital Jena, Jena, Germany

Lil-Sofie Ording Müller Department of Radiology and Nuclear Medicine, Unit for Paediatric Radiology, Oslo University Hospital, Oslo, Norway

Aikaterini Ntoulia Department of Radiology, Children's Hospital of Philadelphia, Philadelphia, PA, USA

Josef Oswald Department of Pediatric Urology, Hospital of the Sisters of Charity, Linz, Austria

Frederica Papadopoulou Pediatric Ultrasound Center Thessaloniki, Thessaloniki, Ioannina, Greece

Radiology, Ioannina University, Ioannina, Greece

Rene-Hilaire Priso Department of Pediatric Imaging, Jeanne de Flandre Hospital, Lille University Hopsitals, Lille, France

Wolfgang Rascher Kinder- und Jugendklinik, Universitätsklinikum Erlangen, Erlangen, Germany

Michael Riccabona Department of Radiology, Division of Pediatric Radiology, LKH University Hospital, Graz, Austria

Ekkehard Ring (Retired) Department of Pediatrics, Division of General Pediatrics, University Hospital Graz, Graz, Austria

Wolfgang H. Rösch Department of Pediatric Urology, University Medical Center Regensburg, Regensburg, Germany

Sabine Rudnik Sektion Humangenetik, Medizinische Universität Innsbruck, Innsbruck, Austria

Carrie Schaefer Department of Medical Imaging, Phoenix Children's Hospital, Phoenix, AZ, USA

Annette Schröder Department of Pediatric Urology, University Medical Center Regensburg, Regensburg, Germany

Gisela Schweigmann Section of Pediatric Radiology, Medical University of Innsbruck, Innsbruck, Austria

Anne Smets Department of Radiology, Academic Medical Center, Amsterdam, The Netherlands

Erich Sorantin Department of Radiology, Division of Pediatric Radiology, Medical University Graz, Graz, Austria

Gundula Staatz Department of Radiology, Section of Pediatric Radiology, Medical Center of the Johannes Gutenberg University, Mainz, Germany

Samuel Stafrace Sidra Medical and Research Center, Doha, Qatar

Marianne Tondeur Department of Radio-Isotopes, CHU Saint-Pierre, Brussels, Belgium

Richard Towbin Phoenix Children's Hospital, Phoenix, AZ, USA

Pierre-Hugues Vivier Service de Radiologie, CHU Charles-Nicolle, Rouen Cedex, France

X-Ray Expert, Maison Médicale, Hôpital Privé de l'Estuaire, Le Havre, France

Klaus Zerres Institute of Humangenetics, RWTH Aachen University, Aachen, Germany

Part I

Diagnostic Procedures

Diagnostic Procedures: Excluding MRI, Nuclear Medicine and Video Urodynamics

Aikaterini Ntoulia, Jean-Nicolas Dacher, and Michael Riccabona

Contents

1	**Introduction**	3
2	**Kidneys-Ureter-Bladder Radiograph**	4
2.1	Introduction	4
2.2	Indications	4
2.3	Equipment	6
2.4	Acquisition Technique	6
3	**Ultrasound**	7
3.1	Introduction	7
3.2	Indications	7
3.3	Equipment	11
3.4	Preparation	12
3.5	Scanning Technique	12
4	**Contrast-Enhanced Ultrasonography**	15
4.1	Introduction	15
4.2	Contrast-Enhanced Voiding Urosonography	15
4.3	Contrast-Enhanced Ultrasonography with Intravenous Administration of Ultrasound Contrast Agents	18
5	**Sono-elastography**	19
6	**Voiding Cystourethrography**	20
6.1	Introduction	20
6.2	Indications	20
6.3	Equipment	21
6.4	Preparation	21
6.5	Procedure	21
7	**Retrograde Urethrography**	24
8	**Intravenous Urography**	24
9	**Computed Tomography of the Urinary Tract (uro-CT)**	25
9.1	Introduction	25
9.2	Indications	25
9.3	Preparation	26
9.4	Acquisition Technique	26
	Conclusion	28
	References	28

1 Introduction

In the introduction of his course on Pediatric Uroradiology at Harvard Medical School, Prof. Robert L. Lebowitz cited the following sentence by LL. Weed: "Just as important as doing the thing right is doing the right thing". This is an excellent introduction to this chapter.

Imaging of the urinary tract is among the most commonly requested examinations in

A. Ntoulia, MD, PhD
Department of Radiology, Children's Hospital of Philadelphia, Philadelphia, PA, USA

J.-N. Dacher
Department of Radiology, University Hospital of Rouen, Rouen, France

M. Riccabona (✉)
Department of Radiology, Division of Pediatric Radiology, LKH University Hospital, Graz, Austria
e-mail: michael.riccabona@meduni-graz.at

paediatric radiology practice. In children, the lack of specificity of abdominal symptoms and the high prevalence of renal and urinary tract disease justify the high volume of these requests. Recent technological advances have significantly improved the diagnostic capabilities of existing imaging modalities and have further introduced advanced imaging applications in routine clinical practice, maximising the diagnostic yield. From a radiologists' perspective, it is important to know the clinical indications for the requested examination and what the referring physician expects of its results, so that the appropriate examination will be undertaken. Direct communication with the referring physician is always recommended, especially if there is any discrepancy between the examination request form, the medical records and the parents/children's interview.

This chapter aims to give a comprehensive overview of the diagnostic imaging procedures most commonly used for evaluation of the paediatric urinary tract. We hope it will provide the background for understanding the indications and the strategies on how to perform properly each examination and refresh some basic understanding of the anatomy as necessary for properly performing and reading these studies. X-ray procedures, conventional ultrasound and advanced ultrasound applications (e.g. Doppler techniques, extended field of view, harmonic imaging, contrast-enhanced ultrasound, sono-elastography) as well as computed tomography are described. Intravenous urography will only be mentioned briefly, as it has largely been replaced by magnetic resonance urography and is less frequently performed in children today, though in some, particularly low resource settings, it still may be the only available tool, and some potential indications still exist. Each subsection starts with the main indications for the study concerned, followed by updated technical and procedural recommendations and imaging strategies. Normal findings and clinical background as well as established query-defined imaging algorithms are discussed in the respective chapters of the book.

2 Kidneys-Ureter-Bladder Radiograph

2.1 Introduction

A plain film of the abdomen, known as kidneys-ureter-bladder (KUB) radiograph, is a widely available and relatively inexpensive imaging modality, frequently requested for initial evaluation of various abdominal pathologies and conditions (Dorfman et al. 2011). It is an anteroposterior radiograph, obtained in supine position and coned to include the abdomen from the diaphragm to the symphysis pubis, flank to flank.

2.2 Indications

A KUB film can provide preliminary overview information in children with suspected congenital, obstructive, traumatic, inflammatory or neoplastic processes and might be useful in differentiating gastrointestinal from urological conditions. However, it is important to mention that although KUB films are frequently and easily requested as a baseline imaging examination, they yield low diagnostic outcome in terms of accurately characterising intra-abdominal pathology. For this reason, KUB films have largely been supplanted in paediatric diagnostic practice by ultrasound as a highly sensitive and radiation-free first-line imaging modality. Other common queries for KUB films include evaluation of catheters, stents, drains and other medical device positioning, as well as search for foreign bodies (Rothrock et al. 1992).

Designated evaluation of the urinary tract on a KUB film warrants careful assessment of kidneys' soft tissue densities that provides basic information regarding their size, shape

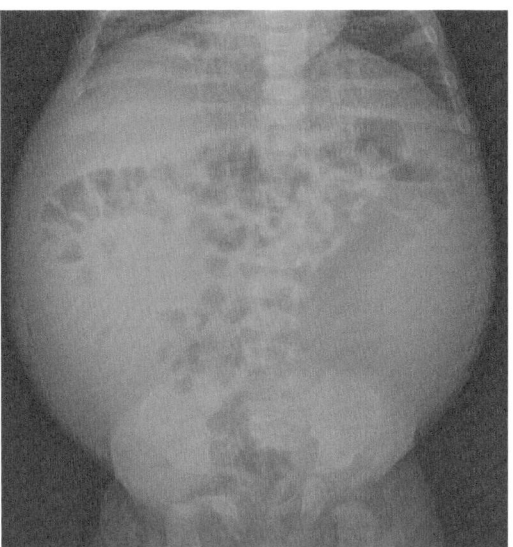

Fig. 1 KUB radiograph, in a neonate with autosomal recessive polycystic kidney disease (ARPKD). Distention of the abdomen with bulging of both flanks, central distribution of bowel loops and medial deviation of the descending colon are highly indicative of bilateral massive renal enlargement

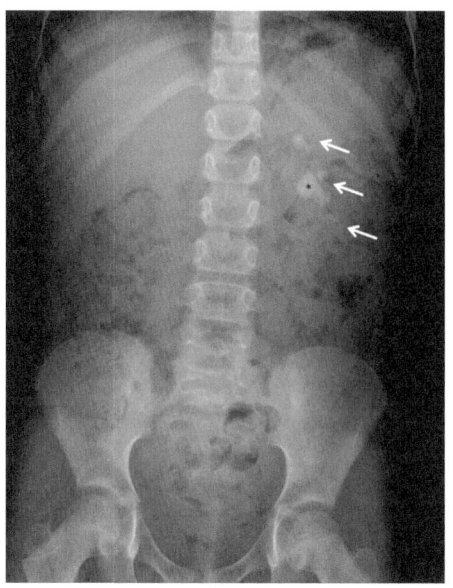

Fig. 2 KUB radiograph, in a 7-year-old female with persistent urinary tract infection from *Proteus mirabilis*. Partial staghorn calculus within the left kidney, forming a cast of the renal pelvis (*asterisk*) and branching within at least three major calyces (*arrows*)

and position and may reveal related abnormalities (Fig. 1). The transverse processes of the lumbar vertebrae act as anatomic landmarks for the course of the ureters. The latter insert into the urinary bladder at the level of the ischial spines.

A KUB film can reveal radiopaque stones along the urinary tract and reassess their size and position after urologic interventions (Fig. 2). Additionally it can demonstrate cortical or medullary calcifications related to a variety of metabolic, genetic or acquired pathologic conditions (Fig. 3) (Habbig et al. 2011). Urolithiasis and nephrocalcinosis should be differentiated from extra-urinary calcifications such as adrenal calcifications, appendicoliths or pelvic phleboliths (Rothrock et al. 1992) (Fig. 4). The presence of irregular calcifications associated with a soft tissue mass and bowel displacement is indicative of a neoplastic process and further dedicated imaging is typically performed for further diagnosis and staging (Fig. 5).

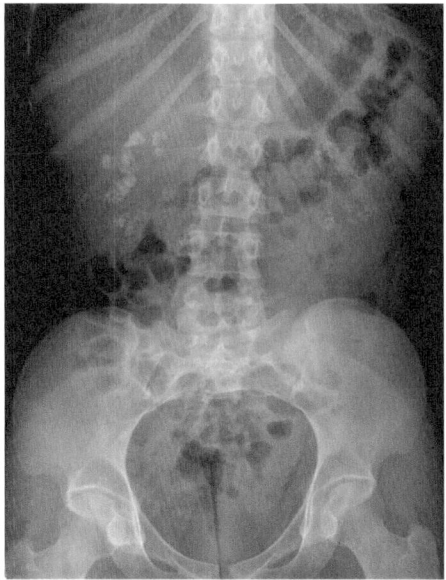

Fig. 3 KUB radiograph in a 16-year-old female with systemic lupus erythematosus and hypercalcaemia. Clusters of calcifications are deposited centrally within both kidneys, corresponding to the shape and position of the renal pyramids, consistent with medullary nephrocalcinosis

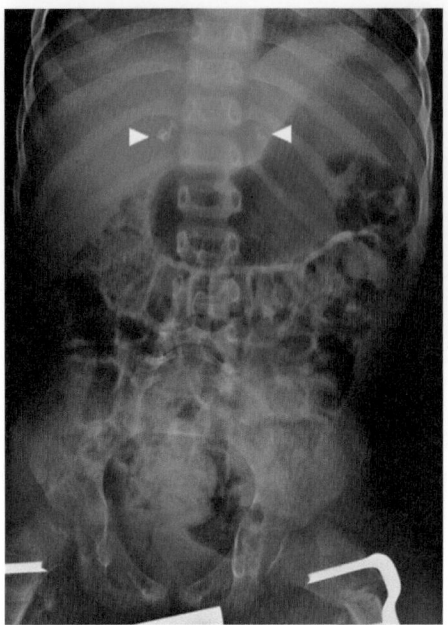

Fig. 4 KUB radiograph, in a 5-year-old male with prenatal history of asphyxia. Adrenal calcifications: bilateral dense calcifications, with triangular configuration, located in the region of the adrenal glands, adjacent to the spine

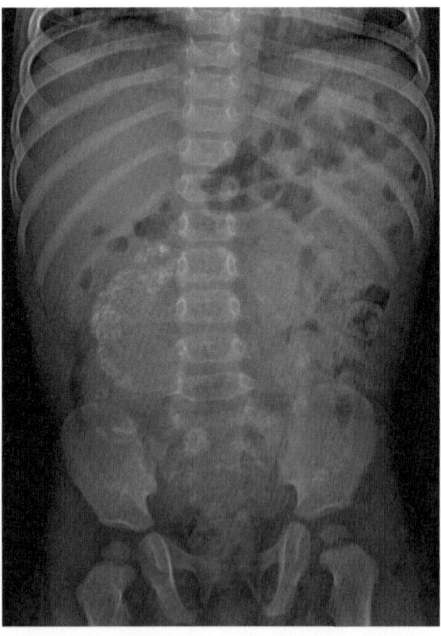

Fig. 5 KUB radiograph, in a 13-month-old male with palpable abdominal mass. The presence of abundant amorphous calcifications, associated with soft tissue density mass located centrally within the abdomen and extending to the level of the upper pelvis, causing displacement of bowel loops. Further diagnostic workup confirmed that the mass was consistent with neuroblastoma

Interpretation of KUB films should also include careful evaluation of the visualised skeletal structures of the spine, pelvis and lower ribs. Vertebral and genitourinary abnormalities are frequently associated due to the skeletal-genitourinary embryologic link at the early stages of development. Additionally, in cases of poor renal function, slip of the femoral epiphysis may occur, or renal osteodystrophy may become obvious.

2.3 Equipment

Significant technological innovations have resulted in the development of high-end digital radiography systems with many advantages over the traditional film-screen-based technology. The latter has been replaced in many radiology departments, although may still be present in lower resource settings. Modern radiography systems, including direct digital radiography and computed radiography, acquire images of high contrast and resolution and achieve also dose reduction, provided that the settings, filters and algorithms are adapted to paediatric needs and patients' age (Korner et al. 2007; Sorantin 2008; Don et al. 2011). Obtained radiographs are transferred to dedicated workstations and can be electronically archived and retrieved for future reference without loss of image quality. These can be further configured with advanced post-processing techniques to achieve optimal imaging display on a case-required basis. Moreover images can be readily accessible by other physicians within the hospital network and be even remotely distributed, contributing to significant workflow efficiency, provided the respective viewing stations have a diagnostically sufficient monitor resolution.

2.4 Acquisition Technique

Prior to KUB examination, all clothes should be removed, since contained metallic zippers, buttons and other clothing parts might obscure substantial findings if projected within the examined area. Diapers should also be removed, particularly if wet, in order to avoid the overlying appearance of the characteristic coalescent, nodular, radio-dense artefact caused due to urine absorption by the diaper polymer (Markowitz et al. 2009). This artefact may significantly interfere with imaging of the lower pelvis structures. Hospital gowns, if available, should be provided.

The child is positioned supine on the examination bed and is temporarily immobilised, usually with the help of the parents who can be present during the examination, with special attention to avoid overlying of artifactual densities within the imaged field of view.

Local lead shields should be used to protect radiosensitive organs, such as the thyroid, eyes, breast buds and gonads, whenever it is feasible, particularly if not interfering with the region of interest.

The wide range of paediatric body sizes plays a significant role in the radiographic technique. Selection of the appropriate image receptor size relative to the child's body size is necessary to improve image quality and decrease the amount of scattered radiation. Most KUB radiographs are obtained at 110–115 cm source image distance (SID). Proper beam collimation is required for all patients to limit the exposure to the anatomic area of interest. The use of grids, although can effectively eliminate scatter radiation in adults, is not suggested in small children. However it should be considered an option in adult-size adolescents and obese children, with body parts more than 10–12 cm in thickness (Willis 2009). Similarly, the use of automatic exposure control (AEC) sensors, although is typically preferred to deliver consistent exposure in adults, is not suggested in children, as these sensors tend to remain partially or completely uncovered and thus inactive in small-size children, leading to noise-degraded images (Goske et al. 2011). Therefore, manual selection of kVp and mAs settings in children is suggested, tailored to patient size and clinical indication, with low kVp techniques (60–75 kVp) being generally preferable depending on the detector specifications (Willis 2009; Goske et al. 2011; Don et al. 2013).

The exposure should be taken when the child is still, to avoid blurred images and potentially repeated examination. Images should be reviewed for diagnostic quality before the patient is released.

Take Away
A KUB film provides baseline overview evaluation of various abdominal pathologies and conditions, however, with quite low diagnostic yield in characterising intra-abdominal pathology. It has been largely supplanted in most of its indications with ultrasound.

3 Ultrasound

3.1 Introduction

Ultrasound (US) is a non-invasive, highly sensitive, widely available and cost-effective imaging modality that is routinely used as the first-line examination for the diagnosis of several developmental and acquired conditions and diseases of the urinary tract in children (Muller-Ording 2014; Riccabona 2014a, b). The lack of ionising radiation and the excellent anatomic resolution owing to the small amount of fat in children make US an outstanding technique for paediatric population.

Technological progress has significantly improved the diagnostic capabilities of conventional US and contributed to the development of novel US applications, such as harmonic imaging, high-resolution techniques, speckle and motion reduction filters, the various Doppler sonography options, extend field of view imaging, contrast-enhanced US imaging and sono-elastography, that have further expanded imaging potentials in clinical and research settings.

3.2 Indications

US imaging of the urinary tract is performed for a wide range of clinical indications (Riccabona et al. 2008; Muller-Ording 2014; Riccabona

2014a, b). A considerable number of children are referred for US due to a prenatal finding, most commonly urinary tract dilatation detected during maternal-foetal US. Postnatally, depending on whether or not the child requires immediate intervention, the first US is performed during the first day(s) of life or can be delayed until after 1 week of age. Therefore, in newborns with prenatally detected high-grade urinary tract dilatation, particularly if bilateral, if involving a single kidney, if associated with dysplastic renal parenchyma or if posterior urethral valves are suspected, an early US examination is recommended (Fig. 6). Other reasons for an early study are detection of a suspected ectopic kidney and complex urogenital malformations before excessive overlying bowel gas obscures the deeper structures (see respective chapters). Otherwise, in newborns with mild-to-moderate prenatal urinary tract dilatation, postnatal US can be performed later after birth (usually a period of at least 4–5 days is recommended), when the physiological immaturity and the relative dehydration of the neonatal kidney have been resolved (see chapters "Congenital Anomalies of the Renal Pelvis and Ureter" and "Upper Urinary Tract Dilatation in Newborns and Infants and the Postnatal Work up of Congenital Uro-nephropathies"). US can identify an underlying dilating abnormality of the urinary tract, often caused by obstructive uropathy (see chapters "Congenital Urinary Tract Dilatation and Obstructive Uropathy" and "Upper Urinary Tract Dilatation in Newborns and Infants and the Postnatal Work Up of Congenital Uro-nephropathies"). Alternatively, if vesicoureteral reflux (VUR) is suspected, additional imaging studies [voiding cystourethrography (VCUG) or contrast-enhanced voiding urosonography (ce-VUS)] can be further scheduled (see chapter "Vesicoureteric Reflux"). In the follow-up of children with either obstructive or refluxing abnormalities, including children who underwent surgical intervention, US can assess interval renal growth and the degree of the collecting system dilatation (Riccabona et al. 2009) (see chapters "Surgical Procedures and Indications for Surgery" and "Postoperative Imaging and Findings").

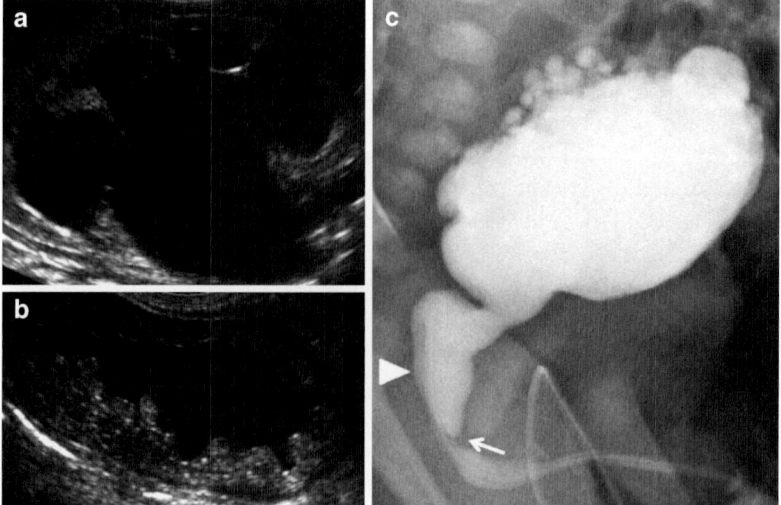

Fig. 6 Postnatal ultrasound in a neonate with prenatal diagnosis of urinary tract dilatation. (**a, b**) Greyscale ultrasound, performed in the first day of life, shows marked pelvicaliectasis with cortical thinning and decreased corticomedullary differentiation in both kidneys (here only the right kidney is shown), as well as diffuse bladder wall thickening and trabeculation, indicative of bladder outlet obstruction. (**c**) Voiding cysteourethrography, revealed the presence of posterior urethral valves, seen as linear filling defects in the flow of contrast during voiding (*arrow*), causing disproportional dilation of the posterior urethra (*arrowhead*) compared to the normal calibre anterior urethra. The bladder wall trabeculation and the multiple diverticula are again visualised

Urinary tract infection (UTI) is another common indication for renal US. Determination of renal involvement is of utmost importance to identify if a given patient should require intensive treatment and further imaging evaluation. The markedly improved US technology and up-to-date scanning protocols with high-resolution imaging including colour/power Doppler sonography techniques have contributed to a significant increase in US sensitivity to effectively and reliably detect early and subtle renal abnormalities in cases of UTI. These findings include focal or generalised renal enlargement, increased echogenicity of the renal parenchyma with reduced corticomedullary differentiation and focal or diffuse areas of decreased perfusion (Fig. 7). US can also play a significant role in the follow-up of these cases to confirm response to treatment or to rule out abscess formation and to search for long-term complications such as renal scarring (Dacher et al. 1996) (for details see chapters "UTI and VUR" and "Imaging in Urinary Tract Infections").

US is also very helpful in establishing the initial diagnosis of various nephropathies in children as well in the follow-up of these patients (Avni et al. 2012; Riccabona et al. 2012). US can detect the majority of nongenetic and genetic cystic kidney diseases, including cystic/multicystic dysplastic kidney, and autosomal dominant (ADPKD) or recessive polycystic kidney disease (ARPKD), respectively, and guide renal biopsy and evaluate for potential associations or complications (see chapters "Congenital Anomalies of the Renal Pelvis and Ureter", "Imaging in Prune Belly Syndrome and Other Syndromes Affecting the Urogenital Tract", and "Imaging in Renal Agenesis, Dysplasia, Hypoplasia and Cystic Diseases of the Kidney").

In children with palpable abdominal mass, US and plain abdominal films are usually sufficient to establish the diagnosis, which is then confirmed and staged by contrast-enhanced MRI or CT (see chapter "Neoplasms of the Genitourinary System"). In children with spontaneous haematuria, US can often rule out significant urolithiasis or malignancy.

In cases of acute renal failure, US can find or exclude (major) thrombosis of renal vessels (Fig. 8) or infectious disease (Hibbert et al. 1997; Moudgil 2014) (see chapters "Renal Failure and Renal Transplantation", "Neurogenic Bladder in Infants and Children" and "Imging in Renal Parenchymal Disease"). Haemolytic-uremic syndrome is one of the main causes of acute renal failure, especially in children, and US can confirm the diagnosis and monitor the recovery of these patients (Igarashi et al. 2014).

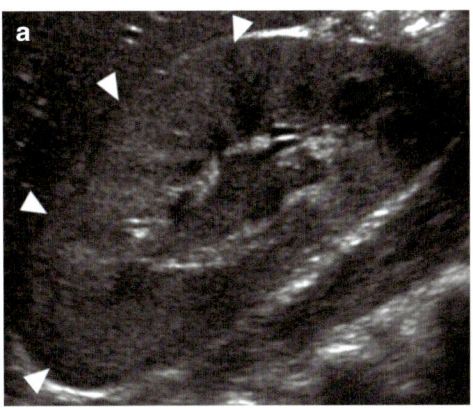 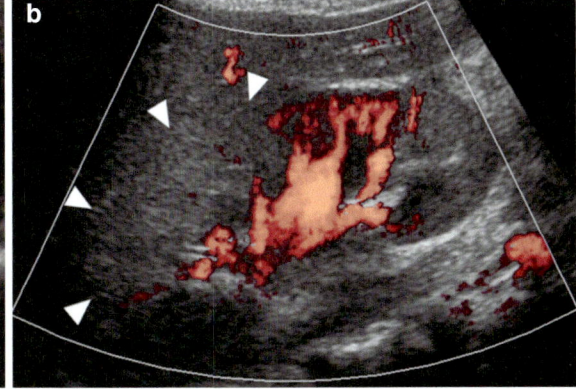

Fig. 7 Ultrasound examination in an 8-year-old female presented with fever and emesis. (**a**) Greyscale renal ultrasound. Diffusely increased echogenicity, with loss of corticomedullary differentiation, is noted in the middle and upper pole of the right kidney (*arrowheads*). (**b**) Power Doppler mode reveals decreased perfusion in the respective area of the right kidney. The constellation of these findings is suggestive of acute pyelonephritis

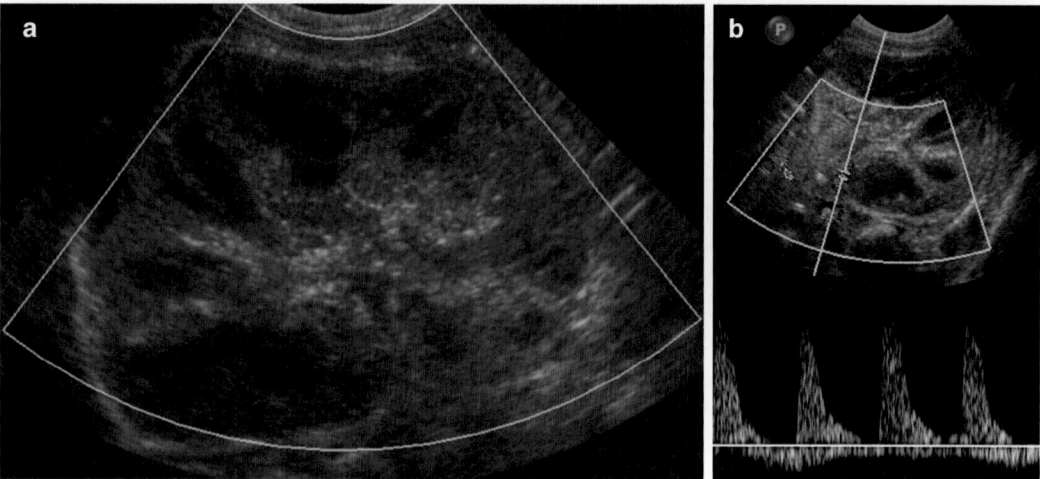

Fig. 8 Acute main renal vein thrombosis. (**a**) Power Doppler ultrasound, longitudinal plane. The kidney is enlarged with diffusely hyperechoic cortex and the absence of blood flow on power Doppler mode within the main renal vein, suggestive of acute renal vein thrombosis. (**b**) Spectral Doppler mode, transverse scan at the level of the renal hilum, reveals diminished flow into a segmental branch of the main renal artery with increased peak systolic flow velocities, indirect signs of renal vein thrombosis

In patients with arterial hypertension, US can detect renal scarring, hypoplasia or nephropathy. Colour/power Doppler sonography of renal vessels and parenchyma can orient the diagnosis toward vascular cause (see chapter "Renovascular Hypertension"); however, the variable cooperation of children may limit the contribution of Doppler sonography, and therefore renal angiography remains the reference examination.

After blunt abdominal trauma, haematuria is very common, and its grade does not correlate with the severity of the injury. Multi-detector CT is the unanimous gold-standard examination in cases of severe and multiple trauma. However, when US is optimally performed, it seems able to exclude severe renal injury and detect most relevant findings, reducing the need for CT in moderate trauma (Fig. 9) (see chapter "Urinary Tract Trauma") (Amerstorfer et al. 2015). For follow-up, US and/or MRI should be used for radiation protection issues.

Periodic US screening is recommended in children with characteristics that are known to be associated with benign or malignant renal tumours, including aniridia, hemihypertrophy, Denys-Drash syndrome, Beckwith-Wiedemann syndrome and tuberous sclerosis (Fig. 10). In patients with malformations highly associated with renal abnormality, such as the VA(C)TER(L) association, imperforate anus, internal genital anomalies and Fanconi anaemia, US examination of the urinary tract is recommended for completing a comprehensive diagnosis.

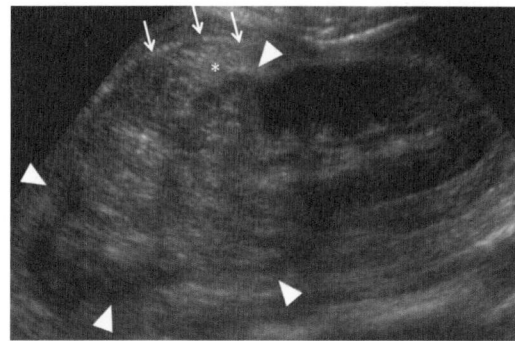

Fig. 9 Greyscale ultrasound in a 16-year-old female with history of blunt abdominal trauma. Significant disruption of the parenchymal architecture in the middle aspect and upper pole of the right kidney (*arrowheads*) is consistent with kidney laceration. The heterogeneously echogenic region (*asterisk*) extending from the subcapsular area along the Gerota's fascia (*arrows*) represents an associated perinephric haematoma

Ultrasound imaging before and after renal transplantation is important for the evaluation of

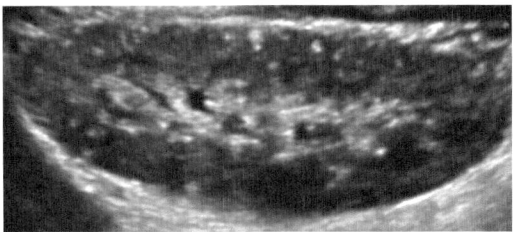

Fig. 10 Greyscale ultrasound of the right kidney, longitudinal plane, prone position. Multiple echogenic foci noted within the renal parenchyma are in keeping with angiomyolipomas in this patient with history of tuberous sclerosis

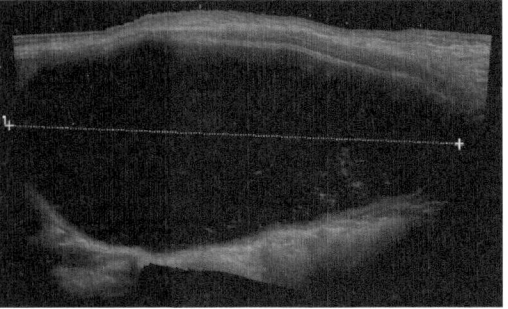

Fig. 11 Greyscale ultrasound. Extended field of view. Extended field of view for accurate measurement of bladder size thus enabling a reliable depiction of the increased capacity in this case of bladder function disorder with the presence of internal echogenic debris

the donor and the recipient (see chapter "Imaging in Renal Failure, Neonatal Oligoanuria, and Renal Transplantation"). Non-invasive, longitudinal evaluation of renal allografts is based on serial US and colour/spectral Doppler examinations and measurement of resistance and perfusion indices (Riccabona et al. 2012).

Ultrasound can estimate bladder wall morphology and bladder capacity in children with neurogenic bladder or other non-neurogenic voiding dysfunction (see chapters "Urinary Problems Associated with Imperforate Anus", "Epispadias-Exstrophy Complex", "Non-neurogenic Bladder-Sphincter Dysfunction ("Voiding Dysfunction")", and "Neurogenic Bladder in Infants and Children").

Finally, US can be used as a guide for interventional procedures. Renal biopsy, nephrostomy tube placement and abscess drainage can be performed using real-time US guidance (Feneberg et al. 1998; Lungren et al. 2014) (see chapter "Pediatric Genitourinary Intervention").

3.3 Equipment

Advances in US technology have significantly improved the quality of an US image (Riccabona et al. 2008; Muller-Ording 2014; Riccabona 2014a, b). The availability of a wide variety of curved and linear array transducers with broad bandwidth frequency range including also higher frequencies up to 18 MHz allows high-resolution imaging and adequate penetration over the entire spectrum of children ages, body sizes and body compartments ranging from small preterm babies to adolescents and even including obese patients. Curved array transducers are usually selected for orienting morphologic evaluation of the urinary tract and in older children, while linear transducers enable further detailed, high-resolution imaging and exquisite imaging in neonates. The examiner must select the appropriate transducer according to the age and size of the patient, the anatomic location and the tissue composition of the depicted structure and adjust image parameters in order to optimise image quality, including depth of view display, output energy and gain, focus number and zone, depth gain compensation and zoom (Muller-Ording 2014; Riccabona 2014a).

Tissue harmonic imaging is an imaging mode available in most modern US scanners and is used to increase contrast resolution reducing noise and artefacts. Thus, the image clarity is significantly improved, enabling more conspicuous visualisation of the internal echotexture and the borders of the examined structure (Bartram and Darge 2005; Darge and Heidemeier 2005). The panoramic or extended field of view imaging option can be selected if a lengthy field of view in a single scanplane is required, such as in cases of enlarged polycystic kidneys or renal transplants (Fig. 11). Application of motion mode (M-mode) may allow evaluation and quantification of movement changes over time such as ureteral peristalsis (Fig. 12) (Riccabona et al. 1998). Power Doppler sonography (also named amplitude-coded colour

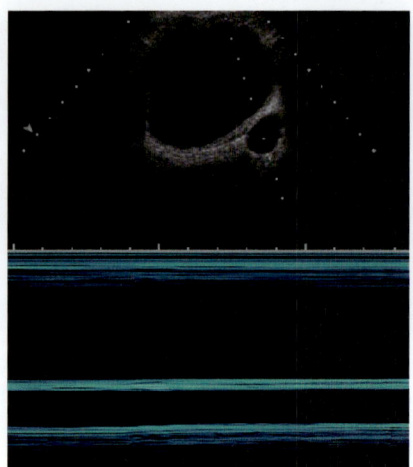

Fig. 12 M-mode sonography. In M-mode sonography, the variation of echoes motion through a single line of information is continuously displayed over time. In this case, M-mode through the plane of the dilated left retrovesical megaureter (*dotted line*) convincingly demonstrates the absence of peristaltic motion

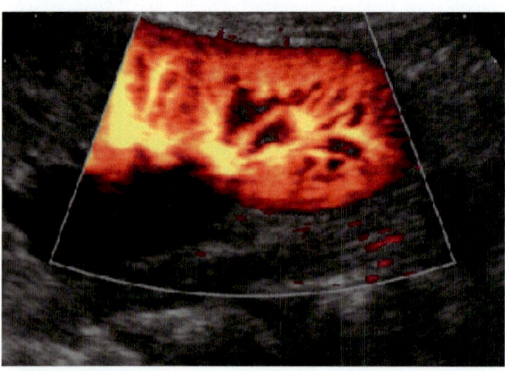

Fig. 13 Power Doppler sonography. Normal peripheral pararenchymal vascularisation at the level of the lower half of the left kidney

Doppler sonography) allows identification of blood flow within an operator-defined region of interest (Fig. 13) (Riccabona 2000; Riccabona et al. 2001). Colour Doppler sonography enables visualisation of blood flow directionality as an assigned colour in a colour-coded map superimposed into a B-mode US image. Spectral analysis based on pulsed wave Doppler sonography can be further applied, if measurements of blood flow velocities and analysis of the flow spectrum are required. These measurements include peak systolic, end diastolic, systolic/diastolic ratio or resistive and pulsatility indices. All currently available transducers have available colour and power Doppler sonography modes integrated.

3.4 Preparation

The child should be well hydrated before the examination for adequate distension of the collecting system and for proper assessment of the bladder. Oral uptake of clear liquids should be performed prior to the visit. Parents are encouraged to be present during the whole examination. Every study should start with an explanation to the parents and to the child if he or she is old enough to understand.

In case the US examination is performed in the intensive care unit, radiologists and technologists should follow basic rules of neonatal and intensive care. Incubator doors should be kept closed as much as possible, and extreme caution should be taken to prevent any catheter or tube contamination or withdrawal. Examinations should be performed as quickly and silently as possible, without omitting or missing essential aspects only for time reasons.

3.5 Scanning Technique

A generous amount of coupling agent (gel) should be applied along the entire area to be scanned, preferably prewarmed to body temperature to increase child's tolerability and comfort during the exam. Hygiene measures should be taken to avoid bacterial or fungal overgrowth.

3.5.1 Lower Urinary Tract

US examination should start with imaging of the bladder, especially in newborns and infants, since reflex micturition is frequent when the transducer is placed on the abdominal wall. Examination of the full bladder includes analysis of urine echogenicity and the bladder wall morphology. Normal bladder content should be anechoic, and the bladder wall should be smooth, with a maximum 3 mm thickness when full and 6 mm when empty (Jequier and Rousseau 1987). It is extremely important to look for dilated ureter(s) behind the bladder or an ureterocele inside it (Fig. 14). In children with normally shaped bladders, bladder capacity can be assessed by the ellipsoid equation: Volume (ml) =0.53 × D × H × W (D, depth; H, height; W, width in centimetres) (refer to chapter "Normal Values" for normal values) (Roehrborn and Peters 1988). Embedded software can automatically and accurately estimate bladder capacity and residual urine after micturition, provided the bladder has an ovoid shape – otherwise the correction factor has to be adapted. These estimations are particularly important in patients with neurogenic bladders or any kind of voiding dysfunction.

Ureteral jets are depicted with colour Doppler sonography "or modern non-Doppler-based flow imaging technique such as "B-flow"(GE Healthcare) or Superb Micro-Vascular Imaging, namely "SMI" (Toshiba) (Fig. 15)". Although their clinical significance has been a subject of literature debate, visualisation may be helpful in order to ascertain a degree of renal function, indicate the absence of acute obstruction or confirm the opening of a ureteral orifice within the bladder. Finally, the transperineal approach can be used to visualise the urethra, particularly in cases of posterior urethra valves in boys, and to assess lower urogenital tract malformations in girls (Fig. 16) (Teele and Share 1997; Berrocal et al. 2002; Schoellnast et al. 2004; Riccabona 2014a).

3.5.2 Upper Urinary Tract

Real-time scanning of the kidneys and ureters should then follow. Adequate access of the examined structure is obtained with the child in supine and prone positions. Curved and linear array transducers can be used alternatively during both positions, although the lower penetration of linear transducers makes prone position most preferable. In cooperative, older children instructions for inspiration and breath holding may further improve the acoustic window. However, in a moving, playing or crying child, a variety of positions, sometimes unconventional as the opportunity arises, are often necessary for the examination.

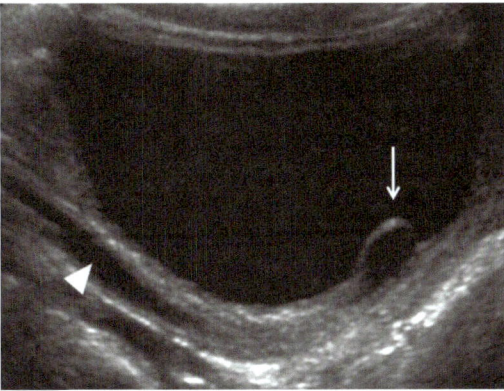

Fig. 14 Postnatal ultrasound in a neonate with prenatal diagnosis of lower urinary tract obstruction. Greyscale ultrasound shows dilation of the distal ureter (*arrowhead*) which ends into a thin-walled saccular outpouch prolapsing into the bladder, consistent with ureterocele

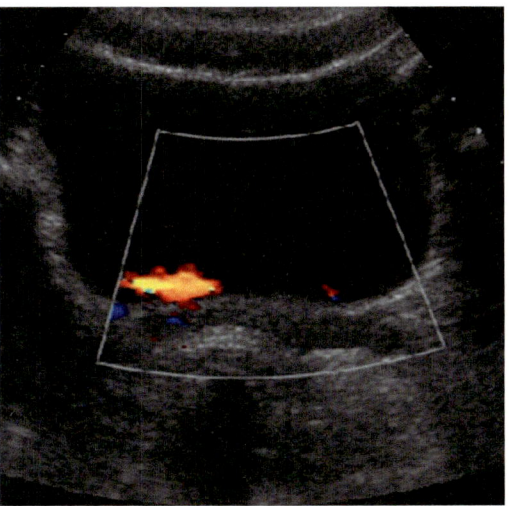

Fig. 15 Colour Doppler sonography. Transverse scanning of the bladder. Bilateral ureteral jets. Colour Doppler sonography enables the detection of urine flow arising from the ureteral orifices bilaterally – note the asymmetry

Morphologic evaluation of kidneys includes measurements of the longitudinal and transverse dimensions and calculation of the overall renal volume. The latest has been considered more sensitive to reflect changes in size compared to measurement of the length alone and can be assessed by the ellipsoid equation: Volume (ml)=0.53 × D × H × W (D, depth; H, height; W, width in centimetres) (refer to chapter "Normal Values" for normal values). In most modern US scanners,

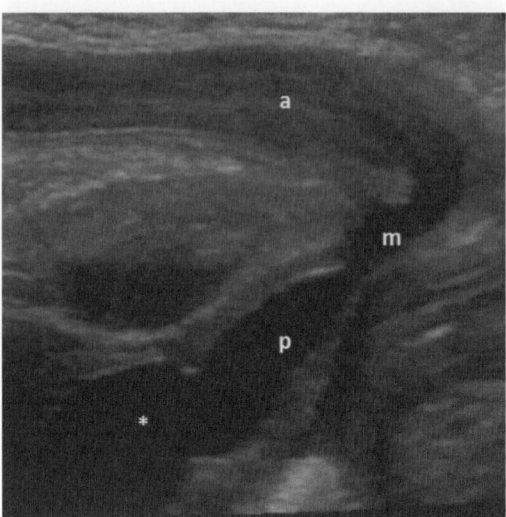

Fig. 16 Greyscale US in tissue harmonic imaging mode. Transperineal scanning of the urethra in a male neonate during voiding attempt. Normal configuration of the prostatic (*p*), membranous (*m*) and anterior (*a*) urethra during voiding. Bladder neck (*asterisk*). Note the indention at the level of the pelvic floor – not to be mistaken for a urethral valve

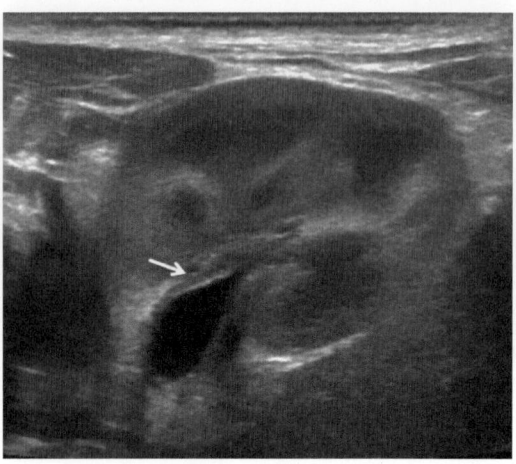

Fig. 17 Greyscale US in tissue harmonic imaging mode using a high-resolution linear transducer. Urothelial thickening sign. Transverse scan at the level of the renal pelvis reveals thickening of the urothelium with increased mucosal echogenicity (*arrow*)

incorporated software can automatically generate renal volumes, which are reliable as long as the kidney has an ellipsoid shape. Results have to be compared to those of prior examinations (sonographic, prenatal or others) as well as to normal values. Measurement of the anteroposterior/axial diameter of the renal pelvis is performed in transverse plane (refer to chapter "Normal Values" for normal values). Variability and peristaltic motion should be recorded if present. Moreover, evaluation of the urothelial thickness at the level of the renal pelvis using high-frequency linear transducers has been shown to be of diagnostic value in the setting of inflammatory processes involving the kidney and may further indicate an obstructive or refluxing condition (Fig. 17) (Sorantin et al. 1997). Echogenicity of the cortex and medulla is assessed in comparison to that of the adjacent liver and spleen. Knowledge of the physiologic changes in echogenicity of the cortex and medulla between newborns and older children is essential for accurate interpretation of the imaging findings.

Evaluation of renal vasculature and perfusion of the kidney can be performed in colour and power Doppler sonography modes, respectively.

Colour Doppler sonography enables differentiation between prominent hilar vessels from dilated renal pelvis, provided provided adequate setting of the scale also for low flow velocities. In some cases, pulsed wave duplex sonography is performed for spectral analysis to evaluate renal arterial flow waveforms, and measurements are obtained at three kidney parts (upper and lower pole as well as middle aspect) and in three sites along the renal arteries' course (proximal, middle, distal site in relation to the aorta) using the best accessible patient's position.

Labelled serial static images and video clips can be obtained and saved in dedicated archiving systems to be available for retrospective review.

> **Take Away**
> Ultrasonography performed in a comprehensive fashion using modern techniques as well as standardised approach and scanning protocol is an outstanding modality with high diagnostic yield in detection, potential differentiation and follow-up of urinary tract pathologies in children.

4 Contrast-Enhanced Ultrasonography

4.1 Introduction

Contrast-enhanced ultrasonography (ce-US) has been gaining increasing use in the field of diagnostic imaging (Claudon et al. 2008; Piscaglia et al. 2012; Piskunowicz et al. 2012; Riccabona 2012; Claudon et al. 2013). It is performed with US and use of a dedicated US contrast agent (UCA) that can be administered intravenously or intracavitarily. There are two distinct intracavitary applications of ce-US performed either with UCA administration into physiological cavities or with UCA injection into non-physiological cavities and fistulas. In paediatrics, ce-US with the intravesical UCA administration, namely, contrast-enhanced voiding urosonography, is the most common ce-US application.

Since their introduction in diagnostic practice, UCAs have been strikingly evolved to become clinically and commercially applicable. A real breakthrough took place with the development of the first generation of stabilised UCAs. These agents comprised of air microbubbles encapsulated within a stable outer shell of different composition, generally comprised of proteic, lipidic or polymeric materials. Currently, the first-generation air-filled UCAs have been commercially replaced by the second-generation UCAs comprised of gas-filled microbubbles. Their improved physic-chemical properties, combined with the remarkable advances in US technology, further increased microbbubles detection in real time (Darge 2010). Most modern US scanners use contrast harmonic imaging softwares and low mechanical index (MI) technology that is based on the nonlinear oscillation of the UCA microbubbles and the transmission of an amplified US signal without causing microbubbles destruction. Selection among several display modes can further improve microbubbles visualisation, including contrast enhancement mode only, contrast enhancement as a colour overlay on the grey scale image and background subtraction options. Moreover, most US scanners are equipped with the dual display mode, where the image can be split into two parts and the examined area can be displayed side-by-side in contrast imaging and greyscale mode, providing the anatomic landmark information to ensure in plane scanning.

The most commonly used UCAs in paediatric applications are SonoVue® (Bracco, Milan, Italy) comprised of sulphur hexafluoride gas microbubbles stabilised within a shell of phospholipids (registered and approved as Lumason® in the USA) and Optison™ (General Electric Healthcare, Princeton, NJ) comprised of perflutren gas microbubbles stabilised within a human serum albumin outer shell. Sonazoid® (Daiichi Sankyo, Tokyo, Japan; GE Healthcare) composed of perfluorobutane gas within a phospholipid shell has been widely used in adult population in Japan (Piscaglia et al. 2012; Claudon et al. 2013).

It is important to note that at the time that the current chapter was prepared, none of the commercially available second-generation UCAs was approved for paediatric intraveous indication in Europe; however, in the USA, since 2016, the second-generation UCA Lumason® (Bracco, Milan, Italy) has been approved for pediatric intravesical and intravenous liver applications and in Europe, SonoVue was approved for intravesical use in childhood. The indications that will be described below are partially still performed off-label in children in Europe, though a broader approval for paediatric applications is expected. That means that currently parents/legal guardians and/or children themselves, if applicable, should be thoroughly informed regarding the risks and benefits of the examination and should provide their consent prior to the examination.

4.2 Contrast-Enhanced Voiding Urosonography

Contrast-enhanced voiding urosonography (ce-VUS) is a highly sensitive, radiation-free imaging modality for the detection and grading of vesicoureteral reflux (VUR) in children. It entails bladder catheterization and intravesical UCA administration (Darge 2008a, b). Ce-VUS has become integrated into routine diagnostic practice, and in many institutions it is used as the primary diagnostic option for VUR imaging, replacing conventional ionising modalities such as voiding cystourethrography (VCUG) and scintigraphy. Several comparative studies have been conducted so far, all demonstrating the high diagnostic accuracy of ce-VUS when compared to its ionising counterparts. Most importantly, ce-VUS has been shown not only to be more sensitive to detect more cases of VUR but also of higher grade, hence of higher clinical significance (Papadopoulou et al. 2007).

No serious adverse events have been described so far regarding the intravesical use of UCAs in children. A few complaints, mainly dysuria, have been reported, but these are most likely related to the inevitable catheterisation process, rather than the contrast agent itself (Riccabona 2012; Darge et al. 2013b; Papadopoulou et al. 2014).

4.2.1 Procedure

Urine analysis should be performed prior to ce-VUS to ensure that urine is sterile. If the patient is being treated for UTI, antibiotics must be completed, and urine analysis should be repeated prior to ce-VUS. The use of prophylactic antibiotics has also been recommended in the immediate period before and after ce-VUS. However, there is ongoing discussion on when to give therapeutic and when to give prophylactic antibiotics, and this is often individualised according to the clinical history and the patient's age.

Before proceeding with the examination, it is important to take time and inform the parents – and the child if he or she is old enough – about the examination. Psychological consequences of urethral catheterisation should not be underestimated. Post-procedural minor discomfort can occur, and it seems less worrisome when announced. Discussion with trained health professionals might be of help to prepare children and families to better cope with the overall stress of the examination.

The patient is positioned supine on the examination table. Initially, a baseline US examination of the urinary tract is performed. Then, experienced personnel catheterise the bladder under aseptic conditions. In some institutions, the catheter is already placed at the paediatric ward allowing the child (and the bladder) to adapt to the situation. A four to eight French feeding tube is recommended. Local anaesthetic, e.g. lidocaine gel, should be used to decrease patient discomfort and lubricate the urethra. The suprapubic approach can be alternatively used in neonates with posterior urethral valves and in children in whom catheter placement may be difficult or painful (urethral trauma, hypospadias, cloacal malformation, religious aspects). After catheter placement, the bladder is completely emptied, and a sterile urine specimen is used to confirm the absence of active inflammation and may be retained for culture if clinically indicated.

The UCA dose is related to the bladder filling capacity, which is age dependent and is calculated by the Koff formula as follows: Volume (mL) = [child's age + 2] × 30 (Koff 1983). The most commonly reported dosage schemes for the second-generation UCAs range from 0.5 to 1 % of UCA per bladder filling volume, although a lower dose of 0.2 % has also been shown to be adequate; this may also depend agent itself and the contrast visualization technique available visualisation technique available (Riccabona et al. 2014). The company recommendation is a dose of 1 ml.

Two techniques have been described for UCA intravesical administration. The first technique requires partial filling of the bladder with saline by drip infusion, up to approximately one third of the age-related bladder capacity. Then UCA is directly injected into the bladder through a three-way valve, with no filters in place, and the bladder is filled with saline up to the maximum age-related bladder capacity; potentially, fractionated administration of the total UCA dose may be an option to avoid obscuring the far field (Darge 2008a). Alternatively, UCA can be directly injected into a plastic bag of saline, and the resultant UCA/saline solution is subsequently infused into the bladder via gravity (Duran et al. 2012). In the latter case, use of a pressure gauge or periodic direct injection of normal saline through the three-way valve might be necessary to produce homogenous distribution of the microbubbles within the bag or the bladder, respectively. Regardless of whether UCA is diluted with saline inside or outside the bladder, the common principle of both techniques is to avoid direct contact and potential interaction of the UCA, in its concentrated form, with the bladder uroepithelium.

The plastic bottle with normal saline or the UCA/saline solution is usually hanged approximately 40 cm above the level of the bladder to enable a physiologic filling pressure, especially in cases of recent bladder or urethral surgery.

Once UCA is introduced into the bladder, scanning of the bladder and the retrovesical space is performed with the patient in supine position. Then, scanning of the kidneys is performed alternatively and continuously in supine or prone position. The dual-screen display mode is preferably used to confirm anatomic scanning. VUR diagnosis is established if echogenic microbubbles are present in the ureters, renal pelvis and/or the calyces (Fig. 18); VUR in ce-VUS is graded into five grades in a similar manner to the international grading system for VUR applied with VCUG (Darge and Troeger 2002). However, additional information can be acquired with ce-VUS, such as the presence of VUR into a previously dilated or non-dilated collecting system as well as the presence of intrarenal reflux, which has been associated with increased risk of associated parenchymal damage.

The whole ce-VUS procedure can be repeated in a cyclic manner, with the aim to increase VUR detection rate (Novljan et al. 2003; Papadopoulou et al. 2006). In this case, multiple cycles of bladder filling and voiding, usually two to three times, with the catheter remaining in place are performed. This is due to the intermittent nature of the VUR phenomenon, and therefore the prolonged real-time US imaging without the issue of ionising without the issue of ionizing exposure, thus further increasing the possibility to detect VUR. The last cycle is dedicated to urethra imaging during voiding. Transperineal and/or transabdominal approach and high-resolution linear multifrequency transducers are used to delineate the urethral lumen and detect urethral pathology (such as posterior urethral valves, urethral diverticulum or stenosis of the urethra lumen) (Fig. 19) (Berrocal et al. 2005; Duran et al. 2009; Durán Feliubadaló et al. 2015). While performing ce-VUS, sterile precautions are extremely important in all patients. The whole procedure usually lasts around up to 20–30 min.

Recently, novel ce-VUS applications have been increasingly explored in children. The availability

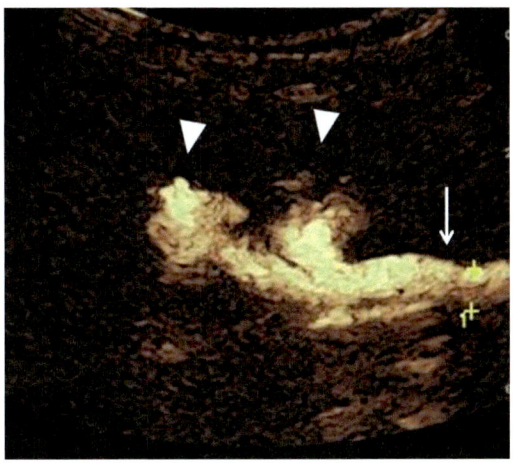

Fig. 18 Contrast-enhanced voiding urosonography (ce-VUS) in contrast harmonic imaging mode. Grade III vesicoureteral reflux. Echogenic microbubbles are seen refluxing within the ureter (*arrow*) and the bifid renal pelvis of the right kidney (*arrowhead*) with mild dilation and blunted configuration of the lower calyces (Image courtesy of Dr. Frederica Papadopoulou, University of Ioannina and Pediatric Ultrasound Center, Thessaloniki, Greece)

of three-dimensional (3D) and four-dimensional (4D) contrast-enhanced US imaging techniques enabled acquisition of 3D image datasets that allow for multiplanar reconstructions, volumetric rendering and spatial rotation display options even in real time. These techniques provide volumetric visualisation of the refluxing collecting system and may be proved of added value in a more precise evaluation of VUR grade, and a more comprehensive representation of the imaging findings that is easier appreciated by the clinicians (Wozniak et al. 2014b).

In addition, ce-VUS can be performed intraoperatively to directly assess the effectiveness of endoscopic injection of anti-reflux bulking agents, potentially increasing operative success rates and reducing the number of reoperations (Wozniak et al. 2014a).

> **Take Away**
> Ce-VUS is a radiation-free and highly sensitive alternative imaging modality for the detection and grading of VUR and imaging of urethra morphology in children.

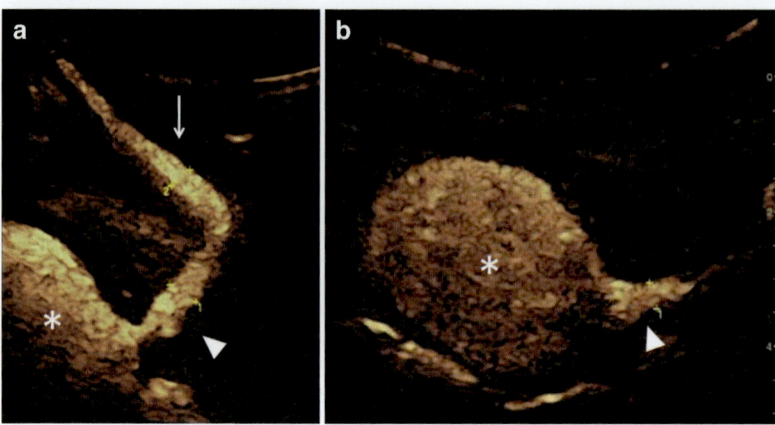

Fig. 19 Contrast-enhanced voiding urosonography (ce-VUS) in contrast harmonic imaging mode. Scanning during micturition. (**a**) Normal male urethra. Echogenic microbubbles are seen within the bladder (*asterisk*) and the urethra lumen, with normal dimensions of the posterior (*arrowhead*) and anterior (*arrow*) urethra. (**b**) Normal female urethra. The stream of microbubbles during voiding delineates the conical configuration of the normal female urethra (*arrowhead*) (Image courtesy of Dr. Frederica Papadopoulou, University of Ioannina and Pediatric Ultrasound Center, Thessaloniki, Greece)

4.3 Contrast-Enhanced Ultrasonography with Intravenous Administration of Ultrasound Contrast Agents

Contrast-enhanced ultrasonography (ce-US) with intravenous (IV) UCA administration has been gaining increasing use in a variety of oncologic, traumatic or inflammatory indications (Valentino et al. 2008; Catalano et al. 2009; Mccarville et al. 2012; Piskunowicz et al. 2012; Quaia et al. 2012; Jacob et al. 2013; Ripolles et al. 2013; Coleman et al. 2014; Menichini et al. 2015). IV ce-US does not involve radiation exposure, permits real-time scanning and enables accurate depiction of any rapid changes in enhancement patterns. Also, the study may be repeated if necessary, and renal impairment does not contradict the IV use of UCAs (refer to Fig. 37.5). Liver applications and trauma imaging are the most commonly reported indications in paediatric patients.

Particularly in the field of paediatric uroradiology, the most frequently reported indication of IV ce-US is imaging of the kidneys as an integral or targeted part of abdominal IV ce-US examination in the clinical setting of trauma (Valentino et al. 2008; Catalano et al. 2009). It can be performed as bedside examination, in haemodynamically stable patients, with minimal to moderate low-energy trauma as initial examination and/or as follow-up examination of known injuries that are treated conservatively. It can also be proved useful in the diagnostic workup of trauma patients with negative baseline US and persistent clinical and/or laboratory suspicion of solid organ injury (Riccabona et al. 2014). Other less frequent indications of IV ce-US in paediatric uroradiology include detection and characterisation of renal lesions and evaluation of treatment response after chemotherapy sessions as well as renal transplant evaluation (Correas et al. 1999; Coleman et al. 2014).

4.3.1 Procedure

Prior to IV ce-US, no blood or urine tests are required to assess renal function. An IV line with adequate flow should be established for UCA administration and in anticipation of any potential adverse events that may require fluid or IV medication infusion; any bacterial filter must be avoided. Monitoring of vital signs during the procedure is recommended.

The United States Federal Drug Adminstration (FDA) approved dose of Lumason® for pediatric liver IV ce-US applications is 0.03 mL/Kg up to a maximum of 2.4 mL per injection. Before Lumason® approval, variable dosage schemes have been reported in the literature, depending on the UCA type, US equipment, patient's age and clinical indication (please refer to chapter "Contrast Agents in Childhood: Application and Safety Considerations") (Riccabona et al. 2014). Regarding SonoVue®, the most frequently used single dose is that of a 2.4 ml, in school-age children (as recommended for adults) which might be repeated, if needed.

Initially a baseline pre-contrast abdominal US examination is performed. In every case, the examination needs to be tailored to the specific clinical query. A single UCA dose is administered one for each abdominal side, with a repeated dose if necessary (after the UCA has dissolved, usually within 15 min after initial injection). Examination may start from the side of increased clinical concern or side with "positive" findings after the baseline US. In each side, the kidney is the first organ to be scanned, because of its quick parenchymal enhancement pattern. There is approximately a 2–3 min adequate scanning window from the onset of enhancement and throughout the phase of homogeneous renal parenchyma enhancement. Transverse and longitudinal views with the patient in supine position, using additional lateral and dorsal approaches, when possible, are acquired. Imaging of the liver and spleen may follow on each side, depending on the clinical query (Valentino et al. 2008; Catalano et al. 2009). Static images and particularly video clips should be obtained during the examination and stored in order to be available for retrospective review.

As with any contrast agent that is used in radiology practice, adverse events might occur with UCA administration. These events, although extremely rare, may vary from mild discomfort to life-threatening emergencies. Minor and moderate adverse events may include but are not limited to nausea, vomiting, cough, headache, itching, pallor, flushing and chills. Serious adverse events include hypersensitivity, allergic or anaphylactic reaction with tachycardia/bradycardia or cardiac arrest, bronchospasm, laryngeal oedema, angio-oedema and hypotensive shock. These events mostly occur acutely (within minutes up to 1 h following injection), theoretically also subacutely (within the next 24 h) or delayed (after 24 h). The radiologist in charge should be trained to recognise the onset and type of any potential adverse event related to UCA administration, and precautionary measures should be taken. They include careful patient selection, adequate monitoring of vital signs and available resuscitation equipment. So far, a few extremely rare episodes of serious anaphylactic reactions after IV UCA administration have been reported in children, as well as some cases of minor, transient, self-limited adverse events (Riccabona 2012; Darge et al. 2013b; Piskunowicz et al. 2015; Rosado and Riccabona 2016).

Take Away
Intravenous ce-US can provide high diagnostic yield as an alternative or problem-solving radiation-free imaging modality in specific clinical settings in children, often obviating the need for further imaging or other invasive procedures.

5 Sono-elastography

Sono-elastography is an advanced US application that provides non-invasive information regarding the inherent elasticity properties of biological tissues. It has been predominantly performed in the liver to assess pathological alterations related to hepatic fibrosis and cirrhosis (Bamber et al. 2013; Goya et al. 2014; Ozkan et al. 2014; Pico Aliaga et al. 2014; Stenzel and Mentzel 2014). In the field of uroradiology, two types of renal pathology might be detected and quantified by US elastography: first, localised changes in elasticity properties produced by neoplasm, infection, scarring and/or infarction and second and most commonly, diffuse changes of cortical fibrosis in renal transplants and chronic kidney nephropathies (Grenier et al. 2013). This might be of utmost clinical importance since current laboratory and imaging methods are non-specific or not sensitive enough in detecting slowly evolving disease.

There is a wide variety of technologies available for sono-elastography performance, and even more new technologies are constantly being developed. The basic principle is that the propagation velocity of an US wave through a biological tissue is directly related to its elastic properties. These properties are associated with the ability of the tissue to restore the displacement that its elements undergo after application of a deformation force (shear wave). Tissue deformation can be caused mechanically or by US-induced forces.

Static or strain elastography is one of the first developed elastography techniques that uses compression forces to generate mechanical tissue excitation. These forces are applied either actively by gentle pressure of the transducer or passively by physiological motion (cardiovascular, breathing movements). This technique directly depends on the appropriate application of mechanical pressure to the examined tissue; thus, the objectivity and the reproducibility are largely operator dependent.

A newer technique of sono-elastography is dynamic and transducer-immanent elastography. This technique employs automatically generated acoustic radiation force impulses (ARFIs) that induce shear waves within a freely selectable targeted region of interest (ROI). The velocity of this shear wave propagation is measured in metre per seconds (m/s) and is directly related to the stiffness (kPA) of the tissue within this ROI. The stiffer the tissue, the higher is the shear wave velocity. By measuring tissue element displacements, shear wave elastography is able to provide objective qualitative and quantitative information on tissue stiffness that can be also displayed in colour-coded maps (Fig. 10).

> **Take Away**
> Sono-elastography can provide additional information regarding the elastic properties of a tissue, enabling qualitative and quantitative evaluation of the underlying pathology; however, at present this is only applied in research settings.

6 Voiding Cystourethrography

6.1 Introduction

Voiding cystourethrography (VCUG) has been for decades a frequently performed fluoroscopic procedure in paediatric radiology departments and is considered a reliable diagnostic option for detection and grading of VUR and urethral imaging in children. VCUG, however, uses ionising radiation that in addition to the overall somatic exposure involves direct irradiation of the gonads, particularly in girls. Moreover, due to the intermittent nature of VUR phenomenon, prolonged examination times may be required, raising even higher the overall radiation exposure.

In the last decades, evidenced-based data emerged regarding the association of VUR with UTI pathogenesis has turned the diagnostic interest into identifying children at risk for renal scarring, whether or not VUR is present (the so-called "top-down" approach). This new scientific knowledge coupled with the increasing awareness of the radiation risks for diagnostic purposes and the availability of ce-VUS as a highly sensitive, radiation-free imaging alternative have all contributed to a more critical approach regarding the role of VCUG in diagnostic imaging algorithms (Pohl and Belman 2009). Evaluation of clinical indications, respect of the As Low As Reasonably Achievable (ALARA) principles and choice of alternative procedures, if available, continue to be of great significance in daily practice to avoid unnecessary radiation exposure of paediatric population (Riccabona 2002; Riccabona et al. 2008).

6.2 Indications

Most recent recommendations indicate that VCUG can be performed after the first episode of febrile UTI – if US reveals urinary tract dilatation, scarring or other findings that would suggest either high-grade VUR or lower obstructive uropathy such as posterior urethral valves or urethral diverticulum, as well as in other atypical or complex clinical circumstances and workup of malformations, e.g. a dilated ureter. Patients with cloacal anomalies, ambiguous genitalia or imperforate anus can also be explored with VCUG (see chapters "Female Genital Anomalies and Important Ovarian Conditions", "Urinary Problems Associated with Imperforate Anus" and "Epispadias-Exstrophy Complex").

6.3 Equipment

Major innovation in fluoroscopic equipment allowed significant radiation dose reduction while maintaining and at times even improving image quality (Cleveland et al. 1992). Such innovations include digital X-ray equipment and use of pulsed fluoroscopy with last-image hold technique (Fig. 20). This technique captures the last fluoroscopic frame or even a series of frames in a cine-loop-like video enabling adequate documentation without creation of additional images. This modern equipment has advantageously replaced the film-screen combination that should no longer be used to perform VCUG in children.

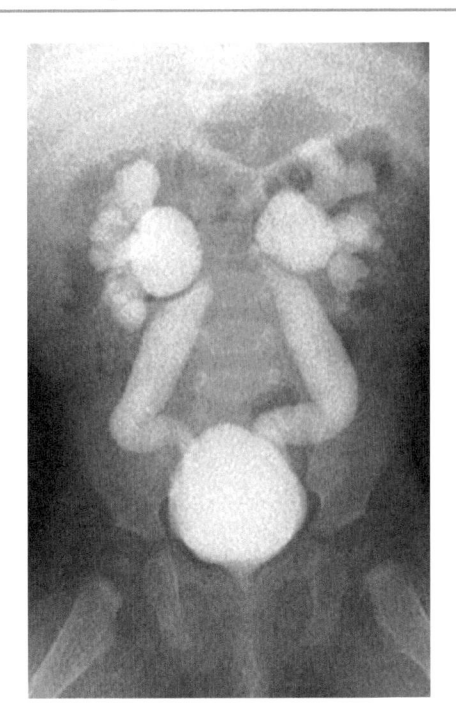

Fig. 20 VCUG. Pulsed fluoroscopy with "last-image hold" feature and inversion of image contrast. Bilateral grade IV vesicoureteral reflux. "Last-image hold" feature enables the last frame of fluoroscopic image to be displayed on the monitor and be captured, even when the fluoroscopy has been terminated

6.4 Preparation

No diet restrictions or preparation with enema is recommended prior to VCUG, with some promoting reduced fluid input to increase VUR detection rate. Regarding urine analysis and use of prophylactic antibiotics, similar principles to those applied for ce-VUS are also recommended for VCUG (see above). The addition of Refobacin (gentamicin-based antibiotic) into the contrast drip has also been suggested to prevent the initiation or exacerbation of existing infections during the VCUG procedure.

The use of light sedation can be used for VCUG performance. It might be applied in uncooperative toddlers or in cases of major anxiety and should preferably be organised in collaboration with the department of anaesthesiology. In these cases, e.g. midazolam can offer minimal light sedation during which the child is in a relaxed state but awake and able to respond. Midazolam® is usually administered orally (0.5–0.6 mg/kg, maximum 15 mg) or intranasally (0.2 mg/kg, maximum 15 mg). Inhalation of an equimolecular mixture of nitrous oxide and oxygen (Entonox®) in fasting children is also being routinely used in many institutions (Schmit and Sfez 1997).

6.5 Procedure

While performing VCUG, sterile precautions are extremely important in all patients. Same principles regarding bladder catheterisation apply with ce-VUS and VCUG. Recommendations have been issued to allow for a standardised procedure (Riccabona et al. 2008). The patient is positioned supine on the examination table, and the bladder is completely emptied after the catheter placement. Radiopaque (low concentration if available) contrast agent is instilled via gravity into the bladder under intermittent pulsed fluoroscopic observation. Documentation is mostly sufficiently achieved by using the last-image hold

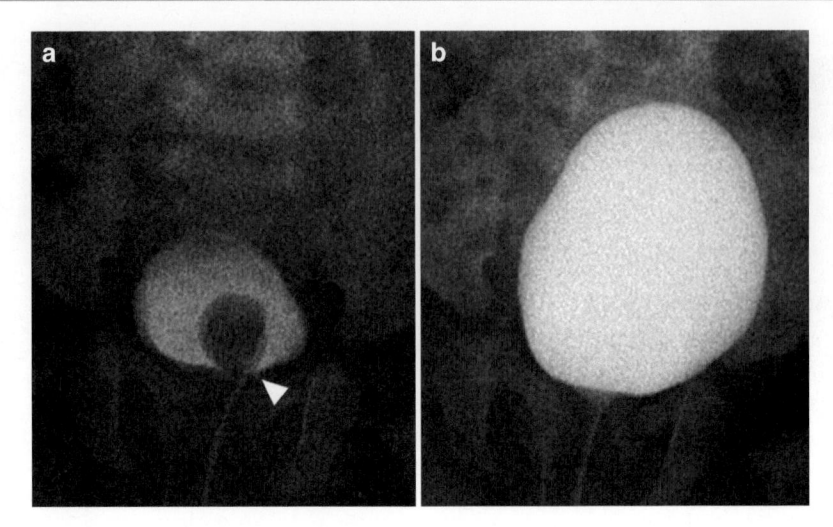

Fig. 21 VCUG. Pulsed fluoroscopy and "last-image hold" feature and inversion of image contrast. Ureterocele. (**a**) A smooth round filling defect is seen within the bladder, consistent with ureterocele (*arrowhead*). (**b**) With continuing bladder filling, the ureterocele collapses and cannot be further visualised

technique. However, for high-resolution, detailed images of subtle pathology (e.g. intrarenal reflux, urethral pathology), normal exposures may become necessary. The bottle with the contrast agent can be hanged approximately 30 to 40 cm above the level of the bladder to enable a somewhat physiologic filling pressures. Bladder filling capacity is age related and is calculated by the Koff formula: Volume (mL)=[child's age+2] × 30 (Koff 1983). Typically, the bladder is filled up to the maximum for age volume; however, in cases of megabladder, the actual filling volume may exceed the expected for age maximum filling bladder capacity.

Observation of the contrast dripping pattern may disclose valuable information regarding the presence of bladder dysfunction (Fotter et al. 1986). (See chapter "Video-Urodynamics" and "Non-neurogenic Bladder-Sphincter Dysfunction ("Voiding Dysfunction")", where the details of this modified VCUG technique are described). Interruption or back flow can be due to contractions of the detrusor muscle when an unstable bladder is present.

In both genders, early-filling last-image capture of the bladder is required and may reveal an intravesical ureterocele as a smooth rounded filling defect. Ureteroceles may collapse if the bladder is completely filled and thus cannot be seen or their visualisation becomes obscured due to the projecting strong contrast of filled large bladder (effacement) (Fig. 21). Later on, under maximal intravesical pressure, a ureterocele may become everted outside the bladder through the para-ureteric fossa (eversion) – sometimes only detectable by oblique views (Fig. 22). Anteroposterior views of the bladder and the renal fossae should be obtained to demonstrate if VUR is present, which side is affected and to what degree, as well as to look for intrarenal reflux (Fig. 23) (Lebowitz et al. 1985). These views are also helpful to analyse the anatomy of the excretory system, including VUR into the lower or upper pole of a duplex system, and association of VUR and pelvi-ureteric junction obstruction in the same renal unit. Right and left oblique or lateral views are necessary to search for retrovesical refluxing ureters and to reveal the ureterovesical junction anatomy, disclosing the presence of periosteal diverticula or potentially refluxing ectopic ureters.

Cyclic filling is helpful to increase VUR detection rate, particularly in infants and young children who tend to void at lower filling volumes (Paltiel et al. 1992; Papadopoulou et al. 2002; Kadioglu et al. 2006). The bladder volume at the time of VUR and the VCUG cycle should be recorded.

For imaging of the urethra, the catheter may or may not be removed during voiding. In gen-

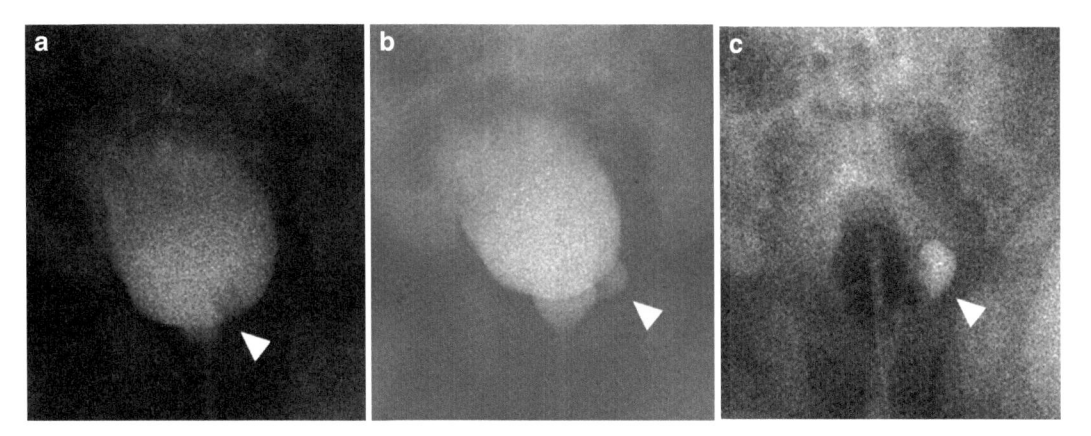

Fig. 22 VCUG. Ureterocele eversion. Pulsed fluoroscopy and "last-image hold" feature and inversion of image contrast. (**a**) Left-side ureterocele (*arrowhead*). (**b**) With continuing bladder filling, the ureterocele is everted and filled with contrast. (**c**) After micturition, contrast remains within the everted ureterocele, while the bladder is completely emptied

visualisation of posterior urethral valves or the diagnosis of other significant urethral pathology (Lebowitz 1996). During voiding, lateral views of the urethra in boys and anteroposterior (centred, but sometimes also oblique) views of the urethra in girls are adequate to reveal any urethral pathology. Anteroposterior views of the bladder and the renal fossae should be obtained after voiding to assess contrast drainage from the kidney, if VUR was present. Moreover, a 5-min delayed view is also valuable to evaluate contrast clearance in refluxing systems with some obstructive component, as VUR associated with prolonged stasis is thought to increase the risk of severe infection.

Estimators of radiation exposure, such as fluoroscopic parameters used and fluoroscopy time, should be documented for calculation of the overall exposure dose.

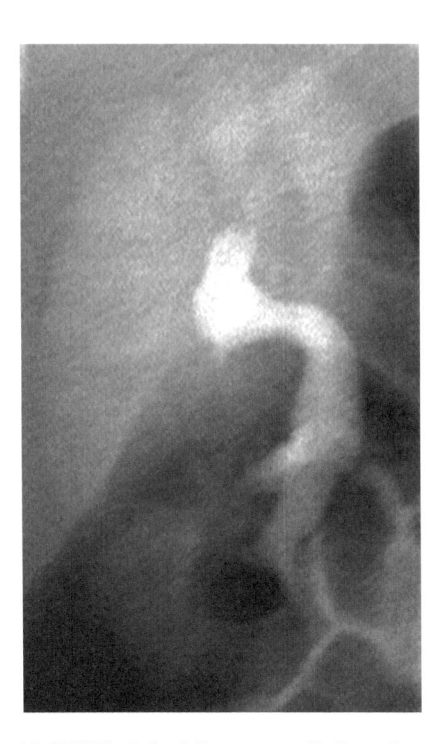

Fig. 23 VCUG. Pulsed fluoroscopy. Reflux of contrast material into the right collecting system, which appears dysmorphic, with significant intrarenal reflux throughout the entire kidney. These findings indicate high-grade vesicoureteral reflux

eral, removal of the catheter is suggested to facilitate free voiding unless another VCUG cycle will follow. However, the presence of the small, properly sized catheter should not inhibit

Take Away
VCUG is a well-established imaging modality for VUR detection and grading as well as for urethral imaging in children and – when performed with modern technology and according to appropriate acquisition techniques – can achieve high diagnostic yield with significantly reduced radiation exposure.

7 Retrograde Urethrography

Retrograde urethrography has been traditionally used for imaging of the anterior urethra. The most common indication is to rule out traumatic urethral injury. This type of injury occurs predominantly in male adolescents, in the setting of high-energy trauma to the perineum, mainly during a direct blow or straddle injury or during vehicle accidents such as falling on the saddle or handlebars of a bicycle. Other less common indications for retrograde urethrography are suspected congenital urethral anomalies including dilatations of the anterior urethra such as saccular or diffuse megalourethra before and after surgical reconstruction, as well as evaluation of post-traumatic, post-inflammatory or post-surgical complications such as urethral strictures or fistulas.

Recently, a standardised recommendation on how to perform these studies in children has been issued (Riccabona et al. 2015). For performing the study, an age-appropriate Foley catheter is selected. It is important to flush the catheter with the contrast agent before placement in order to remove any existing amount of air. Under sterile conditions, the catheter is partially inserted in the urethral meatus, potentially under fluoroscopic guidance. When the tip is at the level of the fossa navicularis, the balloon is gently inflated with 1–2 ml of saline or air to ensure stabilisation. A small amount of lidocaine gel can be used as local anaesthesia to alleviate discomfort, but excessive amount might cause poor balloon stabilisation.

The patient is positioned in oblique position with the penis mildly stretched, in order to achieve visualisation of the full urethra length avoiding overlap with the femur. Water-soluble contrast material is slowly injected into the urethra in a retrograde fashion via the catheter under fluoroscopic guidance. The contrast flow allows distension of the penile, bulbar and membranous urethra. In most instances, the posterior urethra is not opacified. This should not be considered abnormal, since it is caused by the action of the intrinsic sphincter. Lateral and oblique images are obtained (Fig. 24).

The catheter may be further inserted into the bladder, and subsequent VCUG examination may follow, allowing for additional evaluation of the urethra during voiding. After the completion of the examination, the balloon of the catheter is deflated, and the catheter is subsequently removed.

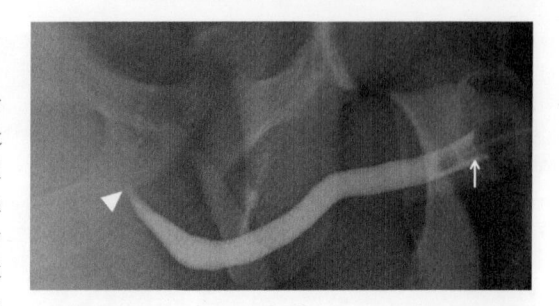

Fig. 24 Retrograde urethrogram. The tip of the catheter is inserted into the distal urethra (*arrow*), and its balloon tip is inflated. Contrast is injected into the urethra in a retrograde fashion distending the normal-appearing urethra, with no evidence of a stricture or wall irregularity. The smooth tapering of the urethral lumen at the junction of membranous-prostatic urethra is normal

> **Take Away**
> Retrograde urethrography is indicated for evaluation of congenital, traumatic, inflammatory and post-surgical anterior urethra pathology and should be performed in a standardised fashion by experienced radiologists.

8 Intravenous Urography

Intravenous urography (IVU) was for decades an important imaging modality that was used for delineation of the urinary tract anatomy and evaluation of renal function and urinary excretion and drainage. With the advent of US, MRI and nuclear medicine, the role of IVU has been substantially diminished in routine practice. However, it can still be the one and only available method in areas with restricted resources and can still be indicated in cases of ureteral or calyceal pathology, such as suspected ectopic ureteral insertion or calyceal diverticula, in cases of urolithiasis (if US is not available or insufficient for decision-making) as well as in cases of suspected renal or ureteral trauma as a delayed KUB view complementary to preceding CT or if CT is not available at all. In these clinical settings, IVU can be used as the initial imaging examination and/or as follow-up examination when the primary diagnosis is known and specific queries decisive for patients' management are to be determined (Riccabona et al. 2010).

Due to the immaturity of the newborn kidney, IVU is typically performed after the first 4–6 weeks of life. Knowledge of creatinine levels is required in all cases, and appropriate hydration is essential to avoid renal damage. Food and fluid uptake are not withheld from infants except for the feeding just prior to the examination. Bowel preparation is also not required in infants and small children but can be suggested in older children and adolescents. This usually includes administration of bisacodyl suppositories (Dulcolax®) a few hours before the examination.

An intravenous line should be established prior to the examination. The volume of the administered iodinated contrast agent should be age and weight adapted. The recommended dose ranges from 2.5 ml/kg, for children 1-year-old, to 1.0 ml/kg, for children >4 years old (Riccabona et al. 2010). Following the IV administration of contrast agent, sequential evaluation of the renal parenchyma, pelvicalyceal system, ureters and bladder is performed. Modifications of the standard IVU acquisition technique, regarding the number, timing and regions of exposures, are acceptable when individually tailored to obtain specific information (Riccabona et al. 2010). Acquisition of an early renal view 5 min following injection and a single late KUB film at 15–20 min is usually sufficient.

> **Take Away**
> IVU under specific circumstances remains an important diagnostic option to obtain anatomic and functional information of the urinary tract; however, it has to be adapted, focussed and well indicated – and is not any longer a generally and routinely used imaging option in the paediatric urinary tract.

9 Computed Tomography of the Urinary Tract (uro-CT)

9.1 Introduction

Computed tomography of the urinary tract (uro-CT) has become the mainstay in the field of adult uroradiology, for investigation of haematuria, abdominal trauma and complicated inflammatory or infectious conditions. In children, a number of factors need to be carefully weighted when considering or performing a CT examination. Children's developing tissues are more sensitive to the effects of ionising radiation compared to adults, and their longer life expectancy increases the possibility to manifest a radiation-induced malignancy. Therefore, CT examinations particularly in the urinary tract can be conducted in children only if diagnostically and clinically thoroughly justified, and if there is no other imaging alternative, and should be performed with special attention to minimise exposure while providing examinations of diagnostic quality (Riccabona et al. 2010; Damasio et al. 2013; Darge et al. 2013a; Riccabona 2013; Amerstorfer et al. 2015).

9.2 Indications

Uro-CT should never be performed as a first-line investigation of the urinary tract in a child, with the exception of high-energy abdominal or polytrauma settings; however, non-ionising imaging examinations (US, MRI, IV ce-US) when feasible should be considered first. Additionally, children with complicated cases of urolithiasis (see also chapter "Imaging of Urolithiasis and Nephrocalcinosis"), unusual or severe urinary tract infections and renal or bladder masses may be investigated with uro-CT, only if prior dedicated US is inconclusive or if MRI is not available. Renal CT angiography can be an option to assess renovascular disease in children with a low disease probability who are not directly referred to catheter angiography (Riccabona et al. 2010).

9.3 Preparation

If contrast agent administration is planned, measurements of creatinine levels are of fundamental importance to ensure normal kidney function. An IV line is necessary, most preferably placed at a peripheral vein of the upper extremity. The largest possible size is chosen. Central lines should not be routinely used. However, in some patients with malignancy, peripheral veins are severely damaged, and a central catheter is the only possible venous access. A fasting period is only required for sedated children (not for contrast agent injection). It should be limited to 2 h in young children and to 3 h in older ones, and dehydration should always be prevented –potentially by an intravenous infusion.

Natural sleep is a relatively safe option to avoid undesirable patient's movement during CT. Sleep deprivation is often successful, particularly if unenhanced CT is performed and immobilisation is also strongly recommended. However, natural sleep is, not infrequently, disturbed in a busy and noisy CT room, and children tend to wake up or at least move particularly when the power contrast injection is performed. In general, if IV contrast is administered, sedation and immobilisation are strongly recommended. The most commonly used medications for sedation in children include midazolam, fentanyl, propofol and pentobarbital (Meyer et al. 2007). Anaesthesiologists should preferably provide the sedation protocol and vital signs including heart rate; breathing rate and pulse oxymetry need to be closely monitored during the procedure and later to ensure patient's safety (American Academy on Pediatrics and Dentistry 2008). The venous access needs to be maintained visible.

Nonionic iodinated contrast agents are preferred because they have been shown to decrease the incidence of minor events. Weight-dependent dose schemes are applied ranging from 1.0 to 2.5 ml/kg (see also chapter "Contrast Agents in Childhood: Application and Safety Considerations" on contrast agents). Oral administration of water-soluble contrast agents or diluted barium sulphate (the child's preferred liquid is recommended for dilution) can be used to mark the gastrointestinal tract and is given about 45 min prior to the scan (Sorantin et al. 2013).

A child with a proven history of a severe adverse event with iodinated contrast agent should be referred to an anaesthesiologist with allergology skills who will make medical decisions about any further injection. If contrast injection is mandatory, a different contrast agent has to be selected. Patients with common allergies or asthma can be given an antihistamine medication for 24 h before examination. Latex allergy is a relative frequent occurrence in children with a history of multiple surgical procedures; latex-free materials and gloves should be used in such patients.

Adverse reactions are rare in paediatric practice. However, preventive measures should be taken, and any reactions that do occur should be managed in collaboration with anaesthesiologists. Adverse events justify the presence of at least two persons during any examination with contrast agent injection (one to take care of the patient and one to call the anaesthesiologist). Severe allergic accidents can occur (tachycardia, severe hypotension), and radiologists and technicians should be aware of first-aid principles (good venous access, perfusion of saline solution, oxygen, preparation of a syringe of diluted adrenaline). The emergency phone number should be visible from anywhere in the CT suite and dialled as soon as possible. Adrenaline can induce severe side effects. For this reason, it would be safer to have only anaesthesiologists administer it. Mild allergic accident (itching, urticaria) can be treated by corticoids and an antihistaminic medication.

9.4 Acquisition Technique

The As Low As Reasonably Achievable (ALARA) principle should be a priority in paediatric CT. Size-, age- and organ-specific protocols in quality-controlled CT equipment should be applied. The variability of technical features in commercially available CT scanners (e.g. number of detector rows, detector sensitivity, rotation speeds, tube current, bore size) should be taken into consideration when designing paediatric CT protocols. However, some practical dose reduction strategies can be partially applied (Stover and Rogalla 2008; Nievelstein et al. 2010).

Most vendors have available default paediatric scan protocols organised by body region. Selection of these protocols and even further optimisation, when possible, can achieve significant dose reduction. Local lead shields should be used to protect radiosensitive organs, such as thyroid, eyes, breast buds and gonads, particularly if not interfering with the scanning region – provided there is no "on the flight" automated dose adaptation. Centring of the patient within the gantry and the scanned field of view is essential for dose reduction and image quality. CT parameters must be adjusted to minimise dose exposure and decrease scanning times: the scan region should be limited to the smallest necessary size and lower kVp and mAs settings, and increased pitch, higher rotation speed and wider collimation are suggested but should be balanced with image quality. If non-contrast scanning is planned, further dose decreasing can be achieved without affecting diagnostic reliability. In general there is a simple rule: if the images are very nice with a low noise level, one can try to reconstruct the dataset in a smaller slice thickness – if the images still turn out of diagnostic quality, one can reduce the dose usually by at least 20–30 % (Sorantin et al. 2013).

Efforts should be made to tailor protocols to query (according to clinical indication and the results of preceding examinations). In the majority of cases, a single-scanning phase is sufficient (Riccabona et al. 2010; Damasio et al. 2013). Selection between an unenhanced, arterial, nephrographic or excretory phase can be performed according to the indication and the known findings from preceded examinations, usually US. A nephrographic phase is always informative (Fig. 25). In the setting of suspected injury of the collecting system, additional scanning during excretory phase might be necessary (Fig. 26). Alternatively, split-bolus technique should be considered an option for synchronous imaging during nephrographic and excretory phases while reducing the radiation dose. In this technique, splitting the contrast bolus in two parts, injecting

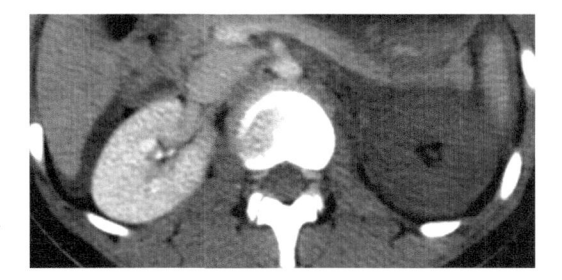

Fig. 25 Contrast-enhanced CT. Grade V laceration of the left kidney. Nephrographic phase. The left kidney appears enlarged with complete lack of parenchymal enhancement, indicative of kidney devascularisation

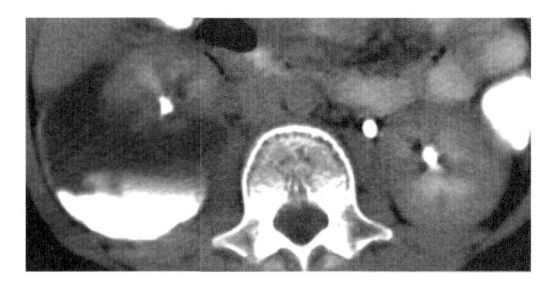

Fig. 26 Contrast-enhanced CT. Grade IV laceration of the right kidney. Excretory phase. Grade IV laceration of the right kidney, involving the renal cortex, medulla and the collecting system, with a large low-attenuation collection in the perinephric space representing a urinoma. Leek of contrast is noted within the dependent part of this fluid collection

at two different time points and obtaining a single image acquisition can provide simultaneously the required information from both phases (Darge et al. 2013a).

The use of power injection provides an excellent examination quality, and the continuous flow decreases the risk of extravascular passage. Injection speed can be adjusted to 1–4 ml/s; faster injection rates are usually not achievable in children and hardly necessary. The injection should be visually monitored and stopped in case of extravascular passage. However, depending on the location, size and type of IV access, child size and weight, underlying disease and the clinical query, the contrast agent can be hand injected.

The radiologist should check the acquired images for quality and diagnostic completeness and decide if additional images are needed before the child leaves the CT room.

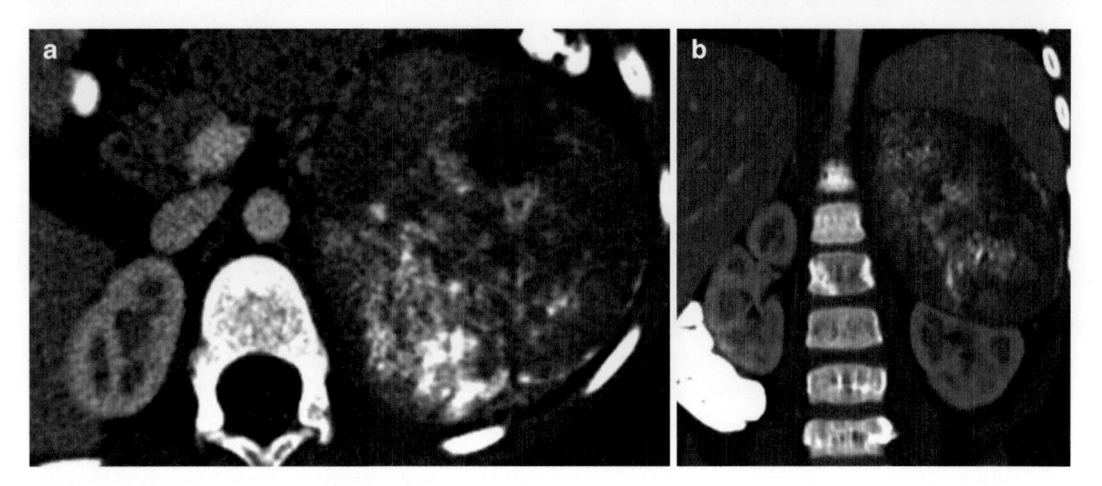

Fig. 27 Contrast-enhanced CT. Five-year-old male with abdominal distention. (**a**) Axial scan. A large, well-circumscribed, solid and heterogeneously enhancing mass is seen in the left upper quadrant. The mass contains multiple calcifications and areas of low attenuation consistent with necrosis. (**b**) Coronal reconstruction. The mass displaces inferiorly and compresses the left kidney, as well as abuts the inferior surface of the spleen, suggestive of adrenal origin

Multiplanar reformatting is particularly useful in evaluating renal traumatic injuries or retroperitoneal tumours (Fig. 27). Maximal intensity projection (MIP) images in coronal and sagittal planes are also useful for angiographic studies. Volume rendering techniques allow better representation of the urinary tract. The CT dose index and dose length product should be mentioned in the report.

Take Away

Uro-CT in children is the imaging choice in cases of high-energy trauma, complicated urolithiasis (or rarely also infections) and neoplasm staging, if preceding non-irradiating imaging is not diagnostic and MRI is not available or not able to answer the query.

Conclusion

A wide variety of imaging examinations are available in clinical paediatric uroradiology practice. The radiologist should be well familiar with the indications, the technical parameters and the procedural skills to perform a diagnostically reliable examination. In addition to performing a good imaging examination, it is important to minimise irradiation, pain and risk; the chosen technique must also be well adapted to the patient (age, condition, disease) and the question posed by the referring physician. US is the mainstay of uroradiological imaging throughout childhood and should be available 24/7/356. US is often complemented by KBU or VCUG (unless ce-VUS or MRI is performed). IVU is hardly used nowadays, and CT should be avoided whenever possible for its radiation burden but should never be withheld from a patient if there is a valid indication with no other accessible or diagnostically reliable imaging option such as, e.g. severe and multiple trauma.

References

American Academy on Pediatrics, and American Academy on Pediatric Dentistry (2008) Guideline for monitoring and management of pediatric patients during and after sedation for diagnostic and therapeutic procedures. Pediatr Dent 30(7 Suppl):143–159

Amerstorfer EE, Haberlik A, Riccabona M (2015) Imaging assessment of renal injuries in children and adolescents: CT or ultrasound? J Pediatr Surg 50(3):448–455. doi:10.1016/j.jpedsurg.2014.07.006

Avni FE, Garel C, Cassart M, D'Haene N, Hall M, Riccabona M (2012) Imaging and classification of congenital cystic renal diseases. AJR Am J Roentgenol 198(5):1004–1013. doi:10.2214/AJR.11.8083, 198/5/1004 [pii]

Bamber J, Cosgrove D, Dietrich CF, Fromageau J, Bojunga J, Calliada F, Cantisani V et al (2013) EFSUMB guidelines and recommendations on the clinical use of ultrasound elastography. Part 1: Basic principles and technology. Ultraschall Med 34(2):169–184. doi:10.1055/s-0033-1335205

Bartram U, Darge K (2005) Harmonic versus conventional ultrasound imaging of the urinary tract in children. Pediatr Radiol 35(7):655–660. doi:10.1007/s00247-005-1415-9

Berrocal T, Lopez-Pereira P, Arjonilla A, Gutierrez J (2002) Anomalies of the distal ureter, bladder, and urethra in children: embryologic, radiologic, and pathologic features. Radiographics 22(5):1139–1164. doi:10.1148/radiographics.22.5.g02se101139

Berrocal T, Gaya F, Arjonilla A (2005) Vesicoureteral reflux: can the urethra be adequately assessed by using contrast-enhanced voiding US of the bladder? Radiology 234(1):235–241. doi:10.1148/radiol.2341031503

Catalano O, Aiani L, Barozzi L, Bokor D, De Marchi A, Faletti C, Maggioni F et al (2009) CEUS in abdominal trauma: multi-center study. Abdom Imaging 34(2):225–234. doi:10.1007/s00261-008-9452-0

Claudon M, Cosgrove D, Albrecht T, Bolondi L, Bosio M, Calliada F, Correas JM et al (2008) Guidelines and good clinical practice recommendations for contrast enhanced ultrasound (CEUS) – update 2008. Ultraschall Med 29(1):28–44. doi:10.1055/s-2007-963785

Claudon M, Dietrich CF, Choi BI, Cosgrove DO, Kudo M, Nolsoe CP, Piscaglia F et al (2013) Guidelines and good clinical practice recommendations for Contrast Enhanced Ultrasound (CEUS) in the liver – update 2012: A WFUMB-EFSUMB initiative in cooperation with representatives of AFSUMB, AIUM, ASUM, FLAUS and ICUS. Ultrasound Med Biol 39(2):187–210. doi:10.1016/j.ultrasmedbio.2012.09.002, doi:S0301-5629(12)00543-1 [pii]

Cleveland RH, Constantinou C, Blickman JG, Jaramillo D, Webster E (1992) Voiding cystourethrography in children: value of digital fluoroscopy in reducing radiation dose. AJR Am J Roentgenol 158(1):137–142. doi:10.2214/ajr.158.1.1727340

Coleman JL, Navid F, Furman WL, McCarville MB (2014) Safety of ultrasound contrast agents in the pediatric oncologic population: a single-institution experience. AJR Am J Roentgenol 202(5):966–970. doi:10.2214/AJR.13.12010

Correas J, Helenon O, Moreau JF (1999) Contrast-enhanced ultrasonography of native and transplanted kidney diseases. Eur Radiol 9(Suppl 3):S394–S400

Dacher JN, Pfister C, Monroc M, Eurin D, LeDosseur P (1996) Power Doppler sonographic pattern of acute pyelonephritis in children: comparison with CT. AJR Am J Roentgenol 166(6):1451–1455. doi:10.2214/ajr.166.6.8633462

Damasio MB, Darge K, Riccabona M (2013) Multidetector CT in the paediatric urinary tract. Eur J Radiol 82(7):1118–1125. doi:10.1016/j.ejrad.2011.12.005, S0720-048X(11)00838-2 [pii]

Darge K (2008a) Voiding urosonography with ultrasound contrast agents for the diagnosis of vesicoureteric reflux in children. I. Procedure. Pediatr Radiol 38(1):40–53. doi:10.1007/s00247-007-0529-7

Darge K (2008b) Voiding urosonography with US contrast agents for the diagnosis of vesicoureteric reflux in children. II. Comparison with radiological examinations. Pediatr Radiol 38(1):54–63. doi:10.1007/s00247-007-0528-8; quiz 126-127

Darge K (2010) Voiding urosonography with US contrast agent for the diagnosis of vesicoureteric reflux in children: an update. Pediatr Radiol 40(6):956–962. doi:10.1007/s00247-010-1623-9

Darge K, Heidemeier A (2005) Modern ultrasound technologies and their application in pediatric urinary tract imaging. Radiologe 45(12):1101–1111. doi:10.1007/s00117-005-1248-4

Darge K, Troeger J (2002) Vesicoureteral reflux grading in contrast-enhanced voiding urosonography. Eur J Radiol 43(2):122–128, doi:S0720048X02001146 [pii]

Darge K, Higgins M, Hwang TJ, Delgado J, Shukla A, Bellah R (2013a) Magnetic resonance and computed tomography in pediatric urology: an imaging overview for current and future daily practice. Radiol Clin North Am 51(4):583–598. doi:10.1016/j.rcl.2013.03.004, S0033-8389(13)00023-7 [pii]

Darge K, Papadopoulou F, Ntoulia A, Bulas DI, Coley BD, Fordham LA, Paltiel HJ et al (2013b) Safety of contrast-enhanced ultrasound in children for non-cardiac applications: a review by the Society for Pediatric Radiology (SPR) and the International Contrast Ultrasound Society (ICUS). Pediatr Radiol 43(9):1063–1073. doi:10.1007/s00247-013-2746-6

Don S, Goske MJ, John S, Whiting B, Willis CE (2011) Image Gently pediatric digital radiography summit: executive summary. Pediatr Radiol 41(5):562–565. doi:10.1007/s00247-010-1966-2

Don S, Macdougall R, Strauss K, Moore QT, Goske MJ, Cohen M, Herrmann T et al (2013) Image gently campaign back to basics initiative: ten steps to help manage radiation dose in pediatric digital radiography. AJR Am J Roentgenol 200(5):W431–W436. doi:10.2214/AJR.12.9895

Dorfman AL, Fazel R, Einstein AJ, Applegate KE, Krumholz HM, Wang Y, Christodoulou E, Chen J, Sanchez R, Nallamothu BK (2011) Use of medical imaging procedures with ionizing radiation in children: a population-based study. Arch Pediatr Adolesc Med 165(5):458–464. doi:10.1001/archpediatrics.2010.270, archpediatrics.2010.270 [pii]

Durán Feliubadaló C, Beltrán Salazar VP, Martin C, Riera L, Artacho I, Preciado Borreguero D, Consola B (2015) Tips and tricks to evaluate the urethra through serial voiding urosonography (VUS): making it easy. Paper presented at the ECR 2015, Vienna

Duran C, Valera A, Alguersuari A, Ballesteros E, Riera L, Martin C, Puig J (2009) Voiding urosonography: the study of the urethra is no longer a limitation of the technique. Pediatr Radiol 39(2):124–131. doi:10.1007/s00247-008-1050-3

Duran C, del Riego J, Riera L, Martin C, Serrano C, Palana P (2012) Voiding urosonography including urethrosonography: high-quality examinations with an optimised procedure using a second-generation US contrast agent. Pediatr Radiol 42(6):660–667. doi:10.1007/s00247-012-2360-z

Feneberg R, Schaefer F, Zieger B, Waldherr R, Mehls O, Scharer K (1998) Percutaneous renal biopsy in children: a 27-year experience. Nephron 79(4): 438–446

Fotter R, Kopp W, Klein E, Hollwarth M, Uray E (1986) Unstable bladder in children: functional evaluation by modified voiding cystourethrography. Radiology 161(3):811–813. doi:10.1148/radiology.161.3.3786739

Goske MJ, Charkot E, Herrmann T, John SD, Mills TT, Morrison G, Smith SN (2011) Image Gently: challenges for radiologic technologists when performing digital radiography in children. Pediatr Radiol 41(5):611–619. doi:10.1007/s00247-010-1957-3

Goya C, Hamidi C, Ece A, Okur MH, Tasdemir B, Cetincakmak MG, Hattapoglu S, Teke M, Sahin C (2014) Acoustic radiation force impulse (ARFI) elastography for detection of renal damage in children. Pediatr Radiol. doi:10.1007/s00247-014-3072-3

Grenier N, Gennisson JL, Cornelis F, Le Bras Y, Couzi L (2013) Renal ultrasound elastography. Diagn Interv Imaging 94(5):545–550. doi:10.1016/j.diii.2013.02.003, S2211-5684(13)00038-7 [pii]

Habbig S, Beck BB, Hoppe B (2011) Nephrocalcinosis and urolithiasis in children. Kidney Int 80(12):1278–1291. doi:10.1038/ki.2011.336, ki2011336 [pii]

Hibbert J, Howlett DC, Greenwood KL, MacDonald LM, Saunders AJ (1997) The ultrasound appearances of neonatal renal vein thrombosis. Br J Radiol 70(839):1191–1194. doi:10.1259/bjr.70.839.9536915

Igarashi T, Ito S, Sako M, Saitoh A, Hataya H, Mizuguchi M, Morishima T et al (2014) Guidelines for the management and investigation of hemolytic uremic syndrome. Clin Exp Nephrol 18(4):525–557. doi:10.1007/s10157-014-0995-9

Jacob J, Deganello A, Sellars ME, Hadzic N, Sidhu PS (2013) Contrast enhanced ultrasound (CEUS) characterization of grey-scale sonographic indeterminate focal liver lesions in pediatric practice. Ultraschall Med 34(6):529–540. doi:10.1055/s-0033-1355785

Jequier S, Rousseau O (1987) Sonographic measurements of the normal bladder wall in children. AJR Am J Roentgenol 149(3):563–566. doi:10.2214/ajr.149.3.563

Kadioglu A, Mihmanli I, Kantarci F, Tekes A, Uysal O (2006) Cyclic voiding cystourethrography without the use of fluoroscopic monitoring. Eur J Radiol 57(1):138–147. doi:10.1016/j.ejrad.2005.06.012

Koff SA (1983) Estimating bladder capacity in children. Urology 21(3):248

Korner M, Weber CH, Wirth S, Pfeifer KJ, Reiser MF, Treitl M (2007) Advances in digital radiography: physical principles and system overview. Radiographics 27(3):675–686. doi:10.1148/rg.273065075, doi:27/3/675 [pii]

Lebowitz RL (1996) Voiding cystourethrography in boys: the presence of the catheter does not obscure the diagnosis of posterior urethral valves but prevents estimation of the adequacy of transurethral fulguration. AJR Am J Roentgenol 166(3):724–725. doi:10.2214/ajr.166.3.8623666

Lebowitz RL, Olbing H, Parkkulainen KV, Smellie JM, Tamminen-Mobius TE (1985) International system of radiographic grading of vesicoureteric reflux. International Reflux Study in Children. Pediatr Radiol 15(2):105–109

Lungren MP, Patel MN, Racadio JM, Johnson ND (2014) Ultrasound-guided interventions in children. Eur J Radiol 83(9):1582–1591. doi:10.1016/j.ejrad.2014.04.021, S0720-048X(14)00221-6 [pii]

Markowitz RI, Altes TA, Jaramillo D (2009) What causes the "wet diaper" artifact? Computed tomography and magnetic resonance observations. Clin Imaging 33(3):226–230. doi:10.1016/j.clinimag.2008.09.013, S0899-7071(08)00314-8 [pii]

McCarville MB, Kaste SC, Hoffer FA, Khan RB, Walton RC, Alpert BS, Furman WL, Li C, Xiong X (2012) Contrast-enhanced sonography of malignant pediatric abdominal and pelvic solid tumors: preliminary safety and feasibility data. Pediatr Radiol 42(7):824–833. doi:10.1007/s00247-011-2338-2

Menichini G, Sessa B, Trinci M, Galluzzo M, Miele V (2015) Accuracy of contrast-enhanced ultrasound (CEUS) in the identification and characterization of traumatic solid organ lesions in children: a retrospective comparison with baseline US and CE-MDCT. Radiol Med. doi:10.1007/s11547-015-0535-z

Meyer S, Grundmann U, Gottschling S, Kleinschmidt S, Gortner L (2007) Sedation and analgesia for brief diagnostic and therapeutic procedures in children. Eur J Pediatr 166(4):291–302. doi:10.1007/s00431-006-0356-0

Moudgil A (2014) Renal venous thrombosis in neonates. Curr Pediatr Rev 10(2):101–106

Muller-Ording LS (2014) Ultrasound of the paediatric urogenital tract. Eur J Radiol 83(9):1538–1548. doi:10.1016/j.ejrad.2014.04.001, S0720-048X(14)00173-9 [pii]

Nievelstein RA, van Dam IM, van der Molen AJ (2010) Multidetector CT in children: current concepts and dose reduction strategies. Pediatr Radiol 40(8):1324–1344. doi:10.1007/s00247-010-1714-7

Novljan G, Kenig A, Rus R, Kenda RB (2003) Cyclic voiding urosonography in detecting vesicoureteral reflux in children. Pediatr Nephrol 18(10):992–995. doi:10.1007/s00467-003-1228-8

Ozkan F, Menzilcioglu MS, Duymus M, Yildiz S, Avcu S (2014) Acoustic radiation force impulse elastography for evaluating renal parenchymal stiffness in children. Pediatr Radiol. doi:10.1007/s00247-014-3174-y

Paltiel HJ, Rupich RC, Kiruluta HG (1992) Enhanced detection of vesicoureteral reflux in infants and children with use of cyclic voiding cystourethrography. Radiology 184(3):753–755. doi:10.1148/radiology.184.3.1509062

Papadopoulou F, Efremidis SC, Oiconomou A, Badouraki M, Panteleli M, Papachristou F, Soteriou I (2002) Cyclic voiding cystourethrography: is vesicoureteral reflux missed with standard voiding cystourethrography? Eur Radiol 12(3):666–670. doi:10.1007/s003300101108

Papadopoulou F, Tsampoulas C, Siomou E, Tzovara J, Siamopoulou A, Efremidis SC (2006) Cyclic contrast-enhanced harmonic voiding urosonography for the evaluation of reflux. Can we keep the cost of the examination low? Eur Radiol 16(11):2521–2526. doi:10.1007/s00330-006-0253-y

Papadopoulou F, Anthopoulou A, Fotopoulos A, Siomou E, Bokhrhli JA, Papastefanaki M, Bellou S, Efremidis E (2007) Is reflux missed on fluoroscopic voiding cysteourethrography and demonstrated only by contrast-enhanced voiding urosonography clinically important? Pediatr Radiol 37(Suppl 2):S105–S118

Papadopoulou F, Ntoulia A, Siomou E, Darge K (2014) Contrast-enhanced voiding urosonography with intravesical administration of a second-generation ultrasound contrast agent for diagnosis of vesicoureteral reflux: prospective evaluation of contrast safety in 1,010 children. Pediatr Radiol 44(6):719–728. doi:10.1007/s00247-013-2832-9

Pico Aliaga SD, Muro Velilla D, Garcia-Marti G, Sanguesa Nebot C, Marti-Bonmati L (2014) Acoustic radiation force impulse imaging elastography is efficacious in detecting hepatic fibrosis in children. Radiologia 57(4):314–320. doi:10.1016/j.rx.2014.04.005. S0033-8338(14)00065-4 [pii]

Piscaglia F, Nolsoe C, Dietrich CF, Cosgrove DO, Gilja OH, Bachmann Nielsen M, Albrecht T et al (2012) The EFSUMB Guidelines and Recommendations on the Clinical Practice of Contrast Enhanced Ultrasound (CEUS): update 2011 on non-hepatic applications. Ultraschall Med 33(1):33–59. doi:10.1055/s-0031-1281676

Piskunowicz M, Kosiak W, Batko T (2012) Intravenous application of second-generation ultrasound contrast agents in children: a review of the literature. Ultraschall Med 33(2):135–140. doi:10.1055/s-0031-1281936

Piskunowicz M, Kosiak W, Batko T, Piankowski A, Polczynska K, Adamkiewicz-Drozynska E (2015) Safety of intravenous application of second-generation ultrasound contrast agent in children: prospective analysis. Ultrasound Med Biol 41(4):1095–1099. doi:10.1016/j.ultrasmedbio.2014.11.003

Pohl HG, Belman AB (2009) The "top-down" approach to the evaluation of children with febrile urinary tract infection. Adv Urol 783409. doi:10.1155/2009/783409

Quaia E, De Paoli L, Stocca T, Cabibbo B, Casagrande F, Cova MA (2012) The value of small bowel wall contrast enhancement after sulfur hexafluoride-filled microbubble injection to differentiate inflammatory from fibrotic strictures in patients with Crohn's disease. Ultrasound Med Biol 38(8):1324–1332. doi:10.1016/j.ultrasmedbio.2012.04.008, doi:S0301-5629(12)00220-7 [pii]

Riccabona M (2000) Amplitude-coded color Doppler ultrasonography in pediatrics. Ultraschall Med 21(6):273–283. doi:10.1055/s-2000-9121

Riccabona M (2002) Cystography in infants and children: a critical appraisal of the many forms with special regard to voiding cystourethrography. Eur Radiol 12(12):2910–2918. doi:10.1007/s00330-002-1430-2

Riccabona M (2012) Application of a second-generation US contrast agent in infants and children--a European questionnaire-based survey. Pediatr Radiol 42(12):1471–1480. doi:10.1007/s00247-012-2472-5

Riccabona M (2013) CT in children: why and what to consider for CT in children. Eur J Radiol 82(7):1041–1042. doi:10.1016/j.ejrad.2011.11.039

Riccabona M (2014a) Basics, principles, techniques and modern methods in paediatric ultrasonography. Eur J Radiol 83(9):1487–1494. doi:10.1016/j.ejrad.2014.04.032, S0720-048X(14)00234-4 [pii]

Riccabona M (2014b) Diagnostic ultrasonography in neonates, infants and children-Why, when and how. Eur J Radiol 83(9):1485–1486. doi:10.1016/j.ejrad.2014.04.010, S0720-048X(14)00210-1 [pii]

Riccabona M, Sorantin E, Ring E (1998) Application of M-mode sonography to functional evaluation in pediatric patients. Eur Radiol 8(8):1457–1461. doi:10.1007/s003300050575

Riccabona M, Ring E, Schwinger W, Aigner R (2001) Amplitude coded-colour Doppler sonography in paediatric renal disease. Eur Radiol 11(5):861–866. doi:10.1007/s003300000665

Riccabona M, Avni FE, Blickman JG, Dacher JN, Darge K, Lobo ML, Willi U (2008) Imaging recommendations in paediatric uroradiology: minutes of the ESPR workgroup session on urinary tract infection, fetal urinary tract dilatation, urinary tract ultrasonography and voiding cystourethrography, Barcelona, Spain, June 2007. Pediatr Radiol 38(2):138–145. doi:10.1007/s00247-007-0695-7

Riccabona M, Avni FE, Blickman JG, Dacher JN, Darge K, Lobo ML, Willi U (2009) Imaging recommendations in paediatric uroradiology. Minutes of the ESPR uroradiology task force session on childhood obstructive uropathy, high-grade fetal urinary tract dilatation, childhood haematuria, and urolithiasis in childhood. ESPR Annual Congress, Edinburgh, UK, June 2008. Pediatr Radiol 39(8):891–898. doi:10.1007/s00247-009-1233-6

Riccabona M, Avni FE, Dacher JN, Damasio MB, Darge K, Lobo ML, Ording-Muller LS, Papadopoulou F, Willi U (2010) ESPR uroradiology task force and ESUR paediatric working group: imaging and procedural recommendations in paediatric uroradiology, part III. Minutes of the ESPR uroradiology task force minisymposium on intravenous urography, uro-CT and MR-urography in childhood. Pediatr Radiol 40(7):1315–1320. doi:10.1007/s00247-010-1686-7

Riccabona M, Avni FE, Damasio MB, Ording-Muller LS, Blickman JG, Darge K, Lobo ML, Papadopoulou F, Vivier PH, Willi U (2012) ESPR Uroradiology Task Force and ESUR Paediatric Working Group--Imaging recommendations in paediatric uroradiology, part V: childhood cystic kidney disease, childhood renal transplantation and contrast-enhanced ultrasonography in children. Pediatr Radiol 42(10):1275–1283. doi:10.1007/s00247-012-2436-9

Riccabona M, Vivier PH, Ntoulia A, Darge K, Avni F, Papadopoulou F, Damasio B et al (2014) ESPR uroradiology task force imaging recommendations in paediatric uroradiology, part VII: standardised terminology, impact of existing recommendations, and update on contrast-enhanced ultrasound of the paediatric urogenital tract. Pediatr Radiol 44(11):1478–1484. doi:10.1007/s00247-014-3135-5

Riccabona M, Darge K, Lobo ML, Ording-Muller LS, Augdal TA, Avni FE, Blickman J et al (2015) ESPR Uroradiology Taskforce-imaging recommendations in paediatric uroradiology, part VIII: retrograde urethrography, imaging disorder of sexual development and imaging childhood testicular torsion. Pediatr Radiol 45(13):2023–2028. doi:10.1007/s00247-015-3452-3

Ripolles T, Rausell N, Paredes JM, Grau E, Martinez MJ, Vizuete J (2013) Effectiveness of contrast-enhanced ultrasound for characterisation of intestinal inflammation in Crohn's disease: a comparison with surgical histopathology analysis. J Crohns Colitis 7(2):120–128. doi:10.1016/j.crohns.2012.03.002, doi:S1873-9946(12)00103-1 [pii]

Roehrborn CG, Peters PC (1988) Can transabdominal ultrasound estimation of postvoiding residual (PVR) replace catheterization? Urology 31(5):445–449

Rosado E, Riccabona M (2016) Off-label use of ultrasound contrast agents for intravenous applications in children: Analysis of the existing literature. J Ultrasound Med 35(3):487–496

Rothrock SG, Green SM, Hummel CB (1992) Plain abdominal radiography in the detection of major disease in children: a prospective analysis. Ann Emerg Med 21(12):1423–1429, doi:S0196-0644(05)80053-8 [pii]

Schmit P, Sfez M (1997) Management of anxious and painful manifestations in pediatric uroradiology. J Radiol 78(5):367–372. doi:MDOI-JR-05-1997-78-5-0221-0363-101019-ART85 [pii]

Schoellnast H, Lindbichler F, Riccabona M (2004) Sonographic diagnosis of urethral anomalies in infants: value of perineal sonography. J Ultrasound Med 23(6):769–776

Sorantin E (2008) Soft-copy display and reading: what the radiologist should know in the digital era. Pediatr Radiol 38(12):1276–1284. doi:10.1007/s00247-008-0898-6

Sorantin E, Fotter R, Aigner R, Ring E, Riccabona M (1997) The sonographically thickened wall of the upper urinary tract system: correlation with other imaging methods. Pediatr Radiol 27(8):667–671. doi:10.1007/s002470050208

Sorantin E, Weissensteiner S, Hasenburger G, Riccabona M (2013) CT in children--dose protection and general considerations when planning a CT in a child. Eur J Radiol 82(7):1043–1049. doi:10.1016/j.ejrad.2011.11.041, S0720-048X(11)00819-9 [pii]

Stenzel M, Mentzel HJ (2014) Ultrasound elastography and contrast-enhanced ultrasound in infants, children and adolescents. Eur J Radiol 83(9):1560–1569. doi:10.1016/j.ejrad.2014.06.007, S0720-048X(14)00325-8 [pii]

Stover B, Rogalla P (2008) CT examinations in children. Radiologe 48(3):243–248. doi:10.1007/s00117-007-1600-y

Teele RL, Share JC (1997) Transperineal sonography in children. AJR Am J Roentgenol 168(5):1263–1267. doi:10.2214/ajr.168.5.9129424

Valentino M, Serra C, Pavlica P, Labate AM, Lima M, Baroncini S, Barozzi L (2008) Blunt abdominal trauma: diagnostic performance of contrast-enhanced US in children--initial experience. Radiology 246(3):903–909. doi:10.1148/radiol.2463070652

Willis CE (2009) Optimizing digital radiography of children. Eur J Radiol 72(2):266–273. doi:10.1016/j.ejrad.2009.03.003, S0720-048X(09)00112-0 [pii]

Wozniak MM, Osemlak P, Pawelec A, Brodzisz A, Nachulewicz P, Wieczorek AP, Zajaczkowska MM (2014a) Intraoperative contrast-enhanced urosonography during endoscopic treatment of vesicoureteral reflux in children. Pediatr Radiol 44(9):1093–1100. doi:10.1007/s00247-014-2963-7

Wozniak MM, Pawelec A, Wieczorek AP, Zajaczkowska MM, Nachulewicz P, Borzcka H (2014b) The usefulness of 3D/4D techniques during voiding urosonography (VUS) in the diagnostics and monitoring of treatment of vesicoureteral reflux in children. In: ecr2014. Vienna

MR of the Urogenital Tract in Children

J. Damien Grattan-Smith and Richard A. Jones

Contents

1 Introduction.. 33
2 **MR Urography Technique**........................... 34
2.1 Core Protocol.. 34
2.2 Optional Sequences.................................. 38
2.3 MR Contrast Agents................................. 40
3 **Post-processing**.. 41
4 **Clinical Applications**................................ 45
4.1 Evaluation of Urinary Tract Dilatation...... 45
4.2 Congenital Anomalies of the Kidney and Urinary Tract (CAKUT)............................. 64
4.3 Pyelonephritis and Renal Scarring............ 68
4.4 MR for VUR Assessment: MR VCUG...... 70
4.5 MR Genitography..................................... 72
4.6 MR Imaging of Renal Tumors.................. 77
4.7 MR Imaging in Renal Trauma.................. 80
4.8 MR Imaging in Renal Transplantation...... 81

Conclusion.. 83

References... 83

J.D. Grattan-Smith, MBBS (✉)
Department of Radiology, Children's Healthcare of Atlanta, 1001 Johnson Ferry Road, Atlanta, GA 30342, USA,
e-mail: Damien.grattan-smith@choa.org

R.A. Jones, PhD
Department of Radiology, Emory University School of Medicine, Atlanta, GA, USA

1 Introduction

MR urography comprehensively evaluates the urinary tract in a single examination that does not use ionizing radiation (Grattan-Smith and Jones 2008; MD et al. 2010; Vivier et al. 2010b; Jones et al. 2011; Zhang et al. 2013b; Boss et al. 2014; Claudon et al. 2014). MR urography utilizes both static and dynamic imaging, taking advantage of the intrinsically high spatial and contrast resolution to provide high-resolution anatomic images. Additionally, dynamic imaging after administration of intravenous contrast medium is used to obtain functional information about the enhancement, concentration, and excretion of the kidneys using both qualitative and quantitative analysis. The signal changes related to perfusion, concentration, and excretion of the contrast agent can be evaluated sequentially as the contrast agent passes through the renal cortex, the medulla, and then into the collecting systems. Urinary tract anatomy is assessed using a combination of both T2-weighted and contrast-enhanced images. MR urography is similar to intravenous urography but has greater intrinsic contrast, spatial, and temporal resolution. The functional information obtained is comparable to renal scintigraphy but with the important distinction that anatomic images allow the signal originating from the renal parenchyma to be separated from those originating in the collecting system. As a result, the analysis of signal intensity versus time changes in the renal parenchyma can be isolated from those occurring in the collecting system.

Several groups have described different approaches to MR urography with variations both in the imaging protocols and methods used to perform functional analysis (Bokacheva et al. 2008; Khrichenko and Darge 2009; Vivier et al. 2010a; Jones et al. 2011; Boss et al. 2014). Variations in imaging technique differ in the approach to sedation, timing of furosemide administration, as well as the administration and dose of contrast agent. Another key difference in the various approaches to MR urography is based on the use of 3D versus 2D acquisition of data for functional analysis. The 3D sequences provide greater spatial resolution, whereas the 2D sequences have greater temporal resolution. The greater temporal resolution is advantageous in the evaluation of renal function. These techniques are currently being refined and assessed. No consensus protocol has been established although we prefer 3D techniques.

The primary indication for MR urography in children is the evaluation of UTD. Other indications for MR of the pediatric urogenital tract include evaluation of congenital malformations and dysplasia, diagnosis of pyelonephritis and renal scarring, identification of ectopic ureters in children with urinary incontinence, and the evaluation of disorders of sexual differentiation. Furthermore, transplant kidney imaging and imaging of renal vasculature, after renal trauma, and of urogenital tract tumors are accepted indications (see Chaps. 34, 35, 36, and 37). Additionally, the improved anatomic and functional information obtained with MR urography provides new insights into the underlying pathophysiology of urinary tract disorders. As a result, it is likely that MR of the pediatric urogenital tract will become the primary tool in the evaluation of complex urogenital tract disorders in children.

2 MR Urography Technique

2.1 Core Protocol

We mainly describe and discuss our imaging protocol – there are others that differ slightly (Darge et al. 2010; Renjen et al. 2010; Vivier et al. 2010b; Jones et al. 2011). Recommendations on the anatomic MR study have been issued by the ESPR urogenital imaging task force (Riccabona et al. 2010). The imaging protocols used for clinical studies consist of coronal T1 FLAIR, multiplanar FSE T2-weighted sequences prior to contrast administration, and dynamic 3D gradient echo sequences after contrast administration (Perez-Brayfield et al. 2003; Grattan-Smith et al. 2003; Jones et al. 2005, 2011) (Figs. 1, 2, and 3). The images are routinely acquired on a 1.5 T Siemens Avanto scanner fitted with a standard gradient system. The patient is positioned supine on the scanner and the spine coils and one or two body coils, depending on the size of the patient, are used for signal reception. There is a fundamentally complex relationship between signal intensity and gadolinium concentration, with T1 effects predominating at lower concentrations and T2* effects at higher concentrations which may lead to signal loss. Phantom studies have shown that the relationship between signal intensity and gadolinium concentration is relatively linear at low concentrations (Jones et al. 2005). To stay within this linear portion of the curve, we keep the gadolinium concentration low by hydrating the patient, by giving furosemide 15 min before the contrast is administered, and by infusing the contrast agent slowly for the dynamic series.

For our protocols, all children are hydrated prior to the study with an intravenous infusion of lactated Ringer's solution; for sedated children the volume infused is calculated to replace the NPO deficit, otherwise the volume is calculated using a guideline of 10 ml/kg. Typically, all children less than 7 years of age require sedation for the examination, and the department's standard sedation procedures are followed. A bladder catheter is placed to eliminate the possibility of reflux and to ensure free drainage of the bladder. Once the patient is positioned in the scanner, scout images are acquired to determine both the positioning of the kidneys and bladder and the combination of spine coil elements required to optimize the signal-to-noise ratio (SNR) for these anatomical structures. After the scout images were completed, axial T2-weighted (TR 6000, TE 144, ETL = 23) TSE images with high spatial

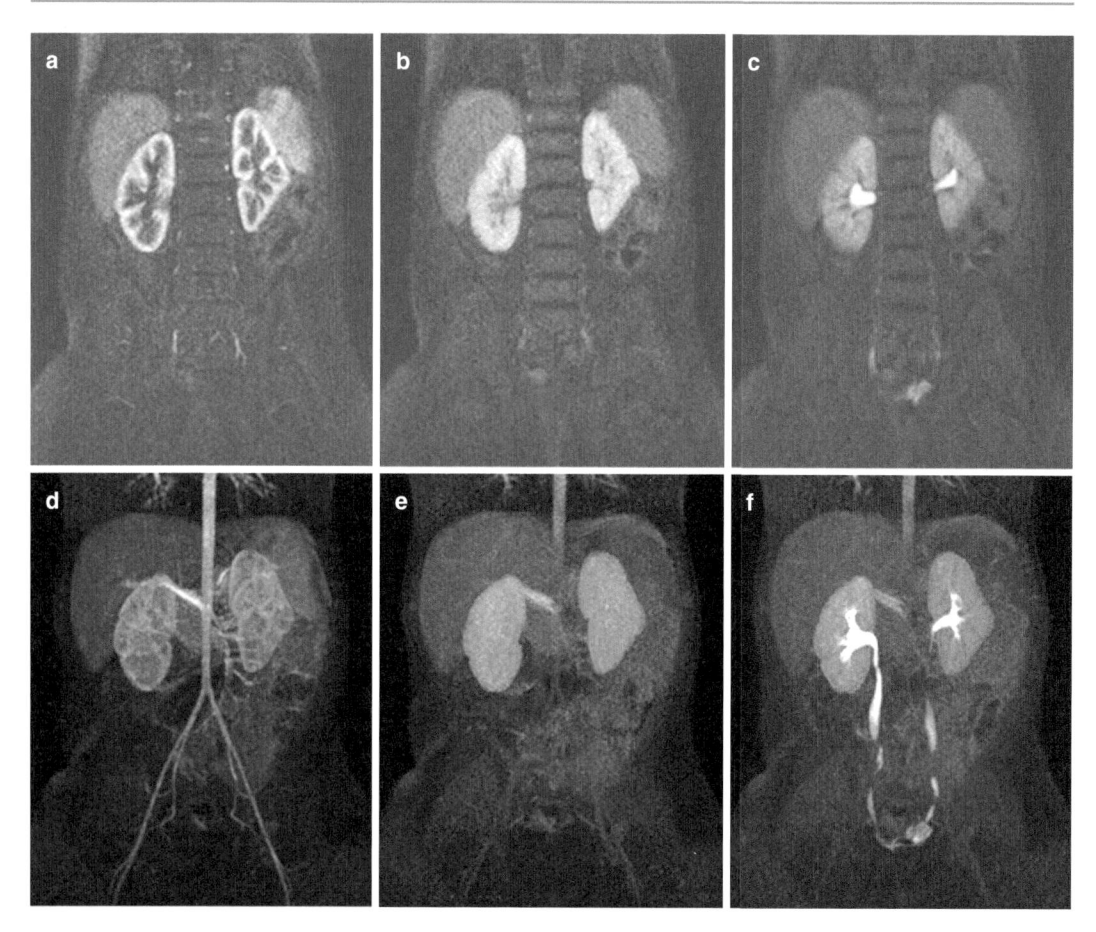

Fig. 1 Normal MR urogram in a 3-month-old boy with antenatal UTD. Images (**a–c**) show the same slice from each of three separate volume acquisitions, whereas (**d–f**) show MIP projections derived from the same three separate time points. **a** and **d** show the cortical phase. **b** and **e** were acquired 60 s later and demonstrate enhancement of both the cortex and medulla with the signal intensity of the medulla exceeding the cortex. **c** and **f** were acquired 115 s after the vascular phase and show excretion into the calyces, renal pelvis, and ureters. The renal transit time was 2 min and 20 s bilaterally, and the volumetric DRF was 51:49

resolution that are acquired through the kidneys are obtained.

Furosemide (1 mg/kg, max. 20 mg) is then administered intravenously. We administer furosemide 15 min before we inject the contrast for three reasons: (1) the urinary tract is subjected to a fluid challenge to unmask evidence of obstruction, (2) the gadolinium concentration is diluted which reduces the susceptibility artifacts and helps maintain the contrast-induced signal changes to within the range where they are linearly related to contrast agent concentration, and (3) the examination time is shortened (Jones et al. 2005). The majority of our patients are in the age range that requires sedation, and the protocol for these patients is outlined below. For non-sedated patients, images with similar contrast are acquired, but breath-hold acquisitions are used for some of the sequences. Coronal, 2D, flow compensated, respiratory-gated T1-weighted FLAIR (TR = 2000, TE = 9, TI = 950), and coronal 2D, T2-weighted (TR = 6000, TE = 2001, ETL = 27) series, and a coronal respiratory-gated, heavily T2-weighted 3D sequence (TE = 354, TR = respiratory period ETL = 122) and an axial T2-weighted sequence through the bladder(TR = 4100, TE = 70) are then acquired. The 2D series served to provide detailed anatomical reference scans, while the heavily T2-weighted 3D scan provided the basis for a pre-contrast maximum intensity projection (MIP) of the collecting

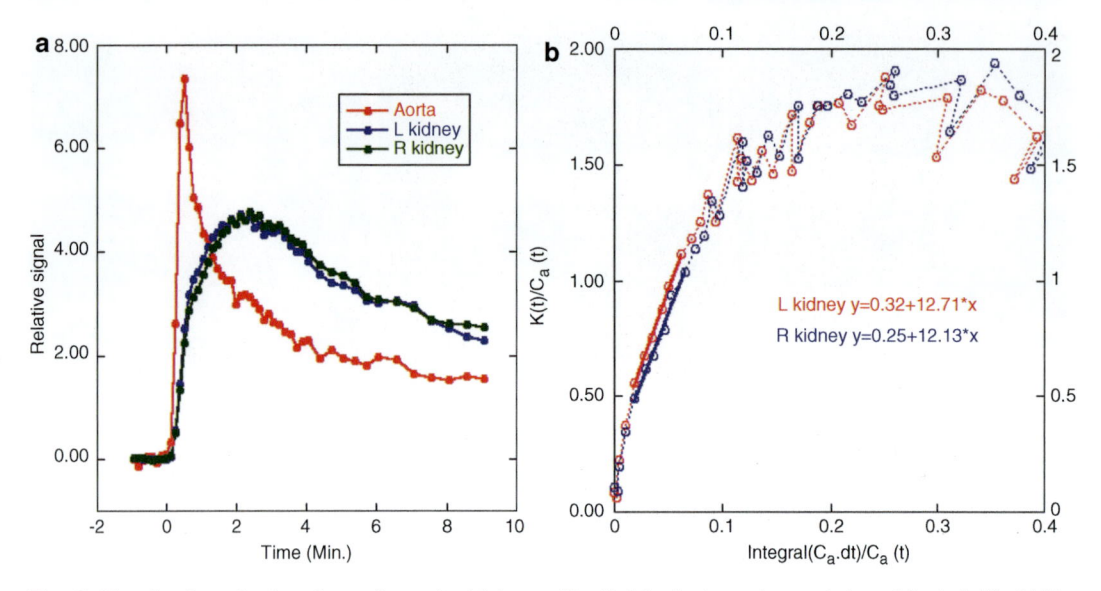

Fig. 2 Functional evaluation for a 3-month-old boy shown in Fig. 1. (**a**) Relative signal intensity versus time curve showing curves for the aorta and both kidneys. Note the symmetric parenchymal curves with equivalent perfusion, concentration, and excretion of contrast agent. (**b**) The Patlak plot is used as an index of the individual kidney GFR. The slope of each plot reflects the GFR of each kidney (12.7 ml/min on left and 12.1 ml/min on right). The y intercept represents the fractional blood volume of each kidney. The Patlak DRF was calculated at 50:50

system, ureters, and bladder. In order to create the MIP, other T2 structures with long T2 relaxation times, such as CSF and the gallbladder, are manually edited out from the images. The T2-weighted images are particularly useful to define the anatomy of nonfunctioning or poorly functioning systems. These systems are generally associated with marked UTD or cystic changes, and heavily T2-weighted images are able to delineate the anatomy even if little contrast excretion occurs. Volume-rendered images from the T2 data sets are used to delineate the anatomy of complex hydronephrotic systems (Fig. 3).

Once the above sequences are complete, the acquisition of a 3D, coronal, dynamic, gradient echo sequence (TR=3.4 ms, TE=1.5 ms, flip angle=30°) orientated along the axis of the kidneys and including the bladder begins (Fig. 3). The start of the dynamic series is approximately 15 min after the injection of furosemide, which coincides with the maximum effect of the furosemide (Brown et al. 1992). There is significant diuretic effect from about 5–30 min after injection so there is considerable latitude in the timing of the furosemide administration. All patients have a serum creatinine-based GFR estimation performed prior to the MRU, and patients with a GFR in excess of 60 ml/min/1.73 m^2 a dose of 0.1 mmol/kg Gd-DTPA (Magnevist; Berlex laboratories, Wayne, NJ, USA) has been used; today linear Gd-compounds are obsolete at least in Europe for pediatric use and replaced by Dotarem (Guerbet AG, Zürich, Switzerland) or Gadovist (Baayer, Berlin Germany) are slowly infused using a power injector. For patients with a GFR in the range of 30–60 ml/min/1.73 m^2, the same dose of ProHance (Bracco Diagnostics, Princeton, NJ, USA) or other cylic cGd contrast agents such as Gadovist or Dotarem are used due to its superior safety profile with respect to nephrogenic systemic fibrosis (NSF). No contrast is given if the serum creatinine-based GFR is below 30 ml/min/1.73 m^2. Previously, we had administered a compact bolus of contrast, but this results in an aortic signal well above the linear range of gadolinium concentration. We now instill the contrast typically at a rate of 0.25 ml/s so that the injection lasts more than 30 s. Each time point of the dynamic sequence consisted of 36–44 slices, with the outer three slices on each side being discarded in order to limit variations in the flip angle related to the slice profile and also to limit wraparound

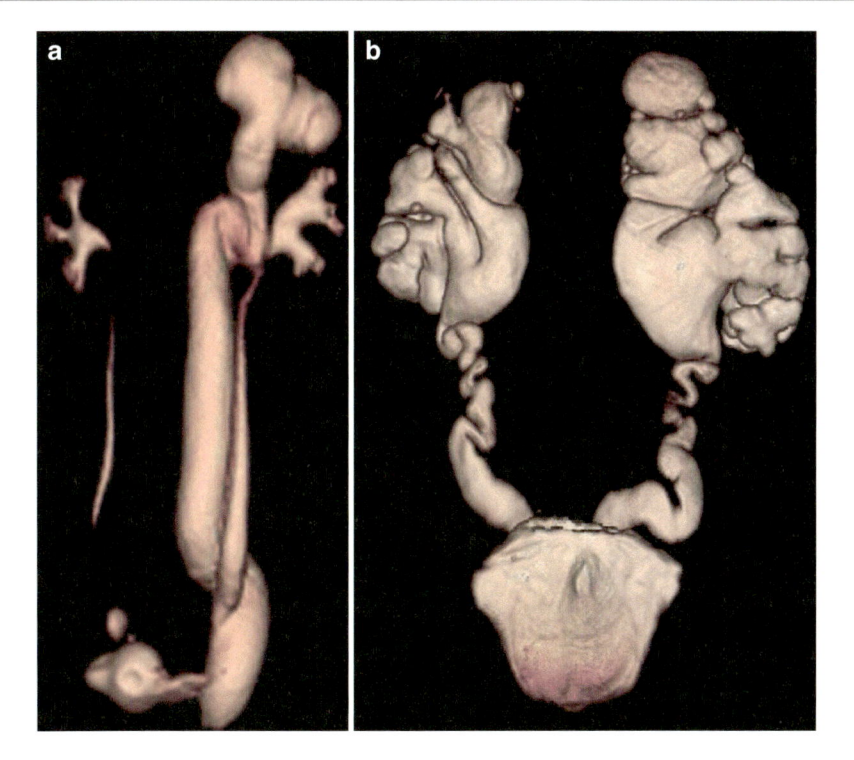

Fig. 3 Volume-rendered T2-weighted images. (**a**) Volume-rendered T2 images of duplex system with poorly functioning and obstructed upper pole moiety. Despite minimal excretion of contrast agent, anatomic images of the duplex system can be obtained with T2-weighted images that show the ectopic distal insertion of the upper pole ureter. (**b**) Volume-rendered T2 images of poorly functioning hydronephrotic kidneys in a boy with posterior urethral valves. Even with poor renal function, exquisite anatomical images are easily obtained

artifacts. Parallel imaging with an "acceleration factor" of 2 is used to reduce the acquisition time per volume to approximately 9 s. The scans are acquired contiguously for the first 3 min; subsequently, intervals of progressively increasing duration are inserted between the scans. The total duration for the acquisition of 60 dynamic scan is 10 min. For each volume acquisition, a maximum intensity projection (MIP) of the whole volume is automatically generated. If both ureters are clearly visualized 10 min after the injection of contrast media, no further dynamic series are acquired. Otherwise, the acquisition of dynamic images is continued for a further 5 min at 1 min intervals. After the completion of the dynamic series, sagittal, axial, and coronal 3D images with high spatial resolution are acquired for the purpose of reformatting and volume rendering on a 3D workstation. These images provide exquisite anatomic evaluation of the kidneys and ureters. In cases where poor drainage from the renal pelvis means that no contrast is seen in the ureters during the 15 min of dynamic scanning, the patient may be turned prone to promote mixing of the contrast agent in the collecting system prior to the acquisition of high spatial resolution coronal and sagittal images. The total imaging time for non-obstructed patients is typically 45 min; for poorly draining kidneys, the imaging time is typically 1 h. An abbreviated protocol is used for the evaluation of renal masses as well as renal scarring and pyelonephritis. If there is a concern for ectopic ureteric insertion or calyceal diverticulum, images delayed by several hours are sometimes helpful.

The MIP images from each volume acquisition are placed in a single cine sequence to provide a rapid overview of the transit of the contrast agent through the kidney. The delayed high-resolution anatomic images are particularly valuable in the evaluation of congenital malformations including ureteric strictures and ectopic ureteric insertion as well as complex postoperative anatomy (Adeb et al. 2013; Arlen et al. 2014; Figueroa et al. 2014).

> **Take Away**
> Reproducible high-quality MR urography requires meticulous attention to a standardized protocol with particular emphasis on patient hydration, sedation, and sequence acquisition. Using these techniques, exquisite and comprehensive anatomical and functional evaluation of the entire genitourinary tract can be performed routinely.

2.2 Optional Sequences

2.2.1 Diffusion-Weighted Imaging (DWI)

DWI is an MR sequence which uses strong, bipolar gradients to create a sensitivity of the signal to the thermally induced Brownian (or random walk) motion of water molecules. By acquiring images with two or more different diffusion weightings or b factors (with the b factor being determined by the strength, duration, and spacing of the bipolar gradients), the apparent diffusion coefficient (ADC) can be calculated from DWI images. The term ADC reflects the fact that in tissue, the water molecules cannot freely diffuse, rather their motion is impeded by cellular structures such as membranes and organelles. In addition, the ADC is also dependent on capillary perfusion and water diffusion in the extravascular space. Le Bihan et al. first described the dependency of the ADC on perfusion effects at lower b-values ($b < 200$ s/mm^2) in their works on intra-voxel incoherent motion (IVIM) (Le Bihan et al. 1986; Le Bihan 2013). These effects of pseudodiffusion can be excluded when high b-values ($b > 400$ s/mm^2) are applied to obtain true diffusion measurements. Some authors have tried to quantify the perfusion information from DWI of the kidneys using a bi-exponential fit of the ADC curve and calculating the perfusion fraction to evaluate renal function (Ichikawa et al. 2013). However, as the intravascular fraction is rather small, it has been shown that very high signal-to-noise ratio is required for this kind of bi-exponential fitting to be accurate, and in general, the required signal levels cannot be achieved with a resolution that permits the differentiation of the main renal structures (Pekar et al. 1992). However, the use of a low b-value, rather than zero in the standard diffusion acquisition, has the advantage of suppressing the signal from flowing blood and hence improving the contrast in the ADC images.

The ADC of the kidneys is higher than the ADC of other abdominal organs, most likely due to the high water content and the high blood supply of the kidneys and possible contributions of the flow in the tubular system. In general the cortical ADC has been found to be higher than that of the medulla, possibly because of the higher perfusion component (Ries et al. 2001). Measurements of renal ADC have been detailed in various studies, showing that DWI is a feasible approach for the characterization of renal diseases and lesions (Thoeny et al. 2005; Ries et al. 2001). Because diffusion measurements are sensitive to the microscopic motion of water, macroscopic effects such as patient motion, respiration, and pulsatility of the kidney will be several orders of magnitude larger than the water diffusion and will render the DWI images useless. Thus DWI is typically acquired using ultrafast, single-shot echo-planar imaging (EPI) sequences, which effectively freeze bulk motion. Parallel imaging is also generally used in conjunction with abdominal DWI as it allows increased resolution and acquisition speed with negligible alteration of diffusion values. Moreover, distortion artifacts caused by magnetic field inhomogeneities are reduced because of shorter echo train length. While there is general consensus on DWI parameters for clinical brain imaging, there is little consensus on the optimal parameters for DWI of the kidney, with maximal b-values ranging from 200 to 800 s/mm (Erbay et al. 2012; Chuck et al. 2013). Similarly, some institutions use breath-hold acquisitions for DWI measurements, others use respiratory triggering, and some use neither but rely on averaging to smooth out the effects of respiration. Diffusion-weighted imaging in the kidneys is usually performed to assess renal transplants, to diagnose acute pyelonephritis, and to better characterize renal masses such as Wilm's tumors and nephroblastomatosis (Gee et al. 2013; Vivier et al. 2013; Abou-El-Ghar et al. 2012; Zhang et al. 2013a).

2.2.2 Arterial Spin Labeling (ASL)

Arterial spin labeling (ASL) uses magnetically labeled blood as an endogenous "contrast agent" and can be used to measure renal perfusion (i.e., local blood flow) rather than the global perfusion obtained by measuring the blood flow in the renal artery. ASL has been widely used for studies of cerebral perfusion with the data typically being acquired using an echo-planar imaging sequence. However, in the abdomen the use of EPI sequences is complicated by greater magnetic field inhomogeneity and shorter T_2^* relaxation times, resulting in increased image distortion and a reduced signal-to-noise ratio. The kidneys are highly perfused, receiving about 20 % of the cardiac output, compared to 14 % for the brain, and the blood flow per gram of renal tissue in a normal adult is about 4 ml/min, compared to 0.5 ml/min in the brain. There are significant variations in the flow rates within the kidney, with the flow in the renal cortex being roughly five times greater than that in the outer medulla and 20 times greater than that in the inner medulla. Despite this high flow, the signal difference due to blood flow between the control and tag phases of the ASL experiment is still only a few percent. Hence, multiple acquisitions (averages) are required, leading to a typical acquisition time of between tens of seconds and several minutes. Because the total acquisition time is much longer than the respiratory cycle, ASL in the kidney has to contend not only with patient movement but also with the periodic motion of the kidneys during the respiratory cycle. As a control for the effect of motion, images from the same phase (e.g., control) can be subtracted. Even when these show no discernable motion artifacts, the signal difference on subtraction may be of the order of a few percent, i.e., of the same order of magnitude as that expected from perfusion when subtracting tag images from the control images in the absence of motion. Hence, great care must be taken both to minimize the effects of motion and to reduce the signal differences caused by residual motion. As outlined above, the use of EPI sequences, which are ubiquitous for ASL in the brain, for renal studies is complicated by increased magnetic field inhomogeneity and shorter T_2^* relaxation times. One approach to addressing these problems has been to reduce the sensitivity of EPI to these effects by using combinations of high (>2) acceleration factors, partial k-space sampling, and increased sampling bandwidths, which serve to reduce the duration of the EPI echo train and speed up the traversal of k-space (Gardener and Francis 2010). These measures reduce EPI's sensitivity to these effects. While reducing the number of phase-encoding steps or increasing the bandwidth will nominally reduce the SNR, this is offset by a shorter echo time and reduced signal decay during the echo train. Alternatively, other groups have used TrueFISP or HASTE sequences as an alternative readout method to EPI (Martirosian et al. 2004; Robson et al. 2009). Both TrueFISP (also known as FIESTA or balanced SSFP) and HASTE (also known as single-shot FSE with partial ky-acquisition) are less affected by the effects mentioned above; however, they require longer acquisition times (which reduces the number of slices that can be acquired) and generally have lower SNR than EPI sequences.

2.2.3 Contrast-Enhanced MR Angiography (CE-MRA)

If renal artery stenosis (RAS) is suspected, then either a contrast-enhanced MRA (CE-MRA) or a non-contrast MRA of the renal arteries can be performed. In the case that a functional evaluation of the kidneys will be performed as well, then a non-contrast MRA is preferred in order to avoid having contrast present when the second injection for the functional analysis is performed. For a CE-MRA the protocol typically uses a compact bolus of contrast, preferably injected using a power injector and a rapid, dynamic gradient echo scan aligned along the descending aorta to monitor the arrival of contrast. The progress of the contrast agent down the aorta is monitored, and when the contrast nears the renal arteries, the dynamic sequence is halted, the patient is instructed to perform a breath-hold, and a 3D data set is acquired using a short TE gradient echo sequence. The duration of the volumetric sequence is short enough to keep both the duration of the breath-hold within reasonable limits and to minimize the possibility of venous contamination. CE-MRA has generally been found to have a high specificity and sensitivity compared to digital subtraction angiography (DSA) which, while invasive, serves as the gold standard for the assessment of RAS. For example, Soulez et al. performed a multicenter trial comparing CE-MRA on 1.5 T scanners with DSA for depicting RAS which enrolled 268 patients, 178 of whom had significant RAS (Soulez et al. 2008). They found that sensitivity, specificity, and accuracy for CE-MRA for detecting >50 % stenosis were 60–84 %, 89–95 %, and 80–87 %, respectively. The above study used MultiHance (gadobenate dimeglumine) as the contrast agent, which is generally the contrast agent of choice for CE-MRA as it has higher T1 relaxivity due to transient protein binding (Prokop et al. 2005); however this agent has been withdrawn for pediatric use (only some dedicated applications particularly in the liver are still approved in Europe mostly for adults) and must be replaced by cyclic Gd contrast agents such as Gadovist, Dotarem or Prohance. It should also be noted that the quality of CE-MRA is further improved on 3 T scanners compared to 1.5 T scanners. CE-MRA was probably the method of choice for assessing RAS prior to the discovery of nephrogenic systemic fibrosis (NSF) which, while rare and more strongly associated with specific contrast agents, has led to patients with severe chronic or acute renal insufficiency being carefully evaluated before being approved for such studies. A second consideration is the fact that the CE-MRA is a relatively expensive study. These concerns have led to development of non-contrast techniques for contrast-free MRA of the renal arteries. The exact details of the sequences used for non-contrast MRA of the renal arteries vary between manufacturers, but the general principle is to use a steady-state free precession (SSFP) which has high signal from the vessels in conjunction with an inversion pulse. The delay between the inversion pulse and the pulse sequence is chosen to maximize the attenuation of the background tissue while allowing sufficient time for non-attenuated blood to flow into the imaged volume. Additional saturation pulses are used to attenuate the venous signal and motion artifacts originating from the abdominal wall. These techniques are combined with either a respiratory trigger or a navigator pulse to minimize motion artifacts. In a recent study, non-contrast MRA was shown to have a sensitivity of 74 %, specificity of 93 %, and accuracy of 90 % compared to contrast-enhanced CT angiography (CTA) (Albert et al. 2015). It should be noted that the non-contrast techniques take considerably longer (typically ~5 min) than a CE-MRA; however, the acquisition of a non-contrast MRA has no effect on a subsequent study of renal function.

> **Take Away**
> Advanced imaging techniques such as DWI, ASL, and CE-MRA continue to increase the capabilities of MR urography by analyzing the anatomy and function of the kidney with demonstration of both renal perfusion and diffusion at a microstructural level.

2.3 MR Contrast Agents

Gadolinium-based contrast agents (GBCAs) were first associated with nephrogenic systemic fibrosis (NSF) in January 2006 when five end-stage renal failure patients undergoing MRA developed signs of NSF 2–4 weeks after GBCAs administration (Grobner 2006; Marckmann 2006). Subsequently, there have been reports of

NSF associated with other GBCAs, and this issue has been subject to close regulatory reviews.

The US Food and Drug Administration (FDA), the American College of Radiology (ACR), and the European Medicines Agency (EMA) all consider three of these agents (Magnevist, Omniscan, and Optimark) to be high risk for NSF. The FDA and ACR confine their warning to patients with acute kidney injury or with chronic, severe kidney disease (GFR < 30 mL/min/1.73 m^2, though the ACR extends this to 40 mL/min/1.73 m^2 because of the inherent variability in the measurement of GFR) (see also Chap. 6). The EMA uses a broader recommendation; specifically, "they must not be used in patients with severe kidney problems, in patients around the time of liver transplantation, and in newborn babies less than 4 weeks of age, who are known to have immature kidneys." All three agencies recommend the screening of patients to identify patients with renal problems prior to using these agents. It should be noted that for the three "high-risk" agents, there is evidence that the risk is higher with Omniscan than with Magnevist (Altun et al. 2009). The FDA does not differentiate between the other agents, while the EMA considers MultiHance and Ablavar to be medium risk and Dotarem, ProHance, and Gadavist to be low risk. In contrast, the American College of Radiology policy defines MultiHance, Dotarem, ProHance, and Gadavist to be medium risk and Ablavar to be low risk (Table 1).

More recently it has been reported that deposits of GBCAs remain in the brains of some patients who undergo multiple contrast-enhanced MRI scans long after the last administration (Kanda et al. 2014). Currently, it is not known whether these gadolinium deposits are harmful or can lead to adverse health effects. While this is still an area of active research, recent studies indicate that the same agents that are classified as having a higher risk for NSF are also associated with more significant deposition of GBCA in the brain (Kanda et al. 2015b; Radbruch et al. 2015; Kanda et al. 2015a). According to the newest recommendations these linear GD contrast agents should thus NOT be used in children any longer.

> **Take Away**
> MR contrast agents have been associated with NSF, and more recently GBCAs have been found to leave significant deposits of gadolinium in the brain. Cyclic GBCAs are thought to be more stable and are recommended for MR urography in children.

3 Post-processing

Differential renal function (DRF) is among the most widely used measure of renal function. The DRF as measured by dynamic renal scintigraphy (DRS) is based on the integration of the tracer curve over a range of time points at which the tracer is assumed to be located predominately in the parenchyma (Durand 2014). Due to the limited spatial resolution of DRS studies, fixed time points are used since the exact location of the tracer cannot be confirmed by visual inspection of the images. Since DRS measurements are based on projection images of the

Table 1 MR contrast agents

Brand name	Generic name	Acronym	Excretion pathway	Structure
Magnevist	Gadopentetate dimeglumine	Gd-DTPA	Kidney	Linear
Omniscan	Gadodiamide	Gd-DTPA-BMA	Kidney	Linear
Optimark	Gadoversetamide	Gd-DTPA-BMEA	Kidney	Linear
MultiHance	Gadobenate dimeglumine	Gd-BOPTA	97 % kidney, 3 % bile	Linear
Ablavar	Gadofosveset trisodium	Gd-DTPA	91 % kidney, 9 % bile	Linear
ProHance	Gadoteridol	Gd-HP-DO3A	Kidney	Cyclic
Gadavist	Gadobutrol	Gd-BT-DO3A	Kidney	Cyclic
Dotarem	Gadoterate meglumine	Gd-DOTA	Kidney	Cyclic

whole kidney, they measure the activity in the whole kidney. The majority of techniques developed for measuring the DRF with MRI have attempted to duplicate this approach by combining the area under the time-intensity curve obtained from either a single slice, or a few slices, with a separate volume measurement (Huang et al. 2004; Vivier et al. 2010b; Artunc et al. 2010; Boss et al. 2014). We use a slightly different approach since the 3D volumes we use cover the full extent of both kidneys and the uptake of the contrast in each kidney can be followed volumetrically. We make the assumption that voxels represent either functional or nonfunctional tissue and that by summing the voxels that show a significant uptake of contrast, one can calculate the functional volume of each kidney and hence the split renal function. The dynamic series are visually inspected to determine the volumes in which contrast is first seen in the collecting system of each kidney; the volume prior to this is then used for the calculation of the functional volume of each kidney (Fig. 4). In this way, possible differences between the two kidneys are taken into account, and it is not necessary to assume a particular time point, or range of times, for the calculation. In previous studies several authors have shown that the calculation differential renal function based on renal volume agrees well with the DRF calculated using nuclear medicine (Heuer et al. 2003; Claudon et al. 2014; Grattan-Smith et al. 2003; Cerwinka et al. 2014). The volume of functioning tissue has also been shown to be well correlated with creatinine clearance rates. For the dose of contrast and the pulse sequence parameters used in our studies, the segmentation of the kidneys at this homogeneous enhancement phase is straightforward and can be performed using semiautomatic segmentation. While the renal volume can be estimated from T1- or T2-weighted images, this is much more user intensive (Bakker et al. 1999; Lee et al. 2003). The methodology presented here makes a clear distinction between functioning and nonfunctioning tissue and accounts for the effects of cortical scarring or patchy enhancement, such as that seen in uropathic or dysplastic kidneys. In the evaluation of duplex kidneys, MR urography can separate the boundaries between the upper and lower pole moieties by delineating the column of cortex separating the upper and lower poles so that the relative contributions of the upper and lower poles can be calculated.

We generate signal intensity versus time curves for each kidney (Fig. 3). Although it is possible to generate separate curves for the cortex and medulla, this is too time-consuming for routine studies. The global curves for each kidney describe the perfusion, concentration, and excretion of the contrast agent over time. The two kidneys are easily compared and contrasted which is especially helpful when one kidney is normal. The signal versus time curves are converted to relative signal versus time curves by calculating $(S_t-S_0)/S_0$, where S_0 is the mean precontrast signal, for each time point. The relative signal has a linear relationship with contrast agent concentration over a limited range of concentrations and compensates for spatial variations in the background signal, facilitating comparison of the two kidneys (Jones et al. 2005).

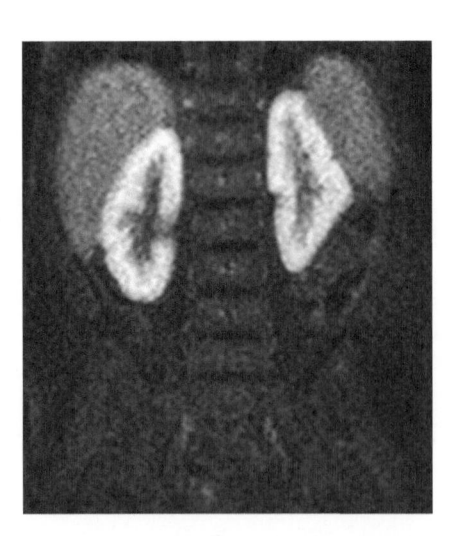

Fig. 4 Volumetric differential function. The time point for calculation of renal volumes is determined visually by defining the time when the kidneys have enhanced maximally and before contrast has been excreted into the collecting systems. At this time the kidneys are easily separated from the background with semiautomated techniques that produce volume calculations for each kidney depending on a user-defined threshold

The most widely used non-imaging clinical test of renal function is to measure the serum creatinine level. However, this test is a relatively insensitive measure of decreased glomerular filtration rate (GFR) and only measures the global, rather than single kidney, function. Although GFR can be accurately measured using techniques such as inulin clearance, such tests are invasive and are not feasible in a clinical setting. Several methods have been developed for estimating the GFR from dynamic nuclear medicine data, but all of these are hampered by the poor counting statistics of such dynamic studies and the problem of accounting for the extrarenal component of the signal. More recently several groups have applied the methods developed for nuclear medicine to dynamic MRI data acquired in conjunction with an injection of the contrast agent Gd-DTPA (Lee et al. 2003; Hackstein et al. 2003). When applying these techniques to MRI data, several issues have to be addressed: firstly, while nuclear medicine directly measures the activity, and hence the concentration, of the contrast agent, the MRI contrast agents change signal by altering the relaxation times of the tissue, and this produces a linear relationship with the concentration only over a limited range of concentrations. Secondly, the exact relationship between the signal and concentration depends on the flip angle used, and, since the flip angle varies across the slice in 2D studies, time-consuming corrections are required for 2D data, making these unsuitable for routine clinical applications. Thirdly, in order to obtain adequate signal-to-noise ratio, it is generally necessary to use surface array coils for the reception of the signal, which in turn can lead to local variations in signal intensity which complicate the analysis of the data. Our approach addresses these problems by using a slow injection of contrast in order to limit the arterial concentration, by using a 3D technique and discarding the outer slices to ensure a uniform flip angle, and by using the pre-contrast signal to correct for spatial variations in the signal intensity.

To estimate the GFR, we use the Rutland-Patlak technique which is based on a two-compartment model with unilateral flow of tracer from the first compartment (vasculature) into the second compartment (nephrons) (Rutland 1979; Patlak and Blasberg 1985; Peters 1994) (Fig. 3). With this model the GFR is measured as the transfer of the contrast agent from arterial blood to the renal tubules and the fact that the kidney includes both vascular and tubular components is taken into account. The amount of contrast agent in any one kidney at a time point t, $C_k(t)$, prior to the excretion of the contrast agent can be expressed as the sum of the contrast agent in the vascular space and nephrons. Assuming that the plasma concentration of the contrast agent in the vascular space is proportional to the plasma concentration in the aorta, $c_p(t)$, then, defining the constants k_1 and k_2 to represent the vascular volume within the kidney and the clearance of the contrast agent from the vascular space, respectively, one can write

$$C_k(t) = k_1 c_p(t) + k_2 \cdot \int_0^t c_p(u)\,du \qquad (1)$$

where $t=0$ is the arrival time of the contrast agent. The values for $C_p(t)$ and $C_k(t)$ are derived from the AIF and renal curves, respectively. Equation 1 can be rewritten in the form of a linear equation, and values for k_1 and k_2 are derived from the plot of this equation. However, this requires the choice of a start point (time when contrast agent is uniformly distributed in the vasculature) and an end point (excretion of contrast) for the plot, and it is simpler to apply a nonlinear fit of Eq. 4 to all the data points between the arrival and the excretion of the contrast agent in order to derive values for k_1 and k_2 (Buckley et al. 2006). The pre-contrast relaxation times of, and the relaxivity of the contrast agent in, the blood and kidneys are different; similarly, these quantities also differ between the sub-compartments within each of these compartments (e.g., plasma and red cells). A correction for the difference in relaxation rates can be estimated from phantom studies (Rusinek et al. 2001; Hackstein et al. 2005) or from mathematical simulations based on the measured signal (Pedersen et al. 2004), but these do not accurately reflect the in vivo situation where exchange effects between different compartments (e.g., plasma and red cells) contribute to the observed relaxivity. For this reason we use the relative signal, as opposed to a measurement of the relaxation time, which may lead to errors in the Patlak analysis but is simpler and can be regarded as a GFR index, rather than an absolute measure of the GFR. When the Patlak DRF is calculated, such effects are assumed to be common to both kidneys and can hence be ignored. Other possible sources of error in the Rutland-Patlak analysis include the fact that the interstitial space is neglected, that pulsation of the descending aorta may distort the measurement of the vascular signal and the T2* shortening effects of the contrast agent may distort the relative signal measurements.

Typically one measures the average concentration of the contrast agent within the kidney, thus k_2 represents the clearance per unit volume of tissue, which we refer to as the unit GFR. We believe this quantity is related to the single-nephron GFR and have noted that this quantity is reduced in decompensated, as well as dysplastic and uropathic kidneys. An estimate of the single-kidney GFR (SK-GFR) can be obtained by multiplying k_2 by the renal volume (V_r). The Patlak model breaks down after a certain time because it fails to take account of the onward transport of the contrast agent (i.e., the drop in signal seen at later time points in the parenchymal curves). Annet et al. developed a model which includes an additional term which accounts for the onward transport of the contrast agent and hence allows the whole time course to be modeled (Annet et al. 2004). Their equation is of the form

$$C_k(t) = k_1 c_p(t) + k_2 \cdot \int_0^t c_p(u) \cdot \exp(K_{ep}(t-u)) du \quad (2)$$

In their original article, Annet et al. confined their analysis to the renal cortex, and the term k_{ep} represented the rate constant of the onward transport of the contrast agent. We apply the model to the whole kidney, and in this context, k_{ep} is the rate constant of the excretion of the contrast agent from the kidney which we refer to as the tubular output. A nonlinear fit of Eq. 2 can be applied to all the points acquired after the arrival of the contrast agent, and hence no preselection of the range of data points is required. In addition Annet et al. also modified C_p by including a delay time (δ) to account for the transit time from the arterial ROI to the renal parenchyma and a term to account for the dispersion of the contrast agent during this time. If only the delay term is incorporated, then $C_p(t)$ is replaced by a time-shifted plasma concentration $C_p(t-\delta)$. Because the transit times are exponentially distributed, the dispersion term can be expressed as a convolution of the time-shifted plasma concentration with the mean transit time of the plasma compartment (MTT$_p$) (Annet et al. 2004). The plasma concentration corrected for delay and dispersion (C_p') is given by

$$C_p'(t) = C_p(t-\delta) \otimes \frac{1}{\mathrm{MTT}_p} \exp\left(\frac{-t}{\mathrm{MTT}_p}\right) \quad (3)$$

The vascular contribution is determined primarily by the aortic concentration scaled by the plasma fractional volume, and if dispersion is not accounted for, then an artificially low plasma volume is often derived in order to achieve the required scaling of the arterial concentration. This results in a vascular component with a low peak and a low "tail," causing most of the rest of the renal curve to be attributed to glomerular filtration. When dispersion is accounted for, the vascular component is broader with a more pronounced tail leading to less of the curve being attributed to glomerular filtration. Thus, accounting for dispersion is expected to result in more accurate GFR values; however, due to the less stable fitting caused by the introduction of the convolution and the extra terms (δ and MTT$_p$) to the fitting process, combined with the limited temporal resolution used in our studies, we currently do not model the dispersion and use a fixed delay.

For each patient the key features derived from MR urography include calculation of differential renal function (both volume and Patlak), the unit GFR for each kidney, and the inverse of the term k_{ep} from the Annet model, which corresponds to the mean transit time of the contrast through the kidney. Differential renal function calculated using MR urography techniques show excellent correlation with differential function calculations using renal scintigraphy (Perez-Brayfield et al. 2003; Cerwinka et al. 2014). Signal versus time curves for the kidneys and the aorta, plots of the fits for the Patlak and Annet models to the time-intensity curves, and an asymmetry index are also generated for each patient. It is important to understand that we have two methods to determine the differential renal function: one based on volume and one based on the individual kidney GFR as determined by the Patlak and/or Annet plot. In most cases the volumetric and Patlak differential function are symmetric; however, when there is a difference in these two measures of DRF, it implies a change in renal pathophysiology that occurs in response to the fluid and diuretic challenge.

> **Take Away**
> The functional parameters routinely assessed by MR urography include the vDRF and pDRF, asymmetry index, mean transit times, renal and calyceal transit times, as well as signal intensity versus time curves. No single parameter is sufficient to categorize renal disease so each parameter must be used in conjunction with the overall anatomic diagnosis to arrive at the clinically relevant diagnosis.

4 Clinical Applications

4.1 Evaluation of Urinary Tract Dilatation

4.1.1 The Diagnosis of Obstruction

All systems with urinary tract dilatation have some impairment of renal drainage, and the goal of imaging is to distinguish urinary tract dilatation (UTD) secondary to stasis from UTD caused by physiologically significant obstruction (see also Chaps. 14 and 26). The definition of obstruction is difficult clinically and is usually defined in one of two ways: either as a restriction to urinary outflow that, when left untreated, will cause progressive renal deterioration or as a condition that hampers optimal renal development (Peters and Chevalier 2012). Unfortunately, these are retrospective definitions that make it difficult to identify prospectively which children may benefit from surgery. Obstructive uropathy occurs in a subset of children with UTD and refers to damage to the renal parenchyma caused by obstruction of urine flow from the kidney to the bladder (O'Reilly 2002; Becker and Baum 2006). The consequences of urinary tract obstruction occur secondarily to a complex syndrome resulting in alterations of both glomerular hemodynamics and tubular function caused by the interaction of a variety of vasoactive factors and cytokines (Chevalier 2007; Chevalier et al. 2010; Klein et al. 2010). The initiating event for the cascade of vasoactive factors is stretching of the renal pelvis in response to increase in intrapelvic pressure (Chevalier et al. 2010). The effects of obstruction on the developing kidney depend on the time of onset, location, and degree of obstruction (Chevalier et al. 2010).

Probably a more useful definition of obstruction is based on the pressure-flow relationship between the urine production and drainage. Whitaker in 1982 defined urinary tract obstruction as a condition that "impairs urinary drainage from the pelvicalyceal system and leads to increased pressure and reduced urine flow rate" (Whitaker et al. 1982). Chevalier et al. have demonstrated that it is the stretching and distension of the renal pelvis secondary to the increased intrapelvic pressure that releases the vasoactive factors and cytokines that may lead to renal damage (Chevalier et al. 2010). The diagnosis of obstruction has been extensively studied using intravenous urography (Saxton 1969; Sherwood 1971; Dawson 1990). This knowledge can be applied to MR urography as the same pathophysiologic changes occur in response to obstruction. MR urography is a more powerful tool than intravenous urography because it provides nephrotomography with 2 mm thick slices every 8 s through the entire urinary tract. The enhancement, concentration, and excretion of the contrast agent are demonstrated with much greater spatial, contrast, and temporal resolution than could be obtained with intravenous urography (IVU). The hallmark of acute obstruction on IVU as well as MR urography is the delayed and dense nephrogram (Anigstein et al. 1972; O'Reilly 1982; Davies 1988; Samin and Becker 1991) (Fig. 5). The findings of acute obstruction on IVU or MR urography include:

1. The immediate nephrogram is usually normal or mildly diminished (reflecting normal RBF).
2. The nephrogram becomes increasingly dense over time.
3. There is delayed excretion of contrast agent into the collecting system.
4. There is variable dilation of collecting system proximal to point of obstruction.

The obstructed nephrogram is the result of increased pressure within the renal pelvis transmitted in a retrograde fashion throughout the nephron (Brenes et al. 1966; Korobkin 1972; Dyer et al. 1986). The increased pressure in the nephron is transmitted across Bowman's space and results in prolonged transit of the contrast agent from the level of the glomerulus to the collecting system. Glomerular filtration continues but at a reduced rate (Anigstein et al. 1972). The tubular system continues to reabsorb electrolytes and fluid but does not reabsorb the contrast agent. This results in an ever-increasing concentration of the contrast media in the excreted urine within the tubular lumen. The nephrogram is initially delayed and subsequently becomes more and more intense before fading as unopacified urine replaces opacified urine (Samin and Becker 1991). This delayed and dense nephrogram is not unique to an obstructive process and may be seen with other causes of prolonged

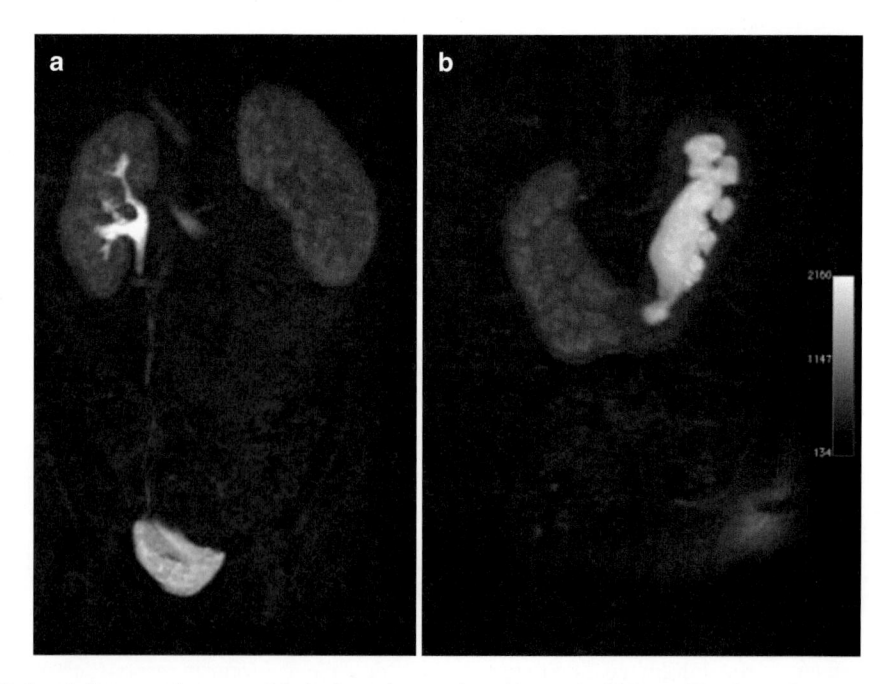

Fig. 5 Delayed dense nephrogram. (**a**) A five-minute MIP image following contrast administration in a 3-year-old girl with a physiologically significant PUJ obstruction manifested as a delayed dense nephrogram on the left. On the non-obstructed side, contrast is seen in the pelvicalyceal system and ureter. On the obstructed left side, the contrast medium has not yet reached the calyces. (**b**) A three-minute MIP image following contrast administration in a 12-month-old boy with a horseshoe kidney shows a delayed dense nephrogram on the right. The medulla is dense, but no excretion is seen into the calyceal system resulting in clear demarcation between the parenchyma of the obstructed as opposed to the non-obstructed side. The delayed and dense nephrogram is caused by increased pressure in the renal pelvis which is transmitted along the nephron and decreases individual kidney GFR

transit time of urinary filtrate through the nephron such as arterial hypotension or renal vein thrombosis (Brenes et al. 1966; Dyer et al. 1986). However, there is rarely clinical confusion with these conditions when evaluating children with UTD.

In 1980 Davies and Price described the urographic signs of *acute on chronic obstruction* of the kidney (Davies and Price 1980). This is particularly germane to pediatric uroradiology because in children with UTD, the obstruction is usually both chronic and partial (Koff 2007). The partial obstruction results in equilibrium between urine production, impaired outflow, and pelvic reservoir capacity (Koff 2007). A steady state is reached between the amount of urine produced and the volume of the renal pelvis so that the pressure in the renal pelvis remains in the normal range. Koff has elegantly shown that UTD is a protective measure against increases in pressure and that chronic partially obstructed kidneys typically have normal or low pressure within the renal pelvis and collecting system.

With MR urography, the kidneys are evaluated after a fluid and diuretic challenge in order to unmask partial obstruction and to provoke an acute on chronic obstruction of the kidney. If the production of urine exceeds the drainage capacity of the renal pelvis, the equilibrium is deranged. This loss of balance results in transient increase in pelvic pressure with dilatation and stretching of the renal pelvis. It is this stretching of the renal pelvis that stimulates the potentially deleterious cascade of cytokines and vasoactive factors that can lead to permanent renal damage (Chevalier et al. 2010). The increased intrapelvic pressure is transmitted back through the nephron. The physiologic response to elevated intrapelvic pressure is for the GFR to decrease as glomerular filtration depends on the difference in hydrostatic pressure between the glomerulus and Bowman's space. Increased pressure in the nephron is manifested as reduced GFR and delayed calyceal excretion. The signs of acute obstruction are nephrographic and are manifested by a delayed and increasingly dense nephrogram (Fig. 5). The signs of chronic obstruction are a dilated pelvicalyceal system with a normal or low-intensity nephrogram. Acute on chronic obstruction results in a combination of these signs (Davies and Price 1980). The hallmark of an acute on chronic obstruction is the delayed nephrogram in a dilated system. In the setting of UTD, delayed calyceal excretion of contrast indicates increased intrapelvic pressure. Delayed excretion is easy to assess visually when the contralateral kidney is normal but can be challenging in children with a single functioning kidney or in cases of bilateral UTD.

Urinary tract obstruction is a spectrum, and the change in intrapelvic pressure that occurs after a fluid challenge is a continuum from unchanged to marked increase in pressure. It is unknown what degree of obstruction and what increase in pelvic pressure will lead to subsequent renal damage. However by simply dividing hydronephrotic systems into those with elevated intrapelvic pressure from those that do not have increased pressure, more precise prospective evaluation of children with UTD may be performed. It seems logical that children without increased pressure following a fluid and furosemide challenge will not suffer further damage and therefore do not require surgery. The degree of obstruction and the amount of increased pressure that necessitates surgical intervention have yet to be defined.

4.1.2 Congenital UTD

The most common indication for MR urography has been the evaluation of UTD, especially in infants and young children. The evaluation and treatment of congenital UTD remain a clinical conundrum. Congenital UTD may be transient, stable, or lead to progressive renal damage. It is one of the most commonly identified anomalies and is seen on antenatal ultrasound in approximately 1 % of all pregnancies (Vemulakonda et al. 2014). Most experts currently advocate primary conservative management for infants with UTD with close follow-up and surgery only if there is evidence of decreased renal function or progressive UTD (Csaicsich et al. 2004; Eskildjensen et al. 2005; Peters and Chevalier 2012). Infants with moderate to severe antenatal UTD should undergo routine postnatal imaging with both anatomical and functional tests (Vemulakonda et al. 2014). Typically between 25 and 50 % of children with antenatal UTD ultimately require surgery (Ulman et al. 2000; Chertin et al. 2006).

Traditionally children with congenital UTD were evaluated with renal ultrasound and diuretic renal scintigraphy to establish baseline renal function. Follow-up studies were used to identify increasing UTD or loss of renal function. Unfortunately diuretic renal scintigraphy has significant limitations when evaluating congenital UTD. Impaired drainage on diuretic scintigraphy has been shown not to represent obstruction particularly in neonates, infants, and young children (Amarante et al. 2003). Additionally neither the degree of UTD nor the impairment of differential function nor the quality of the response to furosemide can define which kidney is in danger of further deterioration (Piepsz 2007; Piepsz 2011; Ismaili and Piepsz 2013). Furthermore diuretic scintigraphy cannot predict which kidneys may demonstrate improved renal function following pyeloplasty (Piepsz 2011).

MR urography is being used more often as the primary modality to evaluate children with congenital UTD (McMann et al. 2006; Boss et al. 2014). The anatomic information obtained with MR urography includes grading the UTD, identification of transition in caliber of the ureter, evaluation of underlying causes of obstruction such as kinks, strictures, or crossing vessels and provides a morphologic assessment of the quality of the renal parenchyma (Fig. 6). Both the T2-weighted and the delayed post-contrast images are used synergistically to define the pelvicalyceal and ureteric anatomy. The T2-weighted images are particularly helpful in children with severe UTD and/or poorly functioning systems. The volumetric T2 and post-contrast images can be used to generate exquisite volume-rendered images of the pelvicalyceal systems and ureters. Changes in ureteric caliber are useful indicators of the level of obstruction although they may simply reflect kinks in a tortuous and redundant ureter.

MR urography is useful in determining the prognosis by preoperatively evaluating the renal parenchyma and identifying permanent renal

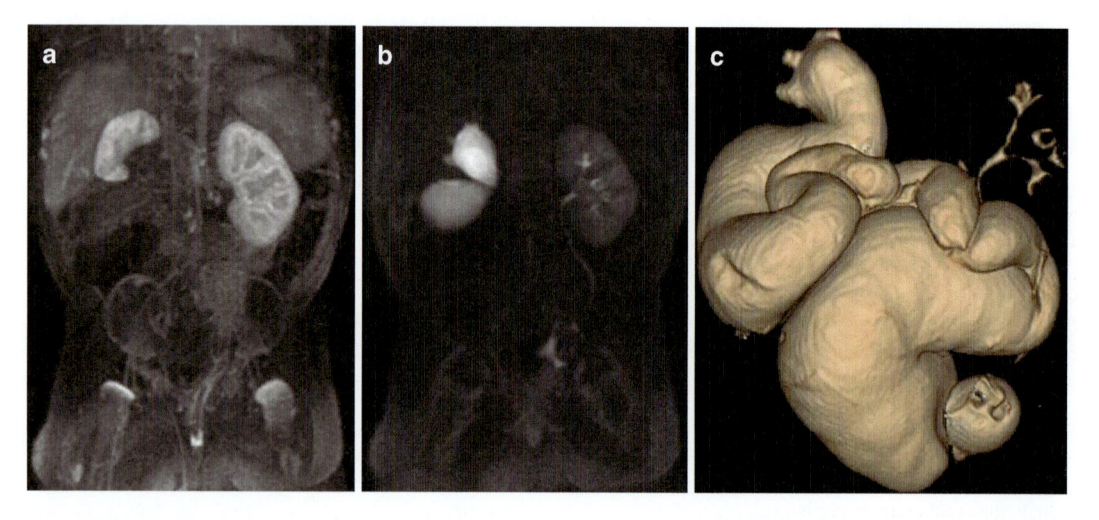

Fig. 6 Synergistic evaluation of massive UTD in a 6-month-old boy using a combination of contrast-enhanced and T2-weighted images. (**a**) The nephrographic phase shows that the right kidney is small and the lower pole is rotated laterally. (**b**) After 10 min, contrast is seen in the proximal right ureter, but the anatomy of the distal ureter is not defined. (**c**) The T2-weighted MIP images show the massive hydroureteronephrosis with the distal right ureter inserting ectopically below the bladder base. Also note how there are only three calyces in the right kidney and that they are simple and dysmorphic

damage. The quality of the renal parenchyma is assessed both on the high-resolution T2-weighted images and during the parenchymal phase of the nephrogram. The renal parenchyma is typically classified as normal, edematous, or uropathic (Figs. 7 and 8). On the T2-weighted images,

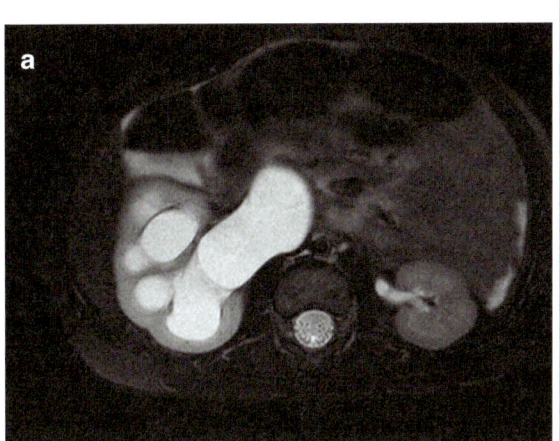

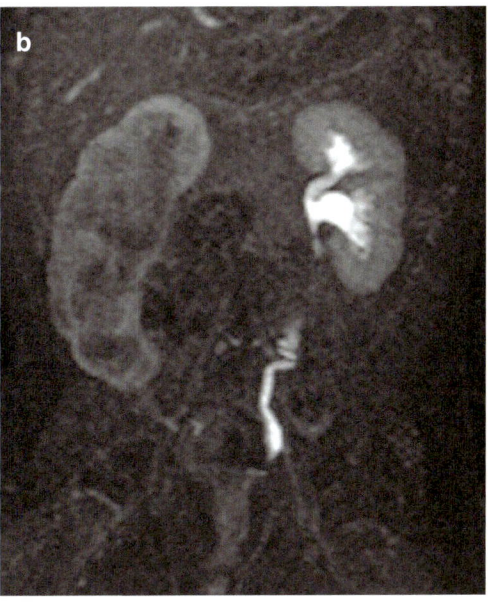

Fig. 7 A three-month-old boy with acute decompensated UTD and parenchymal edema. (**a**) On the axial T2-weighted image, the marked UTD with renal enlargement is noted. The signal intensity of the parenchyma is greater than the contralateral non-obstructed left kidney as a result of parenchymal edema. (**b**) The 5 min MIP image after contrast again demonstrates the enlarged right kidney with a markedly delayed and dense nephrogram. The delayed and dense nephrogram indicates that there is significant recoverable function if a pyeloplasty is performed

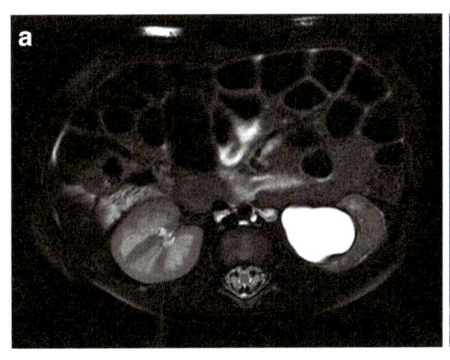

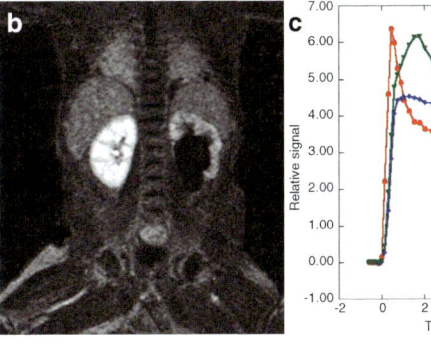

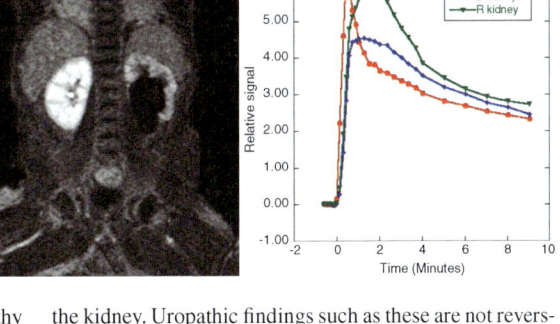

Fig. 8 A nine-month-old girl with significant uropathy and renal damage. (**a**) The axial T2-weighted image shows moderate UTD. When compared with the normal right kidney, the renal architecture is distorted with loss of the corticomedullary differentiation. Additionally there are innumerable small subcapsular cysts. (**b**) The coronal source image during the nephrographic phase demonstrates the decreased enhancement of the left kidney. The decreased enhancement indicates both decreased perfusion and concentration related to microvascular damage to the kidney. Uropathic findings such as these are not reversible, and there will be no significant improvement in renal function following pyeloplasty. (**c**) Signal intensity versus time curve for the left kidney demonstrates decreased amplitude and prompt washout from the renal parenchyma. The kidney is perfused but no significant concentration occurs. These findings are typical findings of uropathy and can be contrasted with the normal signal intensity time curve for the right kidney

signs that indicate underlying uropathy and permanent damage include decrease in renal size, architectural disorganization with loss of the corticomedullary differentiation, small subcortical cysts, and low cortical T2 signal intensity. The nephrogram in these cases usually shows dim and patchy contrast enhancement reflecting damage to the microvasculature as well as glomeruli and tubules. These imaging findings reflect the histological changes of renal damage based on reduced glomerular number, glomerular hyalinization, cortical cysts, and interstitial inflammation and fibrosis (Elder et al. 1995; Huang et al. 2006). In contrast to uropathic kidneys, edematous kidneys are large and typically show increased signal intensity on the T2-weighted images. The preoperative diagnosis of uropathy is important as these changes are permanent and will not be reversed following successful pyeloplasty. Parenchymal edema resolves following successful pyeloplasty.

Initially, MR urography was used to evaluate urinary tract dilatation and obstruction by calculating the renal transit time (RTT), which was defined as the time it takes for the contrast agent to pass from the renal cortex to the ureter below the lower pole of the kidney (Jones et al. 2004). Although the RTT calculation is similar to DRS for categorizing dilated systems, it has become apparent from the high-resolution anatomic images that renal drainage is dependent on the anatomy of the pelviureteric junction (PUJ), particularly the site of insertion of the ureter into the renal pelvis (Perez-Brayfield et al. 2003). For drainage to occur down the ureter, the contrast agent has to reach the level of the PUJ. The ureteric insertion is variable and may be high on the renal pelvis, anteriorly or posteriorly located (Kaneyama et al. 2006). As the contrast agent macromolecule is heavier than water, the contrast agent layers in the dependent portions of the kidney especially when there is marked UTD and stasis. It is important to realize that the RTT is simply a measure of renal drainage, that prolonged renal transit times simply indicate poor drainage, and that stasis of urine is manifested by fluid levels (Fig. 9). The RTT is most valuable when it occurs in less than 4 min

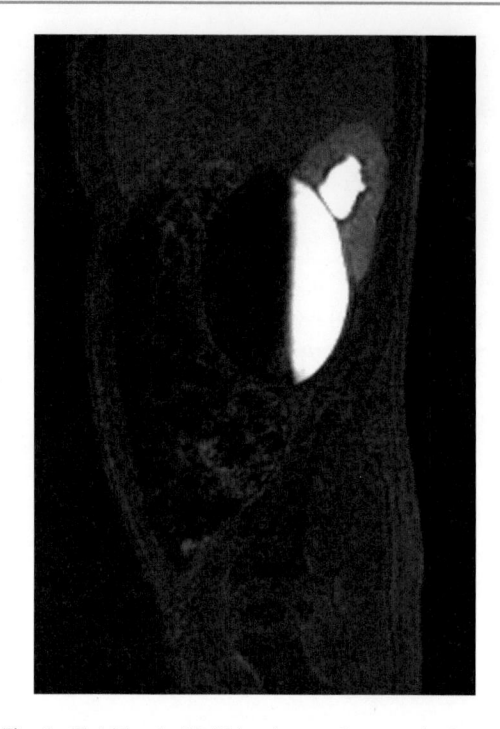

Fig. 9 Fluid levels. Fluid levels are often seen in the setting of marked UTD and are an indicator of stasis within the collecting system with the heavier contrast material layering along the dependent portions. Stasis does not necessarily mean obstruction but is generally associated with impaired drainage

demonstrating that there is no significant obstruction.

More recently, the focus of MR urography as well as renal scintigraphy has shifted toward pathophysiologic changes occurring within the kidney itself as opposed to a simple evaluation of renal drainage. Using DRS some authors have used the cortical transit time defined as the absence of activity in the subcortical structures within three minutes of tracer injection on diuretic renogram to predict functional deterioration (Schlotmann et al. 2009; Sfakianakis et al. 2009; Piepsz et al. 2011; Harper et al. 2013) (Duong et al. 2013). Delayed cortical transit was predictive of DRF improvement postoperatively, and it seems the best criterion for identifying children for whom pyeloplasty is warranted (Duong et al. 2013). Delayed parenchymal transit as a marker of urinary tract obstruction was first described by Whitfield in 1978, but DRS is limited by its poor spatial resolution and has been unreliable when trying to separate renal parenchyma from collecting system especially in markedly dilated systems (Whitfield et al. 1978; Sfakianakis et al. 2009). The delayed cortical transit time described by renal scintigraphy represents the same pathophysiology as the delayed nephrogram seen on IVU and MR urography. The hallmark is delayed calyceal excretion which indicates elevated intrapelvic pressure.

With MR urography, the diagnosis of acute on chronic obstruction is made more easily because there is clear demarcation of contrast in the renal parenchyma from contrast in the collecting system. This difference is readily identified on visual inspection. The dilated kidney is challenged by both a fluid and diuretic challenge prior to contrast administration using the F-15 approach. How the kidney responds to this challenge determines the appearance of the MR nephrogram. The calyceal transit time is the time it takes for the contrast to pass through the kidney, i.e., from the initial enhancement of the cortex until it first appears as high signal intensity in the dependent calyces. The calyceal transit time is analogous to the cortical transit time derived from renal scintigraphy (Schlotmann et al. 2009; Harper et al. 2013). A delayed calyceal or cortical transit time represents delayed transit of Tc-MAG3 or Gd-DTPA through the renal parenchyma and in the setting of UTD is indicative of acute on chronic obstruction. The elevated intrapelvic pressure causes a decrease in the GFR, while the effective renal plasma flow is maintained. These pathophysiologic changes cause a decreased washout of Tc-MAG3 or Gd-DTPA from the renal parenchyma. Delayed cortical transit is analogous to the delayed nephrogram and occurs when the intrapelvic pressure increases, indicating physiologically significant obstruction. The decrease in GFR can be quantitated by the Patlak differential function when there is a discrepancy between the pDRF and the vDRF. Normally, the volumetric and Patlak differential functions are similar but with acute obstruction, the Patlak number decreases. The greater the decrease in Patlak number, the more severe the obstruction. The great advantage of MR urography over renal scintigraphy is the much greater inherent spatial and contrast resolution so that identification of delayed excretion is apparent and straightforward even in markedly hydronephrotic systems.

An early physiologic indicator of acute obstruction and increased intrapelvic pressure is reduction in GFR. Logically the agent most sensitive to obstruction would be an agent excreted by glomerular filtration. Changes in glomerular filtration secondary to increased pressure in the nephron are better demonstrated by MR urography than MAG3 scintigraphy because of the different pathways of tracer elimination. Excretion of 99mTc-MAG3 is predominantly tubular, whereas Gd-DTPA is excreted almost exclusively by glomerular filtration. MAG3 is highly protein bound, its excretion is related to relative effective plasma flow, and it is cleared almost exclusively by tubular secretion (Itoh 2001). For this reason DTPA may be more sensitive than MAG3 in detecting acute obstruction (Boss et al. 2014).

A useful concept when analyzing MR urograms is to define UTD as either compensated or decompensated in response to the Lasix and fluid challenge (Aaronson 1980; Jones et al. 2011) (Figs. 10 and 11). If there are symmetric changes in signal intensity of the nephrogram, and symmetric or rapid calyceal transit time, it is classified as a compensated dilated system – the fluid challenge has been accommodated without increasing the pressure in the pelvicalyceal system. However, when the signal intensity changes are asymmetric and the calyceal transit time is delayed, they most often indicate acute on chronic obstruction – the fluid challenge has exceeded the capacity for renal drainage and the pressure in the collecting system rises. These are classified as decompensated dilated systems. Near-normal renal blood flow, glomerular filtration, and tubular function are required to develop an obstructive nephrogram and so the findings of decompensation usually indicate significant recoverability of renal function. Signs associated with decompensation on MR urography include

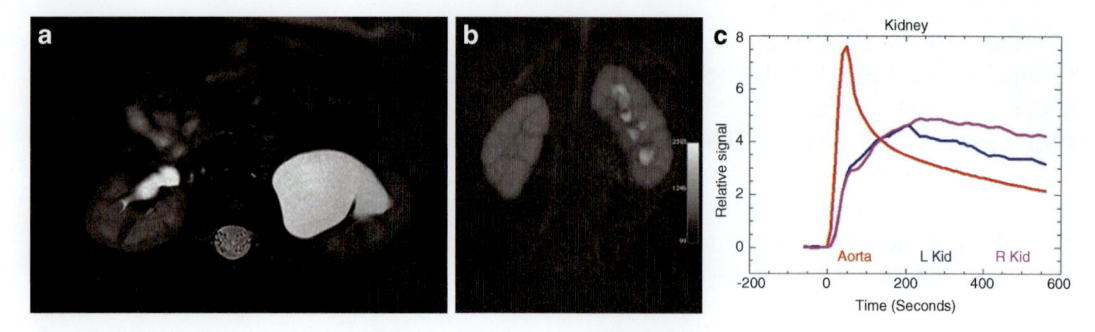

Fig. 10 A 6-month-old boy with "compensated UTD." (**a**) There is moderate UTD and caliectasis on the left with preservation of the corticomedullary differentiation. (**b**) Coronal post-contrast MIP images show that there has been rapid excretion of contrast material into the pelvicalyceal system. This rapid excretion indicates that there has been no increase in intrapelvic pressure and that there is an underlying concentration defect in the left kidney. (**c**) Signal intensity versus time curve demonstrates symmetric perfusion but impaired concentration with decreased peak enhancement on the left. There is good washout of the contrast agent from the renal parenchyma. The volumetric and Patlak differential functions were equivalent. All these parameters indicate that the left-sided dilated kidney can accommodate the fluid challenge without increasing intrapelvic pressure. Therefore, it is categorized as a compensated system that is unlikely to deteriorate and can be followed conservatively

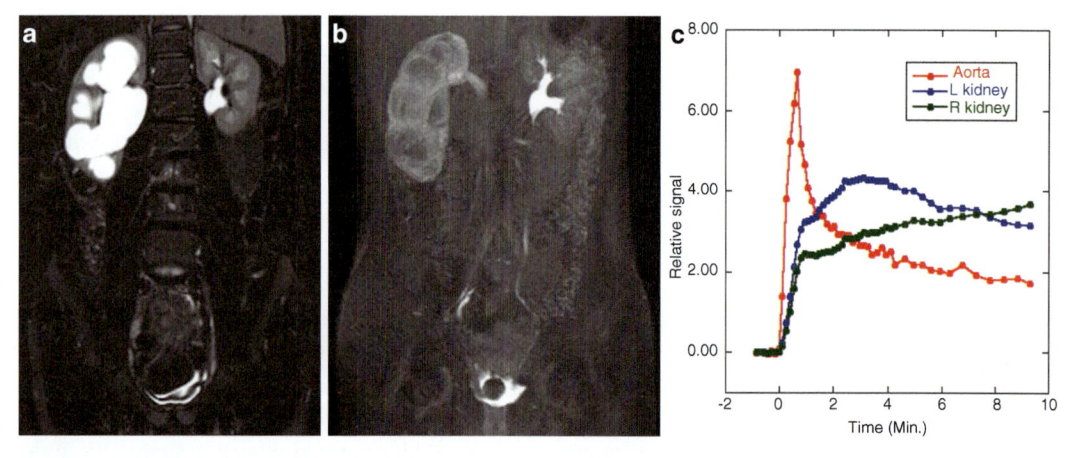

Fig. 11 A 2-year-old boy with decompensated UTD. (**a**) Coronal T2-weighted images showing marked UTD and parenchymal loss on the right with loss of the medullary pyramids. (**b**) Coronal MIP from the dynamic series showing normal excretion on the left. The right kidney is large and has a delayed dense nephrogram with delayed calyceal transit time. (**c**) Signal intensity versus time curves demonstrating asymmetric concentration and excretion of contrast agent. The curve for the left kidney is normal and on the right represents the delayed increasingly dense nephrogram. The vDRF was 47 % on the right, and the pDRF was 37 %, indicating a significant change in the GFR related to acute increase in intratubular pressure secondary to the fluid challenge. This is classified as a decompensated UTD and will demonstrate improved function following a successful pyeloplasty

parenchymal edema on the T2-weighted images, delayed calyceal transit time, a delayed and increasingly dense nephrogram, and discrepancy between the vDRF and the pDRF. These changes can also be used to grade the severity of the obstruction. These two patterns have different prognostic implications – little improvement in renal function can be expected following pyeloplasty in compensated or severely uropathic systems – but significant improvement is seen in decompensated UTD (Little et al. 2007). Once the obstruction is relieved by a successful pyeloplasty, the previously demonstrated delayed nephrogram resolves, and there is typically rapid calyceal excretion on the formerly obstructed side (Fig. 12). The rapid calyceal excretion following pyeloplasty is thought to occur as a result of a concentration defect caused by prior medullary injury.

It is important to remember that obstruction is a spectrum and the delay in the nephrogram ranges from minimal to marked prolongation reflecting the severity of the obstruction. Further work will determine what threshold of obstruction should be treated. The degree of underlying uropathy or congenital dysplasia will determine not only the size and appearance of the kidney but also its ability to concentrate and excrete the contrast agent. In most cases of uropathy without obstruction, there is an underlying concentration defect that results in a dim and patchy nephrogram with rapid excretion of contrast into the calyces. However, when uropathy is combined with physiologically significant obstruction, rather than rapid excretion, the excretion may be slightly delayed with symmetrical CTT, mimicking a compensated UTD (Fig. 13). By first evaluating the renal parenchyma on T2-weighted images, the degree of medullary volume loss, and the appearance of the nephrogram, it is possible to assess the presence or absence of underlying uropathy. Such kidneys are classified as being both decompensated and uropathic. Kidneys with mild uropathic changes may benefit from pyeloplasty, whereas those with severe uropathy rarely show functional improvement although relief of obstruction may prevent further injury to the kidney (Little et al. 2007).

Currently the calculation of DRF by renal scintigraphy is one of the key determinants in the decision when to operate in children with UTD. This is an overly simplistic approach to a complex problem as a kidney providing 35 % of total renal function may indicate uropathic, compensated, or decompensated UTD with significant obstruction. With MR urography the DRF is calculated on the basis of a number of parameters as described earlier. The vDRF represents the functioning renal mass. Since a threshold is used for segmentation of the kidneys, the vDRF tends to underestimate the function of very poorly enhancing kidneys. The same renal segmentation is used

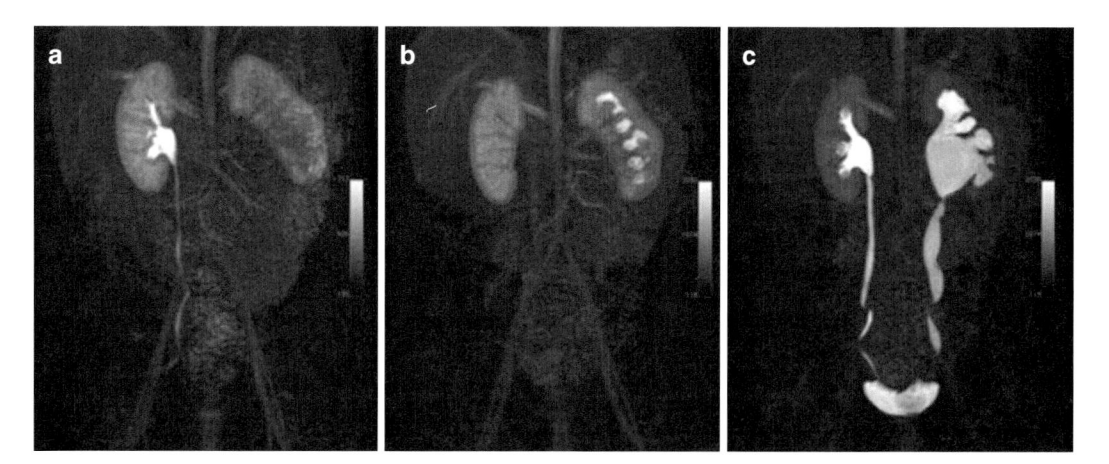

Fig. 12 Successful pyeloplasty in a 9-month-old infant. (**a**) Preoperative coronal MIP from the dynamic series demonstrating a delayed dense nephrogram on the left secondary to PUJ obstruction. (**b**) Postoperative coronal MIP image demonstrates rapid calyceal excretion on the left following pyeloplasty. In almost all successful pyeloplasties, there is a decrease in the degree of UTD and rapid calyceal transit on the operated side. If the calyceal transit is delayed, this is usually an early indicator of a failed pyeloplasty. (**c**) Coronal MIP from late in the dynamic series demonstrating delayed RTT (8 min) but with a wide open and straight border to the PUJ. The vDRF and pDRF are now equivalent

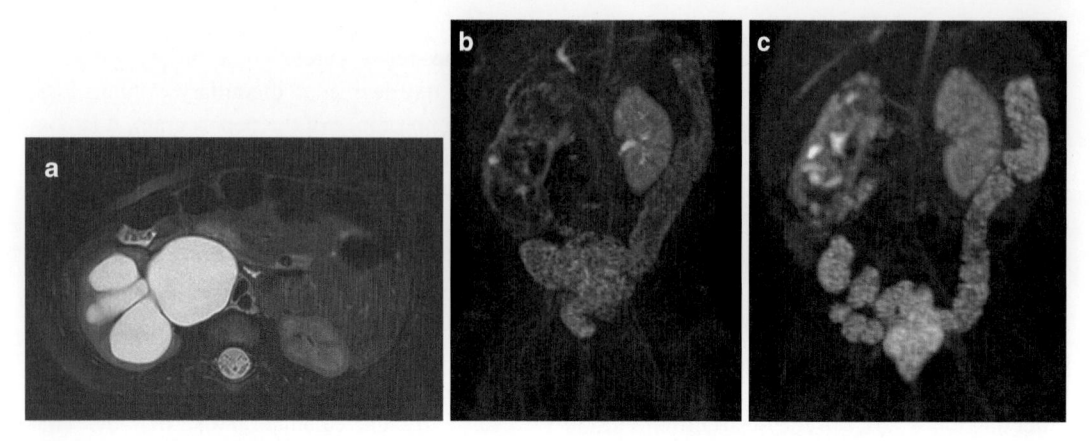

Fig. 13 Successful pyeloplasty in a 1-year-old girl with underlying uropathy. (**a**) The T2-weighted axial image shows the marked UTD on the right with loss of renal parenchyma. There is loss of medullary volume compared with the normal left kidney. (**b**) Coronal MIP image after contrast administration demonstrates symmetric calyceal excretion in the markedly enlarged, dilated right kidney. With the amount of uropathy seen on the T2-weighted images, rapid calyceal excretion of contrast would be expected if the pressure in the collecting system stayed low. (**c**) Following successful pyeloplasty, the coronal MIP image after contrast administration demonstrates rapid calyceal excretion of contrast indicating that the underlying PUJ obstruction that caused increased pressure on the prior study has resolved. Also note that the size of the kidney is smaller with less distension of the renal pelvis and parenchyma

in the calculation of the Patlak index, and hence the pDRF also tends to underestimate the function of very poorly functioning kidneys. In this context the pDRF is generally a more useful parameter since it is independent of the renal volume. In decompensated systems there is significant asymmetry in the pDRF, with the degree of asymmetry being more pronounced in severely decompensated systems.

Although it is relatively straightforward to determine if a system is not obstructed on the basis of the renal transit time, no single parameter is adequate to fully characterize obstruction. With MR urography we can now discriminate between compensated and decompensated dilated systems and identify uropathic changes. This classification has important prognostic implications: following a technically successful pyeloplasty, there is little change in function for compensated PUJ obstruction, there is improvement in function in decompensated PUJ obstruction, and minimal improvement is seen in uropathic kidneys. MR urography provides a wealth of information in the evaluation of obstructive uropathy that provides a nuanced evaluation that helps select those patients most likely to benefit from surgical intervention and to predict outcome in individual patients.

One of the perceived limitations of MR urography has been the lack of widely available programs to perform quantitative functional analysis. However, the intrinsic high contrast and spatial resolution of MR urography combined with rapid temporal resolution produce images that enable robust semiquantitative analysis. Simply by analyzing the images visually, the size, quality, and function of the kidneys can be assessed, and by evaluating the passage of contrast through the kidneys, physiologically significant obstruction can be identified as a delayed nephrogram. Most importantly the preoperative MR urogram is predictive of the postoperative appearance following successful pyeloplasty and can identify children who will benefit from surgery (Little et al. 2007; Jones et al. 2011).

Take Away
The diagnosis of urinary tract obstruction is challenging because it represents a continuum. Using MR urography dilated systems can be classified as compensated or decompensated based on the excretion of contrast material into the collecting system. Knowledge gained from prior studies of IVU provides physiological insights into MR urography. The preoperative MR urogram is predictive of the postoperative appearance following successful pyeloplasty.

4.1.3 PUJ Obstruction

PUJ obstruction is a complex and temporally dynamic process that comprises a spectrum from reversible UTD to severe parenchymal changes that may necessitate pyeloplasty or nephrectomy (Rosen et al. 2008; Ismaili and Piepsz 2013). Each child with a PUJ obstruction is unique. PUJ obstruction may be idiopathic, secondary to a neuromuscular defect at the ureteropelvic junction, or associated with abnormalities such as aberrant lower pole vessels, kinks, adhesions, or abnormal angulations (Hashim and Woodhouse 2012; Rodriguez 2014). In many cases it may be multifactorial (Williams et al. 2007). There are two distinct populations of PUJ obstruction: young infants diagnosed with antenatal UTD who are usually asymptomatic and older children who present with symptoms related to abdominal pain or infection. The decision to operate is usually straightforward in the symptomatic population.

The aorta and main renal arteries are routinely visualized during the early dynamic imaging phase. Accessory and crossing vessels are commonly seen, and the 3D images from early and late data sets can be superimposed to delineate the relationship of these vessels to the anatomic change in caliber (Fig. 14). Although PUJ obstruction related to crossing vessels is typically seen in older children, crossing vessels are often seen in association with PUJ obstruction in young infants (Krepkin et al. 2014).

There has been debate in the literature about whether there is improvement in renal function following pyeloplasty (Shokeir et al. 1999; Castagnetti et al. 2008; Wu et al. 2012; Bhat et al. 2012; Harraz et al. 2013). Pediatric pyeloplasty is considered a very successful procedure for PUJ obstruction with success rates as high as 98 % although the criterion for success is vari-

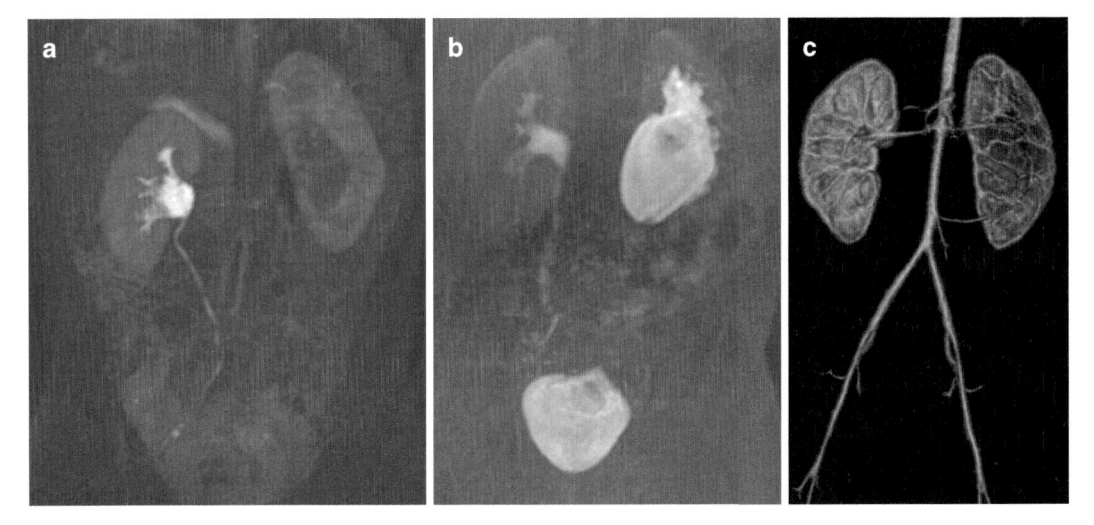

Fig. 14 PUJ obstruction secondary to crossing vessel in a 12-year-old boy. (**a**) Coronal MIP image after contrast administration demonstrates a delayed dense nephrogram on the left. (**b**) Delayed post-contrast image shows a rounded configuration to the inferior aspect of the renal pelvis. (**c**) Arterial MIP image obtained from early volumetric acquisition shows the lower pole accessory artery crossing at the level of the PUJ

able (Pohl et al. 2001). Because most children with PUJ obstruction are asymptomatic, the aim of surgery is preservation of renal function. Residual dilatation may persist for years. Amling et al. reported that at 1 month after pyeloplasty, 92 % of renal ultrasounds are similar or worse than preoperative studies although 91 % showed improvement by 8 years. Postoperative imaging following pyeloplasty is important to demonstrate that the surgery was successful especially in infants and children who were asymptomatic preoperatively. The definition of successful pyeloplasty is variable and ranges from stable to decrease in UTD and/or improvement in function or drainage demonstrated by renal scintigraphy (Pouliot et al. 2010). The problems posed by preoperative evaluation with scintigraphy are also problematic following pyeloplasty (Amarante et al. 2003; Piepsz 2011; Ismaili and Piepsz 2013). Postoperative ultrasound may produce misleading results if not performed under standardized hydration (Pohl et al. 2001; Riccabona 2010).

The postoperative evaluation of a pyeloplasty with MR urography is straightforward and is able to discriminate a successful pyeloplasty from an equivocal or failed pyeloplasty (Little et al. 2007). On MR urography a successful pyeloplasty is characterized by rapid calyceal transit time, symmetric nephrograms, and almost equivalent pDRF and vDRF. The PUJ is shown to be widely patent. The preoperative delayed calyceal excretion secondary to increased intrapelvic pressure resolves and rapid calyceal excretion occurs as a result of an underlying concentration defect in a system with low intrapelvic pressure. Preoperative functional discrepancies typically resolve, and the degree of UTD is typically improved, although dilation and calyceal clubbing persist. The renal transit time often remains prolonged, indicating stasis and poor mechanical drainage (Kirsch et al. 2006; Little et al. 2007). Those children who have decompensated systems have significant improvement in renal function following pyeloplasty, whereas in those with compensated systems, there is little change in renal function. An equivocal pyeloplasty shows improved but persistent delay in calyceal excretion with narrowed PUJ. A failed pyeloplasty shows findings of persistent acute obstruction (Fig. 15).

> **Take Away**
> MR urography can identify children with significant physiological obstruction secondary to PUJ obstruction and in some cases identify the cause. MR urography is useful in the postoperative evaluation by demonstrating rapid calyceal excretion which is the hallmark of a successful pyeloplasty.

4.1.4 Ureteric Anomalies That May Mimic PUJ Obstruction

An advantage of MR urography over other modalities is the ability to identify ureters reliably in most children using the combination of T2 and post-contrast images. By delineating the ureteric anatomy, conditions which may mimic PUJ obstruction are readily diagnosed. Persistent fetal folds can be differentiated from mid-ureteric strictures. Fetal folds are typically seen in young infants with numerous small kinks or folds seen in the upper and mid-ureters. The UTD is compensated, and there is a classical corkscrew appearance to the upper ureter. Persistent fetal folds are considered a normal variant in that the UTD tends to be mild and self-limited, and there is no or only minimal impairment of renal function.

Children with ureteric strictures typically present with antenatal UTD but may present with pain, incontinence, or urinary tract infection (Arlen et al. 2014). The ureteric strictures typically occur in the mid-ureter but may be distal or rarely proximal (Fig. 16). Associated anomalies are common and include MCDK, duplication of the collecting system, paraureteral diverticulum, and ectopic ureterocele.

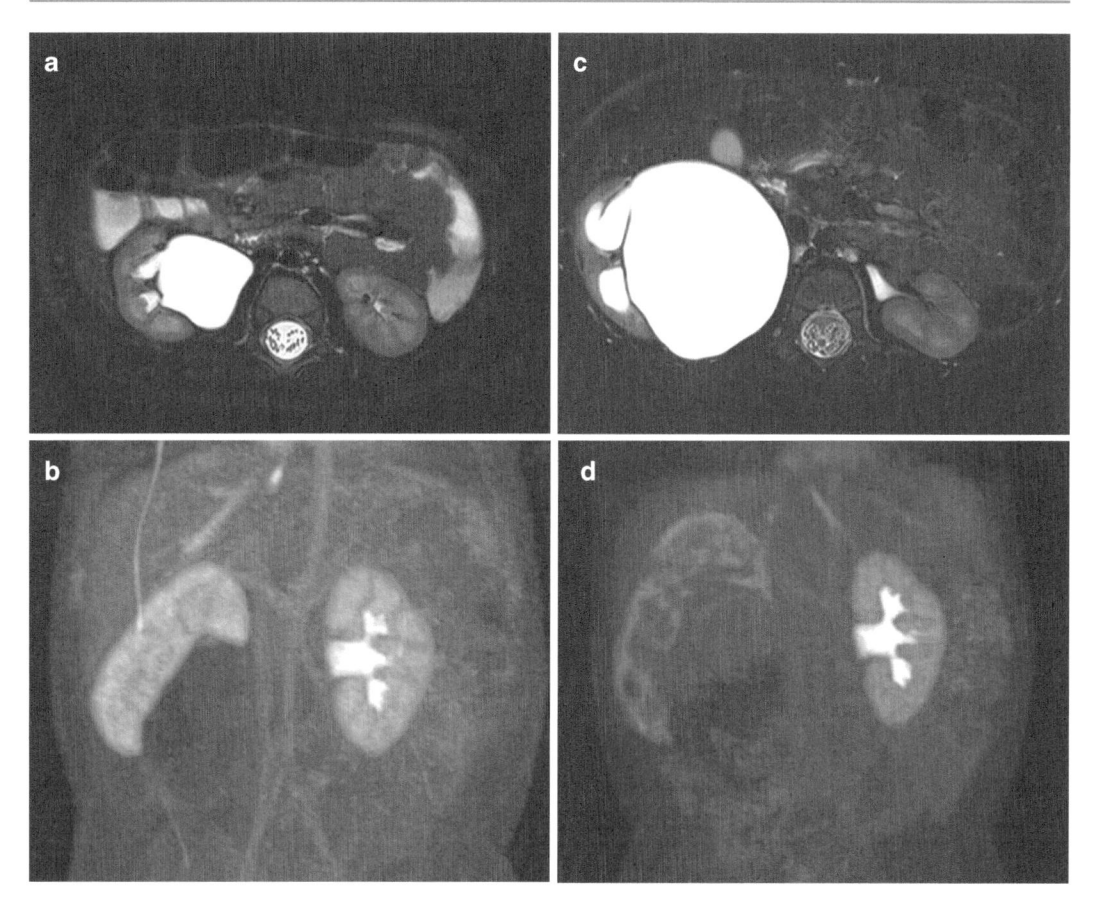

Fig. 15 Failed pyeloplasty in a 6-month-old boy with PUJ obstruction. (**a**) Axial T2-weighted image shows a dilated right renal pelvis with only mild caliectasis. There is preservation of the corticomedullary differentiation. (**b**) Coronal MIP image after contrast administration demonstrates a delayed and dense nephrogram on the right. The lower pole of the kidney is rotated laterally. (**c**) Following pyeloplasty the degree of UTD has increased with greater dilatation of the calyces. (**d**) Coronal MIP image after contrast administration demonstrates persistent delayed and dense nephrogram on the right. The nephrogram is also patchy indicating developing uropathy as a result of the failed pyeloplasty

Mid-ureteric strictures are often misdiagnosed by ultrasound and renal scintigraphy (Hwang et al. 2005). Preoperative diagnosis of ureteric strictures is important as the surgical approach varies depending on the location of the stricture. The combination of transition in ureteric caliber with decompensated UTD is the key feature in the diagnosis of mid-ureteric stricture. Although mid-ureteric strictures have been considered a rare anomaly in children, they are readily diagnosed by MR urography, and this condition has probably been underdiagnosed by traditional modalities (Arlen et al. 2014).

Fibroepithelial polyps may be seen in up to 0.5 % of children with PUJ obstruction and have been notoriously difficult to diagnose preoperatively (Shive et al. 2012). They are more commonly seen in boys and on the left side (Niu et al. 2007). The polyps are usually in the upper ureter and may prolapse into the renal pelvis and mimic PUJ obstruction (Fig. 17). Fibroepithelial polyps are readily diagnosed by MR urography as

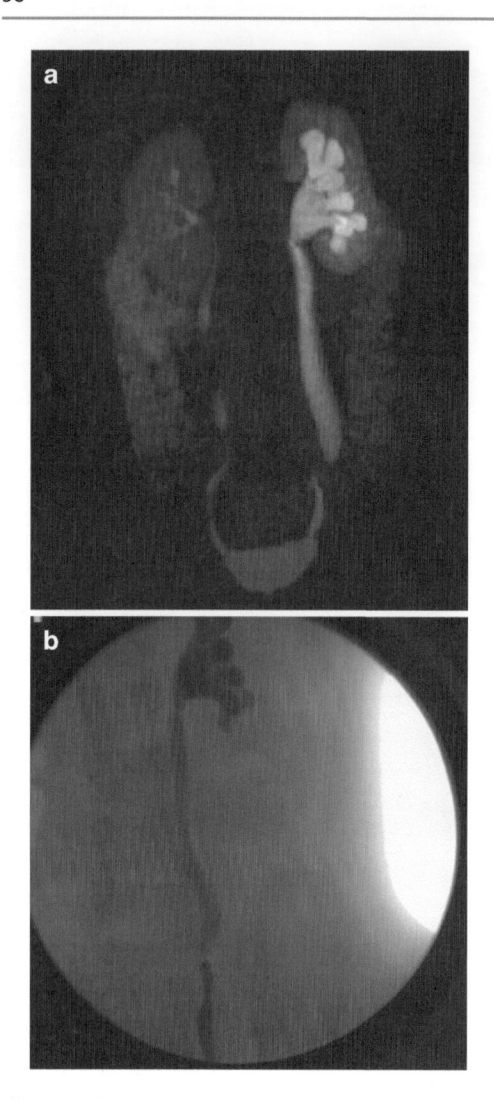

Fig. 16 Mid-ureteric stricture in a 5-year-old girl with recurrent left-sided abdominal pain. (**a**) Delayed coronal MIP image after contrast administration demonstrates moderate left-sided hydroureteronephrosis with transition in caliber in the distal third of the ureter. Note the delayed and dense nephrogram on the left. (**b**) Retrograde pyelogram confirms the ureteric stricture

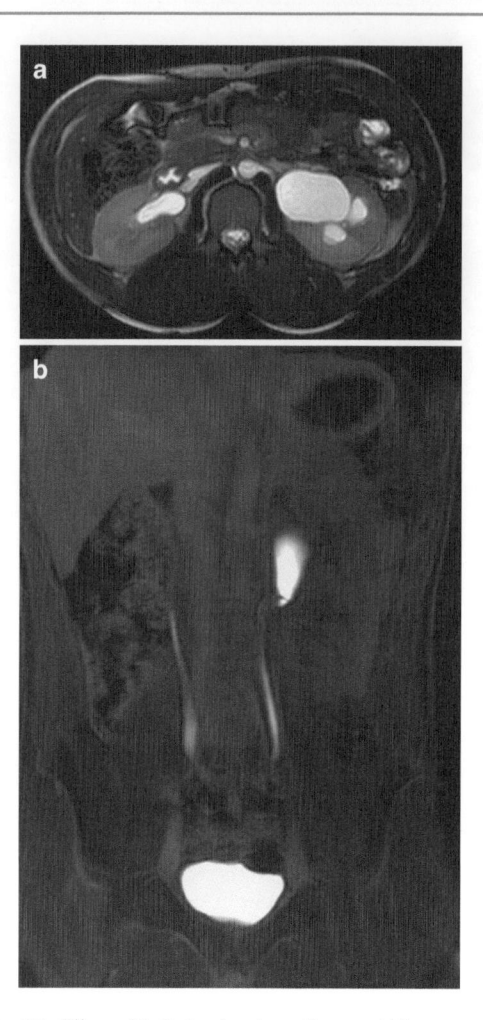

Fig. 17 Fibroepithelial polyp in an 8-year-old boy causing left-sided PUJ obstruction. (**a**) Axial T2-weighted image showing moderate left-sided pelvicaliectasis. (**b**) Coronal MIP image after contrast administration demonstrates an irregular and serpiginous filling defect extending from the renal pelvis into the proximal left ureter

elongated filling defects in the ureter (TKK Lai 2008; Patheyar et al. 2011). Retrocaval ureter is a developmental anomaly that rarely presents in children (Barker and Soundappan 2004; Acharya et al. 2009; González et al. 2011). It is more common in boys and usually on the right side. They typically present with pain, UTI, or hematuria and have a high incidence of developing calculi (Acharya et al. 2009). With MR the dilated upper ureter can be demonstrated curving upward and medially (Uthappa et al. 2002).

> **Take Away**
> MR urography is useful in identifying abnormalities that mimic PUJ obstruction. These include persistent fetal folds, mid-ureteric strictures, fibroepithelial polyps, and retrocaval ureter.

4.1.5 Megaureter and the Ureterovesical Junction (UVJ) Obstruction

Any dilatation of the distal ureter 7 mm or greater is abnormal (Farrugia et al. 2014). Megaureters were initially classified by Smith into four categories, obstructed, refluxing, refluxing with obstruction, and nonrefluxing/non-obstructed, which was later subdivided into primary and secondary by King (Smith et al. 1977; King 1980). Almost all children with primary megaureter measuring less than 10 mm resolve spontaneously although it may take up to 5 years (Ranawaka and Hennayake 2013). If the diameter is >15 mm, spontaneous resolution occurs rarely (Gimpel et al. 2010). Most cases of megaureter are nonobstructive and nonrefluxing (Hodges et al. 2010). Ultimately, only about 20% of children with megaureter will undergo surgery (Hodges et al. 2010; Gimpel et al. 2010; Arena et al. 2012).

Traditionally, children with megaureter have been followed conservatively, and surgery is reserved for cases that have an initial DRF<40% especially when associated with massive UTD or failure of conservative treatment (breakthrough UTIs, pain, worsening dilatation, or deteriorating DRF over time (Farrugia et al. 2014). Some cases with a DRF <40% have renal hypo-/dysplasia (Gimpel et al. 2010). Underlying renal dysplasia or uropathy can be readily identified on the MR scans showing disorganized renal parenchyma and dysmorphic calyceal anatomy.

The key to correct classification of megaureter is to evaluate the ureteric insertion for ureterocele or ectopia, to determine if physiologically significant obstruction is present, and to identify associated renal dysplasia or damage. Ultrasound is the primary method to identify the child with megaureter, and voiding cystourethrography should be obtained to demonstrate VUR or a cause of bladder outlet obstruction such as posterior urethral valves. Once VUR and bladder outlet obstruction are excluded, a functional test is used to identify obstruction at the UVJ. Interpretation of MAG3 renogram in the presence of a megaureter can be difficult because of the large capacity of the ureter (Gordon 2001). The washout curve should be evaluated with caution, and decisions to operate are typically based on decrease in the differential renal function.

The distal ureteric anatomy is well demonstrated with MR urography (Avni et al. 2001). Ectopic ureteric insertion either in single systems or in combination with duplex systems can usually be delineated on the delayed post-contrast images or on the T2-weighted images even when dealing with markedly dilated or poorly functioning system (Fig. 18). Axial and sagittal T2-weighted images of the bladder can be helpful in identifying anomalies of the distal ureter in dilated systems and delayed contrast-enhanced images in non-obstructed systems. The diagnosis of primary megaureter is made when the ureter measures more than 7 mm in diameter and the ureteric insertion into the bladder is normally located. The appearance of megaureter ranges from marked hydroureter with severe UTD to mild hydroureter more pronounced in the distal ureter without UTD. MR urography is superior to other modalities in the ability to delineate the dilated ureter as well as to differentiate it from other causes of a dilated ureter such as distal ureteric strictures and ectopic insertion of the ureter.

Using MR urography, the differentiation of obstructed from non-obstructed megaureter is made on the basis of physiologic changes demonstrated by the excretion of the contrast by the kidneys identical to the criteria used for PUJ obstruction. Most cases of megaureter are not obstructed and appear as compensated UTD with rapid or symmetric calyceal transit times (Fig. 19). When the calyceal excretion is delayed, it indicates physiologically significant obstruction (Fig. 20). Again, focusing on the changes that occur in the kidney is crucial in identifying children who may benefit from surgery. In most children with obstructed primary megaureter, there is only mild delay in calyceal excretion due to the reservoir effect of the large ureter so that little pressure increase is transmitted back to the kidneys. A markedly delayed

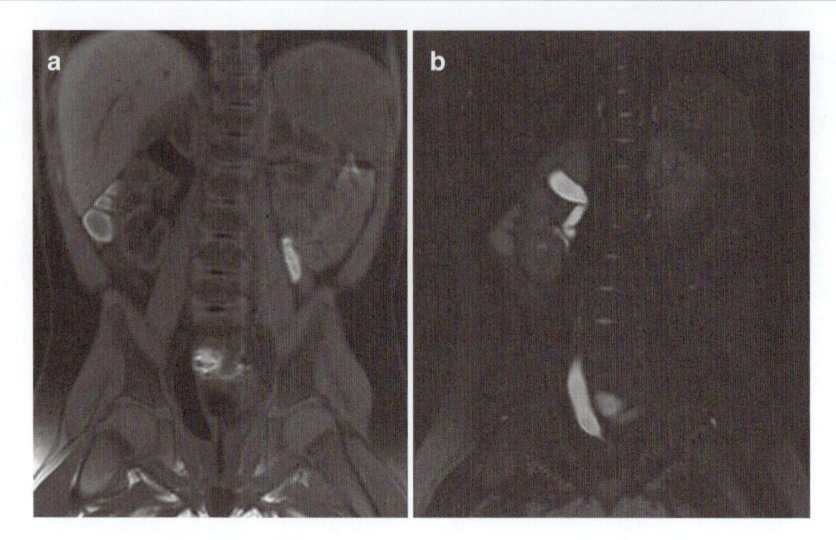

Fig. 18 Ectopic upper pole insertion associated with duplex collecting system. (**a**) Coronal T1 flair image prior to contrast administration shows the mild dilatation of the upper pole ureter on the right. The distal ureter tapers and inserts directly into the urethra. (**b**) Coronal T2-weighted image again demonstrates the ectopic ureteric insertion into the urethra. There is minimal renal dysplasia of the upper pole parenchyma

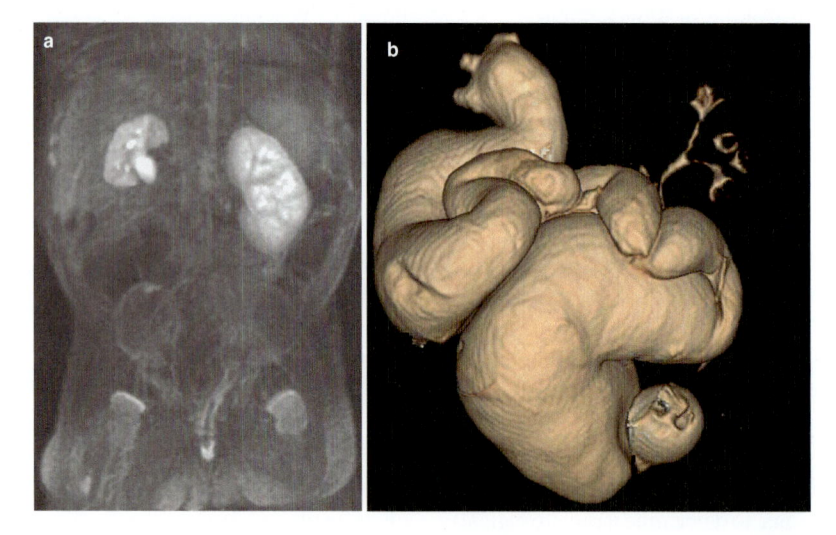

Fig. 19 Renal hypoplasia associated with massive hydroureteronephrosis in a 3-month-old boy. (**a**) Coronal MIP image after contrast administration demonstrates a small right kidney with relatively rapid excretion into the renal pelvis when compared to the normal left kidney. The rapid excretion is related to underlying uropathy associated with a concentration defect. (**b**) Volume-rendered T2-weighted image demonstrates the marked hydroureteronephrosis. The ureter inserted into the posterior urethra. Note the simplified and dysplastic calyceal anatomy of the hypoplastic right kidney

dense nephrogram with primary megaureter is rare, and if there is evidence of high-grade obstruction, careful analysis should be performed to try to identify a combined PUJ and UVJ obstruction.

MR urography is the best technique to reveal subtle duplication with infrasphincteric insertion in girls with incontinence. Ectopic insertion occurs with abnormal ureteric bud migration and usually results in caudal ectopia. In girls, the

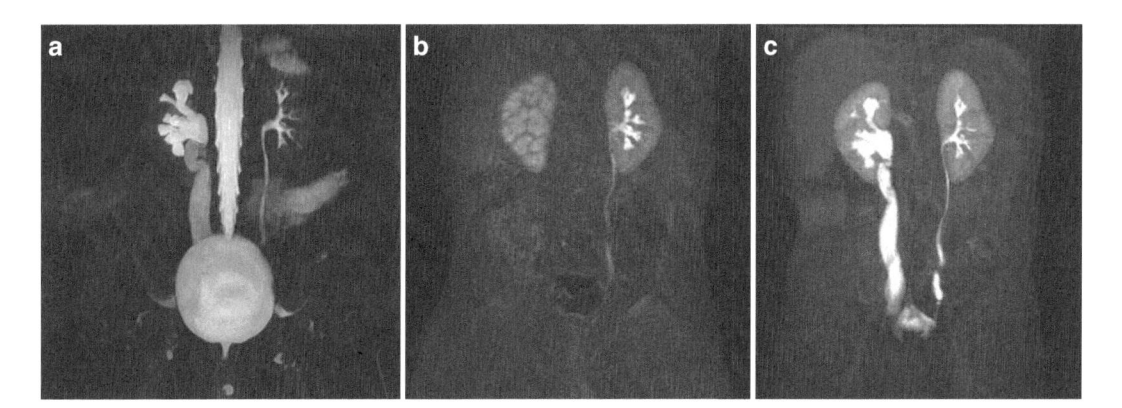

Fig. 20 Obstructive megaureter in a 6-month-old boy. (**a**) Coronal T2 MIP demonstrates the dilated upper system on the right. (**b**) Coronal MIP image after contrast administration demonstrates a delayed dense nephrogram with pronounced concentration in the renal medulla. (**c**) Delayed coronal MIP image after contrast administration demonstrates the right-sided UTD with normal insertion of the distal ureter into the bladder

ureter may insert into the lower bladder, urethra, vestibule, or vagina. Rarely, it can empty into the uterus or a Wolffian duct remnant such as a Gartner duct or cyst. In boys it may empty into the lower bladder, posterior urethra, seminal vesicle, vas deferens, or ejaculatory duct (Berrocal et al. 2002). The fundamental difference is that in females, ectopic ureters may insert distal to the external sphincter and be associated with incontinence, whereas in boys it always inserts above the external urethral sphincter. The upper pole of a duplex kidney may remain unrecognized until late in childhood. MR is able to demonstrate small dysplastic or cystic upper poles which may be invisible on ultrasound (Avni et al. 2001). The amount of functioning kidney parenchyma may be small and the calyces hypoplastic (Fig. 21). If there is a suspicion of a duplex kidney with ectopic ureteric insertion, MR should be used to evaluate the anomaly.

Occasionally, an ectopic ureter can drain a single kidney, but 70 % are associated with complete ureteral duplication. In boys an ectopic ureter drains a single system more commonly, and they can be bilateral in 10 % (Fig. 22). The most frequent anomaly associated with an ectopic ureter is hypoplasia or dysplasia of the renal moiety. In ectopic insertion of a single collecting system, the involved kidney is usually small and dysplastic. When an ectopic ureter drains outside the urinary system, the ectopic insertion may not be seen on VCUG. Bilateral single ectopic ureters are rare and are usually associated with a poorly developed bladder and bladder neck. Associated genital and renal anomalies are common and are associated with renal dysplasia and UTD (Fig. 22) (see also Chaps. 7, 9, and 26). They usually present with UTD or urinary tract infection.

> **Take Away**
> In the evaluation of megaureter, MR urography is used to evaluate the ureteric insertion for ureterocele or ectopia, to determine if obstruction is present, and to identify associated renal dysplasia or uropathy. MR urography is the optimum method to evaluate suspected ectopic ureters in patients with incontinence.

4.1.6 Ureteroceles

Ureteroceles are a common congenital malformation seen mostly in Caucasians and more frequently in girls (Shokeir and Nijman 2002). Ureteroceles are defined as cystic dilatation of the intravesical submucosal ureter. They are categorized as intravesical ureteroceles or as ectopic when some portion involves the bladder

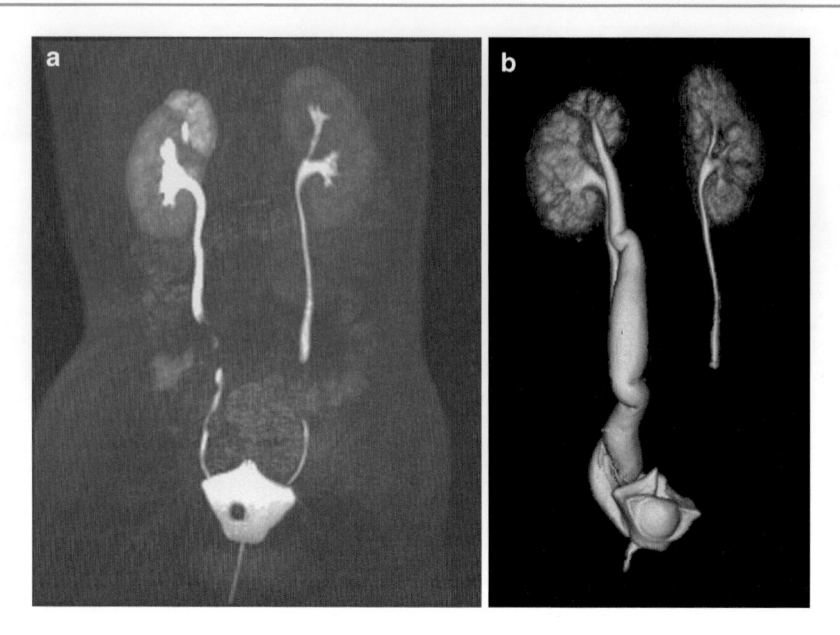

Fig. 21 Ectopic ureteric insertion in an 8-year-old girl with incontinence. Previous renal ultrasounds were normal. (**a**) Coronal MIP image after contrast administration demonstrates a delayed and dense nephrogram of the upper pole moiety with a small dysplastic calyx. The filling defect in the bladder is the balloon from the urethral catheter. (**b**) T2 volume-rendered image shows the pronounced dilatation of the upper pole ureter distally with an ectopic insertion below the bladder base

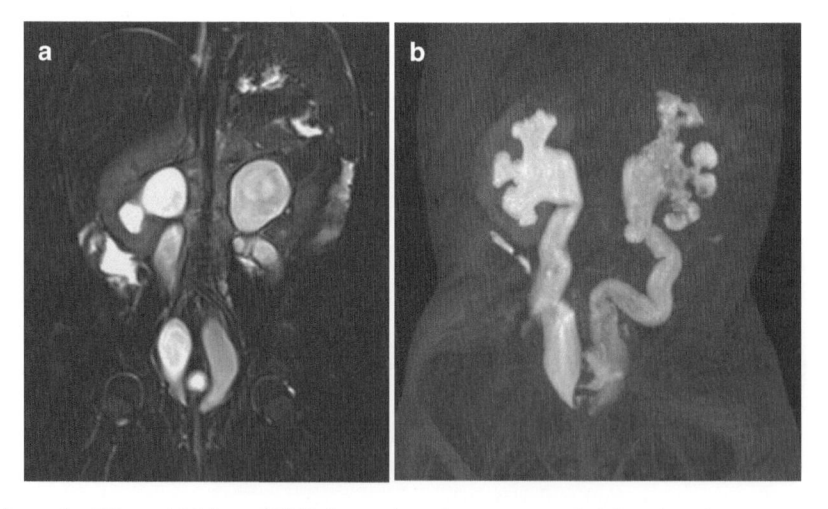

Fig. 22 A six-week-old boy with bilateral UTD detected antenatally. (**a**) Coronal T2-weighted image shows bilateral hydroureteronephrosis with the ureters inserting into the posterior urethra. (**b**) Delayed coronal MIP image after contrast administration demonstrates the bilateral hydroureteronephrosis with dysplastic pelvicalyceal systems. Filling defects in the left renal pelvis are secondary to pyonephrosis

neck or urethra. Ectopic ureteroceles are more common and usually associated with duplex systems. Ureteroceles range in size from small cystic dilatation to large cyst-like spaces filling the bladder in a balloon-like fashion. Ureteroceles associated with the upper pole of a duplex system are commonly associated with renal dysplasia (Fig. 23). The management of ureteroceles depends on associated obstruction, VUR, continence, and renal function. On MR

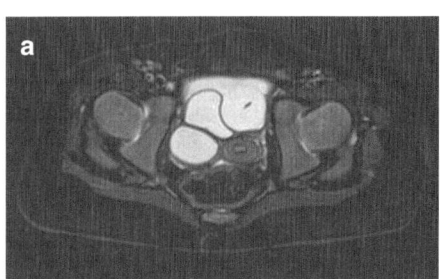

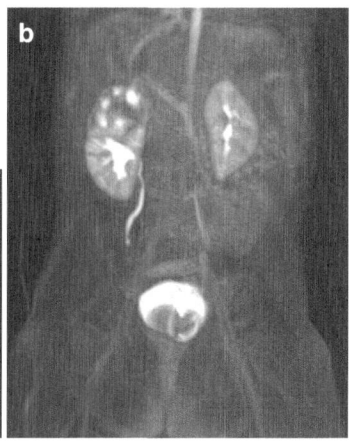

Fig. 23 Duplex system with ectopic ureterocele. (**a**) Axial T2-weighted image shows the dilated distal right ureter with the ureterocele at the right bladder base. Balloon from urethral catheter is seen on the left side of the bladder. (**b**) Delayed coronal MIP image after contrast administration demonstrates a duplex right kidney with upper pole UTD. The upper pole nephrogram is dim and patchy indicating renal dysplasia. Note the bilobed filling defect at the bladder base representing both the ureterocele and the balloon of the urethral catheter

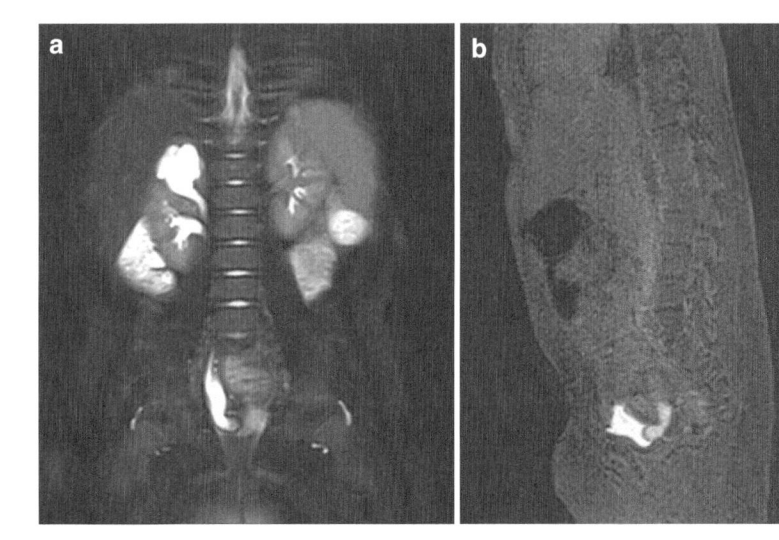

Fig. 24 Duplex system with orthotopic ureterocele. (**a**) Coronal T2-weighted image shows the duplex right kidney hydroureteronephrosis of the upper pole ureter. Note the "cobra head" appearance of the upper pole ureteric insertion. (**b**) Sagittal T1-weighted image shows contrast medium filling the distal right ureter again defining the orthotopic ureterocele

imaging ureteroceles appear as round, cyst-like structures in the bladder with a thin and smooth well-defined wall. A ureterocele should not be confused with the balloon of a urinary catheter. Virtual MR cystography is a recently described technique which has been shown to be most sensitive in detection of ureterocele extension and its precise anatomy, particularly in bilateral and ectopic types (Esfahani et al. 2011).

A characteristic "cobra head" deformity of the distal ureter is produced when opacified urine in the ureterocele is surrounded by the halo that represents the walls of the ureterocele (Fig. 24). Occasionally an ectopic ureter inserting into the urethra can elevate the floor of the bladder sufficiently to mimic a ureterocele. This is referred to as a "pseudoureterocele." Single system, usually orthotopic, ureteroceles are associated with better function and less UTD than the more common, usually ectopic, ureteroceles of duplex systems.

> **Take Away**
> On MR urography, ureteroceles appear as round, cyst-like structures in the bladder with a thin, smooth, and well-defined wall.

4.2 Congenital Anomalies of the Kidney and Urinary Tract (CAKUT)

Congenital anomalies of the kidney and urinary tract describe a wide range of structural malformations (Pope et al. 1999; Miyazaki and Ichikawa 2003; Sanna-Cherchi et al. 2009; Vivante et al. 2014; Rodriguez 2014; Soares dos Santos Junior et al. 2014). Abnormalities in urinary tract development occur in approximately 10 % of the population (Bonsib 2010). Some of these disorders are detected as part of a syndrome affecting multiple organ systems or in children with a positive family history. Most however are sporadic and confined to the urinary tract. The pathology of CAKUT occurs secondarily to a disturbance in normal nephrogenesis and can be due to genetic abnormalities in renal development (Miyazaki and Ichikawa 2003; Rodriguez 2014). CAKUT includes renal agenesis, renal malformations such as horseshoe and crossed fused kidneys, hypodysplasia, multicystic dysplastic kidneys (MCDK), UTD, PUJ obstruction, megaureter, duplication of the urinary tract, VUR, and posterior urethral valves. They account for up to 50 % of children with chronic renal disease. CAKUT may arise from mutations in a multitude of different single-gene causes (Vivante et al. 2014). MR urography offers an opportunity to study these malformations in vivo and to detect subtle abnormalities in the contralateral kidney (Kalisvaart et al. 2011). Abnormalities of calyceal anatomy are a useful indicator of underlying developmental abnormalities and are best demonstrated by MR urography on 3D volume-rendered images (Fig. 25). The calyces develop from the ureteric

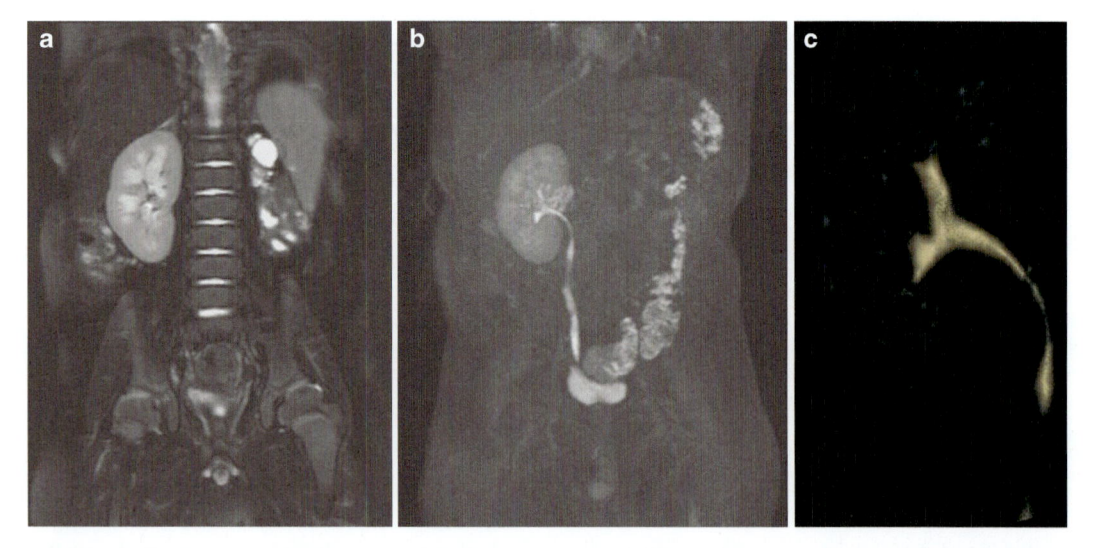

Fig. 25 Renal hypodysplasia contralateral to multicystic dysplastic kidney. (**a**) Coronal T2-weighted image shows multicystic dysplastic kidney on the left with apparently normal renal parenchyma on the right. (**b**) Delayed coronal MIP image after contrast administration demonstrates no evidence of renal function on the left. Close inspection of the right kidney shows a very simplified pelvicalyceal system indicating renal hypodysplasia. (**c**) T2 volume-rendered image confirms the markedly simplified pelvicalyceal system on the right with only two formed calyces

bud in a complex process of growth, branching, and remodeling termed branching morphogenesis (Blake and Rosenblum 2014; Bohnenpoll and Kispert 2014). Each successive division of the ureteric bud is binary until the entire collecting system is formed. Abnormal calyceal development is almost universally associated with small kidneys and reflects abnormal interaction between the ureteric bud and metanephric mesenchyme and is a useful marker of CAKUT (see also Chaps. 7 and 26).

Currently, the diagnosis of renal dysplasia is based on the histological identification of primitive tubules surrounded by stroma, smooth muscle collars, metaplastic cartilage, dysmorphic nerves and vessels, and erythropoietic cells (Greenbaum 2007). It is a descriptive term of a heterogeneous group of disorders with diverse etiologies and represents one of the most common causes of end-stage renal disease in children. However, because the diagnosis is made only after biopsy, nephrectomy, or autopsy, there is no practical or clinically useful classification. There are two main theories regarding dysplasia (Woolf 2004). It is thought to occur either as a result of failure of primary ureteric bud interaction with the metanephric mesenchyme or occur secondary to urinary tract obstruction. The appearance of dysplasia secondary to obstruction is thought to be related to both the timing and the severity of the obstruction. The various forms of renal dysplasia include multicystic dysplastic kidney (MCDK), cystic obstructive dysplasia, hypodysplasia, and solid renal dysplasias (Glassberg 2002). Mackie and Stephens suggested that renal dysplasia is closely correlated with an abnormal ureteral orifice location (Mackie and Stephens 1975). A laterally positioned ureteric bud provides an embryological explanation for VUR. The mismatch between the laterally positioned ureteric bud and the metanephros during early gestation results in dysplasia as well as VUR. Risdon has described hypoplasia and dysplasia in a large majority of boys with gross reflux (Risdon 1993). The typical imaging features associated with dysplastic kidneys include small size, disorganized architecture with loss of normal corticomedullary differentia-

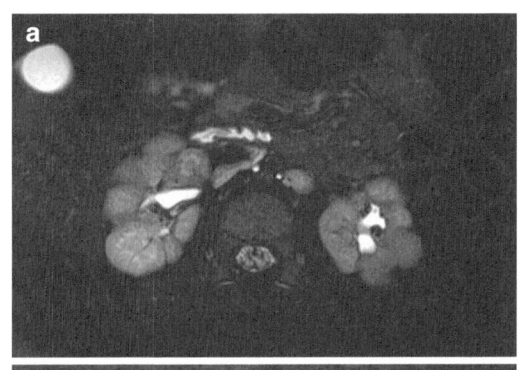

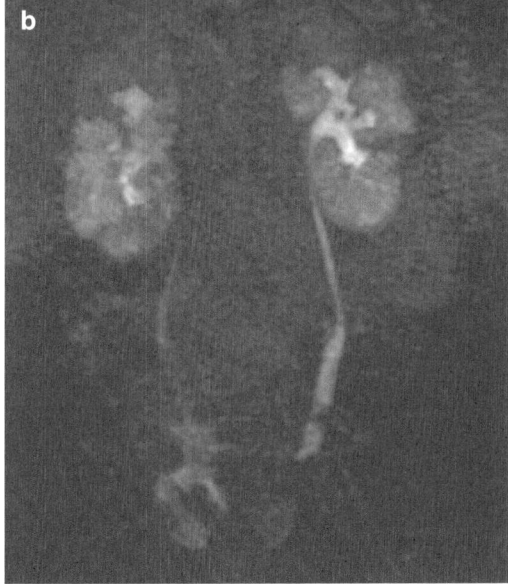

Fig. 26 Bilateral renal dysplasia. (**a**) Axial T2-weighted image showing lobulated outline to both kidneys with heterogeneous signal intensity and loss of corticomedullary differentiation. (**b**) Delayed coronal MIP image after contrast administration demonstrates patchy and irregular contrast enhancement most marked in the upper poles bilaterally. The calyces are deformed and reduced in number

tion, small subcortical cysts, decrease in signal intensity on T2-weighted images, and poor perfusion manifested as a dim and patchy nephrogram with dysmorphic calyces (McMann et al. 2006; Grattan-Smith et al. 2007; Grattan-Smith et al. 2010) (Fig. 26). These are similar to the features previously described as representing uropathy in children with antenatally diagnosed PUJ obstruction (Fig. 27).

Children born with a solitary functioning kidney have a greater predisposition to develop renal

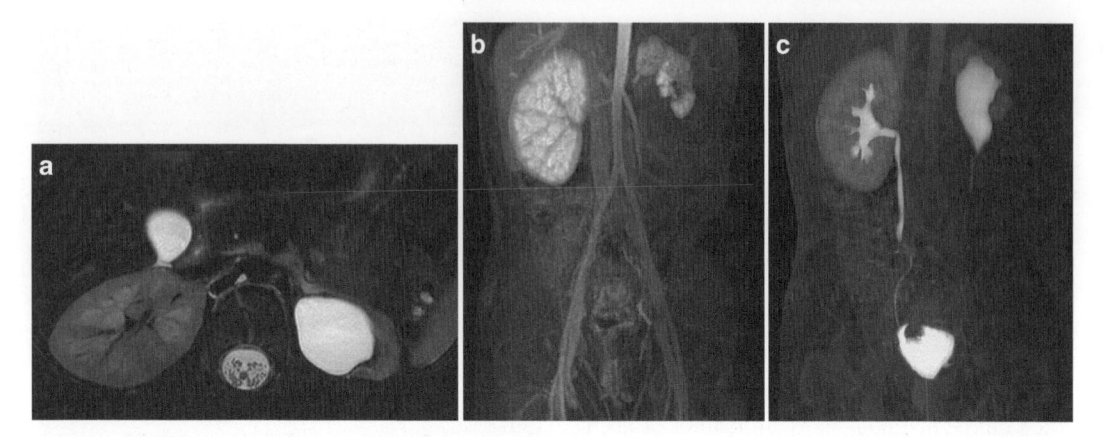

Fig. 27 Unilateral renal dysplasia with contralateral compensatory hypertrophy. (**a**) Axial T2-weighted image shows a small left kidney with loss of corticomedullary differentiation. Several small subcortical cysts are present. (**b**) Coronal MIP image after contrast administration demonstrates the small left kidney with rapid calyceal excretion secondary to underlying uropathy and dysplasia. The right kidney is enlarged and shows normal concentration within the renal medulla. (**c**) Delayed coronal MIP image after contrast administration demonstrates and shows the small left kidney with dysmorphic and simplified pelvicalyceal system

insufficiency and hypertension in early adult life due to reduced nephron mass (Chevalier 2009; Schreuder 2012; Westland et al. 2013; Lankadeva et al. 2014). The majority of congenitally small kidneys also exhibit evidence of renal dysplasia. Ultrasound is unable to discriminate hypoplasia from dysplasia. Severe reduction in nephron numbers that are characteristic of renal hypoplasia/dysplasia is the leading cause of ESRD in children (Cain et al. 2010). There is a significantly poorer outcome for patients carrying bilateral renal hypodysplasia, solitary kidneys, and posterior urethral valves compared with other categories. By 30 years of age, nearly 50 % of patients with a solitary kidney may be on dialysis (Chevalier 2009; Sanna-Cherchi et al. 2009). Children with contralateral abnormalities are at increased risk of hyperfiltration injury. MR urography can detect renal hypodysplasia on the basis of reduced number of calyces similar to prior studies using intravenous urography (Risdon et al. 1975) (Fig. 28).

Anomalies of renal position and rotation are well demonstrated by the high-resolution anatomic images. Horseshoe and ectopic kidneys can be easily separated from the background and overlying tissues (Fig. 29). Ectopic kidneys are usually in the pelvis and rarely in the thorax. They are often small, lobulated with abnormal rotation and dysmorphic extrarenal calyces (Fig. 30). There is an increased incidence of PUJ obstruction in ectopic kidneys. If the two developing kidneys come into contact, fusion anomalies such as horseshoe, crossed fused kidneys, or lump kidneys result. MR urography provides superior anatomical delineation of the structural abnormality as well as being able to characterize associated anomalies such as PUJ obstruction. Accurate anatomic delineation is important when surgery is contemplated as the approach may be retroperitoneal or transperitoneal. Hypoplastic kidneys associated with ureteric ectopia and supernumerary kidneys, which have been difficult to demonstrate with other imaging modalities, can usually be demonstrated even if there is minimal renal function (Fig. 31).

Anomalies of the calyces have been considered rare but are commonly visualized using MR urography. In the normal kidney, there are between 7 and 14 calyces on each side. Congenital calyceal anomalies include calyceal diverticula,

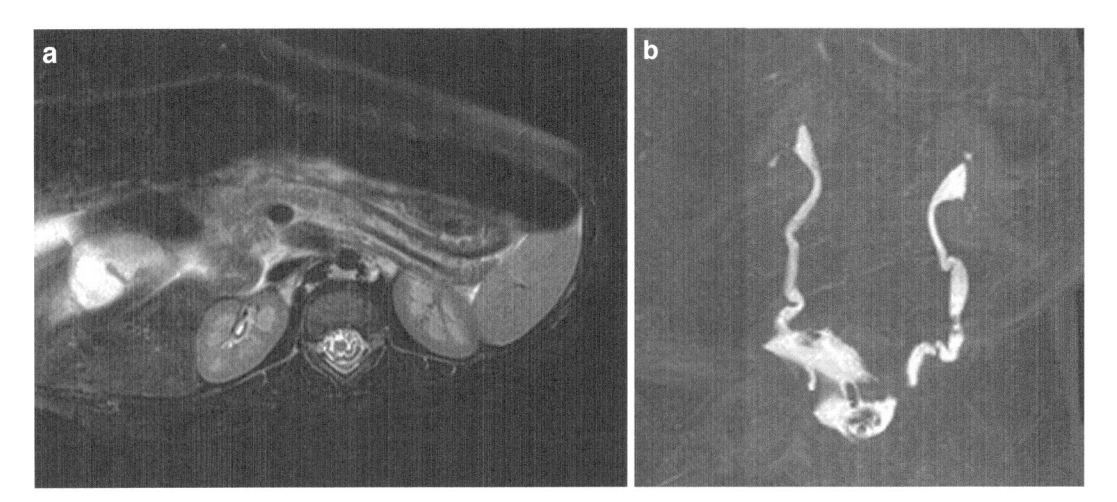

Fig. 28 Prune belly syndrome with dysplastic calyces. (**a**) Axial T2-weighted image demonstrates two normal-appearing kidneys without significant UTD. There is preserved corticomedullary differentiation. Note the deformity of the abdomen related to underlying prune belly syndrome. (**b**) Delayed coronal MIP image after contrast administration demonstrates bilateral simplified and dysmorphic pelvicalyceal systems with redundant ureters. The bladder is large and irregularly shaped

hydrocalyx and Fraley's syndrome, megacalyces, polycalycosis, and infundibular stenosis. Calyceal diverticula are outpouches from the calyces and are often complicated by development of renal stones (Waingankar et al. 2014). The diverticula communicate with the main collecting system via a narrow channel and fill passively with urine (Fig. 32). They are often peripelvic in location and usually seen as small round cystic structures on ultrasound. Delayed imaging with MR urography is diagnostic by identifying progressive filling of the calyceal diverticulum.

Hydrocalyx may be caused by extrinsic or intrinsic anomalies (Fig. 33). Fraley's syndrome is a rare condition characterized by severe flank pain and is caused by a vessel obstructing an upper pole calyx. The hydrocalyx is demonstrated on the T2 and delayed post-contrast images, while the crossing vessel is defined on the vascular phase of the MR urogram. Congenital infundibular stenosis is rare and characterized by progressive narrowing of the infundibulum with progressive dilatation of the calyx (Lucaya et al. 1984; Nurzia et al. 2002). It may be localized or diffused. The renal pelvis is often small and stenotic. Infundibular stenosis has been reported contralateral to multicystic dysplastic kidney (Dally et al. 2011).

Megacalycosis is characterized by dilated, malformed calyces without obstruction (Redman and Neeb 2005; Pieretti-Vanmarcke et al. 2008). It is usually unilateral and more frequent in males. Rarely it is bilateral. Additionally, the number of calyces may be increased. Megacalycosis is characterized by hypoplastic medullary pyramids, and the calyces are often polyclonal and faceted rather than the blunted calyces typically associated with obstruction. Usually there is disproportion between the dilatation of the calyces and the normal size of the renal pelvis and ureter. Although megacalycosis is not typically associated with obstruction, some cases have been noted (Whitaker and Flower 1981) (Fig. 34). MR urography is recommended to differentiate megacalycosis from infundibular stenosis or other obstructive entities.

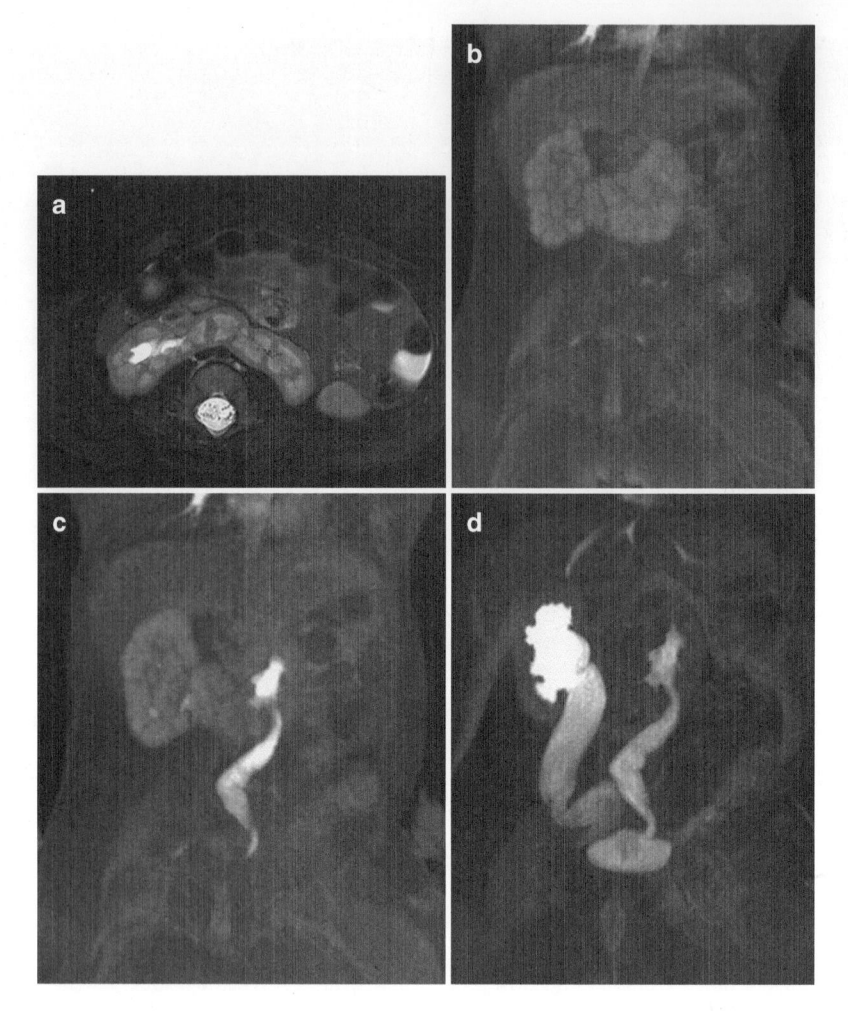

Fig. 29 Horseshoe kidney with bilateral megaureter. (**a**) Axial T2-weighted image shows the isthmus connecting the lower poles of both kidneys across the midline. (**b**) Coronal MIP image after contrast administration demonstrates symmetric enhancement and medullary concentration of the horseshoe kidney. (**c**) There is relatively rapid excretion of the contrast into the left pelvicalyceal system and ureter indicating an obstructive component on the right. (**d**) Delayed coronal MIP image after contrast administration demonstrates the bilateral hydroureteronephrosis more marked on the right than the left

Take Away
MR urography characterizes congenital abnormalities of the urinary tract including abnormalities of calyceal development more precisely than other modalities. It is important to evaluate the entire urinary tract as these abnormalities are often multiple and may be overlooked.

4.3 Pyelonephritis and Renal Scarring

Although urinary tract infection (UTI) is common in childhood, the imaging workup remains controversial (see also Chaps. 13 and 30). Various strategies have been used including ultrasonography, VCUG, and DMSA to diagnose and detect complications of UTI. With the

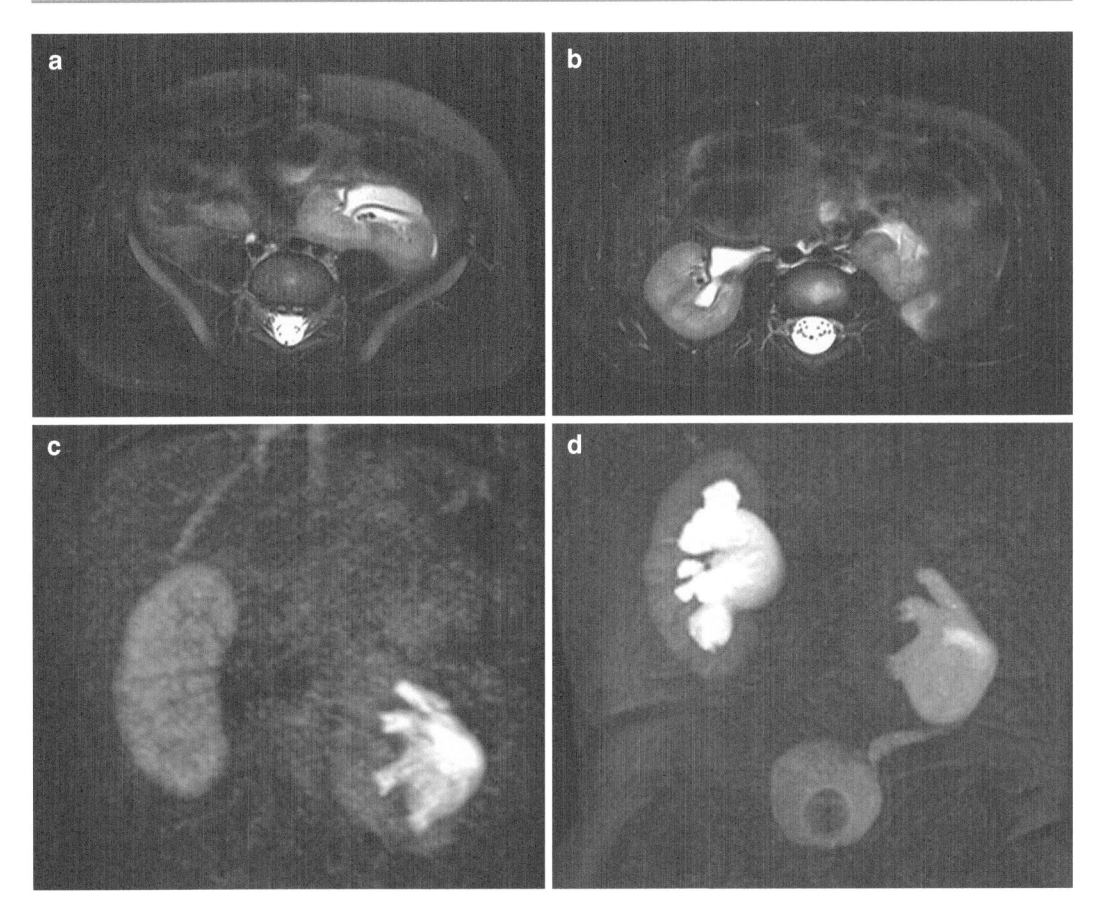

Fig. 30 Malrotated, ectopic kidney with contralateral PUJ obstruction. (**a**) Axial T2-weighted image through the pelvis demonstrates the ectopic left kidney with the renal pelvis rotated anteriorly. (**b**) Axial T2-weighted image at the level of the renal fossa shows a normally positioned right kidney with only mild UTD. (**c**) Coronal MIP image after contrast administration demonstrates a delayed dense nephrogram on the right with the malrotated ectopic kidney on the right. (**d**) Delayed coronal MIP image after contrast administration demonstrates ballooning of the renal pelvis with distention of the calyces in response to the fluid and diuretic challenge. The changes are more pronounced on the right

addition of DWI, MR imaging is now the most accurate way to identify acute pyelonephritis and differentiate acute pyelonephritis from renal scarring (Weiser et al. 2003; Kavanagh et al. 2005; Grattan-Smith et al. 2007; Martina et al. 2010; De Pascale et al. 2013; Vivier et al. 2013; Faletti et al. 2013; Cerwinka et al. 2014). MR urography is able to differentiate areas of acute pyelonephritis from developed renal scars on the basis of mass effect and inflammatory changes. Acute pyelonephritis is associated with edema, loss of corticomedullary differentiation, and patchy contrast enhancement (Fig. 35). On DWI images areas of pyelonephritis restrict diffusion with high signal on DWI images and decreased ADC values compared to noninfected parenchyma. The restricted diffusion is probably related to edema in the renal parenchyma and accumulation of inflammatory cells within the renal tubules. DWI is more sensitive to noncomplicated pyelonephritis, and contrast-enhanced MR is more useful in diagnosing renal

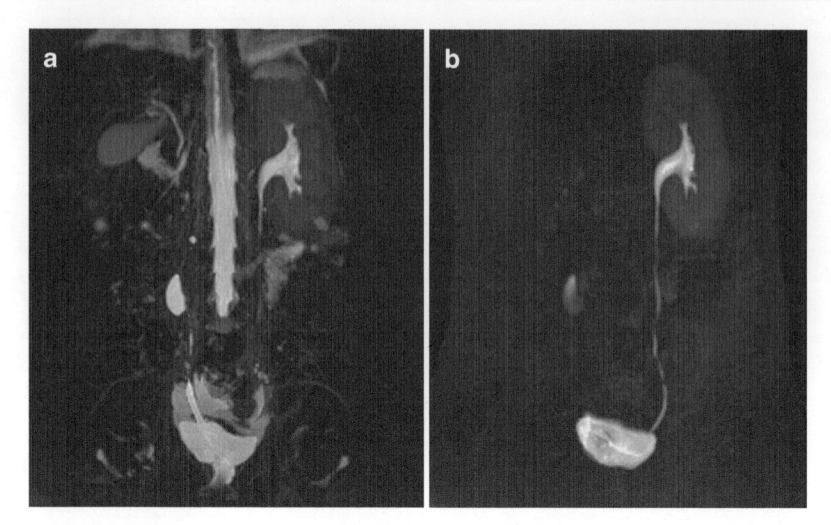

Fig. 31 An 11-year-old girl with incontinence and hypoplastic ectopic right kidney. (**a**) Coronal T2 MIP image demonstrates a normal left kidney and no appreciable parenchyma in the right renal fossa. There is a small right kidney with dilated renal pelvis located at the pelvic brim. The dilated right ureter can be traced below the bladder base. (**b**) Delayed coronal MIP image after contrast administration demonstrates compensatory hypertrophy of the left kidney. There is minimal excretion into the ectopic hypoplastic right kidney. The anatomic information provided is important in surgical planning

abscess (Faletti et al. 2013). The duration of restricted diffusion after acute pyelonephritis is as yet unknown and will be important to understand if DWI is used to follow pyelonephritic lesions (Martina et al. 2010; Vivier et al. 2013). Fluid-debris levels may be seen with pyonephrosis.

Cortical scars are seen as focal areas of volume loss with deformity of the renal contour (Fig. 36). The underlying calyx is often deformed. The use of the cortical phase of the dynamic post-contrast scan demonstrates cortical perfusion defects similar to those seen on CT. Mature scars are characterized by volume loss and contour defects of the kidney on T2-weighted images and perfusion defects on the dynamic contrast-enhanced images and exhibit dilatation of the adjacent calyx, indicating transmural parenchymal loss. Affected regions demonstrate no appreciable contrast enhancement reflecting fibrosis and microvascular damage. When the scarring is diffuse, there is significant loss of renal function which is readily quantifiable with MR urography. In the evaluation of renal scarring, MR urography shows greater interobserver reliability than DMSA scintigraphy, and some now regard it as the gold standard (Cerwinka et al. 2014).

> **Take Away**
> MR urography is superior to DMSA scanning in the evaluation of renal scarring and pyelonephritis and is now the most accurate way to identify acute pyelonephritis and to differentiate acute pyelonephritis from renal scarring.

4.4 MR for VUR Assessment: MR VCUG

Several authors have explored the accuracy and feasibility of MR VCUG in depicting VUR (Hekmatnia et al. 2013; Rodríguez et al. 2001; Takazakura et al. 2007; Johnin et al. 2013; Arthurs et al. 2013). Both direct and indirect MR VCUG have been evaluated (Johnin et al. 2013). In direct MR VCUG, dilute Gd-based contrast agent is instilled via a urethral catheter. With the indirect

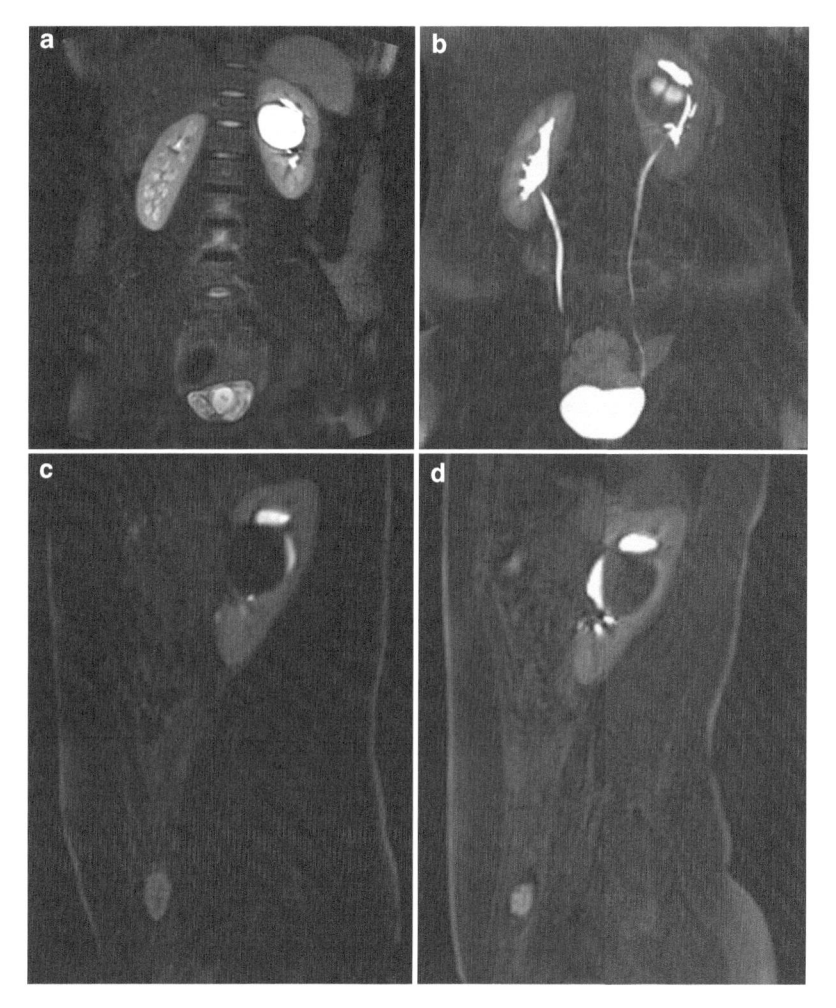

Fig. 32 Large calyceal diverticulum. (**a**) Coronal T2-weighted image shows large peripelvic cyst on the left. (**b**) Delayed coronal MIP image after contrast administration shows accumulation of contrast medium into the cystic structure with displacement and deformity of the surrounding calyces. (**c**) Sagittal T1-weighted image after contrast administration demonstrates layering of contrast within the cyst, confirming its communication with the pelvicalyceal system. (**d**) Further confirmation of excreted contrast within the diverticulum can be obtained by turning the patient prone and identifying the dependent fluid level. Delayed images are required when evaluating calyceal diverticula

MR VCUG, diuretics are used to promote filling of the bladder (Hekmatnia et al. 2013; Johnin et al. 2013). The voiding part of the examination was performed with various MR fluoroscopic techniques. One study successfully examined young infants without sedation (Arthurs et al. 2013). Most other studies used intravenous sedation. Failure rates were higher in toddlers usually related to issues with sedation or secondary to inability to void during the study (Johnin et al. 2013). The studies all demonstrate significant accuracy in the diagnosis of high-grade VUR as well as visualizing urethral abnormalities. The major advantage of MR is the ability to assess the anatomy of the kidney and identify renal scars, dysplasia, or malformations without ionizing radiation (Rodríguez et al. 2001). However, most children will need sedation, catheterization, or administration of diuretics. Other disadvantages of MR VCUG include its high cost.

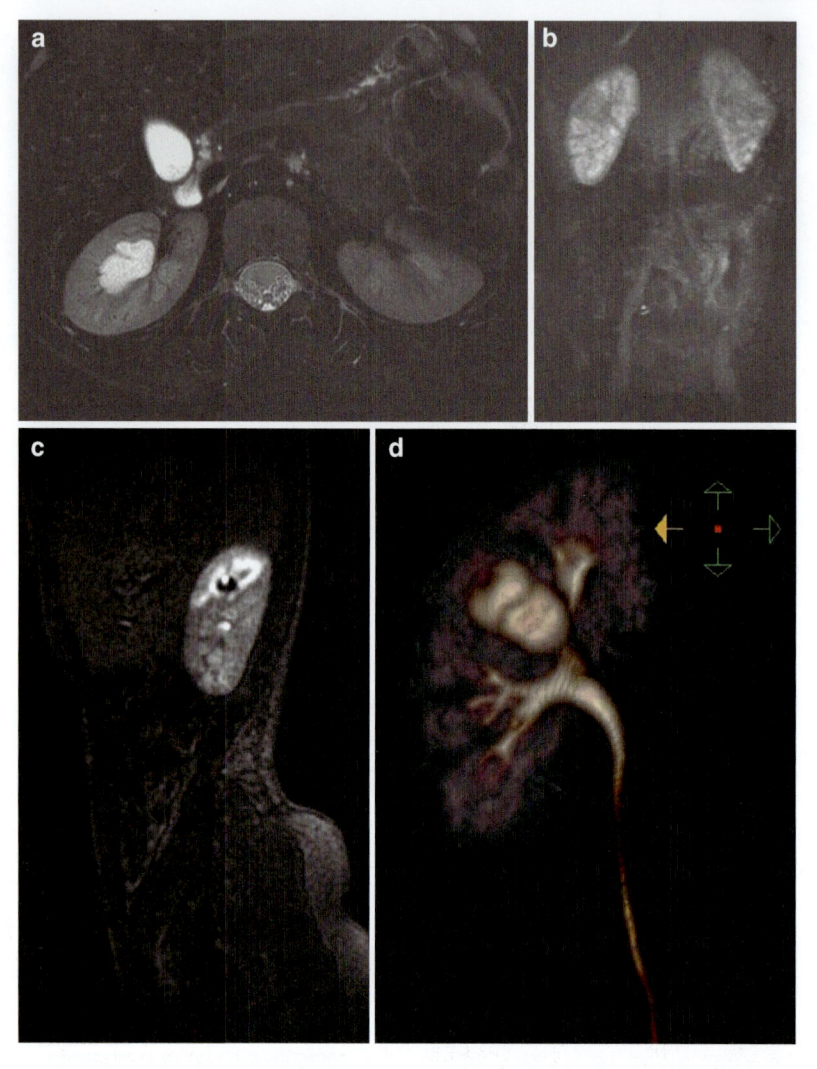

Fig. 33 Infundibular stenosis with hydrocalyx. (**a**) Axial T2-weighted image showing a peripelvic cyst on the right. (**b**) Coronal MIP image after contrast administration demonstrates a focal area of decreased enhancement of the upper mid-pole of the right kidney. (**c**) Sagittal T1-weighted image shows a wedge-shaped area of the right kidney representing a focally delayed dense nephrogram associated with the dilated calyx. (**d**) Volume-rendered image of the right kidney demonstrates the dilated calyx with stenosis of its infundibulum

> **Take Away**
> Although MR VCUG is feasible, the disadvantages compared with traditional VCUG will limit its widespread application.

4.5 MR Genitography

Disorders of sexual development (DSD) are defined as conditions in which chromosomal sex is not consistent with phenotypic sex or in which the phenotype is not classifiable as either male or female (Mansour et al. 2012) (see also Chaps. 7, 19, 20, and 21). The male or female configuration of the genitalia normally evolves in fetal life and is determined by the genetic, gonadal, and hormonal sex (Grinspon and Rey 2014; Hughes 2002). Disorders of sex development occur when the male hormone (androgens and anti-Mullerian hormone) secretion or action is insufficient in the 46 XY fetus or when there is androgen excess in the 46 XX fetus. DSD with ambiguous genitalia is typically diagnosed clinically in the newborn

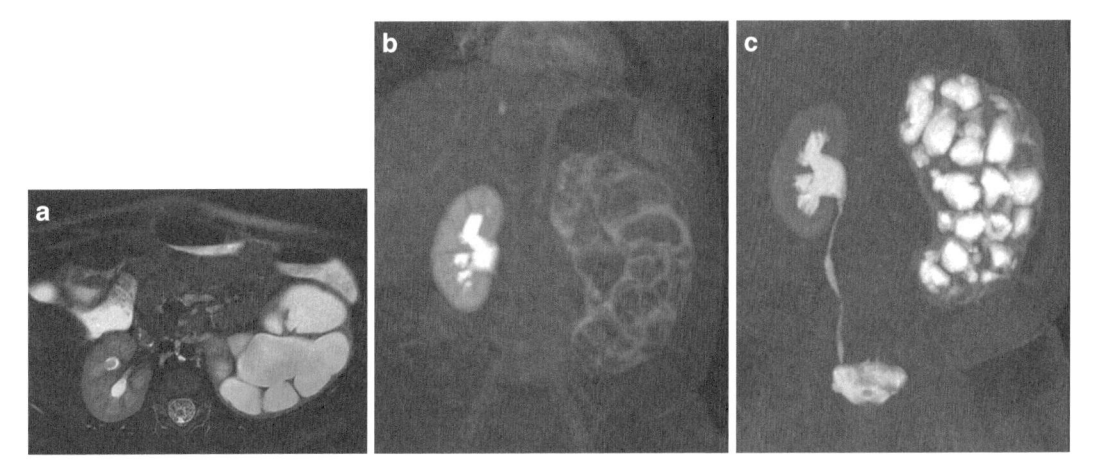

Fig. 34 Unilateral megacalycosis with obstruction. (**a**) Axial T2-weighted image showing marked dilation of the pelvicalyceal system on the left with thinning of the renal parenchyma. (**b**) Coronal MIP image after contrast administration demonstrates an enlarged left kidney with delayed and dense nephrogram. (**c**) Delayed coronal MIP image after contrast administration demonstrates the marked increase in number of calyces. Most cases of megacalycosis do not demonstrate obstruction

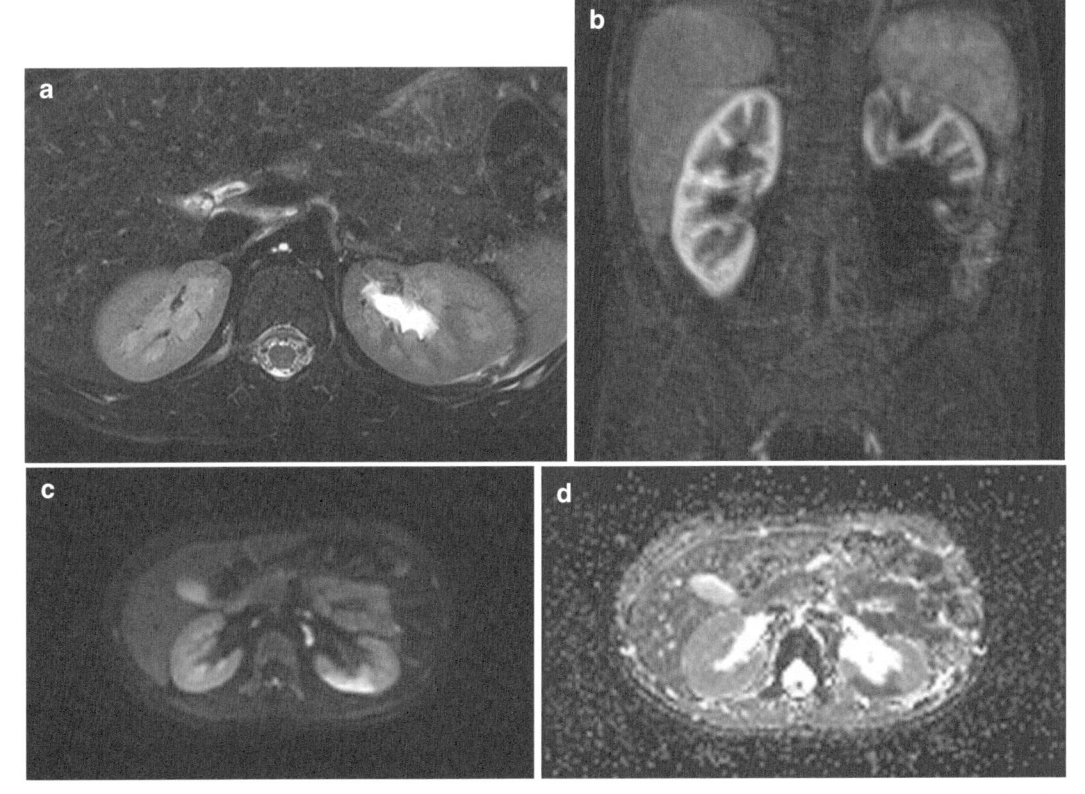

Fig. 35 Acute pyelonephritis superimposed on previously scarred kidney. (**a**) Axial T2-weighted image shows mild swelling of the upper pole of the left kidney with blurring of the corticomedullary junction. The changes are subtle on the T2-weighted images, but there is no evidence of volume loss. Note the small amount of perinephric fluid. (**b**) Early perfusion phase following contrast administration demonstrates normal cortical enhancement of the right kidney. There are multifocal areas of decreased cortical perfusion on the left. There is volume loss associated with the lower pole indicating prior scarring. (**c**) Axial trace image from the diffusion-weighted sequence shows increased signal involving the mid-pole of the left kidney. (**d**) ADC map confirms the focal area of acute restricted diffusion indicating acute pyelonephritis. Diffusion-weighted imaging is a very sensitive method for detecting acute pyelonephritis

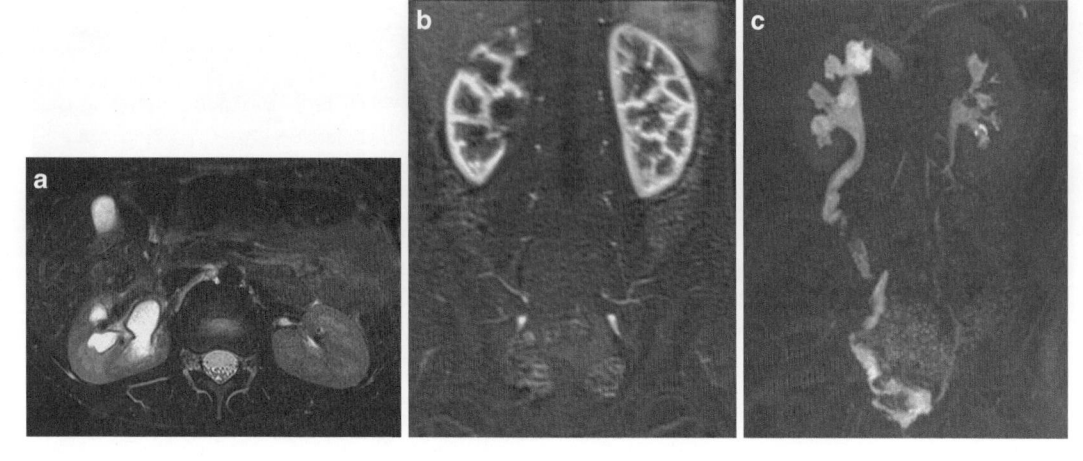

Fig. 36 Multifocal renal scarring. (**a**) Axial T2-weighted image showing irregular calyceal dilatation on the right. There is flattening of the posterior aspect of the right kidney with decreased signal intensity indicating scarring and fibrosis. (**b**) Coronal perfusion image after contrast administration demonstrates multifocal areas of scarring involving the upper pole of the left kidney. Identifying volume loss is key in differentiating renal scarring from acute pyelonephritis. (**c**) Delayed coronal MIP image after contrast administration demonstrates irregularity and dilatation of the calyces on the right indicating transmural volume loss. The right ureter is dilated, and the child had a history of grade IV vesicoureteric reflux on the right

period, whereas those associated with male and female phenotypes may not present until adolescence. Patients with pure gonadal dysgenesis or complete androgen insensitivity usually are phenotypic females who present at puberty with primary amenorrhea.

Diagnosis and classification of these disorders are complex, and the role of imaging in infants is to identify a uterus and/or cervix, to locate the gonads, and to define the anatomy of cloacal malformations, Mullerian duct anomalies, urinary tract anomalies as well as anorectal and spine malformations (Riccabona et al. 2015). Ultrasound has been the primary modality to identify the internal organs, and occasionally fluoroscopic genitography and VCUG are used to assess the vagina, urethra, and any fistulas or complex tracts. MR genitography is being used more often in the evaluation of these anomalies especially in defining the anatomy of the urogenital tract and anorectal malformations and to identify otherwise occult gonads (Baughman et al. 2007; Jarboe et al. 2012; Podberesky et al. 2013a; Ehammer et al. 2011). MR genitography is similar to traditional fluoroscopic genitography in that contrast material is used to demonstrate the anatomy of the various cavities. However, the complex communications are better defined using both T1- and T2-weighted 3D imaging sequences. Although various contrast agents have been used including mineral oil and ultrasound gel, we prefer to use diluted (1:1000) gadolinium-based contrast agent.

When performing a genitogram, it is important to ensure that all perineal orifices are examined (Shopfner 1964). It is also important to preserve the morphological appearance by only inserting the catheters a short distance (Wright et al. 1995). The goal is to define a male or female urethral configuration and identify any fistulous communication with the vagina or rectum. Demonstration of the level at which the vagina opens into a urogenital sinus and its relationship to the external sphincter are important in surgical planning (Figures 37 and 38). The vagina is evaluated to determine its presence or absence, its relationship to the urethra and to identify the uterus. The presence of hydrocolpos associated with ambiguous genitalia and two perineal orifices confirms the presence of a urogenital sinus. In the presence of a large hydrocolpos, the bladder may be displaced anteriorly, making it difficult to see, so care is needed to make sure a fluid-filled vagina is not confused with the urinary bladder. The uterus often is identified capping the vagina, and the distended vagina often contains a fluid-debris level. In cloacal malformations, the genital, urinary, and gastrointestinal tracts open into a single common channel classically located at the expected site of the urethra (Jaramillo et al. 1990; Winkler 2012). It is almost exclusively seen in girls. Cloacal malformations are divided into two groups depending on the length of the common channel. A common channel less than 3 cm is more easily repaired and has a lower incidence of associated anomalies.

Mullerian duct anomalies are a broad and complex spectrum of anomalies that often present with primary amenorrhea in adolescents. MR is the imaging method of choice in defining these anomalies (Junqueira et al. 2009; Marcal et al. 2011; Behr et al. 2012; Yoo et al. 2013; Hall-Craggs et al. 2013a). The uterus, fallopian tubes, cervix, and upper two thirds of the vagina are derived from the Mullerian ducts. The ovaries are embryologically separate and not typically involved in Mullerian duct anomalies. In patients with Mullerian duct anomalies, renal and ureteric anomalies are common (Hall-Craggs et al. 2013a). In addition to the well-known association with renal agenesis which is found in up to 30%, there is also a high incidence of ectopic, malrotated, or dysplastic kidneys (see also Chap. 19). Additionally, 25% of patients with renal agenesis have distal ureteric remnants or ectopic ureteric insertion. These ureteric remnants may become distended by menstrual blood leading to abdominal pain and infection or present with urinary incontinence and recurrent UTI. All patients with Mullerian duct anomalies need assessment of the

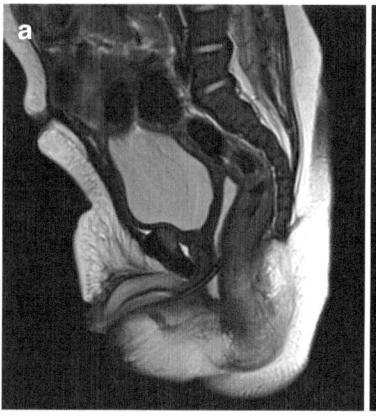

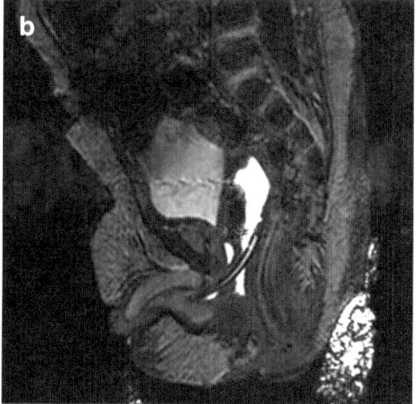

Fig. 37 MR genitogram demonstrating a urogenital sinus. (**a**) Sagittal T2-weighted image shows fluid in both the urinary bladder and the vagina. The urethral catheter passes into the vagina demonstrating the level at which the urethra and vagina communicate. (**b**) T1 sagittal GRE image with contrast administered via the catheter again outlines the communication between the vagina and urethra which is important for surgical planning

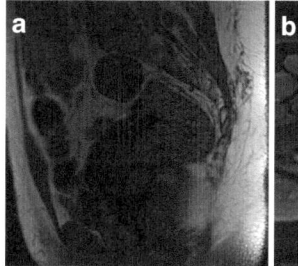

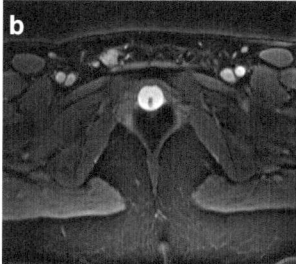

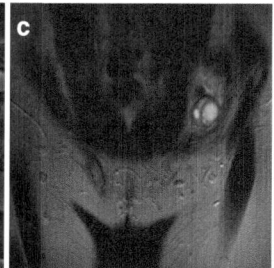

Fig. 38 Mayer-Rokitansky-Kuster-Hauser syndrome. (**a**) Sagittal T1-weighted image with a urethral catheter in place demonstrates the close proximity of the rectum and urethra. The vagina is absent. (**b**) Axial T2 with fat suppression again shows the close proximity of the urethral catheter and rectum. (**c**) Coronal T2-weighted image shows an ectopic left ovary within the left inguinal canal

urinary tract to identify renal agenesis, ectopic ureters, or ureteric stumps – as well as vice versa.

Mayer-Rokitansky-Kuster-Hauser syndrome is a heterogeneous disorder characterized by ureterovaginal atresia in 46 XX girls (Fig. 38) (see also Chap. 21). Abnormalities of the genital tract may range from upper vaginal atresia to total Mullerian agenesis with associated urinary tract anomalies. The external genitalia are normal (Kara et al. 2012; Yoo et al. 2013; Hall-Craggs et al. 2013b; Preibsch et al. 2014). Rudimentary uteri are seen in up to 93% of patients (Hall-Craggs et al. 2013b). Cyclical abdominal pain due to endometrial tissue or even hematometra in the rudimentary uterus may be a cause of clinical confusion. The ovaries are ectopic in 40% of cases and are readily identified on preoperative MR imaging (Hall-Craggs et al. 2013b; Preibsch et al. 2014). Herlyn-Werner-Wunderlich syndrome is characterized by uterus didelphia and unilateral hematocolpos related to an obstructed hemivagina with unilateral renal agenesis or sometimes a dysfunctional renal bud, a MCDK, or an ectopic cystic dysplastic kidney (Yavus et al. 2015). They are often diagnosed early in infancy but may present in adolescence with hematocolpos, hematometra, or hematosalpinx (Fig. 39). The diagnostic dilemma in these patients is that most

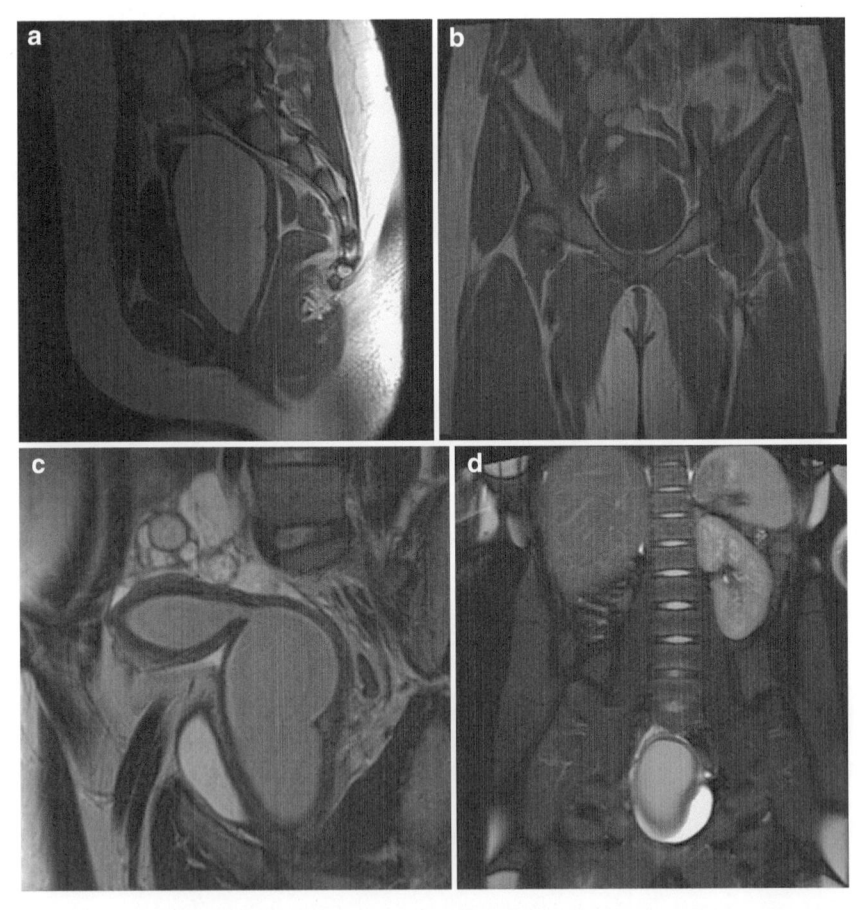

Fig. 39 Herlyn-Werner-Wunderlich syndrome. (**a**) Sagittal T1-weighted image showing a markedly dilated hemivagina with T1 shortening due to presence of blood products. (**b**) Coronal T1-weighted image show uterus didelphia with right-sided hematometra. (**c**) Oblique T2-weighted image demonstrates the communication of the right hematometra with the unilateral hematocolpos due to an obstructed hemivagina. (**d**) Coronal T2-weighted image shows congenital absence of the right kidney

have regular menstruation because one uterus is not obstructed. Therefore early sonographic search for the syndrome is indicated in newborn girls with MCDK or renal agenesis before the physiologically stimulated genital tract involutes.

> **Take Away**
> The diagnosis and classification of disorders of sexual differentiation are complex. The role of imaging in infants is to identify a uterus and/or cervix, to locate the gonads, and to define the anatomy of cloacal malformations, Mullerian duct anomalies, urinary tract anomalies as well as anorectal and spine malformations. Mullerian duct anomalies often present with primary amenorrhea in adolescents. MR is the imaging method of choice in defining these anomalies.

4.6 MR Imaging of Renal Tumors

Malignant renal tumors represent 6% of childhood cancer with 90% being Wilms' tumors (Swinson and McHugh 2011). MR is being used to evaluate pediatric renal tumors more often because the superior contrast resolution and advanced imaging techniques such as DWI and perfusion imaging add crucial information and avoid exposure to ionizing radiation. In one study over half the patients imaged with CT or MR, additional information in the local staging of Wilms' tumor was gained (McDonald et al. 2013). When evaluating renal masses, we use a slight variation of our standard MR imaging protocol. To minimize susceptibility artifacts from concentrated gadolinium in the collecting system, the patient is hydrated in the usual manner, but furosemide is not administered. A bladder catheter is not needed. The protocol is shorter with dynamic imaging used for the first 5 min to assess both the patency of the renal vein and characterize perfusion of the tumor mass and its microvascular environment (Smith 2013). Dynamic MR images can be used as a quantitative technique to assess tissue vascularity and membrane permeability (Fig. 40). The gadolinium-based contrast agents diffuse quickly into the extracellular space and then wash out slowly. Malignant tumors have disorganized vasculature that results in slow leakage of contrast agents into the extravascular space. The amount of leakage is determined by tissue perfusion, vessel wall permeability, and the rate of diffusion. This results in a gradual accumulation of contrast agent in the tumor.

The aim at initial imaging workup is to identify local extension, metastases, and involvement of the contralateral kidney (Brisse et al. 2008). MR can be used to characterize and delineate the primary tumor, as well as identify adenopathy, liver metastases, tumor thrombus, and signs of rupture. Wilms' tumor is the most common renal tumor in childhood, but others include nephrogenic rests and nephroblastomatosis, renal cell carcinoma, clear cell sarcoma, rhabdoid tumor, ossifying renal tumor of infancy, congenital mesoblastic nephroma, multilocular cystic renal tumor, and medullary cell carcinoma, angiomyolipoma, leukemia and lymphoma, and nephrogenic adenofibroma. MR is used for diagnosis and staging, but imaging cannot reliably distinguish between the renal masses.

The management of Wilms' tumors varies in Europe and North America. In Europe initial chemotherapy is followed by surgery. A biopsy is recommended if there are unusual imaging or clinical features. In North America, surgery is advocated before chemotherapy except when there are bilateral tumors, tumors in a solitary or horseshoe kidney, extension of tumor thrombus above the intrahepatic vena cava, or extensive metastatic disease (Kembhavi et al. 2013).

MR imaging can help distinguish Wilms' tumor from nephrogenic rests and nephroblastomatosis (Fig. 41). Wilms' tumor is typically heterogeneous because it contains a mixture of blood, tissue necrosis, fat, and cysts. The tumor enhances inhomogeneously (Smith 2013; Geller and Kochan 2011). Nephrogenic rests and nephroblastomatosis have decreased signal intensity on all sequences when compared to renal cortex. Nephrogenic rests are homogeneous, may be sclerotic, and often

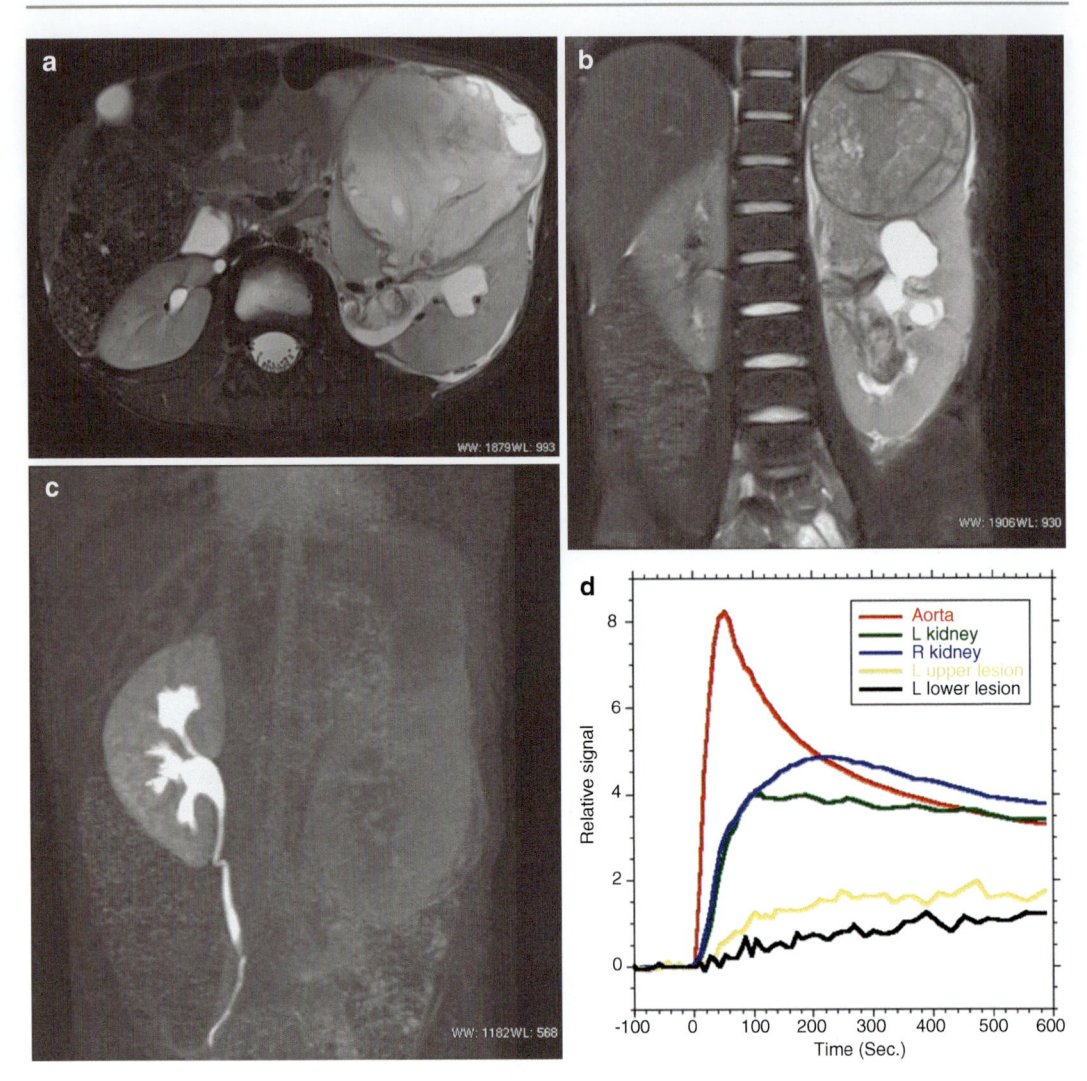

Fig. 40 Multicentric Wilms' tumor. (**a**) Axial T2-weighted image at the level of the renal pelvis showing a heterogeneous solid and cystic mass in the left kidney with invasion of the collecting systems. Perinephric fluid suggests rupture. (**b**) Coronal T2-weighted image showing second mass with well-defined capsule in the upper pole. Tumor related to the mid-pole mass is seen invading the renal pelvis and calyces with resultant UTD. (**c**) Delayed post-contrast T1-weighted image shows some parenchymal enhancement of the residual left-sided parenchyma without excretion. Relative decreased enhancement is seen in the upper pole mass. (**d**) Dynamic contrast-enhanced imaging can characterize enhancement patterns of the different regions. The right kidney curve is normal. The left kidney curve is flat, indicating that it is perfused but does not concentrate nor excrete. The two Wilms' tumors are poorly perfused but gradually accumulate contrast secondary to the disorganized vasculature of malignant tumors that results in slow leakage of contrast agents into the extravascular space

have a lenticular shape (Lonergan et al. 1998). A nephrogenic rest that grows and becomes rounder or more heterogeneous is suspicious for malignant degeneration. Nephroblastomatosis can be suspected on the basis of their typical distribution (perilobar, intralobar, or diffuse]. Nephroblastomatosis that is dark on T2-weighted images is usually sclerotic or regressing, whereas hyperplastic nephroblastomatosis can enlarge and is usually bright on T2-weighted images. The key feature of nephroblastomatosis at MR imaging is its

MR of the Urogenital Tract in Children

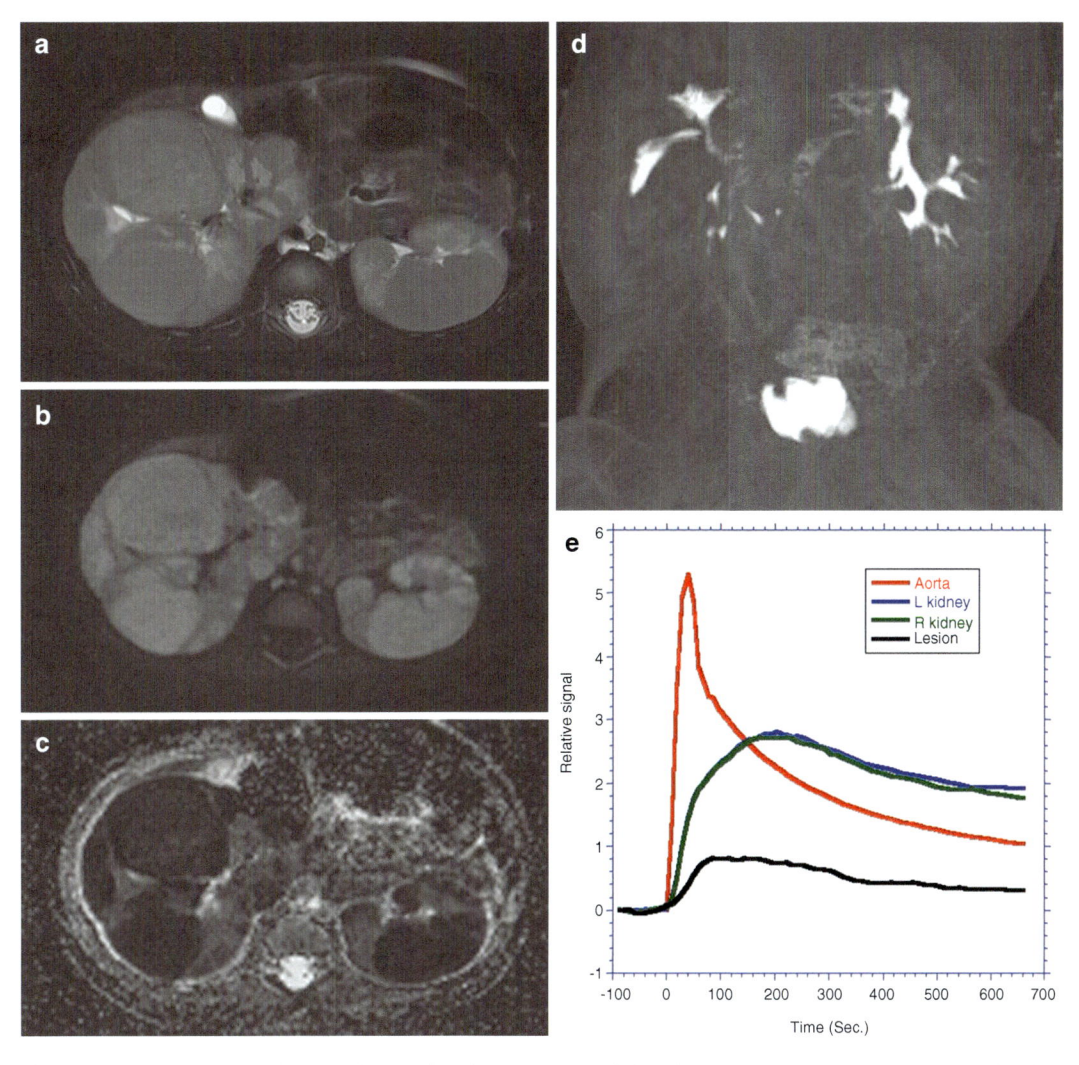

Fig. 41 Nephroblastomatosis. (**a**) Axial T2-weighted image showing multiple masses of varying size in both kidneys. Little normal renal parenchyma can be identified. The masses are homogeneous in signal characteristics and hypointense relative to normal parenchyma. (**b**) Trace DWI image demonstrating that the masses are homogeneous and distinct from normal renal parenchyma. (**c**) ADC map confirms that the masses restrict diffusion homogenously. (**d**) Delayed contrast-enhanced T1-weighted image shows that both kidneys function, but there is marked calyceal deformity caused by the multifocal masses. (**e**) The signal intensity versus time curves shows normal characteristics for both kidneys. The areas of nephroblastomatosis show decreased perfusion compared with normal renal parenchyma. However, there is normal washout from the nephroblastomatosis because the vasculature is intact helping to differentiate nephroblastomatosis from Wilms' tumor

homogeneity on all pulse sequences including diffusion imaging. Perfusion imaging also shows characteristic features with the contrast agent diffusing quickly into the extracellular space and then washing out slowly. This pattern reflects the intact vascular membrane which is disrupted in malignancies.

Take Away
MR is used for diagnosis and staging of renal tumors, but imaging cannot reliably distinguish between the renal masses.

4.7 MR Imaging in Renal Trauma

Blunt abdominal trauma is the main cause of renal trauma in children (Santucci et al. 2004; Buckley and McAninch 2006). Most renal trauma is minor and is managed conservatively with successful outcomes in greater than 98% (Buckley and McAninch 2004). Even high-grade lesions can be managed conservatively. The rate of healing and amount of scarring correlate with the initial grade of renal injury. Contusions and small lacerations heal quickly, whereas grade IV and V injuries result in variable amounts of renal loss (Abdalati et al. 1994). In children with grade IV or V injuries (shattered kidney or major vascular injury), renal salvage is possible in 78% (Eassa et al. 2010). However, complications are greater with higher-grade injuries with some patients showing significant loss of renal function (Keller et al. 2004; Eassa et al. 2010). Long-term complications include loss of renal function, renal scarring, and hypertension, with rare vascular complications such as pseudoaneurysms and arteriovenous fistula (Buckley et al. 2006; Eassa et al. 2010).

Imaging acutely after injury is typically with ultrasound or CT (Riccabona et al. 2011; Amerstorfer et al. 2015). MR urography has no role in the acute evaluation but is reserved for cases requiring problem-solving and to assess long-term outcomes. The purpose of repeat imaging is to identify patients with worsening urinary extravasation, ongoing significant hemorrhage, and rarer complications such as pseudoaneurysms (Santucci et al. 2004). Repeat imaging with contrast medium is recommended 36–48 h after initial scanning for grade IV and V injury to identify injuries to the collecting system and assess traumatic urinomas (Buckley and McAninch 2004). Imaging is also recommended when the patient has unexplained fever, flank pain, flank mass, or bleeding. Repeat CT scanning has been traditionally used in these circumstances, but MR urography is being used more often in the subacute phase. MR urography is excellent at depicting the severity of the renal injury, as well as perinephric hematoma. Because MR urography provides multiple phases, the perfusion as well as the excretion can be assessed (Fig. 42).

The specific MR imaging findings of hemorrhage depend on the age of the hemorrhage. The signal intensity changes over time due to degradation of the hematoma and subsequent changes in the magnetic properties of the hemoglobin molecule (Hammond et al. 2015). In the acute phase (less than 2 days), there is breakdown of hemoglobin to intracellular deoxyhemoglobin which produces hypointense signal on both T1- and T2-weighted images. In the early subacute phase (2–7 days), the paramagnetic effects of intracellular methemoglobin result in hyperintense T1 signal and hypointense T2 signal. In the late subacute phase (7–14 days), further breakdown results in extracellular methemoglobin causing hyperintensity on both T1- and T2-weighted images. A chronic hematoma demonstrates peripheral low T1 and T2 signal due to intracellular hemosiderin with central T2 hyperintensity and T1 isointensity (Hammond et al. 2015).

Long-term decrease in renal function is directly correlated with the grade of injury and independent of the mechanism of injury (Tasian et al. 2010). All grade IV or V renal injuries should have follow-up imaging at 1–3 months to document adequate healing and function (Keller et al. 2004; Buckley and McAninch 2004). Follow-up with MR urography can be used in place of repeat CT or DMSA scanning to demonstrate resolution of the renal and perinephric injury and to quantify the parenchymal scarring as well as assessment of differential renal function (Fig. 42). MR urography has been shown to be equivalent to DMSA scanning in the identification and quantification of renal scarring but has the additional advantage of dynamic assessment of the renal perfusion and the vascularity (Cerwinka et al. 2014).

> **Take Away**
> MR urography has no role in the acute evaluation of renal trauma but is reserved for cases requiring problem-solving and to assess long-term outcomes.

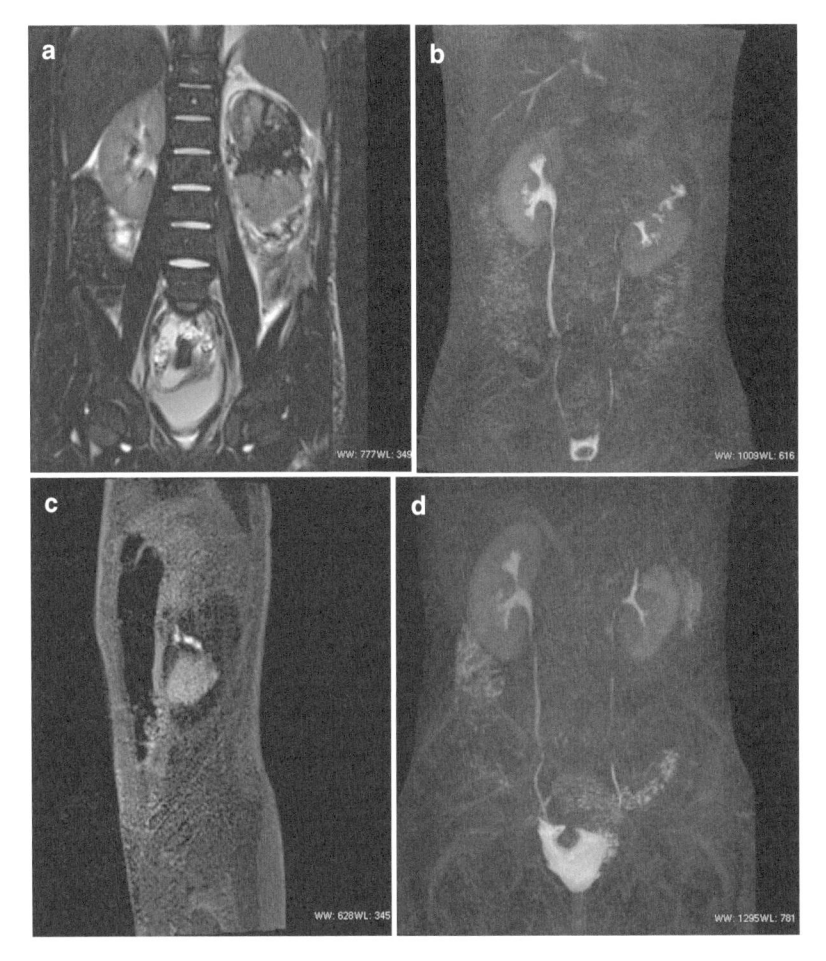

Fig. 42 Renal trauma. (**a**) Coronal T2-weighed image obtained 48 h after severe renal injury shows a fracture of the left kidney with acute blood products in the defect. Perinephric fluid has contrasting signal characteristics. (**b**) Delayed coronal contrast-enhanced T1-weighted MIP image showing absent perfusion of the left upper pole with apparent contrast extravasation above the visualized calyces. The left kidney represented 30% of total renal function. (**c**) Sagittal delayed contrast-enhanced T1-weighted image through the lateral aspect of the left kidney demonstrates the contrast extravasation extending above the residual functioning kidney. The upper pole is not perfused. (**d**) Follow-up scan 3 months after conservative treatment shows that the contrast extravasation has resolved. Only the residual left lower pole functions contributing 30% of total renal function

4.8 MR Imaging in Renal Transplantation

Kidney transplantation is the treatment of choice for children and adolescents with end-stage renal disease (Peruzzi 2014; Patel 2014; Van Arendonk et al. 2014) (see also Chap. 34). Kidney transplant dysfunction is often nonspecific presenting with rising serum creatinine, with decreasing urine output, or with pain and tenderness over the graft (Sharfuddin 2014). Vascular complications are a common cause for morbidity and mortality and include transplant renal artery stenosis (TRAS), AV fistulas, pseudoaneurysms as well as arterial or venous thrombosis. Nonvascular complications include urologic complications such as ureteral obstruction and urinary leak, pyelonephritis, and perigraft fluid collections including hematoma, abscess, urinoma, and lymphocele. Intrinsic conditions leading to renal parenchymal injury, such as acute rejection, acute tubular necrosis (ATN), and drug toxicity, are more difficult to diagnose because the clinical symptoms, laboratory data, and image findings of these diseases often overlap. Therapeutic strategies are radically different depending on the etiology of the graft dysfunction. Percutaneous renal transplant biopsy is used to distinguish between causes of acute graft dysfunction but can be complicated by bleeding, infection, and, rarely, graft loss.

A noninvasive and accurate assessment of transplant renal function is critical to guide postoperative management. Ultrasound is the primary imaging modality used to identify complications associated with renal transplantation but provides no assessment of renal function (Sharfuddin 2011; Nixon et al. 2013; Riccabona et al. 2012; Sharfuddin 2014). MR urography demonstrates structural abnormalities including urinary tract obstruction and urologic complications as well as functional data related to GFR and renal blood flow (Sharfuddin 2014; Wang 2015). Dynamic CE-MR imaging provides information about renal perfusion, function, and ureteric drainage. The combination of T2-weighted images with contrast-enhanced images allows characterization of perinephric fluid collections as well as differentiating global from segmental disease. MR angiography defines the vascular anatomy of the renal transplant identifying vascular complications. Advanced MR urography techniques can define new parameters (Eisenberger et al. 2009; Thoeny and De Keyzer 2011; Liu et al. 2014). DWI imaging provides information about renal perfusion and diffusion simultaneously. BOLD imaging evaluates intrarenal oxygen bioavailability by measuring the concentration of deoxyhemoglobin. These advanced imaging techniques explore different tissue properties and provide complimentary information that can be used to monitor graft function during therapy and show promise in the evaluation of intrinsic causes of graft dysfunction.

Multicompartment kinetic modeling analyzes dynamic contrast-enhanced images and distinguishes parameters derived from the vascular and tubular compartments of the kidney (Martin et al. 2008; Bokacheva et al. 2009; Sourbron 2010; Yamamoto et al. 2011). These techniques use the tracer transit through the kidneys to quantify physiologic parameters such as GFR and calculate the mean transit time. The GFR and the mean transit time are significantly lower in patients with acute renal dysfunction when compared to normally functioning transplants, and these parameters may be able to discriminate between acute rejection and acute tubular necrosis (Yamamoto et al. 2011). Diffusion-weighted imaging is able to detect pyelonephritis (Fig. 43).

Transplant renal artery stenosis (TRAS) usually presents in the first 3 months to 2 years after transplantation (Bruno 2004). Catheter angiography is considered the gold standard for the diagnosis of TRAS, but because of associated complications, it is used only when there is high suspicion for significant TRAS demonstrated on nonvascular imaging (Gaddikeri et al. 2014). CE-MR angiography is similar to

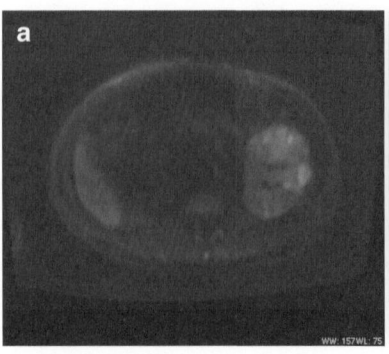

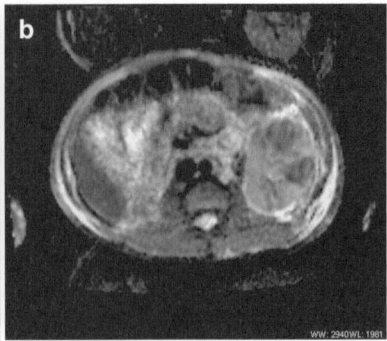

Fig. 43 Pyelonephritis in transplanted kidney. (**a**, **b**) Trace diffusion-weighted image and ADC map of failing transplanted kidney demonstrates multifocal areas of restricted diffusion typical for pyelonephritis. Non-contrast MR imaging can identify complications associated with renal transplantation

CT angiography for the assessment of hemodynamically significant TRAS (Gaddikeri et al. 2014). CE-MRA can accurately depict arterial anatomy, detect and grade renal artery stenosis, and identify renal vein thrombosis as well as pseudoaneurysms. CE-MR angiography is preferred to CTA due to the lack of ionizing radiation and nephrotoxic iodinated contrast agent. However, susceptibility artifacts owing to surgical clips at the anastomosis may limit diagnostic ability of MRA.

> **Take Away**
> MR urography shows promise as a noninvasive and comprehensive method to asses transplant renal function as well as associated complications that are critical to guide postoperative management.

Conclusion

MR urography is a comprehensive evaluation of the urinary tract in children, providing an unprecedented level of anatomic information combined with quantitative functional evaluation of each kidney individually. MR urography provides clinically useful assessment of obstructive uropathy and provides predictive information about which children will benefit from surgery. MR urography will improve our ability to categorize renal malformations in vivo and contribute significantly to our understanding of renal dysplasia. With the addition of DWI, MR urography is the imaging modality of choice in the evaluation of pyelonephritis and renal scarring. There is an ever-increasing role for MR urography in the evaluation of urinary tract disorders including renal tumors, disorders of sexual differentiation, renal trauma, and renal transplantation.

References

Aaronson IA (1980) Compensated obstruction of the renal pelvis. Br J Urol 52:79–83

Abdalati H, Bulas DI, Sivit CJ et al (1994) Blunt renal trauma in children: healing of renal injuries and recommendations for imaging follow-up. Pediatr Radiol 24:573–576

Abou-El-Ghar ME, El-Diasty TA, El-Assmy AM et al (2012) Role of diffusion-weighted MRI in diagnosis of acute renal allograft dysfunction: a prospective preliminary study. Br J Radiol 85:e206–e211. doi:10.1259/bjr/53260155

Acharya SK, Jindal B, Yadav DK et al (2009) Retrocaval ureter: a rare cause of hydronephrosis in children. J Pediatr Surg 44:846–848. doi:10.1016/j.jpedsurg.2008.11.053

Adeb M, Darge K, Dillman JR et al (2013) Magnetic resonance urography in evaluation of duplicated renal collecting systems. Magn Reson Imaging Clin NA 21:717–730. doi:10.1016/j.mric.2013.04.002

Albert TSE, Akahane M, Parienty I et al (2015) An international multicenter comparison of time-SLIP unenhanced MR angiography and contrast-enhanced CT angiography for assessing renal artery stenosis: the renal artery contrast-free trial. Am J Roentgenol 204:182–188. doi:10.2214/AJR.13.12022

Altun E, Martin DR, Wertman R et al (2009) Nephrogenic systemic fibrosis: change in incidence following a switch in gadolinium agents and adoption of a gadolinium policy—report from Two U.S. Universities 1. Radiology 253:689–696. doi:10.1148/radiol.2533090649

Amarante J, Anderson PJ, Gordon I (2003) Impaired drainage on diuretic renography using half-time or pelvic excretion efficiency is not a sign of obstruction in children with a prenatal diagnosis of unilateral renal pelvic dilatation. J Urol 169:1828–1831. doi:10.1097/01.ju.0000062640.46274.21

Amerstorfer EE, Haberlik A, Riccabona M (2015) Imaging assessment of renal injuries in children and adolescents: CT or ultrasound? J Pediatr Surg 50:448–455. doi:10.1016/j.jpedsurg.2014.07.006

Anigstein R, Elkin M, Roland P, Schulz RJ (1972) The obstructive nephrogram--microradiographic studies. Invest Radiol 7:24–32

Annet L, Hermoye L, Peeters F et al (2004) Glomerular filtration rate: assessment with dynamic contrast-enhanced MRI and a cortical-compartment model in the rabbit kidney. J Magn Reson Imaging 20:843–849. doi:10.1002/jmri.20173

Arena S, Magno C, Montalto AS et al (2012) Long-term follow-up of neonatally diagnosed primary megaureter: rate and predictors of spontaneous resolution. Scand J Urol Nephrol 46:201–207. doi:10.3109/00365599.2012.662695

Arlen AM, Kirsch AJ, Cuda SP et al (2014) Magnetic resonance urography for diagnosis of pediatric ureteral stricture. J Pediatr Urol 10:1–7. doi:10.1016/j.jpurol.2014.01.004

Arthurs OJ, Edwards AD, Joubert I et al (2013) Interactive magnetic resonance imaging for paediatric vesicoureteric reflux (VUR). Eur J Radiol 82:e112–e119. doi:10.1016/j.ejrad.2012.10.024

Artunc F, Yildiz S, Rossi C et al (2010) Simultaneous evaluation of renal morphology and function in live kidney donors using dynamic magnetic resonance imaging. Nephrol Dial Transplant 25:1986–1991. doi:10.1093/ndt/gfp772

Avni FE, Nicaise N, Hall M et al (2001) The role of MR imaging for the assessment of complicated duplex kidneys in children: preliminary report. Pediatr Radiol 31:215–223

Bakker J, Olree M, Kaatee R et al (1999) Renal volume measurements: accuracy and repeatability of US compared with that of MR imaging. Radiology 211:623–628. doi:10.1148/radiology.211.3.r99jn19623

Barker AP, Soundappan SVS (2004) Retrocaval ureter in children: a report of two cases. Ped Surg Int 20:158–160. doi:10.1007/s00383-003-1038-x

Baughman SM, Richardson RR, Podberesky DJ et al (2007) 3-Dimensional magnetic resonance genitography: a different look at cloacal malformations. J Urol 178:1675–1678. doi:10.1016/j.juro.2007.03.196; discussion 1678–1679

Becker A, Baum M (2006) Obstructive uropathy. Early Hum Dev 82:15–22. doi:10.1016/j.earlhumdev.2005.11.002

Behr SC, Courtier JL, Qayyum A (2012) Imaging of Müllerian duct anomalies. RadioGraphics 32:E233–E250. doi:10.1148/rg.326125515

Berrocal T, López-Pereira P, Arjonilla A, Gutiérrez J (2002) Anomalies of the distal ureter, bladder, and urethra in children: embryologic, radiologic, and pathologic features. RadioGraphics 22:1139–1164

Bhat GS, Maregowda S, Jayaram S, Siddappa S (2012) Health outcomes research. Urology 79:321–325. doi:10.1016/j.urology.2011.10.018

Blake J, Rosenblum ND (2014) Renal branching morphogenesis: morphogenetic and signaling mechanisms. Semin Cell Develop Biol 36:2–12. doi:10.1016/j.semcdb.2014.07.011

Bohnenpoll T, Kispert A (2014) Ureter growth and differentiation. Semin Cell Develop Biol 36:21–30. doi:10.1016/j.semcdb.2014.07.014

Bokacheva L, Rusinek H, Zhang JL, Lee VS (2008) Assessment of renal function with dynamic contrast-enhanced MR imaging. Magn Reson Imaging Clin N Am 16:597–611. doi:10.1016/j.mric.2008.07.001

Bokacheva L, Rusinek H, Zhang JL et al (2009) Estimates of glomerular filtration rate from MR renography and tracer kinetic models. J Magn Reson Imaging 29:371–382. doi:10.1002/jmri.21642

Bonsib SM (2010) The classification of renal cystic diseases and other congenital malformations of the kidney and urinary tract. Arch Pathol Lab Med 134:554–568

Boss A, Martirosian P, Fuchs J et al (2014) Dynamic MR urography in children with uropathic disease with a combined 2D and 3D acquisition protocol—comparison with MAG3 scintigraphy. Br J Radiol 87:20140426. doi:10.1259/bjr.20140426

Brenes LG, Forlano H, Koutouratsas N, Stauffer HM (1966) Mechanism of the nephrographic effect during urinary stasis. Acta Radiol Diagn (Stockh) 4:14–20

Brisse HJ, Smets AM, Kaste SC, Owens CM (2008) Imaging in unilateral Wilms tumour. Pediatr Radiol 38:18–29. doi:10.1007/s00247-007-0677-9

Brown SC, Upsdell SM, O'Reilly PH (1992) The importance of renal function in the interpretation of diuresis renography. Br J Urol 69:121–125

Bruno S (2004) Transplant renal artery stenosis. J Am Soc Nephrol 15:134–141. doi:10.1097/01.ASN.0000099379.61001.F8

Buckley JC, McAninch JW (2004) Pediatric renal injuries: management guidelines from a 25-year experience. JURO 172:687–690. doi:10.1097/01.ju.0000129316.42953.76

Buckley JC, McAninch JW (2006) The diagnosis, management, and outcomes of pediatric renal injuries. Urol Clin NA 33:33–vi. doi:10.1016/j.ucl.2005.11.001

Buckley DL, Shurrab AE, Cheung CM et al (2006) Measurement of single kidney function using dynamic contrast-enhanced MRI: comparison of two models in human subjects. J Magn Reson Imaging 24:1117–1123. doi:10.1002/jmri.20699

Cain JEJ, Di Giovanni VV, Smeeton JJ, Rosenblum NDN (2010) Genetics of renal hypoplasia: insights into the mechanisms controlling nephron endowment. Pediatr Res 68:91–98. doi:10.1203/PDR.0b013e3181e35a88

Castagnetti M, Novara G, Beniamin F et al (2008) Scintigraphic renal function after unilateral pyeloplasty in children: a systematic review. BJU Int 102:862–868. doi:10.1111/j.1464-410X.2008.07597.x

Cerwinka WH, Grattan-Smith JD, Jones RA et al (2014) Comparison of magnetic resonance urography to dimercaptosuccinic acid scan for the identification of renal parenchyma defects in children with vesicoureteral reflux. J Pediatr Urol 10:344–351. doi:10.1016/j.jpurol.2013.09.016

Chertin B, Pollack A, Koulikov D et al (2006) Conservative treatment of ureteropelvic junction obstruction in children with antenatal diagnosis of hydronephrosis: lessons learned after 16 years of follow-up. Eur Urol 49:734–739. doi:10.1016/j.eururo.2006.01.046

Chevalier RL (2007) Chronic partial ureteral obstruction and the developing kidney. Pediatr Radiol 38:35–40. doi:10.1007/s00247-007-0585-z

Chevalier RL (2009) When is one kidney not enough? Kidney Int 76:475–477. doi:10.1038/ki.2009.244

Chevalier RL, Thornhill BA, Forbes MS, Kiley SC (2010) Mechanisms of renal injury and progression of renal disease in congenital obstructive nephropathy. Pediatr Nephrol 25:687–697. doi:10.1007/s00467-009-1316-5

Chuck NC, Steidle G, Blume I et al (2013) Diffusion tensor imaging of the kidneys: influence of b-value and number of encoding directions on image quality and diffusion tensor parameters. Clin Imaging Sci 2013(3):53

Chung CHS, Chin ACW, Szeto PS et al. (2008). Magnetic resonance imaging for ureteral fibroepithelial polyp. Hong King Med J 2008;14:408–10

Claudon M, Durand E, Grenier N et al (2014) Chronic urinary obstruction: evaluation of dynamic contrast-enhanced MR urography for measurement of split renal function. Radiology 273:801–812. doi:10.1148/radiol.14131819

Csaicsich D, Greenbaum LA, Aufricht C (2004) Upper urinary tract: when is obstruction obstruction? Curr Opin Urol 14:213–217. doi:10.1097/01.mou.0000135075.19968.d9

Dally EA, Raman A, Webb NR, Farnsworth RH (2011) Unilateral multicystic dysplastic kidney with progressive infundibular stenosis in the contralateral kidney: experience at 1 center and review of literature. JURO 186:1053–1058. doi:10.1016/j.juro.2011.05.001

Darge K, Grattan-Smith JD, Riccabona M (2010) Pediatric uroradiology: state of the art. Pediatr Radiol 41:82–91. doi:10.1007/s00247-010-1644-4

Davies P (1988) Obstructive uropathy. BMJ 297:68–68

Davies P, Price H (1980) The urographic signs of acute on chronic obstruction of the kidney. Clin Radiol 31:205–213. doi:10.1016/S0009-9260(80)80163-2

Dawson P (1990) Intravenous urography revisited. Br J Urol 66:561–567

De Pascale A, Piccoli GB, Priola SM et al (2013) Diffusion-weighted magnetic resonance imaging: new perspectives in the diagnostic pathway of non-complicated acute pyelonephritis. Eur Radiol 23:3077–3086. doi:10.1007/s00330-013-2906-y

Duong HP, Piepsz A, Collier F et al (2013) Pediatric urology predicting the clinical outcome of antenatally detected unilateral pelviureteric junction stenosis. URL 82:691–696. doi:10.1016/j.urology.2013.03.041

Durand E (2014) Comparison of magnetic resonance imaging with radionuclide methods of evaluating the kidney. Semin Nucl Med 44:82–92. doi:10.1053/j.semnuclmed.2013.10.003

Dyer RB, Munitz HA, Bechtold R, Choplin RH (1986) The abnormal nephrogram. RadioGraphics 6:1039–1063

Eassa W, El-Ghar MA, Jednak R, El-Sherbiny M (2010) Nonoperative management of grade 5 renal injury in children: does it have a place? Eur Urol 57:154–163. doi:10.1016/j.eururo.2009.02.001

Ehammer T, Riccabona M, Maier E (2011) High resolution MR for evaluation of lower urogenital tract malformations in infants and children: feasibility and preliminary experiences. Eur J Radiol 78:388–393. doi:10.1016/j.ejrad.2010.01.006

Eisenberger U, Thoeny HC, Binser T et al (2009) Evaluation of renal allograft function early after transplantation with diffusion-weighted MR imaging. Eur Radiol 20:1374–1383. doi:10.1007/s00330-009-1679-9

Elder JS, Stansbrey R, Dahms BB, Selzman AA (1995) Renal histological changes secondary to ureteropelvic junction obstruction. J Urol 154:719–722

Erbay G, Koc Z, Karadeli E et al (2012) Evaluation of malignant and benign renal lesions using diffusion-weighted MRI with multiple b values. Acta Radiol 53:359–365

Esfahani SA, Kajbafzadeh A-M, Beigi RS et al (2011) Precise delineation of ureterocele anatomy: virtual magnetic resonance cystoscopy. Abdom Imaging 36:765–770. doi:10.1007/s00261-011-9695-z

Eskildjensen A, Gordon I, Piepsz A, Frokiar J (2005) Congenital unilateral hydronephrosis: a review of the impact of diuretic renography on clinical treatment. J Urol 173:1471–1476. doi:10.1097/01.ju.0000157384.32215.fe

Faletti R, Cassinis MC, Fonio P et al (2013) Diffusion–weighted imaging and apparent diffusion coefficient values versus contrast–enhanced mr imaging in the identification and characterisation of acute pyelonephritis. Eur Radiol 23:3501–3508. doi:10.1007/s00330-013-2951-6

Farrugia M-K, Hitchcock R, Radford A et al (2014) British Association of Paediatric Urologists consensus statement on the management of the primary obstructive megaureter. J Pediatr Urol 10:26–33. doi:10.1016/j.jpurol.2013.09.018

Figueroa VH, Chavhan GB, Oudjhane K, FARHAT W (2014) Utility of MR urography in children suspected of having ectopic ureter. Pediatr Radiol 44:956–962. doi:10.1007/s00247-014-2905-4

Gaddikeri S, Mitsumori L, Vaidya S et al (2014) Comparing the diagnostic accuracy of contrast-enhanced computed tomographic angiography and gadolinium-enhanced magnetic resonance angiography for the assessment of hemodynamically significant transplant renal artery stenosis. Curr Probl Diagn Radiol 43:162–168. doi:10.1067/j.cpradiol.2014.03.001

Gardener AG, Francis ST (2010) Multislice perfusion of the kidneys using parallel imaging: image acquisition and analysis strategies. Magn Reson Med 63:1627–1636. doi:10.1002/mrm.22387

Gee MS, Bittman M, Epelman M et al (2013) Magnetic resonance imaging of the pediatric kidney. Magn Reson Imaging Clin NA 21:697–715. doi:10.1016/j.mric.2013.06.001

Geller E, Kochan PS (2011) Renal neoplasms of childhood. Radiol Clin NA 49:689–709. doi:10.1016/j.rcl.2011.05.003

Gimpel C, Masioniene L, Djakovic N et al (2010) Complications and long-term outcome of primary obstructive megaureter in childhood. Pediatr Nephrol 25:1679–1686. doi:10.1007/s00467-010-1523-0

Glassberg KI (2002) Normal and abnormal development of the kidney: a clinician's interpretation of current knowledge. JURO 167:2339–2331

González PAL, Cubillana PL, Pastor GS et al (2011) Retrocaval ureter in children. Case report and bibliographic review. Arch Esp Urol 64:461–464

Gordon I (2001) Diuretic renography in infants with prenatal unilateral hydronephrosis: an explanation for the controversy about poor drainage. BJU Int 87:551–555. doi:10.1046/j.1464-410X.2001.00081.x

Grattan-Smith JD, Jones RA (2008) MR urography: technique and results for the evaluation of urinary obstruction in the pediatric population. Magn Reson Imaging

Clin N Am 16:643–660, viii–ix. doi:10.1016/j.mric.2008.07.003

Grattan-Smith JD, Perez-Bayfield MR, Jones RA et al (2003) MR imaging of kidneys: functional evaluation using F-15 perfusion imaging. Pediatr Radiol 33:293–304. doi:10.1007/s00247-003-0896-7

Grattan-Smith JD, Little SB, Jones RA (2007) Evaluation of reflux nephropathy, pyelonephritis and renal dysplasia. Pediatr Radiol 38:83–105. doi:10.1007/s00247-007-0668-x

Grattan-Smith JD, Jones RA, Little S, Kirsch AJ (2010) Bilateral congenital midureteric strictures associated with multicystic dysplastic kidney and hydronephrosis: evaluation with MR urography. Pediatr Radiol 41:117–120. doi:10.1007/s00247-010-1799-z

Greenbaum LA (2007) Renal dysplasia and MRI: a clinician's perspective. Pediatr Radiol 38:70–75. doi:10.1007/s00247-007-0586-y

Grinspon RP, Rey RA (2014) When hormone defects cannot explain it: malformative disorders of sex development. Birth Defect Res C 102:359–373. doi:10.1002/bdrc.21086

Grobner T (2006) Gadolinium--a specific trigger for the development of nephrogenic fibrosing dermopathy and nephrogenic systemic fibrosis? Nephrol Dial Transplant 21:1104–1108. doi:10.1093/ndt/gfk062

Hackstein N, Heckrodt J, Rau WS (2003) Measurement of single-kidney glomerular filtration rate using a contrast-enhanced dynamic gradient-echo sequence and the Rutland-Patlak plot technique. J Magn Reson Imaging 18:714–725. doi:10.1002/jmri.10410

Hackstein N, Kooijman H, Tomaselli S, Rau WS (2005) Glomerular filtration rate measured using the Patlak plot technique and contrast-enhanced dynamic MRI with different amounts of gadolinium-DTPA. J Magn Reson Imaging 22:406–414. doi:10.1002/jmri.20401

Hall-Craggs MA, Kirkham A, Creighton SM (2013a) Renal and urological abnormalities occurring with Mullerian anomalies. J Pediatr Urol 9:27–32. doi:10.1016/j.jpurol.2011.11.003

Hall-Craggs MA, Williams CE, Pattison SH et al (2013b) Mayer-Rokitansky-Kuster-Hauser syndrome: diagnosis with MR imaging. Radiology 269:787–792. doi:10.1148/radiol.13130211

Hammond NA, Lostumbo A, Adam SZ et al (2015) Imaging of adrenal and renal hemorrhage. Abdom Imaging 40:1–14. doi:10.1007/s00261-015-0453-5

Harper L, Bourquard D, Grosos C et al (2013) Cortical transit time as a predictive marker of the need for surgery in children with pelvi-ureteric junction stenosis: preliminary study. J Pediatr Urol 9:1054–1058. doi:10.1016/j.jpurol.2013.03.002

Harraz AM, Helmy T, Taha D-E et al (2013) Changes in differential renal function after pyeloplasty in children. J Urol 190:1468–1473. doi:10.1016/j.juro.2013.01.004

Hashim H, Woodhouse CRJ (2012) Ureteropelvic junction obstruction. Eur Urol Suppl 11:25–32. doi:10.1016/j.eursup.2012.01.004

Hekmatnia A, Merrikhi A, Farghadani M et al (2013) Diagnostic accuracy of magnetic resonance voiding cystourethrography for detecting vesico-ureteral reflux in children and adolescents. J Res Med Sci 18:31–36

Heuer R, Sommer G, Shortliffe LD (2003) Evaluation of renal growth by magnetic resonance imaging and computerized tomography volumes. J Urol 170:1659–1663. doi:10.1097/01.ju.0000085676.76111.27

Hodges SJ, Werle D, McLorie G, Atala A (2010) Megaureter. Scientific World J 10:603–612. doi:10.1100/tsw.2010.54

Huang AJ, Lee VS, Rusinek H (2004) Functional renal MR imaging. Magn Reson Imaging Clin N Am 12:469–486. doi:10.1016/j.mric.2004.04.001

Huang W-Y, Peters CA, Zurakowski D et al (2006) Renal biopsy in congenital ureteropelvic junction obstruction: evidence for parenchymal maldevelopment. Kidney Int 69:137–143. doi:10.1038/sj.ki.5000004

Hughes IA (2002) Intersex. BJU Int 90:769–776. doi:10.1046/j.1464-410X.2002.02920.x

Hwang AH, McAleer IM, Shapiro E et al (2005) Congenital mid ureteral strictures. J Urol 174:1999–2002. doi:10.1097/01.ju.0000176462.56473.0c

Ichikawa S, Motosugi U, Ichikawa T et al (2013) Intravoxel incoherent motion imaging of the kidney: alterations in diffusion and perfusion in patients with renal dysfunction. Magn Reson Imaging 31:414–417. doi:10.1016/j.mri.2012.08.004

Ismaili K, Piepsz A (2013) The antenatally detected pelvi-ureteric junction stenosis: advances in renography and strategy of management. Pediatr Radiol 43:428–435. doi:10.1007/s00247-012-2505-0

Itoh K (2001) 99mTc-MAG3: review of pharmacokinetics, clinical application to renal diseases and quantification of renal function. Ann Nucl Med 15:179–190. doi:10.1007/BF02987829

Jaramillo D, Lebowitz RL, Hendren WH (1990) The cloacal malformation: radiologic findings and imaging recommendations. Radiology 177:441–448. doi:10.1148/radiology.177.2.2217782

Jarboe MD, Teitelbaum DH, Dillman JR (2012) Combined 3D rotational fluoroscopic-MRI cloacagram procedure defines luminal and extraluminal pelvic anatomy prior to surgical reconstruction of cloacal and other complex pelvic malformations. Ped Surg Int 28:757–763. doi:10.1007/s00383-012-3122-6

Johnin K, Takazakura R, Furukawa A et al (2013) Magnetic resonance voiding cystourethrography (MRVCUG): a potential alternative to standard VCUG. J Magn Reson Imaging 38:897–904. doi:10.1002/jmri.24052

Jones RA, PEREZ-BRAYFIELD MR, Kirsch AJ, Grattan-Smith JD (2004) Renal transit time with MR urography in children1. Radiology 233:41–50. doi:10.1148/radiol.2331031117

Jones RA, Easley K, Little SB et al (2005) Dynamic contrast-enhanced MR urography in the evaluation of pediatric hydronephrosis: part 1, functional assessment. Am J Roentgenol 185:1598–1607. doi:10.2214/AJR.04.1540

Jones RA, Grattan-Smith JD, Little S (2011) Pediatric magnetic resonance urography. J Magn Reson Imaging 33:510–526. doi:10.1002/jmri.22474

Junqueira BLP, Allen LM, Spitzer RF et al (2009) Müllerian duct anomalies and mimics in children and adolescents: correlative intraoperative assessment with clinical imaging1. RadioGraphics 29:1085–1103. doi:10.1148/rg.294085737

Kalisvaart J, Bootwala Y, Poonawala H et al (2011) Comparison of ultrasound and magnetic resonance urography for evaluation of contralateral kidney in patients with multicystic dysplastic kidney disease. JURO 186:1059–1064. doi:10.1016/j.juro.2011.04.105

Kanda T, Ishii K, Kawaguchi H et al (2014) High signal intensity in the dentate nucleus and globus pallidus on unenhanced T1-weighted MR images: relationship with increasing cumulative dose of a gadolinium-based contrast material. Radiology 270:834–841. doi:10.1148/radiol.13131669

Kanda T, Fukusato T, Matsuda M et al (2015a) Gadolinium-based contrast agent accumulates in the brain even in subjects without severe renal dysfunction: evaluation of autopsy brain specimens with inductively coupled plasma mass spectroscopy. Radiology 276:228–232. doi:10.1148/radiol.2015142690

Kanda T, Osawa M, Oba H et al (2015b) High signal intensity in dentate nucleus on unenhanced T1-weighted mr images: association with linear versus macrocyclic gadolinium chelate administration. Radiology 275:803–809. doi:10.1148/radiol.14140364

Kaneyama K, Yamataka A, Someya T et al (2006) Magnetic resonance urographic parameters for predicting the need for pyeloplasty in infants with prenatally diagnosed severe hydronephrosis. J Urol 176:1781–1785. doi:10.1016/j.juro.2006.03.122

Kara T, Acu B, Beyhan M, Gokce E (2012) Magnetic resonance imaging in diagnosis of the mayer-rokitansky-kuster-hauser syndrome. Diagn Interv Radiol. doi:10.4261/1305-3825.DIR.6341-12.1

Kavanagh EC, Ryan S, Awan A et al (2005) Can MRI replace DMSA in the detection of renal parenchymal defects in children with urinary tract infections? Pediatr Radiol 35:275–281. doi:10.1007/s00247-004-1335-0

Keller MS, Eric Coln C, Garza JJ et al (2004) Functional outcome of nonoperatively managed renal injuries in children. J Trauma Injury Infect Crit Care 57:108–110. doi:10.1097/01.TA.0000133627.75366.CA

Kembhavi SA, Qureshi S, Vora T et al (2013) Understanding the principles in management of Wilms. Clin Radiol 68:646–653. doi:10.1016/j.crad.2012.11.012

Khrichenko D, Darge K (2009) Functional analysis in MR urography – made simple. Pediatr Radiol. doi:10.1007/s00247-009-1458-4

King LR (1980) Megaloureter: definition, diagnosis and management. JURO 123:222–223

Kirsch AJ, McMann LP, Jones RA et al (2006) Magnetic resonance urography for evaluating outcomes after pediatric pyeloplasty. J Urol 176:1755–1761. doi:10.1016/j.juro.2006.03.115

Klein J, Gonzalez J, Miravete M et al (2010) Congenital ureteropelvic junction obstruction: human disease and animal models. Int J Exp Pathol 92:168–192. doi:10.1111/j.1365-2613.2010.00727.x

Koff SA (2007) Requirements for accurately diagnosing chronic partial upper urinary tract obstruction in children with hydronephrosis. Pediatr Radiol 38:41–48. doi:10.1007/s00247-007-0590-2

Korobkin M (1972) Physiology and significance of the prolonged nephrogram. Calif Med 117:55–56

Krepkin K, Won E, Ramaswamy K et al (2014) Dynamic contrast-enhanced MR renography for renal function evaluation in ureteropelvic junction obstruction: feasibility study. Am J Roentgenol 202:778–783. doi:10.2214/AJR.13.11321

Lankadeva YR, Singh RR, Tare M et al (2014) Loss of a kidney during fetal life: long-term consequences and lessons learned. AJP: Renal Physiol 306:F791–F800. doi:10.1152/ajprenal.00666.2013

Le Bihan D (2013) Apparent diffusion coefficient and beyond: what diffusion MR imaging can tell us about tissue structure. Radiology 268:318–322. doi:10.1148/radiol.13130420

Le Bihan D, Breton E, Lallemand D et al (1986) MR imaging of intravoxel incoherent motions: application to diffusion and perfusion in neurologic disorders. Radiology 161:401–407. doi:10.1148/radiology.161.2.3763909

Lee VS, Rusinek H, Noz ME et al (2003) Dynamic three-dimensional mr renography for the measurement of single kidney function: initial experience1. Radiology 227:289–294. doi:10.1148/radiol.2271020383

Little SB, Jones RA, Grattan-Smith JD (2007) Evaluation of UPJ obstruction before and after pyeloplasty using MR urography. Pediatr Radiol 38:106–124. doi:10.1007/s00247-007-0669-9

Liu G, Han F, Xiao W et al (2014) Detection of renal allograft rejection using blood oxygen level-dependent and diffusion weighted magnetic resonance imaging: a retrospective study. BMC Nephrol 15:158. doi:10.1007/s11547-008-0248-7

Lonergan GJ, Martínez-León MI, Agrons GA et al (1998) Nephrogenic rests, nephroblastomatosis, and associated lesions of the kidney. RadioGraphics 18: 947–968

Lucaya J, Enriquez G, Delgado R, Castellote A (1984) Infundibulopelvic stenosis in children. AJR Am J Roentgenol 142:471–474. doi:10.2214/ajr.142.3.471

Mackie GG, Stephens FD (1975) Duplex kidneys: a correlation of renal dysplasia with position of the ureteral orifice. JURO 114:274–280

Mansour SM, Hamed ST, Adel L et al (2012) Does MRI add to ultrasound in the assessment of disorders of sex development? Eur J Radiol 81:2403–2410. doi:10.1016/j.ejrad.2011.12.036

Marcal L, Nothaft MA, Coelho F et al (2011) Mullerian duct anomalies: MR imaging. Abdom Imaging 36:756–764. doi:10.1007/s00261-010-9681-x

Marckmann P (2006) Nephrogenic systemic fibrosis: suspected causative role of gadodiamide used for contrast-enhanced magnetic resonance imaging. J Am Soc Nephrol 17:2359–2362. doi:10.1681/ASN.2006060601

Martin DR, Sharma P, Salman K et al (2008) Individual kidney blood flow measured with contrast-enhanced first-pass perfusion MR imaging. Radiology 246:241–248. doi:10.1148/radiol.2461062129

Martina MC, Campanino PP, Caraffo F et al (2010) Dynamic magnetic resonance imaging in acute pyelonephritis. Radiol Med 115:287–300. doi:10.1007/s11547-009-0468-5

Martirosian P, Klose U, Mader I, Schick F (2004) FAIR true-FISP perfusion imaging of the kidneys. Magn Reson Med 51:353–361. doi:10.1002/mrm.10709

McDonald K, Duffy P, Chowdhury T, McHugh K (2013) Added value of abdominal cross-sectional imaging (CT or MRI) in staging of Wilms. Clin Radiol 68:16–20. doi:10.1016/j.crad.2012.05.006

McMann LP, Kirsch AJ, Scherz HC et al (2006) Magnetic resonance urography in the evaluation of prenatally diagnosed hydronephrosis and renal dysgenesis. J Urol 176:1786–1792. doi:10.1016/j.juro.2006.05.025

Miyazaki Y, Ichikawa I (2003) Ontogeny of congenital anomalies of the kidney and urinary tract, CAKUT. Pediatr Int 45:598–604. doi:10.1046/j.1442-200X.2003.01777.x

Niu ZB, Yang Y, Hou Y et al (2007) Ureteral polyps: an etiological factor of hydronephrosis in children that should not be ignored. Ped Surg Int 23:323–326. doi:10.1007/s00383-007-1884-z

Nixon JN, Biyyam DR, Stanescu L et al (2013) Imaging of pediatric renal transplants and their complications: a pictorial review. RadioGraphics 33:1227–1251. doi:10.1148/rg.335125150

Nurzia MJ, Costantinescu AR, Barone JG (2002) Childhood infundibular stenosis. Urology 60:344–344. doi:10.1016/S0090-4295(02)01714-4

O'Reilly PH (1982) Role of modern radiological investigations in obstructive uropathy. Br Med J (Clin Res Ed) 284:1847–1851

O'Reilly PH (2002) Obstructive uropathy. The quarterly journal of nuclear medicine: official publication of the Italian Association of Nuclear Medicine (AIMN)[and] the International Association of Radiopharmacology (IAR) 46:295–303

Patel UD (2014) Outcomes after pediatric kidney transplantation improving: how can we do even better?Pediatrics133:734–735.doi:10.1542/peds.2014-0124

Patheyar V, Venkatesh SK, Siew E et al (2011) MR imaging features of fibroepithelial ureteral polyp in a patient with duplicated upper urinary tract. Singapore Med J 52:e45–e47

Patlak CS, Blasberg RG (1985) Graphical evaluation of blood-to-brain transfer constants from multiple-time uptake data. Generalizations J Cereb Blood Flow Metab 5:584–590. doi:10.1038/jcbfm.1985.87

Pedersen M, Shi Y, Anderson P et al (2004) Quantitation of differential renal blood flow and renal function using dynamic contrast-enhanced MRI in rats. Magn Reson Med 51:510–517. doi:10.1002/mrm.10711

Pekar J, Moonen CT, van Zijl PC (1992) On the precision of diffusion/perfusion imaging by gradient sensitization. Magn Reson Med 23:122–129. doi:10.1002/mrm.1910230113

Perez-Brayfield MR, Kirsch AJ, Jones RA, Grattan-Smith JD (2003) A prospective study comparing ultrasound, nuclear scintigraphy and dynamic contrast enhanced magnetic resonance imaging in the evaluation of hydronephrosis. J Urol 170:1330–1334. doi:10.1097/01.ju.0000086775.66329.00

Peruzzi L (2014) Challenges in pediatric renal transplantation. WJT 4:222. doi:10.5500/wjt.v4.i4.222

Peters AM (1994) Graphical analysis of dynamic data: the Patlak-Rutland plot. Nucl Med Commun 15:669–672

Peters CA, Chevalier RL (2012) Chapter 113 – Congenital urinary obstruction: pathophysiology and clinical evaluation, 10th edn. Elsevier Inc., Philadelphia. http://doi.org/10.1016/j.ucl.2010.03.007

Piepsz A (2007) Antenatally detected hydronephrosis. Semin Nucl Med 37:249–260. doi:10.1053/j.semnuclmed.2007.02.008

Piepsz A (2011) Antenatal detection of pelviureteric junction stenosis: main controversies. Semin Nucl Med 41:11–19. doi:10.1053/j.semnuclmed.2010.07.008

Piepsz A, Tondeur M, Nogarède C et al (2011) Can severely impaired cortical transit predict which children with pelvi-ureteric junction stenosis detected antenatally might benefit from pyeloplasty? Nucl Med Commun 32:199–205. doi:10.1097/MNM.0b013e328340c586

Pieretti-Vanmarcke R, Pieretti A, Pieretti RV (2008) Megacalycosis: a rare condition. Pediatr Nephrol 24:1077–1079. doi:10.1007/s00467-008-1039-z

Podberesky DJ, Towbin AJ, Eltomey MA, Levitt MA (2013) Magnetic resonance imaging of anorectal malformations. Magn Reson Imaging Clin NA 21:791–812. doi:10.1016/j.mric.2013.04.010

Pohl HG, Rushton HG, Park JS et al (2001) Early diuresis renogram findings predict success following pyeloplasty. J Urol 165:2311–2315

Pope JC, Brock JW, ADAMS MC et al (1999) How they begin and how they end: classic and new theories for the development and deterioration of congenital anomalies of the kidney and urinary tract, CAKUT. J Am Soc Nephrol 10:2018–2028

Pouliot F, Lebel MH, Audet J-F, Dujardin T (2010) Determination of success by objective scintigraphic criteria after laparoscopic pyeloplasty. J Endourol 24:299–304. doi:10.1089/end.2009.0134

Preibsch H, Rall K, Wietek BM et al (2014) Clinical value of magnetic resonance imaging in patients with Mayer-Rokitansky-Küster-Hauser (MRKH) syndrome: diagnosis of associated malformations, uterine rudiments and intrauterine endometrium. Eur Radiol 24:1621–1627. doi:10.1007/s00330-014-3156-3

Prokop M, Schneider G, Vanzulli A et al (2005) Contrast-enhanced MR Angiography of the renal arteries: blinded multicenter crossover comparison of gadobenate dimeglumine and gadopentetate dimeglumine1. Radiology 234:399–408. doi:10.1148/radiol.2342040023

Radbruch A, Weberling LD, Kieslich PJ et al (2015) Gadolinium retention in the dentate nucleus and globus pallidus is dependent on the class of contrast agent. Radiology 275:783–791. doi:10.1148/radiol.2015150337

Ranawaka R, Hennayake S (2013) Resolution of primary non-refluxing megaureter: an observational study. J Pediatr Surg 48:380–383. doi:10.1016/j.jpedsurg.2012.11.017

Redman JF, Neeb AD (2005) Congenital megacalycosis: a forgotten diagnosis? Urology 65:384–385. doi:10.1016/j.urology.2004.09.058

Renjen P, Bellah R, Hellinger JC, Darge K (2010) Pediatric urologic advanced imaging: techniques and applications. Urol Clin NA 37(2):307–318. http://doi.org/10.1016/j.ucl.2010.03.007

Riccabona M (2010) Obstructive diseases of the urinary tract in children: lessons from the last 15 years. Pediatr Radiol 40:947–955. doi:10.1007/s00247-010-1590-1

Riccabona M, Avni FE, Dacher J-N et al (2010) ESPR uroradiology task force and ESUR paediatric working group: imaging and procedural recommendations in paediatric uroradiology, part III. Minutes of the ESPR uroradiology task force minisymposium on intravenous urography, uro-CT and MR-urography in childhood. Pediatr Radiol 40:1315–1320. doi:10.1007/s00247-010-1686-7

Riccabona M, Avni F, Dacher JN, Damasio B, Darge K, Lobo ML, Ording-Müller LS, Papado-poulou F, Vivier P, Willi U (2011) ESPR uroradiology task force and ESUR paediatric working group: imaging recommendations in paediatric uroradiology, Part IV Minutes of the ESPR urora-diology task force minisymposium on imaging in childhood renal hypertension and imaging of renal trauma in children. Pediatr Radiol 41:939–944. doi:10.1007/s00247-011-2089-0

Riccabona M, Avni F, Damasio B, Ordning-Mueller LS, Lobo ML, Darge K, Papadopoulou F, Willi U, Blickmann J, Vivier PH (2012) ESPR Uroradiology Task Force and ESUR Paediatric Working Group – Imaging recommendations in Paediatric Uroradiology, Part V: Childhood cystic kidney disease, childhood renal transplantation, and contrast-enhanced ultrasound in children. Pediatr Radiol 42:1275–1283. doi:10.1007/s00247-012-2436-9

Riccabona M, Darge K, Lobo M-L et al (2015) ESPR Uroradiology Taskforce—imaging recommendations in paediatric uroradiology, part VIII: retrograde urethrography, imaging disorder of sexual development and imaging childhood testicular torsion. Pediatr Radiol 45:2023–2028. doi:10.1007/s00247-015-3452-3

Ries M, Jones RA, Basseau F et al (2001) Diffusion tensor MRI of the human kidney. J Magn Reson Imaging 14:42–49. doi:10.1002/jmri.1149

Risdon RA (1993) The small scarred kidney in childhood. Pediatr Nephrol 7:361–364

Risdon RA, Young LW, Chrispin AR (1975) Renal hypoplasia and dysplasia: a radiological and pathological correlation. Pediatr Radiol 3:213–225

Robson PM, Madhuranthakam AJ, Dai W et al (2009) Strategies for reducing respiratory motion artifacts in renal perfusion imaging with arterial spin labeling. Magn Reson Med 61:1374–1387. doi:10.1002/mrm.21960

Rodriguez MM (2014) Congenital anomalies of the kidney and the urinary tract (CAKUT). Fetal Pediatr Pathol 33:293–320. doi:10.3109/15513815.2014.959678

Rodríguez LV, Spielman D, Herfkens RJ, Shortliffe LD (2001) Magnetic resonance imaging for the evaluation of hydronephrosis, reflux and renal scarring in children. JURO 166:1023–1027. doi:10.1016/S0022-5347(05)65910-1

Rosen S, Peters CA, Chevalier RL, Huang W-Y (2008) The kidney in congenital ureteropelvic junction obstruction: a spectrum from normal to nephrectomy. J Urol 179:1257–1263. doi:10.1016/j.juro.2007.11.048

Rusinek H, Lee VS, Johnson G (2001) Optimal dose of Gd-DTPA in dynamic MR studies. Magn Reson Med 46:312–316. doi:10.1002/mrm.1193

Rutland (1979): Rutland MD. A single injection technique for subtraction of blood background in 131I-hippuran renograms. Br J Radiol 1979;52:134–137

Samin A, Becker JA (1991) CT nephrogram in acute obstructive uropathy. Urol Radiol 12:178–180

Sanna-Cherchi S, Ravani P, Corbani V et al (2009) Renal outcome in patients with congenital anomalies of the kidney and urinary tract. Kidney Int 76:528–533. doi:10.1038/ki.2009.220

Soares dos Santos Junior AC, Marques de Miranda D, Simões e Silva AC (2014) Congenital anomalies of the kidney and urinary tract: an embryogenetic review. Birth Defect Res C. doi:10.1002/bdrc.21084

Santucci RA, Wessells H, Bartsch G et al (2004) Evaluation and management of renal injuries: consensus statement of the renal trauma subcommittee. BJU Int 93:937–954. doi:10.1111/j.1464-4096.2004.04820.x

Saxton HM (1969) Review article: urography. Br J Radiol 42:321–346

Schlotmann A, Clorius JH, Clorius SN (2009) Diuretic renography in hydronephrosis: renal tissue tracer transit predicts functional course and thereby need for surgery. Eur J Nucl Med Mol Imaging 36:1665–1673. doi:10.1007/s00259-009-1138-5

Schreuder MF (2012) Safety in glomerular numbers. Pediatr Nephrol 27:1881–1887. doi:10.1007/s00467-012-2169-x

Sfakianakis GN, Sfakianaki E, Georgiou M et al (2009) A renal protocol for all ages and all indications: mercapto-acetyl-triglycine (MAG3) with simultaneous injection of furosemide (MAG3-F0): a

17-year experience. Semin Nucl Med 39:156–173. doi:10.1053/j.semnuclmed.2008.11.001

Sharfuddin A (2011) Grattan-Smith09102015. YSNEP 31:259–271. doi:10.1016/j.semnephrol.2011.05.005

Sharfuddin A (2014) Renal relevant radiology: imaging in kidney transplantation. Clin J Am Soc Nephrol 9:416–429. doi:10.2215/CJN.02960313

Sherwood T (1971) The physiology of intravenous urography. Sci Basis Med Annu Rev 336–348

Shive ML, Baskin L, Harris C et al (2012) Ureteral fibroepithelial polyp causing urinary obstruction. Radiol Case. doi:10.3941/jrcr.v6i7.1076

Shokeir AA, Nijman RJM (2002) Ureterocele: an ongoing challenge in infancy and childhood. BJU Int 90:777–783. doi:10.1046/j.1464-410X.2002.02998.x

Shokeir AA, Provoost AP, Nijman RJ (1999) Recoverability of renal function after relief of chronic partial upper urinary tract obstruction. BJU Int 83:11–17. doi:10.1046/j.1464-410x.1999.00889.x

Shopfner CE (1964) Genitography in intersexual states. Radiology 82:664–674

Smith EA (2013) Advanced techniques in pediatric abdominopelvic oncologic magnetic resonance imaging. Magn Reson Imaging Clin NA 21:829–841. doi:10.1016/j.mric.2013.06.002

Smith ED, Cussen LJ, Glenn J et al (1977) Report of working party to establish an international nomenclature for the large ureter. Birth Defects Orig Artic Ser 13:3–8

Soulez G, Pasowicz M, Benea G et al (2008) Renal artery stenosis evaluation: diagnostic performance of gadobenate dimeglumine–enhanced MR angiography—comparison with DSA 1. Radiology 247:273–285. doi:10.1148/radiol.2471070711

Sourbron S (2010) Compartmental modelling for magnetic resonance renography. Zeitschrift fuer Medizinische Physik 20:101–114. doi:10.1016/j.zemedi.2009.10.010

Swinson S, McHugh K (2011) Urogenital tumours in childhood. Cancer Imaging 11:S48–S64. doi:10.1102/1470-7330.2011.9009

Takazakura R, Johnin K, Furukawa A et al (2007) Magnetic resonance voiding cystourethrography for vesicoureteral reflux. J Magn Reson Imaging 25:170–174. doi:10.1002/jmri.20822

Tasian GE, Aaronson DS, McAninch JW (2010) Trauma/reconstruction/diversion/evaluation of renal function after major renal injury: correlation with the American Association for the Surgery of Trauma Injury Scale. JURO 183:196–200. doi:10.1016/j.juro.2009.08.149

Thoeny HC, De Keyzer F (2011) Diffusion-weighted MR imaging of native and transplanted kidneys. Radiology 259:25–38. doi:10.1148/radiol.10092419

Thoeny HC, De Keyzer F, Oyen RH, Peeters RR (2005) Diffusion-weighted MR imaging of kidneys in healthy volunteers and patients with parenchymal diseases: initial experience1. Radiology 235:911–917. doi:10.1148/radiol.2353040554

Ulman I, Jayanthi VR, Koff SA (2000) The long-term followup of newborns with severe unilateral hydronephrosis initially treated nonoperatively. J Urol 164:1101–1105

Uthappa MC, Anthony D, Allen C (2002) Case report: retrocaval ureter: MR appearances. Br J Radiol 75:177–179

Van Arendonk KJ, Boyarsky BJ, Orandi BJ et al (2014) National trends over 25 years in pediatric kidney transplant outcomes. Pediatrics 133:594–601. doi:10.1542/peds.2013-2775

Vemulakonda V, Yiee J, Wilcox DT (2014) Prenatal hydronephrosis: postnatal evaluation and management. Curr Urol Rep 15:430. doi:10.1007/s11934-014-0430-5

Vivante A, Kohl S, Hwang D-Y et al (2014) Single-gene causes of congenital anomalies of the kidney and urinary tract (CAKUT) in humans. Pediatr Nephrol 29:695–704. doi:10.1007/s00467-013-2684-4

Vivier P-H, Dolores M, Taylor M, Dacher J-N (2010a) MR urography in children. Part 2: how to use ImageJ MR urography processing software. Pediatr Radiol 40:739–746. doi:10.1007/s00247-009-1536-7

Vivier P-H, Dolores M, Taylor M et al (2010b) MR urography in children. Part 1: how we do the F0 technique. Pediatr Radiol 40:732–738. doi:10.1007/s00247-009-1538-5

Vivier P-H, Sallem A, Beurdeley M et al (2013) MRI and suspected acute pyelonephritis in children: comparison of diffusion-weighted imaging with gadolinium-enhanced T1-weighted imaging. Eur Radiol 24:19–25. doi:10.1007/s00330-013-2971-2

Waingankar N, Hayek S, Smith AD, Okeke Z (2014) Calyceal diverticula: a comprehensive review. Rev Urol 16:29–43. doi:10.3909/riu0581

Wang Y-T (2015) Functional assessment of transplanted kidneys with magnetic resonance imaging. WJR 7:343. doi:10.4329/wjr.v7.i10.343

Weiser AC, Amukele SA, Leonidas JC, Palmer LS (2003) The role of gadolinium enhanced magnetic resonance imaging for children with suspected acute pyelonephritis. J Urol 169:2308–2311. doi:10.1097/01.ju.0000068082.91869.29

Westland R, Schreuder MF, Ket JCF, Van Wijk JAE (2013) Unilateral renal agenesis: a systematic review on associated anomalies and renal injury. Nephrol Dial Transplant 28:1844–1855. doi:10.1093/ndt/gft012

Whitaker RH, Flower CD (1981) Megacalices--how broad a spectrum? Br J Urol 53:1–6

Whitaker RH, Bullock KN, Buxton-Thomas MS et al (1982) Role of modern radiological investigations in obstructive uropathy. Br Med J (Clin Res Ed) 285:211

Whitfield HN, Britton KE, Hendry WF et al (1978) The distinction between obstructive uropathy and nephropathy by radioisotope transit times. Br J Urol 50:433–436

Williams B, Tareen B, Resnick MI (2007) Pathophysiology and treatment of ureteropelvic junction obstruction. Curr Urol Rep 8:111–117. doi:10.1007/s11934-007-0059-8

Winkler NS, Kennedy AM, Woodward PJ (2012) Cloacal malformation. Embyrology, Anatomy and prenatal imaging features. J Ultrasound Med 31: 1843–1855

Woolf AS (2004) Evolving concepts in human renal dysplasia. J Am Soc Nephrol 15:998–1007. doi:10.1097/01.ASN.0000113778.06598.6F

Wright NB, Smith C, Rickwood AM, Carty HM (1995) Imaging children with ambiguous genitalia and intersex states. Clin Radiol 50:823–829

Wu AK, Tran TC, Sorensen MD et al (2012) Relative renal function does not improve after relieving chronic renal obstruction. BJU Int 109:1540–1544. doi:10.1111/j.1464-410X.2011.10788.x

Yamamoto A, Zhang JL, Rusinek H et al (2011) Quantitative evaluation of acute renal transplant dysfunction with low-dose three-dimensional MR renography. Radiology 260:781–789. doi:10.1148/radiol.11101664

Yavus A, Bora A, Kurdoglu M et al (2015) Herlyn-Werner-Wunderlich Syndrome: merits of sonographic and magnetic resonance imaging for accurate diagnosis and patient management in 13 cases. J Pediatr Adolesc Gynecol 28:47–52. doi:10.1016/j.jpag.2014.03.004

Yoo R-E, Cho JY, Kim SY, Kim SH (2013) Magnetic resonance evaluation of Müllerian Remnants in Mayer-Rokitansky-Küster-Hauser Syndrome. Korean J Radiol 14:233. doi:10.3348/kjr.2013.14.2.233

Zhang JL, Morrell G, Rusinek H et al (2013a) New magnetic resonance imaging methods in nephrology. Kidney Int 85:768–778. doi:10.1038/ki.2013.361

Zhang JL, Rusinek H, Chandarana H, Lee VS (2013b) Functional MRI of the kidneys. J Magn Reson Imaging 37:282–293. doi:10.1002/jmri.23717

Nuclear Medicine

Marina Easty and Isky Gordon

Contents

1 Introduction 94
2 Static Renal Scan 94
3 Common Indication for DMSA 95
4 Dynamic Renography 99
5 Indications for MAG3 Tc^{99m} Renography 99
6 Isotope Cystography 105
6.1 Direct Radioisotope Cystography (DIC) 106
6.2 Indirect Radioisotope Cystography 106
7 Functional Imaging in Paediatric Nephro-urological Tumours and in Paediatric Post-transplant Lymphoproliferative Disorder (PTLD) 109
Conclusion 110
References 110

With thanks to Professor Isky Gordon, Consultant Paediatric Radiologist (retired), Great Ormond Street Hospital for Children NHS Foundation Trust for his reproduced input from the 2nd Edition

M. Easty (✉) • I. Gordon
Department of Diagnostic Imaging, Great Ormond Street Hospital for Children NHS Foundation Trust, Great Ormond Street, London, WC1N 3JH, UK
e-mail: Marina.Easty@gosh.nhs.uk

Abbreviations

CT	Computerised Tomography
DIC	Direct isotope cystogram
DMSA	Di-mercapto-succinic acid
EANM	European Association of Nuclear Medicine
FDG PET-CT	Fluorodeoxyglucose positron emission tomography Computerised Tomography
IRC	Indirect radionuclide cystogram
MAG3	Mercapto-acetyl-tri-glycine
MBq	Megabecquerels
MRI	Magnetic resonance imaging
mSv	Millisievert
NORA	Normalised residual activity
PEE	Pelvic excretion efficiency
PM	Post-micturition
PTLD	Post-transplant lymphoproliferative disorder
RDF	Renal differential function
ROE	Renal output efficiency
ROI	Region of interest
SPECT	Single-photon emission Computerised Tomography
TAC	Time-activity curve
US	Ultrasound
UTI	Urinary tract infection
VCUG	Voiding cystourethrogram
VUR	Vesicoureteric reflux

1 Introduction

Paediatric renal radionuclide imaging is used for accurate assessment of renal function and the drainage pattern. The increase in functional MRI has overtaken radionuclide functional assessment in only a small number of establishments due to the requirement for patient cooperation, reasonably long scanning times and the possible need for general anaesthetic in order to undertake the MRI study. The availability of MRI scanning time also plays a significant contribution. Static renal scintigraphy with technetium-99m di-mercapto-succinic acid (Tc-99m DMSA) is used to image renal parenchymal detail, most commonly to assess for the presence of renal scarring following a complicated urinary tract infection.

The dynamic renogram using Tc^{99m} mercapto-acetyl-tri-glycine (Tc-99m MAG3) is used in the assessment of renal function and drainage with excellent correlation with renal differential function (RDF) assessed on DMSA studies (Ritchie et al. 2008). In addition, when the child is continent and able to cooperate, an indirect radionuclide cystogram (IRC) to assess for the presence of reflux may be performed, thus providing a cystogram without catheterisation. The IRC is the only physiological method to assess for reflux. Occasionally, a low-dose direct isotope cystogram (DIC) may be required where fluoroscopic facilities are poor (newer fluoroscopic machines with pulsed radiation have very low doses, and therefore DICs are now rarely required).

Nephro-urological tumours such as bladder and prostate rhabdomyosarcomas may require staging by functional imaging using fluorine-18-fluorodeoxyglucose positron emission tomography/Computerised Tomography (FDG PET-CT). Increasingly, with the availability of new MRI hybrid PET scanners, there can be a low-dose functional and diagnostic 'one stop shop' in the assessment of paediatric tumours.

2 Static Renal Scan

Technetium-99m DMSA binds to the proximal convoluted tubules of the kidney, with only approximately 10 % of the tracer excreted in the urine. The remaining bound tracer provides an unchanging image of functioning renal tissue and demonstrates an accurate parenchymal outline. The image can be obtained many hours after injection, as Tc^{99m} has a half-life of approximately 6 hours.

The majority of paediatric DMSA scans are requested to assess renal parenchymal abnormalities following severe urinary tract infection (UTI) (Baumer and Jones 2007). DMSA imaging in UTI is a sensitive test to assess the appearance of cortical abnormalities, namely, inflammatory change in acute infection and scarring as a sequel of UTI. Although extremely sensitive, the test is not specific. Photopenic defects may be seen in dysplastic kidneys, with renal masses such as abscess, cyst or tumour, post-traumatic or postsurgical change (including post angioplasty in children with renal artery stenosis), with congenital renal variants and also with dilatation of all, or part of the renal collecting system. In view of this lack of specificity, contemporaneous ultrasound (US) plus clinical information is essential. DMSA studies performed acutely to assess for UTI are no longer routinely performed in most of Europe, as clinical assessment, high-quality modern US and urinalysis are likely to lead to a diagnosis. The abnormalities seen on the early scan may be transient, and thus a follow-up scan is warranted. The radiation burden from a DMSA study of 0.7–1.0 mSv in children is not insubstantial, and therefore a delayed DMSA at least 4–6 months after the urinary tract infection is better recommended to assess permanent renal parenchymal abnormalities, rather than both early and late studies (Fig. 1) (Mandell et al. 1997a, b; Piepsz et al. 2001).

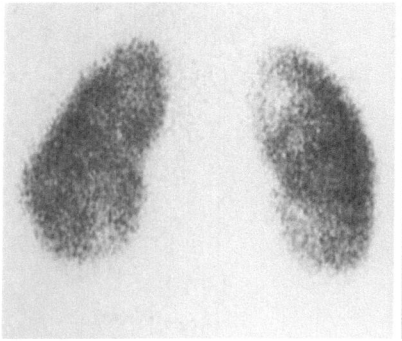

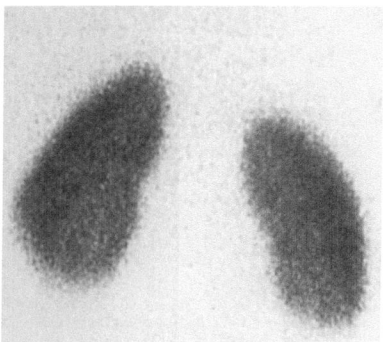

Fig. 1 Urinary tract infection with defect in acute phase with normal final outcome. This 4-year-old girl was being investigated for a urinary tract infection; the US was normal. The Tc-99m DMSA scan on the left was undertaken 1 week after the diagnosis of the urinary tract infection. There are multiple defects in the right kidney with a defect in the lower pole of the left kidney. The Tc-99m DMSA scan on the right undertaken 6 months later is now normal. Although most defects that return to normal do so within the first 3 months after urinary tract infection, approximately 15 % will take up to 6 months to return to normal (Reproduced from *Pediatric Uroradiology*, 2nd Edition, Fotter)

3 Common Indication for DMSA

1. UTI
2. Ectopic kidney
3. Anatomical variant
4. Assessment of dysplastic renal tissue
5. Severely dilated kidneys where drainage assessment by MAG3 renography is not possible and renal differential function (RDF) is needed, for example, in posterior urethral valves where a MAG3 study may be inaccurate
6. Functioning renal tissue with bilateral renal tumours (e.g. stage V Wilms' tumour), where nephron-sparing surgery is indicated
7. Before abdominal radiotherapy to assess renal function and to plan radiation field
8. Following renal trauma
9. Pre- and post renal angioplasty in hypertensive patients with renal artery stenosis
10. Post renal transplant where there is an unused bladder and the risk of UTI is high
11. Rarely in children with calculi prior to intervention (Figs. 1 and 2).

Preparation and Sedation Sedation is not used in standard DMSA acquisitions as the parents assist in immobilisation. Sandbags may be placed by the side of the child and Velcro straps, or similar means are used to maintain position (Fig. 3). The environment should be child-friendly, with toys, games and interactive wall decorations, ideally with television and film-viewing facilities. Trained imaging staff will engage children in play and enable quality scans without sedation.

There are a group of children who may require a DMSA SPECT Computerised Tomography (CT) study, for example, small children with bilateral Wilms tumours before nephron-sparing surgery. These children usually require a general anaesthetic in order to obtain a diagnostic, registered SPECT CT dataset. Older children can usually lie still by watching films.

Precautions Tubular defects such as the Fanconi syndrome may result in poor renal visualisation due to defective binding of the isotope within the tubular cell and consequent high urinary excretion. If there is a significant urinary tract dilatation (UTD), a MAG3 study may be necessary to give a more accurate RDF, although a delayed DMSA image may be useful in this situation.

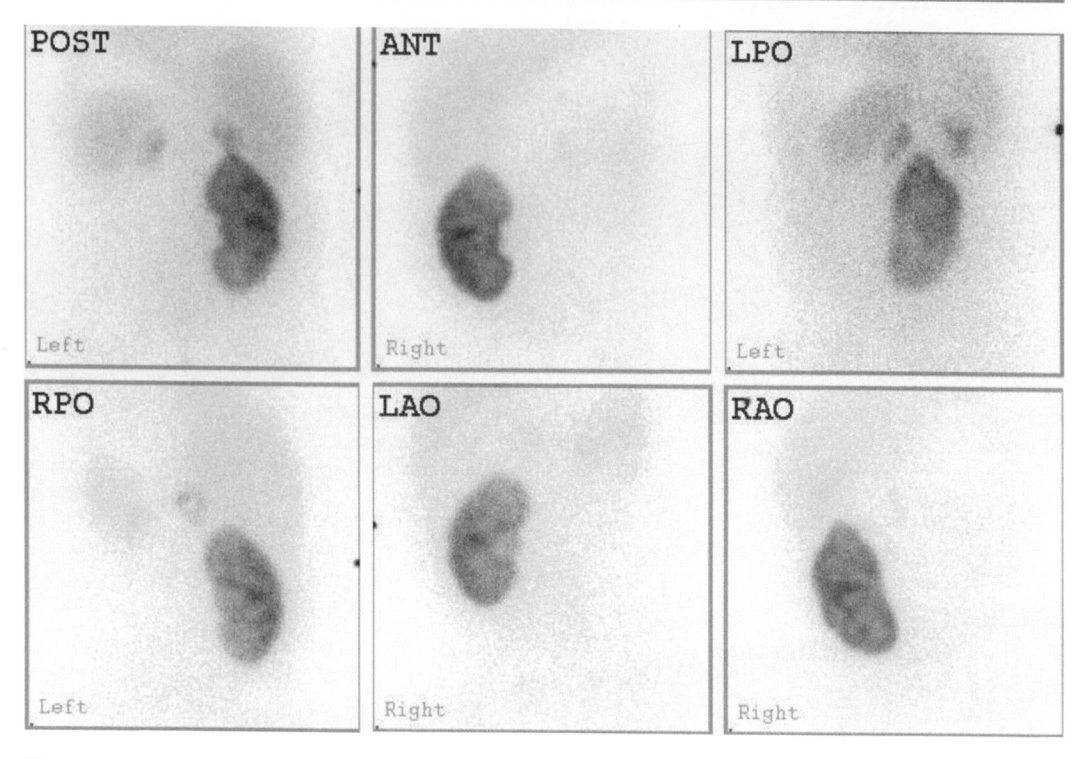

Fig. 2 Live-related donor transplant in a 4-year-old boy with posterior urethral valves (PUV). The shrunken native kidneys are demonstrated above the transplant in the right flank. Six views of the transplant kidney are obtained to exclude focal defects. The DMSA study was performed as a baseline study as silent UTI's are common in children with abnormal bladder function, such as in boys with PUV. The DMSA shows no focal defects and clear internal architecture

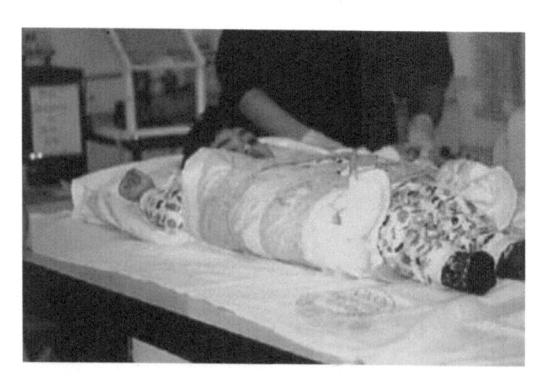

Fig. 3 Immobilisation. The child is lying directly on the collimator surface as the strengthened perspex bed has a hole cut out, thus the child is as close to the camera as possible. This clearly improves image quality (see below). The child has sandbags attached with Velcro straps on either side of the body, thus reducing movement (Reproduced from *Pediatric Uroradiology*, 2nd Edition, Fotter)

Radiopharmaceutical A dose schedule using a minimum dose of 18.5 MBq and a maximum dose of 100 MBq scaled on a body surface basis is advised (Lassmann and Treves 2014). The child can attend the department for anaesthetic cream application approximately 45 min prior to the study if required. The tracer should be injected using a small calibre needle. The effective dose is a maximum of approximately 0.9 mSv per examination, regardless of the age of the child, providing that the dose is selected according to body surface area.

Image acquisition should begin between 2 and 3 h after tracer injection. The camera should be collimator side up, using a high- or ultra-high-resolution collimator (Figs. 3 and 4) (Piepsz et al. 2001). The child should be placed supine on the camera face so that a posterior view and both posterior oblique views may be obtained. The anterior view is required for a congenital variant kidney such as a horseshoe, where there is an ectopic kidney, when hunting for a 'missing kidney', or when a spinal abnormality such as a sco-

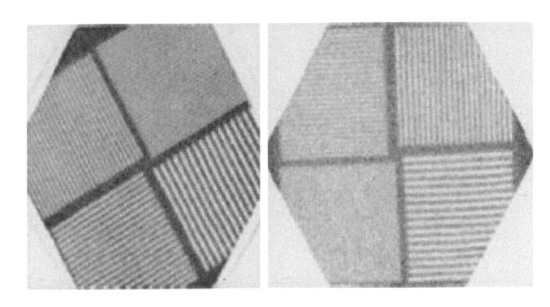

Fig. 4 Effect of distance on image quality. The two images are of the same line bar phantom showing how one may degrade the image quality by simply increasing the distance between the gamma camera face and the phantom. In the image on the left with the phantom on the camera face, the lines are clearly seen in all four segments. When the phantom is placed on the imaging bed 1 cm above the camera and as close to the camera as possible, the lines are clearly seen in only three segments (Reproduced from *Pediatric Uroradiology*, 2nd Edition, Fotter)

liosis may distort the anatomy causing a kidney to be more anteriorly positioned. When scanning a transplant kidney, the anterior view and both anterior and posterior oblique views are required due to the superficial position of the transplant and possible anatomical distortion due to the large donor kidney in a paediatric patient (Fig. 2).

The computer acquisition set-up should include a pixel size between 1.8 and 2.5 mm; this can be achieved with a 128×128 matrix plus zoom at acquisition or a 256×256 matrix. At least 300,000 counts or 5-min counting per image is necessary.

SPECT The use of SPECT for Tc-99m DMSA scintigraphy in children has increased over the last few years particularly in the assessment of congenital renal variants such as cross-fused ectopic kidneys and in the renal transplant kidney. The increased scanning time may lead to the need for general anaesthetic for the procedure. The amount of administered radioactivity should not routinely be increased.

Processing The differential renal function (DRF) is calculated by drawing a region of interest (ROI) around each kidney, delineated on a highly contrasted image. An ectopic kidney, such as a pelvic kidney, will require an anterior image in order to calculate the DRF by the geometric mean, thereby taking into account the more anterior position of the ectopic kidney (Yapar et al. 2005).

Interpretation Normal values of DRF are between 45 and 55 % uptake. Values outside this range may be seen when there is an uncomplicated unilateral duplex kidney, which may contribute 57 or 58 % to total renal function. Values within the normal range may be seen with bilateral small kidneys or with abnormal kidneys symmetrically affected by disease. UTD, as in a pelvi-ureteric junction anomaly, may cause 'supra-normal' DRF in the affected kidney which may persist following surgery, and thus a contemporaneous renal ultrasound scan should always be assessed when interpreting the image.

Images Normal appearances include sharp renal outlines with clear delineation of the medullary pyramids from the higher uptake in the proximal tubules (Fig. 5). There are many anatomical variants, including flattening and compression of the superolateral contour of the left kidney by the spleen and more bulbous or pear-shaped kidneys. The renal cortex shows more avid uptake than the renal medulla. The number and size of the columns of Bertin differ from patient to patient (variable thickness of the cortical rim) and may cause false interpretation of the image. An uncomplicated duplex kidney may have a more vertical lie, pointing towards the ipsilateral shoulder of the patient rather than the contralateral shoulder as is usual in a simplex kidney. Attention should be paid to the presence of foetal lobulation, and careful review of the ultrasound is essential in order not to misinterpret this as scarring.

When an abnormal pattern is seen, the number, size and location of areas of cortical loss should be noted. Loss of the outline may or may not be present. Differentiation between acute lesions, which will improve or disappear, and chronic lesions (scars) is not always possible in the acute phase of a UTI (Fig. 1). A polar photopenic area with an intact renal outline will

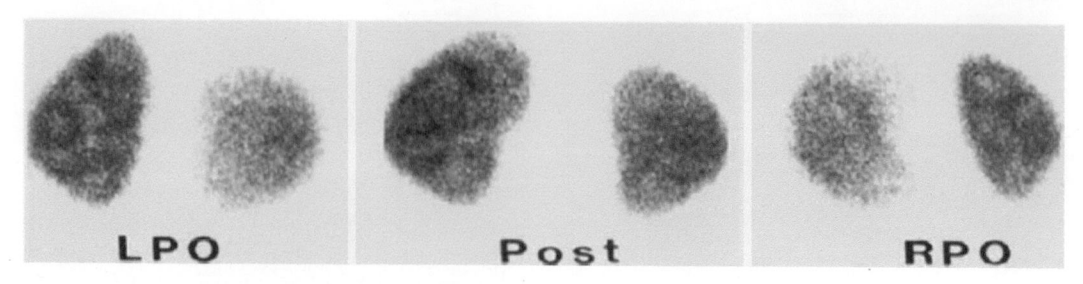

Fig. 5 Normal Tc-99m DMSA scan. This 3-year-old was undergoing investigation for a urinary tract infection. Note the clarity in the outline of both kidneys. The internal architecture is clearly seen in both kidneys. For the right kidney, this is better on the right posterior oblique projection (*RPO*), while for the left kidney, this is best seen on the left posterior oblique projection (*LPO*) (Reproduced from *Pediatric Uroradiology*, 2nd Edition, Fotter)

generally heal; marked localised deformity of the outlines or volume loss generally corresponds to a permanent scar. To assess renal scars after UTI, Tc-99m DMSA scintigraphy should be performed at least 6 months after acute infection.

Image quality is assessed prior to the child leaving the department as poor studies can lead to under-interpretation of pathology. Movement will cause blurring of the outline of the kidneys or a double outline.

The advantage of Tc-99m DMSA scans is the high sensitivity in the detection of parenchymal pathology and quantification especially for the ectopic kidney; differential renal function is more reliably assessed than with the dynamic Tc-99m MAG3. The disadvantages include the 2 h wait between injection and scan, and each image requires approximately 5 min to obtain, and therefore technicians and radiographers with training in handling children are necessary. The radiation burden is higher than for a Tc-99m MAG3, so Tc-99m DMSA is not advocated solely for assessment of DRF. In the presence of dilatation of the renal pelvis, the Tc-99m DMSA may accumulate in the pelvis and result in a falsely high estimation of the function of the hydronephrotic kidney, although supra normal values may also be seen in the affected kidney.

In the estimation of DRF, there is close correlation between the results of Tc-99m MAG3 and Tc-99m DMSA (Fig. 6.). If only DRF is required, then a Tc-99m MAG3, with the lower radiation burden, should be performed.

If the clinical question is whether there is evidence of scarring following a severe urinary tract infection, the DMSA study will be the investigation of choice, particularly if there is no associated collecting system dilatation.

> **Take Away**
> Tc^{99m} DMSA scintigraphy is used to assess DRF, and internal architecture may be demonstrated on a high-quality study. Focal parenchymal defects will be detected.

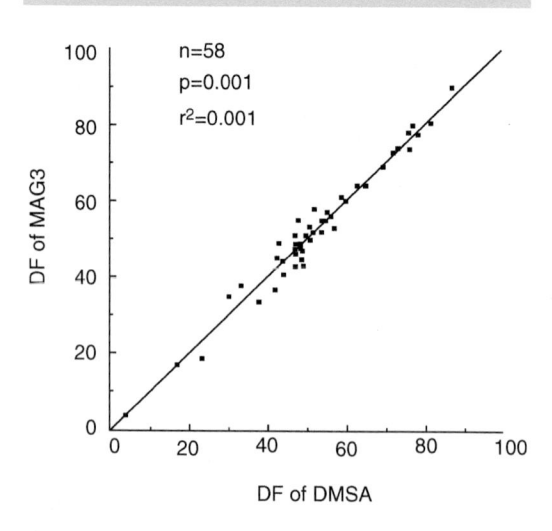

Fig. 6 Differential renal function using Tc-99m DMSA and Tc-99m MAG3 in the same children. The studies were done within 4 weeks of each other. There is close correlation between the two tracers (Reproduced from *Pediatric Uroradiology* 2nd Edition, Fotter)

4 Dynamic Renography

The use of dynamic renography has been well established; however, quality studies need to be performed in the paediatric population, and therefore Tc^{99m} MAG3 studies should be performed in a child-friendly environment by staff experienced in handling children.

Dynamic renography allows estimation of three parameters of renal function: blood flow to the kidney; renal clearance (Piepsz et al. 1998; Prigent et al. 1999; Rutland 1985), i.e. the extraction of a tracer from the blood, when estimation of relative clearance occurs as in DRF; and the drainage function or excretion from the kidney.

Blood flow estimation must be undertaken during the first few seconds and is only indicated following renal transplantation in paediatric nephro-urology. The native Paediatric kidney is too small to estimate the blood flow accurately. DRF estimation is best undertaken approximately 1–2 min after tracer injection. After 2 min, the tracer may already have reached the collecting system, thus invalidating the DRF estimation. Background correction is particularly important in estimation of DRF when there is asymmetrical renal function or decreased overall function. Drainage or disappearance of the tracer from the kidney can simply be estimated by inspecting the renogram time-activity curve (TAC): an early peak followed by a rapidly descending phase is typical for normal excretion. Delay in excretion is characterised by a continuously ascending curve. Several techniques have been proposed for quantifying the transit of tracer through the kidney. These range from simple descriptive parameters such as the time to reach the maximum of the curve, T_{max}, to more sophisticated parameters, such as deconvolution analysis, output efficiency (OE)/pelvic excretion efficiency (PEE) (Anderson et al. 1997; Chaiwatanarat et al. 1993) or normalised residual activity (NORA) (Piepsz et al. 2000). Sufficient information is provided by the shape of the TAC and the T_{max} to discriminate between normal transit (T_{max} around 3 min) or very delayed transit (T_{max} of 20 min). There is no proof that in clinical practice the more sophisticated techniques can improve the information obtained. When dilatation of the collecting system exists, the standard renogram is generally characterised by a continuously rising curve, reflecting poor drainage of the kidney while in the supine position. In cases of dilatation, furosemide should be injected (diuretic renography), which increases urinary flow and may distinguish between good and impaired drainage; the data acquired post-furosemide must include a series following a change of posture and micturition (see Post-micturition Images, below).

Tracers Used Tc-99m MAG3 is the tracer almost solely used in Europe as it relies on tubular extraction. Tc-99m MAG3 has a greater renal extraction than Tc-99m DTPA which depends on filtration, resulting in a lower background activity and a higher kidney to background ratio than Tc-99m DTPA.

The kidney of the young infant is immature, and the renal clearance, even corrected for body surface, progressively increases until approximately 2 years of age. Therefore, renal uptake of tracer is particularly low in infants, with a high background activity.

Indications These include all pathology where an assessment of DRF and drainage is required. Renography in children is almost invariably performed following diuretic injection which provokes diuresis and therefore improves tracer drainage from a dilated and capacious collecting system.

5 Indications for MAG3 Tc^{99m} Renography

1. Pelvi-ureteric junction (PUJ) anomaly
2. Vesicoureteric junction (VUJ) anomaly
3. Drainage in boys with posterior urethral valves
4. Complicated duplex kidneys
5. DRF and drainage of congenital renal variants or ectopic kidneys

6. Following trauma
7. Following renal transplantation to assess for urinary leak or abnormal drainage
8. Bladder dysfunction

There are limitations to renography if renal function is poor or if the collecting system is dilated and drainage is poor. The drainage image, following a change in posture and micturition, if possible, will improve drainage with the effect of gravity and is an essential component for a complete study. There are no contraindications. Diuretic administration is avoided if the child has pain from an acute obstructive episode, such as with a renal calculus. The strengths of dynamic renography lie in the ability to routinely quantify DRF and drainage; serial renography is also reliable. There is a low radiation burden, especially with the use of tubular agents such as MAG3.

The optimal technique includes a well-hydrated child prior to the injection of tracer, which is accomplished by offering fluids freely before the injection. Anaesthetic cream should be applied at the injection sites; this requires a 30–45-min wait for the cream to have its effect and so provides an opportunity to ensure good hydration. The maximum recommended injected activity of Tc-99m MAG3 is 80 MBq, scaled on a body surface basis using the EANM paediatric dosage card (Lassmann and Treves 2014). The minimum recommended injected activity is Tc-99m MAG3, 15 MBq (Gordon et al. 2011). For Tc-99m MAG3, the effective dose in a 5-year-old lies between 0.20 and 0.38 mSv or around 1–2 months of background radiation in London, England, respectively (Stabin and Gelfand 1998).

Images should be acquired with the child lying supine on the camera in all circumstances except following renal transplantation when the scan is done with the camera positioned anteriorly (due to the more anterior position of the transplant kidney). Placing the child supine reduces movement, and supporting the child with sandbags plus straps around the child further stabilises the patient. When possible the child should lie directly on the collimator face. The heart, kidneys and bladder are all included in the field of view. The heart is important if analysis of the renogram will use the curve from the cardiac ROI (see below). The blood flow phase requires a rapid frame rate (0.5 s/frame for 40 s). A rate of one frame every 10 or 20 s is suggested for the standard and diuretic renogram. The DRF estimation is independent of frame time and will be the same using either 10 s or 20 s frames. The duration of the study should be a minimum of 20 min.

Diuretic administration using furosemide should be 1 mg/kg with a maximum dose of 20 mg. There are various regimes for the timing of furosemide administration; however, we favour administration soon after tracer injection in case venous access is lost later in the study. Post-furosemide acquisition parameters should use the same frame rate, zoom factor and matrix size as for the renogram.

Post-micturition (PM) Images The renogram is obtained with the patient in the supine position; thus, gravity has not had its normal effect. To allow the renogram to be analysed including the effect of gravity, the infant should be placed erect (on the carer's shoulder for 5 min), or the older child should be allowed to walk around the play area and be sent to the toilet to void. Following the administration of furosemide, almost all infants and children will void during this period. Following the void or the waiting period, the child should return to the gamma camera, and data should be acquired for 1 min in exactly the same way as for the renogram. For consistency, PM images should be acquired within 60 min after the injection of tracer. Each institution should ensure that there is an attempt to standardise the entire renogram including the time of the post-micturition image. This will allow for comparison with sequential studies as well as comparison between different children.

To analyse the renogram data from the images, the curves as well as the numerical data derived from the curves must be used together. Three parameters can be estimated: blood flow (only done for renal transplants), DRF and drainage.

Both renal and background ROIs should be drawn on all acquisition data; background ROIs should be perirenal, including the upper, outer and inferior aspects of the kidney. In the presence of gross pelvic dilatation in the young infant, a complete perirenal background may not be possible since the kidneys may extend to the edge of the body contour. In such circumstances, a background ROI above and below the kidney might be the best compromise. Background-corrected curves should be created for each acquisition series and used for analysis.

Images should include a summed image of all the frames during the clearance or uptake phase, i.e. 60–120 s after the peak of the cardiac curve (vascular phase). This image reflects the regional parenchymal function and may allow the detection of regional abnormalities. Differential function should be visually assessed on this image and compared to the DRF estimated from the curves to ensure that there is congruity of results. In addition, a series of timed images over the duration of the study should be created. The optimum is to combine frames into 1-min images covering the duration of the study, including the PM images. All images, including the post-diuretic and PM images, should be displayed with the same scaling factor. Functional images during the early phase may be useful, especially if one can create an image of pure proximal tubular function using a tubular agent, as this may allow focal parenchymal abnormalities to be seen more easily than on a summated image (giving an image similar to a posterior view from a DMSA study).

Blood flow estimation is analysis of the images where one looks for the appearance of tracer in the kidney relative to the aorta (Figs. 7 and 8). Numerical estimation is to quantify the activity in the kidney relative to either the percentage of cardiac output or the activity arrival in the aorta or iliac vessel. This is still performed in renal transplant patients, more frequently now with MAG3 rather than DTPA.

Quantification should include DRF, the relative function of each kidney expressed as a percentage of the sum of the right and left kidneys. It is computed between 60 and 120 s from the peak of the cardiac (vascular) curve. No renal depth correction is required in children. The International Scientific Committee on Radionuclides in Nephrourology has recommended either the integral method or the Patlak-Rutland plot method. The integral method uses the area under the background-corrected renograms, representing the cumulative uptake during the selected time interval (Fig. 9). The Patlak-Rutland plot method is the mean slope of the ascending portion of the curve plotting the background-corrected kidney ROI counts [R (t)] divided by the cardiac ROI counts [H (t)] as a function of the integral of the cardiac ROI counts divided by [H (t)] (Fig. 10).

For the estimation of excretion or drainage, numerous methods have been proposed. The simplest method is inspection of the curve: normal excretion (early peak with a rapidly descending curve) as well as slightly delayed excretion is readily distinguished from very abnormal excretion (continuously rising curve). Adequate assessment of the response to the diuretic must include the analysis of the PM images and also take into account the function of the kidney. This can be achieved by expressing the activity in the PM image as a percentage of the activity taken up at 2–3 min or as a ratio of the radionuclide taken up by the kidney, giving the pelvic excretion efficiency (PEE) (see Fig. 11). There are, however, no cut-off values available to differentiate between partial and poor emptying. Assessment of the diuretic response must be clearly distinguished from the interpretation of the result. Simple analysis of the post-diuretic curve is inadequate (Reproduced from *Pediatric Uroradiology*, 2nd Edition, Fotter).

Normal DRF values are between 45 and 55 % uptake. DRF values within the normal range will be seen where there is bilateral, symmetrical renal damage or in the presence of chronic renal failure. Values outside this normal range may be seen when there is an uncomplicated unilateral duplex kidney as well as in unilateral renal damage. The function of an ectopic kidney will be underestimated on dynamic

Blood flow images @ 2.5 sec each

Summared images @ 1 minute each

Functional image between 60-120 seconds representing glomerular filtration

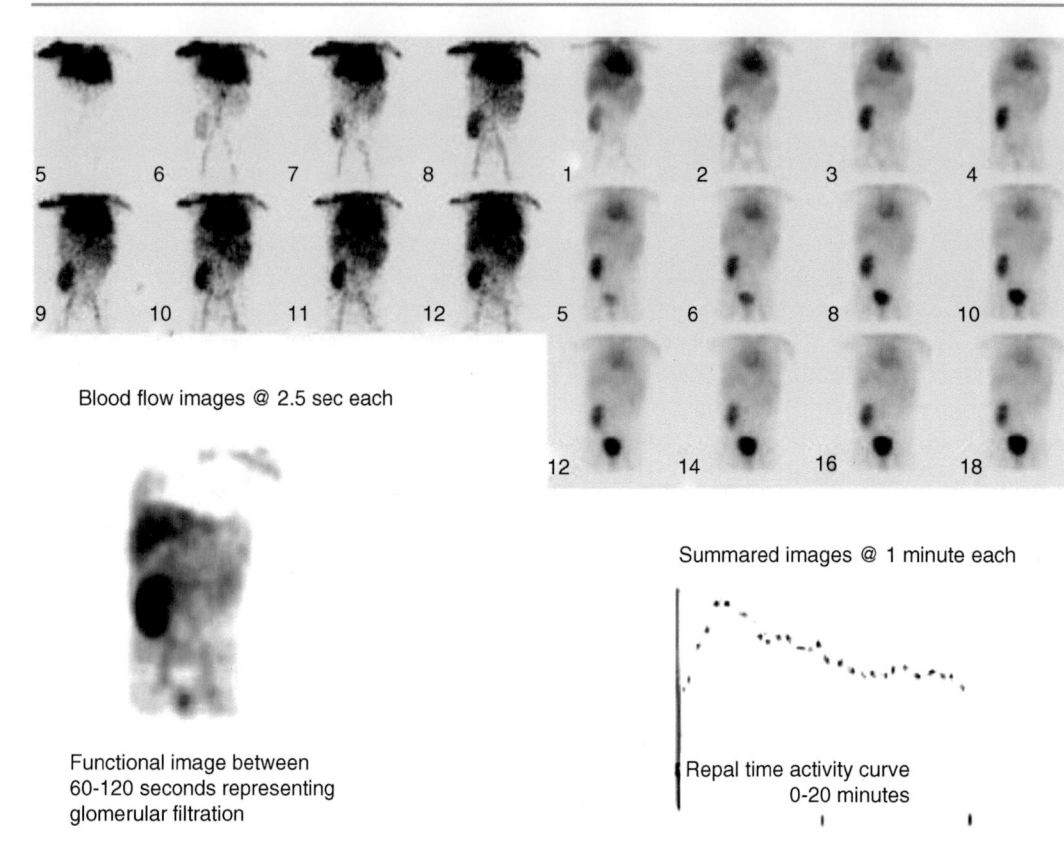

Repal time activity curve 0-20 minutes

Fig. 7 Normal Tc-99m DTPA renogram in a 6-year-old boy 4 days after a renal transplant. The eight images at upper left (labelled 5–12) represent the blood flow phase after the bolus injection of tracer. The aorta is just visible on the first frame but easily identified on the second frame; the kidney is clearly seen on the second frame representing good perfusion. The 12 images at top right are summated images over 18 min; each image represents 1 min. Note how the isotope moves from the renal parenchyma on the early images into the calyces and finally into the pelvis. The image at lower left is the functional image during the period 60–120 s, which, when using Tc-99m DTPA, represents glomerular filtration; this is normal. The renogram curve shows minimal delay in drainage. This is a normal study (Reproduced from *Pediatric Uroradiology*, 2nd Edition, Fotter)

renography: correct evaluation requires a Tc-99m DMSA scan with both posterior and anterior images. Images may show a focal renal defect on early images: dilated calyces and renal pelvis or a dilated ureter may be evident. Comparison between the renogram and PM images is important to assess the effect of a change of posture and micturition (Fig. 12).

Adequate hydration is important; this is readily achieved by including the need for good fluid intake in the information letter received prior to the study. Furthermore, since an anaesthetic cream is applied to many children and this takes up to 45 min to be fully effective, there is a second opportunity to encourage oral fluid intake. Infants could receive an additional feed, while older children could be encouraged to drink fluids (250–500 ml). The interpretation of impaired drainage is debated, and its relationship to surgery does not meet universal agreement.

Advantages of Tc-99m MAG3 renography include the ability to quantify DRF reliably, assess parenchymal abnormalities, visualise the collecting systems and assess drainage. The high extraction by the kidneys from the blood gives a low background and thus facilitates the analysis

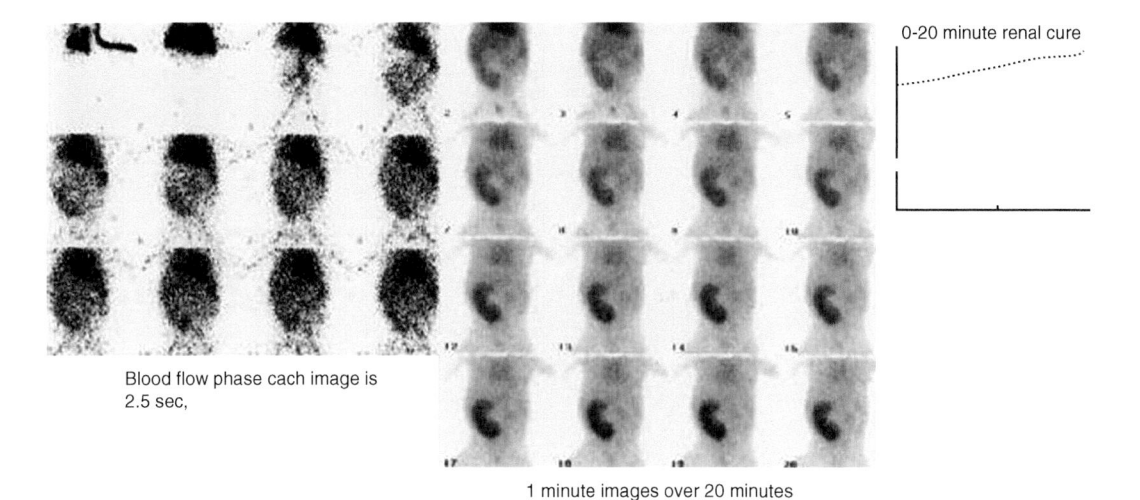

Fig. 8 Four days after renal cadaveric transplant in a 3-year-old boy with no urine output due to clot obstruction at the lower end of the ureter. The ultrasound examination including power Doppler was normal (not shown). The 12 images on the left represent the blood flow phase after the bolus injection of tracer. The aorta is seen on the third frame; the kidney is seen with difficulty on the fourth and fifth frames, showing that perfusion is present but reduced. The images on the right are 1-min images over the 20-min study; there is progressive increase in the kidney with no isotope in the bladder by the end of the 20-min period. This is reflected in the progressively rising curve. These features could represent acute tubular necrosis (ATN) or an acute obstruction; however, in this clinical situation where there was haematuria (no clots), a diagnosis of clot obstruction was suspected and proved on an antegrade study. In ATN one would expect better perfusion and filtration than is seen in this child. The clinicians were anxious that the cause of the loss of urine output was renal artery and venous pathology. This study not only excluded the possibility but also suggested the true cause (Reproduced from *Pediatric Uroradiology*, 2nd Edition, Fotter)

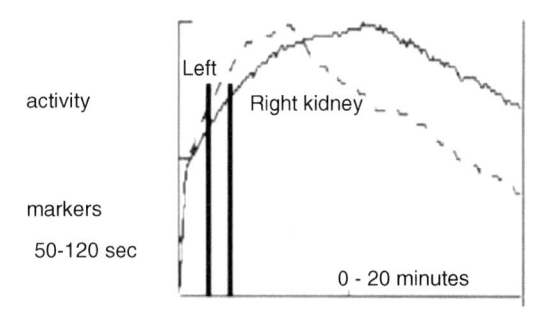

Fig. 9 Integral technique for estimation of DRF

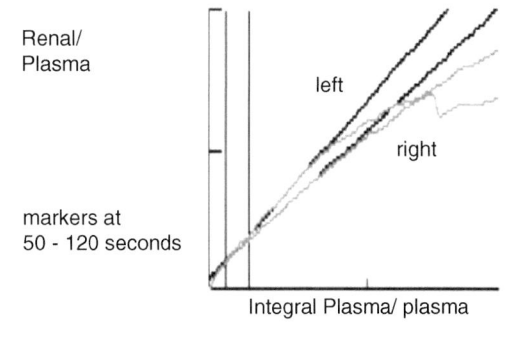

Fig. 10 Patlak plot technique for estimation of DRF

of the infant's kidneys and also reduces the radiation burden. It allows physiological assessment of the bladder and the collecting systems when an indirect radionuclide cystogram (IRC) is undertaken. The disadvantages include the fact that the child should lie still for 20 min and that movement makes analysis more difficult. There is controversy in the interpretation of the diuretic response; this is not the fault of the technique, however, but rather shows the difficulty of having an appropriate reference technique to judge infant renal pelvic dilatation.

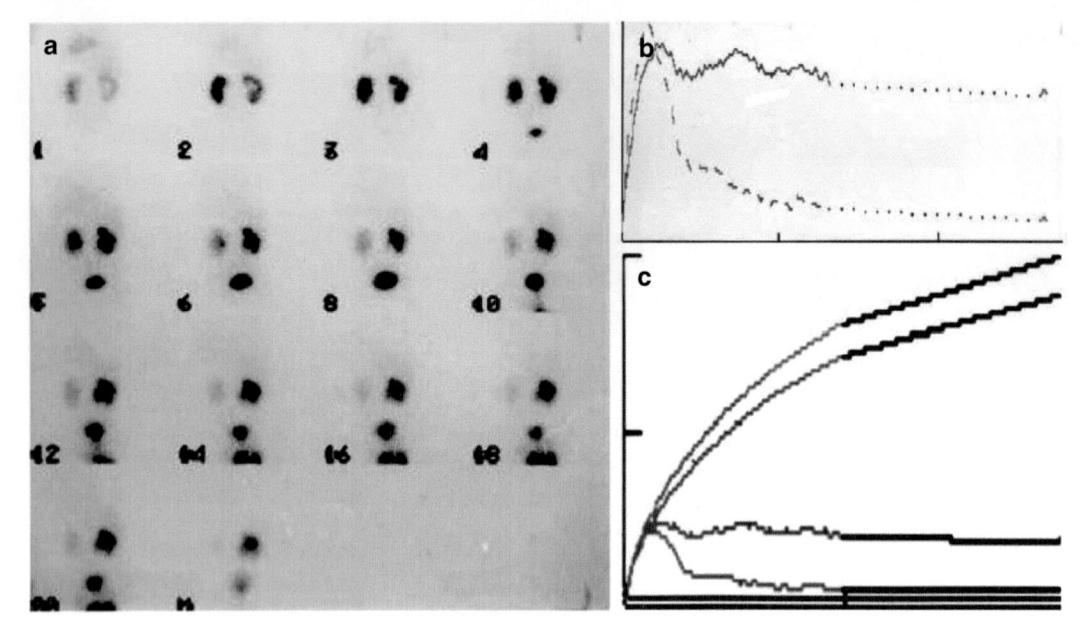

Fig. 11 Pelvic excretion efficiency (PEE). Unilateral PUJ hold-up in a 12-month-old boy with prenatal diagnosis of unilateral hydronephrosis found postnatally to have isolated right pelvic dilatation with good drainage. The diuretic Tc-99m MAG3 renogram with furosemide injected 2 min after the Tc-99m MAG3. One-minute images for the duration of the study including the post-micturition image at 40 min shows good function of both kidneys (DRF left 53 %, right 47 %), with normal drainage on the left and poor drainage on the right until 20 min, but the post-micturition image shows little isotope in the renal pelvis. (**b**) The background subtracted renogram curves over the entire study show good uptake by both kidneys and good drainage on the left. The right renal curve is almost flat from approximately 5 min onward. (**c**) These curves represent the principle of the PEE. The two lower curves represent the actual activity in each kidney over the duration of the study. The upper curves start with the actual curves but are then extrapolated as if nothing left the kidney for the duration of the study, i.e. as if the kidneys were completely obstructed. The difference between the upper and lower curve for each kidney then represents the amount of isotope, which has come into the kidney and has left the kidney. As seen in these curves, there is very good drainage from both kidneys despite the rather flat curve of the right kidney in Fig. 9b

Fig. 12 Value of post-micturition image series. Tc-99m MAG3 diuretic renogram with consecutive images over 20 min is shown. Both kidneys show prompt uptake of tracer with poor drainage by 20 min. The post-micturition image at 40 min (M) reveals little tracer in the renal pelvis on both sides. Note the bladder is also now empty. This was reflected in the curves and numerical analysis (PEE) (Reproduced from *Pediatric Uroradiology*, 2nd Edition, Fotter)

Diuretic renogram including the Post-Micturition view at 40 minutes

Note how there has been complete emptying of both collecting systems simply by adding this one additional series (see text fot details).

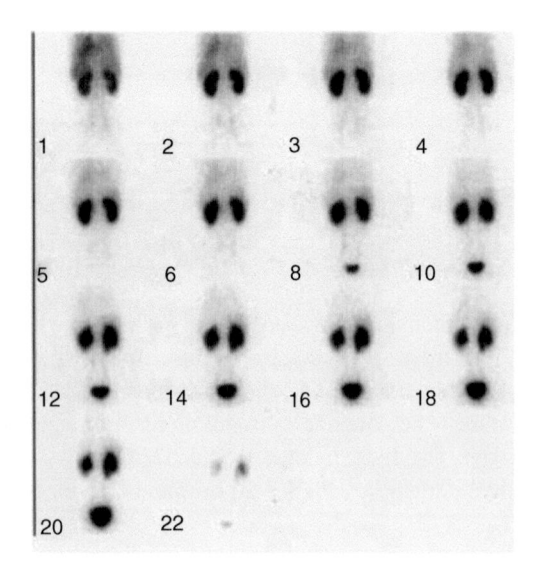

> **Take Away**
> Dynamic renography assesses renal blood flow, differential function and drainage. A post-micturition image is an essential component of the study. Full analysis includes images, numbers and curves.

6 Isotope Cystography

The voiding cystourethrogram (VCUG) is the reference technique for vesicoureteric reflux (VUR), yet VUR may be seen on one examination and not another. Figure 13 demonstrates how one may see VUR bilaterally in a child at one moment and a short while later find unilateral VUR suggesting the transient nature of reflux. All children and their parents find bladder catheterisation unpleasant, and it should be avoided if possible. In older children, it can cause both psychological and physical trauma. A reliable and accurate, non-traumatic way to assess VUR is provided by the indirect radionuclide cystogram (IRC).

There are at least four different methods for undertaking cystography in children; only the IRC with Tc-99m MAG3 precludes bladder catheterisation and is wholly physiological. In toilet-trained children, the IRC is the method of choice to detect VUR.

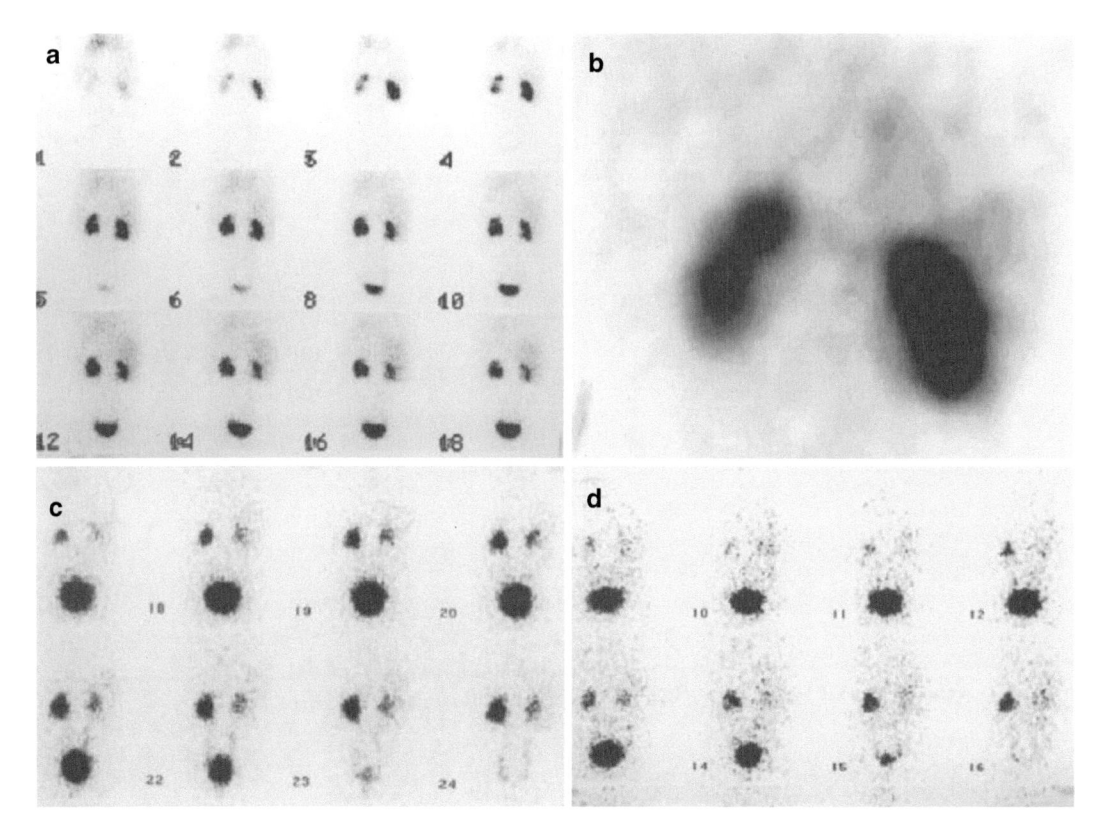

Fig. 13 (**a**–**d**) A 5-year-old girl followed up for recurrent urinary tract infections. Tc-99m MAG3 + IRC with intermittent VUR. (**a**) Images 0–18 min of the dynamic Tc-99m MAG3 renogram showing good uptake by the right kidney and good drainage. There is reduced function in the left kidney (23 % of overall function) with only moderate drainage by 18 min. (**b**) The functional image from the Tc-99m MAG3 renogram shows the damaged left kidney to better advantage. (**c**) The first micturition of the IRC shows complete bladder emptying with isotope refluxing into the left kidney before micturition and into the right kidney with micturition. (**d**) The second micturition 30 min later again shows complete bladder emptying with reflux only into the left kidney during micturition (Reproduced from *Pediatric Uroradiology*, 2nd Edition, Fotter)

6.1 Direct Radioisotope Cystography (DIC)

The use of DIC (Mandell et al. 1997a) in female infants (<1 year of age) with a severe UTI and a normal ultrasound has dwindled due to the marked reduction in radiation burden from fluoroscopic VCUG.

The advantages of the DIC are its high sensitivity for VUR because of continuous monitoring and low radiation exposure: the effective dose is approximately 0.3 mSv. The disadvantage is that bladder catheterisation is required and the anatomy and grading of VUR may be difficult, although with a contemporaneous ultrasound, the anatomy should be correctly interpreted.

The technique and procedure are similar to conventional VCUG (Fig. 14). Following bladder catheterisation, Tc-99m pertechnetate (20 MBq) is instilled followed by warm normal saline until the bladder is full, when micturition should occur. The entire procedure is carried out with double disposable diapers on the infant who is lying on top of the gamma camera linked to a computer system. Both renal areas and the bladder are kept in the field of view (Godley et al. 1990; Kuzmanovska et al. 1996).

> **Take Away**
> The DIC is a low-radiation technique to identify VUR; however, its use is falling out of favour due to a reduced radiation burden in fluoroscopic VCUG.

6.2 Indirect Radioisotope Cystography

Indirect radioisotope cystography (IRC) may be undertaken in any child who is toilet trained and cooperative (van der Vis-Melsen et al. 1989). The IRC is done following a dynamic

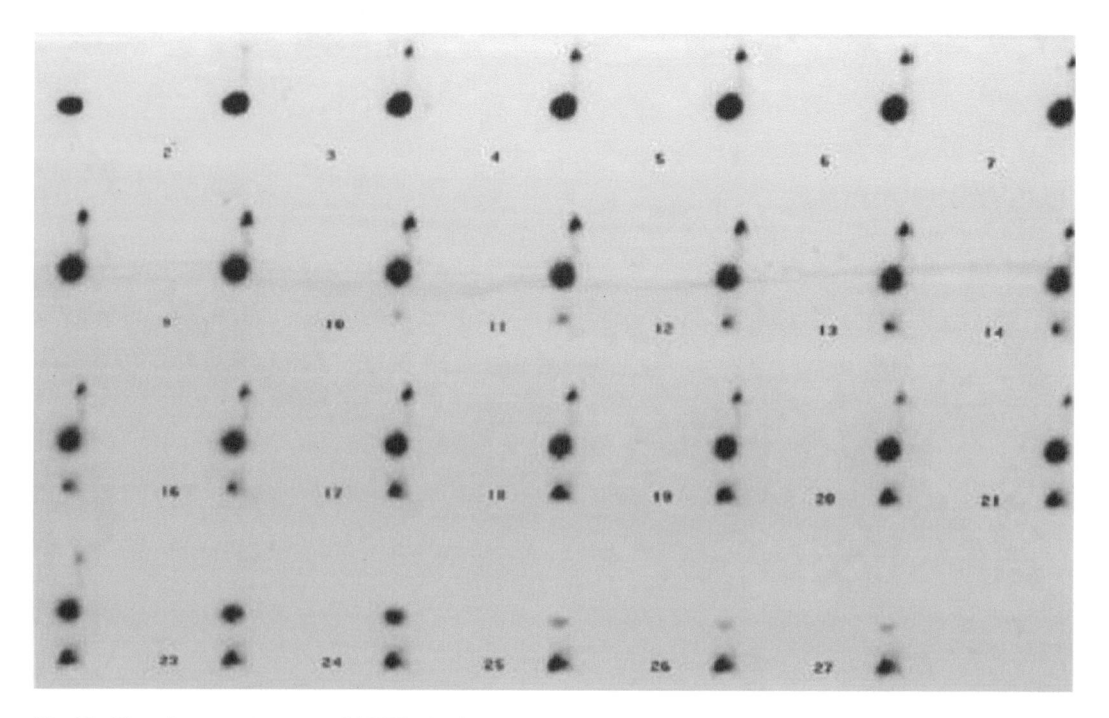

Fig. 14 Direct isotope cystogram with VUR. A 15-month-old boy with prenatal diagnosis of unilateral hydronephrosis. Postnatally the only abnormality was right VUR on VCUG. This follow-up cystogram at 15 months of age shows ongoing right renal reflux in the filling phase of this DIC (Reproduced from *Pediatric Uroradiology*, 2nd Edition, Fotter)

renogram whenever the child wishes to void. All children are adequately hydrated for the renogram and are offered drinks freely following the dynamic study so that most children do not require encouragement to void. Of note, furosemide is not given to promote diuresis unless there is a very dilated collecting system. Micturition takes place in front of the gamma camera. If at the end of micturition isotope is still noted in the bladder or kidneys, then the child should be offered more to drink and asked to return to the gamma camera room when he wishes to void again. A quiet room with few additional people and adequate privacy screens helps for a short successful examination. This is a physiological study that does not require a bladder catheter.

Detection of VUR An increase of activity in the kidney during the study indicates VUR. The filling phase of the bladder, studied with VCUG or DIC, cannot be studied with IRC. Thus, VUR present only in the filling phase will be missed by IRC. VUR is an intermittent phenomenon for which the incidence varies even using the same examination on different occasions (Fig. 13.) Evaluating any technique for the detection of VUR will remain difficult since there is no absolute reference method. There is agreement that IRC is contributory only when positive, whereas a negative examination cannot exclude VUR. This argument holds true, however, for all cystogram techniques. IRC is a valuable screening technique for the detection of reflux reaching the kidney and observation of physiological micturition; this is especially important when one is dealing with a difficult case, e.g. the older girl with recurrent UTI who has a normal ultrasound examination, normal Tc-99m DMSA, but remains symptomatic and may have bladder dysfunction (Figs. 15 and 16).

Indications for IRC include whenever VUR must be excluded in the toilet-trained older child (Figs. 13, 15 and 16); ureteric dilatation, again in the toilet-trained older child; potentially in older children with known bladder dysfunction (includ-

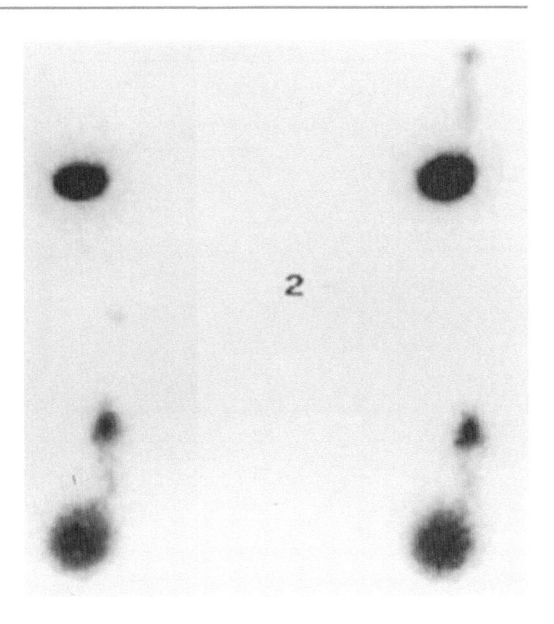

Fig. 15 IRC for recurrent urinary tract infection in a 4-year-old girl. VUR into right kidney is noted on this IRC despite the fact that there was no micturition. This suggests the diagnosis of an unstable bladder that was confirmed on further investigation (Reproduced from *Pediatric Uroradiology*, 2nd Edition, Fotter)

ing posterior urethral valve) (Dinneen et al. 1994); and girls with recurrent UTI and normal ultrasound and Tc-99m DMSA scans, in whom the entire nephro-urological system can be evaluated.

The strength of the IRC lies in the fact that the procedure has a low radiation burden; there is no increase in radiation dose above the routine renogram. Encouraging voiding will reduce the radiation burden since the bladder is the target organ. The Tc-99m MAG3 + IRC provides information about renal function and drainage with a full and empty bladder and also permits assessment of bladder function. When bladder dysfunction is suspected, this is the only physiological cystogram as it does not entail bladder catheterisation.

The weakness of IRC includes the need for the child to be toilet trained. Renal and upper ureteric reflux will be detected, but only the voiding phase of micturition is examined. When there is a high urinary flow rate, as seen after the administration of a diuretic, renal reflux may not be detectable. In the context of hydronephrosis or

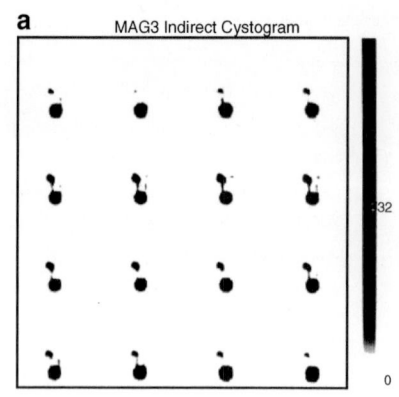

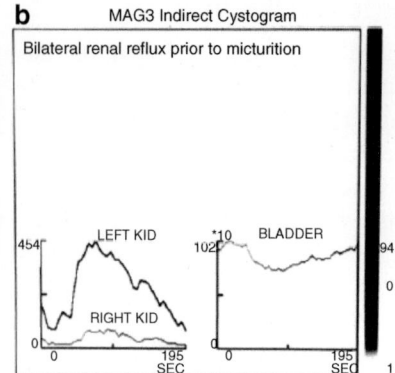

Fig. 16 Bilateral VUR prior to micturition, first on the left and then on the right. (**a**) The images are of 5-s duration; the left kidney is seen on the first image, but on the second there is little activity in the kidney. The activity however becomes obvious again by 20 s. (**b**) The *curves* show that the VUR is more marked into the left kidney than into the right kidney (Reproduced from *Pediatric Uroradiology*, 2nd Edition, Fotter)

hydroureter, reflux into a dilated, poorly draining system may be difficult to evaluate. Anatomical detail of the vesicoureteric junction is poor. The urethra is not demonstrated. The presence of a low or ectopic kidney makes the detection of VUR difficult or impossible if the kidney lies completely or in part behind the bladder. This is the case in transplant kidneys, and therefore the IRC is not helpful in detecting VUR in these children (unless there is an intraperitoneal kidney, transplanted into the very young child, rather than the more routine transplant into the iliac fossae in the older child). Comparison studies between IRC and either VCUG or DIC show variable results, with many institutions having a close correlation and others unable to achieve agreement.

Method After the routine Tc-99m MAG3 study for 20 min, the child is asked to return to the waiting room until they need to void. On return to the gamma camera room, the child voids when she is in front of the camera, which has been turned to a vertical position (the child sits on a commode with their back to the camera). Although boys prefer to stand erect, they should be encouraged to sit with their back to the gamma camera so as to reduce movement to a minimum during micturition. Acquisition should include a 30 s period both before and after micturition. The data should be collected on a computer with a fast frame rate of 1 frame/s. The processing includes viewing, regrouping the data into 5 s frames, and reviewing this data in both cine mode as well as drawing ROI over the bladder and kidneys and generating curves from these ROIs. In addition, a compressed image of the raw data should be created. The diagnosis of VUR should only be made when there is a clear increase in activity in the renal areas. If the curves suggest an increase in activity, then this must be seen either on the cine or compressed images or both. Noting only an increase on the curves is not sufficient to diagnose VUR as movement may be the cause of false abnormal curves.

There are no contraindications to IRC; however, caution should be exercised in excluding VUR when there is dilatation with poor drainage of the upper tracts. Also in the presence of a pelvic transplant kidney or a low ectopic kidney, the full bladder may obscure the kidney.

Take Away
No bladder catheterisation is required for the IRC. The Tc-99m MAG3-IRC study assesses renal function, bladder function as well as VUR in a physiological fashion.

7 Functional Imaging in Paediatric Nephro-urological Tumours and in Paediatric Post-transplant Lymphoproliferative Disorder (PTLD)

Wilms' tumour is the second most common paediatric solid tumour. Prognosis is good although higher stage disease carries significant mortality and treatment-related morbidity. DMSA SPECT CT may be useful in the assessment of functional renal tissue prior to nephron-sparing surgery (Fig. 17).

F-18-Fluorodeoxyglucose positron emission tomography/computerised tomography (FDG PET-CT) in Wilms' tumour is not usually performed; however, it may occasionally be useful in high-risk cases or in children with bilateral disease (Begent et al. 2011). FDG PET-CT is now indicated in staging and follow-up of prostate and bladder rhabdomyosarcoma (Eugene et al. 2012). Imaging using FDG PET-MRI will further improve the staging of these paediatric malignancies.

PET studies involve relatively high radiation burdens, ranging from around 8 to 13 mSv for a whole-body examination (Alessio et al. 2009). They require the child to stay still during both the PET dataset and the CT component, and thus general anaesthetic is required for the majority of cases due to the young age of patients with rhabdomyosarcoma.

Post-transplant lymphoproliferative disease (PTLD) is seen in between 1 and 10 % of all paediatric renal transplant recipients (Shroff and Rees 2004). It is an unusual entity that has many features of an immune system malignancy. It is characterised by uncontrolled proliferation of lymphoid cells, typically B cells, in a context of post-transplant immunosuppression. In some situations, reducing the immunosuppression can reverse this proliferation, thus differentiating it from truly irreversible malignancies (Cleper et al. 2012). Most PTLD cases have a strong relationship with Epstein-Barr virus (EBV). The single most important risk factor for PTLD is the lack of previous exposure to EBV in the transplant recipient, with seronegativity conferring a threefold to 33-fold higher risk of developing PTLD. Clinical presentation is variable, but an acute illness with malaise, fever, weight loss and lymphadenopathy within a year of transplant, particularly where a seronegative recipient received a seropositive kidney, is a common scenario. Diagnosis rests on assessment of viral DNA load in the blood and biopsy of an area of disease. Viral load monitoring is therefore routine following renal transplantation in a child. The usual imaging modalities of US, MRI and CT are utilised to assess and stage PTLD; however, in complex or unusual disease, 18F-FDG PET-CT imaging may be an essential step in diagnosis and staging, particularly when a site for biopsy is not forthcoming from usual cross-sectional imaging modalities. Adolescent renal transplant recipients who were EBV-naïve recipients have a slightly worse outcome than younger children with PTLD.

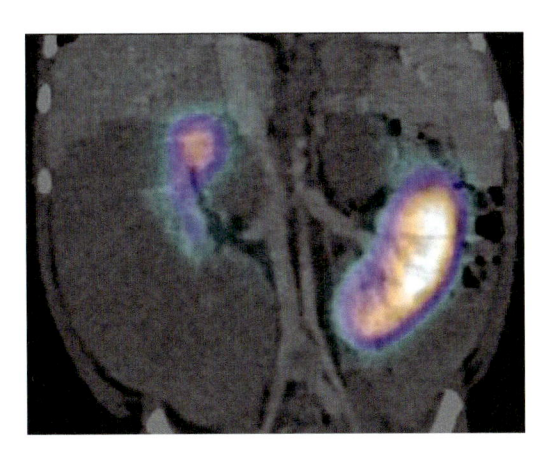

Fig. 17 DMSA SPECT CT in a 2-year-old child with nephroblastomatosis who may be a candidate for nephron-sparing surgery following chemotherapy. The SPECT DMSA was done prior to chemotherapy to assess the DRF. Contrast was administered for the low-dose CT study to delineate the vascular anatomy in relation to the kidneys distorted by the perilobar nephroblastomatosis. The coronal reformat demonstrates better function in the left kidney

> **Take Away**
> FDG PET-CT and, increasingly, FDG PET-MRI functional imaging have a role to play in diagnosis, staging and treatment options in nephro-urological malignancies and PTLD following renal transplantation.

Conclusion

Functional imaging of the renal tract is still the most common reason for a child to be referred to the nuclear medicine department.

Imaging of the kidneys to assess DRF and the extent of renal parenchymal damage by Tc-99m DMSA and Tc-99m MAG3 renography to determine DRF and drainage patterns in dilated renal collecting systems are the most common reasons to request nephro-urological studies. The IRC is extremely useful in the assessment of VUR in the toilet-trained child.

Hybrid imaging is increasingly being used in staging nephro-urological tumours in children, and this will increase in the future, with PET-MRI imaging providing a 'one stop shop' for functional nephro-urological imaging, with a reduction in radiation burden. In all radioisotope studies in children, training in handling children, immobilisation techniques and attention to detail in image processing are essential in order to provide exquisite, easily interpretable functional studies.

References

Alessio AM, Kinahan PE, Manchanda V, Ghioni V, Aldape L, Parisi MT (2009) Weight-based, low-dose pediatric whole-body PET/CT protocols. J Nucl Med: Off Pub Soc Nucl Med 50(10):1570–1577

Anderson PJ, Rangarajan V, Gordon I (1997) Assessment of drainage in PUJ dilatation: pelvic excretion efficiency as an index of renal function. Nucl Med Commun 18(9):823–826

Baumer JH, Jones RW (2007) Urinary tract infection in children, National Institute for Health and Clinical Excellence. Arch Dis Child Educ Pract Ed 92(6):189–192

Begent J, Sebire NJ, Levitt G, Brock P, Jones KP, Ell P, Gordon I, Anderson J (2011) Pilot study of F(18)-Fluorodeoxyglucose Positron Emission Tomography/computerised tomography in Wilms' tumour: correlation with conventional imaging, pathology and immunohistochemistry. Eur J Cancer 47(3):389–396

Chaiwatanarat T, Padhy AK, Bomanji JB, Nimmon CC, Sonmezoglu K, Britton KE (1993) Validation of renal output efficiency as an objective quantitative parameter in the evaluation of upper urinary tract obstruction. J Nucl Med: Off Pub Soc Nucl Med 34(5):845–848

Cleper R, Ben Shalom E, Landau D, Weissman I, Krause I, Konen O, Rahamimov R, Mor E, Bar-Nathan N, Frishberg Y et al (2012) Post-transplantation lymphoproliferative disorder in pediatric kidney-transplant recipients - a national study. Pediatr Transplant 16(6):619–626

Dinneen MD, Duffy PG, Lythgoe MF, Ransley PG, Gordon I (1994) Mercapto-acetyltriglycine (MAG 3) renography and indirect radionuclide cystography in posterior urethral valves. Br J Urol 74(6):785–789

Eugene T, Corradini N, Carlier T, Dupas B, Leux C, Bodet-Milin C (2012) (1)(8)F-FDG-PET/CT in initial staging and assessment of early response to chemotherapy of pediatric rhabdomyosarcomas. Nucl Med Commun 33(10):1089–1095

Godley ML, Ransley PG, Parkhouse HF, Gordon I, Evans K, Peters AM (1990) Quantitation of vesico-ureteral reflux by radionuclide cystography and urodynamics. Pediatr Nephrol 4(5):485–490

Gordon I, Piepsz A, Sixt R, and Auspices of Paediatric Committee of European Association of Nuclear M (2011) Guidelines for standard and diuretic renogram in children. Eur J Nucl Med Mol Imaging 38(6):1175–1188

Kuzmanovska D, Tasic V, Sahpazova E (1996) Detection of vesicoureteral reflux with radionuclide cystography. Srpski arhiv za celokupno lekarstvo 124(Suppl 1):78–81

Lassmann M, Treves ST (2014) Pediatric Radiopharmaceutical Administration: harmonization of the 2007 EANM Paediatric Dosage Card (Version 1.5.2008) and the 2010 North American Consensus guideline. Eur J Nucl Med Mol Imaging 41(8):1636

Mandell GA, Eggli DF, Gilday DL, Heyman S, Leonard JC, Miller JH, Nadel HR, Treves ST (1997a) Procedure guideline for radionuclide cystography in children. Society of Nuclear Medicine. J Nucl Med: Off Pub Soc Nucl Med 38(10):1650–1654

Mandell GA, Eggli DF, Gilday DL, Heyman S, Leonard JC, Miller JH, Nadel HR, Treves ST (1997b) Procedure guideline for renal cortical scintigraphy in children. Society of Nuclear Medicine. J Nucl Med: Off Pub Soc Nucl Med 38(10):1644–1646

Piepsz A, Arnello F, Tondeur M, Ham HR (1998) Diuretic renography in children. J Nucl Med: Off Pub Soc Nucl Med 39(11):2015–2016

Piepsz A, Colarinha P, Gordon I, Hahn K, Olivier P, Roca I, Sixt R, van Velzen J, and Paediatric Committee of the

European Association of Nuclear M (2001) Guidelines for 99mTc-DMSA scintigraphy in children. European journal of nuclear medicine 28(3):BP37–41

Piepsz A, Tondeur M, Ham H (2000) NORA: a simple and reliable parameter for estimating renal output with or without frusemide challenge. Nucl Med Commun 21(4):317–323

Prigent A, Cosgriff P, Gates GF, Granerus G, Fine EJ, Itoh K, Peters M, Piepsz A, Rehling M, Rutland M et al (1999) Consensus report on quality control of quantitative measurements of renal function obtained from the renogram: International Consensus Committee from the Scientific Committee of Radionuclides in Nephrourology. Semin Nucl Med 29(2):146–159

Ritchie G, Wilkinson AG, Prescott RJ (2008) Comparison of differential renal function using technetium-99m mercaptoacetyltriglycine (MAG3) and technetium-99m dimercaptosuccinic acid (DMSA) renography in a paediatric population. Pediatr Radiol 38(8):857–862

Rutland MD (1985) A comprehensive analysis of renal DTPA studies. I Theory and normal values. Nucl Med Commun 6(1):11–20

Shroff R, Rees L (2004) The post-transplant lymphoproliferative disorder-a literature review. Pediatr Nephrol 19(4):369–377

Stabin MG, Gelfand MJ (1998) Dosimetry of pediatric nuclear medicine procedures. O J Nucl Med: Off Pub Ital Assoc Nucl Med 42(2):93–112

van der Vis-Melsen MJ, Baert RJ, Rajnherc JR, Groen JM, Bemelmans LM, De Nef JJ (1989) Scintigraphic assessment of lower urinary tract function in children with and without outflow tract obstruction. Br J Urol 64(3):263–269

Yapar AF, Aydin M, Reyhan M, Yapar Z, Sukan A (2005) The conditions for which the geometric mean method revealed a more accurate calculation of relative renal function in 99mTc-DMSA scintigraphy. Nucl Med Commun 26(2):141–146

Video Urodynamics

Erich Sorantin, Katrin Braun, and Richard Fotter

Contents

1. Introduction 113
2. The Procedure 114
3. Findings, Applications, and Indications 115

References 116

1 Introduction

In several conditions of the lower urinary tract, a combined anatomical and functional assessment is essential. Video Urodynamics (VUD), a combination of urethrocystometry and voiding cystourethrography (VCUG), fulfills these requirements. The combination of these two methods dates back to the 1950s and underwent further development during the following decades (Enhornig et al. 1964; Bates et al. 1970; Hinman and Earl 1979; Marks and Goldman 2014). Until the 1980s there was no widespread utilization (Marks and Goldman 2014). The name was given since an analog portable fluoroscopy unit (C-arm) was used in combination with an oscilloscope for pressure recordings. Using appropriate electronic devices, both signals (fluoroscopy and pressure recordings) could be displayed on the same screen – hence the name Video Urodynamics (Marks and Goldman 2014).

Basically a double lumen catheter is placed within the bladder for contrast medium instillation as well as intravesical pressure recordings, another one in the rectum for measuring the intra-abdominal pressure – for the same purpose a catheter can be placed within the colostomy or a nasogastric tube used in case of imperforate anus.

The difference between the intravesical and intra-abdominal pressure corresponds to detrusor pressure and is calculated online.

E. Sorantin, MD (✉) • R. Fotter, MD (Retired)
Department of Radiology, Division of Pediatric Radiology, Medical University Graz, Auenbruggerplatz 34, A-8036 Graz, Austria
e-mail: Erich.Sorantin@medunigraz.at

K. Braun, MD
Department of Pediatric and Adolescent Surgery, Medical University Graz, Auenbruggerplatz 34, A-8036 Graz, Austria
e-mail: karin.braun@medunigraz.at

For assessment of the sphincter and pelvic floor activity, skin electrodes are placed on the perineum in order to obtain electromyography (EMG) tracings. Additionally the volume of contrast medium as instillation to the bladder is recorded. All signals are connected to a PC interface; the software allows displaying all signals and images simultaneously. It is the author's personal experience that fluoroscopy time is not increased as compared to VCUG. Figure 1 displays – as an example – the tracings of an unstable bladder, thus depicting the basic urodynamic patterns.

The procedure sounds rather complicated but the opposite is true – it is basically simple. The only thing to consider is that information from both modalities (fluoroscopy and urodynamics) has to be aggregated into one report. For example, VUD enables detection of vesicoureteral reflux (VUR) episodes during the filling phase caused by unstable contractions – thus enabling identification of treatable conditions which otherwise can hardly be detected.

The Procedure

In the beginning of the study, all catheters are put in place and pressure transducers getting calibrated. In addition, a check for correct transmission of fluoroscopy images is necessary. Pressure and EMG recordings are continuous, whereas pulsed fluoroscopy is used intermittently especially in episodes of detrusor contractions and voiding – the images are last-image hold captures to be stored together with all the other data and recorded information. A paper towel is put between the legs of the patient in order to assess urine loss. During micturition uroflow is recorded in addition and residual volume estimated either by fluoroscopy or ultrasound. At the end of the examination, bladder catheter removal is used for execution of a "pull-through measurement" in order to determine the urethral pressure profile. Figure 2 depicts findings in a child with neurogenic bladder.

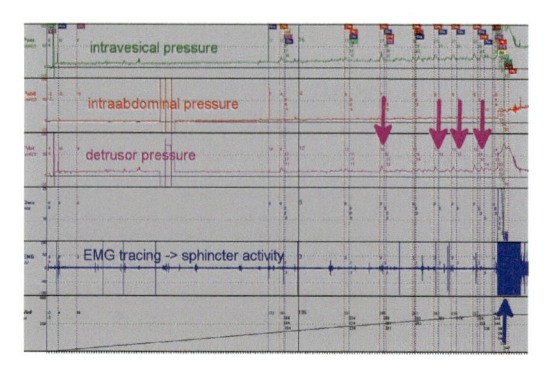

Fig. 1 Time on the *x*-axis from left to right; VUD recordings correspond to different colored lines – *green* intravesical pressure, *red* intra-abdominal pressure, *pink* detrusor pressure (equals intravesical pressure minus intra-abdominal pressure), *blue* EMG activity, and *gray* installed volume. As it can be seen at the end of the filling (*right side of the image*), there are spikes at the pressure recordings of the intravesical pressure as well as detrusor pressure (marked by *pink arrows*); intra-abdominal pressure does not change during these episodes. This is a typical pattern of unstable detrusor contractions. At micturition EMG tracings exhibit massive sphincter activity (*blue upward arrow*) – thus representing sphincter detrusor dyssynergia. Final diagnosis: unstable bladder and sphincter detrusor dyssynergia during micturition

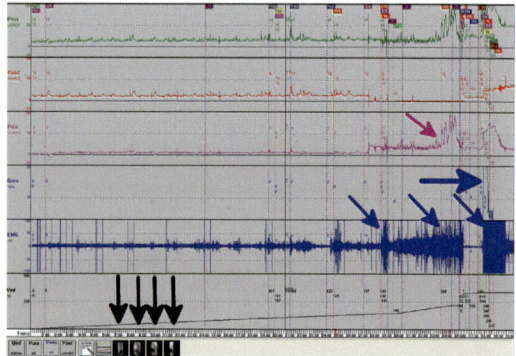

Fig. 2 VUD from a child with imperforate anus, intraspinal lipoma, and neurogenic bladder. As in Fig. 1 – *green line* intravesical pressure, *red* intra-abdominal pressure, *pink* detrusor pressure, and *blue* uroflow and sphincter activity; *black arrows* mark the saved fluoroscopy images. As it can be seen at the end of the filling, there are unstable detrusor contractions (*pink arrows*) and a burst in sphincter activity (*oblique blue arrows*). At voiding (*horizontal blue arrow*) massively increased sphincter activity is depicted. The concomitant acquired fluoroscopy images did not exhibit VUR in these phases. Final diagnosis: neurogenic bladder, contractile detrusor, and sphincter detrusor dyssynergia during micturition

3 Findings, Applications, and Indications

The findings are composed of two aspects – those from the urodynamic study and those from VCUG.
Parameters that can be obtained from the urodynamic study are:

- Detrusor pressure: difference of intravesical and rectal (intra-abdominal) pressure
  - Estimated during filling, micturition, and during unstable contractions
- Compliance: equals volume change by pressure change – $\Delta V/\Delta p$
- Safe storage volume: filling volume where intravesical pressure is lower than 40 cm H_2O, since in higher values damage of the upper urinary tract, particularly the renal parenchyma, is more likely
- Leak point pressure: the detrusor pressure in the moment where passive urine loss occurs (sphincter weakness incontinence) reflects passive urethral resistance
- Frequency, time point of occurrence, and pressure gradient of unstable detrusor contractions: per definition detrusor contractions are counted if pressure gradient changes by 10 cm H_2O from baseline. This is particularly important during VUR episodes
- Detrusor pressure during voiding: together with an increased activity at the electromyographic tracings, sphincter detrusor dyssynergia can be diagnosed in combination with a typical appearance at fluoroscopy, where the external sphincter is closed
- Uroflow and urethral pressure profile

The features obtained by fluoroscopy are:

- Bladder wall contour morphology – smooth, trabeculated, diverticulum
- Possibly persisting/recanalized urachus
- Behavior of the bladder neck
- VUR episodes and assessment of the vesico-ureteral angle
- For definition of the leak point pressure: demonstration of urine loss in addition to wetting of the paper towel between the patient's legs
- Sphincter detrusor dyssynergia during voiding
- Inability to void due to passive sphincter obstruction: even low-amplitude sphincter fasciculations lead to sphincter muscle hypertrophy, which acts as a barrier in patients with only weak detrusor contractions
- Estimation of residual post-void volume (if not measured by ultrasound)
- Pelvic floor palsy

Conclusion and Take Away
VUD is the combination of VCUG with pressure/flow/electromyographic studies of the lower urinary tract. It is the gold standard for the assessment of children with neurogenic bladder dysfunction and only a second-step study in children with non-neurogenic bladder sphincter dysfunction (voiding dysfunction).

All the abovementioned diagnostic markers have to be aggregated into a conclusive report, thus delivering all relevant information for further patient management. According to our experience and that of others, VUD is the gold standard for investigating children with neurogenic bladder, whenever and wherever it is available. For children with non-neurogenic bladder-sphincter dysfunction, VUD only is a second-step investigation. VUD should be performed in cases where a ("modified") VCUG study is indistinct or when complex dysfunctional patterns can be expected from (e.g., non-neurogenic/neurogenic bladder dysfunction), which need comprehensive and complex management (see also chapters "Urinary Problems Associated with Imperforate Anus", "Epispadias-Exstrophy Complex", "Non-neurogenic Bladder-Sphincter Dysfunction ("Voiding Dysfunction")", and "Neurogenic Bladder in Infants and Children").

References

Bates CP, Whiteside CG, Turner-Warwick RT (1970) Synchronous cine pressure flow cysto-urethrography, with special reference to stress and urge incontinence. Br J Urol 42:714–722

Enhornig G, Miller ER, Hinman F Jr (1964) Urethral closure studied with cineroentgenography and simultaneous bladder-urethra pressure recording. Surg Gynecol Obstet 118:507–511

Hinman F Jr, Earl R (1979) Miller: an appreciation. Urol Clin North Am 6:3–6

Marks BK, Goldman HB (2014) Videourodynamics: indications and technique. Urol Clin North Am 41(3):383–391, vii–viii

Nomenclature and Reporting

Pierre-Hugues Vivier and Freddy Avni

Contents

1	Introduction	117
2	**How to Report**	118
2.1	General Consideration	118
2.2	Number of Kidneys	118
2.3	Location of Kidneys	118
2.4	Renal Size	118
2.5	Renal Parenchymal Morphology	119
2.6	Pelvicaliceal Dilatation	120
2.7	Urinary Bladder	121
2.8	Urethra	121
2.9	Conclusion of the Report = Interpretation of Findings	121
Conclusion		121
References		122

P.-H. Vivier (✉)
Service de radiopédiatrie, CHU Charles-Nicolle, 1, rue de Germont, 76031 Rouen cedex, France

X-Ray expert, Maison médicale, Hôpital Privé de l'Estuaire, 505, rue Irène-Joliot-Curie, 76620 Le Havre, France
e-mail: pierrehuguesvivier@yahoo.fr

F. Avni, MD, PhD
Department of Pediatric Radiology, Jeanne de Flandre Hospital, Lille University Hospital, 59037 Lille, France
e-mail: favni@skynet.be

1 Introduction

Reports in uroradiology should be well structured with a systematic description of normal findings and potential pathology. Reports have to be understandable by all physicians who may have to manage children with urologic or nephrologic disorders. To achieve this goal, terms have to be standardized and accepted by the medical community in general. The European Society of Pediatric Radiology uroradiology task force is currently working on harmonizing and standardizing uroradiologic terminology in cooperation with European urologists and nephrologists.

Whatever the imaging modality, a classical report should include a description and eventually an interpretation; the description should address the following items (if applicable):

- Number, location, size
- Renal parenchyma morphology
- Potential dilatation of urinary cavities
- All relevant bladder features including ostia and distal ureters, and (if applicable) the urethra, the perirenal and perivesical space need to be included

2 How to Report

2.1 General Consideration

When referring to the anatomy of the urogenital tract, the natural flow of urine from the kidney to the urethra has to be considered. *Proximal* means close to the arriving urine unlike *distal* which means downstream. For example, the proximal ureter is close to the kidney, whereas the distal part is close to the bladder. Furthermore, the terms used in the report should be consistent, and a standardized fashion including relevant measurements should be respected.

2.2 Number of Kidneys

Usually two kidneys are present. In case of a solitary kidney, the term *renal agenesis* should be avoided as imaging cannot determine the cause of the missing kidney (shrinkage or renal agenesis) or some remnants may not be depictable. The radiological absent kidney may correspond to a real renal agenesis or more often results from an involution of dysplastic kidney tissue or an ectopic renal bud difficult to visualize (Zaffanello et al. 2009). In this context, ipsilateral Müllerian or Wolffian anomalies are frequently associated. Therefore, genital abnormalities have to be screened and reported.

Supernumerary kidneys are exceptional. The supernumerary kidney is a definitive accessory organ with its own collecting system, blood supply, and distinct encapsulated parenchyma. It should not be confused with a duplex kidney which is much more frequent. A *duplex kidney* corresponds to a renal unit with a single capsule, containing two pyelocalyceal systems associated with either a single or double ureters. In case of two ureters, a complete duplicated (separated) set of ureters can be observed with two ureterovesical junctions and ostia, or the ureters can fuse (anywhere) on its course and drain by a single ostium. The former malformation is called *duplicated ureter* and is often associated with disease; the latter is called *bifid ureter* and is often just an anatomic variant. If a parenchymal renal bridge is present without pyelocalyceal dilatation and without vesical abnormality, ultrasound (US) is generally not able to differentiate both entities, except if the two ostia (with two separate urinary inflow jets) can be depicted.

The term *double kidney* has an unclear meaning and should be avoided.

2.3 Location of Kidneys

Kidneys are normally located in the lumbar fossae. Embryologically, they migrate cephalad from the pelvis to the level of the adrenal glands. An *ectopic kidney* is defined by its location elsewhere than in the lumbar fossa and results from a failure of the normal migration (see chapters "Urinary Tract Embryology, Anatomy and Anatomical Variants" and "Anomalies of Kidney Rotation, Position and Fusion"). It is generally located below (*pelvic kidney*, *iliac kidney*, *horseshoe kidney*) or on the opposite side (*crossed renal ectopia* with or without fusion with the other kidney) of its usual position. Exceptionally, the cephalad migration of the kidney can be excessive prior to the diaphragmatic closure or in combination with delayed diaphragmatic closure, then even resulting in an intrathoracic location.

2.4 Renal Size

The size of both kidneys should be reported in every report when kidneys are measurable. Kidney volume is usually correlated with the single kidney glomerular filtration rate. Kidney length is generally considered as a surrogate measurement of kidney volume. The long axis has to be compared to age-related normal values (Dinkel et al. 1985; Kadioglu 2010; Konus et al. 1998; Rosenbaum et al. 1984). Nomograms should be easily accessible when reporting; patient age/size/weight must be available. Normal values are included within the interval range: mean ± 2 standard deviations.

However, it should be kept in mind that the correlation between kidney length and kidney volume is quite poor (Bakker et al. 1999; Emamian et al. 1993; van den Dool et al. 2005).

In case of pelvicaliceal dilatation, the kidney often increases in size due to the urine accumulation although the kidney parenchymal volume may be decreased. Moreover, the variability in sonographic measurement of renal length is comparable to the expected annual increase in length during childhood (2–6 mm per year). Also renal length in the same patient may vary in a small amount, up to 4.3%, with the hydration status (Peerboccus et al. 2013). Therefore, caution is suggested when using sonography to evaluate renal growth in children during a year's time.

Some authors have reported the use of the ellipsoid formula (kidney volume = length × width × thickness × 0.5) to estimate kidney volume. However, the volumes are underestimated by the ellipsoid formula to up to 20% with a large variability that does not allow a systematic correction (Bakker et al. 1999). The inaccuracy occurs because the kidney is not a true ellipsoid and because errors in measurements in the three dimensions can be additive (Emamian et al. 1995).

Other authors proposed to measure renal parenchymal area (Cost et al. 1996) on an oblique coronal view or the parenchymal thickness (Emamian et al. 1995). Both methods have shown to have a poor reproducibility and are considered unwieldy in a clinical setting (Brandt et al. 1982; Jeon 2013).

Semiautomatic renal volume measurement techniques have been developed with (3D) US, CT, and MRI (Breau et al. 2013; Riccabona et al. 2005; Vivier et al. 2008). The results are promising, but these algorithms are time consuming or not widely available and not used for routine examinations.

Despite its limitations, kidney length is the most important measurement in daily practice. Comparison of measured values with the previous ones is key when reporting.

2.5 Renal Parenchymal Morphology

- *Thickness*: This parameter is also an indirect estimate of kidney volume. Age-related renal parenchymal thickness values have been published (Kadioglu 2010). However, in case of pelvicaliceal dilatation, the thickness can be decreased due to a tissular stretching rather than to a real parenchymal volume shrinkage.
- *Corticomedullary differentiation:* US and MRI allow for observing the corticomedullary differentiation without contrast injection. For consistency, the echogenicity of the cortex has to be compared to the adjacent spleen and liver. It should be mentioned in every report, even if normal.

  Note that a transient increase in the echogenicity of the pyramids is commonly seen in neonates and is the result of physiologic events in the postnatal period. The maximal hyperechogenicity is located at the apex of the pyramids near/in the papillae. This increased echogenicity is transient and usually resolves in a few days when the infants have been hydrated and urine output reaches the standard rate. The cause of this transient increase in echogenicity in neonates remains uncertain, but seems to be independent from the deposition of Tamm-Horsfall protein as suggested formerly.

  Corticomedullary differentiation can be increased (for instance, in the neonatal period and in hemolytic and uremic syndrome or in acute cortical necrosis) (Kraus et al. 1990), decreased, or reversed. A decreased differentiation is often but not always suggestive of a poor single kidney function (Mercado-Deane et al. 2002). In this case, the term *renal dysplasia* should be avoided by radiologists as it is a histological term corresponding to undifferentiated and metaplastic tissues (see chapter "Imaging in Renal Agenesis, Dysplasia, Hypoplasia and Cystic Diseases of the Kidney"). The simple description of *loss of corticomedullary differentiation* is recommended. A reversed corticomedullary differentiation is seen, for example, in medullary nephrocalcinosis (see chapters "Urolithiasis and Nephrocalcinosis" and "Imaging of Urolithiasis and Nephrocalcinosis").
- *Scarring:* Visualization of cortical scarring is common with MRI and CT, but it can be observed also with US. It should not be confused with *junctional parenchymal defect* or

line (corresponding to the fusion of fetal lobulations) that appears as a triangular echogenic focus peripherally without cortical loss and between pyramids, unlike scarring that develops in front of pyramids.

- *Cysts:* They can be sporadic, acquired, or inherited. Their absence at birth does not preclude their appearance during childhood. The number, size, features, and location of cysts should be described. They can be located in the cortex (mainly subcapsular or not) or medulla, at their junction, or in all of these and parapelvic. In case of renal cysts, the liver, spleen, and pancreas have to be evaluated for cysts. For proper interpretation of these findings, the medical history of the patient and the knowledge of a family history of cystic disease are of utmost importance (see chapters "Renal Agenesis, Dysplasia, Hypoplasia and Cystic Diseases of the Kidney" and "Imaging in Renal Agenesis, Dysplasia, Hypoplasia and Cystic Diseases of the Kidney").

- *Tumors/space occupying and other focal lesions:* The size, location, content (tissue, calcifications, fat, liquid, or necrosis), vascularization, borders, local and distal extension, as well as relation to surrounding structures have to be described. Differentiation against a parenchymal bridge needs to be considered as well as other pseudotumoral (inflammatory) lesions; a potential membrane-like containment may indicate an abscess. Patency of the renal vein and inferior vena cava has to be systematically imaged. Note that nonhemorrhagic peritoneal effusion is often present without peritoneal rupture (Brisse et al. 2008) (see chapter "Neoplasms of the Genitourinary System").

In case of *acute obstruction*, dilatation of the urinary cavities is often absent within the first hours.

Chronic dilatation of the collecting system does not necessarily indicate obstruction. The current definition of *chronic obstruction* in practice is the one described by Peters and Koff (Koff 1987; Peters 1995) and is based on functional deterioration and loss of growth potential rather than morphologic changes. Based on this definition, none of the terms describing an upper urinary tract dilatation should have an "obstruction" connotation. As a result, the term "obstruction" should be avoided by radiologists in case of chronic dilatation.

Dilatation of the pelvis and calices is sometimes referred to as *hydronephrosis*. However, this term has been used with different meanings. Depending on physicians and institutions, a notion of chronic obstruction can be included in this term. That is the reason why the use of *hydronephrosis* should be avoided, and simple and descriptive terms such as *pelvicaliceal dilatation* should be preferred. This has been also recently addressed by a consensus statement from the USA where a new suggestion for grading urinary tract dilatation has been proposed, in addition to or replacing the existing "hydronephrosis" grading schemes (Nguyen et al. 2014). Furthermore, the ESPR abdominal imaging task force has also changed its terminology and grading of former "hydronephrosis" to "pelvicaliceal distentions / dilatation (PCD)" and issued a respective statement (Riccabona et al. 2017).

A *ureteral dilatation* should not be described as a *megaureter* as this term may be misleading. It should always be prefaced with the terms

2.6 Pelvicaliceal Dilatation

It should be emphasized that the anteroposterior diameter of the intrarenal pelvis (Fig. 1) is more important than the extrarenal diameter. Dilatation of calices and their shape should be described. The diameter of the proximal and distal ureter should be reported whenever possible, also addressing peristalsis and ureteral or pelvic wall thickening. On US, M-mode can be used to document peristalsis.

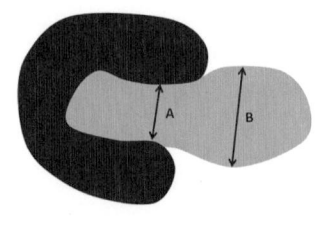

Fig. 1 Measurement of anteroposterior (AP) renal pelvis diameter on a true axial view of the kidney. This view has to be orthogonal to the long axis of the kidney. The classical AP diameter has to be measured in the intrarenal portion, between the hilar lips (**A**). If an additional measure of the extrarenal pelvis (**B**) is performed, it should be mentioned that this measurement is "extrarenal"

primary, *secondary*, *obstructive*, or *refluxing*. Note that a combination of both mechanisms can occasionally coexist. It can be shown by a post-micturition evaluation for "trapped" urine above the ureterovesical junction. When describing a dilated ureter without knowing the etiology, the term *megaureter* should be avoided. If the cause is unknown, the term *ureteral dilatation* (or *ureteropelvicaliceal dilatation* if any) should be used.

2.7 Urinary Bladder

The bladder wall and its content should be described. Mobile debris is sometimes visible and not systematically associated with urinary tract infection.

Urologists sometimes request *post-void residual urine* measurement. Healthy infants and toddlers have shown not to empty the bladder completely with every micturition, but they do so at least once during a four-hour observation. Normal residual urine volume is zero, while 20 ml or more on repeat measurements is pathological. Values between these two measurements represent a possible clinical relevant amount of residual urine. In older children, an easy and useful definition is the presence of a residual urine volume higher than 10% of the *expected/actual bladder capacity* (Jansson et al. 2000; Neveus et al. 2006). In practice, the definition of the *expected bladder capacity* is the one of the *expected maximum voided volume* calculated via the formula [30 + (age in years × 30)], in mL. For US measurement of this volume, an individually adapted correction factor has to be applied depending on the bladder shape (Knorr et al. 1990, see also chapter "Normal Values").

The morphology of the bladder wall should be described, especially if it is regular or not or if there are diverticula, trabeculations, or focal or global thickening. The bladder thickness is difficult to evaluate as it depends on the filling status. The thickness of the bladder wall decreases continuously as the bladder fills. Bladder wall thickness measurement seems to be more reproducible when nearly empty (Jequier and Rousseau 1987; Kaefer et al. 1997).

2.8 Urethra

If applicable, difficulties in catheterization have to be reported, as usually some sort of filling is required for assessing the urethra either fluoroscopically or by perineal and penile US. The entire urethra must be imaged because disease can occur anywhere from the bladder base to the urethral meatus.

In case of opacification, steep oblique imaging is optimal, especially in male to avoid superimposition of penile urethra and posterior urethra.

Precise location of abnormalities has to be described. The male urethra is divided into anterior and posterior portions. The *posterior urethra* is composed of the *prostatic* and *membranous urethra* (through the urogenital diaphragm). The *anterior urethra* is composed of the *bulbar* and *penile urethra*.

2.9 Conclusion of the Report = Interpretation of Findings

A conclusion must be drawn at the end of every report. It should not repeat the previous reported findings but should provide a comprehensive diagnosis deducted from the findings described above. Ideally, the primary abnormality should be mentioned at first with its consequences thereafter. The conclusion should include other data from the clinical history or from other imaging modalities. For example, if unilateral ureteropelvicaliceal dilatation is found at US and that a previous VCUG did not show VUR, the conclusion should suggest a primary megaureter as the diagnosis. Furthermore, any limitations of the study (e.g., some parts not visible, artifacts, etc.) need to be mentioned. And a recommendation on further complementing imaging should be stated if deemed necessary.

> **Conclusion**
>
> Use of rigorous imaging technique, systematic reporting, standardized terminology, and a comprehensive conclusion improves the quality of the examination and avoids potential misunderstandings.

References

Bakker J, Olree M, Kaatee R, de Lange EE, Moons KG, Beutler JJ, Beek FJ (1999) Renal volume measurements: accuracy and repeatability of US compared with that of MR imaging. Radiology 211(3): 623–628

Brandt TD, Neiman HL, Dragowski MJ, Bulawa W, Claykamp G (1982) Ultrasound assessment of normal renal dimensions. J Ultrasound Med 1(2):49–52

Breau RH, Clark E, Bruner B, Cervini P, Atwell T, Knoll G, Leibovich BC (2013) A simple method to estimate renal volume from computed tomography. Can Urol Assoc J 7(5-6):189–192

Brisse HJ, Schleiermacher G, Sarnacki S, Helfre S, Philippe-Chomette P, Boccon-Gibod L, Peuchmaur M, Mosseri V, Aigrain Y, Neuenschwander S (2008) Preoperative Wilms tumor rupture: a retrospective study of 57 patients. Cancer 113(1):202–213

Cost GA, Merguerian PA, Cheerasarn SP, Shortliffe LM (1996) Sonographic renal parenchymal and pelvicaliceal areas: new quantitative parameters for renal sonographic followup. J Urol 156(2 Pt 2):725–729

Dinkel E, Ertel M, Dittrich M, Peters H, Berres M, Schulte-Wissermann H (1985) Kidney size in childhood. Sonographical growth charts for kidney length and volume. Pediatr Radiol 15(1):38–43

Emamian SA, Nielsen MB, Pedersen JF (1995) Intraobserver and interobserver variations in sonographic measurements of kidney size in adult volunteers. A comparison of linear measurements and volumetric estimates. Acta Radiol 36(4):399–401

Emamian SA, Nielsen MB, Pedersen JF, Ytte L (1993) Kidney dimensions at sonography: correlation with age, sex, and habitus in 665 adult volunteers. AJR Am J Roentgenol 160(1):83–86

Jansson UB, Hanson M, Hanson E, Hellstrom AL, Sillen U (2000) Voiding pattern in healthy children 0 to 3 years old: a longitudinal study. J Urol 164(6):2050–2054

Jeon HG (2013) Estimating renal volume from CT: Is this is easiest way? Can Urol Assoc J 7(5-6):193–194

Jequier S, Rousseau O (1987) Sonographic measurements of the normal bladder wall in children. AJR Am J Roentgenol 149(3):563–566

Kadioglu A (2010) Renal measurements, including length, parenchymal thickness, and medullary pyramid thickness, in healthy children: what are the normative ultrasound values? AJR Am J Roentgenol 194(2):509–515

Kaefer M, Barnewolt C, Retik AB, Peters CA (1997) The sonographic diagnosis of infravesical obstruction in children: evaluation of bladder wall thickness indexed to bladder filling. J Urol 157(3):989–991

Koff SA (1987) Problematic ureteropelvic junction obstruction. J Urol 138(2):390

Konus OL, Ozdemir A, Akkaya A, Erbas G, Celik H, Isik S (1998) Normal liver, spleen, and kidney dimensions in neonates, infants, and children: evaluation with sonography. AJR Am J Roentgenol 171(6):1693–1698

Kraus RA, Gaisie G, Young LW (1990) Increased renal parenchymal echogenicity: causes in pediatric patients. Radiographics 10(6):1009–1018

Mercado-Deane MG, Beeson JE, John SD (2002) US of renal insufficiency in neonates. Radiographics 22(6):1429–1438

Neveus T, von Gontard A, Hoebeke P, Hjalmas K, Bauer S, Bower W, Jorgensen TM, Rittig S, Walle JV, Yeung CK, Djurhuus JC (2006) The standardization of terminology of lower urinary tract function in children and adolescents: report from the Standardisation Committee of the International Children's Continence Society. J Urol 176(1):314–324

Peerboccus M, Damry N, Pather S, Devriendt A, Avni F (2013) The impact of hydration on renal measurements and on cortical echogenicity in children. Pediatr Radiol 43(12):1557–1565

Peters CA (1995) Urinary tract obstruction in children. J Urol 154(5):1874–1883; discussion 1883–1874

Riccabona M, Fritz GA, Schollnast H, Schwarz T, Deutschmann MJ, Mache CJ (2005) Hydronephrotic kidney: pediatric three-dimensional US for relative renal size assessment--initial experience. Radiology 236(1):276–283

Riccabona M, Lobo M-L, Ording-Muller L-S, Thomas Augdal A, Fred Avni E, Blickman J, Bruno C, Damasio B, Darge K, Ntoulia A, Papadopoulou F, Vivier P-H (2017) European Society of Paediatric Radiology Abdominal imaging task force recommendations in paediatric uroradiology, part IX: imaging in anorectal and cloacal malformation, imaging in childhood ovarian torsion, and efforts in standardising paediatric uroradiology terminology. Pediatr Radiol 47(10):1369–1380

Rosenbaum DM, Korngold E, Teele RL (1984) Sonographic assessment of renal length in normal children. AJR Am J Roentgenol 142(3):467–469

van den Dool SW, Wasser MN, de Fijter JW, Hoekstra J, van der Geest RJ (2005) Functional renal volume: quantitative analysis at gadolinium-enhanced MR angiography--feasibility study in healthy potential kidney donors. Radiology 236(1):189–195

Vivier PH, Dolores M, Gardin I, Zhang P, Petitjean C, Dacher JN (2008) In vitro assessment of a 3D segmentation algorithm based on the belief functions theory in calculating renal volumes by MRI. AJR Am J Roentgenol 191(3):W127–134

Vivier P-H, Augdal TA, Avni FE, Bacchetta J, Beetz R, Bjerre AK, Blickman J, Cochat P, Coppo R, Damasio B, Darge K, El-Ghoneimi A, Hoebeke P, Läckgren G, Leclair M-D, Lobo M-L, Manzoni G, Marks SD, Mattioli G, Mentzel H-J, Mouriqu P, Nevéus T, Ntoulia A, Ording-Muller L-S, Oswald J, Papadopoulou F, Porcellini G, Ring E, Rösch W, Teixeira AF, Riccabona M (2017) Standardization of pediatric uroradiological terms: a multidisciplinary European glossary. Pediatr Radiol. https://doi.org/10.1007/s00247-017-4006-7

Zaffanello M, Brugnara M, Zuffante M, Franchini M, Fanos V (2009) Are children with congenital solitary kidney at risk for lifelong complications? A lack of prediction demands caution. Int Urol Nephrol 41(1):127–135

Contrast Agents in Childhood: Application and Safety Considerations

Michael Riccabona and Hans-Joachim Mentzel

Contents

1	Introduction...	123
2	**Ultrasound (US) Contrast Agents**............	124
3	**Radiopaque Iodine-Based Contrast Agents**..	125
3.1	Intracavitarily Applied Radiopaque Iodine-Based Contrast Agents...............	125
3.2	Intravascularly Applied Radiopaque Iodine-Based Contrast Agents (CA).......	126
4	**Gadolinium (Gd)-Based MR Contrast Agents**..	127
5	**Summary and Conclusion**........................	129
	References...	129

M. Riccabona, MD (✉)
Department of Radiology, Division of Pediatric Radiology, University Hospital Graz, Auenbruggerplatz 34, A – 8036 Graz, Austria
e-mail: michael.riccabona@meduni-graz.at

H.-J. Mentzel, MD
Section of Paediatric Radiology, Institute of Diagnostic and Interventional Radiology, University Hospital Jena, Erlanger Allee 101, D – 0774 Jena, Germany
e-mail: Hans-Joachim.Mentzel@med.uni-jena.de

1 Introduction

Contrast agents are essential for a number of radiological studies in children; most of them are handled and excreted by the kidney. This chapter tries to summarize the relevant contrast agents that are used in childhood imaging, to give some considerations toward age and weight-adapted dose, and to discuss safety issues including precautions helpful to avoid complications or their sequelae. Contrast agents and applications outside the genitourinary tract as well as those not primarily handled by the kidney are not addressed – a comprehensive summary of all potential applications and risks can be found in the book entitled *Contrast Media: Safety Issues and ESUR Guidelines* (Thomsen et al. 2014).

In general, basic rules as in adults apply also in children. In older children and adolescents, there is no significant difference to adult use, application, and handling. However, particularly in early childhood, specific physiologic phenomena have to be considered such as renal immaturity and the respective impact on contrast handling and dose in neonates, the higher relative circulating blood volume (up to 120 ml/kg body-weight – compared to adults with around 80 ml/kg bodyweight), the different tissue composition (with less fat necessitating contrast for studies which might be diagnostic in adults without using an intravenous contrast agents), or a faster heart rate with shorter distances causing shorter circulation time and impacting delay time in CT and MRI.

Orally and rectally applied contrast agents are usually not or only in small portions absorbed, and thus these do not pose a realistic threat to the kidney – these will not be addressed. The following will focus on the three main groups used for intravascular or intracavitary opacification – ultrasound contrast agents, radiopaque iodine-based contrast agents, and gadolinium (Gd)-based contrast agents.

During pregnancy ultrasound and MRI should be preferred as urogenital tract imaging methods for queries in adolescents/young adults. Contrast agents should be avoided if possible, especially in the first trimester. If a contrast-enhanced study is necessary, macrocyclic gadolinium-based agents have to be used for MRI. There are no reported restrictions with contrast-enhanced ultrasound during pregnancy; however, it should be used with caution (Webb 2014). If any contrast application (iodinated or gadolinium-based agents) is necessary in breastfeeding mothers, there is no evidence that oral ingestion of contrast agents by an infant (less than 1 % of the ingested contrast agent is absorbed by the gastrointestinal tract) would cause any toxic effects. Thus, and also according to ESUR recommendations, it is safe for infant and mother to continue breastfeeding after receiving such an agent, though some centers still advocate a 24 h breastfeeding brake.

> **Take Away**
> Contrast agents are also used for imaging neonates, infants, and children. Though general similar rules apply, there are some differences, particularly in terms of renal handling and body physiology – impacting contrast agent use and application. These aspects need to be considered when applying contrast agents in childhood.

2 Ultrasound (US) Contrast Agents

Intravenously applied US contrast agents are metabolized by the liver using physiologic pathways for the various carrier molecules; the micro-gas bubbles are eliminated by the lung (Calliada et al. 1998; ter Haar 2009). These agents are not handled by the kidney and therefore can be used also in renal failure. However, at present there is no US contrast agent available that is registered for intravascular pediatric use in Europe – and therefore all those pediatric applications are off-label (i.e., will need a profound indication and validation for the study, as well as an informed consent). Only recently, the intravenous use of the US contrast agent "Lumason®" (Bracco, Milan, Italy) was approved for pediatric liver applications (and use in the pediatric bladder for VUR assessment) in the USA; a broader approval for pediatric applications is expected in Europe (it was recently approved for pediatric intravesical use by the EMA). Nevertheless, US contrast agents are used for imaging children and – to the author's opinion – these need to be promoted, especially due to their huge potential to reduce the need for studies with radiation burden or methodically sophisticated studies as MRI and as these US contrast agents appear to be relatively safe (Darge et al. 2013; Papadopoulou et al. 2014; Piscaglia and Bolondi 2006; Piskunowicz et al. 2012; Riccabona 2012). As rarely more severe reactions have been observed with intravenous applications, respective precautions have to be taken (Stenzel and Mentzel 2014; Piskunowicz et al. 2011; Torzilli 2005). Diagnostically, particularly using modern contrast imaging techniques, US contrast agents are reliable and particularly valuable – not only for lesion detection but also for lesion characterization (as dynamic evaluation is easily feasible without increasing any risk or burden to the patient) (McCarville 2011; Piskunowicz et al. 2012; Stenzel 2013; Valentino et al. 2008). There are no official dose-finding studies; however, suggestions of how to adapt the dose for the various pediatric age groups exist (Table 1) (Riccabona et al. 2012, 2014). Nevertheless, the specific requirements for off-label use of these agents in the different countries have to be respected (Schreiber-Dietrich and Dietrich 2012; Esposito et al. 2012).

A specific pediatric application in uroradiology of US contrast agents is its intravesical use for assessment of vesicoureteric reflux called contrast-enhanced voiding urosonography (ce-VUS). This method has been well validated, is safe and reliable, has high diagnostic accuracy, and helps to reduce conventional fluoroscopic voiding cystourethrography with its considerable radiation burden (Ascenti et al. 2004; Berrocal et al. 2001; Mentzel et al. 1999; Darge 2010; Papadopoulou et al. 2014; Valentini et al. 2002). With the intravesical use, its safety profile is even better than for the intravenous applications (Papadopoulou et al. 2014; Riccabona 2012). It has also been shown that ce-VUS is reliable for assessing urethral pathology when using a perineal approach (Duran et al. 2009; Berrocal et al. 2005; Bosio and Manzoni 2002) – thus also this aspect is no longer a limitation of the technique, and it has helped to reduce the use of ionizing studies (Darge et al. 2001). Therefore – this has become an important method which is described in more detail in chapter "Diagnostic Procedures: Excluding MRI, Nuclear Medicine and Video-Urodynamics" and where procedural recommendations are available describing this technique that by now has been fairly standardized (Darge 2008; Riccabona et al. 2008; Riccabona 2002, 2014).

Table 1 Dose suggestions for pediatric ultrasound contrast agent applications (using SonoVue®, Bracco, Italy – the most commonly available drug, particularly in Europe), based on individual experiences, several reports, and extrapolation from adult dose taking the child's circulating blood volume (which is relatively higher in neonates than in older children) into account (as there are no dose finding studies available, except for a small series for ce-VUS) (see also Riccabona 2014; Riccabona et al. 2012; Darge 2010)

ce-VUS: 0.2–0.5–1 % of actual bladder filling volume dose partially also depends on imaging technique used	
iv.-CEUS (maximum single dose – often lower dose at around 50 % sufficient):	
Neonates	0.1–0.15 ml/kg b.w.
Infants	0.08–0.1 ml/kg b.w.
Older children (>20 kg b.w.)	0.05–0.08 ml/kg b.w.
Adolescents: Like adults	2.4–4.8 ml (~0.025/0.05 ml/kg b.w.)
Some use the formula 0.1 ml/year of age	
Repetition possible as soon as old bolus has dissolved/vanished (usually within 15–20 min.)	

ce-VUS contrast-enhanced voiding urosonography, *iv.-CEUS* intravenous contrast-enhanced ultrasound, *b.w.* body weight, *min.* minute. The recently issued compay recommendations (Lumason/Sonovue by Bracco) for pediatric dosage are 0.03 ml/kg for intravenous use (USA) and 1 mg for intravesical use (USA and Europe) (see www.drugs.com/dosage/lumason.html - last visited Nov 18th 2017)

Take Away
Presently available US contrast agents are not licensed for intravascular pediatric use in Europe. However, they have been applied both intravenously as well as intracavitarily (e.g., ce-VUS, which now is an approved application both in Europe and in the USA). It has been shown that they are reliable and safe, and they can be applied after (informed) consent has been retrieved – helping to reduce the need for other particularly irradiating investigations thus reducing radiation burden to our pediatric patients.

3 Radiopaque Iodine-Based Contrast Agents

3.1 Intracavitarily Applied Radiopaque Iodine-Based Contrast Agents

Iodine-based contrast agents are used for antegrade or retrograde pyelography/urethrography, voiding cystourethrography, and – sometimes – orally administered bowel contrast in abdominal CT. Furthermore, these can be used for interventional procedures such as abscess drainage. In the bladder usually hyperosmolar contrast agents are used; these ionic agents even have the benefit of being antiseptic and antimicrobial (Dawson et al. 1983; Speck 1999). In any application where there is a risk for contact to the peritone cavity or vessels, barium-based contrast agents should be avoided, and water-soluble low- (or iso-)osmolar nonionic contrast agents as used for intravenous studies should be administered (Zerin 1992; Hiorns 2011) (see below). The concentration usually is in the 150–200 mg/ml range, and sometimes they are diluted, particularly for CT – here usually diluted low-osmolar radiopaque contrast agents in a 2 % solution are used, with age-adapted volume (Table 2) (Sorantin 2012).

3.2 Intravascularly Applied Radiopaque Iodine-Based Contrast Agents (CA)

Intravascularly applied iodine-based contrast agents (CA) are commonly used for a number of procedures and usually given intravenously, particularly and most commonly for CT; sometimes and in exceptional cases (or if no access to other modern imaging is available, e.g., in low-resource settings), IVU or a catheter angiography needs to be performed using these agents. After the first years of life, radiopaque iodine-based CA are handled by the kidney similarly as in adults. But in neonates and infants, there are very little hard data and facts on details about renal handling of these agents; additionally the physiologic renal immaturity in newborns and side effects from osmolarity and concentration need to be considered. Furthermore, adverse reactions, particularly allergic, and (though rarely) even anaphylactic reactions exist also in childhood (Mikkonen et al. 1995; Brasch 2008). The other major complication of iodine-based radiopaque CA is contrast-induced nephropathy (CIN), a phenomenon that may occur in children too just as in adults, particularly in those with impaired renal function and with poor hydration. This aspect is undergoing refinements – probably CIN is less relevant than previously considered and needs to be only considered in patients with a glomerular filtration rate (GFR) below 40 ml/min/1.73 m^2, in combination with other nephrotoxic agents or diseases with renal involvement, and most important with poor hydration (Garfinkle et al. 2015; Davenport et al. 2013; Newhouse et al. 2008); however, no data on this exist in children and particularly in neonates till now. A final important aspect is the risk of iodine-induced hypothyreosis in neonates after oral, rectal, intra-arterial, or intravenous application of iodinated CA – thus in these patients thyroid function should be tested after iodine applications (Thaker et al. 2014). All these aspects need to be considered when indicating, planning, and performing a contrast-enhanced study.

To address all these aspects, the general consensus within pediatric radiology is first to try to avoid using contrast-enhanced examinations that carry a radiation burden following the ALARA principle whenever possible – often these can be replaced by modern detailed US (including Doppler sonography and potentially US contrast agents) and MR imaging. Sometimes non-enhanced studies such as an abdominal plain film or an unenhanced CT may suffice in conjunction with the other options. If a contrast agent is necessary, iso- or low-osmolar nonionic contrast agents should be preferred, and adequate (physiologic) hydration should be granted; if possible, additional particularly native unenhanced CT acquisitions should be avoided. The dose needs to be corrected according to body weight and age – with some variability depending on the studied object. Furthermore, patients should be checked for renal disease or functional impairment, and if there is any potential risk, renal functional tests by measuring creatinine and calculating GFR must be

Table 2 Recommendation for age-adjusted amount of oral contrast for paediatric CT (low-osmolar radiopaque contrast agents at 200–300 mg J/ml in a 2 % solution)

Age	CM amount (ml)
Under 6 months	100
6 months–1 year	200
1–3 years	300
3–10 years	700
Older than 10 years	1000

undertaken. It needs to be remembered that creatinine values are age dependent and may differ significantly from adult values and that GFR is calculated by a slightly different equation than in adults (see chapter "Normal Values").

Premedication – to avoid allergic/anaphylactic reaction to the contrast media as well as treatment of these events – differs, depending on age as well as on institution. As a general rule, corticosteroid and antihistamine premedication can be used as a prophylactic tool in children with known allergy to iodine-based contrast media (see American College of Radiologists – Recommendation 2012); the treatment of an adverse event depends on severity and usually is defined in cooperation with the anesthesiologists by the individual institution.

The actual contrast agent dose depends on age as well as the iodine load and concentration of the individual CA: the younger the child, the lower the concentration – starting from 150 to 200 mg iodine per ml in neonates and gradually increasing with age up to 350 mg iodine per ml in older children. Particularly in CTA, a lower relative iodine load can be advocated, as CTA is often performed at lower kV settings (e.g., 80–100 kV) that yield a higher contrast effect, additionally helping to reduce the CT dose. As a rule of a thumb, the dose suggestion is 2.5 ml/kg body weight (to a maximum of 3 ml/kg body weight) in neonates and 2 ml/kg body weight in infants; thereafter usually 1–1.5 ml/kg body weight is sufficient (Pärtan 2014; Sorantin et al. 2002, 2013; Sorantin 2013) (Table 3). However, for some exams a larger contrast amount may be necessary, particularly if a dual or split bolus technique is used, such as in some trauma protocols or for CT urography. Nevertheless, higher contrast doses are associated with a higher risk of CIN, and thus the risk to benefit relation has to be carefully assessed (Frush 2008; Kurian et al. 2013; Heran et al. 2010). In neonates with an immature renal function in the first weeks of life, radiopaque contrast agents should be avoided unless there is a "vital" indication for the study with no other imaging alternatives and emergent therapeutic impact.

Table 3 Recommendations on weight- and age-dependent dose and concentration for pediatric intravenous radiopaque iodine-based contrast agent applications

Age	Iodine concentration[a] (mg/ml)	Dose[b] (ml/kg b.w.)
Less than 1 year	150–200	2.5
Between 1 and 2 years	200–250	2.0
Older than 2 years	250–300	1.5
Older than 6 years	300–350	1–1.5
Adolescents As in adults	300–400	0.5–1 Depending on protocol and indication

Try to avoid administration of more than 100 ml (Adapted from Sorantin et al. 2013)
b.w. body weight, mg/kg milligram per kilogram, mg/ml milligram per milliliter
[a]Use higher concentration for smaller and more peripheral vessels
[b]For some specific applications, 0.5–1 ml may need to be added (e.g., split bolus technique). Sometimes (e.g., for CTA, using ultrafast and most modern devices with low KV and sensitive detectors) even a reduction of 30–50% can be sufficient

Take Away
Iodine-based radiopaque contrast agents are safe for application in childhood – age-adapted dose and concentration need to be used, and low- or iso-osmolar drugs should be administered. Nevertheless, though rarer than in adults, complications and adverse reactions as well as (relative) contraindications exist, too. These have to be respected and respective precautions have to be taken.

4 Gadolinium (Gd)-Based MR Contrast Agents

Basically similar statements apply as in adults for the use of Gd-based MR contrast agents in children. However, there is little information about pharmacokinetics and safety data available for the use of these contrast agents in children (Hahn et al. 2009), particularly in neonates and infants less than 1 year. But there is a (though small) risk of inducing nephrogenic systemic fibrosis (NSF) (Foss et al. 2009; Jain et al. 2004). Basically, the same general rules apply as in adults (Karcaaltincaba et al. 2009; Thomson and Webb 2014). Particularly renal insufficiency, poor hydration (that impairs Gd excretion and leads to a longer Gd circulation time), as well as acidosis pose major risk factors (Dharnidharka et al. 2007; Mendichovszky et al. 2008; Thomson and Webb 2014). At present practically all proven incidents of NSF (particularly in children) have been observed with linear compounds (Morcos 2007; Penfield and Reilly 2008; Riccabona 2014). Therefore the Guidelines from the American Working Group of Radiologists, the ESUR Contrast Media Safety Committee, the ESPR Uroradiology Task Force, and the ESUR Paediatric Working Group as well as the respective EC committees and agencies propose to avoid linear compounds in children, particularly in infants and neonates, and to take precautions to assure a normal renal function by measuring creatinine and calculating GFR at least in all those children, who have a potential risk of impaired renal function. Additionally, the EMA has issued a statement that obviates the use of non-linear Gd-based contrast agents in Europe and particularly in Pediatrics (EMA 2017). Age-adapted reference values of GFR have to be used (see chapter "Normal Values"). Additionally, acidosis should be corrected, and proper (physiologic) hydration should be granted before an intravenous Gd application, the latter also for preventing Gd accumulation in the tubules with a consecutive phenomenon similar to contrast-induced nephropathy (Kalmar and Riccabona 2013).

As no data are available on the handling of Gd by the neonatal kidney, the respective recommendations are extrapolated from adult physiology; but in general Gd should be avoided unless there is a serious indication – after assessing the risk to benefit relation rating the gadolinium-enhanced MR as the most adequate imaging approach and consultation with the pediatric nephrologist (Mendichovszky et al. 2008; Riccabona et al. 2009). In general, particularly for MR angiography, non-enhanced MR techniques such as time of flight or arterial spin labeling techniques or diffusion weighted imaging should be considered first (Mannelli et al. 2012, Penfield and Reilly 2008), and alternative imaging approaches (e.g., by US) should be exploited (Mendichovszky et al. 2008; Riccabona 2014). The dose is calculated by the body weight – the respective dose suggestions from the manufacturers should be followed; usually a range from 0.05 to 0.1 ml/kg body weight are recommended by the companies, with some variance depending on the drug and the application and using the lowest possible dose that still grants a diagnostically reliable enhancement/contrast.

If there is renal function impairment, Gd is not completely contraindicated. However, there must be a compelling indication, no alternative substitute imaging option with less risk, and proper preparation by hydration, correcting acidosis and similar measures – then, after retrieving an informed consent of the parents and consulting the pediatric nephrologist, Gd may be an accepted option. As repeated administration of Gd potentially leads to higher cumulative systemic dose and may be a possible risk factor for (irreversible long term) Gd deposits in some body compartments, repeated investigations within a short time should be avoided. Note that this Gd accumulation on several body compartments such as the brain (e.g., dentate nucleus) or the bone marrow has recently been shown even in patients with a normal renal function but repeated Gd applications (McDonald et al. 2015) – no knowledge exists to date on the long-term impact of these phenomena or specific pediatric implications, but this phenomenon has been also observed in pediatric patients. It is therefore even more obvious that the patient's cumulative dose should be recorded in the patients' file or register, and its use and indication should be handles with caution based on a thorough justification, i.e., should be avoided if not necessary. The latter will not only help to monitor the patient but also create more evidence for future analysis and more profound recommendations. Additionally, as a general rule, double-dose administration should be avoided, although at present there is no direct evidence that this is harmful. Furthermore, the European medicines agency has just recently issued a recommendation that linear compounds should be generally avoided and not used particularly in childhood. As in some countries no cyclic Gd-based contrast agent is registered for use in neonates and the first year of life, an off-label application may be and often is considered safer than the use of a potentially registered linear compound, provided there is a thorough indication and consent from the parents – particularly, as the lack of approval is mostly only based on missing phase III studies which are rarely done in very young children.

are tested and licensed in children of all ages in accordance with the rules of the various medicine agencies and different countries. However, this does not mean that untested and officially unapproved contrast agents cannot be used in childhood – but in these cases an informed consent must be obtained and the indication for the study must be thoroughly validated. Only if there is an absolute contraindication a contrast agent cannot be used even with informed consent.

> **Take Away**
> Gd-based MR contrast agents are used in children and follow similar rules as in adults; the dose however must be adapted to age and weight of the patient. Though rarer, side effects exist and need to be considered – particularly for NSF prevention, cyclic compounds should be used throughout childhood and particularly in infancy, even if this implies an off-label application. Patient registers that allow following the individual Gd exposure will hopefully in future provide more evidence on childhood-specific aspects.

> **Take Away**
> Contrast agents play a major role also for imaging children, but safety considerations have to be respected. The dose must be adjusted to the patient age and weight, renal function parameters must be observed – considering the different normal values for the various age groups – and other precautions such as proper hydration should be taken.

5 Summary and Conclusion

Contrast agents play a major role also for imaging children. However, safety considerations have to be respected and are similar but not always quite the same as in adults. The dose must be adjusted to the patient age and weight, and renal function parameters must be observed considering the different normal values for the various age groups (see chapter "Normal Values"). And other precautions such as proper hydration and correcting acidosis should be taken.

For radiography, fluoroscopy, and CT, nonionic iodine-based contrast agents should be used with a lower concentration in younger children. For MRI, linear Gd compounds should be avoided in children and replaced by cyclic contrast agents. The Summary of Product Characteristics should be consulted, particularly since not all contrast agents

References

American College of Radiology – ACR 2012/manual on contrast media v8 – contrast media in children. http://www.acr.org/Quality-Safety/Resources/Contrast-Manual

Ascenti G, Zimbaro G, Mazziotti S et al (2004) Harmonic US imaging of vesicoureteric reflux in children: usefulness of a second generation US contrast agent. Pediatr Radiol 34:481–487

Berrocal T, Gaya F, Arjonilla A et al (2001) Vesicoureteral reflux: diagnosis and grading with echo-enhanced cystosonography versus voiding cystourethrography. Radiology 221:359–365

Berrocal T, Gaya F, Arjonilla A (2005) Vesicoureteral reflux: can the urethra be adequately assessed by using contrast-enhanced voiding US of the bladder? Radiology 234:235–241, 650

Bosio M, Manzoni GA (2002) Detection of posterior urethral valves with voiding cysto-urethrosonography with echo contrast. J Urol 168:1711–1715

Brasch RC (2008) Contrast media toxicity in children. Pediatr Radiol 38(S2):S281–S284

Calliada F, Campani R, Bottinelli O, Bozzini A, Sommaruga MG (1998) Ultrasound contrast agents: basic principles. Eur J Radiol 27(S2):S157–S160

Darge K (2008) Voiding urosonography with ultrasound contrast agents for the diagnosis of vesicoureteric reflux in children. I. Procedure. Pediatr Radiol 38:40–53

Darge K (2010) Voiding urosonography with US contrast agent for the diagnosis of vesicoureteric reflux in children: an update. Pediatr Radiol 40:956–962

Darge K, Zieger B, Rohrschneider W et al (2001) Reduction in voiding cystourethrographies after the introduction of contrast enhanced sonographic reflux diagnosis. Pediatr Radiol 31:790–795

Darge K, Papadopoulou F, Ntoulia A, Bulas DI, Coley BD, Fordham LA, Paltiel HJ, McCarville B, Volberg FM, Cosgrove DO, Goldberg BB, Wilson SR, Feinstein SB (2013) Safety of contrast-enhanced ultrasound in children for non-cardiac applications: a review by the Society for Pediatric Radiology (SPR) and the International Contrast Ultrasound Society (ICUS). Pediatr Radiol 43:1063–1073

Davenport MS, Khalatbari S, Dillman JR, Cohan RH, Caoili EM, Ellis JH (2013) Contrast material-induced nephrotoxicity and intravenous low-osmolality iodinated contrast material. Radiology 267:94–105. doi:10.2214/AJR.14.13761

Dawson P, Becker A, Holton JM (1983) The effect of contrast media on the growth of bacteria. Br J Radiol 56:809–815

Dharnidharka VR, Wesson SK, Fennell RS (2007) Gadolinium and nephrogenic fibrosing dermopathy in pediatric patients. Pediatr Nephrol 22:1395

Duran C, Valera A, Alguersuari A et al (2009) Voiding urosonography: the study of the urethra is no longer a limitation of the technique. Pediatr Radiol 39:124–131

EMA's final opinion confirms restrictions on use of linear gadolinium agents in body scans (2017). EMA/457616/2017, last visited April 2018. http://www.ema.europa.eu/docs/en_GB/document_library/Referrals_document/gadolinium_contrast_agents_31/Opinion_provided_by_Committee_for_Medicinal_Products_for_Human_Use/WC500231824.pdf

Esposito F, Di Serafino M, Sgambati P, Mercogliano F, Tarantino L, Vallone G, Oresta P (2012) Ultrasound contrast media in paediatric patients: is it an off-label use? Regulatory requirements and radiologist's liability. Radiol Med 117:148–159

Foss C, Smith JK, Ortiz L, Hanevold C, Davis L (2009) Gadolinium-associated nephrogenic systemic fibrosis in a 9-year-old boy. Pediatr Dermatol 26:579–582

Frush DP (2008) Pediatric abdominal CT angiography. Pediatr Radiol 38(S2):S259–S266

Garfinkle MA, Stewart S, Basi R (2015) Incidence of ct contrast agent–induced nephropathy: toward a more accurate estimation. AJR Am J Roentgenol 204:1146–1151. doi:10.2214/AJR.14.13761

Hahn G, Sorge I, Gruhn B et al (2009) Pharmacokinetics and safety of gadobutrol-enhanced magnetic resonance imaging in pediatric patients. Invest Radiol 44:776–783

Heran MK, Marshalleck F, Temple M et al. Society of Interventional Radiology Standards of Practice Committee; Society of Pediatric Radiology Interventional Radiology Committee (2010) Joint quality improvement guidelines for pediatric arterial access and arteriography: from the Societies of Interventional Radiology and Pediatric Radiology. Pediatr Radiol 40:237–250

Hiorns MP (2011) Gastrointestinal tract imaging in children: current techniques. Pediatr Radiol 41:42–54

Jain SM, Wesson S, Hassanein A et al (2004) Nephrogenic fibrosing dermopathy in pediatric patients. Pediatr Nephrol 19:467–470

Kalmar P, Riccabona M (2013) Intramedulläre Gadoliniumresiduen in Nieren pädiatrischer Onkologie-Patienten – ein Wort zur Vorsicht. 50. GPR Jahrestagung, Jena, September 2013. Fortschr Röntgenstr (RöFo) 185:893 (abstract)

Karcaaltincaba M, Oguz B, Haliloglu M (2009) Current status of contrast-induced nephropathy and nephrogenic systemic fibrosis in children. Pediatr Radiol 39(S3):S382–S384

Kurian J, Epelman M, Darge K et al (2013) The role of CT angiography in the evaluation of pediatric renovascular hypertension. Pediatr Radiol 43:490–501

Mannelli L, Maki JH, Osman SF et al (2012) Non-contrast functional MRI of the kidneys. Curr Urol Rep 13:99–107

McCarville MB (2011) Contrast-enhanced sonography in pediatrics. Pediatr Radiol 41(S1):S238–S242

McDonald RJ, McDonald JS., Kallmes DF, Jentoft ME, Murray DL, Thielen KR, Williamson EE, Eckel LJ (2015) Intracranial gadolinium deposition after contrast-enhanced MR imaging. Radiology 275:772–7782. doi:http://dx.doi.org/10.1148/radiol.15150025

Mendichovszky IA, Marks SD, Simcock CM, Olsen OE (2008) Gadolinium and nephrogenic systemic fibrosis: time to tighten practice. Pediatr Radiol 38:489–496

Mentzel HJ, Vogt S, Patzer L, Schubert R, John U, Misselwitz J, Kaiser WA (1999) Contrast-enhanced sonography of vesicoureteral reflux in children: preliminary results. Am J Roentgenol 173:737–740

Mikkonen R, Kontkanen T, Kivisaari L (1995) Late and acute adverse reactions to iohexol in a pediatric population. Acta Radiol 35:350–352

Morcos SK (2007) Nephrogenic systemic fibrosis following the administration of extracellular gadolinium based contrast agents: is the stability of the contrast agent molecule an important factor in the pathogenesis of this condition? Br J Radiol 80:73–76, Erratum in: Br J Radiol 2007;80:586

Newhouse JH, Kho D, Rao QA, Starren J (2008) Frequency of serum creatinine changes in the absence of iodinated contrast material: implications for studies of contrast nephrotoxicity. AJR Am J Roentgenol 191:376–382. doi:10.2214/AJR.14.13761

Papadopoulou F, Ntoulia A, Siomou E, Darge K (2014) Contrast-enhanced voiding urosonography with intravesical administration of a second-generation ultrasound contrast agent for diagnosis of vesicoureteral reflux: prospective evaluation of contrast safety in 1,010 children. Pediatr Radiol 44:719–728

Pärtan G (2014) Radiography and fluoroscopy. In: Riccabona M (ed) Pediatric imaging essentials.

Thieme, Stuttgart/New-York, pp 10–19. ISBN 987-3-13-166191-3
Penfield JG, Reilly RF (2008) Nephrogenic systemic fibrosis risk: is there a difference between gadolinium-based contrast agents? Semin Dial 21:129–134
Piscaglia F, Bolondi L (2006) The safety of Sonovue in abdominal applications: retrospective analysis of 23188 investigations. Ultrasound Med Biol 32:1369–1375
Piskunowicz M, Kosiak W, Irga N (2011) Primum non nocere? Why can't we use second generation ultrasound contrast agents for the examination of children? Ultraschall Med 32:83–86
Piskunowicz M, Kosiak W, Batko T (2012) Intravenous application of second-generation ultrasound contrast agents in children: a review of the literature. Ultraschall Med 33:135–140
Riccabona M (2002) Cystography in infants and children: a critical appraisal of the many forms with special regard to voiding cystourethrography. Eur Radiol 12:2910–2918
Riccabona M (2012) Application of a second-generation US contrast agent in infants and children – a European questionnaire-based survey. Pediatr Radiol 42:1471–1480
Riccabona M (2014) Contrast media use in pediatrics: safety issues. In: Thomsen HS, Webb JAW (eds) Contrast media. Safety issues and ESUR guidelines, 3rd edn. Springer, Heidelberg/New-York/Dordrecht/London, pp 245–253. ISBN 978-3-642-36723-6
Riccabona M, Avni FE, Blickman JG et al (2008) Imaging recommendations in paediatric uroradiology: minutes of the ESPR workgroup session on urinary tract infection, fetal hydronephrosis, urinary tract ultrasonography and voiding cystourethrography. Barcelona, Spain, June 2007. Pediatr Radiol 38:138–145
Riccabona M, Avni FE, Blickman JG, Dacher JN, Darge K, Lobo ML, Willi U, Members of the ESUR Paediatric Paediatric Recommendation Work Group and ESPR Paediatric Uroradiology Work Group (2009) Imaging recommendations in paediatric uroradiology, part II: urolithiasis and haematuria in children, paediatric obstructive uropathy, and postnatal work-up of foetally diagnosed high grade hydronephrosis. Minutes of a mini-symposium at the ESPR annual meeting, Edinburg, June. Pediatr Radiol 39:891–898
Riccabona M, Avni F, Damasio B et al (2012) ESPR Uroradiology Task Force and ESUR Paediatric Working Group: imaging recommendations in paediatric uroradiology, part V: childhood cystic kidney disease, childhood renal transplantation and contrast-enhanced ultrasound in children. Pediatr Radiol 42:1275–1283
Schreiber-Dietrich D, Dietrich CF (2012) Contrast enhanced ultrasound (CEUS) and off-label use (in children). Ultraschall Med 33:295–296
Sorantin E, Weissensteiner S, Hasenburger G, Riccabona M. CT in children - dose protection and generalconsiderations when planning a CT in a child. Eur Radiol 2013; 82 (7): 1043-1049.
Sorantin E (2013) Special aspects of computed tomography in children. In: Riccabona M (ed) Pediatric imaging essentials. Thieme, Stuttgart/New-York, pp 22–28. ISBN 987-3-13-166191-3
Sorantin E, Zsivcsec B, Zebedin D, Fotter R (2002) Optimierung von i.v. Kontrastmittel-applikatonen für pädiatrische Spiral-CT Untersuchungen (Optimisation of i.v. contrast application for pediatric spiral-CT). Radiologe 45:683–684
Sorantin E, Weissensteiner S, Hasenburger G, Riccabona M (2013) CT in children – dose protection and general considerations when planning a CT in a child. Eur J Radiol 82:1043–1049
Speck U (1999) Kontrastmittel: Übersicht, Anwendung und pharmazeutische Aspekte [Contrast Media. overview, use and pharmaceutical aspects]. Springer, Berlin, pp 16–17. ISBN 978-3-540-65712-5
Stenzel M (2013) Intravenous contrast-enhanced sonography in children and adolescents – a single center experience. J Ultrason 13:133–144
Stenzel M, Mentzel HJ (2014) Ultrasound elastography and contrast-enhanced ultrasound in infants, children and adolescents. Eur J Radiol 83:1560–1569
ter Haar G (2009) Safety and bio-effects of ultrasound contrast agents. Med Biol Eng Comput 47:893–900
Thaker VV, Leung AM, Braverman LE, Brown RS, Levine B (2014) Iodine-induced hypothyroidism in full-term infants with congenital heart disease: more common than currently appreciated? J Clin Endocrinol Metab 99:3521–3526. doi:10.1210/jc.2014-1956
Thomsen HS, Webb JAW (eds) (2014) Contrast media. Safety issues and ESUR guidelines, 3rd edn. Springer, Heidelberg/New-York/Dordrecht/London. ISBN 978-3-642-36723-6
Torzilli G (2005) Adverse effects associated with SonoVue use. Expert Opin Drug Saf 4:399–401
Valentini AL, De Gaetano AM, Destito C et al (2002) The accuracy of voiding urosonography in detecting vesico-ureteral reflux: a summary of existing data. Eur J Pediatr 161:380–384
Valentino M, Serra C, Pavlica P et al (2008) Blunt abdominal trauma: diagnostic performance of contrast-enhanced US in children – initial experience. Radiology 246:903–909
Webb JAW (2014) Pregnancy and lactation: intravascular use of contrast media. In: Thomsen HS, Webb JAW (eds) Contrast media: safety issues and ESUR guidelines, 3rd edn. Springer, Heidelberg/New-York/Dordrecht/London, pp 113–121. ISBN 978-3-642-36723-6
Zerin JM (1992) Contrast studies of the gastrointestinal tract in the neonate. Semin Pediatr Surg 1:284–295

Part II

Fetal Findings, Embryology, Anatomy, Normal Variants

Urinary Tract Embryology, Anatomy, and Anatomical Variants

Aikaterini Ntoulia, Frederica Papadopoulou, and Gabriele Benz-Bohm

Contents

1	Embryology	135
1.1	Development of the Kidneys and the Ureters	135
1.2	Development of the Urinary Bladder	137
1.3	Development of the Urethra	137
2	**Anatomy and Variants**	138
2.1	The Kidneys	138
2.2	The Pelvicalyceal System and the Ureters	145
2.3	The Urinary Bladder	146
2.4	The Male Urethra	147
2.5	The Female Urethra	148
Conclusion		149
References		149

A. Ntoulia, MD, PhD (✉)
Department of Radiology, Children's Hospital of Philadelphia, Philadelphia, PA, USA
e-mail: ntouliaa@email.chop.edu

F. Papadopoulou
Pediatric Ultrasound Center Thessaloniki, Thessaloniki, Ioannina, Greece

G. Benz-Bohm, MD, (Retired)
Department of Radiology, The Children's Hospital of Philadelphia, Philadelphia, PA, USA
e-mail: g.benz-bohm@t-online.de

1 Embryology

1.1 Development of the Kidneys and the Ureters

The normal embryonic development of the human kidney has been studied in detail (Potter 1972). Understanding this process is essential in the evaluation of the various structural malformations of the kidney.

During the development of the human kidney, there are three successive ontogenetic stages: the pronephros, the mesonephros, and the metanephros (Fig. 1). Although the pronephros and the mesonephros are transitory organs, they are essential for the development of the definitive kidney, the metanephros. All three systems are of mesodermal origin and develop from the nephrogenic cord.

Near the end of the 3 week after conception, the pronephros begins to form. The proximal ends form nephrostomes, which open into the coelomic cavity, and the distal ends of successive tubules coalesce to form the pronephric ducts. The cephalic segments regress before the caudal parts form and all degenerate by the 5 week. The pronephros appears to be nonfunctional in humans, but is important in giving rise to the mesonephric ducts.

The mesonephros develops in the 4 week after conception, caudal to the last of the pronephric tubules. Whereas the pronephros is a cervical organ, the mesonephros is a thoracic organ. Each mesonephric unit consists of a glomerular structure, a proximal tubule segment that is secretory in nature, and a distal tubule segment that ends in the mesonephric duct. These represent the first true nephron units in renal development. In the female, most of the mesonephros regresses in the third month of gestation with the epoophoron, the paroophoron, and Gartner's duct remaining as vestigial structures. In the male, the mesonephric tubules and the mesonephric duct continue to develop to form the excretory ducts of the male reproductive system.

The definitive kidney is the metanephros and has a dual origin. The glomeruli and tubules arise from a mesenchyme called metanephric blastema in the nephrogenic cord, caudal to the mesonephros. The excretory segments, including the collecting ducts, calyces, pelvis, and ureter, develop from a branch of the mesonephric duct called the ureteric bud (Fig. 1). This structure arises during the 4 and 5 weeks and grows dorsally and cephalad until it contacts the nephrogenic cord. The metanephric blastema surrounds the dividing ureteric bud as a condensation of cells. Branches of the ureteric bud must come into contact with the metanephric blastema in order for the kidney to develop properly.

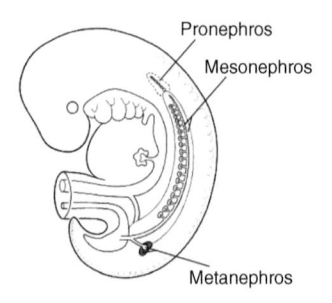

Fig. 1 Topography of the pronephros, mesonephros, and metanephros

At 7–8 weeks, the first nephrons with well-developed glomeruli are formed from the metanephric blastema. The first three to five generations of branches of the ureteric bud form the renal pelvis. The terminal portions of the next generation of branches remain somewhat constricted and form the infundibula, which connect the calyces with the pelvis. The early calyces are formed at 10 weeks, and by 13–14 weeks the cuplike shape of the calyx is established. It has been estimated that the papillary collecting ducts are developed from the seventh to eleventh generations from the original ureteric bud. Rapid branching continues with the formation of collecting tubules until about 14–15 weeks.

Nephron formation begins in about the 8 week in small foci of metanephric blastema adjacent to the ampulla of the ureteric bud. Approximately one million nephrons at different stages of maturation are present in the kidney at birth. Although maturation of the nephrons proceeds after birth, no new nephrons are formed. Growth in the kidney continues until adult life, mainly as a result of elongation of the proximal convoluted tubules and loops of Henle and an increase in the size of the interstitium.

The kidneys undergo cephalad migration from their site of origin. The ascent of the kidney occurs due to true migration and also secondary to differential somatic growth of the lumbar portion of the body. They reach their final level by the end of the eighth week of fetal life. During their ascent from the pelvis, the kidneys normally undergo medial rotation of roughly 90° around their longitudinal axis before they assume their final position. During ascent, each kidney receives its blood supply from the neighboring vessels. Initially, this is from the middle sacral artery, then the common iliac and inferior mesenteric arteries, and finally the aorta (Clapp and Tisher 1989; Kissane

1983; Moore and Persaud 1998; Netter 1983; Deeg et al. 1997).

> **Take Away**
> The definitive kidney, the metanephros, has a dual mesoderm origin. The glomeruli and tubules arise from metanephric blastema and the excretory segments from the ureteric bud.

1.2 Development of the Urinary Bladder

The cloaca is divided by the urorectal septum into a dorsal rectum and a ventral urogenital sinus (Fig. 2). The urogenital sinus is divided into a cranial vesical part that is continuous with the allantois, a middle pelvic part, and a caudal phallic part that grows toward the genital tubercle. The pelvic part becomes the bladder neck and the prostatic part of the male urethra and the entire female urethra. The bladder develops mainly from the vesical part. The trigone region, however, is derived from the caudal ends of the mesonephric ducts. The allantois becomes a thick fibrous cord, the urachus. It extends from the apex of the bladder to the umbilicus. As the bladder enlarges, distal parts of the mesonephric ducts are incorporated into its posterior wall. As the mesonephric ducts are absorbed, the ureters come to open separately into the urinary bladder. The orifices of the ureters move superolaterally – partly due to the ascent of the kidneys – and the ureters enter obliquely through the base of the bladder. The orifices of the mesonephric ducts move close together and enter the prostatic part of the urethra as their caudal ends become the ejaculatory ducts. In females, the distal end of the mesonephric ducts degenerate (Moore and Persaud 1998).

> **Take Away**
> The bladder develops mainly from the vesical part of the urogenital sinus. The trigone region is derived from the caudal end of the mesonephric ducts.

1.3 Development of the Urethra

The epithelium of most of the male urethra and the entire female urethra derive from the endoderm of the urogenital sinus. The distal part of the male urethra is derived from the glandular-urethral plate. This ectodermal plate grows, becomes canalized, and joins the rest of the spongy urethra. Therefore, the epithelium of the terminal part of the urethra is derived from surface ectoderm. The connective tissue and smooth muscle of the urethra in both sexes derive from the adjacent splanchnic mesenchyme (Moore and Persaud 1998).

> **Take Away**
> The epithelium of most of the male urethra and the entire female urethra is derived from the endoderm of the urogenital sinus. The distal part of the male urethra derives from an ectodermal plate, called the urethral plate.

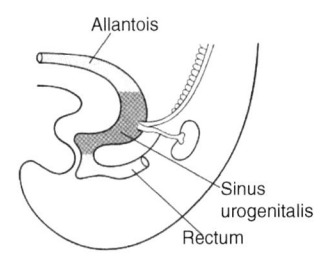

Fig. 2 Diagram of urogenital sinus, lateral view

2 Anatomy and Variants

2.1 The Kidneys

2.1.1 Position and Anatomical Relationship

The kidneys, bean-shaped organs situated in the retroperitoneum, extend from the 12th thoracic to the third lumbar vertebra, with the right kidney usually slightly more caudal in position in approximately two-thirds of people. The difference in position relative to the spine usually corresponds to the height of one vertebral body (Currarino et al. 1993). The upper pole of each kidney is usually more medial and posterior than the lower pole. The hilum of each kidney is rotated anteriorly on the psoas major muscle, and there is posterior rotation of the convex lateral renal margin – best seen on CT or MRI – near the level of the second lumbar vertebra. The kidney is surrounded by a thin fibrous capsule that is adherent to the pelvis at the hilum, where the vessels pass in or out of the kidney. The posterior surface of the kidney is partly in contact with the diaphragm above the posterior costophrenic sinus. This anatomical relationship explains how a pleural effusion, for example, at the level of the posterior costophrenic sinus above the diaphragm, may cause a downward displacement of the kidney, most often left, simulating an adrenal mass. Intraperitoneally, in front of the right kidney and the proximal descending duodenum is a posterior extension of the infrahepatic recess termed the Morrison pouch, an important space for fluid collection.

The right kidney is slightly less mobile than the left. The degree of mobility usually corresponds to the height of one vertebral body.

2.1.2 Shape, Size, and Measurement

In the newborn, it is possible to recognize the renal lobes by the presence of grooves surrounding them on the subcapsular surface (Figs. 3 and 4). As the kidney matures, the grooves tend to disappear. They are absent in most adult kidneys, but persistence of fetal lobulation is possible. Campbell (1970) found fetal lobulation at autopsy in 17.6 % of children and in 3.9 % of adults. It should be recognized as a variant of normal renal form without clinical importance. Radiographically, this may

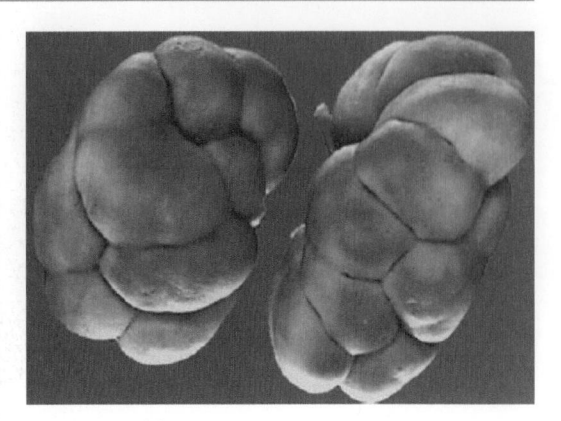

Fig. 3 Kidneys from a newborn showing characteristic fetal lobulation by grooves on the surface (Courtesy of the Department of Anatomy, University of Cologne)

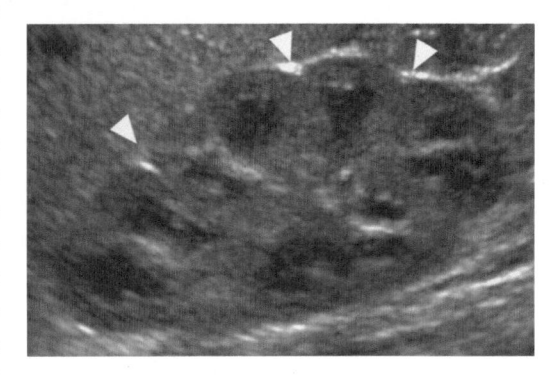

Fig. 4 Right kidney in longitudinal view. Typical sonographic appearance of the normal neonatal kidney, demonstrating multiple grooves (*arrowheads*) on the surface, increased differentiation between the echogenic cortex and the prominent anechoic pyramids, and reduced echoes in central renal sinus

appear as small notches in the renal margin placed midway between normal-appearing calyces. In contrast, cortical scars correspond to a calyx or group of calyces.

Related to the fetal lobulations is the junctional parenchymal defect (JPD) (Fig. 5). This defect consists of a thin triangular echogenic notch in the anterosuperior or posteroinferior aspect of the kidney mimicking a cortical scar. It is sometimes connected with the hilum of the kidney by an echogenic line called the junctional parenchymal line or interrenicular septum (Hoffer et al. 1985; Richter and Lierse 1990; Currarino et al. 1993). The finding is due to incomplete fusion of two embryonic parenchymatous masses – subkidneys – called renunculi or reniculi and is more commonly seen on the right kidney (Yeh et al.

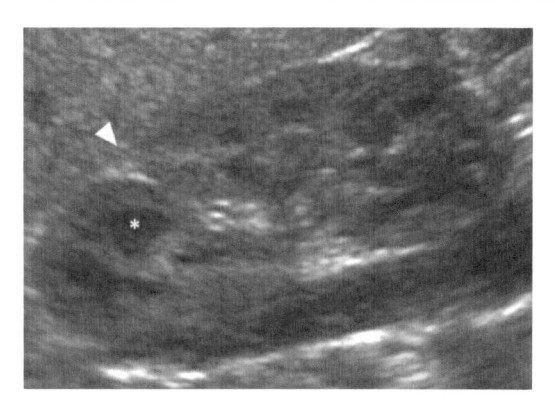

Fig. 5 Sonogram of 1-month-old boy. Right kidney in longitudinal view. The junctional parenchymal (or upper parenchymal junction line) (*arrowhead*) is seen as an echogenic triangular area in the anterior-superior aspect of the kidney. Its location between the renal pyramids (*asterisk*) allows its differentiation from a true renal scar which typically overlies the pyramid

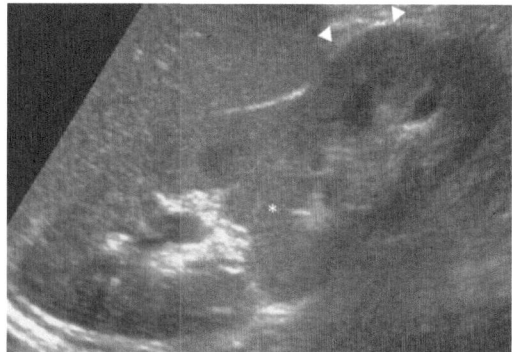

Fig. 7 Sonogram of a 4.7-year-old girl. Left kidney in longitudinal view. There is a focal smooth bulge (*arrowheads*) on the lateral aspect of the left kidney, dromedary hump, as a result of renal contour adaptation to the available space next to the spleen. *Asterisk* shows a hypertrophic column of Bertin

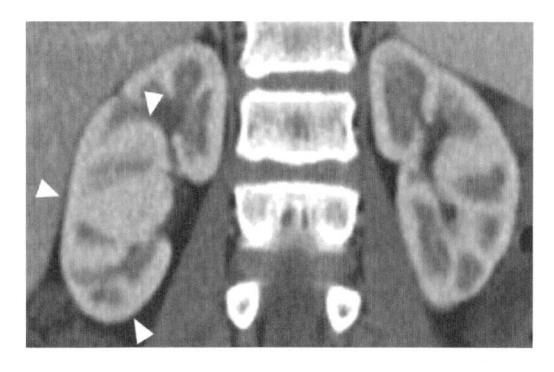

Fig. 6 Contrast-enhanced CT of the abdomen. Coronal reconstruction. Incidental finding: incomplete fusion and overlap of the two embryonic parenchymatous masses (subkidneys) with prominence of the polar parenchyma of the inferior subkidney (*arrowheads*)

1992; Hoffer et al. 1985; Carter et al. 1985; Dalla Palma and Rossi 1982; Richter and Lierse 1990; Currarino et al. 1993). Occasionally, incomplete fusion of the two embryonic subkidneys may result in the partial overlap of their parenchymatous masses. In that case, the overlapping portion either in the lower pole of the superior subkidney or in the upper pole of the inferior subkidney may not be fully resorbed and thus remain apparent. The presence of a papilla trapped at the site of the fusion, known as "engulfed" or "imprisoned" papilla, allows differentiation from a hypertrophic column of Bertin, which is composed only of renal cortex (Fig. 6) (Lafortune et al. 1986; Yeh et al. 1992).

In infants, the kidney is more rounded and relatively broader than in adults, and its poles are folded into a narrower renal sinus.

The weight and size of the kidney are proportional to body habitus. The two kidneys represent 1/80 and 1/240 of the total body weight in the newborn and in the adult, respectively (Olsson 1986). The left kidney tends to be slightly larger than the right, and the superior pole of each kidney is thicker and rounder than the inferior pole. Additionally, along the lateral-middle aspect of the left kidney, a focal cortical bulge may be incidentally encountered. This is a normal variant, produced by developmental adaptation of the renal contour to the available space next to the spleen. It is usually referred as a dromedary or splenic hump (Fig. 7) (Williams 2007).

Compensatory hypertrophy following unilateral nephrectomy is usually complete within 2 years. Compensatory hypertrophy is more rapid in infants than in children or adults. In a congenitally solitary kidney or in a congenitally functionally solitary kidney, compensatory hypertrophy is not present at birth, but develops rapidly thereafter. Measurements can be made by US or on urographic supine films. The length of the kidney corresponds to the height of the first four lumbar vertebral bodies with their three interspaces ±1 cm, except for the first 1, and a half year of life (on plain film or IVU images). At this age the kidneys are relatively larger, corresponding to the height of 4.5 lumbar vertebral bodies, or five vertebral bodies in the newborn. The left kidney is slightly longer than the right. Duplex kidneys are also slightly longer than normal kidneys.

The width of the kidney is approximately 50 % of the kidney length and is relatively greater in newborns than in older children. The kidney lengths obtained by US are generally slightly lower than those derived from the urographic films at all ages, being slightly less than 1 cm in the first 5 years and a little more than 1 cm afterwards. The simplified short version of the ellipsoid formula is used to be applied for the calculation of the kidney volume (most commonly based on US), which is as follows:

$$V = L \times W \times AP \times 0.52$$

where L is the maximal length in longitudinal scan and W and AP are the maximal width and anteroposterior diameter in a transverse section (Currarino et al. 1993). These volume standards are correlated with body weight (for normal values, please refer to chapter "Normal Values") (Dinkel et al. 1985). However, most modern US scanners have incorporated software for automatic calculations of the renal volume providing useful numbers as long as the kidney maintains its normal shape.

2.1.3 Internal Anatomy

A coronal section of the kidney reveals an outer zone, or cortex, and an inner zone, or medulla. The medulla is composed of 8–18 pyramids that terminate in the renal papillae at the level of the calyces. Two or more pyramids may share the same papilla as confluent papillae. The cortex extends into the space between adjacent pyramids as the septa or column of Bertin. Each half of the septa of Bertin receives its blood supply from a separate artery, and each half makes up the lateral margin of adjacent lobes. The septa of Bertin extend downward to the renal sinus, into which they project as ridges (Fig. 8). It is along these ridges that the interlobar arteries are arranged. Occasionally, a column of Bertin may be unusually enlarged simulating a mass-like lesion. Careful examination will reveal that this cortical projection is typically located between the pyramids and has similar characteris-

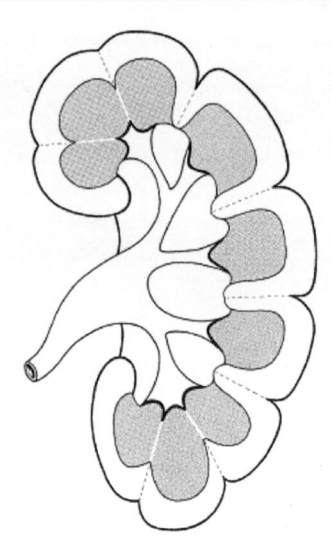

Fig. 8 Diagram of lobar architecture in the kidney. In the mid-zone the septa of Bertin reach down to the renal sinus. In the polar regions, they are smaller, due to pyramidal fusion

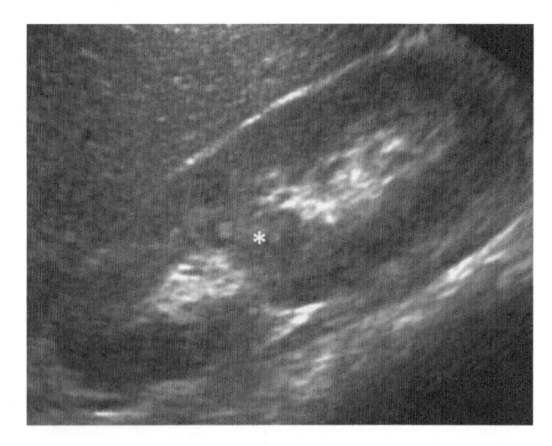

Fig. 9 Sonogram of a 2-year-old girl. Right kidney in longitudinal view. The column of Bertin extends within the renal sinus, exhibiting similar echogenicity with the renal cortex without distorting its normal architecture

tics to the adjacent cortex without distorting its normal architecture (Fig. 9); in doubtful cases, a follow-up study may be advisable to rule out a different etiology. The hypertrophic column of Bertin may protrude deeply into the renal sinus, bifurcating the renal pelvis into two pyelocalyceal systems, with a characteristic pincerlike splaying of the normal renal vasculature around the enlarged column (Fig. 10) (el-Galley and Keane 2000; Dalla Palma et al. 1990).

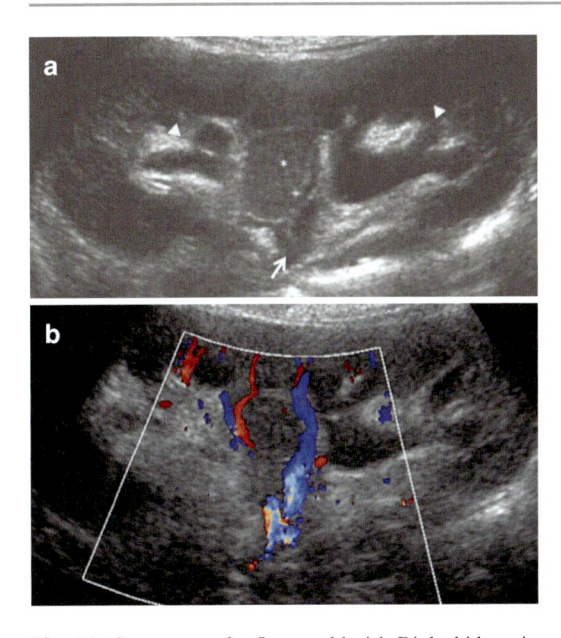

Fig. 10 Sonogram of a 5-year-old girl. Right kidney in longitudinal view. (**a**) A hypertrophic column of Bertin (*asterisk*) extends to the level of the renal sinus bifurcating the renal pelvis into two pyelocalyceal systems (*arrowheads*) which join at the level of the ureteropelvic junction (*arrow*). (**b**) Doppler sonography: characteristic pincerlike splaying of the normal renal vasculature around the enlarged column of Bertin

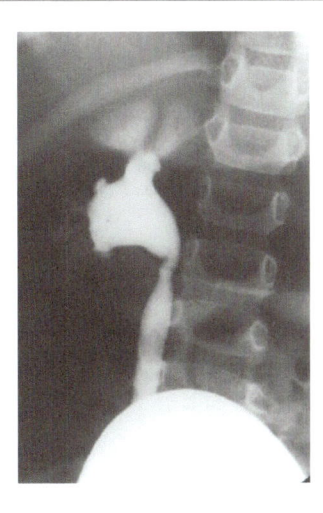

Fig. 11 VCUG in a 2-year-old girl. Intrarenal reflux predominantly at the upper pole

The pyramid with its surrounding cortex makes up a lobe. There are fourteen lobes or more per kidney. In the mid-zone of the kidney, the lobes are simple and conform to the description already given, but at the poles, they tend to be fused and complex (Hodson 1978). In these areas, the septa of Bertin project downward for only short distances. The papillae at the poles may also share in this fusion, and a compound papilla may drain as many as three once separate lobes. This is the type of papilla that allows urine to reflux into the medullar tubuli (Fig. 11) (Ransley 1977; Ransley and Risdon 1975). There are faint striations in the cortex, which are referred to as the medullary rays. They contain the collecting tubules, the thick ascending limbs, and the terminal straight parts of the proximal convoluted tubule. The cortex is made up of glomeruli and a large number of tubules, mainly proximal and distal convoluted segments. The medulla is made up of two zones: the inner zone, which is synonymous with the papilla and contains collecting ducts, thin limbs, loops of Henle, and vasa recta, and the outer zone, which is made up of the outer and inner stripes. The main component of the outer stripe is the terminal straight part of the proximal convoluted tubules, while the main constituents of the inner stripe are thick ascending limbs and collecting tubules (Fig. 12) (Madsen and Tisher 1986).

The specific structural and functional unit of the kidney is the nephron. The nephron consists of the Malpighian corpuscle, glomerulus, and Bowman's capsule, connected to an elongated tubule component composed of the proximal tubule, the thin limbs, and the distal convoluted tubule. A transitional segment, the connecting tubules, joins the nephron to the collecting duct system.

The cortex and even more the medulla are relatively hypoechoic and are usually well differentiated in newborns and infants by US, less clearly in older patients (see Sect. 2.1.5). The cortico-medullary differentiation is generally well demonstrated by MRI and contrast-enhanced CT. They cannot be differentiated by IVU, although stasis of contrast material in the pyramids can be detected in some cases.

2.1.4 Blood Supply

For purposes of its vascular supply, each kidney is regarded as made up of five segments: the apical, upper, middle, lower, and posterior segments. Each of these is supplied by a segmental artery (Fig. 13) (Graves 1954). The main renal artery, as a rule, divides into anterior and posterior parts in the hilum, one passing in front of the pelvis and the other behind. The anterior part generally divides into three segmental branches, the upper, the middle, and the lower, to supply the corresponding segments. The posterior part continues backward before giving rise to several branches that supply the posterior segment. The apical segment has a variable blood supply, but the artery usually takes its origin from the proximal part of the upper segmental artery. There is no evidence of collateral circulation between these segmental arteries; therefore, ligation of a segmental artery in the belief that it is an accessory vessel will lead to necrosis of the corresponding segment (Clapp and Tisher 1989). The intrarenal veins do not follow a segmental arrangement, and there are free anastomoses of the veins throughout the kidney.

The segmental arteries divide several times, finally forming interlobar arteries, which enter the kidney parenchyma between adjacent renal lobes. They extend forward to the cortex on either side of a renal pyramid. At the junction between the cortex and medulla, the interlobar arteries divide dichotomously into arcuate arteries, which follow a curved course between the cortex and medulla. The arcuate arteries undergo several further divisions. From each of these branches, a series of interlobular arteries arise, which finally ascend radially through the cortex. Most of the interlobular arteries terminate within the cortex. Only about five in each kidney, called perforating arteries, reach the surface of the kidney, where they may anastomose with capsular branches derived from the inferior suprarenal, renal, and gonadal arteries (Fig. 14) (Netter 1983).

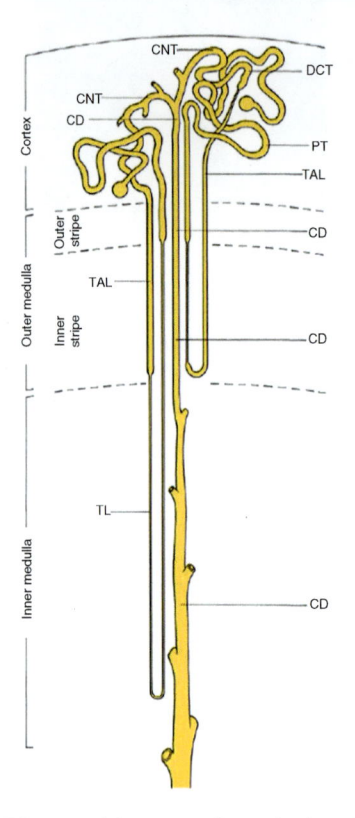

Fig. 12 Diagram of the structural organization of the kidney and its relationships to the zones of the kidney. *CD* collecting duct, *CNT* collecting tubule, *DCT* distal convoluted tubule, *PT* proximal tubule, *TAL* thick ascending limb, *TL* thin limb of Henle's loop

The intrarenal veins accompany the arteries. There are two types of interlobular veins draining the cortex. One type originates at the surface of the kidney as stellate veins draining the most superficial parts of the renal cortex. Most interlobular veins are of the second type, which originates in the cortex as a result of the joining of venules from the peritubular plexus. Both types accompany interlobular arteries and drain in arcuate veins. The arcuate veins join to form interlobar veins. These finally form several veins that join in a simple renal vein (Clapp and Tisher 1989; Heptinstall 1983; Lemley and Kriz 1989).

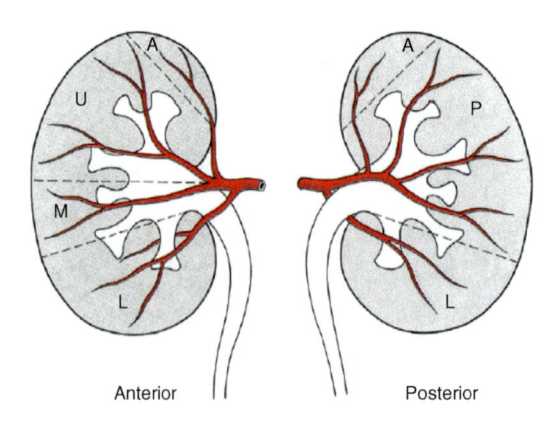

Fig. 13 Diagram of the vascular supply of the kidney. Apical (*A*), lower (*L*), middle (*M*), posterior (*P*), upper (U) segment and segmental branches of the main renal artery a variaty of variations exist

There is a wide variability in the number and course of the renal vessels in relation to the aorta and the inferior vena cava (IVC). Regarding renal arteries, the most frequently encountered variations are related to the number of the main renal arteries and the course of the right renal artery. Two or more main renal arteries can be unilaterally or bilaterally seen in up to 25% of population (Kawamoto et al. 2004; Bouali et al. 2012). Moreover, accessory renal arteries provide frequently additional blood supply to the upper, or, most commonly, the lower pole of the kidneys with a reported prevalence of 25–40% (Satyapal et al. 2001). These arteries may arise from the aorta, the iliac, the superior mesenteric, suprarenal, testicular, or ovarian arteries (Fig. 15). Typically, the right renal artery courses posterior to the IVC, but it can also be found anteriorly. The prevalence of the precaval right renal artery has been reported to be between 0.8 and 9% (Bouali et al. 2012). Early renal arterial branching (i.e., prehilar branching) is another common variant with a reported prevalence in up to 10% of the population (Kawamoto et al. 2004).

Regarding the renal veins, in 5–25% of population, multiple renal veins can be encountered bilaterally or unilaterally (Satyapal et al. 1995). The left renal vein typically courses anterior to the aorta and drains into the IVC on the right. However, anatomic variations in the position of the left renal vein have commonly been described in up to 9% of the population (Sheth and Fishman 2007; Bouali et al. 2012). A retroaortic left renal vein, passing behind the aorta is a common anatomic variant with a prevalence of 7–9% (Fig. 16) (Sheth and Fishman 2007). A circumaortic left renal vein can be found incidentally in as many as 8% of the population and is characterized by the presence of two left renal veins, one preaortic and one retroaortic, forming a collar around the abdominal aorta and draining into the IVC (Fig. 17) (Sheth and Fishman 2007). Most of these variations are found incidentally, although they have been

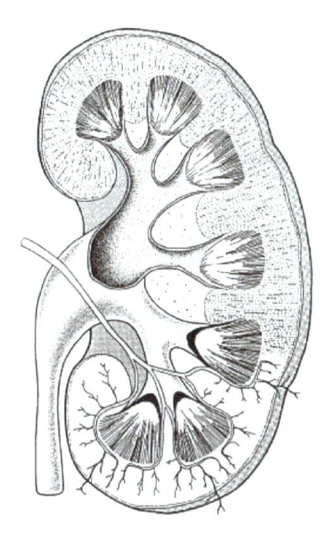

Fig. 14 Cut surface of the right kidney in different levels. The lower half with arteria renalis and its branches

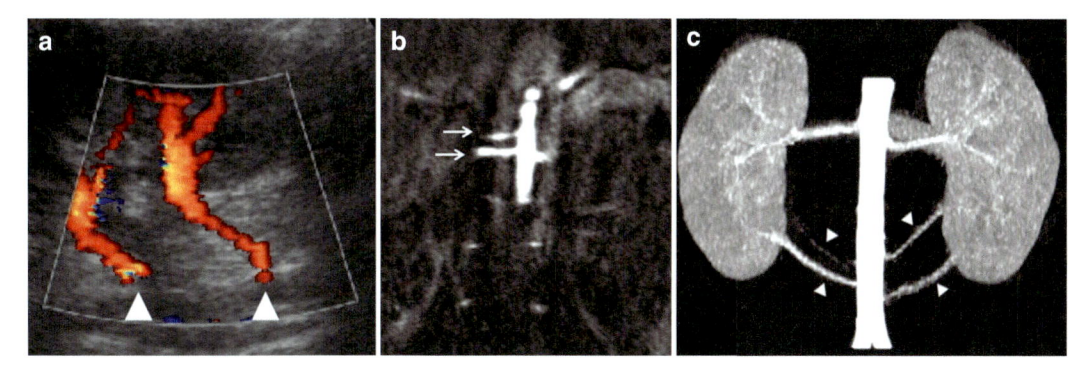

Fig. 15 Renal vasculature variants, incidental findings. (**a**) Color Doppler ultrasound. Two main renal arteries (*arrowheads*) originating from the abdominal aorta supply the right kidney. (**b**) Magnetic resonance angiography. Similarly, two main renal arteries (*arrows*) originating from the abdominal aorta are seen on the right. (**c**) Contrast-enhanced CT. Incidental finding: two accessory renal arteries are seen bilaterally, originating from the abdominal aorta and supplying the lower pole of both kidneys. The more cranially originating right accessory renal artery is smaller in caliber compared to the contralateral and ipsilateral ones

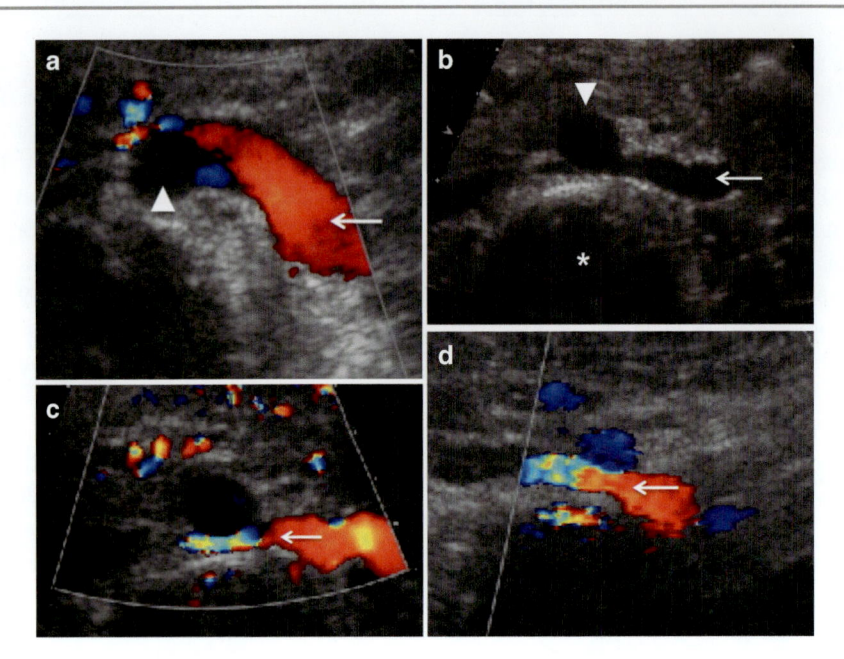

Fig. 16 Left renal vein. Normal course and anatomic variants. (**a**) Colour Doppler sonography. Normal left renal vein (*arrow*) crosses anterior to the aorta and drains into the inferior vena cava on the right. (**b**) Gray scale image of a retroaortic left renal vein, located between the aorta (*arrowhead*) and a lumbar vertebra (*asterisk*). (**c**) Corresponding colour Doppler sonography image demonstrates the retroartic course of the left renal vein with caliber narrowing (*arrow*) and colour aliasing effect, indicative of turbulent and accelerated blood flow within the compressed vessel. This patient had developed mild symptoms of "posterior nutcracker syndrome." (**d**) Colour Doppler sonography in a different patient incidentally demonstrates the retroartic course of the left renal vein without significant narrowing of its lumen. No symptoms of "posterior nutcracker syndrome" were clinically evident

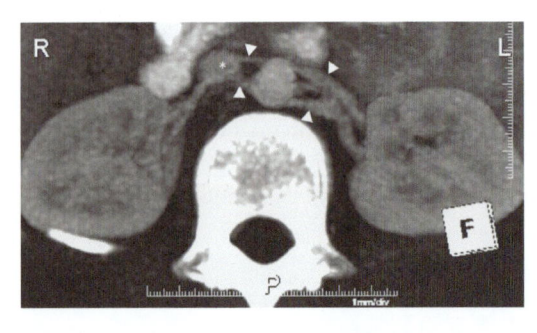

Fig. 17 CT of the abdomen, Maximum intensity projection (MIP) image in oblique transverse plane. Circumaortic left renal vein, an incidental finding. Two left renal vein branches encircle the aorta circumferentially from anterior and posterior (*arrowheads*), draining into the inferior vena cava (*asterisk*)

associated with deep venous thrombosis of the common femoral or iliac veins, and higher risk for development of varicocele in males or pelvic varices/pelvic congestion syndrome in females (Spentzouris et al. 2014). Moreover, they may pose specific challenges during renal or retroperitoneal surgery (Nam et al. 2010). Compression of the retroaortic renal vein between the aorta and lumbar vertebrae may lead to venous drainage impairment on the left kidney, which may clinically be presented with flank pain, hematuria, proteinuria, and hypertension, and is known as "posterior nutcracker syndrome" (Waseem et al. 2012; Alaygut et al. 2013). Another common variant is extrahilar confluence of the renal venous branches.

2.1.5 Neonatal Kidney by Ultrasonography

The US of the neonatal kidney is characterized by typical findings (Fig. 4):

- The increased cortical echogenicity: the echogenicity is usually equal to that of the adjacent liver and spleen; an increased cortical echogenicity in older children usually indicates renal parenchymal disease.

- The medullary pyramids are prominent and relatively hypo- or even nearly anechoic. Furthermore, a transient increase of the echogenicity of the distal medullae and (pre-) papillary region due to physiologic tubular deposits is a normal finding known as transient renal medullary, hyperechogenicity earlier used to be called "Tamm Horsfall Syndrome" (Howlett et al. 1997) (see also chapter "Diagnostic Procedures: Excluding MRI, Nuclear Medicine and Video-Urodynamics").
- Central sinus echoes are absent or reduced.
- Grooves (renculation residuals) are on the surface.

Morphometric studies provide an anatomic basis for understanding this sonographic appearance (Hricak et al. 1983; Dunnill and Halley 1973; McRory 1978).

- Glomeruli occupy proportionally a much greater volume of the renal cortex during the first 2 months of life than at any later time. The number of glomeruli reaches a maximum at 36 gestational weeks. In the normal kidney, the number of nephrons remains constant from 36 weeks of gestational age to 40 years of age. In the neonatal period, the glomeruli occupy 18% of the volume of the cortex as compared with the mean volume of 8.9% in the adult kidney. Furthermore, in mature neonates, 20% of the loops of Henle are still present within the cortex of the kidney at birth. Thus, the cortex usually appears broader than later in life.
- In the neonate, the medulla occupies a proportionally larger cortico-medullary volume than it does later in life. The hypoechoic appearance of the medulla might also be a relative impression secondary to increased cortical echogenicity.
- A lack or paucity of adipose tissue as determined at gross and microscopic inspection would readily explain the absent or reduced dense central sinus echoes.
- The fetal lobulation is still present.

This sonographic appearance of the neonatal kidney can be seen up to the age of 6 months. By 7 months, the renal parenchyma shows the adult pattern. The central sinus echoes gradually increase with age, and a high-intensity adult pattern is seen in most teenagers (Han and Babcock 1985).

Take Away

The junctional parenchymal defect should not be mistaken for a renal scar. The segmental arteries have no collateral circulation. The sonographic appearance of the kidneys for the first months differs from that later in life.

2.2 The Pelvicalyceal System and the Ureters

The renal pelvis varies in size. The pelvis may lie entirely within the renal sinus–intrarenal pelvis – or almost entirely outside it – extrarenal pelvis. An extrarenal pelvis can be found in approximately 10% of the population and is considered a normal anatomic variant without clinical significance (Katzir et al. 2005). However, given the fact that an extrarenal pelvis is not confined by the structures of the renal hilum, it can be more distensible compared to the intrarenal pelvis, thus mimicking obstructive pathology, parapelvic cyst, or collection. In that case careful examination will reveal the coalescence of the renal calyces outside the borders of the renal hilum (Fig. 18). In newborns and small infants, the pelvis is often small and intrarenal and usually points medially instead of downwards.

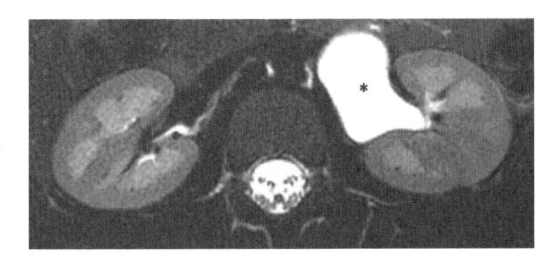

Fig. 18 MRI. T2-weighted sequence with fat suppression. The renal pelvis projects outside the renal hilum (*asterisk*) without any calyceal dilatation being noted

There is a great variation in the configuration of the pelvicalyceal system. The pelvi-ureteric junction (PUJ) is sometimes sharply defined, sometimes difficult to localize. Filling defects or narrowing at the PUJ without pelvicaliceal dilatation due to transient contractions or mild and insignificant narrowing is common findings. A persistence of normal fetal characteristics is sometimes encountered in unobstructed ureters of newborns and infants as mild ureteral elongation and tortuosity, mild widening of the mid-ureter, and short kinks or intraluminal mucosal folds in the proximal ureter.

The ureters in children may be highly mobile and can be displaced by distended bowel loops. Because of continuous peristaltic activity, a normal ureter is not commonly seen in its entirety on a single urographic film. The normal ureter courses obliquely within the bladder wall through the bladder musculature and then submucosally to end in the lateral upper corner of the trigone (Currarino et al. 1993).

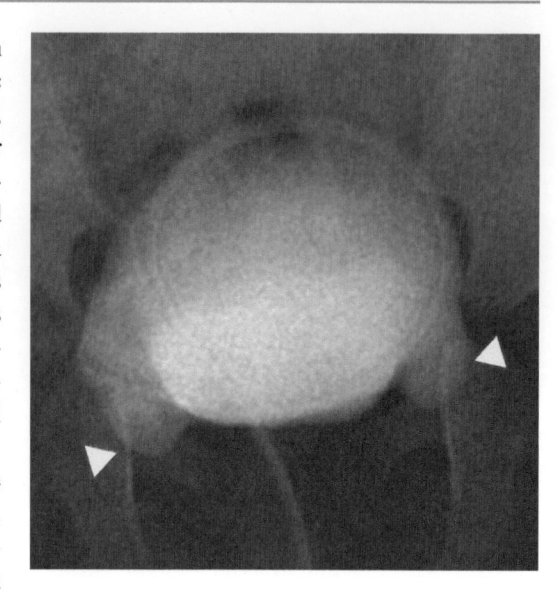

Fig. 19 VCUG in a 4-month-old female. Pulsed fluoroscopy with "last image hold" feature and image contrast inversion. Bladder ears. Bilateral herniation of the urinary bladder into the inguinal canal (*arrowheads*)

2.3 The Urinary Bladder

The bladder is divided into the vertex, body, and fundus. The trigone is the posterior aspect of the bladder base. This triangular space is formed by the two ureteral orifices superolaterally and by the internal urethral meatus inferiorly in the midline. The trigonal or interureteral ridge, the transverse ridge between the two ureteral orifices, may produce a transverse linear defect in the frontal projection when the bladder is incompletely filled with contrast material.

An incompletely filled bladder in infants occasionally shows a transient unilateral or bilateral herniation of its inferolateral wall into a dilated internal inguinal ring. This condition has been observed during VCUGs in up to 10% of infants and is known as "bladder ears" (Fig. 19) (Allen and Condon 1961). These "bladder ears" disappear when the bladder is fully distended. Its occurrence is probably related to the musculature immaturity coupled with the fact that in infants and children the urinary bladder, even when empty, is predominantly located within the abdomen and thus in a close proximity to the internal inguinal ring. With aging the bladder assumes a true pelvic position and this condition resolves by itself. The bladder begins to enter the greater pelvis at about 6 years of age, but it does not enter the lesser pelvis and become a pelvic organ until after puberty (Moore 1992). The same phenomenon has also been detected with the adnexal structures in the lateral-posterior compartment and is usually better depicted by US than by VCUG.

The bladder neck is the poorly delineated junction between the bladder and urethra at the level of the internal urethral sphincter. At the beginning of voiding, the bladder floor descends and becomes funnel-shaped and in continuity with the proximal urethra. At the end of voiding, the bladder base ascends to its normal position. A wide bladder neck and a dilated proximal urethra during voiding (wide bladder neck anomaly and spinning top urethra, respectively) are variants that will be discussed in the chapter on non-neurogenic bladder-sphincter dysfunction (functional disorders of the lower urinary tract).

> **Take Away**
> The bladder begins to descend from the abdomen into the pelvis major at about 6 years of age.

2.4 The Male Urethra

The male urethra is divided into a posterior and an anterior segment (Fig. 20a) (Allen 1970). The posterior (or proximal) urethra is the prostatic urethra, extending from the bladder neck to and through the urogenital diaphragm. This part is surrounded by the prostate and lowers by the external urethral sphincter. In the posterior urethra, there are a number of anatomical landmarks: (1) The verumontanum is an oval swelling of approximately half a centimeter in length. (2) Inferiorly, two thin folds, or fins, can encircle the urethra, completely simulating mild posterior urethral valves. (3) A thin horizontal mucosal fold in the anterior wall of the urethra opposite the verumontanum is called the incisura (Fig. 21). (4) At the apex of the verumontanum, a small diverticulum of the urethra corresponds to the prostatic utricle. (5) Numerous openings of the prostatic ducts are on the wall of the posterior urethra; sometimes contrast material refluxes into the prostatic ducts without distal urethral obstruction. (6) Slightly below there are the openings of the two ejaculatory ducts; sometimes reflux also occurs here without a known cause. (7) The urogenital diaphragm normally causes a circumferential narrowing at the distal end of the posterior urethra (Fig. 2.22). Beyond this narrowing is the membranous urethra, a poorly defined zone, tending to be less distensible than the more dilated bulbous portion below it.

The anterior (or distal) urethra is the cavernous or spongy urethra, divided by the suspensory ligament of the penis into a proximal, bulbar urethra and a distal, pendulous, or penile urethra. On the floor of the bulbar urethra are the two openings of the ducts of the Cowper

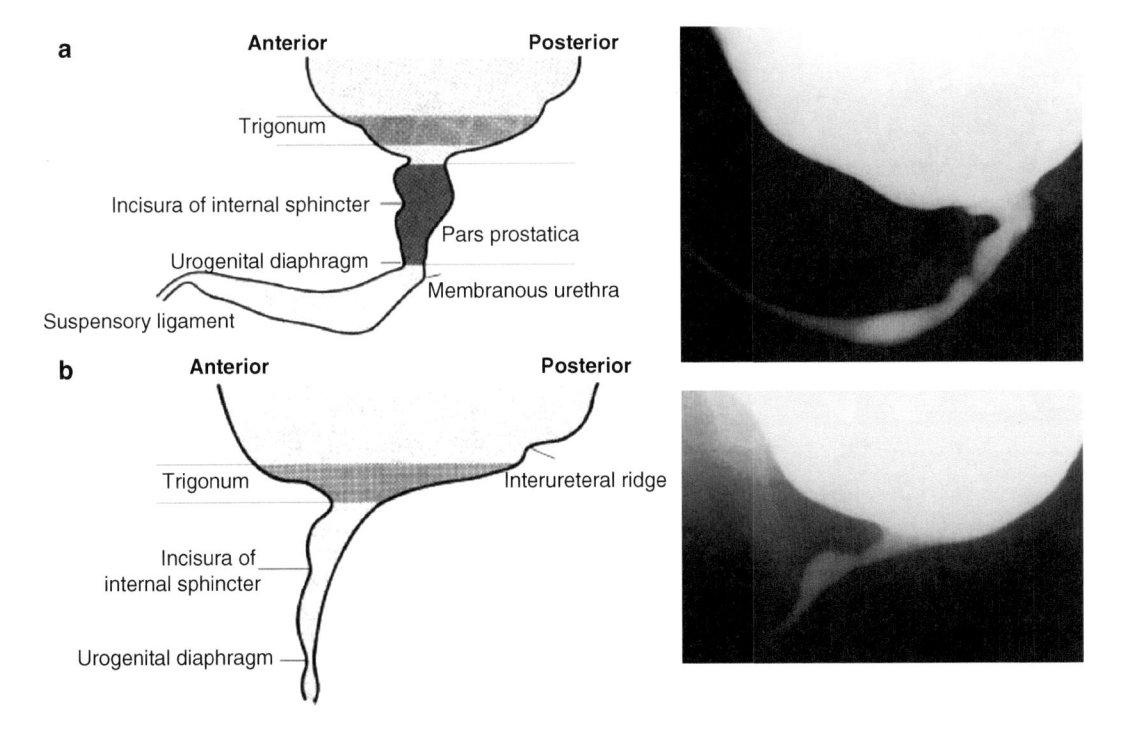

Fig. 20 Diagram of urethrogram and fluoroscopic urethrogram (during voiding on VCUG) showing landmarks of normal structures. (**a**) Male, (**b**) female

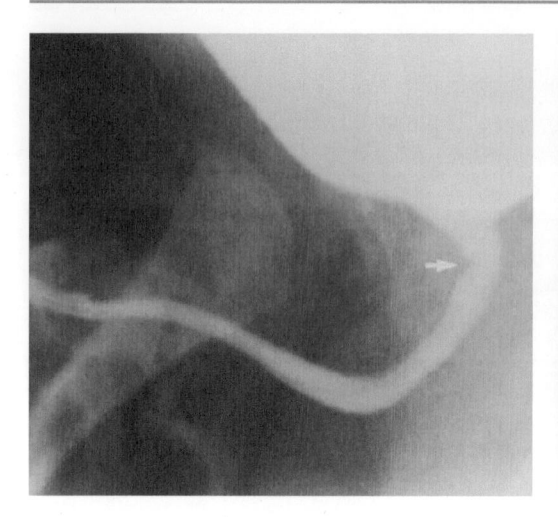

Fig. 21 Voiding image during VCUG in an 8-week-old boy with a normal urethra. The incisura (*arrow*) in the anterior wall is a common anatomical variant

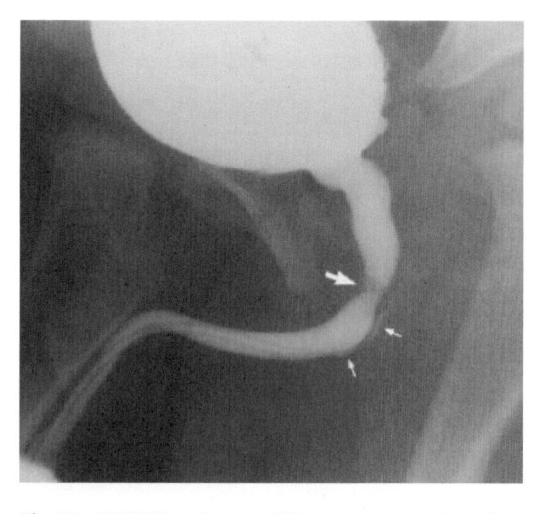

Fig. 22 VCUG in a 2-year-old boy with a normal urethra. The slight narrowing (*large arrow*) at the junction between the posterior and the anterior urethra corresponds to the urogenital diaphragm. The duct of one Cowper gland is visualized by reflux (*double arrow*)

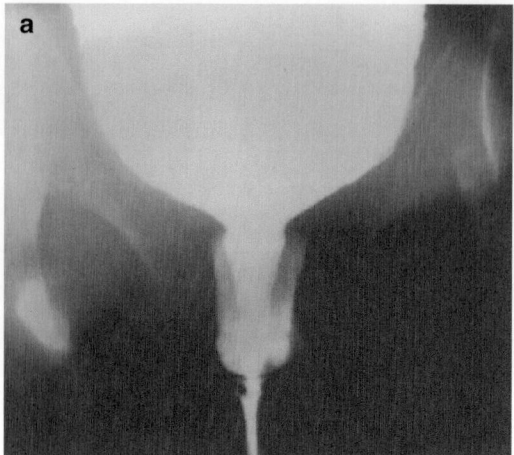

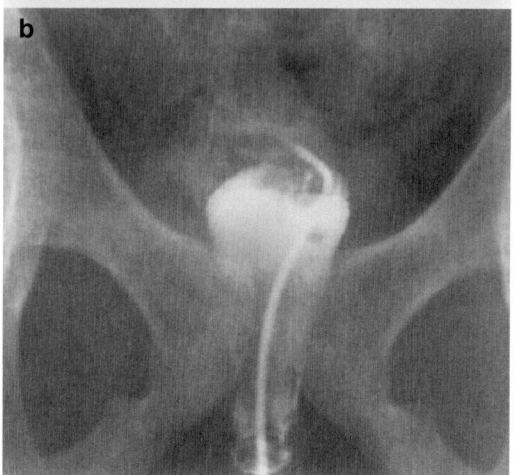

Fig. 23 VCUG in a 9-year-old-girl. (**a**) Influx of contrast material into the vagina during micturition. (**b**) Vaginogram after micturition

glands. Reflux into these openings during VCUG in normal children is possible (Fig. 22). Throughout the anterior urethra are numerous openings of the urethral glands of Littré and the lacunae of Morgagni, seldom seen radiographically. During VCUG in uncircumcised patients, contrast material may accumulate between the glans penis and the prepuce with a typical radiographic pattern.

2.5 The Female Urethra

A diagram of the female urethra is shown in Fig. 20b (Allen 1970). The female urethra has many variations in its normal appearance, depending on the degree of relaxation of the external urethral sphincter and musculature of the pelvic floor during micturition. Influx of contrast material into the vagina during micturition is a very frequent finding without significance – although it may explain some clinical findings in some girls with "recurrent infections" or may lead to a thorough clinical inspection eventually reveling a labial synechia, as such this finding needs to be mentioned in the report (Fig. 23) (Allen 1970; Currarino et al. 1993).

Conclusion

The normal male urethra shows variations in caliber in the different segments. The female urethra varies in appearance on VCUs.

References

Alaygut D, Bayram M, Soylu A, Cakmakci H, Turkmen M, Kavukcu S (2013) Clinical course of children with nutcracker syndrome. Urology 82(3):686–690

Allen RP (1970) The lower urinary tract. In: Kaufmann HJ (ed) Progress in pediatric radiology, genito-urinary tract, vol 3. Karger, Basel, pp 139–163

Allen RP, Condon VR (1961) Transitory extraperitoneal hernia of the bladder in infants (bladder ears). Radiology 77:979–983

Bouali O, Labarre D, Molinier F, Lopez R, Benouaich V, Lauwers F, Moscovici J (2012) Anatomic variations of the renal vessels: focus on the precaval right renal artery. Surg Radiol Anat 34(5):441–446

Campbell MF (1970) Anomalies of the kidney. In: Campbell MF, Harrison JH (eds) Urology, vol 2, 3rd edn. Saunders, Philadelphia, p 1416

Carter AR, Horgan JG, Jennings TA, Rosenfield AT (1985) The junctional parenchymal defect: a sonographic variant of renal anatomy. Radiology 154:499–502

Clapp WL, Tisher CC (1989) Gross anatomy and development of the kidney. In: Tisher CC, Brenner BM (eds) Renal pathology with clinical and functional correlations, vol 1. Lippincott, Philadelphia, pp 67–89

Currarino G, Wood B, Majd M (1993) The genitourinary tract and retroperitoneum. Normal findings and anatomical variants. In: Silverman FN, Kuhn JP (eds) Caffey's pediatric X-ray diagnosis: an integrated imaging approach, vol 2, 9th edn. Mosby, St Louis, pp 1201–1221

Dalla Palma L, Rossi M (1982) Advances in radiological anatomy of the kidney. Br J Radiol 55:404–412

Dalla Palma L, Bazzocchi M, Cressa C, Tommasini G (1990) Radiological anatomy of the kidney revisited. Br J Radiol 63(753):680–690

Deeg KH, Peters H, Schumacher R, Weitzel D (1997) Die Ultraschalluntersuchung des Kindes, 2nd edn. Springer, Berlin/Heidelberg/New York, pp 458–462

Dinkel E, Ertel M, Dittrich M, Peters H, Berres M, Schulte-Wissermann H (1985) Kidney size in childhood. Sonographical growth charts for kidney length and volume. Pediatr Radiol 15(1):38–43

Dunnill MS, Halley W (1973) Some observations on the quantitative anatomy of the kidney. J Pathol 110:113–121

el-Galley RE, Keane TE (2000) Embryology, anatomy, and surgical applications of the kidney and ureter. Surg Clin North Am 80(1):381–401, xiv. Review

Graves FT (1954) The anatomy of the intrarenal arteries and its application to segmental resection of the kidney. Br J Surg 42:132–139

Han BK, Babcock DS (1985) Sonographic measurements and appearance of normal kidneys in children. Am J Roentgenol 145:611–616

Heptinstall RH (1983) Anatomy. In: Heptinstall RH (ed) Pathology of the kidney, 3rd edn. Little, Brown, Boston, pp 1–60

Hodson CJ (1978) The renal parenchyma and its blood supply. Curr Probl Diagn Radiol 7:5–32

Hoffer FA, Hanabergh AM, Teele RL (1985) The interrenicular junction: a mimic of renal scarring on normal pediatric sonograms. Am J Roentgenol 145:1075–1078

Howlett DC, Greenwood KL, Jarosz JM, MacDonald LM, Saunders AJ (1997) The incidence of transient renal medullary hyperechogenicity in neonatal ultrasound examination. Br J Radiol 70:140–143

Hricak H, Slovis TL, Callen CW, Callen PW, Romanski RN (1983) Neonatal kidneys: sonographic anatomic correlation. Radiology 147:699–702

Katzir Z, Witzling M, Nikolov G, Gvirtz G, Arbel E, Kohelet D, Boaz M, Smetana S, Lorberboym M (2005) Neonates with extra-renal pelvis: the first 2 years. Pediatr Nephrol 20(6):763–767

Kawamoto S, Montgomery RA, Lawler LP, Horton KM, Fishman EK (2004) Multi-detector row CT evaluation of living renal donors prior to laparoscopic nephrectomy. Radiographics 24(2):453–466

Kissane JM (1983) Development of the kidney. In: Heptinstall RH (ed) Pathology of the kidney, 3rd edn. Little, Brown, Boston, pp 61–81

Lafortune M, Constantin A, Breton G, Vallee C (1986) Sonography of the hypertrophied column of Bertin. AJR Am J Roentgenol 146(1):53–56

Lemley KV, Kriz W (1989) Structure and function of the renal vasculature. In: Tisher CC, Brenner BM (eds) Renal pathology with clinical and functional correlations, vol 2. Lippincott, Philadelphia, pp 926–964

Madsen KM, Tisher CC (1986) Structural-functional relationships along the distal nephron. Am J Physiol 250(Renal Fluid Electrolyte Physiol 19):F1–F15

McRory WW (1978) Embryonic development and prenatal maturation of the kidney. In: Edelmann CM Jr (ed) Pediatric kidney disease. Little, Brown, Boston, pp 23–25

Moore KL (1992) Clinically oriented anatomy, 3rd edn. Williams & Wilkins, Baltimore

Moore KL, Persaud TVN (1998) The developing human. Clinically oriented embryology, 6th edn. Saunders, Philadelphia

Nam JK, Park SW, Lee SD, Chung MK (2010) The clinical significance of a retroaortic left renal vein. Korean J Urol 51(4):276–280

Netter FH (1983) Farbatlanten der Medizin, vol 2, Niere und Harnwege. Thieme, Stuttgart

Olsson CA (1986) Anatomy of the upper urinary tract. In: Walsh PC, Gittes RF, Perlmutter AD, Stamey TA (eds) Campbell's urology, 5th edn. Saunders, Philadelphia, pp 12–46

Potter EL (1972) Normal and abnormal development of the kidney. Year Book, Chicago

Ransley PG (1977) Intrarenal reflux. I. Anatomical, dynamic and radiological studies. Urol Res 5:61–69

Ransley PG, Risdon RA (1975) Renal papillary morphology and intrarenal reflux in the young pig. Urol Res 3:105–109

Richter E, Lierse W (1990) Radiologische Anatomie des Neugeborenen. Urban & Schwarzenberg, Munich

Satyapal KS, Rambiritch V, Pillai G (1995) Additional renal veins: incidence and morphometry. Clin Anat 8(1):51–55

Satyapal KS, Haffejee AA, Singh B, Ramsaroop L, Robbs JV, Kalideen JM (2001) Additional renal arteries: incidence and morphometry. Surg Radiol Anat 23(1):33–38

Sheth S, Fishman EK (2007) Imaging of the inferior vena cava with MDCT. AJR Am J Roentgenol 189(5):1243–1251

Spentzouris G, Zandian A, Cesmebasi A, Kinsella CR, Muhleman M, Mirzayan N, Shirak M, Tubbs RS, Shaffer K, Loukas M (2014) The clinical anatomy of the inferior vena cava: a review of common congenital anomalies and considerations for clinicians. Clin Anat 27(8):1234–1243. doi:10.1002/ca.22445

Waseem M, Upadhyay R, Prosper G (2012) The nutcracker syndrome: an underrecognized cause of hematuria. Eur J Pediatr 171(8):1269–1271

Williams H (2007) Renal revision: from lobulation to duplication – what is normal? Arch Dis Child Educ Pract Ed 92(5):ep152–ep158

Yeh HC, Halton KP, Shapiro RS, Rabinowitz JG, Mitty HA (1992) Junctional parenchyma: revised definition of hypertrophic column of Bertin. Radiology 185(3):725–732

Urogenital Fetal Imaging: US and MRI

Marie Cassart

Contents

1	Introduction	151
2	**The Normal Aspects of the Urinary Tract**	152
2.1	Ultrasound (US)	152
2.2	Fetal Magnetic Resonance Imaging (MRI)	152
3	**Fetal Uropathies**	154
3.1	Obstructive Uropathies	154
3.2	Uretero-pelvic Duplication	156
3.3	Refluxing Uropathy/Vesicoureteric Reflux	157
4	**Fetal Nephropathies**	158
4.1	Multicystic Dysplastic Kidneys (MCDK)	158
4.2	Polycystic Kidneys	159
4.3	Renal Dysplasia	160
4.4	Renal Vein Thrombosis	160
5	**Fetal Bladder Anomalies**	161
5.1	Megabladder	161
5.2	Bladder Exstrophy	162
6	**Complex Lower Urinary Tract Malformations**	163
6.1	Urogenital Sinus Anomalies	163
6.2	Cloacal Dysgenesis	164
	Conclusion	165
	References	165

M. Cassart, MD, PhD
Department of Fetal and Pediatric Imaging,
Etterbeek-Ixelles Hospital, Brussels, Belgium
e-mail: MCASSART@his-izz.be

1 Introduction

Congenital abnormalities of the kidneys and urinary tract (CAKUT) represent the most frequently encountered malformations in the fetus. They can affect the renal parenchyma or the urinary tract very early in the fetal development and lead to chronic renal failure in early childhood. The more systematic use of obstetrical US has led to the discovery of many fetal malformations. Abnormalities of the kidney and urinary tract represent the largest group of congenital anomalies leading to neonatal and pediatric care. The affected population represents 0.2–2 % of all newborns (Wiesel et al. 2005). The complementary use of fetal magnetic resonance imaging (MRI) is a step forward that may improve diagnostic assessment of structural urinary tract abnormalities (Pico et al. 2014). The aim of prenatal diagnosis is to entail a better management of these patients pre- and postnatally. Even in asymptomatic patients, a preventive treatment can sometimes be established in order to improve the long-term prognosis of some uro-nephropathies (Ismaili et al. 2005a, b, 2006).

2 The Normal Aspects of the Urinary Tract

2.1 Ultrasound (US)

Depending on the acoustic quality of an ultrasound examination, the fetal kidneys can be seen at around 12 weeks with transabdominal probes. During the first trimester, the kidneys appear as hyperechoic oval structures at both sides of the spine (Fig. 1) (Avni et al. 2002, 2007). This echogenicity will progressively decrease, in parallel with the visualization of a cortico-medullary differentiation that will begin around 14–15 weeks, which should always be visible in fetuses older than 18 weeks (Fig. 2) (Devriendt et al. 2013). The kidneys will grow in size, and – as a rule – a normal kidney grows at a rate of 1.1 mm per week of gestation (length). Measurements should be referred to the tables (van Vuuren et al. 2012). An axial scan centered on the hilum of the kidneys is performed in order to measure the renal pelvis.

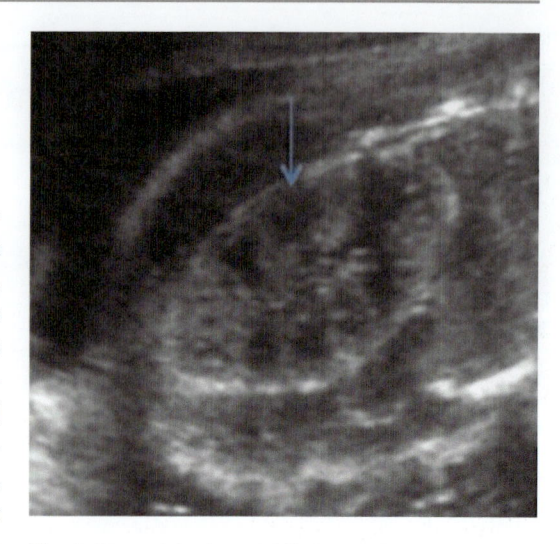

Fig. 2 Normal fetal renal US. Parasagittal US scan of a well-differentiated kidney at 28 weeks of gestational age. Notice the hypoechoic aspect of the pyramids allowing depiction of cortico-medullary differentiation (*arrow*)

The pelvis measurement should not exceed 4 mm in the second and 7 mm in the third trimester. The bladder is visible from the ninth week of gestation, thanks to its own fetal urinary production. It is seen as a small anechoic structure surrounded by the two umbilical arteries in the fetal pelvis (Fig. 3). The bladder should always be seen during sonographic examinations, and its filling-emptying cycle is around 25 min (Lee et al. 2010).

> **Take Away**
> The sonographer should be aware of the physiological developmental changes of the kidneys during pregnancy.

2.2 Fetal Magnetic Resonance Imaging (MRI)

Fetal MRI is mostly performed later in pregnancy. In the second trimester, US has a better spatial resolution. In the third trimester, secondary to the increase in fetal volume and decrease in its mobility, MRI becomes a very performing tool for imaging the fetal urinary

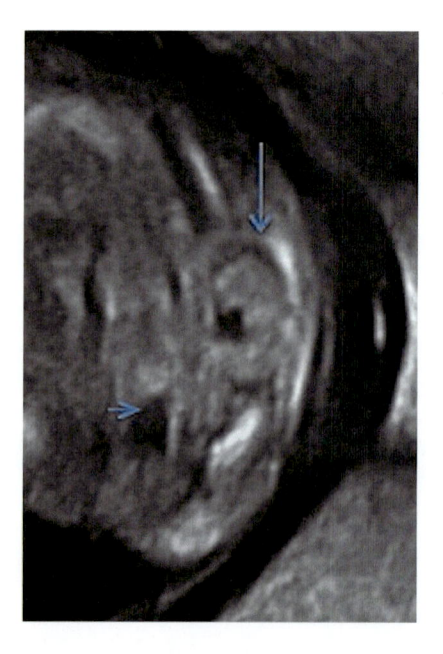

Fig. 1 Normal fetal renal US in early pregnancy. Parasagittal US scan of the abdomen of a 14-week-old fetus. The kidney appears like a hyperechoic mass (*arrow*) and the bladder like a pelvic liquid structure (*arrowhead*)

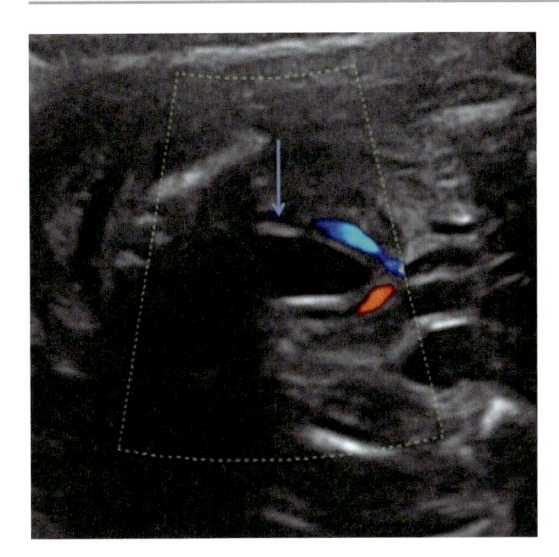

Fig. 3 Normal fetal bladder US. Axial US scan centered on the bladder (*arrow*) of a 22-week-old fetus. The bladder is surrounded by the two umbilical arteries encoded in *blue* and *red* on color Doppler sonography

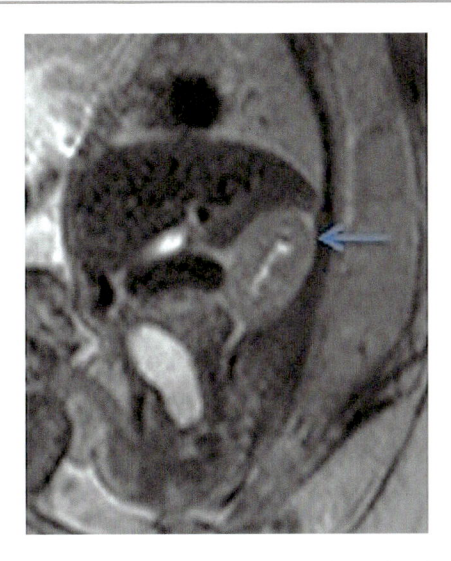

Fig. 4 Normal fetal kidney – MRI. Sagittal T2-weighted MR image centered on a normal right kidney (*arrow*) in a 31-week-old fetus. The cortico-medullar differentiation is not depictable

tract, thanks to its large field of view and excellent contrast resolution (Cassart et al. 2004a, b). Still, it is only performed in cases for which US has not completely elucidated the malformation. The sequences used are mostly T2 weighted. They are performed in three orthogonal planes according to the fetus. The parameters of the TSE sequence are as follow (TE, 80 ms; TR, 8130 ms; slice thickness, 3.5 mm; acquisition time, 16 s.) On these sequences, the kidneys appear like intermediate signal structures (Fig. 4). The cortico-medullar differentiation is presently not or only poorly visible on MRI. On the contrary, the renal cavities and the bladder, filled with urine, are easily seen as hyperintense structures (Fig. 5). Diffusion sequences in conjunction with anatomical sequences can be interesting in cases of sus-

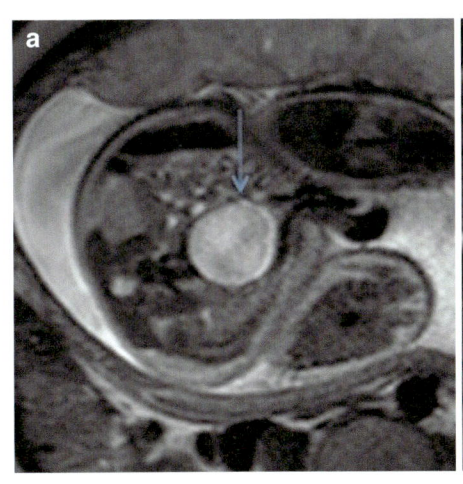

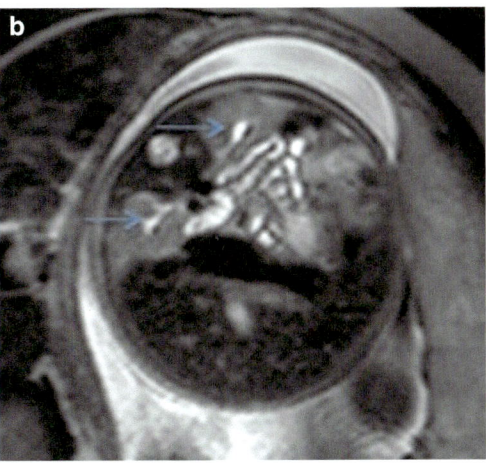

Fig. 5 Normal fetal urinary tract – MRI. (**a**) Axial T2-weighted MR image on the pelvis of a 30-week-old fetus. The bladder appears like a hyperintense pelvic structure (*arrow*). (**b**) Axial T2-weighted MR image on the abdomen of the same fetus. The normal renal cavities filled with urine appear hyperintense (*arrows*)

pected nephropathies or parenchymal insults (renal vein thrombosis, dysplasia), as well as poorly depictable ectopic kidneys (Chaumoitre et al. 2006; Witzani et al. 2006). MRI, better than US, allows the differentiation of the urinary tract from the digestive tract (Fig. 6), as both present a specific signal due to their respective urine or meconium contents: on T1-weighted sequences, meconium appears hyperintense helping to identify the digestive tract; the parameters of the FFE T1-weighted sequence preferably performed during breath hold are TR/TE of 152/4.6, slice thickness of 4 mm, and acquisition time of 17 s. This may be of great interest in complex malformations involving both urinary and digestive tracts such as cloacal dysgenesis.

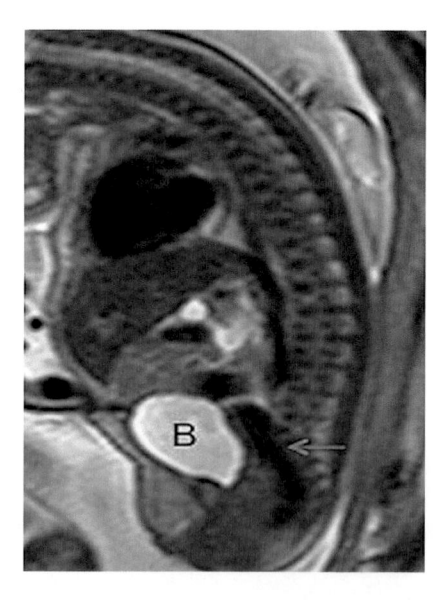

Fig. 6 Normal fetal pelvic – MRI. Sagittal T2-weighted MR images performed on a 32-week-old fetus showing the normal spontaneous different signal of the bladder (*B*) and rectosigmoid (*arrow*)

Take Away
MRI is a helpful complementary tool to US in imaging the fetal urinary tract, thanks to its greater contrast resolution, particularly helpful in difficult case or equivocal US results.

3 Fetal Uropathies

3.1 Obstructive Uropathies

3.1.1 Pelvi-ureteric Junction Obstruction

This malformation consists in a functional or anatomical obstruction to the urine flow between the renal pelvis and the ureter. It may be secondary to an intrinsic anomaly (collagen, muscle) or an extrinsic compression (crossing vessels, tumor, etc.). It occurs in 13 % of children with antenatal diagnosis of renal pelvis dilatation (Ismaili et al. 2004). On prenatal US, the renal pelvis is enlarged without dilatation of the ureters or bladder. It should be suspected in case with moderate (10–15 mm) or severe (larger than 15 mm) dilatation, when the renal calices appear round shaped, or in the presence of a perirenal urinoma (Ismaili et al. 2005a, b) (Fig. 7). Prognosis may be poor in bilateral cases associated with oligohydramnios. The aspect of the renal parenchyma is important for the prognosis: cortical hyper-echogenicity, reduced renal parenchymal thickness, and parenchymal cysts are predictors of a poorer outcome.

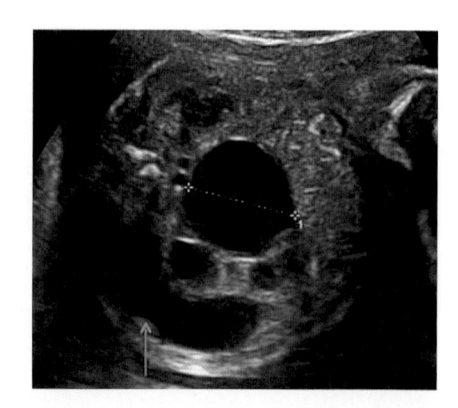

Fig. 7 Fetal US in pelvi-ureteric junction obstruction. Axial US scan showing the dilated round-shaped pelvic cavity of the right kidney (+ +) in a pelvi-ureteric junction stenosis in a 26-week-old fetus. Adjacent to the kidney, an urinoma is present due to the pelvic rupture (*arrow*)

3.1.2 Ureterovesical Junction Obstruction (Megaureter)

In utero, under normal conditions, the fetal ureters should not be visualized. On US, an enlarged "megaureter" presents like a serpentine fluid-filled structure potentially associated with dilated renal cavities (Fig. 8). The ureter may be dilated because of mechanical obstruction or because of a (segmentally) dysplastic wall of the ureter at the level of the ureterovesical junction. Nonobstructive etiologies such as high-grade vesicoureteric reflux (VUR) are secondary to a lack of normal valve-like mechanism or normal ureteral tonus and peristalsis at the ureterovesical junction. In the fetus, the differential diagnosis between the two entities is difficult. In both cases, the renal cavities can be dilated. Megaureter can also be encountered in fetuses with urethral obstruction (posterior urethral valves) because of associated uni- or bilateral VUR (also see chapters "UTI and VUR" and "Vesicoureteric Reflux)". The etiology of the dilated ureter will be clarified after birth on voiding cystography that will confirm or exclude a VUR.

3.1.3 Urethral Obstruction

In the fetus, an obstacle on the urethra can be suspected when the bladder appears constantly enlarged. When encountered in the first trimester, the most common causes are prune belly syndrome and fibro-urethral stenosis (Fig. 9). A significant proportion of these cases is associated with chromosomal and/or multiple congenital anomalies and carry a poorer prognosis (Jouannic et al. 2003). In the second trimester, the most common cause of lower urinary tract obstruction in male fetuses is a posterior urethral valve (PUV) which is an abnormal mucosal fold between the lateral urethral wall and the distal end of the verumontanum. On US, failure of the bladder to empty during a lasting examination, a thickened bladder wall, abnormal kidneys and oligohydramnios must raise the suspicion of a PUV. Under favorable US conditions, the dilated proximal urethra may take the aspect of a keyhole (Fig. 10). This sign is suggestive but not specific of PUV. In some cases, urinary ascites and urinoma may be seen secondary to bladder or renal collecting system rupture (Fig. 10). This phenomenon was thought to be a protective pop-off mechanism, although recent reports critically discuss this aspect (Spaggiari et al 2013).

In many cases, there is only a partial urinary obstruction, and amniotic fluid volume can be maintained throughout pregnancy. Sometimes spontaneous rupture of valves may occur prena-

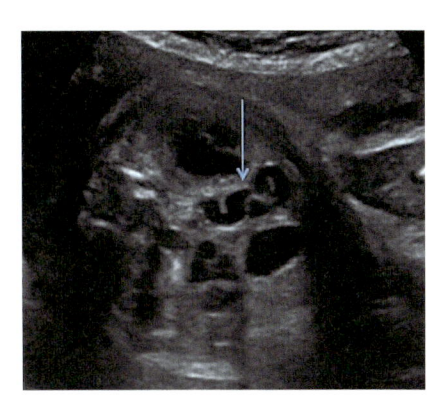

Fig. 8 Fetal US in megaureter. Axial US scan on the abdomen of a 28-week-old fetus showing a serpentine fluid-filled structure corresponding to the dilated ureter (*arrow*)

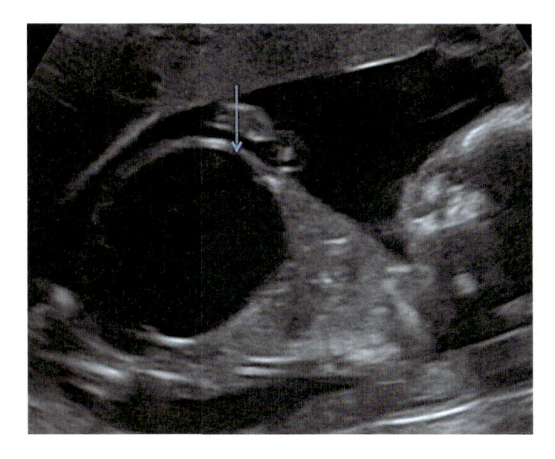

Fig. 9 Fetal US in prune belly syndrome. Sagittal US scan of a 16-week-old fetus with distended bladder (*arrow*) in a context of prune belly syndrome (confirmed on postmortem examination)

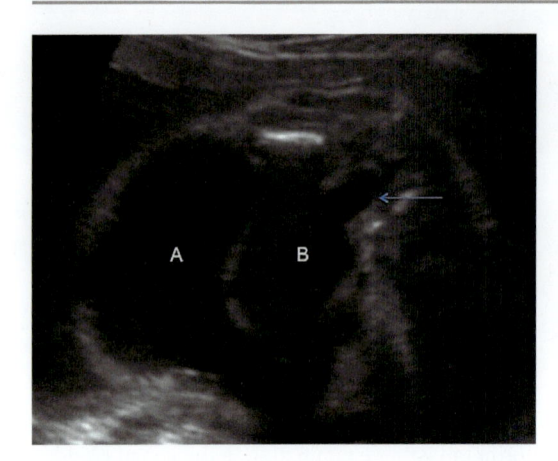

Fig. 10 Fetal US of the proximal urethra in PUV. Axial US scan centered on the pelvis of a 30-week-old fetus presenting a urethral valve. There is ascites (*A*). The posterior dilated urethra is visible (*arrow*) below the bladder (*B*)

tally with the reappearance of a normal cyclical bladder emptying. Diagnosis before 24 weeks, oligohydramnios, and increased renal cortical echogenicity with the absence of cortico-medullary differentiation are the most reliable indicators for a poor prognosis (Morris et al. 2009). Renal parenchymal lesions are secondary to the obstruction (dysplasia) but also to the frequently associated high-grade VUR (see below).

> **Take Away**
> Whatever the level of the obstruction and the coexistence of a possible associated VUR, the main prognostic factors are the aspect of the renal parenchyma and the amount of amniotic fluid.

3.2 Uretero-pelvic Duplication

The term renal duplication includes a complete or partial duplication of the kidney and ureters. The kidney presents two pelvi-caliceal systems drained either by a complete duplicated set of ureters or a bifid ureter with two proximal ureters that fuse somewhere above the ureterovesical junction. On fetal US, the kidney presents two sinuses separated by a parenchymal bridge (Whitten and Wilcox 2001). Cases with non-dilated cavities have no renal functional impairment and are considered as normal variants; these may be more difficult to depict. However, a proportion of duplex kidneys may be associated with significant pathology, due to the presence of associated VUR and/or obstruction (Fig. 11). Vesicoureteral reflux usually occurs into the lower pole ureter and can be of a high grade. Obstruction mostly involves the upper moiety. It may be associated with an obstructive ureterocele although obstruction of the upper pole may also occur secondary to an ectopic insertion or an isolated vesicoureteric junction obstruction, with a high incidence of parenchymal dysplasia (Whitten and Wilcox 2001). On fetal US, these "complicated" duplications should be suspected in the presence of two separate noncommunicating renal pelves, dilated ureters, cystic structures within one pole (more frequently the upper pole), and a cystic dilatation of the distal ureter seen within the bladder corresponding to the uretero-cele (Fig. 12). In very complex cases (huge dilatation, renal dysplasia, ectopic ureteral insertion) when US is unclear, MRI may help in the understanding of the malformation (Cassart et al.

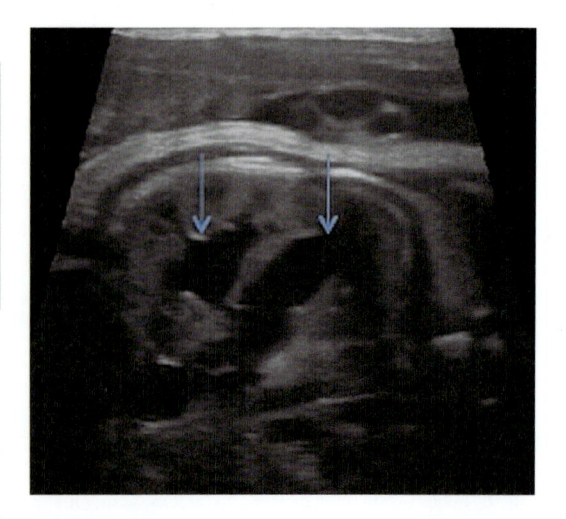

Fig. 11 Fetal US in duplication. Coronal US scan of a duplex kidney in a 32-week-old fetus. The two pelvic cavities are dilated (*arrows*) – this is a complicated duplication

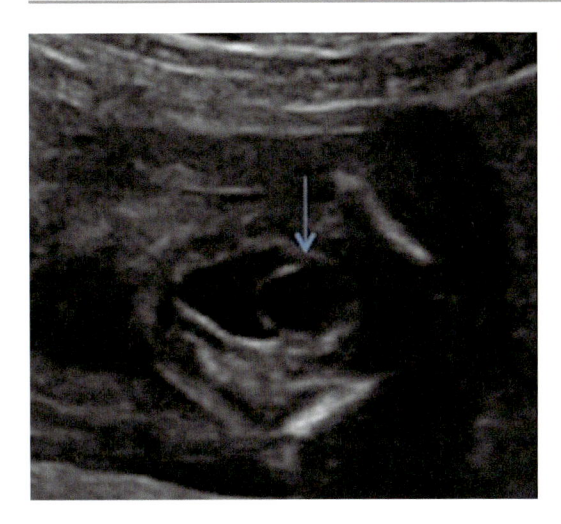

Fig. 12 Fetal US of an ureterocele. Axial US scan performed on the bladder of a 20-week-old fetus with a duplex kidney. The scan shows a cystic dilatation of the distal ureter seen within the bladder corresponding to an ureterocele (*arrow*)

2004a). In cases with huge ureteral dilatation, the differentiation with dilated bowel may be difficult on US. Thanks to the specific T2 hypersignal of their liquid content, the ureters can more easily be identified on MRI; sometimes also their ectopic insertion can be diagnosed (Fig. 13).

> **Take Away**
> MRI better than US may help in depicting the precise anatomy of complex duplicated systems.

3.3 Refluxing Uropathy/ Vesicoureteric Reflux

Vesicoureteric reflux (VUR) is defined as the retrograde flow of urine from the bladder upward into the ureters, sometimes the renal pelvis, calyces, and even intrarenally into the collecting ducts. It is secondary to an anomaly of the ureterovesical junction or secondary to an ectopic insertion of the ureter in cases of ureteral duplication (the respective ostium is usually seen more lateralized and more cranially). On fetal US, VUR should be suspected in cases of a dilated renal pelvis at the second or third trimester (more than 4 or 7 mm, respectively), particularly if associated with varying axial diameter. Fetal renal pelvis dilatation is secondary to VUR in 11–30 % of cases (Ismaili et al. 2004). Some additional sonographic find-

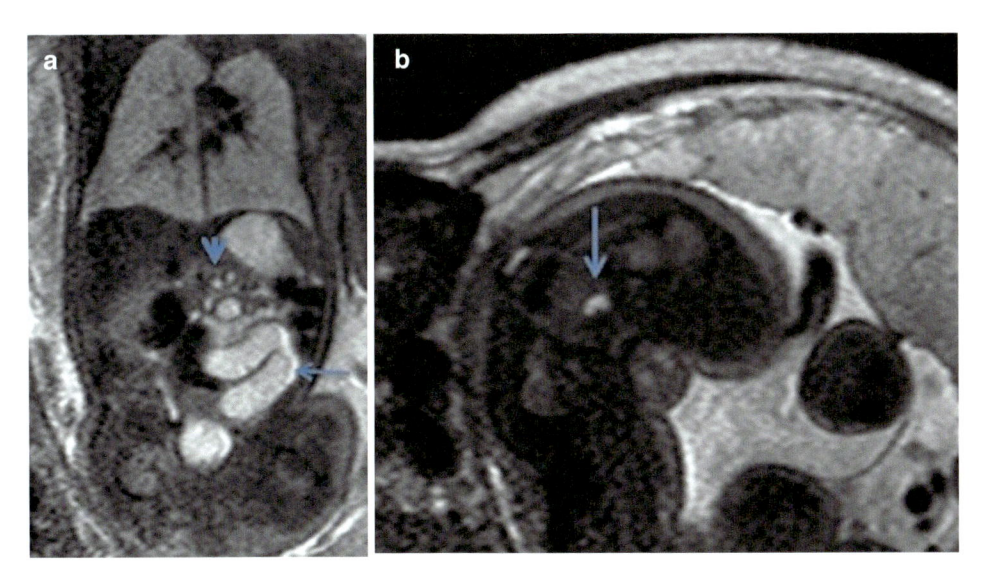

Fig. 13 Fetal MRI of a complicated renal duplication. (**a**) Coronal T2-weighted MR image of a 30-week-old female fetus with left duplex kidney. The upper pole is dysplastic with cysts (*arrowhead*) and drained by a megaureter (*arrow*). (**b**) More caudal axial T2-weighted MR image on the pelvis of the same fetus, the ureter is seen under the bladder neck suggesting an ectopic (vaginal) insertion, which was confirmed after birth

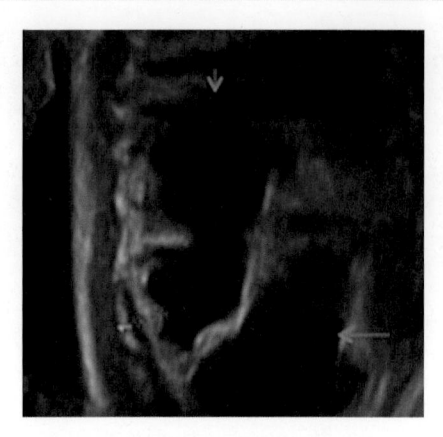

Fig. 14 Fetal US in reflux. Sagittal US scan performed on a 32-week-old fetus. The bladder is enlarged (*arrow*). The kidney presents dilated cavities (*arrowhead*) and a thinned hyperechoic parenchyma (+ +). High-grade VUR was confirmed after birth

ings may support the diagnosis of VUR; those signs include variable renal collecting system dilatation during real-time scanning, pelvi-caliceal wall thickening, ureteral enlargement, and megabladder (without wall thickening) (Grazioli et al. 2010). The arguments supporting the importance of antenatal diagnosis of VUR derive from an increased risk of postnatal infection and progressive functional decline in untreated newborns and children with high-grade VUR and urinary tract infections, although some fetuses already have renal lesions due to the disease, namely, associated congenital dysplasia. Those cases may be detected on prenatal US, and the renal parenchyma then appears thinned, hyperechoic, and undifferentiated (Fig. 14).

> **Take Away**
> Refluxing uropathy may be suspected on prenatal US, however the diagnosis should always be confirmed on postnatal imaging as prenatal findings are not specific.

4 Fetal Nephropathies

4.1 Multicystic Dysplastic Kidneys (MCDK)

Multicystic dysplastic kidneys result from an aberrant development of nephrogenic and ductal structures in which the underlying etiology seems to be a very early urinary tract obstruction. In MCDK, the kidney is composed of undifferentiated and metaplastic tissues in association with cysts (Fig. 15). The kidney is often increased in size during fetal life and often shrinks during the first years of life. The ipsilateral ureter is commonly abnormal: atretic, absent, ectopic, with or without ureterocele, or dilated due to a possible urinary tract obstruction. There is an increased risk of associated genital malformations. MCDK may also develop in the upper part of a duplex system or be located in an ectopic position. Because MCDK are nonfunctional, careful examination of the contralateral kidney is essential because there is a higher incidence of associated pathologies (Fig. 16) (Ismaili et al. 2005c).

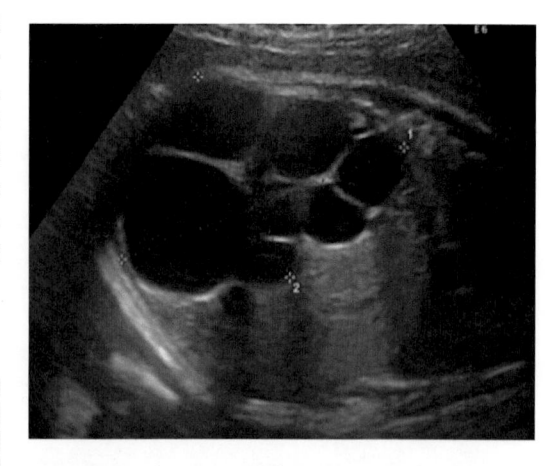

Fig. 15 Fetal US in MCDK. Sagittal US scan performed on a 34-week-old fetus. The multicystic kidney (+ +) is large and almost fills the entire abdominal cavity. There is no renal parenchyma and no renal cavities (Courtesy Dr.L.Tecco)

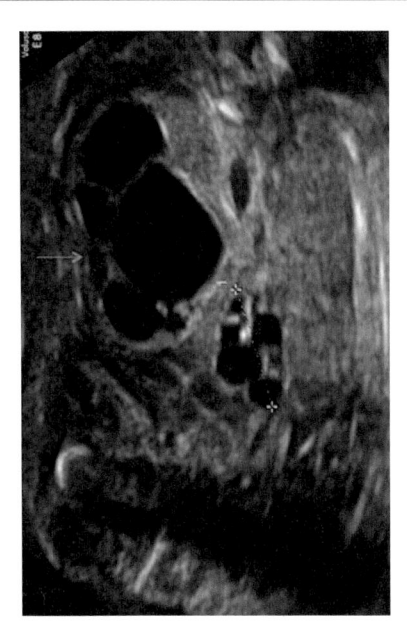

Fig. 16 Fetal US in ectopic MCDK. Coronal US scan performed on a 24-week-old fetus. The small multicystic kidney is in a pelvic location (+ +). The contralateral kidney presents with huge pelvi-caliceal dilatation (*arrow*), which worsens the prognosis

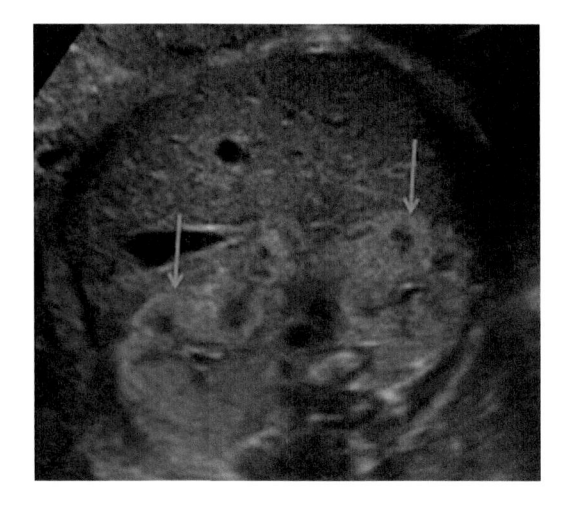

Fig. 17 Fetal US in ADPKD. Axial US scans performed on a 31-week-old fetus. The kidneys are enlarged with increased echogenicity of the cortex (compared to the adjacent liver). The mother is affected by ADPKD. The mutation (PKD1) was confirmed in the newborn (Courtesy Dr. A.Cogan)

> **Take Away**
> MCDK is a dysplastic nonfunctioning kidney resulting from early urinary tract obstruction. The normality of the contralateral kidney is determinant in the prognosis.

4.2 Polycystic Kidneys

Polycystic kidneys are congenital renal malformations of hereditary origin with dominant or recessive transmission (Avni et al. 2012).

4.2.1 Autosomal Dominant Polycystic Kidney Disease (ADPKD)

ADPKD is a common hereditary kidney disease. The abnormality consists of a cystic dilatation of any parts of the nephron, which causes the kidneys to enlarge (Wilson 2004). Although usually there is a late age of clinical onset of this disorder, early detection in the prenatal period has been reported (Brun et al. 2004). The most common presentation in utero consists in slightly enlarged kidneys with increased cortico-medullary differentiation due to cortical hyper-echogenicity (Fig. 17). Cysts are unusual but can occur in utero. According to this pattern and the family history, the diagnosis of recurrence can be suspected and the mutation searched. Another pattern similar to the one of the recessive type has also been described with poorer prognosis.

4.2.2 Autosomal Recessive Polycystic Kidney Disease (ARPKD)

ARPKD is another hereditary kidney disease that belongs to the family of cilia-related disorders. The disease is characterized by dilated collecting tubules in the medulla. The cortex is less affected since it contains fewer tubules. The classical in utero US pattern of ARPKD includes markedly enlarged (>4 SD) hyperechoic kidneys without cortico-medullary differentiation. This appearance can be observed in the second trimester. The patterns may evolve to a reversed cortico-

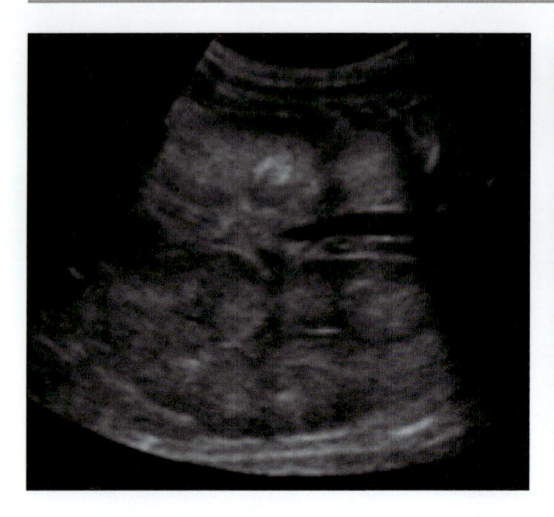

Fig. 18 Fetal US in ARPKD. Coronal US scan performed on a 33-week-old fetus showing enlarged kidneys with cortico-medullar inversion and oligohydramnios. This association is suggestive of ARPKD. The diagnosis was confirmed on histological data (Courtesy Dr. C. Garel)

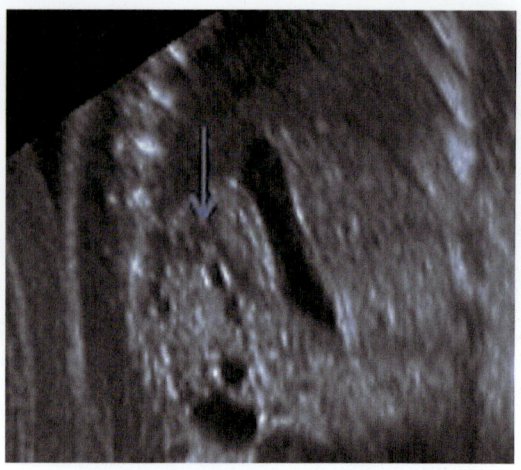

Fig. 19 Fetal US of a renal cystic dysplasia. Parasagittal US scan of a cystic dysplastic kidney (*arrow*) in a 31-week-old fetus. The contralateral kidney is normal

medullary differentiation due to the presence of material within the dilated tubules (Wilson 2004) (Fig. 18) in the third trimester. If associated, oligohydramnios and lung hypoplasia significantly worsen the prognosis. Differential diagnoses include several syndromes like Bardet-Biedl syndrome in which polydactyly is present (Cassart et al. 2004b).

> **Take Away**
> The prenatal sonographic diagnosis of a polycystic renal disease should lead to familial and genetical enquiries in order to establish a precise diagnosis.

4.3 Renal Dysplasia

In renal dysplasia, the parenchyma presents abnormal differentiation and organization. Hypoplasia corresponds to a reduction of the number of nephrons in small kidneys (below −2 SD) (Ismaili et al. 2001). Both hypoplasia and dysplasia often coexist. They may be inherited or secondary to congenital causes (obstruction, VUR, etc.) (see above). On US, the kidneys appear small, sometimes hyperechoic (related to the amount of dysplasia), and sometimes with cystic structures (cystic dysplasia) (Fig. 19). Again, the prognosis in utero relies on the contralateral kidney; cases with oligohydramnios usually have bilateral disease and have the poorest outcome (Winyard and Chitty 2001).

4.4 Renal Vein Thrombosis

Renal vein thrombosis is the most common vascular condition that may affect the fetal kidney. It mostly concerns the left kidney and the male fetus. Predisposing factors in utero are maternal conditions like diabetes, polycythemia, prothrombotic abnormalities (protein C or S deficiency, factor V Leiden mutation, lupus anticoagulant, and antithrombin III deficiency) or twin pregnancies (Marks et al. 2005; Weber et al. 2014), and fetal conditions like ascites or digestive occlusion. However, the origin of the thrombosis is not always obvious. Sonographically, the fetal kidney appears enlarged with an undifferentiated hyperechoic cortex (Fig. 20). Pathognomonic vascular

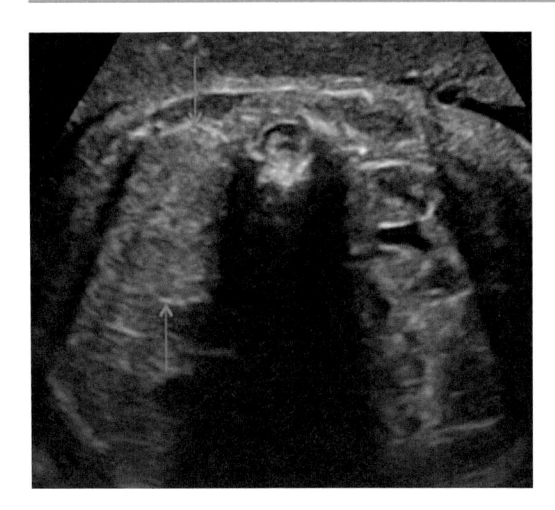

Fig. 20 Fetal US in a renal vein thrombosis. Axial US scan performed on the pelvic cavities of a 34-week-old fetus. The right kidney is undifferentiated, enlarged, and hyperechoic (*arrows*), whereas the left appears normal, with only mild pelvic distention. The diagnosis of renal vein thrombosis was suggested because of acuteness and unilaterality of the affection. The factor V Leiden mutation was found in the father

streaks (possibly representing hemorrhagic infarctions or thrombotic parts) may be visible in the interlobar areas. Thrombus in the inferior vena cava should be searched as well as associated adrenal hemorrhage that appears like a suprarenal mass. Color and pulsed Doppler US may be used in the early stages of renal vein thrombosis, intrarenal and renal venous flow and pulsatility may be absent, and renal arterial diastolic flow may be decreased or even inverted, with a raised resistive index. Collateral vessels develop very rapidly, and in most cases, the kidney quickly recovers a normal aspect with no consequences on further renal development (60–80 %). In unfavorable outcomes, the kidney shrinks and its function is altered (Has et al. 2014).

> **Take Away**
> Renal vein thrombosis should be suspected in cases of acute (most frequently unilateral) changes in renal size and aspect.

5 Fetal Bladder Anomalies

5.1 Megabladder

In the first trimester, a bladder is considered enlarged if superior to 10 mm in height on a sagittal long-axis scan. As previously mentioned, at this gestational age, such finding carries a poor prognosis because they are frequently associated with chromosomal anomalies or part of a syndrome (such as prune belly) (also see chapter "Imaging in Prune Belly Syndrome and Other Syndromes Affecting the Urogenital Tract"). Later in pregnancy, a megabladder is defined as a cephalocaudal diameter superior to three cm in the second trimester and to five cm in the third trimester. At this age, megabladders are mainly due to outflow obstruction or to a major bilateral VUR (Pinette et al. 2003; Osborne et al. 2011).

In cases of outflow obstruction, the bladder wall is thickened and irregular, the posterior urethra is enlarged ("key hole" sign) (Fig. 10), and the upper urinary tract may be dilated. The obstruction can be secondary to a urethral valve (male fetus) or to an obstructive ureterocele (in a context of duplication).

In case of high-grade VUR, the bladder wall is thin and often the upper urinary tract is dilated (see previous paragraph). It is often difficult to make a clear distinction between both etiologies, as they may be simultaneously present and therefore associated with mixed imaging characteristics.

In megacystis-microcolon hypoperistalsis (MMH) syndrome, the megabladder is of dysplastic origin. It is a degenerative affection of the smooth muscle that affects the bladder but also the digestive tract. This autosomal recessive syndrome mostly concerns female fetuses and carries a very poor prognosis (Muller et al. 2005). It can be excluded by MRI during the third trimester because the colon is well visualized at that time. A normal aspect of the colon reasonably allows exclusion of the diagnosis (Fig. 21).

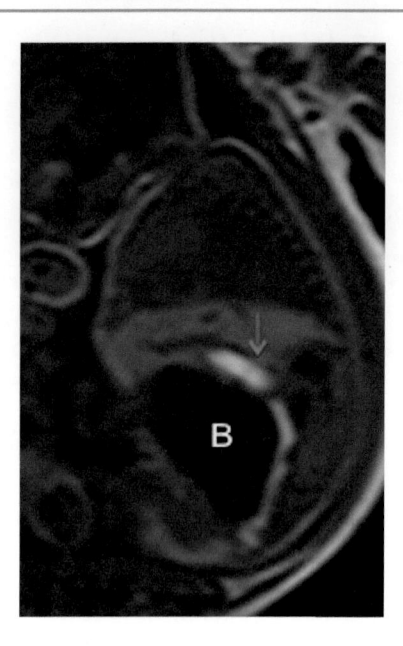

Fig. 21 Fetal MRI of a megabladder. Sagittal T1-weighted MR image. The bladder (*B*) is enlarged, but the hyperintense colon is normal in size, position, and aspect reasonably allowing exclusion of a megacystis-microcolon syndrome

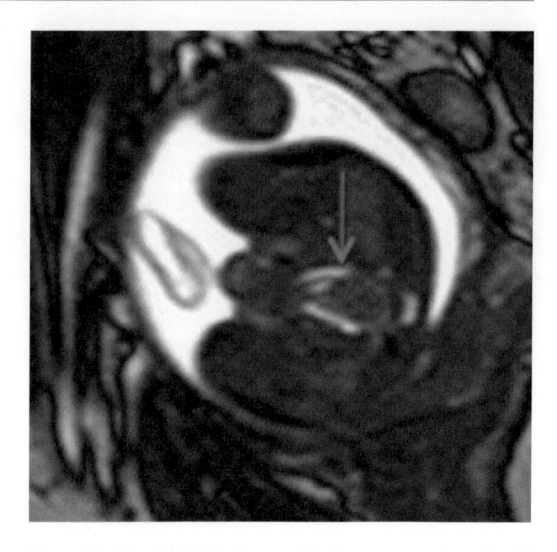

Fig. 22 Fetal MRI in a bladder exstrophy. Axial T2-weighted MR image performed on the pelvis of a 25-week-old fetus. No (fluid-filled, T2 hyperintense) urinary bladder can be seen between the parallelized umbilical arteries (*arrow*). The diagnosis of bladder exstrophy was confirmed on fetopathology

> **Take Away**
> Megabladder is an easy US diagnosis, and the etiologies are numerous. The prognosis relies on the time of discovery, the size of the bladder, and the presence of associated anomalies.

5.2 Bladder Exstrophy

Persistent non-visualization of the bladder during more than 25 min (the normal filling-emptying cycle time) is worrying. It may be due to abnormal urine production in case of renal dysplasia (see above). In this context, the amniotic fluid is reduced.

It can also be secondary to an inability to store urine in the bladder, for example, in cases of bladder or cloacal exstrophy (Wilcox and Chitty 2001). On imaging, no bladder is seen between the two umbilical arteries that appear closer one to the other and parallelized (Fig. 22). The anterior wall of the bladder is absent and the bladder is opened anteriorly. There is no muscle or conjunctive tissue in the abdominal wall. The amniotic fluid and the kidneys are generally normal. It is a congenital malformation of the midline that may affect the abdominal wall, the bladder, the urethra, the genital organs and sometime the spine ("OEIS": malformative complex including omphalocele, exstrophy, anal imperforation, spinal dysraphism). The functional prognosis of all these malformations is very poor. As bladder exstrophy is very rare (1 upon 30,000 live births), fetal MRI may be useful particularly in complex situations to better understand and define the anatomy of the fetal pelvis (Martin et al. 2004).

> **Take Away**
> The absence of visualization of the bladder in a fetus with normal kidneys and normal amniotic fluid should raise the diagnosis of bladder exstrophy.

6 Complex Lower Urinary Tract Malformations

These malformations result from a failure of division between the urinary, Mullerian, and digestive tracts. It may lead to a single common channel (cloaca) or two channels: a common genitourinary channel (urogenital sinus) separated from the digestive tract (Winkler et al. 2012). These malformations can be suspected on US when the normal anatomy of the bladder, uterus, rectum, and anal dimple cannot be displayed, when an abnormal medial pelvic cystic lesion is present (52 %), or when there is a dilatation of the digestive tract or an abnormal echogenicity of its content (Pohl-Schickinger et al. 2006). Yet, the antenatal diagnosis of such malformations is still low (16 %) and the differentiation of the subtypes even more difficult.

Fetal MRI is a very interesting complementary tool in the diagnosis of such malformations (Farhataziz et al. 2005; Calvo-Garcia et al. 2013). It is an excellent technique for documenting the size, signal content, and location of the rectum according to the other pelvic structures. The rectal pouch should normally be seen 10 mm below the bladder neck. It appears hyperintense on T1-weighted sequences and hypointense on T2-weighted sequences (Fig. 6). The normal bladder presents the opposite signal and therefore can easily be differentiated from the digestive tract. Abnormal signal of the digestive tract content (decreased hyperintensity on T1 and increased intensity on T2) suggests a communication with the urinary tract. MRI also helps in the characterization of a cystic pelvic lesion based on its signal and shape, thus improving the differentiation between cysts, isolated hydrocolpos, urogenital sinus, and cloacal dysgenesis (Picone et al. 2007). Meanwhile, the detailed anatomy of the malformation is often not possible to be defined in utero. Neonatal US, MRI, and genital opacifications will be required to precise the anatomy of the malformation.

6.1 Urogenital Sinus Anomalies

Urogenital sinus malformation refers to incomplete separation between the urinary and the genital tract. There is a communication between the two systems, generally between the vagina and the urethra. The urogenital sinus is separated from the hindgut. Ultrasonography demonstrates a retrovesical cystic lesion in the fetal pelvis due to a reflux of urine within the Mullerian structures (Fig. 23a). Urinary ascites is also frequent (Taori et al. 2010). Those malformations are often associated with upper urinary tract anomalies like renal agenesis, ectopia, dysplasia, and pyelocaliceal dilatation.

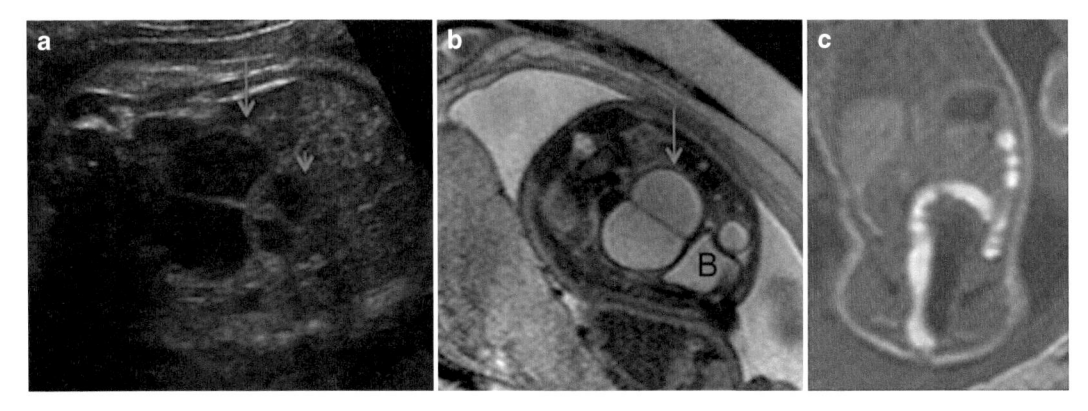

Fig. 23 Fetal US and MRI of a urogenital sinus malformation. (**a**) Axial US scan on the pelvis of a 32-week-old fetus, and there is a four-chamber structure behind the bladder corresponding to duplicated vagina (*arrow*) and duplicated uterus (*arrow head*) filled with urine. It is suggestive of a urogenital fistula with duplicated genital tract. (**b**) Axial T2-weighted image on the same fetus confirming the liquid content of the duplicated vagina (*arrow*) behind the bladder (*B*). (**c**) Coronal T1-weighted image on the same fetus demonstrating the normal recto sigmoid. It confirms that there is no communication with the digestive tract. The final diagnosis was a urogenital sinus with duplicated genital tract

On MRI, the signal and position of the rectosigmoid is normal because the digestive tract is completely separated from the urogenital tract (Fig. 23c). The urogenital sinus appears like a bilobated cystic structure, the bladder anteriorly, and the genital tract posteriorly (Fig. 23b). Often, the anal dimple is anteriorly placed.

> **Take Away**
> Urogenital sinus malformations should be suspected in fetuses with ascites and retrovesical cystic lesion.

6.2 Cloacal Dysgenesis

It is the most complex type of malformation, characterized by direct communication between the gastrointestinal, urinary, and genital structure resulting in a single perineal opening. The cloacal malformation is very rare (1/40,000–50,000 life birth) and exclusively seen in females. The type of communication between the different structures is variable. The most common sonographic findings are ascites (22 % of cases), intrapelvic cystic structures corresponding to distended Mullerian structures by urine reflux, absence of visualization of the rectum, and the anal dimple. These Mullerian structures are often duplicated and appear septated on US (60 % of the cases). There is often associated upper urinary tract dilatation due to perineal outlet obstruction (Fig. 24) (Nitin et al. 2003).

> **Take Away**
> Cloacal dysgenesis is a rare and poor prognosis malformation that should be suspected when the normal pelvic structure cannot be depicted on US. MRI allows a better understanding of these complex malformations.

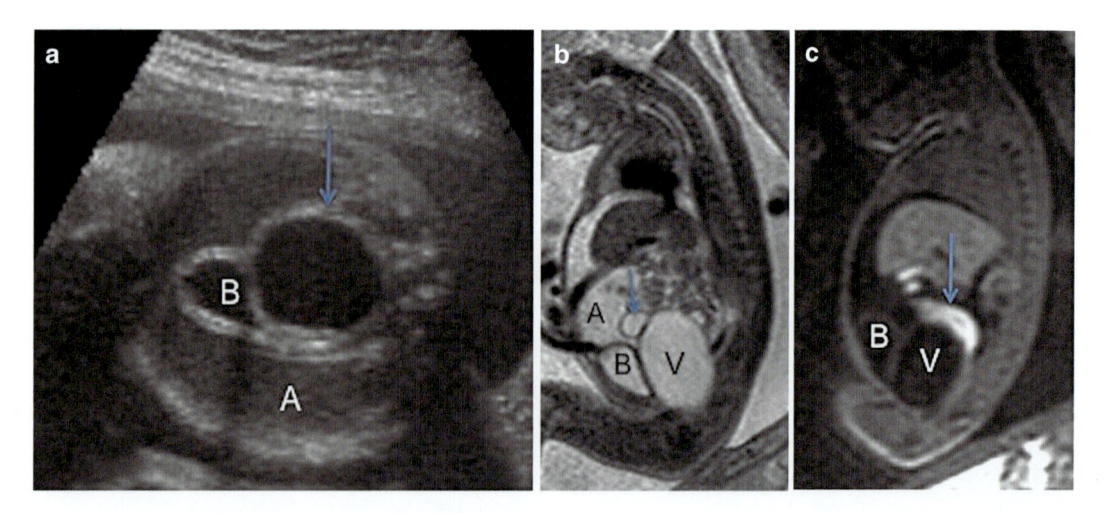

Fig. 24 Fetal US and MRI of a cloacal malformation. (**a**) Axial US scan on the pelvis of a 30-week-old fetus. There is a cystic structure (*arrow*) behind the bladder (*B*). The fetus also presents complex ascites (*A*). (**b**) Sagittal T2-weighted image performed on the same fetus. The cystic structure is the dilated vagina (*V*) with the uterus upward (*arrow*). The Mullerian structures are filled with urine secondary to a fistula to the urinary tract. The ascites (*A*) is due to urine reflux from the Mullerian structures into the peritoneal cavity. (**c**) Sagittal T1-weighted images performed on the same fetus. Notice that a distal colic structure is seen above the distended vagina (*arrow*). A diagnosis of cloacal dysgenesis was confirmed on fetopathology

Conclusion

Fetal urinary tract anomalies are numerous with variable prognosis. The primary insult may occur anywhere in the urinary tract but will have secondary developmental consequences on the whole urinary tract rendering the in utero diagnosis sometimes difficult. The prognostic judgment still mostly relies on additional imaging findings (volume of amniotic fluid, renal parenchyma's aspect, etc.). The aim of prenatal diagnosis is to precisely define the malformation in order to ensure the best prenatal and postnatal management of the fetus and newborn.

References

Avni EF, Garel L, Hall M et al (2002) Perinatal approach in anomalies of the urinary tract, adrenals and genital system. In: Avni FE (ed) Perinatal imaging. From ultrasound to MR imaging. Springer, Berlin/Heidelberg/New York, pp 153–196

Avni EF, Cos T, Cassart M et al (2007) Evolution of fetal ultrasonography. Eur Radiol 17:419–431

Avni EF, Garel C, Cassart M, D'Haene N, Hall M, Riccabona M (2012) Imaging and classification of congenital cystic renal diseases. AJR Am J Roentgenol 198(5):1004–1013

Brun M, Maugey-Laulom B, Eurin D et al (2004) Prenatal sonographic patterns in autosomal dominant polycystic kidney disease: a multicenter study. Ultrasound Obstet Gynecol 24:55–61

Calvo-Garcia MA, Kline-Fath BM, Rubio EI et al (2013) Fetal MRI in cloacal exstrophy. Pediatr Radiol 43:593–604

Cassart M, Massez A, Metens T et al (2004a) Complementary role of MRI after sonography in assessing bilateral urinary tract anomalies in the fetus. AJR Am J Roentgenol 182:689–695

Cassart M, Eurin D, Didier F et al (2004b) Antenatal renal sonographic anomalies and postnatal follow-up of renal involvement in Bardet-Biedl syndrome. Ultrasound Obstet Gynecol 24:51–54

Chaumoitre K, Colavolpe N, Shojai R et al (2006) Diffusion weighted magnetic resonance imaging with apparent diffusion coefficient (ADC) determination in normal and pathological fetal kidneys. Ultrasound Obstet Gynecol 29:22–31

Devriendt A, Cassart M, Massez A et al (2013) Fetal kidneys: additional sonographic criteria of normal development. Prenat Diagn 33:1248–1252

Farhataziz N, Engels JE, Ramus RM et al (2005) Fetal MRI of urine and meconium by gestational age for the diagnosis of genitourinary and gastrointestinal abnormalities. Am J Radiol 184:1891–1897

Grazioli S, Parvex P, Merlini L et al (2010) Antenatal and postnatal ultrasound in the evaluation of the risk of vesicoureteral reflux. Pediatr Nephrol 25:1687–1692

Has R, Corbacioglu Esmer A, Kalelioglu IH et al (2014) Renal failure due to renal vein thrombosis in a fetus with growth restriction and thrombophilia. J Obstet Gynaecol Res 40(4):1124–1127

Ismaili K, Schurmans T, Wissing M et al (2001) Early prognostic factors of infants with chronic renal failure caused by renal dysplasia. Pediatr Nephrol 16:260–264

Ismaili K, Avni FE, Wissing KM et al (2004) Long-term clinical outcome of infants with mild and moderate fetal pyelectasis: validation of neonatal ultrasound as a screening tool to detect significant nephro-uropathies. J Pediatr 144:759–765

Ismaili K, Hall M, Ham H et al (2005a) Evolution of individual renal function in children with unilateral complex renal duplication. J Pediatr 147:208–212

Ismaili K, Hall M, Piepsz A et al (2005b) Insights into the pathogenesis and natural history of fetuses with renal pelvis dilatation. Eur Urol 48:207–214

Ismaili K, Avni FE, Alexander M et al (2005c) Routine voiding cystourethrography is of no value in neonates with unilateral multicystic dysplastic kidney. J Pediatr 146:759–763

Ismaili K, Hall M, Piepsz A et al (2006) Primary vesicoureteral reflux detected among neonates with a history of fetal renal pelvis dilatation: a prospective clinical and imaging study. J Pediatr 148:222–227

Jouannic JM, Hyett JA, Pandya PP et al (2003) Perinatal outcome in fetuses with megacystis in the first half of pregnancy. Prenat Diagn 23:340–344

Lee SM, Jun JK, Lee EJ et al (2010) Measurement of fetal urine production to differentiate causes of increased amniotic fluid volume. Ultrasound Obstet Gynecol 36:191–195

Marks SD, Massicotte P, Steele BT et al (2005) Neonatal renal venous thrombosis: clinical outcomes and prevalence of prothrombotic disorders. J Pediatr 146:811–816

Martin C, Darnell A, Duran C et al (2004) Magnetic resonance imaging of the intra uterine fetal genito-urinary tract. In: Abdominal imaging. Springer, New York

Morris RK, Malin GL, Khan KS et al (2009) Antenatal ultrasound to predict postnatal renal function in congenital lower urinary tract obstruction: systematic review of test accuracy. BJOG 116:1290–1299

Muller F, Dreux S, Vaast P, et al; The Study Group of the French Fetal Medicine Society (2005) Prenatal diagnosis of megacystis-microcolon-intestinal hypoperistalsis syndrome: contribution of amniotic fluid digestive enzyme essay and fetal urinalysis. Prenat Diagn 25:203–209

Nitin C, Manjiri D, Mohit S et al (2003) Calcified meconium. An important sign in the prenatal sonographic diagnosis of cloacal malformation. J Ultrasound Med 22:727–730

Osborne NG, Bonilla-Musoles F, Machado LE et al (2011) Fetal megacystis, differential diagnosis. J Ultrasound Med 30:833–841

Pico H, Dabadie A, Bourlière-Najean B et al (2014) Contribution of foetal uro-MRI in the prenatal diagnosis of uronephropathies. Diagn Interv Imaging 95:573–578

Picone O, Laperelle J, Sonigo P et al (2007) Fetal magnetic resonance imaging in the antenatal diagnosis and management of hydrocolpos. Ultrasound Obstet Gynecol 30:105–109

Pinette M, Blackstone J, Wax J et al (2003) Enlarged fetal bladder: differential diagnosis and outcomes. J Clin Ultrasound 31:328–334

Pohl-Schickinger A, Henrich W, Degenhardt P et al (2006) Echogenic foci in the dilated fetal colon may be associated with the presence of recto urinary fistula. Ultrasound Obstet Gynecol 28:341–344

Spaggiari E, Dreux S, Czerkiewicz I et al (2013) Fetal obstructive uropathy complicated by urinary ascites: outcome and prognostic value of fetal serum β-2-microglobulin. Ultrasound Obstet Gynecol 41:185–189

Taori K, Krishnan V, Sharbidre KG et al (2010) Prenatal sonographic diagnosis of fetal persistent urogenital sinus with congenital hydrocolpos. Ultrasound Obstet Gynecol 36:641–643

van Vuuren SH, Damen-Elias HA, Stigter RH et al (2012) Size and volume charts of fetal kidney, renal pelvis and adrenal gland. Ultrasound Obstet Gynecol 40:659–664

Weber SK, Muller A, Geipel A et al (2014) Prenatal renal vein thrombosis in a dichorionic twin pregnancy. Arch Gynecol Obstet 290(3):587–590

Whitten SM, Wilcox DT (2001) Duplex systems. Prenat Diagn 21:952–957

Wiesel A, Queisser-Luft A, Clementi M, et al; The EUROSCAN Study Group (2005) Prenatal detection of congenital renal malformation by fetal ultrasonographic examination: an analysis of 709 030 births in 12 European countries. Eur J Med Genet 48:131–144

Wilcox DT, Chitty LS (2001) Non visualisations of fetal bladder: aetiology and management. Prenat Diagn 21:977–983

Wilson PD (2004) Polycystic kidney disease. N Engl J Med 350:151–164

Winkler NS, Kennedy AM, Woodward PJ (2012) Cloacal malformation. Embryology, anatomy and prenatal imaging features. J Ultrasound Med 31:1843–1855

Winyard P, Chitty L (2001) Dysplastic and polycystic kidneys: diagnosis, associations and management. Prenat Diagn 21:924–935

Witzani L, Brugger PC, Hormann M et al (2006) Normal renal development investigated with fetal MRI. Eur J Radiol 57(2):294–302

Anomalies of Kidney Rotation, Position, and Fusion

Samuel Stafrace and Gabriele Benz-Bohm

Contents

1   **Anomalies of Rotation**..................................... 167
2   **Anomalies of Position**..................................... 168
2.1 Ectopic Kidney... 168
2.2 Thoracic Kidney... 169
2.3 Supernumerary Kidney.................................... 169
3   **Anomalies of Fusion**....................................... 170
3.1 Horseshoe Kidney.. 170
3.2 Crossed Renal Ectopia..................................... 173
4   **Summary**... 176
References.. 176

S. Stafrace, MD, MRCP (UK), FRCR, FRCP Edin (✉)
Sidra Medical and Research Center, Doha, Qatar
e-mail: sstafrace@sidra.org

G. Benz-Bohm, MD (Retired)
Department of Radiology, The Children's Hospital of Philadelphia, Philadelphia, PA, USA
e-mail: g.benz-bohm@t-online.de

1   Anomalies of Rotation

The fetal kidneys undergo a 90° rotation around their longitudinal axis during their ascent from the pelvis before they reach their final position by the end of the eighth week of fetal life (Moore and Persaud 1998). Campbell (1970) reported only 17 cases of renal malrotation among 32,834 autopsies on adults. However, the true incidence is probably understated because many patients have no clinical symptoms.

Malrotation is most commonly associated with an ectopic or fused kidney, but may also occur in kidneys that undergo complete ascent to the renal fossa. In such a case, the degree of rotation is minimal. The condition may be unilateral or bilateral (Fig. 1). The most common type is an incomplete rotation or non-rotation. The renal pelvis is in the anterior position or in some variation between the anterior and the normal medial position in the adult. Reverse rotation and hyperrotation are other major types of malrotation. In reverse rotation, the renal pelvis rotates laterally and the renal vessels cross the kidney anteriorly to reach the renal hilum. In hyperrotation, the kidney rotates more than 180°, but less than 360°. The pelvis faces laterally, but the renal vessels are carried posteriorly to the kidney. Malrotation is usually discovered by chance during imaging of the kidney or abdomen for other reasons. The calyces are often distorted, even without any associated obstruction (Fig. 2). It is important to establish the correct diagnosis to exclude other pathological conditions that can produce similar distortion of the kidney. Anomalies of rotation may produce partial pelviureteric obstruction (Kissane 1983; Ritchey 1992; Currarino et al. 1993).

Take Away
Malrotation is most commonly associated with an ectopic or fused kidney. Anomalies of rotation may produce partial pelviureteric obstruction.

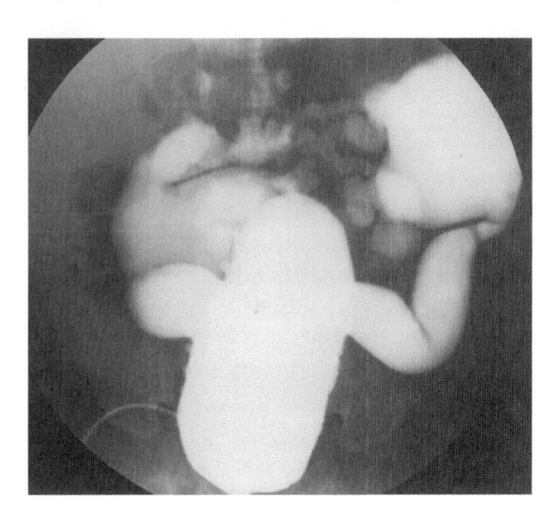

Fig. 1 Voiding cystourethrography (VCUG) in a 2-year-old boy. Vesicoureteric reflux (VUR) in both lumbar ectopic and malrotated kidneys

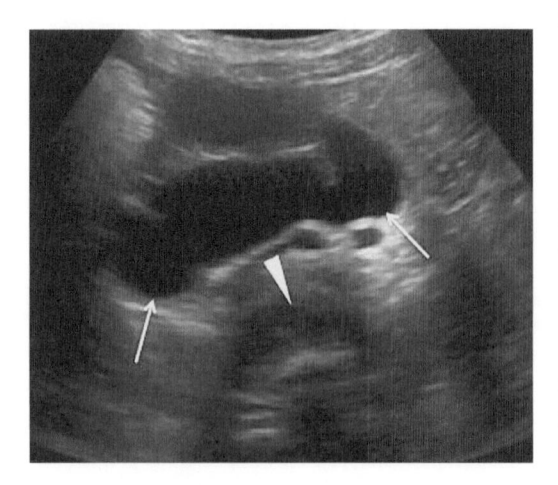

Fig. 2 Axial renal US image: midline malrotated kidney with distended pelvis (*arrows*) facing posteriorly toward the spine (*arrowhead*)

2 Anomalies of Position

2.1 Ectopic Kidney

Renal ectopy is the term for a kidney lying outside the renal fossa. The kidney migrates cephalad early in gestation to arrive at its normal position. Abnormality of the ureteral bud or the metanephric blastema, genetic abnormalities, teratogenic causes, and anomalous vasculature, acting as a barrier to ascent, are reasons for failure of the kidney to complete its ascent (Malek et al. 1971). The incidence of renal ectopy in postmortem studies varies from 1 in 500 (Campbell 1930) to 1 in 1290 (Thompson and Pace 1937). There is a slight predilection for the left side, and 10% of cases are bilateral (Fig. 1).

Simple renal ectopy refers to a kidney that remains in the ipsilateral retroperitoneal space. The most common position is in the pelvis, opposite the sacrum and below the aortic bifurcation as a pelvic or sacral kidney. The lumbar or iliac ectopic kidney is one that is fixed above the iliac crest, but below the level of L3. Malrotation frequently accompanies renal ectopy (Fig. 1) (Kissane 1983; Daneman and Alton 1991; Ritchey 1992; Currarino et al. 1993).

The differentiation between renal ptosis and renal ectopy can be difficult. In renal ptosis, the renal artery arises from the aorta at the normal level and the ureter is of normal length. In renal ectopy, the ureter is short, corresponding to the location of the kidney. Renal ptosis results from hypermobility of the kidney in the retroperitoneal space, usually in obese people who have lost weight rapidly. The ptotic kidney can usually be manipulated into its normal position.

The diagnosis of an ectopic kidney can be made by ultrasonography (US) in most cases. Cross-sectional imaging, mainly MRI, can help in difficult cases. It can also provide information about the vascular supply. The ectopic kidney receives major blood supply from nearby major vessels and such kidneys are often supplied by multiple vessels (Daneman and Alton 1991; Ritchey 1992). Since vesicoureteral reflux (VUR) is frequently associated with an ectopic kidney (Fig. 1), voiding cystourethrography (VCUG) is recommended.

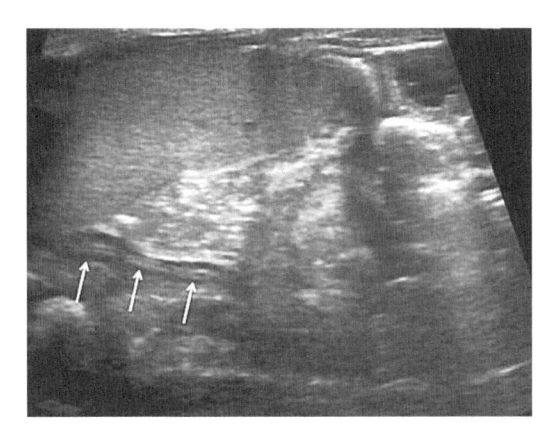

Fig. 3 US of the left renal fossa in a 4-day-old newborn with no left kidney identified in the normal position. A straight adrenal is identified (*arrows*)

2.1.1 Associated Anomalies

The contralateral kidney may be abnormal in up to 50% of patients (Malek et al. 1971). There is a 10% incidence of contralateral renal agenesis. VUR is reported in up to 70% of children with a pelvic kidney. (Kramer and Kelalis 1984). In most cases of renal ectopy, the adrenal gland is in the normal position, though often exhibiting an atypical shape (Fig. 3). Genital anomalies have been described in 15% of males and 75% of females (Thompson and Pace 1937; Downs et al. 1973). Skeletal anomalies are reported in up to 50% of children, cardiovascular lesions in 9 out of 21 children (Malek et al. 1971), and gastrointestinal abnormalities in one-third of patients (Ritchey 1992).

kidney occurs in fewer than 5% of the cases of renal ectopy, with an incidence of 1 in 13,000 autopsies (Campbell 1930). The left side is more commonly involved and there is a male predominance. Occasionally, the condition can be bilateral (N'Guessen et al. 1984). In the supradiaphragmatic kidney, the ureter and hilar vessels enter through the foramen of Bochdalek. In general, the thoracic kidney functions normally, and most patients are asymptomatic. The thoracic kidney is often detected on a routine chest radiograph as a suspected mass (Ritchey 1992) (Fig. 4). The differentiation by US can be possible although cross-sectional imaging is often required particularly for further characterization of potential associated anomalies.

> **Take Away**
> The diagnosis of an ectopic kidney can be made by US in most cases. VUR is frequently associated. The contralateral kidney may be abnormal in up to 50% of patients.

> **Take Away**
> The thoracic kidney is often detected on a routine chest radiograph as a suspected mass and can be differentiated by US.

2.2 Thoracic Kidney

Excessive cranial migration of the kidney results in a thoracic kidney or in a superior ectopic kidney (N'Guessen et al. 1984), lying below a thin membranous portion of the diaphragm. An intrathoracic

2.3 Supernumerary Kidney

There are rarely more than two separate kidneys present. Supernumerary elements are small and often dysplastic. The extrarenal component may be misinterpreted as a malpositioned kidney (Fig. 5). This anomaly is often detected by chance but rarely

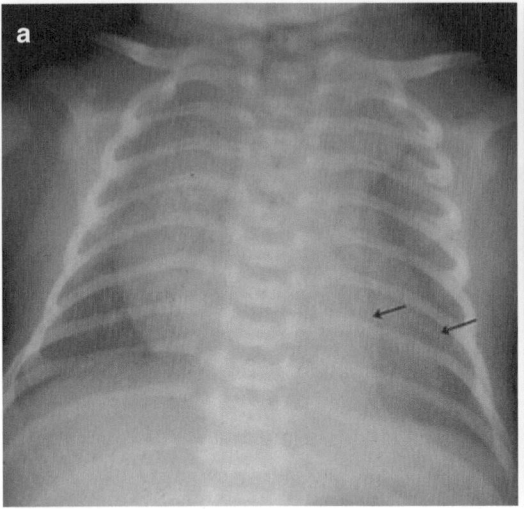

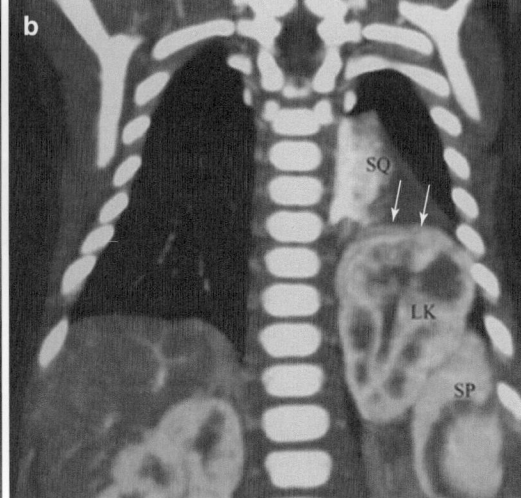

Fig. 4 Thoracic kidney with associated sequestration; (**a**) CXR demonstrating a retrocardiac mass with a double outline of the left side of the mediastinum (*arrows*); (**b**) reformatted coronal CT image demonstrating a sequestration superiorly (*SQ*) above an ectopic intrathoracic left kidney (*LK*) and partially displaced spleen (*SP*) (Courtesy of Prof. Panruethai Trinavarat Chulalongkorn University, Bangkok, Thailand)

by complications such as calculi and infection (Chawla 2013). US, CT, and MRI are all useful to confirm its presence. Functional imaging by isotope studies is also helpful to detect more than two functional renal elements. Dysplastic and poorly functional extrarenal components may, however, not be detected by scintigraphy.

> **Take Away**
> A small malpositioned kidney may represent a supernumerary kidney; therefore further evaluation is required.

3 Anomalies of Fusion

During their ascent, the kidneys cross the umbilical arteries. Malposition of the umbilical arteries may cause the developing nephrogenic blastemas to come together and fuse. Fusion of the nephrogenic masses in the midline results in a horseshoe kidney. This occurs early in embryogenesis, before rotation is complete, and therefore malrotation is present in all such cases (Ritchey 1992).

3.1 Horseshoe Kidney

Horseshoe kidney is the most common type of renal fusion and one of the most frequent renal anomalies. It is usually characterized by fusion of the lower poles across the midline by an isthmus lying anterior, seldom posterior, to the aorta and inferior vena cava (Dajani 1966). Occasionally the lower poles are connected only by fibrous bands. The horseshoe kidney is usually positioned low in the abdomen with the isthmus lying just below the origin of the inferior mesenteric artery from the aorta. The incidence varies from 1 in 400 (Glenn 1959) to 1 in 1800 (Campbell 1970). The abnormality is more common in males.

The diagnosis of a horseshoe kidney can be accidental during imaging of the kidney or the abdomen for other reasons. From a plain radiograph of the abdomen, the diagnosis of a horseshoe kidney may be suspected if one can see the renal outlines in their abnormal position (Fig. 6a). The diagnosis can be confirmed especially by renal US and MRI (Figs. 6 and 7). Features pointing toward a horseshoe kidney are the position of the kidneys – too low, too close to the spine, and more vertically than normal – and the identification of an isthmus (Fig. 6c) (Muttarak and Sriburi

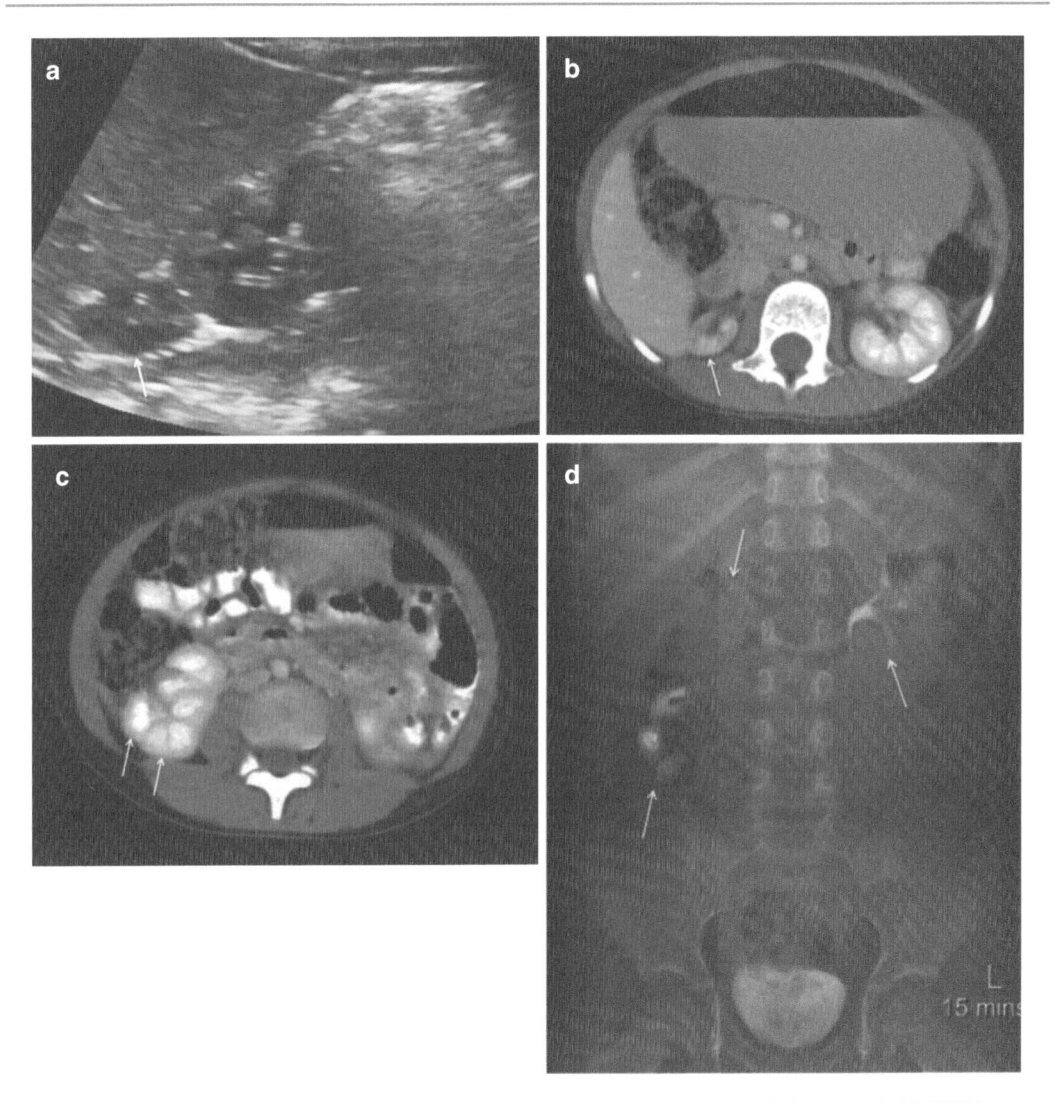

Fig. 5 (**a**) Longitudinal US image demonstrating a small extrarenal element (*arrow*) superior to the right kidney; (**b, c**) contrast-enhanced CT, transverse image; (**b**) shows enhancement of the small right kidney; (**c**) shows a malrotated normal-sized right kidney which is separate to the small kidney located cranially (*arrows*); (**d**) IVU image at 15′ p.i.: contrast excretion in all three renal elements (*arrows*) can be seen (Courtesy of Dr. Annie Paterson, Royal Belfast Hospital for Sick Children, Northern Ireland, UK)

2011). The radiographic appearance of a horseshoe kidney is frequently altered by associated abnormalities such as hydronephrosis and/or diminished renal function. In the majority of cases, there are multiple renal vessels. The blood to the isthmus is often supplied by a separate vessel. This may arise from the aorta, the common iliac, or inferior mesenteric arteries. Before any surgery, it may be necessary to assess the function of the isthmus of the kidneys (Kissane 1983; Ritchey 1992).

3.1.1 Associated Anomalies

The incidence of associated anomalies is much higher if the horseshoe kidney is discovered in the newborn period. In postmortem examinations of 99 infants with horseshoe kidneys, 78 % had malformations of other organ systems such as the central nervous system, the gastrointestinal tract the skeletal and the cardiovascular system (Zondek and Zondek 1964). In another study, one-third of patients with horse-

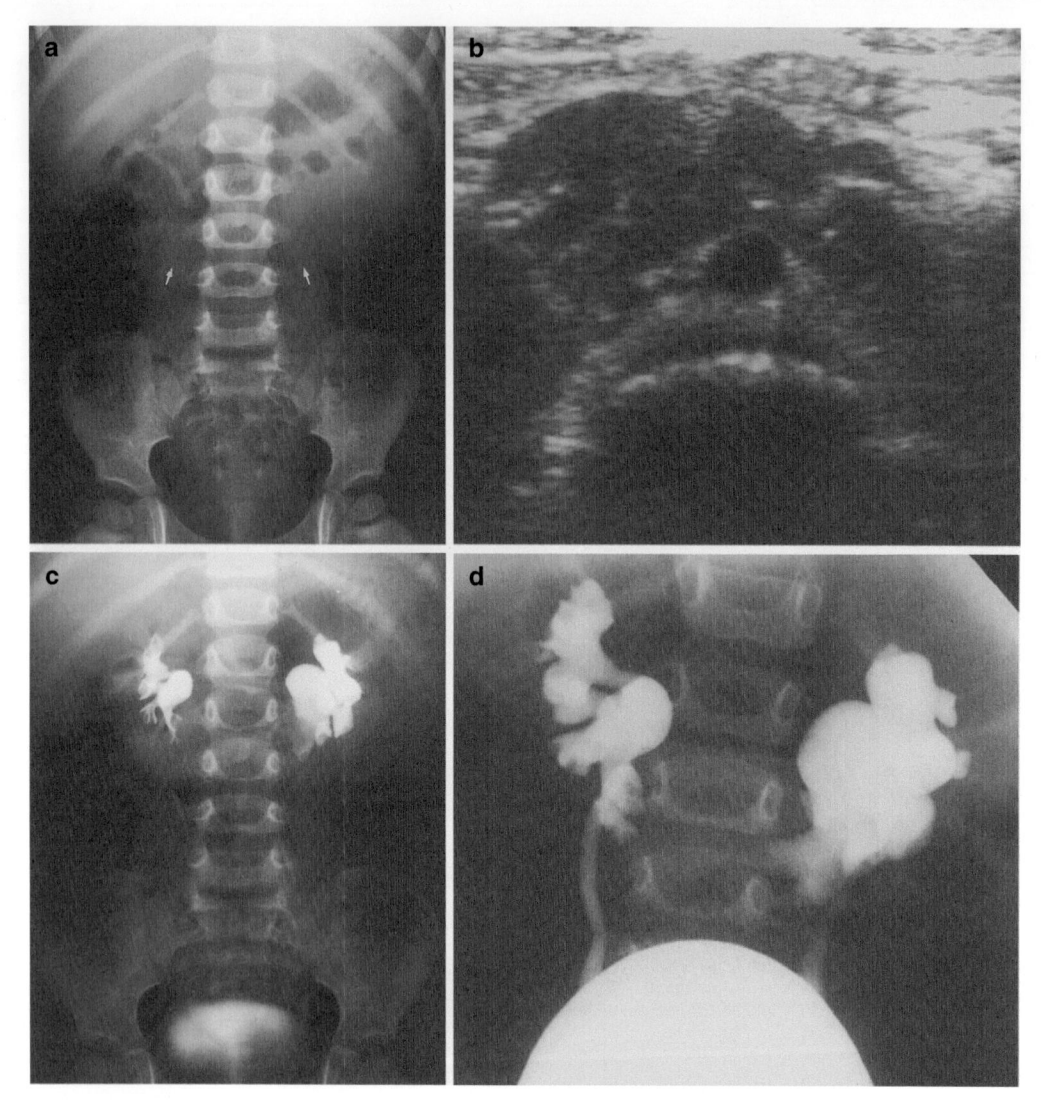

Fig. 6 Typical appearance of horseshoe kidney in a 19-month-old girl: (**a**) on a plain radiograph; (**b**) on US; (**c**) on IVU; (**d**) on VCUG by VUR

shoe kidney had at least one other abnormality (Boatman et al. 1972). Several well-known syndromes are associated with fused kidney: Trisomy 18 has an incidence of 21% (Warkany et al. 1966; Boatman et al. 1972). Lippe et al. (1988) noted horseshoe kidneys on US in seven percent of patients with Turner's syndrome. In patients with neural tube defects, there is also an increased incidence of horseshoe kidneys (Whitaker and Hunt 1987). However, nearly one-third of patients with a horseshoe kidney remain undiagnosed throughout life (Glenn 1959; Pitts and Muecke 1975).

Pelviureteric junction obstruction by a high ureteral insertion or an anomalous renal vessel is the most common cause of hydronephrosis. This occurs in 30% of patients diagnosed with horseshoe kidney during life. Urolithiasis develops in 20% of patients with horseshoe kidney. Stasis secondary to urinary tract dilatation and additional metabolic factors are also other described causes (Evans and Resnick 1981). In all children with horseshoe kidney and some dilatation, VUR should be excluded. The upper urinary tract dilatation may be secondary to VUR (Fig. 6d). More than 100 renal malignancies have been reported

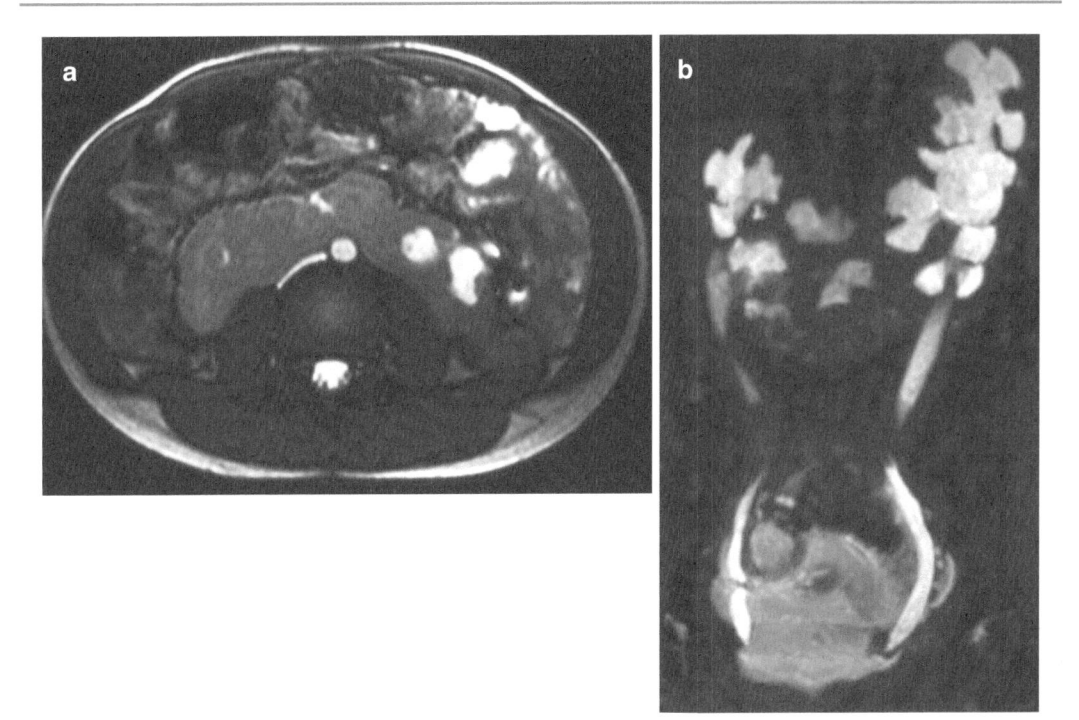

Fig. 7 Horseshoe kidney on transverse (**a**) and coronally reformatted (**b**) heavily T2-weighted MRI sequences. These demonstrate a horseshoe kidney with dilatation and abnormal rotation of both renal components (left more than right). The course of the ureters can be more easily followed on MRI than by other imaging modalities

in patients with horseshoe kidney (Buntley 1976). The risk of developing a Wilms' tumor is increased sevenfold (Fig. 8) (Mesrobian et al. 1985).

> **Take Away**
> The horseshoe kidney is the most common type of renal fusion. Pelvicalyceal dilatation, urolithiasis, and VUR are associated anomalies and effects. The risk of Wilms' tumor is increased.

3.2 Crossed Renal Ectopia

Crossed renal ectopia is the second most common fusion anomaly after horseshoe kidney with an incidence of 1 in 7000 autopsies (Abeshouse and Bhisitkul 1959). The crossed ectopic kidney lies on the opposite side from the ureteral insertion into the bladder. There are four varieties of crossed renal ectopia (Fig. 9) (McDonald and McClellan 1957; Abeshouse and Bhisitkul

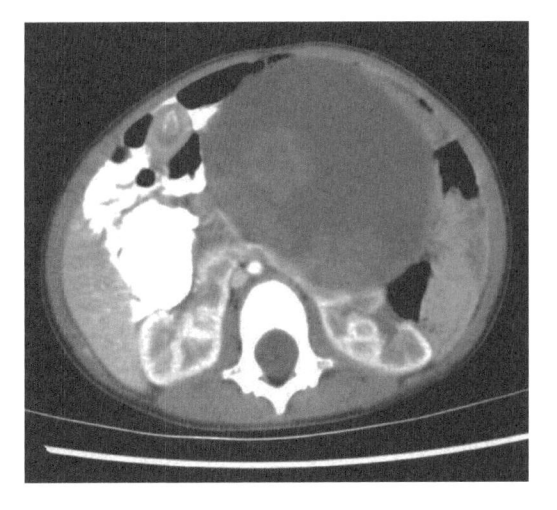

Fig. 8 Wilms' tumor of a horseshoe kidney. Contrast-enhanced CT, transverse image in a 4-year-old child with a midline mass. A mixed cystic and solid tumor is seen arising from the isthmus of this horseshoe kidney

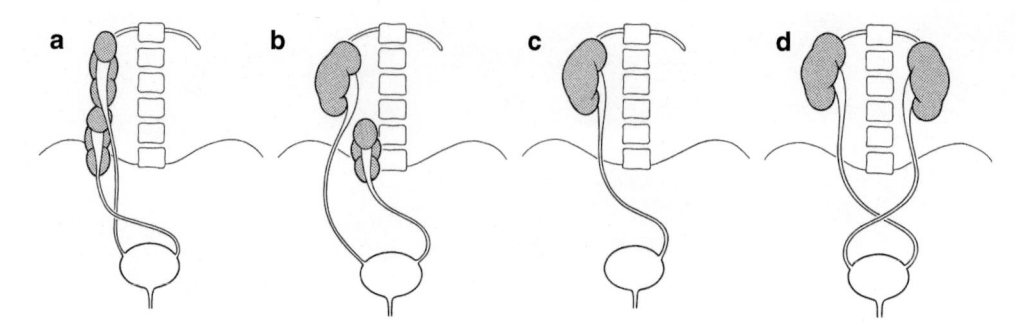

Fig. 9 Four types of crossed renal ectopia: (**a**) with fusion; (**b**) without fusion; (**c**) solitary; (**d**) bilateral

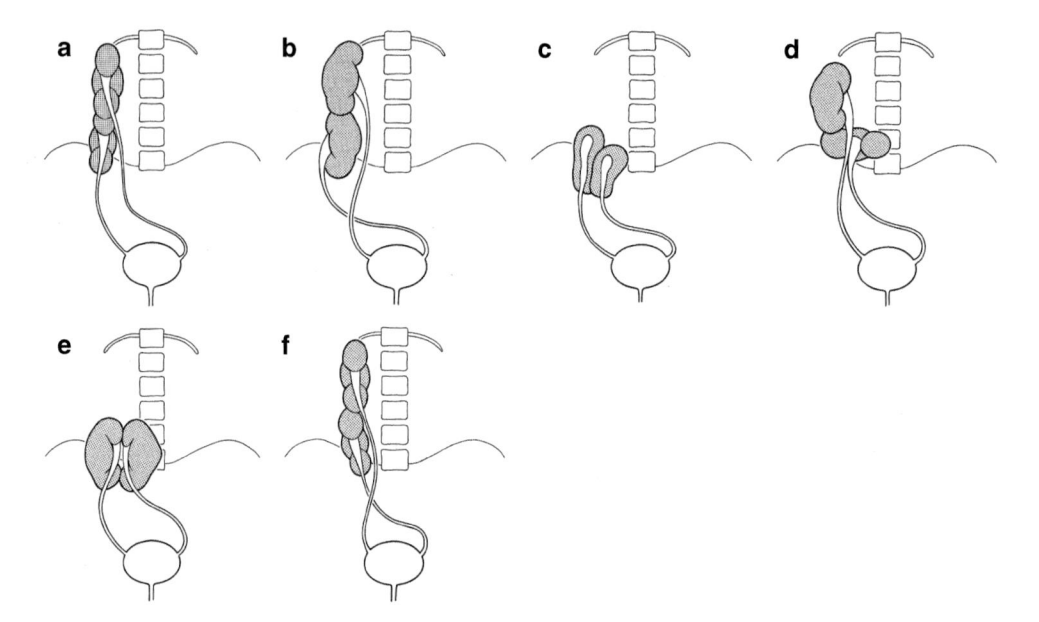

Fig. 10 Six types of crossed renal ectopia with fusion: (**a**) unilateral fused kidney, superior ectopia; (**b**) sigmoid or S-shaped kidney; (**c**) lump kidney; (**d**) L-shaped kidney; (**e**) disk (pancake) kidney; (**f**) unilateral fused kidney, inferior ectopia

1959). Crossed renal ectopia with fusion occurs in 85–90%, without fusion in less than 10%; solitary crossed renal ectopia and bilateral crossed renal ectopia are rare (Kakei et al. 1976). Crossing from left to right occurs more frequently than right to left, and there is a slight male predominance. There are six variations in crossed renal ectopia with fusion (Fig. 10) (McDonald and McClellan 1957; Abeshouse and Bhisitkul 1959). The most common form is the unilateral fused type with inferior ectopia, in which the upper pole of the crossed kidney is fused to the lower pole of the normally positioned kidney. The renal pelves remain in their anterior position, representing failure to complete rotation. The second most common type is the sigmoid or S-shaped kidney with inferior ectopia. In this version, both kidneys have completed their rotation so that the two renal pelves face in opposite directions. The other four types of fusion are less common. In the lump kidney and the disk kidney, the two kidneys are exten-

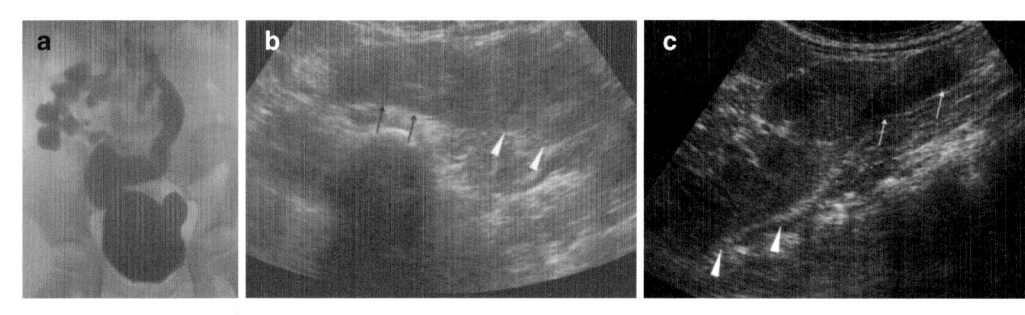

Fig. 11 Crossed renal ectopy. Single image from a VCUG study in a 6-year-old boy. (**a**) High-grade reflux into a crossed fused ectopic kidney with both kidneys draining through the right ureteric system. A distended left ureteric stump is just above the bladder. (**b, c**) US images from a 3-year-old girl, (**b**) axial image. The right kidney (*arrows*) is fused with the medial inferior pole of the left (*arrowheads*) No further renal tissue was detected on the right side. (**c**) Longitudinal image of the left flank. Elongated fused kidneys

sively fused. In the L-shaped kidney, the crossed kidney is in the transverse plane. The superior ectopic kidney lies superior to the normal kidney (Kissane 1983; Ritchey 1992; Currarino et al. 1993).

Generally it is difficult to distinguish between crossed renal ectopy with fusion and crossed renal ectopy without fusion by US (Fig. 11b, c). Cross-sectional imaging mainly MRI is able to establish the correct diagnosis (Fig. 12). It can also provide information about the vascular supply, which is quite variable. Multiple anomalous branches to both kidneys are possible, arising from the aorta or from the common iliac artery. A crossing renal artery to supply the crossed kidney is very rare (Rubinstein et al. 1976). IVU (Fig. 13) may occasionally still be used to delineate the ureteric anatomy although this is now replaced by MRI.

Fig. 12 Coronal T2 MRI image in a neonate. A low-lying midline renal ectopia with fusion, lump kidney (*arrows*), located just above the bladder (Courtesy of Dr. Abdusamea Shabani, Sidra Medical and Research Center, Doha, Qatar)

3.2.1 Associated Anomalies

The most common associated abnormality is VUR; therefore, VCUG should be performed (Fig. 11a) (Kramer and Kelalis 1984; Polak-Jonkisz et al. 2012). Skeletal anomalies, imperforate anus, and cardiovascular anomalies have an increased incidence (Abeshouse and Bhisitkul 1959). Patients with solitary crossed ectopy have a higher incidence of genital abnormalities, probably related to the renal agenesis (Kakei et al. 1976).

> **Take Away**
> Crossed renal ectopia occurs with fusion in 85–90%, without fusion in less than 10%. MRI is the best diagnostic imaging modality. VUR is the most common associated abnormality.

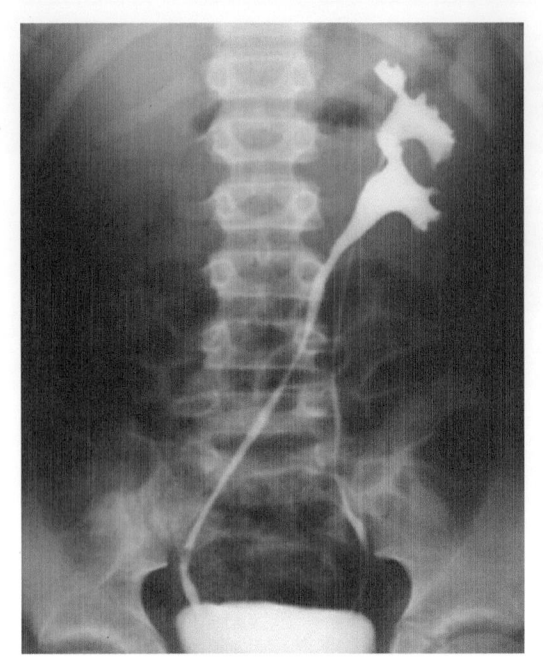

Fig. 13 Selected image from IVU series delineating the ureteric anatomy of the left unilateral fused kidney, inferior ectopia (Courtesy of Dr. Annie Paterson Royal Belfast Hospital for Sick Children, Northern Ireland, UK)

4 Summary

Congenital anomalies of kidney rotation, position, and fusion are very common and are frequently identified by chance. They can be considered as a "normal variant," as long as they do not cause complications or are related to other problems such as urinary drainage impairment, dysplasia, VUR, infection, or other associated malformations. Awareness of these abnormalities and how best to image them is necessary to reduce the complications.

References

Abeshouse BS, Bhisitkul I (1959) Crossed renal ectopia with and without fusion. Urol Int 9:63–91
Boatman DL, Kolln CP, Flocks RH (1972) Congenital anomalies associated with horseshoe kidney. J Urol 107:205–207
Buntley D (1976) Malignancy associated with horseshoe kidney. Urology 8:146–148
Campbell MF (1930) Renal ectopy. J Urol 24:187–198
Campbell MF (1970) Anomalies of the kidney. In: Campbell MF, Harrison JH (eds) Urology, vol 2, 3rd edn. Saunders, Philadelphia, pp 1416–1486
Chawla A (2013) BMJ case reports. doi:10.1136/bcr-2013-201163
Currarino G, Wood B, Majd M (1993) The genitourinary tract and retroperitoneum. Congenital renal anomalies. In: Silverman FN, Kuhn JP (eds) Caffey's pediatric X-ray diagnosis: an integrated imaging approach, vol 2, 9th edn. Mosby, St Louis, pp 1223–1243
Dajani AM (1966) Horseshoe kidney: a review of 29 cases. Br J Urol 38:388–402
Daneman A, Alton DJ (1991) Radiographic manifestations of renal anomalies. Radiol Clin North Am 29:351–363
Downs RA, Lane JW, Burns E (1973) Solitary pelvic kidney: its clinical implications. Urology 1:51–56
Evans WP, Resnick MI (1981) Horseshoe kidney and urolithiasis. J Urol 125:620–621
Glenn JF (1959) Analysis of 51 patients with horseshoe kidney. N Engl J Med 261:684–687
Kakei H, Kondo A, Ogisu BI, Mitsuya H (1976) Crossed ectopia of solitary kidney: a report of two cases and a review of the literature. Urol Int 31:470–475
Kissane JM (1983) Congenital malformations. In: Heptinstall RH (ed) Pathology of the kidney, vol 1, 3rd edn. Little, Brown, Boston, pp 83–140
Kramer SASA, Kelalis PP (1984) Ureteropelvic junction obstruction in children with renal ectopy. J Urol 5:331–336
Lippe B, Geffner ME, Dietrich RB, Boechat MI, Kangarloo H (1988) Renal malformation in patients with Turner's syndrome: imaging in 141 patients. Pediatrics 82:852–856
Malek RS, Kelalis PP, Burke EC (1971) Ectopic kidney in children and frequency of association with other malformations. Mayo Clin Proc 46:461–467
McDonald JH, McClellan DS (1957) Crossed renal ectopia. Am J Surg 93:995–1002
Mesrobian HJ, Kelalis PP, Hrabovsky E, Othersen HB, DeLorimier A, Nesmith B (1985) Wilms' tumor in horseshoe kidneys: a report from the National Wilms' Tumor Study. J Urol 133:1002–1003
Moore KL, Persaud TVN (1998) The developing human. Clinically oriented embryology, 6th edn. Saunders, Philadelphia
Muttarak M, Sriburi T (2011) Congenital renal anomalies detected in adulthood. Biomed Imaging Interv J 8(1):e7
N'Guessen G, Stephens FD, Pick J (1984) Congenital superior ectopic (thoracic) kidney. Urology 24:219–228
Pitts WR Jr, Muecke EC (1975) Horseshoe kidneys: a 40-year experience. J Urol 113:743–746

Polak-Jonkisz D, Fornalczyk K, Musial K et al (2012) Crossed renal ectopia: can it be a diagnostic problem? Postepy Hig Med Dosw 66:201–214

Ritchey M (1992) Anomalies of the kidney. In: Kelalis PP, King LR, Belman AB (eds) Clinical pediatric urology, vol 1, 3rd edn. Saunders, Philadelphia, pp 500–528

Rubinstein ZJ, Hertz M, Shahin N, Deutsch V (1976) Crossed renal ectopia: angiographic findings in six cases. Am J Roentgenol 126:1035–1038

Thompson GJ, Pace JM (1937) Ectopic kidney: a review of 97 cases. Surg Gynecol Obstet 64:935–943

Warkany J, Passarge E, Smith LB (1966) Congenital malformations in autosomal trisomy syndromes. Am J Dis Child 112:502–517

Whitaker RH, Hunt GM (1987) Incidence and distribution of renal anomalies in patients with neural tube defects. Eur Urol 13:322–323

Zondek LH, Zondek T (1964) Horseshoe kidney in associated congenital malformations. Urol Int 18:347–356

Part III

Clinical Statements and Basics: What Every (Pediatric) Uroradiologist Ought to Know

Genetics in Nephrourology

Klaus Zerres, Miriam Elbracht, and Sabine Rudnik

Contents

1 Introduction 181
2 **Formal Genetics** 182
3 **Molecular Genetics** 182
3.1 Conditions with Known Gene Defects 183
3.2 Inherited Disorders with Localized Genes Which Have Not Yet Been Identified 184
3.3 Genetic Counseling 184
4 **Genetics of Important Disorders of the Urogenital System** 186
4.1 Renal Agenesis 186
4.2 Urinary Tract Dilatation 186
4.3 Duplication of Kidneys, Renal Pelvis, and Ureters 188
4.4 Vesicoureteral Reflux (VUR) 188
4.5 Hypospadias 188
4.6 Cystic Kidney Diseases: Ciliopathies 188
4.7 Hereditary Tumors of the Kidney 190
5 **Genetic Basis of Important Nephropathies** 191
5.1 Alport Syndrome (AS) 191
5.2 Bartter Syndrome 192
5.3 Nephrogenic Diabetes Insipidus 192
5.4 Nocturnal Enuresis 192
5.5 Nephrolithiasis 192
5.6 Nephrotic Syndromes 192
5.7 Cystinosis 193
6 **The Use of Databases for Information About the Current Status on Molecular Biology of Hereditary Nephropathies** 193
Conclusion 193
References 193

K. Zerres, MD • M. Elbracht, MD
Institute of Humangenetics, RWTH Aachen University, Pauwelsstrasse 30, D-52074 Aachen, Germany
e-mail: kzerres@ukaachen.de

S. Rudnik, MD (✉)
Sektion Humangenetik, Medizinische Universität Innsbruck, Peter-Mayr-Str. 1/1.OG, A-6020 Innsbruck, Austria
e-mail: sabine.rudnik@i-med.ac.at

1 Introduction

Due to the great number of disorders of the urinary tract and the increasing knowledge about the genetics during the last decades, a comprehensive and complete review on hereditary diseases in nephrology and urology is impossible. Enormous efforts have been spent to disclose the underlying basic defects. Many nephropathies are hereditary and are subject of comprehensive research worldwide. An example for the progress in research is autosomal dominant polycystic kidney disease (ADPKD), but this similarly applies to many others. With an incidence of about 1:1,000, ADPKD is one of the most common hereditary disorders at all. The first gene was mapped on chromosome 16 in 1985 (Reeders et al. 1985) and identified in 1994 (The European Polycystic Kidney Disease Consortium 1994). Including the knowledge of other cystic diseases, experimental in vitro research, and data of numerous animal models, a common pathogenetic theory of cystogenesis allowed the first causal therapeutic trials in the last years; huge research progress can be expected within the next years.

Typical steps on the way to the understanding of the pathogenesis or even suggestions for a rational gene therapy in a future vision are (1) identification of the causal gene; (2) cloning the gene which means disclosing its structure; (3) analyzing mutations and their clinical consequences (genotype/phenotype correlations); (4) studying the gene product, protein structure, and function; and (5) first therapeutic trials based on the understanding of the pathogenesis.

It should be kept in mind, however, that even a specific mutation does usually not allow to predict a certain phenotype since specific consequences are often influenced by other genes or exogenous factors acting as modifiers. Genome-wide association studies (GWASs) to identify these modifying actors are under investigation. Genes which are known to cause rare monogenic kidney disorders are in focus, and in this context, common genetic variants in the uromodulin (UMOD) gene were identified to influence the susceptibility to chronic kidney disease and hypertension (for review, see Trudu et al. 2013; Gorski et al. 2015). In the near future, the list of these modifying actors will grow.

The aim of this contribution is to summarize important information on the genetics of urological and nephrological disorders and to describe the current possibilities and limitations in the diagnosis of hereditary renal disorders by the use of DNA techniques. Because of the complexity of the topic, some major principles will be outlined additionally as a basic introduction.

As the knowledge is constantly growing and the content of this chapter is probably partially outdated by the time of its publication, a detailed list of references is not included; only basic or fundamental texts are listed. Current citations are available in the "Online Mendelian Inheritance in Man" database [(OMIM): http://www.ncbi.nlm.nih.gov/omim/].

2   Formal Genetics

Many hereditary diseases follow defined modes of inheritance and are caused by mutations in single genes. Gene carriers usually present clinical features according to the modes of inheritance. The clinical picture is often variable which is denoted by the term variable expressivity. The related term incomplete penetrance describes the fact that not all gene carriers present clinical features. Beside these monogenic inherited diseases, most conditions have a more complex genetic background. Multifactorial diseases usually have a genetic basis, and additional exogenous factors, most often unknown, are necessary to lead to a clinical manifestation of the disorder. Recurrence risks in this group are usually estimated on an empirical base. Polygenic diseases are caused by the interaction of mutations in more than one gene, e.g., a digenic inherited condition is caused by mutations in two different genes. It can be assumed that in most conditions, however, many genes are involved. The characteristics of the different modes of inheritance are listed in Table 1. For more details, see textbooks of human genetics (e.g., Read and Donnai 2015; Tobias et al 2011; Tumpenny 2012).

3   Molecular Genetics

The identification of the genetic base of a disease is the first step in understanding its physiological and biochemical pathogenesis. Over years, mapping the gene, which means localizing it on a chromosomal region, and sequencing it exon by exon by "Sanger technique" was the main diagnostic approach and is still in well-defined single-gene conditions.

But in many conditions, mutations in more than only one gene can lead to overlapping phenotypes, or the clinical course of a disease cannot be predicted on the basis of a specific mutation. In the last years, new technologies have become available which might enable to solve these problems in the near future. The term next-generation sequencing (NGS) describes techniques of sequencing whole exoms or whole genomes in time- and cost-saving procedures without the need of a clinical hypothesis. Until now the biggest problem of NGS techniques in routine genetic diagnostics is the data evaluation confronted with rare genetic variants of so far

Table 2 Syndromes with renal agenesis (selection)

Syndrome	Major feature	Genetics
Branchio-oto-renal syndrome (BOR1) Melnick-Fraser syndrome (BOR2)	Hearing loss, pinna anomalies, branchial cleft fistulas, preauricular pits	AD (113650), *EYA1* AD (610896), *SIX5*
CHARGE association	Coloboma, heart defect, choanal atresia, mental retardation, genital hypoplasia, ear anomalies, growth impairment, deafness	Most often AD new mutations of *CHD7* (214800), rarely of *SEMA3*
Chromosomal disorders	Depending on the cytogenetic changes additional malformations, facial dysmorphism, mental retardation	Most often de novo, in rare cases consequence of a familial translocation
Cryptophthalmos syndrome (Fraser syndrome)	Cryptophthalmia, cleft lip/palate, genital anomalies, atresia of ear canal, syndactyly	AR (219000), *FRAS1, FREM2, GRIP1*
Hypogonadotropic hypogonadism (HH1-23), Kallmann syndrome	Hypogonadotropic hypogonadism, anosmia, cryptorchism	AD (136350), *FGFR1*, (*FGF8, GNRHR, and others*), AR X-linked (308700), *KAL-1*
Rubinstein-Taybi syndrome types 1 and 2	Broad thumbs and toes, distinctive facial features, mental retardation, microcephaly, cryptorchism, small phallus	Most often (50–70%) de novo microdeletion 16p including the gene *CREBBP*; further cases (3%) with mutations in *CREBBP* (180849), *EP300* (613684)

Table 3 Syndromes with hydronephrosis (selection)

Syndrome	Major features	Renal involvement	Genetics
Chromosomal disorders (e.g., trisomy 8, 13, 18, 18q-, r(18), X0, triploidy)	According to the chromosomal disorder additional malformations, facial dysmorphism, mental retardation	Different types, often only mild changes	Most often de novo, in rare cases consequence of a familial translocation
Bardet-Biedl syndrome (BBS1-19)	Obesity, pigmentary retinopathy, polydactyly, hypogenitalism	Ectopic urethra, cystic kidney	AR (209900), heterogeneous with BBS1-19 identified
Prune belly syndrome	Deficient abdominal muscles, urinary obstruction/distension, cryptorchism, malrotation of the gut, clubfeet, limb reduction anomalies	Urethral atresia, ureteral duplication, bladder distension, hydronephrosis, renal dysplasia	Mostly sporadic (100100), heterogeneous, *CHRM3* mutation in one family
Rubinstein-Taybi syndrome types 1 and 2	Broad thumbs and toes, distinctive facial features, mental retardation, microcephaly, cryptorchism, small phallus	Posterior urethral valves, abnormal bladder shape, absent or extra kidney, double renal pelvis	Most often (50–70%) de novo microdeletion 16p including the gene *CREBBP*; further cases (3%) with mutations in *CREBBP* (180849), *EP300* (613684)
Kaufman-McKusick syndrome	Hydrometrocolpos, transverse vaginal membrane, vaginal septum, postaxial polydactyly, cardiac anomalies, hypospadias	Hydroureter, ureteral duplication, ectopic urethra, urogenital sinus, posterior urethral valves	AR (236700), mutations in Bardet-Biedl type 6 (*BBS6*) gene

known underlying genetic defects are still unknown.

4.3 Duplication of Kidneys, Renal Pelvis, and Ureters

A genetic base is well known, and many reported families indicate autosomal dominant inheritance with variable expressivity and incomplete penetrance. In about 10% of parents and siblings, similar observations can be made, indicating multifactorial inheritance for the majority of cases. According to the general rule of thumb, the recurrence risk doubles with each additionally affected close relative. Duplication malformations can also occur as part of a syndrome, and a selection of such syndromes is given in Table 4.

4.4 Vesicoureteral Reflux (VUR)

Vesicoureteral reflux (VUR, OMIM 193000) is most likely genetically heterogeneous with the majority of cases indicating a multifactorial genesis rather than an autosomal dominant inheritance. At least eight autosomal loci have been identified with evidence for a further X-linked locus. Mutations in the *ROBO2*, *SOX17*, and *TNXB* gene could be detected in respective families. Penetrance rates were about 45% when associated with a gene mutation. Overall – in several systematic studies among first-degree relatives (children, siblings, parents) – about 10–25% showed VUR depending on the different imaging techniques used. Siblings thus should be screened provided there is a therapeutic implication.

4.5 Hypospadias

The genetic nature of hypospadias has been well known for a long time and has been evaluated in several systematic studies. Empiric risk figures for brothers of affected boys are about 7%, and boys of affected fathers probably have a lower risk of approximately 3.5%. These figures indicate a multifactorial base of hypospadias in the majority of cases. In line with this, assumption is the observation that the risk increases according to the grade of hypospadias. The empirical risk for siblings of grade one was 3.5%, for grade two 3.9%, and for grade four 16.6%, respectively. More distant relatives have lower risks: about 2% for second-degree relatives (uncles, nephews, grant parents) and third-degree relatives in only 1%. In rare cases, autosomal dominant inheritance seems possible. An X-linked type with mutations in the *MAMCD1* gene (OMIM 300758) has been described. Rarely, patients with hypospadias showed mutations in the androgen receptor gene responsible for testicular feminization and Kennedy syndrome.

4.6 Cystic Kidney Diseases: Ciliopathies

With the knowledge that dysfunctions of primary cilia play a fundamental role in the pathogenesis of a larger group of hereditary diseases, the term

Table 4 Syndromes with duplication of kidneys, renal pelvis, and ureters (selection)

Close family members should be screened		
Syndrome	Major features	Genetics
Branchio-oto-renal (BOR1) syndrome (Melnick-Fraser syndrome) BOR2	Hearing loss, pinna anomalies, branchial cleft fistulas, preauricular pits	AD (113650), *EYA1* AD (610896), *SIX5*
Chromosomal disorders (e.g., 4p-, 11q-, X0, partial trisomy 3q, trisomy 8 mosaic)	According to the chromosomal disorder additional malformations, facial dysmorphism, mental retardation	Most often de novo, in rare cases consequence of a familial translocation
Nail patella syndrome	Nail hypoplasia, hypoplastic/absent patella	AD (161200), *LMX1B*

of so-called ciliopathies was coined. The ciliary function is fundamentally important for the structure and function of the kidneys, liver, eye, and central nervous system, so that in particular hereditary diseases that are associated with polycystic kidneys can be classified among the ciliopathies.

Autosomal Dominant and Autosomal Recessive Polycystic Kidney Disease (ADPKD and ARPKD)

While the autosomal dominantly inherited types (ADPKD) (OMIM 173910) belong to the most common inherited diseases at all, the recessive type (ARPKD) (OMIM 263200) is mainly important among pediatric patients. Although ADPKD is usually a late-onset disease with clinical signs in adulthood, and ARPKD is often diagnosed in newborns or even prenatally, there is a broad clinical overlap. Therefore, family history, including renal ultrasonography scans of relatives, is still a major criterion for classification of polycystic kidney disease in children.

In ADPKD up to now, two genes could be identified. While about 85% of patients show 16p linkage indicating mutations in the *PKD1* gene, mutations in the *PKD2* gene are responsible for less than 15%. A third gene locus has so far not been identified, if existing. The *PKD1* gene encodes an integral membrane protein, polycystin1, which is involved in cell-cell/cell-matrix interaction. Polycystin2, interacting with polycystin1, shows homologous sequences with polycystin1 as well as to one subunit of a calcium channel. The *PKHD1* gene mutated in ARPKD has 66 exons and encodes a large, receptor-like protein of unclear function.

There is a strong demand for prenatal diagnosis in ARPKD and therefore for mutation detection in contrast to ADPKD where mutation detection is often not necessary (see also Sect. 3.3.1). As about 95% of gene carriers in ADPKD can be identified by renal ultrasonography by the age of 20 years and nearly all gene carriers are detected by the age of 30 years, predictive genetic testing using DNA analysis is usually not necessary. Syndromes with cystic kidneys have always to be excluded (Table 5). The growing availability of preimplantation diagnostics might however change this attitude in the future. Due to the common combination of liver changes in patients with cystic kidneys, the liver morphology is important for clinical classification.

Glomerulocystic Kidney Disease (GCKD)

The genetic basis of autosomal dominant glomerulocystic kidney disease has recently been disclosed with mutations in the *HNF1β*-gene which is the gene mutated in MODY type V also denoted as "renal cysts and diabetes syndrome" (RCAD) (OMIM 137920) (Table 5). The renal disease is highly variable and includes renal cysts, glomerular tufts, aberrant nephrogenesis, primitive tubules, irregular collecting systems, oligomeganephronia, enlarged renal pelvis, abnormal calyces, small kidney, single kidney, horseshoe kidney, and hyperuricemic nephropathy. Affected individuals may also have abnormalities of the genital tract, including vaginal aplasia, rudimentary uterus, bicornuate uterus, epididymal cysts, and atresia of the vas deferens.

Juvenile Nephronophthisis/Medullary Cystic Kidney Disease

This disease group is defined by renal cysts mostly at the cortico-medullary junction and classified into a recessive form (nephronophthisis) and dominant form (medullary cystic kidney disease – MCKD) (OMIM 256100 and 174000). Nephronophthisis is genetically heterogeneous, and 19 genes have been mapped and identified *(NPHP1-19)*. Additional genes can be expected.

Molecular genetic testing can be used for diagnostic classification, as homozygous deletions can be detected in 85% of patients with NPHP1 (juvenile type), thus confirming the diagnosis without renal biopsy. The *NPHP1 gene* encodes the protein nephrocystin and *NPHP2* the protein inversin. Other genes have been identified. Manifestations of nephronophthisis with additional signs like congenital

Table 5 Syndromes with cystic kidneys (selection)

Syndrome	Major features	Renal involvement	Genetics
Chromosomal disorders (e.g., trisomy 10p, 13, 17, XYY, triploidy)	According to the chromosomal disorder additional malformations, facial dysmorphism, mental retardation	Different types, inborn malformations, more often only mild changes	Most often de novo, in rare cases consequence of a familial translocation
Von-Hippel-Lindau syndrome (VHL)	Retinal angiomas, cerebellar hemangioblastomas	Cysts, renal cell carcinoma	AD with incomplete penetrance and variable expressivity (193300), *VHL*
Short-rib thoracic dysplasia syndrome (SRTD1-13) Jeune syndrome (SRTD1)	Small thorax, polydactyly, rhizomelic limb shortening, trident pelvis, biliary dysgenesis and pancreatic dysplasia	Renal dysplasia, juvenile nephronophthisis, hydroureters, multicystic kidneys	AR (208500 & others), heterogeneous, *DYNC2H1*, *NEK1* and further genes
Meckel-Gruber-syndrome (MKS1-12)	Occipital encephalocele, polydactyly, cleft lip/palate, microphthalmia, small or ambiguous genitalia, brain anomalies, biliary dysgenesis, and pancreatic dysplasia	Renal dysplasia or hypodysplasia, ureteral hypoplasia or aplasia, hypoplastic bladder, urethral agenesis	AR (249000 and others), heterogeneous, *MKS1*, *TMEM67*, *CEP290*, *RPGRIP1L* and further genes
Oral-facial-digital syndrome type 1 (OFD1)	Lobulated tongue, median pseudocleft of lip, cleft palate, hypoplastic alae nasi, digital anomalies, mental impairment	Often late-onset polycystic kidney disease	X-linked (311200), *OFD1*
Renal adysplasia (hereditary renal adysplasia, HRA)	Anomalies of internal genitalia, occasional anomalies of the anus, heart, and spine	Renal agenesis, hypodysplasia, dysplasia, ureteral and urethral anomalies	AR (191830), *TGA8*, *RET*, *PAX2*
Tuberous sclerosis	Hypopigmentated macules, adenoma sebaceum, retinal and brain tumors, seizures, mental retardation	Renal angiomyolipomas (40–80 %), renal dysplasia, cortical cysts, renal vascular anomalies, renal cell carcinomas, polycystic kidney disease	AD (191100) new mutations in about 85 % of cases, variable expressivity, incomplete penetrance *TSC1*, *TSC2* (605284)

hepatic fibrosis, retinitis pigmentosa, as well as cerebellar lesions are summarized as Senior-Loken syndrome (OMIM 266900); mutations have been identified in the *NPHP1*, *NPHP4*, *NPHP5*, and *NPHP6* genes. Two genes responsible for autosomal dominant medullary cystic kidney disease, which seems to be rare in Europe, could be mapped on chromosomes 1q21 (*MCKD1*) and 16p12 (*MCKD2*). The *MCKD2* gene encodes the protein uromodulin (UMOD).

Medullary Sponge Kidney

The term medullary sponge kidney (MSK) does not describe a defined clinical entity with a uniform genetic cause. This kidney malformation usually occurs sporadic, and rarely familial cases are observed (Zerres et al 1984). Many case reports describe MSK in combination with other renal and extrarenal malformations. In some cases, a defined genetic entity could be identified; among these there are also ADPKD families (for review, see Fabris et al 2013).

4.7 Hereditary Tumors of the Kidney

Renal tumors are very heterogeneous in their pathogenesis. In 1–5 %, genetic germline alternations play a major role, and tumors can occur as part of a complex genetic disease. Tumors are major manifestations in the two forms of tuberous sclerosis and the von Hippel-Lindau syndrome. The responsible genes are tumor suppressor genes. The two-step hypothesis of Knudson gives an explanation for the great clinical variability.

Wilms tumor is only rarely inherited (about 5 %) and follows an autosomal dominant pattern in these families. The involvement of tumor suppressor gene has been shown. The risk for birth of an affected child of a healthy gene carrier (see below) is approximately 30 %. Bilateral and multifocal tumors can always be regarded as heritable. For practical counseling, the following risks can be given:

- Risks for children of surviving patients with Wilms tumor: 2–4 % in cases of unilateral tumor with no further affected family member and 50 % in cases with bilateral or multifocal occurrence
- Risk for children of non-affected parents in families with known Wilms tumor:
  (a) For relatives of a sporadic case, most likely <1 %
  (b) For children of persons who are carrier (e.g., a sibling and a child is affected or two children are affected), at least 30 %
  (c) For healthy siblings of two affected siblings or of an affected parent and an affected siblings, about 9 %

A Wilms tumor can occur as part of complex disorder like the WAGR syndrome with Wilms tumor, aniridia, genital malformation, and mental retardation. Responsible genes are in close vicinity on chromosome 11 in the regions p13 (*WT1*) and p15.5 (*CDKN1C*). Mutations in the *CDKN1C* gene were found in patients with Beckwith-Wiedemann syndrome, who can exhibit Wilms tumors. Other responsible loci for Wilms tumor have been discussed: 16q (WT3), 17q12–q21 (*WT4*), and (7p15–p11.2). Wilms tumors can also occur as a feature of Denys-Drash syndrome characterized by nephrotic syndrome and diffuse mesangial sclerosis as well as male hermaphroditism. At the DNA level, mutations in the zink finger coding domains of the *WT1* gene on chromosome 11p13 were shown. This is most likely a sporadic disease and only in rare cases consequence of a familial translocation. In cases of Wilms tumor with additional features, especially of the eyes, mutations in the *MET* gene (OMIM 605074) in patients with familial renal carcinoma were found.

> **Take Away**
> Important genetic disorders of the kidney and the urogenital tract can be divided into inborn congenital malformations (CAKUT), cystic kidney diseases/ciliopathies, and tumor syndromes. The congenital malformations are usually multifactorial and part of a broader clinical spectrum, but more rarely they can also occur in the context of a defined malformation syndrome. In contrast, ciliopathies and tumor syndromes usually have a monogenic cause and follow a specific inheritance pattern.

5 Genetic Basis of Important Nephropathies

5.1 Alport Syndrome (AS)

Alport syndrome is genetically heterogeneous with X-linked (OMIM 301050) and autosomal recessive modes (OMIM 203780) of inheritance. About 85 % of cases follow an X-linked pattern and show mutations in the *alpha 5(IV) collagen* (*COL4A5*) gene. Mutation screening is hampered by a complex genomic region and many different mutations. In practice, mutations can be detected only in about 70–80 % of patients with clearly X-linked AS. Mutations in other alpha subunits of the type IV collagen are the genetic basis of the rare autosomal recessive AS (*COL4A4*, *COL4A3*). Benign familial hematuria is a dominant condition with mild features of Alport nephritis; after heterozygous mutations in the *COL4A4* gene were found, it was concluded that benign familial hematuria can be regarded as a heterozygous manifestation of autosomal recessive AS.

If the diagnosis of AS is suspected in a patient, a mutation screening in the responsible collagen genes as a basis for genetic classification and counseling has to be discussed. In patients with a proven mutation, no invasive diagnostic means are necessary, such as renal biopsy,

5.2 Bartter Syndrome

This condition is characterized by hypokalemic metabolic alkalosis, hyperreninism, and hyperaldosteronism – with normal blood pressure. Three different forms following autosomal recessive inheritance can be distinguished: classical Bartter syndrome (OMIM 607364), neonatal form (hyperprostaglandin E syndrome), as well as the mild Gitelman syndrome of adolescence and adulthood. According to the known pathogenesis of salt-losing, mutations of genes involved in NaCl reabsorption can be detected (classical Bartter syndrome, renal chloride channel *CLCNKB*; neonatal Bartter syndrome, furosemide dependent NaK2Cl cotransporter *NKCC2* or renal potassium channel *ROMK*; Gitelman syndrome, thiazide-sensitive NaCl cotransporter). A molecular genetic diagnosis is useful for a presymptomatic testing of children at risk in order to avoid uncontrolled salt-wasting.

5.3 Nephrogenic Diabetes Insipidus

The nephrogenic diabetes insipidus (OMIM 304800, 125800) is characterized by the resistance of the kidney toward the action of vasopressin resulting in the production of large volumes of diluted urine. After previous mapping of the X-linked type, mutations in the *vasopressin V2 receptor* gene were found. Autosomal recessive or dominant have a percentage of about 10% and are caused by mutations of the *water channel aquaporin 2* gene (*AQP2*) on chromosome 12q12–q13. Genetic testing has as yet no therapeutic consequences but can be used for prenatal diagnosis, if requested. The molecular disclosure of basic defects is an impressive confirmation of the known pathogenesis of water transport.

5.4 Nocturnal Enuresis

Positive family history of nocturnal wetting in children older than 7 years is well known affecting about 50% of relatives of index patients and indicating major genetic factors in the pathogenesis. A primary form (PNE) or type I is distinguished from a secondary form, in whom the child has been dry for at least 6 months but enuresis has recurred. Although ENUR1 and ENUR2 have been mapped to chromosomes 13q and 12q, no causal gene has been identified (OMIM 600631).

5.5 Nephrolithiasis

The genetic base of an increasing number of conditions leading to hereditary renal stones has been disclosed. The recently detected mutations in a renal chloride channel gene (*CLCN5*) are responsible for the X-linked nephrolithiasis (OMIM 310468) and Dents disease (with Fanconi syndrome) (OMIM 300009). Autosomal recessive cystinuria (OMIM 220100) type I and type II is caused by allelic mutations of the *membrane transporter* gene *rBAT* for dibasic amino acids (*SCL3A1*). In type III, mutations in the *SCL7A9-AS transporter* gene could be found.

Further genes involved in other conditions responsible for renal stone development among many others could be identified: e.g., osteopetrosis with tubular acidosis type I (xanthine oxidase), hyperoxaluria type I (alanine glyoxylate aminotransferase), adenine phosphoribosyltransferase deficiency (ATRTase), distal tubular acidosis, and primary hypomagnesemia.

5.6 Nephrotic Syndromes

Nephrotic syndrome can also be inherited, following an autosomal recessive or dominant mode in these families. Up to now, the recessive genes responsible for the congenital nephrotic syndrome of the Finnish type (*NPHS1* on chromosome 19q12, gene product nephrin, OMIM 256300) and the gene involved in the steroid-resistant nephrotic syndrome (*NPHS2* on chromosome 1q25, gene product podocin, OMIM 600995) have been be identified. Further genes for the dominant nephrotic syndrome with adult-onset and focal segmental glomerulosclerosis are known (OMIM 603278) (*ACTN4*, *TRPCG*, and haploinsufficiency for the CD2-associated protein).

The involvement of several genes reflects the heterogeneous pathogenesis of the nephrotic syndromes. Pathoanatomical lesions do not indicate a specific genetic entity. Apart from the congenital nephrotic syndrome of the Finnish type, which rarely occurs in non-Finnish populations, genetic testing is not applicable on a routine basis.

5.7 Cystinosis

Patients with cystinosis (OMIM 219800) develop nephritis, cataracts, retinopathy, and hypothyroidism due to an autosomal recessive transport defect of cystin. The responsible gene *CTNS* encodes an integral membrane protein cystinosin.

> **Take Away**
>
> The genetic nephropathies can be distinguished according to the localization and the type of the underlying defect. Defects of the glomerular structure, ion channelopathies, and amino acid transporters have different clinical consequences. Most genetic nephropathies have a monogenic cause, and clinical diagnosis can be confirmed by molecular genetic analysis.

6 The Use of Databases for Information About the Current Status on Molecular Biology of Hereditary Nephropathies

This overview will be outdated with regard to the actual knowledge in molecular biology after publication of this issue. Therefore, the use of databases is important for practitioners as well as for scientists.

The most important database about the current development of inherited diseases, which is updated daily, is Victor McKusick's database "Online Mendelian Inheritance in Man" (OMIM) (http://www.ncbi.nlm.nih.gov/OMIM/). The entries include current references.

A database on diseases is orphanet, dedicated to information on rare diseases and orphan drugs (http://www.orpha.net/).

A database of laboratories in Europe offering DNA diagnoses is available: (http://www.eddnal.com). Addresses of genetic laboratories are usually published through the national societies of human genetics.

> **Conclusion**
>
> Molecular techniques have contributed enormous knowledge about the nature of hereditary diseases. Molecular biology provides new insights into basic mechanisms of the nature and classification of these entities. The understanding of the underlying defects and the pathogenesis of a certain disease may give clues to the development of a future therapy.
>
> The diagnostic facilities also offer new possibilities, but it should be realized that DNA diagnosis differs in many aspects from conventional diagnosis and has certain limitations and consequences which requires a careful application.

References

Fabris A, Anglani F, Lupo A, Gambaro G (2013) Medullary sponge kidney: state of the art. Nephrol Dial Transplant 28(5):1111–1119

Gorski M, Tin A, Garnaas M, McMahon GM et al (2015) Genome-wide association study of kidney function decline in individuals of European descent. Kidney Int 87(5):1017–1029

Reeders ST, Breuning MH, Davies KE et al (1985) A highly polymorphic DNA marker linked to adult polycystic kidney disease on chromosome 16. Nature 317(6037):542–544

The European Polycystic Kidney Disease Consortium (1994) The polycystic kidney disease 1 gene encodes a 14 kb transcript and lies within a duplicated region on chromosome 16. Cell 77(6):881–894

Trudu M, Janas S, Lanzani C et al (2013) Common noncoding UMOD gene variants induce salt-sensitive hypertension and kidney damage by increasing uromodulin expression. Nat Med 19(12):1655–1660

Zerres K, Volpel MC, Weiss H (1984) Cystic kidneys. Genetics, pathologic anatomy, clinical picture, and prenatal diagnosis. Hum Genet 68:104–135

Current citations are available in Online Mendelian Inheritance in Man (OMIM): http://www.ncbi.nlm.nih.gov/omim/

For background information, see textbooks of human genetics e.g.:

Read A, Donnai D (2015) New clinical genetics 3. Scion, Banbury. ISBN 9781907904677

Tobias ES, Connor M, Ferguson-Smith M (eds) (2011) Essential medical genetics, 6th edn. Wiley-Blackwell, Chichester/Hoboken. ISBN 9781405169745

Tumpenny PD (2012) Emery's elements of medical genetics, 14th edn. Elsevier/Churchill Livingstone, Philadelphia. ISBN 9780702040436

Renal Agenesis, Dysplasia, Hypoplasia, and Cystic Diseases of the Kidney

Christoph Mache and Holger Hubmann

Contents

1 Introduction 195
2 **Renal Agenesis** 196
3 **Renal Dysplasia and Hypoplasia** 197
4 **Cystic Kidney Disease** 197
4.1 Autosomal Recessive Polycystic Kidney Disease (ARPKD) 197
4.2 Autosomal Dominant Polycystic Kidney Disease (ADPKD) 198
4.3 Nephronophthisis (NPHP) and Medullary Cystic Kidney Disease (MCKD) 199
4.4 Glomerulocystic Kidney Disease (GCKD) ... 199
4.5 Multicystic Dysplastic Kidney (MCDK) 200
4.6 Medullary Sponge Kidney (MSK) 200
4.7 Simple Renal Cyst 200
4.8 Complicated Renal Cyst, Multiloculated Cyst, and Cystic Renal Tumor 201

Conclusion 202

References 202

C. Mache, MD (✉) • H. Hubmann, MD
Department of Paediatrics, Division of General Paediatrics, Medical University Graz,
8036 Graz, Austria
e-mail: christoph.mache@medunigraz.at

1 Introduction

Congenital anomalies of the kidney and urinary tract (CAKUT) cover a wide range of structural malformations that result from defects in the morphogenesis of the kidney and/or urinary tract (see also chapter "Congenital Anomalies of the Renal Pelvis and Ureter"). CAKUT occur in approximately 1:500 live-born fetuses and are the most common cause of chronic kidney disease in children worldwide (Renkema et al. 2011; Vivante et al. 2014). Congenital anomalies of the kidney include renal agenesis, renal hypo-/dysplasia with or without cysts, and multicystic dysplastic kidneys (Weber 2012). While most CAKUT cases are sporadic, renal abnormalities are found in close relatives in approximately 10% of cases (Winyard and Chitty 2008). Although CAKUT typically occur as isolated malformations, they occasionally develop in association with additional congenital anomalies outside the urinary tract, such as in the renal coloboma syndrome or the renal cysts and diabetes syndrome; they may also be associated with cardiac malformations. Currently, more than 20 monogenic CAKUT-causing genes have been identified, and recent findings suggest that CAKUT may arise from a multitude of different single-gene causes (Vivante et al. 2014). The malformation phenotypes vary from normally appearing kidneys with preserved renal function (i.e., incomplete penetrance) to severe hypo-/dysplasia and end-stage renal disease. Features linked to worse prognosis are (1) bilateral disease, (2) decreased functional mass (which encompasses not just small kidneys but also large ones where cysts replace normal architecture), (3) lower urinary tract obstruction, and (4) anhydramnios or severe oligohydramnios (Winyard and Chitty 2008). Current management of CAKUT includes observation, surgical interventions, prophylaxis and treatment of urinary tract infections, strict blood pressure control, supplements for renal support, and nephroprotective treatment to slower the progression of chronic kidney disease.

Renal cysts are clinically and genetically heterogeneous conditions. Inherited cystic kidney disorders mainly include polycystic kidney diseases and entities comprising the nephronophthisis and medullary cystic kidney disease complex. These diseases are now categorized as ciliopathies – a disease concept characterized by dysfunction of the primary cilium, a hairlike cellular organelle (Hildebrandt et al. 2011). Cilia sense a wide variety of extracellular signals and transduce them into decisions regarding proliferation, polarity, nerve growth, differentiation, or tissue maintenance (Goetz and Anderson 2010). Since cilia are expressed in variable tissues, ciliopathies may affect multiple organs, and numerous pleiotropic human disorders have been attributed to defective cilia formation. It has become increasingly evident that many ciliopathies have a renal cystogenic component, making kidney cyst formation a hallmark feature of ciliopathies (Bergmann 2012). Renal dysplasia may as well occur as a result of defective differentiation during kidney development. Notably, cystic kidneys and renal dysplasia are important features of numerous genetic syndromes, such as the mainly recessively inherited ciliopathies Bardet-Biedl, Joubert, Meckel, and Jeune syndromes or the dominant disorders of tuberous sclerosis, von Hippel-Lindau disease, and branchio-oto-renal syndrome (Bergmann 2015). At present, treatment of ciliopathies still remains symptomatic.

Several medications are being investigated that might influence ciliary function and, for example, also may delay cyst formation and growth in the kidneys or will reduce the future extrarenal disease burden.

Details on imaging appearance and typical findings can be found in chapter "Imaging in Renal Agenesis, Dysplasia, Hypoplasia, and Cystic Diseases of the Kidney" which addresses all aspects of imaging including the respective imaging modalities, particularly focusing on ultrasonography (US) which is the most commonly used and often diagnostically sufficient modality in these entities.

Take Away

Congenital anomalies of the kidney are part of the CAKUT spectrum. Renal ciliopathies are frequently characterized by renal cyst formation; imaging heavily relies on US and is essential for initial evaluation and follow-up.

2 Renal Agenesis

Unilateral renal agenesis is characterized by the one-sided absence of renal tissue resulting from failure of embryonic kidney development (Woolf and Hillman 2007). The general incidence of unilateral renal agenesis has been estimated to be 1 in 2,000 (Westland et al. 2013). Renal agenesis occurs when the ureteric bud fails to form the ureter, renal pelvis, and renal mesenchyma that are necessary for the development of nephrons (Kerecuk et al. 2008). In these patients one frequently finds no ipsilateral ureter, as well as associated aplasia, hypoplasia, or anomalies of genital structures originating from the ipsilateral Wolffian and Mullerian ducts. Associated CAKUT have been identified in ~32 % of unilateral renal agenesis patients, the most common being vesicoureteric reflux (VUR) (24 %) (Westland et al. 2013). Extrarenal anomalies involving the gastrointestinal tract, heart, or musculoskeletal system were reported in 31 % of patients. Injury of the solitary functioning kidney may lead to hypertension, microalbuminuria, and/or a decrease in glomerular filtration rate. Therefore, these patients need nephrological long-term follow-up, particularly in the absence of compensatory hypertrophy of the solitary kidney.

Bilateral renal agenesis occurs in 1 of 3,000 pregnancies and is considered almost uniformly fatal (Woodward et al. 2011). Affected fetuses die in utero from cord compression, or newborns die within hours after birth from severe pulmonary hypoplasia due to anhydramnios.

> **Take Away**
> In unilateral renal agenesis, sonographic evaluation and monitoring of the contralateral kidney are obligatory.

3 Renal Dysplasia and Hypoplasia

Dysplastic kidneys are abnormally developed kidneys with poorly branched or differentiated nephrons and collecting ducts, increased stroma, and, occasionally, cysts and metaplastic tissues, such as cartilage (Woolf et al. 2004). Dysplastic kidneys range in size from large distended kidneys with multiple large cysts to small kidneys with or without cysts (Rosenblum and Salomon 2008). They are common malformations affecting up to 1 in 1,000 of the general population and comprise part of the spectrum of CAKUT (Ichikawa et al. 2002). Renal dysplasia may be the only CAKUT manifestation or be associated with hydronephrosis, UPJO, megaureter, ureter duplex, VUR, and posterior urethral valve (Schedl 2007). Simple renal hypoplasia is defined as a small kidney with a reduced number of nephrons but maintained normal architecture. However, dysplastic features can be detected in most of these kidneys histologically as well (Watkins et al. 1997). As a consequence, a small kidney without cysts but with sonographical signs of dysplasia is often clinically referred to as a hypo-dysplastic kidney.

Apart from isolated cases of CAKUT, combined malformations with various extrarenal manifestations have been observed. More than 500 syndromes involving CAKUT have been described as yet (Weber 2012) (see also chapter "Genetics in Nephrourology"). However, until recently, only a little more than 20 monogenic CAKUT-causing genes have been identified (Vivante et al. 2014). Among them, autosomal dominant mutations in *HNF1β* (renal cysts and diabetes syndrome), *PAX2* (renal coloboma syndrome) and *EYA1* (branchio-oto-renal syndrome) are the most important (Weber et al. 2006). Renal cysts and diabetes syndrome may include renal dysplasia, diabetes mellitus, hyperuricemia, hypomagnesemia, elevated liver function tests, and malformations of female internal genitalia (Ulinski et al. 2006; Adalat et al. 2009). Renal coloboma syndrome is characterized by coloboma of the optic nerve and renal dysplasia with/without VUR (Sanyanusin et al. 1995). Branchio-oto-renal syndrome is genetically heterogeneous and comprises variable combinations of anomalies of the kidneys, brachial arches (cysts or fistulae), and external and inner ear (deafness) (Chang et al. 2004).

> **Take Away**
> Nowadays, renal hypo dysplasia is mostly detected by fetal or postnatal US. Imaging of associated anomalies of the urinary tract as well as potential extrarenal malformations is important for a correct diagnosis as well as for adequate therapeutic decisions and follow-up.

4 Cystic Kidney Disease

4.1 Autosomal Recessive Polycystic Kidney Disease (ARPKD)

ARPKD is a recessively inherited ciliopathy caused by mutations of the *polycystic kidney and hepatic disease 1* gene (Bergmann et al. 2003). The incidence is approximately 1 in 20,000 live births. Its principal manifestations are polycystic kidney disease and congenital hepatic fibrosis (Bergmann et al. 2005).

The majority of patients are severely affected and ARPKD is frequently detected in late pregnancy or at birth. Fetuses with ARPKD display massively enlarged kidneys and oligohydramnios due to fetal renal failure (see also chapter "Urogenital Fetal Imaging: US and MRI"). Approximately 30–50 % of affected neonates die shortly after birth from respiratory failure due to pulmonary hypoplasia and thoracic compression by the excessively enlarged kidneys. Those surviving the neonatal period frequently take a prolonged course and may develop end-stage renal failure in the second decade of life (Guay-Woodford and Desmond 2003). Moderately affected patients without perinatal manifestation may even enter adulthood with preserved renal function (Adeva et al. 2006).

While the early presentation of ARPKD is clearly dominated by renal disease and early-onset hypertension, liver disease with congenital hepatic fibrosis and biliary duct ectasia is also present in every ARPKD patient. The hepatobiliary complications may also dominate the clinical picture, particularly in older patients. Progressive hepatic fibrosis leads to portal hypertension causing hypersplenism with pancytopenia as well as esophageal varices with bleeding complications. ARPDK patients with extensive dilatations of intra- and extrahepatic bile ducts (Caroli's disease) are also at risk of ascending bacterial cholangitis (Kashtan et al. 1999).

> **Take Away**
> In ARPKD imaging should always include monitoring of congenital hepatic fibrosis and its potential complications.

4.2 Autosomal Dominant Polycystic Kidney Disease (ADPKD)

ADPKD is the most frequent life-threatening genetic disease (prevalence 1/500–1/1,000 live births) affecting approximately 12.5 million individuals worldwide (Harris and Torres 2009). About 50 % of ADPKD patients develop end-stage renal failure by the age of 60 years. While clinical symptoms usually only arise in adulthood, there is considerable phenotypic variability even within the same family. In children, diagnosis of ADPKD is frequently made by family screening or as an incidental finding on US. About 60 % of ADPKD children aged less than 5 years have already *one or more* renal cysts detectable by US (Gabow et al. 1997). In general, the finding of even one renal cyst should alert the physician to the possibility of ADPKD because simple cysts are otherwise rare in childhood. Therefore family history and investigation, in particular parental US, are obligatory. In children with parental ADPKD, the finding of one cyst can already be considered diagnostic (Ravine et al. 1994).

About 2 % of ADPKD patients manifest clinically before age 15 years (Bergmann 2012). ADPKD-related symptoms include arterial hypertension, pain, episodes of hematuria, renal calculi, proteinuria, infection, or a palpable mass. Risk factors for a more rapid progression of ADPKD are (1) renal enlargement early in life, (2) having more than ten renal cysts before age of 12 years, and (3) having blood pressures above the 75th percentile for age, height, and gender (Fick-Brosnahan et al. 2001). Occasional ADPKD cases are even associated with significant perinatal morbidity and mortality and may be indistinguishable from severe forms of ARPKD (Fick et al. 1993; Bergmann et al. 2011).

ADPKD is a systemic ciliopathy, and cysts may also arise in other organs, e.g., liver, pancreas, seminal vesicles, and arachnoid membrane (Torres et al. 2007). About 8 % of ADPKD patients develop intracranial aneurysms, particularly those with a positive family history for intracranial aneurysm and/or hemorrhage (Rossetti et al. 2003). Approximately 10 % of first aneurysmal ruptures were reported to occur before age 20 years (Chauveau et al. 1994). Cardiac valve disease, mainly mitral valve prolapse, has been detected in 26 % of ADPKD patients (Lumiaho et al. 2001).

4.3 Nephronophthisis (NPHP) and Medullary Cystic Kidney Disease (MCKD)

Nephronophthisis (NPHP) comprises a clinically and genetically heterogeneous group of autosomal recessive ciliopathies (Hildebrandt et al. 2011). NPHP is the most frequent genetic cause of end-stage renal disease during the first three decades of life (median age 13 years). Renal histopathology is characterized by the triad of (1) tubular basement disruption, (2) tubulointerstitial fibrosis with cell infiltration, and (3) tubular cysts, mainly at the corticomedullary junction (Waters and Beales 2011). Although NPHP is generally referred to as a cystic kidney disease, cysts are not an obligatory feature and frequently occur only after patients have progressed to end-stage renal failure. NPHP manifests clinically with a urinary concentration defect leading to polyuria and polydipsia, as well as anemia and progressive renal failure (Bergmann 2012). Since cilia are found in virtually all organs and serve distinct functions in different tissues, ciliopathies may cause a broad range of organ involvement. In NPHP extrarenal manifestations are frequent and bear a significant comorbidity (Waters and Beales 2011). Ciliopathies may involve the eyes (retinitis pigmentosa, oculomotor apraxia), the brain (cerebellar vermis hypo-/aplasia associated with the "molar tooth sign" on MRI, mental retardation, encephalocele), the liver (cholangiociliopathies with liver fibrosis), and the bones (short ribs, cone-shaped epiphyses, postaxial polydactyly). Based on the pattern of organ involvement, numerous syndromes with high phenotypic variability and considerable overlap have been described.

MCKD is often considered the autosomal dominant variant of NPHP with a usually later onset of renal failure than in the recessive forms. Mutations in the gene encoding the ciliary protein uromodulin (Tamm-Horsfall glycoprotein) can lead to different tubulointerstitial nephropathies including MCKD2, glomerulocystic kidney disease, and familial juvenile hyperuricemic nephropathy (Vylet'al et al. 2006).

> **Take Away**
> In NPHP patients additional imaging of potential extrarenal manifestations involving, for example, the liver, brain, or bones, is essential for a correct and complete diagnosis as well as during follow-up.

4.4 Glomerulocystic Kidney Disease (GCKD)

GCKD is defined histologically by the occurrence of glomerular cysts with dilatation of the Bowman's space and glomerular tufts (Bernstein 1993). GCKD was described, e.g., in various ciliopathies including ADPKD (particularly in young infants), NPHP, and MCKD (type 2), as well as tuberous sclerosis and the renal cysts and diabetes syndrome (Mache et al. 2002). GCKD has also been associated with renal dysplasia and urinary tract obstruction (Bissler et al. 2010).

> **Take Away**
> In the majority of ADPKD patients, renal cysts arise already during childhood, and family history and parental US are mostly the key to diagnosis. Familial clustering of valvular heart disease and intracranial aneurysms must be taken in account.

> **Take Away**
> GCKD is a histological finding in various cystic kidney diseases. Since in most of these patients no renal biopsy is performed, this diagnosis is rarely made and often missed, as there are no specific imaging or laboratory features that would suggest the diagnosis. However, this has no implication on treatment and prognosis.

4.5 Multicystic Dysplastic Kidney (MCDK)

Unilateral MCDK is the most common form of cystic renal dysplasia with an incidence of 1 in 2,200 to 1 in 4,300 live births (Schreuder et al. 2009). The ipsilateral ureter is frequently atretic and sometimes even absent, supporting the theory that MCDK results from early ureteral pathology during nephrogenesis (Woolf 1997). It usually affects the entire kidney, but rarely can also involve only a part of the kidney, e.g., in a duplex system (Jeon et al. 1999). Unilateral MCKD is commonly a sporadic malformation, incidental reports exist on MCDK in siblings, twins and families (Srivastava et al. 1999). Bilateral MCKD is usually incompatible with extrauterine life.

Renal function depends on the solitary functioning contralateral kidney. Abnormalities of the contralateral renal unit may be found in one-third of patients, mainly VUR (Schreuder et al. 2009). In the absence of compensatory hypertrophy, renal hypo-/dysplasia should be suspected. Injury of the solitary kidney may lead to hypertension, microalbuminuria, and/or a decrease in glomerular filtration rate. Furthermore, associated ipsilateral genital anomalies are found in up to 50%, such as cystic dysplasia of the rete testis or the seminal vesicle. Previous concerns about an increased risk of hypertension and malignancy have been allayed based on results from longer follow-up studies and systematic reviews, as well as on some immature blastema found in surgery specimen that hypothetically allows for an increased risk of malignant differentiation later on (Narchi 2005a, b; Aslam et al. 2006).

Clinically, MCDK is commonly detected by fetal US. MCDK is now generally regarded as a benign condition with conservative management and long-term follow-up predominating over surgical removal. Nephrectomy is mostly restricted to cases with continuous growth leading to compression of adjacent structures, infection, hemorrhage, or suspected tumors. Spontaneous involution of MCKD was reported to be 35% by 2 years, 47% by 5 years, and 62% by 10 years of age, respectively (Hayes et al. 2012). Larger postnatal MCDK (>5 cm) are less likely to involute already during the first decade of life than smaller MCDK (Hayes et al. 2012; Poggiali and Oliveira 2012).

> **Take Away**
> The task of imaging is to establish the diagnosis, to evaluate the contralateral renal unit, to detect rare complications, and to monitor the involution of MCKD.

4.6 Medullary Sponge Kidney (MSK)

MSK is a kidney malformation of unknown etiology that generally becomes manifest with nephrocalcinosis, recurrent renal stones, and pre-calyceal duct ectasias (erroneously diagnosed as cysts) (Fabris et al. 2013) (see also chapter "Urolithiasis and Nephrocalcinosis"). Clinically, MSK may present with renal colic, episodes of hematuria, pyelonephritis, or renal failure. Frequent findings are hypercalciuria as well as renal acidification and concentration defects. MSK rarely presents in childhood and may be a familial disease in up to 10% of cases.

> **Take Away**
> In childhood MSK is a rare and mostly sporadic diagnosis suspected and established by the radiologist. Due to its probably heterogeneous etiology, a comprehensive nephrological work-up is mandatory.

4.7 Simple Renal Cyst

Simple renal cysts can occur spontaneously or be familial. They are rare in childhood with a reported incidence of 0.22% (McHugh et al. 1991). Simple cysts do not bare any consequences or associated risks except for a few occasions, when growing cysts lead to hypertension, compression of adjacent structures, or obstruction of the collecting system (Churchill et al. 1975). In adults, cysts are much more common (up to 50 %), and the development of simple renal cysts is seen as a normal aging phenomenon (Baert and Steg 1977; Tada et al. 1983).

Acquired cysts can occur in post-traumatic and post-inflammatory (tuberculous, etc.) settings or spontaneously develop in kidney parenchyma during chronic renal failure and on dialysis (Dunill et al. 1977; Leichter et al. 1988; Hogg 1992). As in end-stage kidneys with acquired cysts malignancy may develop, they need to be monitored (Bretan et al. 1986; Levine 1992).

Simple renal cysts are rare in infancy and childhood. US usually detects them as an incidental finding. Possible manifestation of a polycystic or dysplastic renal disease must be considered, and follow-up is warranted.

> **Take Away**
>
> In children, a renal cyst may be a feature of ADPKD or cystic renal dysplasia and always warrants at least a follow-up US examination.

4.8 Complicated Renal Cyst, Multiloculated Cyst, and Cystic Renal Tumor

"Complicated cyst" is a term coined by descriptive radiology. The exact definition varies depending on the imaging modality applied and the age of the patient. A complicated cyst is defined as a cystic lesion with some abnormalities, therefore not matching all criteria necessary for a simple cyst. These are small size, clear and sharp margins, no echoes or contents in the clear fluid, and no parenchymal rim or inclusion. The radiological changes of a complicated cyst may originate from secondary hemorrhage or sedimentation of proteins and of membrane cells. Calcifications may also occur, or infection may be present. Differentiation of these cysts, usually discovered by US, is essential and achieved in part by CT/MRI, in part in conjunction with clinical and laboratory findings (Table 1).

Table 1 Differential diagnosis of a complicated renal cyst

"Simple cyst" aggravated by:
Secondary hemorrhage
Sedimentation
Infection
Acquired cysts
Posttraumatic
Inflammatory cyst (abscess, tuberculoma)
Infected calyceal cyst with sedimentation and calculi
Partially thrombosed vascular aneurysm
Necrosis after infarction, abscess
Cystic malformation
Segmental MCDK
Dysplastic cysts
Multilocular cyst and multilocular cystic nephroma
Manifestation of polycystic kidney disease (particularly ADPKD)
Cystic renal tumor
Necrotic hamartoma, capillary hemangioma, vascular malformation, bleeding angiomyolipoma, and other cystic benign renal tumors
Cystic Wilms' tumor, cystic mesoblastic nephroma
Cystic carcinoma and other, partially necrotic or cystic, malignant renal tumors

This table lists the most important entities that have to be considered for differential diagnosis of complicated renal cysts

Tumors have to be recognized and imaged/treated appropriately. Many tumor entities can present as a cystic renal tumor; the histologies range from benign renal neoplasms to cystic Wilms' tumor, cystic mesoblastic nephroma, and cystic renal adenocarcinoma (Theissig et al. 1986; Babut et al. 1993; Upadhyay and Neely 1989). Definite diagnosis is often only made histologically as imaging features may not be characteristic in the individual case (see also chapter "Neoplasms of the Genitourinary System").

> **Take Away**
>
> If a renal cyst does not match the criteria of a "simple" cyst on US, further imaging modalities are necessary and determine whether a biopsy is taken or follow-up is scheduled.

Conclusion

Congenital anomalies of the kidney and cystic renal diseases comprise many entities that may be diagnostically challenging. Family history and investigation, clinical presentation and evolution, renal imaging, and searching for extrarenal manifestations are valuable diagnostic tools. In addition, next-generation sequencing-based approaches allow parallel analysis of multiple genes involved in nephrogenesis and ciliary function and increasingly provide accurate genetic diagnoses. An accurate diagnosis is essential for genetic counseling, prenatal diagnostics, and the clinical management of patients and their families.

References

Adalat S, Woolf AS, Johnstone KA et al (2009) HNF1B mutations associate with hypomagnesemia and renal magnesium wasting. J Am Soc Nephrol 20:1123–1131

Adeva M, El-Youssef M, Rossetti S (2006) Clinical and molecular characterization defines a broadened spectrum of autosomal recessive polycystic kidney disease (ARPKD). Medicine (Baltimore) 85:1–21

Aslam M, Watson AR, Trent & Anglia MCDK Study Group (2006) Unilateral multicystic dysplastic kidney: long term outcomes. Arch Dis Child 91:820–823

Babut JM, Bawab F, Jouan H et al (1993) Cystic renal tumors in children–a diagnostic challenge. Eur J Pediatr Surg 3:157–160

Baert L, Steg A (1977) On the pathogenesis of simple renal cysts in the adult. Urol Res 5:103–108

Bergmann C (2012) Ciliopathies. Eur J Pediatr 171:1285–1300

Bergmann C (2015) ARPKD and early manifestations of ADPKD: the original polycystic kidney disease and phenocopies. Pediatr Nephrol 30(1):15–30

Bergmann C, Senderek J, Sedlacek B et al (2003) Spectrum of mutations in the gene for autosomal recessive polycystic kidney disease (ARPKD/PKHD1). J Am Soc Nephrol 13:76–89

Bergmann C, Senderek J, Windelen E (2005) Clinical consequences of PKHD1 mutations in 164 patients with automoal recessive polycystic kidney disease (ARPKD). Kidney Int 67:829–848

Bergmann C, von Bothmer J, Ortiz Brüchle N et al (2011) Mutations in multiple PKD genes may explain early and severe polycystic kidney disease. J Am Soc Nephrol 22:2047–2056

Bernstein J (1993) Glomerulocystic kidney disease – nosological considerations. Pediatr Nephrol 7:464–470

Bissler JJ, Siroky BL, Yin H (2010) Glomerulocystic kidney disease. Pediatr Nephrol 25:2049–2059

Bretan PN Jr, Bush MP, Hricak H et al (1986) Chronic renal failure: a significant risk factor in the development of acquired renal cysts and renal cell carcinoma. Case report and review of the literature. Cancer 57:1871–1879

Chang EH, Menezes M, Meyer NC et al (2004) Branchio-oto-renal syndrome: the mutation spectrum in EYA1 and its phenotypic consequences. Hum Mut 23:582–589

Chauveau D, Pirson Y, Verellen-Dumoulin C et al (1994) Intracranial aneurysms in autosomal dominant polycystic kidney disease. Kidney Int 45:1140–1146

Churchill E, Kimoff R, Pinshy M et al (1975) Solitary intrarenal cyst: correctable cause of hypertension. Urology 6:485–488

Dunill MS, Millard PR, Oliver D (1977) Acquired cystic disease of the kidneys: a hazard of long term intermittent maintenance haemodialysis. J Clin Pathol 30:868–877

Fabris A, Anglani F, Lupo A et al (2013) Medullary sponge kidney: state of the art. Nephrol Dial Transpl 28:1111–1119

Fick GM, Johnson AM, Strain JD et al (1993) Characteristics of very early onset autosomal dominant polycystic kidney disease. J Am Soc Nephrol 3:1863–1870

Fick-Brosnahan GM, Tran ZV, Johnson AM et al (2001) Progression of autosomal dominant polycystic kidney disease in children. Kidney Int 59:1654–1662

Gabow PA, Kimberling WJ, Strain JD (1997) Utility of ultrasonography in the diagnosis of autosomal dominant polycystic kidney disease in children. J Am Soc Nephrol 8:105–110

Goetz SC, Anderson KV (2010) The primary cilium: a signalling centre during vertebrate development. Nat Rev Genet 11:331–344

Guay-Woodford LM, Desmond RA (2003) Autosomal recessive polycystic kidney disease: the clinical experience in North America. Pediatrics 111:1072–1080

Harris PC, Torres VE (2009) Polycystic kidney disease. Annu Rev Med 60:321–337

Hayes WN, Watson AR, Trent & Anglia MCKD Study Group (2012) Unilateral multicystic dysplastic kidney: does initial size matter? Pediatr Nephrol 27:1335–1340

Hildebrandt F, Benzing T, Katsanis N (2011) Ciliopathies. New Engl J Med 364:1533–1543

Hogg RJ (1992) Acquired cystic kidney disease in children prior to the start of dialysis. Pediatr Nephrol 6:176–178

Ichikawa I, Kuwayama F, Pope JC 4th et al (2002) Paradigm shift from classical anatomic theories to contemporary cell biological views of CAKUT. Kidney Int 61:889–898

Jeon A, Cramer BC, Walsh E et al (1999) A spectrum of segmental multicystic renal dysplasia. Pediatr Radiol 29:309–315

Kashtan CE, Primack WA, Kainer G (1999) Recurrent bacteremia with enteric pathogens in recessive polycystic kidney disease. Pediatr Nephrol 13:678–682

Kerecuk L, Schreuder MF, Woolf AS (2008) Renal tract malformations: perspectives for nephrologists. Nat Clin Pract Nephrol 4:312–325

Leichter HE, Dietrich R, Salusky I et al (1988) Acquired cystic kidney disease in children undergoing long-term dialysis. Pediatr Nephrol 2:8–11

Levine E (1992) Renal cell carcinoma in uremic acquired renal cystic disease: incidence, detection and management. Urol Radiol 13:203–210

Lumiaho A, Ikaheimo R, Miettinen R et al (2001) Mitral valve prolapse and mitral regurgitation are common in patients with polycystic kidney disease type 1. Am J Kidney Dis 38:1208–1216

Mache CJ, Preisegger KH, Kopp S et al (2002) De novo HNF-1 beta gene mutation in familial hypoplastic glomerulocystic kidney disease. Pediatr Nephrol 17:1021–1026

McHugh K, Stringer D, Hebert D (1991) Simple renal cyst in children: diagnosis and follow-up with US. Radiology 178:383–385

Narchi H (2005a) Risk of hypertension with multicystic dysplastic kidney disease: a systematic review. Arch Dis Child 90:921–924

Narchi H (2005b) Risk of Wilms' tumor with multicystic dysplastic kidney disease: a systematic review. Arch Dis Child 90:147–149

Poggiali IV, Oliveira EA (2012) Renal size and sonographic involution of multicystic dysplastic kidney. Pediatr Nephrol 27:1601–1602

Ravine D, Gibson RN, Walker RG et al (1994) Evaluation of ultrasonographic diagnostic criteria for autosomal dominant polycystic kidney disease 1. Lancet 343:824–827

Renkema KY, Winyard PJ, Skovorodkin IN et al (2011) Novel perspectives for investigating congenital anomalies of the kidney and urinary tract. Nephrol Dial Transpl 26:3843–3851

Rosenblum ND, Salomon R (2008) Disorders of kidney formation. In: Geary DF, Schaefer F (eds) Comprehensive pediatric nephrology. Mosby Elsevier, Philadelphia, pp 131–141

Rossetti S, Chauveau D, Kubly V et al (2003) Association of mutation position in polycystic kidney disease 1 (PKD1) gene and development of a vascular phenotype. Lancet 361:2196–2201

Sanyanusin P, Schimmenti LA, McNoe LA et al (1995) Mutation of the PAX2 gene in a family with optic nerve colobomas, renal anomalies and vesicoureteral reflux. Nat Genet 9:358–364

Schedl A (2007) Renal abnormalities and their developmental origin. Nature Rev Genet 8:791–792

Schreuder MF, Westland R, van Wijk JAE (2009) Unilateral multicystic dysplastic kidney: a meta-analysis of observational studies on the incidence, associated urinary tract malformations and the contralateral kidney. Nephrol Dial Transpl 24:1810–1818

Srivastava T, Garola RE, Hellerstein S (1999) Autosomal dominant inheritance of multicystic dysplastic kidney. Pediatr Nephrol 13:481–483

Tada S, Yamagishi J, Kobayashi H et al (1983) The incidence of simple renal cysts by computed tomography. Clin Radiol 34:437–439

Theissig F, Hempel J, Schubert J (1986) Multilocular cystic nephroma simulating kidney carcinoma. Ztschr Urol Nephrol 79:263–267

Torres VE, Harris PC, Pirson Y (2007) Autosomal dominant polycystic kidney disease. Lancet 369:1287–1301

Ulinski T, Lescure S, Beaufils S et al (2006) Renal phenotypes related to hepatocyte nuclear factor-1beta (TCF2) mutations in a pediatric cohort. J Am Soc Nephrol 17:497–503

Upadhyay AK, Neely JAC (1989) Cystic nephroma: an emerging entity. Ann R Coll Surg Engl 71:381–383

Vivante A, Kohl S, Hwang DY et al (2014) Single-gene causes of congenital anomalies of the kidney and urinary tract (CAKUT) in humans. Pediatr Nephrol 29:695–704

Vylet'al P, Kublova M, Kalbacova M et al (2006) Alterations of uromodulin biology: a common denominator of the genetically heterogeneous FJHN/MCKD syndrome. Kidney Int 70:1155–1169

Waters AM, Beales PL (2011) Ciliopathies: an expanding disease spectrum. Pediatr Nephrol 26:1039–1056

Watkins SL, McDonald RA, Avner ED (1997) Renal dysplasia, hypoplasia and miscellaneous cystic disorders. In: Barrat MT, Avner ED, Harmon WE (eds) Pediatric nephrology. Lippincott Williams & Wilkins, Baltimore, pp 415–426

Weber S (2012) Novel genetic aspects of congenital anomalies of kidney and urinary tract. Curr Opin Pediatr 24:212–218

Weber S, Moriniere V, Knüppel T et al (2006) Prevalence of mutations in renal developmental genes in children with renal hypodysplasia: results of the ESCAPE study. J Am Soc Nephrol 17:2864–2870

Westland R, Schreuder MF, Ket JCF et al (2013) Unilateral renal agenesis: a systematic review on associated anomalies and renal injury. Nephrol Dial Transplant 28:1844–1855

Winyard P, Chitty LS (2008) Dysplastic kidneys. Semin Fetal Neonatal Med 13:142–151

Woodward PJ, Kennedy A, Sohaey R et al (2011) Diagnostic imaging – obstetrics. Amirsys, Salt Lake City, pp 2–28

Woolf AS (1997) The kidney: embryology. In: Barrat MT, Avner ED, Harmon WE (eds) Pediatric nephrology. Lippincott Williams & Wilkins, Baltimore, pp 1–17

Woolf AS, Hillman KA (2007) Unilateral renal agenesis and the congenital solitary functioning kidney: developmental, genetic and clinical perspectives. BJU Int 99:17–21

Woolf AS, Price KL, Scrambler PJ et al (2004) Evolving concepts in human renal dysplasia. J Am Soc Nephrol 15:998–1007

Renal Parenchymal Disease

Ekkehard Ring and Birgit Acham-Roschitz

Contents

1 Introduction 205
2 **Clinical Presentation and Symptomatology** 205
2.1 Hematuria and Nephritic Syndrome 206
2.2 Proteinuria and Nephrotic Syndrome 206
2.3 Hypertension 207
2.4 Tubular Dysfunction 207
2.5 Renal Failure 207
3 **Specific Entities** 207
3.1 Glomerular Disease 207
3.2 Vascular and Tubulointerstitial Disease 211
3.3 Renal Parenchymal Involvement in Systemic Disease 213

Conclusion 215

References 215

E. Ring, MD (Retired) (✉)
B. Acham-Roschitz, MD
Department of Pediatrics, Division of General Pediatrics, University Hospital Graz, Auenbruggerplatz 34, 8036 Graz, Austria
e-mail: ekkehard.ring@medunigraz.at

1 Introduction

Renal parenchymal disease (RPD) is classified into glomerular, tubular, interstitial, and vascular disease. These various diseases may be congenital (hereditary) or acquired. They exclusively may affect the kidneys or are systemic disorders with a wide range of renal contribution. This chapter focuses on the "classic entities" of RPD like glomerulonephritis (GN) or nephrotic syndrome (NS) showing clinical presentation, pathogenesis, renal histology if renal biopsy is indicated, treatment, and prognosis of the various diseases. References are restricted to important new publications where the interested reader can also find suggestions for further reading. The implications for imaging including ultrasound-guided renal biopsy are described in chapter "Imaging in Renal Parenchymal Disease".

2 Clinical Presentation and Symptomatology

The presentation of RPD is varied: some urinary symptoms such as the red- or brown-colored urine of macrohematuria, the foaming urine of severe proteinuria, polyuria, or oliguria may obviously point to the urinary tract. Weight loss with hypovolemia, weight gain with edema, headache, fatigue, etc. may be general signs as well as cutaneous lesions of Henoch-Schönlein purpura, vasculitis, or systemic lupus erythematosus (SLE). Measurement of blood pressure may unravel arterial hypertension. However, severe renal disease may be asymptomatic only coming to light as a consequence of routine urinalysis, evaluation of recent and family history, or screening programs. Different forms of RPD initially may present nearly identical and just thorough clinical and laboratory evaluation, frequently completed by renal biopsy, and enable the final diagnosis and selected treatment. Lists of differential diagnoses or specific diagnostic algorithms sometimes are helpful. The more frequently encountered modes of presentation of RPD are now discussed.

2.1 Hematuria and Nephritic Syndrome

Microscopic hematuria is found in approximately 1 % of school children in screening programs, and the outcome is benign in the vast majority of cases (Murakami et al. 1991; Vehaskari et al. 1979). Occasionally, microscopic hematuria may be an early sign of severe renal disease like Alport syndrome. If hematuria is found on urine dipstick test, urine microscopy is needed to confirm the presence of intact red blood cells, thereby excluding hemoglobinuria, myoglobinuria, or discoloration of urine by drugs or foods. The presence of urinary red cell deformity (acanthocytes) and urinary red cell casts on urine microscopy are characteristic markers of glomerular bleeding and point to RPD (Koehler et al. 1991). This differentiation between glomerular and non-glomerular bleeding has a great impact on the further diagnostic approach in a child with hematuria. Children with macrohematuria and proteinuria have acute illness and more urgently need clinical and laboratory evaluation than children with microscopic hematuria.

The nephritic syndrome has an acute onset and is defined by hematuria, arterial hypertension, and acute renal failure (ARF) nowadays frequently named acute kidney injury (AKI). Significant proteinuria, oliguria, and volume overload may be additional features. All glomerular disorders may present this way and laboratory investigations are immediately needed to differentiate the various types of GN as treatment differs. Many children present with incomplete nephritic syndrome (e.g., without hypertension or acute kidney injury) or with silent disease not necessarily meaning a better prognosis. Laboratory evaluation of complement status, antinuclear antibodies (ANA), and antineutrophil cytoplasmatic antibodies (ANCA) is mandatory. A low C3 complement points to acute postinfectious GN, membranoproliferative GN, or lupus where ANA also are positive. Positive ANCA titers indicate vasculitis.

2.2 Proteinuria and Nephrotic Syndrome

The glomerular filter consists of the fenestrated endothelium of glomerular capillaries, the three-layered basement membrane, and the foot processes and slit membrane of the podocytes. The filter is freely permeable for molecules up to a molecular weight below 68,000 Dalton exactly being the molecular weight of albumin. Asymptomatic proteinuria is found in 5–15 % of routine urinalyses or in screening programs, but just 0.1 % of children had persistent proteinuria if four urine samples were analyzed (Vehaskari and Rapola 1982; Park et al. 2005). Orthostatic proteinuria is found in many situations (i.e., no proteinuria in morning urine and proteinuria during daytime) and is a benign condition. In contrast, renal biopsy is indicated even in asymptomatic children if proteinuria persists for 6–12 months. Earlier biopsy is needed if hematuria, hypertension, or renal failure is found during observation.

The nephrotic syndrome (NS) is defined by nephrotic range proteinuria (>2 mg/mg creatinine), hypoalbuminemia (<25 g/L), and edema. Ascites with the risk of pneumococcal peritonitis, pleural effusions, shortness of breath, or arterial hypertension may be additional clinical signs. Intravascular hypovolemia may cause AKI, and changes of blood coagulation – in part caused by urinary losses of inhibitors of coagulation – carry the risk of thromboembolic complications. Hyperlipidemia, low immunoglobulins, significant hematuria ("nephritic-nephrotic syndrome"), or an altered complement system may be additional laboratory findings. These and other evaluations primarily must lead to a differentiation of nephrotic children into three groups: either probably suffering from *idiopathic NS*, having a *secondary form of NS* like membranous nephropathy or SLE, or eventually a *genetically determined NS*. This differentiation is essential as the further diagnostic approach, treatment, and prognosis differ significantly. Infants presenting with NS during the first 3 months of life suffer from "congenital NS." Manifestation between fourth and 12th month of life is named "infantile NS."

2.3 Hypertension

Childhood hypertension (HTN) is predominantly caused by RPD or renovascular disease, and the upper limit of normal blood pressure is shown in chapter "Normal Values". HTN in RPD is caused by the inflammatory disease itself and by hypervolemia in renal failure. Activation of the renin-angiotensin-aldosterone system may be present, but treatment with angiotensin-converting-enzyme (ACE) inhibitors or angiotensin-2 (AT2)-receptor antagonists is prohibited in acute RPD as renal function would worsen. Calcium channel blocking agents, diuretics, and α–/ß– blocking drugs can be used. A slow and moderate reduction of blood pressure level is mandatory. Cerebral convulsions eventually combined with visual disturbances are suspicious of posterior reversible encephalopathy syndrome (PRES). This clinico-radiological entity needs to be confirmed rapidly by cerebral MRI (Ishikura et al. 2012).

2.4 Tubular Dysfunction

The renal tubules are responsible for body homeostasis of electrolytes, water, and the acid/base balance. Numerous active and passive mechanisms modify the glomerular ultrafiltrate and form the final urine. Acute kidney injury, chronic renal disease, and hereditary tubular disorders may lead to a mixed picture of renal tubular dysfunction including polyuria, salt wasting, potassium retention or losses, glucosuria, acidosis, aminoaciduria, etc. In contrast to the glomerular pattern of proteinuria with predominantly albuminuria, the tubular proteinuria is characterized by minor losses of albumin but massive excretion of ß2-microglobulin and other low molecular weight proteins and of tubular enzymes like N-acetyl-ß-D-glucosaminidase (NAG).

2.5 Renal Failure

Acute renal failure is defined as the sudden loss of renal function and is reversible in many cases (Lameire et al. 2005); nowadays, the term AKI is preferred. Various pathogenetic processes are involved, and ARF traditionally is classified into prerenal, intrinsic, and postrenal. In the context of RPD, the AKI is intrinsic in most cases where activation of the complement system and direct cell injury can be found. Deposition of immune complexes, cell proliferation, infiltration with neutrophils and macrophages, activation of the coagulation system with deposition of fibrin, and acute tubular necrosis inhibit filtration and lead to destruction of a variable number of nephrons. Therapy aims at stopping the disease process and (if possible) to save the entire renal parenchyma. Additional details of AKI are discussed in chapter "Renal Failure and Renal Transplantation".

> **Take Away**
> Clinical presentation is extremely variable and inconclusive in many situations. Laboratory evaluation is essential enabling differentiation of predominantly nephritic, nephrotic, or tubulointerstitial compromise.

3 Specific Entities

3.1 Glomerular Disease

3.1.1 Alport Syndrome and Thin Basement Membrane Nephropathy

Alport syndrome (AS) belongs to a group of diseases with familial glomerular hematuria where mutations of genes encoding for three of the six Type IV collagen subunits (COL4A3, COL4A4, and COL4A5) are responsible. Type IV collagen constitutes a major component of the glomerular basement membrane (GBM) and is also found in the basement membranes of the inner ear, the eyes, and the skin. The characteristic lesions of the GBM, like irregular thickening, thinning, multilamellation, and splitting are best demonstrated by electron microscopy. Three genetic forms of AS exist. X-linked (XLAS) is responsible for 80% of cases, autosomal recessive (ARAS) for 15%, and autosomal dominant (ADAS) for 5%. All present with microscopic or macroscopic hematuria, later with proteinuria, and hypertension and (aside from females with XLAS) inevitably progress to terminal renal failure. Virtually all females with XLAS have hematuria and most proteinuria. Yet progression to terminal renal failure is rare (Jais et al. 2003). Important extrarenal symptoms of AS are progressive sensorineural deafness and ocular defects like anterior lenticonus or macular lesions. Occasionally diffuse esophageal or vulvar leiomyomatosis are found. No causative treatment exists, but starting early with ACE inhibitors or AT2 receptor blocking agents may delay onset of terminal renal failure (Savige et al. 2013). Three to five percent of males with XLAS – where mutations in COL4A5 are responsible – present with posttransplant anti-GBM disease with a rapid allograft loss (Kashtan 2006). Diagnosis of AS is established by clinical criteria, renal biopsy with electron microscopy, and genetic analysis. Differentiation to the "MYH9 disorders" Epstein syndrome and Fechtner syndrome is necessary. Clinical presentation, progression to end-stage renal failure, and lamellation of the GMB may be identical to AS but macrothrombocytopenia allows differentiation. These disorders are caused by mutations in the nonmuscle myosin heavy chain IIA.

Familial benign hematuria is the historical term for familial occurrence of persistent, usually microscopic hematuria mostly without progression to renal failure and extrarenal manifestations (Gauthier et al. 1989). Diffuse attenuation of the GBM is the typical ultrastructural finding leading to the term "thin basement membrane nephropathy" (TBMN) being preferred nowadays (Savige et al. 2013). Genetic studies of TMBN families showed mutations in COL4A3 or COL4A4 in about 40% of families and 5–7% of adults have elevated serum creatinine (Rana et al. 2005). In general, TMBN patients can be managed without renal biopsy and treatment.

3.1.2 Acute Postinfectious Glomerulonephritis

This entity is one of the classical immunocomplex-mediated renal diseases following a febrile infection of the upper airways or of the skin. Group A ß-hemolytic streptococci are the most common associated organisms, but infections with other types of streptococci, staphylococci, viruses, and parasites were also found. Clinical manifestation with nephritic syndrome is the rule, but there is a wide spectrum from incomplete to complete nephritic syndrome. Presentation as rapidly progressive GN is rare. Laboratory values typically show low levels of C3 complement returning to normal after 6–8 weeks (Eison et al. 2011). The antistreptolysin titer is only elevated in cases associated with streptococcal infections. Differential diagnoses with low levels of C3 complement as a leading feature are membranoproliferative GN and SLE, but there is no indication for renal biopsy in most cases. Therapy is supportive and outcome is excellent even in cases with prolonged microscopic hematuria.

3.1.3 Rapidly Progressive Glomerulonephritis (RPGN)

This very complicated course of disease is possible in virtually all forms of GN. Histologically, it is defined by crescents in more than 50% of glomeruli ("crescentic nephritis"). There is extravasation of fibrin and protein into the Bowman's space and extracapillary proliferation (cellular crescent). In progression of disease, the crescents become fibrous with invariably loss of the glomerulum. Aside from immunocomplex-mediated GN, SLE, "idiopathic" RPGN, and ANCA-positive vasculitis are found in many cases. Pauci-immune GN (microscopic polyarteritis) is restricted to the kidneys. Systemic manifestations are found in Wegener's granulomatosis with sinusitis and pulmonary hemorrhage. The latter symptom is also a hallmark of Goodpasture's syndrome caused by antibodies against the "Goodpasture epitope" of glomerular and pulmonary basement membranes (linear deposition of IgG-anti-GBM-antibodies). Aside from treatment of acute renal failure frequently including dialysis/hemodiafiltration, treatment with i.v. methylprednisolone pulses, plasma exchange, and i.v. cyclophosphamide is necessary. Maintenance therapy may consist of steroids, mycophenolate, or cyclosporine A. Complete recovery depends on the underlying pathology, but terminal renal failure may be expected if more than 80 % crescents have been found.

3.1.4 IgA Nephropathy and Henoch-Schönlein Nephritis

IgA nephropathy (IgAN), originally described by Berger and Hinglais in 1968, is the most common GN worldwide. Initially regarded as a benign disorder, IgAN is a major cause of end-stage renal failure observed in up to 20–30 % of patients after a disease course of 20 years. Diagnosis requires renal biopsy where typical IgA immune complexes are found. The new Oxford classification of IgAN on renal biopsy could identify variables to predict outcome (Cattran et al. 2009). These variables are also valid for childhood IgAN (Coppo et al. 2010). The pathogenesis is not yet completely understood. Aberrantly glycosylated IgA1 polymers seem to be the basic abnormality being deposited as immune complexes within the kidneys and not regularly degraded by hepatic cells. In addition, genetic susceptibility factors may be of importance (WYATT and Julian 2013). Patients predominantly present with painless gross hematuria and a normal renal function during upper respiratory tract infections. Isolated microscopic hematuria is the next frequent finding. Presentation with acute renal failure, hypertension, proteinuria over one gram per day, and NS is a clinical sign of poor prognosis. These cases and children with recurrent macroscopic hematuria need renal biopsy. In contrast, long-term prognosis of patients with minor urinary abnormalities is excellent – these children can be managed without renal biopsy (Gutierrez et al. 2012).

Henoch-Schönlein purpura (HSP) is the most frequent small-vessel vasculitis in childhood affecting the skin, joints, gut, and kidneys. Nephritis in HSP (HSPN) occurs in 30–50 % of cases and usually is milder than IgAN (Pohl 2015). The renal lesions of HSPN and IgAN are identical as well as the pathology of IgA1 indicating that both lesions belong to the same spectrum of disease. Clinical presentation is dominated by the cutaneous lesions but recurrences without purpura are well recognized. The indications for renal biopsy are identical to IgAN.

Therapy of both disorders is similar. No treatment is required in mild cases. ACE inhibitors or AT2-receptor blockers can suppress mild proteinuria and fish oil may be supportive (Radhakrishnan and Cattran 2012). In severe presentations like mentioned above or if there is no improvement during follow-up, a steroid protocol for six months has proven to be successful (Pozzi et al. 2004). Additional immunosuppressants are rarely required. Both disorders may recur after renal transplantation.

3.1.5 Membranoproliferative Glomerulonephritis

A variety of disease processes and pathogenetic mechanisms lead to a uniform pattern of glomerular injury named membranoproliferative GN (MPGN). Children and young adults are predominantly affected mostly presenting with NS (40–70 %) or nephritic syndrome (20–30 %). Yet various manifestations, from RPGN to asymptomatic proteinuria and hematuria, or recurrent gross hematuria, are reported (Alchi and Jayne 2010). Persistent hypocomplementemia is the characteristic laboratory value, and 40 % of patients slowly progress to end-stage renal failure. Traditionally, MPGN is divided into three subtypes (Type I–III) according to the findings on electron microscopy. Type II is characterized by dense deposits within the GBM and is also called dense deposit disease (DDD). Many cases of MPGN are secondary to infections. They may be viral (hepatitis B and C), bacterial (abscesses, endocarditis, "shunt nephritis"), or protozoal (malaria, schistosomiasis). Recent advances in the understanding of the complement system, especially of the alternative pathway and its relationship to MPGN, enabled a new pathogenetic and practical approach to MPGN (Sethi and Fervenza 2011).

Immunocomplex-mediated MPGN is characterized by an activation of the classic complement pathway with immunoglobulin and C3 deposits on renal biopsy. Aside from the above-mentioned infections, autoimmune disorders like SLE and monoclonal gammopathy of malignancies are found. Dysregulation of the alternative pathway caused by mutations or autoantibodies to regulating proteins is found in *complement-mediated MPGN*. C3 deposition but no immunoglobulins are found on renal biopsy. A summary of possible mutations like of Factor H and on antibodies such as C3 nephritic factor was given recently (Sethi and Fervenza 2012). Complement-mediated MPGN further is divided into DDD and C3 glomerulopathy (Barbour et al. 2013).

Treatment of infections, autoimmune disease, and malignancy is warranted in immunocomplex-mediated MPGN. Treatment with eculizumab, an anti-C5 monoclonal antibody inhibiting the terminal complement pathway, is promising in DDD and C3 glomerulopathy (Bomback et al. 2012; Radhakrishnan et al. 2012). MPGN may lead to end-stage renal failure. Recurrence in renal transplants is high and is nearly 100 % in DDD.

3.1.6 Membranous Nephropathy

Membranous nephropathy (MN) is rare during childhood, and diagnosis is made by typical findings on renal biopsy with subepithelial immune deposits. Clinical presentation with steroid-resistant NS or with asymptomatic proteinuria and microscopic hematuria is the rule (Menon and Valentini 2010). Secondary causes of MN are infections like hepatitis B, malaria, or syphilis and autoimmune disorders like SLE. MN may be paraneoplastic or drug induced and is also found in sickle cell disease (Ayalon and Beck 2015). Circulating anti-PLA2R antibodies directed against the phospholipase A2 receptor of podocytes were found in the majority of primary ("idiopathic") cases of MN (Beck et al. 2009). Some children with MN have anti-bovine serum albumin antibodies (Debiec et al. 2011).

Patients with asymptomatic proteinuria frequently achieve spontaneous remission, and no treatment aside from ACE inhibitors is recommended. Children with NS are at risk of progressive disease, and treatment with steroids, cyclophosphamide, or cyclosporine A has to be considered. Treatment of secondary MN is targeted to the underlying disorder.

3.1.7 Idiopathic and Hereditary Nephrotic Syndrome

The definition of idiopathic nephrotic syndrome (INS) and the clinical hallmarks are given above. If secondary NS is excluded, patient's age is between 2 and 14 years, and no extrarenal signs point to a syndromic form, INS can be assumed. Eighty percent of cases will show "minimal changes" on renal histology with effacement of podocyte foot processes and a breakdown of slit membrane on electron microscopy. About 10 % will have focal-segmental glomerulosclerosis (FSGS) and a similar percentage mesangial proliferation. Other histological lesions are rare. Numerous studies have shown remission of INS following a steroid treatment in 80–90 %. Consequently, no renal biopsy is performed before treatment, and the response to steroid therapy is used for further differentiation (Lombel et al. 2013a). Children with steroid-sensitive INS (SSNS) will have relapses in 80 % once again treated with steroids. Steroid-sparing therapy with cyclosporine A (CSA), mycophenolate, rarely cyclophosphamide, or rituximab is indicated in frequent relapsing and steroid-dependent INS (van Husen and Kemper 2011; Gellermann et al. 2013). Nevertheless, prognosis is favorable and just few patients will enter chronic renal failure.

Cases not responding to steroids suffer from steroid-resistant nephrotic syndrome (SRNS)

(Shenoy et al. 2010; Lombel et al. 2013b). They need renal biopsy, genetic evaluation, and intensified therapy with CSA, mycophenolate, or rituximab if mutations are excluded. Especially children with SRNS and FSGS will enter end-stage renal disease. Recurrence of FSGN following renal transplantation is frequent and is a therapeutic challenge causing graft failure in many cases.

Pathogenesis of NS is not completely understood. T cells are involved probably producing circulating permeability factors. Different factors are found in MCNS and FSGS indicating that these two variants may be different diseases and not a continuum of a spectrum (Cara-Fuentes et al. 2014). B cells also seem to be involved. SRNS frequently has a genetic background. The first mutation reported was found in the Finish type of congenital NS (KESTILÄ et al. 1998). Meanwhile an increasing number of mutations was found involving proteins of the slit membrane (like podocin), of the cytoskeleton (like ACT4, INF), of nuclear proteins (mutation in WT1 gene found in Denys–Drash syndrome), and of other structures (Gbadegesin et al. 2013; Akchurin and Reidy 2015). Virtually all cases of congenital and infantile NS have a genetic background (Hinkes et al. 2007). Children with hereditary NS are resistant to all therapies and invariably will progress to end-stage renal failure. Renal transplantation is favorable as the genetic disease will not recur.

> **Take Away**
> Glomerular diseases are characterized by hematuria and/or proteinuria. Blood pressure and renal function are variable and renal biopsy is needed in many cases.

3.2 Vascular and Tubulointerstitial Disease

3.2.1 Vasculitis

Vasculitis means inflammation and partially necrosis of blood vessels, predominantly arteries. It is rare during childhood and classification focuses on vessel size. Childhood large-vessel vasculitis mostly is Takayasu arteritis. Inflammation of the renal arteries may cause renal artery stenosis, but renal parenchymal involvement is not found (Szugye et al. 2014).

Medium-sized vessels are compromised in polyarteritis nodosa (PAN) and in Kawasaki disease (KD). Histologic evidence of necrotizing vasculitis in medium- or small-sized vessels or aneurysms, stenosis, or occlusion on angiography is the mandatory criterion for PAN, and renal involvement is one additional criterion (Ozen et al. 2009). Patients present with fever, malaise, musculoskeletal symptoms, cutaneous lesions and nodules, or peripheral neuropathy. Half of the patients have renal involvement – mostly hematuria, proteinuria, and hypertension. Biopsy tissue from skin lesions, muscles, or nerves can be diagnostically helpful. Renal biopsy usually is not helpful but carries a high risk of bleeding or formation of arteriovenous fistulae (Dillon et al. 2010; Cakar et al. 2008). Laboratory evaluation shows leukocytosis, thrombocytosis, high C-reactive protein, and elevated erythrocyte sedimentation rate; ANCA usually are negative. Induction therapy includes steroids and cyclophosphamide. Low-dose steroids, azathioprine, mycophenolate, methotrexate, and cyclosporine A are used for maintenance therapy. Rituximab is reported to be successful in children unresponsive to standard therapy (Eleftheriou and Brogan 2009). Long-term prognosis seems to be favorable provided treatment starts early in the course of disease. Relapses may occur but permanent remission can be achieved.

KD is a systemic febrile vasculitis with multiple organ involvement. Especially coronary artery lesions are of concern. Renal involvement with proteinuria, hematuria, and most frequently tubulointerstitial nephritis is reported. Hemolytic–uremic syndrome, GN, and NS are rarely found not changing the basic treatment of KD (Watanabe 2013; Krug et al. 2012).

Extensive renal involvement is found in small-vessel vasculitis (SVV). HSP, the most frequent childhood SVV, is discussed together with IgA nephritis (see above). ANCA-associated forms of

SVV can be divided into granulomatous and non-granulomatous. Microscopic polyangiitis (MPA) is non-granulomatous and differs from PAN by the presence of severe glomerular involvement as necrotizing and rapidly progressive pauci-immune GN with positive ANCA (Brogan et al. 2010). MPA may be limited to the kidneys or is systemic with pulmonary capillaritis. Wegener's granulomatosis nowadays renamed as granulomatosis with polyangiitis (GPA) is a necrotizing granulomatous inflammation with or without necrotizing SVV (Lutalo and D'Cruz 2014). Involvement of the upper and lower respiratory tract is the rule and renal disease is similar to MPA. Both diseases are treated with methylprednisolone pulses and frequently plasma exchanges. Rituximab is an alternative to cyclophosphamide and seems to be superior in children and in a relapsing course (Stone et al. 2010; Zand et al. 2014).

3.2.2 Hemolytic–Uremic Syndrome: Renal Thrombotic Microangiopathies

Hemolytic–uremic syndrome (HUS) is characterized by Coombs-negative hemolytic anemia, thrombocytopenia, and AKI. Fragmented red blood cells (schistocytes) in the blood smear and high serum lactate dehydrogenase are additional findings (Noris and Remuzzi 2005). Thrombotic microangiopathy (TMA) with endothelial damage and microthrombi is the characteristic finding on renal histology. About 90% of pediatric cases are associated with hemorrhagic colitis and with Shiga toxin (Stx) producing bacteria like *Shigella* and *E. coli* predominantly with the serotype O157:H7 (Tarr et al. 2005). Children are infected from contaminated cow milk, apple juice, meat, etc. After a prodromal phase of diarrhea, about 15% of infected children proceed to Stx-associated HUS (previously "typical HUS") with AKI and need for renal replacement therapy in 50% of cases. Treatment is supportive and recovery of renal function is good. Long-term prognosis generally is favorable. Yet there is some concern as 30% were found to have arterial hypertension and 7% chronic renal failure after 5 years (Rosales et al. 2012). Aside from Stx-associated HUS, an etiological classification of TMA includes thrombotic thrombocytopenic purpura (TTP), atypical HUS (aHUS), and other forms like infection with neuraminidase-producing streptococcus pneumonia, defective cobalamine metabolism, and various secondary forms induced by drugs, pregnancy, cancer, glomerulopathies like SLE, or solid organ and stem cell transplantation (Besbas et al 2006; Vester and Mache 2014). In TTP, there is a defective ADAMTS13, a metalloprotease cleaving von Willebrand factor polymers, caused by a genetic defect or autoantibodies against ADAMTS13. The clinical presentation is similar to other types of HUS but cerebral involvement is more frequent. Atypical HUS is a mostly complement-mediated disease. Nowadays, hereditary defects of the complement system or autoantibodies to regulating proteins of the alternative complement pathway can be found in many patients. Half of the patients have mutations or autoantibodies against complement factor H (Loirat and Frémeaux-Bacci 2011). The onset of aHUS mostly is acute with a preceding infection. Untreated recurrences lead to chronic renal failure, and severe extrarenal manifestations like myocardial infarction, peripheral gangrene, or cerebral involvement are reported (Malina et al 2013). Aside from supportive therapy including renal replacement therapy, plasma exchanges and plasma infusions were used with some success in TTP and aHUS. Immunosuppression in various combinations was added in aHUS cases with autoantibodies significantly contributing to prolonged renal survival. Since 2009, reports on treatment with eculizumab, a recombinant humanized antibody binding to C5 and blocking the terminal complement pathway, challenged the treatment of aHUS (Mache et al. 2009; Zuber et al. 2012). Prevention of rapid deterioration of renal function and of aHUS recurrence following renal transplantation seems to be possible in many cases. In addition, eculizumab treatment of patients with Stx-associated HUS during outbreaks is promising concerning maintenance or restoration of renal function (Delmas et al. 2014). Application of eculizumab in children with TMA associated with stem cell transplantation seems to be another promising indication (Jodele et al. 2014).

3.2.3 Tubulointerstitial Nephritis

Acute tubulointerstitial nephritis (TIN) is an inflammatory disorder affecting the renal tubules and the interstitial space. Glomeruli and vessels may be affected secondarily, and severe glomerular disease mostly includes tubulointerstitial injury. Cellular infiltration is diffuse or granulomatous and eosinophils may predominate (Joss et al. 2007). Granulomatous TIN with hypercalcemia may lead to sarcoidosis as final diagnosis. Drugs (71 %) and infections (16 %) are the most frequent causes of TIN (Baker and Pusey 2004). A variety of antibiotics, nonsteroidal anti-inflammatory drugs, anticonvulsants, diuretics, and other drugs such as cyclosporine A are involved. Infection-mediated TIN can be divided in cases with direct infection of the renal parenchyma (infectious agents identified in the interstitium such as cytomegalovirus or bacteria causing pyelonephritis) and in reactive (sterile) TIN. Sterile TIN is found associated with various infectious agents like streptococci, *Legionella*, *Yersinia*, EBV, hepatitis B virus, or HIV virus. Idiopathic TIN may be associated with uveitis, named TINU (Jahnukainen et al. 2011). Clinical presentation of TIN is non-specific with fatigue, weight loss, and emesis in most cases; fever and flank pain may be present. Laboratory investigations show acute mostly polyuric renal failure, signs of tubular dysfunction, sterile leukocyturia, microhematuria, and mild proteinuria. Treatment of TIN mostly is supportive aside from stopping drugs and treating infections. Corticosteroids may be required in severe cases, but prognosis is usually excellent.

3.2.4 Tubular Disorders

It is beyond the scope of this chapter to discuss all possible renal tubular disorders. Most have a genetic background, and patients present with dystrophy, weight loss, fatigue, polyuria, and sometimes rickets. Laboratory evaluation may show acidosis, hypokalemia, and hypophosphatemia. Urinalysis can unravel glucosuria, aminoaciduria, and urinary losses of electrolytes. Nephrocalcinosis and renal stones are frequent (Edvardsson et al. 2013). The name "Fanconi syndrome" characterizes a general dysfunction of the proximal renal tubule found in disorders like cystinosis, tyrosinemia, glycogen storage disease, Dent disease, and Lowe syndrome. The Bartter syndromes are salt-wasting nephropathies with hypokalemic alkalosis and hypercalciuria; Gitelman syndrome is characterized by hypomagnesemia (Seyberth and Schlingmann 2011). Other characteristic findings are the hypophosphatemic rickets of X-linked hypophosphatemia or the polyuria of nephrogenic diabetes insipidus. Treatment is dedicated to replace electrolyte losses, to correct acid–base imbalance and further tubular dysfunctions, thereby preventing a progressive renal disease. Genetic evaluation is warranted in most cases.

> **Take Away**
> Different disorders are summarized in this part with sometimes inconclusive acute presentation. Immediate correct diagnosis is often warranted as treatment is urgent.

3.3 Renal Parenchymal Involvement in Systemic Disease

3.3.1 Systemic Lupus Erythematosus and Antiphospholipid Nephropathy

Systemic lupus erythematosus (SLE) is a generalized autoimmune disorder with autoantibodies directed against a variety of cell components and organs. Adolescent girls are mostly affected and childhood SLE (cSLE) represents 20 % of cases. The clinical presentation is variable including non-specific complaints such as fever, weight loss, and malaise. SLE is diagnosed if 4 or more of 11 features (e.g., positive antinuclear antibodies, antibodies against double-stranded DNA, thrombopenia, low C3 complement, and nephritis) are present (Tan et al. 1982; Hochberg 1997).

Lupus nephritis affects more than 80 % of cases with cSLE which is more frequent compared to adult disease. Presentation with nephritic or nephrotic syndrome is variable, not necessarily reflecting the severity of renal involvement. Consequently, renal biopsy is required before therapy. Histologically, lupus nephritis is categorized into six classes subdivided in acute/chronic, focal/generalized, and sclerotic lesions (Weening et al. 2004). Extrarenal involvement may concern the central nervous system, lungs, musculoskeletal system, skin, heart (Libman–Sacks endocarditis), or the gastrointestinal tract. The presence of antiphospholipid antibodies increases the risk of vascular thrombosis and anticoagulation has to be considered. Various treatment protocols for SLE nephritis exist including corticosteroids, cyclophosphamide, mycophenolate, plasma exchanges, and rituximab for initial and maintenance therapy (Tullus 2012; Punaro 2013). There is a trend to reduce toxicity of treatment (Houssiau et al. 2012), thereby avoiding complications like severe infections including sepsis, avascular bone necrosis, reduced fertility, or malignancies. On the other hand, recurrences of SLE nephritis should be kept to a minimum to avoid progression to end-stage renal disease as recurrence of SLE nephritis is reported following renal transplantation.

Antiphospholipid syndrome (APS) is the association of vascular thrombosis with antiphospholipid antibodies and/or circulating lupus anticoagulant. It may be a primary disease but is mostly associated with autoimmune disease predominantly with SLE. Renal involvement in APS is severe with renal infarction, venous thrombosis, or renal artery stenosis and needs to be distinguished from Lupus nephritis. APS nephropathy (APSN) means vascular lesions in the glomeruli and the arterioles like fibrin thrombi and mesangiolysis, the so-called thrombotic microangiopathy (TMA) also seen in HUS (Alchi et al. 2010). Catastrophic APS is the fulminant form with involvement of at least three organ systems within 1 week including renal TMA (Berman et al. 2014). Clinical presentation of APSN is acute renal failure, hypertension, thrombopenia, and proteinuria. Anticoagulation is the basic treatment of APSN and corticosteroids frequently are added. CAPS patients need plasma exchanges and rituximab or cyclophosphamide in SLE-associated CAPS in addition.

3.3.2 Sickle Cell Nephropathy

Sickle cell disease is an autosomal recessive transmitted hemoglobinopathy with various renal manifestations leading to end-stage renal disease in 4–18 % of the patients at a mean age of 23 years (Becker 2011). Sickle cell nephropathy (SCN) starts early in childhood. Red blood cell sickling within the vasa recta of the renal medulla is caused by the hypertonic, acidic, and hypoxic environment resulting in vessel occlusion, ischemia, and infarction. The release of vasodilating substances causes glomerular hyperfiltration ultimately leading to proteinuria, glomerulosclerosis, and progressive chronic renal disease. The clinical findings may start early in infancy with a urinary concentrating defect leading to polyuria, episodes of dehydration, and later nocturnal enuresis (Sharpe and Thein 2011). Various degrees of hematuria, proteinuria, and renal tubular acidosis are additional findings dependent on the stage of renal dysfunction. Treatment of SCN is directed to prevent vaso-occlusive crises and to manage renal complications adequately. Altitudes above 2,500 m without oxygen supply, heavy exercise, and fluid deprivation should be avoided. Bed rest in gross hematuria, early intravenous fluids and transfusions, diuretics, ACE inhibitors, and sometimes hydroxyurea treatment may contribute to a favorable course of disease (McKie et al 2007). Renal transplantation seems to be a viable option in end-stage SCN (Huang et al 2013). Some patients may benefit from hematopoietic stem cell transplantation (Dallas et al 2013).

3.3.3 Renal Manifestations of Metabolic Disorders

A variety of hereditary disorders of the metabolism may affect the kidneys secondarily or as the main organ manifestation. Most renal lesions are not specific but may be pronounced like in hereditary tyrosinemia, glycogen storage diseases, or methylmalonic academia. Hereditary fever syndromes including familial Mediterranean fever (FMF) may cause amyloidosis progressing through proteinuria and nephrotic syndrome to end-stage renal failure. Amyloidosis is systemic and other organs such as the thyroid glands may be involved (Mache et al. 1993). Treatment of FMF with colchicine is effective in prevention of renal amyloidosis, but progression to end-stage renal failure still is possible (Korkmaz 2012). Diabetic nephropathy, the most important single disorder leading to chronic renal failure during adulthood, usually is not seen during childhood. Two disorders with deleterious renal involvement are of major concern; the hyperoxalurias are discussed in chapter "Urolithiasis and Nephrocalcinosis".

Nephropathic cystinosis is an autosomal recessive inherited disorder resulting from the defective lysosomal cystine transporter cystinosin. The CTNS gene has been mapped to chromosome 17p13.2 (Town et al. 1998). Cystinosis is characterized by intracellular accumulation of cystine in the kidneys and nearly all other organs like the bone marrow, leukocytes, the thyroid gland, and the cornea, but the renal symptoms predominate (Nesterova and Gahl 2013). Affected patients mostly have blond hairs and present during infancy with vomiting, dehydration, polydipsia, polyuria, failure to thrive, and rickets. Laboratory evaluation shows proximal tubular dysfunction (Fanconi syndrome). Diagnosis is confirmed by demonstration of an elevated cystine content in leukocytes, by corneal cystine crystals, and by genetic analysis. Treatment includes correction of electrolyte and fluid disturbances, application of adequate nutrition partially including growth hormone therapy, and amelioration of extrarenal organ manifestations. Administration of cysteamine as cystine-depleting drug can reduce the intracellular content of cystine by more than 90 % and improves the overall prognosis of patients dramatically (Emma et al. 2014). Nevertheless, progression to end-stage renal failure is not yet prevented nowadays. Renal transplantation has good results, but accumulation of cystine in other organs continues. Cysteamine therapy has to be continued to ameliorate hypothyroidism, cardiac failure, and cerebral complications.

Take Away
SLE diagnosis and treatment is urgent including renal biopsy. All other disorders need careful examination and immediate treatment is rarely required.

Conclusion
The classical renal parenchymal disorders are extremely variable in clinical presentation, results of the laboratory evaluation, consequences for additional diagnostic measures including renal biopsy, and for therapeutic consequences being urgent in many situations. Prognosis ranges from an excellent outcome to progression to chronic renal failure despite extensive treatment. Disease recurrence following renal transplantation is possible in many cases. Genetic disorders are resistant to all treatment and progress to end-stage renal failure.

References

Akchurin O, Reidy KJ (2015) Genetic causes of proteinuria and nephrotic syndrome: impact on podocyte pathobiology. Pediatr Nephrol 30:221–233

Alchi B, Jayne D (2010) Membranoproliferative glomerulonephritis. Pediatr Nephrol 25:1409–1418

Alchi B, Griffiths M, Jayne D (2010) What nephrologists need to know about antiphospholipid syndrome. Nephrol Dial Transplant 25:3147–3154

Ayalon R, Beck LH Jr (2015) Membranous nephropathy: not just a disease for adults. Pediatr Nephrol 30:31–39

Baker RJ, Pusey CD (2004) The changing profile of acute tubulointerstitial nephritis. Nephrol Dial Transplant 19:8–11

Barbour TD, Pickering MC, Cook HT (2013) Dense deposit disease and C3 glomerulopathy. Semin Nephrol 33:493–507

Beck LH Jr, Bonegio RG, Lambeau G et al (2009) M-type phospholipase A2 receptor as target antigen in idiopathic membranous nephropathy. N Engl J Med 361:11–12

Becker AM (2011) Sickle cell nephropathy: challenging the conventional wisdom. Pediatr Nephrol 26:2099–2109

Berger J, Hinglais N (1968) Les dépôts intercapillaires d'IgA-IgG. J Urol Neprol 74:694–695

Berman H, Rodriguez-Pinto I, Cervera R et al (2014) Pediatric catastrophic antiphospholipid syndrome: descriptive analysis of 45 patients from the "CAPS Registry". Autoimmun Rev 13:157–162

Besbas N, Karpman D, Landau D et al (2006) A classification of hemolytic uremic syndrome and thrombotic thrombocytopenic purpura and related disorders. Kidney Int 70:423–431

Bomback AS, Smith RJ, Barile GR et al (2012) Eculizumab for dense deposit disease and C3 glomerulonephritis. Clin J Am Soc Nephrol 7:748–756

Brogan P, Eleftheriou D, Dillon M (2010) Small vessel vasculitis. Pediatr Nephrol 25:1025–1035

Cakar N, Özcakar ZB, Soy D et al (2008) Renal involvement in childhood vasculitis. Nephron Clin Pract 108:c202

Cara-Fuentes G, Wei C, Segarra A et al (2014) CD80 and suPAR in patients with minimal change disease and focal glomerulosclerosis: diagnostic and pathogenic significance. Pediatr Nephrol 29:1363–1371

Cattran DC, Coppo R, Cook HT et al (2009) The Oxford classification of IgA nephropathy: rationale, clinicopathological correlations, and classification. Kidney Int 76:534–545

Coppo R, Troyanov S, Camilla R et al (2010) The Oxford IgA nephropathy clinicopathological classification is valid for children as well as adults. Kidney Int 77:921–927

Dallas MH, Triplett B, Shook DR et al (2013) Long-term outcome and evaluation of organ function in pediatric patients undergoing haploidentical and matched related hematopoietic cell transplantation for sickle cell disease. Biol Blood Marrow Transplant 19:820–830

Debiec H, Lefeu F, Kemper MJ et al (2011) Early-childhood membranous nephropathy due to cationic bovine serum albumin. N Engl J Med 364:2101–2110

Delmas Y, Vendrely B, Clouzeau B et al (2014) Outbreak of Escherichia coli O104:H4 haemolytic uraemic syndrome in France: outcome with eculizumab. Nephrol Dial Transplant 29:565–572

Dillon MJ, Eleftheriou D, Brogan PA (2010) Medium-size-vessel vasculitis. Pediatr Nephrol 25:1641–1652

Edvardsson VO, Goldfarb DS, Lieske JC et al (2013) Hereditary causes of kidney stones and chronic kidney disease. Pediatr Nephrol 28:1923–1942

Eison TM, Ault BH, Jones DP et al (2011) Post-streptococcal glomerulonephritis in children: clinical features and pathogenesis. Pediatr Nephrol 26:165–180

Eleftheriou D, Brogan PA (2009) Vasculitis in children. Best Pract Res Clin Rheumatol 23:309–323

Emma F, Nesterova G, Langman C et al (2014) Nephropathic cystinosis: an international consensus document. Nephrol Dial Transplant 29:iv87–iv94

Gauthier B, Trachtman H, Frank R et al (1989) Familial thin basement membrane nephropathy in children with asymptomatic microhematuria. Nephron 51:502–508

Gbadegesin R, Winn M, Smoyer WE (2013) Genetic testing in nephrotic syndrome: challenges and opportunities. Nat Rev Nephrol 9:179–184

Gellermann J, Weber L, Pape L et al (2013) Mycophenolate mofetil versus cyclosporin A in children with frequently relapsing nephrotic syndrome. J Am Soc Nephrol 24:1689–1697

Gutierrez E, Zamora I, Ballarin JA et al (2012) Long-term outcomes of IgA nephropathy presenting with minimal or no proteinuria. J Am Soc Nephrol 23:1753–1760

Hinkes BG, Mucha B, Vlangos CN et al (2007) Nephrotic syndrome in the first year of life: two thirds of cases are caused by mutations in 4 genes (NPHS1, NPHS2, WT1, and LAMB2). Pediatrics 119:e907–e919

Hochberg MC (1997) Updating the American College of Rheumatology revisited criteria for the classification of systemic lupus erythematosus. Arthritis Rheum 40:1725

Houssiau FA, Vasconcelos D, D'Cruz D et al (2012) The 10-year follow-up data of the Euro-Lupus Nephritis Trial comparing low-dose and high-dose intravenous cyclophosphamide. Ann Rheum Dis 69:61–64

Huang E, Parke C, Mehrnia A et al (2013) Improved survival among sickle cell kidney transplant recipients in the recent era. Nephrol Dial Transplant 28:1039–1046

Ishikura K, Hamasaki Y, Sakai T et al (2012) Posterior reversible encephalopathy syndrome in children with kidney diseases. Pediatr Nephrol 27:375–384

Jahnukainen T, Ala-Houala M, Karikoski R et al (2011) Clinical outcome and occurrence of uveitis in children with idiopathic tubulointerstitial nephritis. Pediatr Nephrol 26:291–299

Jais JP, Knebelmann B, Giatras I et al (2003) X-linked Alport syndrome: natural history and genotype-phenotype correlations in girls and women belonging to 195 families: A "European Community Alport Syndrome Concerted Action" study. J Am Soc Nephrol 14:2603–2610

Jodele S, Fukuda T, Vinks A et al (2014) Eculizumab therapy in children with severe hematopoietic stem cell transplantation-assiciated thrombotic microangiopathy. Biol Blood Marrow Transplant 20:518–525

Joss N, Morris S, Young B et al (2007) Granulomatous interstitial nephritis. Clin J Am Soc Nephrol 2:222–230

Kashtan CE (2006) Renal transplantation in patients with Alport syndrome. Pediatr Transplant 10:651–657

Kestilä M, Lenkkeri U, Männikkö M et al (1998) Positionally cloned gene for a novel glomerular protein-nephrin-is mutated in congenital nephrotic syndrome. Mol Cell 1:575–582

Koehler H, Wandel E, Brunck N (1991) Acanthocyturia – A characteristic marker for glomerular bleeding. Kidney Int 40:115–120

Korkmaz C (2012) Therapeutic approach to patients with familial Mediterranean fever-related amyloidosis resistant to colchicine. Clin Exp Rheumatol 30(Suppl 72):S104–S107

Krug P, Boyer O, Balzamo E et al (2012) Nephrotic syndrome in Kawasaki disease: a report of three cases. Pediatr Nephrol 27:1547–1550

Lameire N, Van Biesen W, Vanholder R (2005) Acute renal failure. Lancet 365:417–430

Loirat C, Frémeaux-Bacci V (2011) Atypical hemolytic uremic syndrome. Orphanet J Rare Dis 6:60

Lombel RM, Gipson DS, Hodson EM (2013a) Treatment of steroid-sensitive nephrotic syndrome: new guidelines from KDIGO. Pediatr Nephrol 28: 415–426

Lombel RM, Hodson EM, Gipson DS (2013b) Treatment of steroid-resistant nephrotic syndrome in children: new guidelines from KDIGO. Pediatr Nephrol 28:409–414

Lutalo PM, D'Cruz DP (2014) Diagnosis and classification of granulomatosis with polyangiitis (aka Wegener's granulomatosis). J Autoimmun 48–49:94–98

Mache CJ, Schwingshandl J, Riccabona M et al (1993) Ultrasound and MRI findings in a case of childhood amyloid goiter. Pediatr Radiol 23:565–566

Mache CJ, Acham-Roschitz B, Frémeaux-Bacci V et al (2009) Complement inhibitor Eculizumab in atypical hemolytic uremic syndrome. Clin J Am Soc Nephrol 4:1312.1316

Malina M, Gulati A, Bagga A et al (2013) Peripheral gangrene in children with atypical hemolytic uremic syndrome. Pediatrics 131:e331–e335

McKie KT, Hanevold CD, Hernandez C et al (2007) Prevalence, prevention, and treatment of microalbuminuria and proteinuria in children with sickle cell disease. J Pediatr Hematol Oncol 29:140–144

Menon S, Valentini RP (2010) Membranous nephropathy in children: clinical presentation and therapeutic approach. Pediatr Nephrol 25:1419–1428

Murakami M, Yamamoto H, Ueda Y et al (1991) Urinary screening of elementary and junior high-school children over a 13-year period in Tokyo. Pediatr Nephrol 5:50–53

Nesterova G, Gahl WA (2013) Cystinosis: the evolution of a treatable disease. Pediatr Nephrol 28:51–59

Noris M, Remuzzi G (2005) Hemolytic uremic syndrome. J Am Soc Nephrol 16:1035–1050

Ozen S, Pistorio A, Iusan MS et al (2009) The EULAR/PRINTO/PRES criteria for childhood polyarteritis nodosa. Ankara 2008. Ann Rheum Dis 68(Suppl 3):713

Park YH, Choi JY, Chung HS et al (2005) Hematuria and proteinuria in a mass school screening test. Pediatr Nephrol 20:1126–1130

Pohl M (2015) Henoch-Schönlein purpura nephritis. Pediatr Nephrol 30:245–252

Pozzi C, Andrulli S, Del Veccio L et al (2004) Corticosteroid effectiveness in IgA nephropathy: long-term results of a randomized, controlled trial. J Am Soc Nephrol 15:157–163

Punaro MG (2013) The treatment of systemic lupus proliferative nephritis. Pediatr Nephrol 28:2069–2078

Radhakrishnan S, Cattran DC (2012) The KDIGO practice guideline on glomerulonephritis: reading between the (guide)lines-application to the individual patient. Kidney Int 82:840–856

Radhakrishnan S, Lunn A, Kirschfink M et al (2012) Eculizumab and refractory membranoproliferative glomerulonephritis. N Engl J Med 366:1165–1166

Rana K, Wang YY, Buzza M et al (2005) The genetics of thin basement membrane nephropathy. Semin Nephrol 25:163–170

Rosales A, Hofer J, Zimmerhackl LB et al (2012) Need for long-term follow-up in enterohemorrhagic Escherichia coli-associated hemolytic uremic syndrome due to late-emerging sequelae. Clin Inf Dis 54:1413–1421

Savige J, Gregory M, Gross O et al (2013) Expert guidelines for the management of Alport syndrome and thin basement membrane nephropathy. J Am Soc Nephrol 24:364–375

Sethi S, Fervenza FC (2011) Membranoproliferative glomerulonephritis: pathogenetic heterogeneity and proposal for a new classification. Semin Nephrol 31:341–348

Sethi S, Fervenza FC (2012) Membranoproliferative glomerulonephritis – a new look at an old entity. N Engl J Med 366:1119–1131

Seyberth HW, Schlingmann KP (2011) Bartter- and Gitelman-like syndromes: salt-losing tubulopathies with loop or DCT defects. Pediatr Nephrol 26:1789–1802

Sharpe CC, Thein SL (2011) Sickle cell nephropathy – a practical approach. Br J Haematol 155:287–297

Shenoy M, Plant ND, Lewis MA et al (2010) Intravenous methylprednisolone in idiopathic childhood nephrotic syndrome. Pediatr Nephrol 25:899–903

Stone JH, Merkel PA, Spiera R et al (2010) Rituximab versus cyclophosphamide for ANCA-associated vasculitis. N Engl J Med 363:221–232

Szugye HS, Zeft AS, Spalding SJ (2014) Takayasu arteritis in the pediatric population: a contemporary United States-based single center cohort. Pediatric Rheumatology 12:21

Tan EM, Cohen AS, Fries JF et al (1982) The 1982 revised criteria for the classification of systemic lupus erythematosus. Arthritis Rheum 25:1271–1277

Tarr PI, Gordon CA, Chandler WL (2005) Shiga-toxin-producing Escherichia coli and haemolytic uraemic syndrome. Lancet 365:1073–1086

Town M, Jean G, Cherqui S et al (1998) A novel gene encoding an integral membrane protein is mutated in nephropathic cystinosis. Nature Genet 18: 319–324

Tullus M (2012) New developments in the treatment of systemic lupus erythematosus. Pediatr Nephrol 27:727–732

Van Husen M, Kemper MJ (2011) New therapies in steroid-sensitive and steroid-resistant idiopathic nephrotic syndrome. Pediatr Nephrol 26:881–892

Vehaskari VM, Rapola J (1982) Isolated Proteinuria: analysis of a school-age population. J Pediatr 101:661–668

Vehaskari VM, Rapola J, Koskimies O et al (1979) Microscopic hematuria in school children: epidemiology and clinicopathologic evaluation. J Pediatr 95: 676–684

Vester U, Mache CJ (2014) Pharmacologic treatment of atypical hemolytic-uremic syndrome. Exp Opin Orphan Drugs 2:123–135

Watanabe T (2013) Kidney and urinary tract involvement in Kawasaki disease. Int J Pediatr Article ID 831834

Weening JJ, D'Agati VD, Schwartz MM et al (2004) The classification of glomerulonephritis in systemic lupus erythematosus revisited. J Am Soc Nephrol 15:241–250

Wyatt RJ, Julian BA (2013) IgA nephropathy. N Engl J Med 368:2402–2414

Zand L, Specks U, Sethi S et al (2014) Treatment of ANCA-associated vasculitis: new therapies and a look at old entities. Adv Chronic Kidney Dis 21:182–193

Zuber J, Fakhouri F, Roumenina LT et al (2012) Use of eculizumab for atypical hemolytic uremic syndrome and C3 glomerulopathies. Nat Rev Nephrol 8:643–657

UTI and VUR

Rolf Beetz

Contents

1 **Urinary Tract Infection** 219
1.1 Introduction 219
1.2 Definition and Classification 219
1.3 Epidemiology 220
1.4 Etiology and Pathogenesis 220
1.5 Pyelonephritic Damage and Long-Term Consequences of Renal Scarring 222
1.6 Symptoms 222
1.7 Diagnosis 223
1.8 Therapy 224
1.9 Diagnostic Work-Up 226
1.10 Prophylaxis 228

2 **Vesicoureteral Reflux (VUR)** 229
2.1 Introduction 229
2.2 Definition and Classification 229
2.3 Etiology and Pathogenesis 230
2.4 "Reflux Nephropathy" and Renal Scarring ... 230
2.5 Epidemiology and Symptoms 231
2.6 Diagnosis 231
2.7 Therapy 232
2.8 Care After Cessation of VUR 235

Literature 235

R. Beetz
Pediatric Nephrology, Center for Paediatrics and Adolescent Medicine, University Medical Clinic, Langenbeckstr. 1, D – 55131 Mainz, Germany
e-mail: Rolf.beetz@unimedizin-mainz.de

1 Urinary Tract Infection

1.1 Introduction

Urinary tract infections (UTIs) are one of the most common bacterial infections in children (Spencer et al. 2010). Pediatric uroradiologists are frequently confronted with affected children due to the fact that UTI might be the only symptom of renal malformations or abnormalities of the urinary tract.

1.2 Definition and Classification

Urinary tract infection (UTI) is defined as a colonization of the urinary tract with uropathogenic bacteria, which induce a local or systemic inflammatory response.

UTIs can be classified according to localization (urethra, bladder, and kidneys), symptoms, and presence or absence of complicating factors (Table 1). Pyelonephritis is characterized by a segmental or generalized inflammation of the renal parenchyma, whereas cystitis affects the bladder mucosa. This has to be differentiated from asymptomatic bacteria, defined as bacterial colonization without any inflammatory response.

Table 1 Classification of urinary tract infections

According to localization	Urethritis (i.e., *Chlamydia*, *Mycoplasma*) Cystitis Pyelonephritis
According to symptomatology	Asymptomatic UTI (bacteriuria and leukocyturia without symptoms) Symptomatic UTI (symptoms, bacteriuria, and leukocyturia)
According to complications and risk factors	Non-complicated UTI (with normal urinary tract, normal bladder function, normal kidney function, and immunocompetence) Complicated UTI (with congenital anomalies of the kidney and urinary tract, VUR, urinary obstruction, concrements, neurogenic or non-neurogenic bladder dysfunction, imunodeficiency, diabetes mellitus, foreign bodies (i.e., catheter), renal insufficiency, etc.)
According to chronology	First UTI Recurrence, reinfection: a new UTI with an at least serotypically different uropathogen Relapse: anew UTI with the serotypically same uropathogen as in the previous UTI. This is possible (a) with inadequate therapy (i.e., in the case of resistant bacteria, insufficient drug levels, insufficient duration of therapy) and (b) relapse after transient sterility of urine (i.e., in the case of stones or biofilms at foreign bodies, persistence of uropathogens within the bladder mucosa)

1.3 Epidemiology

The incidence of first-time UTI is highest during the first year of life. This is most marked for boys but also evident in girls. By 1 year of age, 2.7% of boys and 0.7% of girls will have had their first UTI (Wettergren et al. 1980). In many aspects, the characteristics of UTI in infants differ from UTIs in children. Its prevalence is higher (Zorc et al. 2005b; Shaikh et al. 2008; Siomou et al. 2009), male gender is affected predominantly (Kanellopoulos et al. 2006), non-*Escherichia coli* infections are more frequent, and there is a higher risk of urosepsis than in older age groups (Magin et al. 2007). However, urosepsis is significantly less frequent in community-acquired than in nosocomial UTI (Sastre et al. 2007).

After the first year of life, the incidence of UTI in girls is up to tenfold higher than in boys. By the age of 6 years, more than 7% of girls and 1.6% of boys will have suffered from at least one symptomatic, culture-confirmed UTI (Marild and Jodal 1998).

> **Take Away**
> Urinary tract infections count among the most frequent bacterial infections in infancy and childhood.

1.3.1 Recurrence and Relapse

After a first symptomatic UTI, the risk of recurrence is up to 20–30%, being highest during the following 2–3 months (Winberg et al. 1975; Kasanen et al. 1983; McCracken 1984; Nuutinen and Uhari 2001). In 20–30% of cases, girls have a new infection within 1 year, some of them presenting with further recurrences over a long time (Beetz et al. 2002; Marchand et al. 2007). The susceptibility for recurrences is highest within the first 2–6 months after a UTI. The recurrence rate is directly correlated with the number of preceding UTIs (McCracken 1984). The longer the infection-free interval, the lower the risk of further recurrences (McCracken 1984).

In boys, early recurrences are as frequent as in girls; later the recurrence rate is much lower in boys than in girls. Recurrent UTIs are rare in boys with a morphologically normal urinary tract (Winberg et al. 1974).

1.4 Etiology and Pathogenesis

Bacterial UTIs occur when specialized (mostly virulent) uropathogenic bacteria invade the urinary tract, multiply faster than they are eliminated, and induce an inflammatory response.

Uropathogenic bacteria are able to colonize the perineal and periurethral region, to invade the urinary tract, to grow in urine, to adhere to uroepithelial cells, and to ascend within the urinary tract. UTIs are predominantly caused by uropathogenic *Escherichia coli* (60–80% of cases), followed by other gram-negative bacteria as *Klebsiella*, *Enterobacter*, *Proteus* which is more common in boys and children with urolithiasis, *Providencia*, *Citrobacter*, *Morganella*, *Serratia*, *Pseudomonas*, and *Salmonella* and gram-positive bacteria (i.e., Staphylococci and Enterococci). The pathogen probability is, however, dependent on age and gender. So the percentage rate of *Enterococcus* infections is higher in early infancy than at a later age (Haller et al. 2004; Gaspari et al. 2005). In a recent study, 20% of uropathogens in boys at the age up to 4 years and 15% in girls at the same age were Enterococci (Gaspari et al. 2005).

Fungal urinary tract infections (i.e., induced by *Candida*) and viral infections (i.e., Adenovirus) are extremely rare.

The human gut microbiome is the main source of uropathogenic bacteria. After colonizing the periurethral region, these bacteria are able to invade the urinary tract by ascension. In *E. coli*, by far the most frequent pathogen, several special virulence factors are prerequisites for this ability, including lipopolysaccharides (O-antigen, up to 80%), capsule antigen (up to 70%), flagellae (facilitating motility), cytotoxic enzymes (alpha- and beta-haemolysines), siderophores (for iron binding as a growth factor), and adhesines (Pili type I and Pap Pili). Pili type I are activated during invasion of the urinary tract and adhere specifically to mannose-containing glycoprotein receptors at the surface of uroepithelial cells. Pap Pili are highly correlated with the capability of *E. coli* to induce pyelonephritis or urosepsis.

However, microbial growth within the urinary tract is constrained by multiple host defense factors, contributing to the "innate system of immunity." As an example, Tamm-Horsefall glycoprotein (uromodulin) act to block bacterial adherence to the uroepithelium by binding of type I-Pili. Several other peptides and proteins, called defensins, are secreted into the fluid layer immediately above the epithelial layer, acting as antimicrobials by producing pores within the bacterial membrane which leads to cell lysis. Once bacteria have attached to the uroepithelium, several specific ligand-receptor interactions are activated. These and further signal-transducing mechanisms result in an inflammatory response.

The normal balance between bacterial virulence factors and host defense factors usually leads to a sterile urinary tract. However, if one or more host defense mechanisms do not work well, virulent bacteria can induce more or less severe infections. Undisturbed urine flow and regular voiding without residual urine is one of the most important host defense mechanisms. If they are altered by urinary obstruction, vesicoureteric reflux (VUR), or bladder dysfunction, the susceptibility to pyelonephritis increases, as these conditions facilitate the ascension of uropathogens to the upper urinary tract and kidney parenchyma.

1.4.1 Risk Factors for Urinary Tract Infections

In children, UTIs are often associated with *bladder dysfunction* (Snodgrass 1991; Koff et al. 1998). Frequently, children with dysfunctional voiding also suffer from constipation and/or encopresis, which lead to the term "dysfunctional elimination syndrome" (DES) (Koff et al. 1998; Nicholson and Smith 2007; Tokgoz et al. 2007) and recently "bladder and bowel dysfunction" (BBD) (Austin et al. 2014). The hypothesis that UTI in early infancy might promote the development of DES/BBD has not been proven (Shaikh et al. 2003).

There is some consideration of *genetic factors* causing an increased susceptibility for UTI. They include genetic polymorphisms for Toll-like receptor 4 (TLR4), which is expressed by uroepithelial cells recognizing lipopolysaccharides in the cell wall of uropathogenic gram-negative bacteria, pro-inflammatory cytokines (i.e., TNF-alpha) or ß-defensins.

Uncircumcised boys bear a ten times higher risk than circumcised boys of having a UTI (Rushton and Majd 1992; Wiswell and Hachey 1993). Colonization with uropathogens such as *E. coli*, *Klebsiella*, *Enterobacter*, *Proteus mirabilis*, and *Pseudomonas aeruginosa* in urethral and periurethral swabs from non-circumcised boys is much more frequent than in circumcised controls (Wiswell et al. 1988).

> **Take Away**
> A disturbed balance of bacterial virulence and host defense factors leads to an increased susceptibility to urinary tract infections.

1.5 Pyelonephritic Damage and Long-Term Consequences of Renal Scarring

Pyelonephritis can progress to renal scarring especially when it remains untreated over several days (Doganis et al. 2007; Hewitt et al. 2008). While it is well known that infants and young children bear a particular risk for pyelonephritic damage (Vernon et al. 1997), renal scars can also develop in later childhood and adolescence (Smellie et al. 1985; Benador et al. 1997; Jakobsson et al. 1999). The preexistence of parenchymal defects further increases this risk (Merrick et al. 1995).

In recent years, it has become obvious that the individual risk for pyelonephritic scars might at least be partially genetically determined (Miller and Findon 1985; Ozen et al. 1999). With the presence of VUR, the risk of persistent renal damage rises more than threefold (Faust et al. 2009). Generally, after pyelonephritis with renal parenchymal damage documented by DMSA-scintigraphy, 40 % of affected kidneys develop persistent scarring (Faust et al. 2009). Significant delays in initiating antibacterial therapy increase the risk of renal scarring in experimental as well as in clinical settings (Miller and Phillips 1981; Ransley and Risdon 1981; Slotki and Asscher 1982; Smellie et al. 1985; Glauser et al. 1987; Hiraoka et al. 2003). Early diagnosis and immediate therapy of UTI might be one of the most effective strategies in the prevention of renal scarring in patients with UTI (Doganis et al. 2007).

Pyelonephritic scarring and reflux nephropathy belong to the main causes of arterial hypertension in youth and young adulthood. In adolescent patients with renal scarring, prevalence of arterial hypertension was found to be 11–14 % (Wallace et al. 1978; Beetz et al. 1989; Jacobson et al. 1989). The prevalence increases with the extent of damage, with bilateral manifestation, and with increasing age (Lama et al. 2003; Simoes e Silva et al. 2007).

> **Take Away**
> Pyelonephritic episodes may result in persistent focal or global parenchymal damage.

1.6 Symptoms

Newborns and very young infants with pyelonephritis can present with nonspecific symptoms, i.e., with failure to thrive, poor feeding, jaundice, hyperexcitability or lethargy, and often without any fever (Ghaemi et al. 2007; Sastre et al. 2007). Among young febrile infants younger than 8 weeks of age, the prevalence of UTI has been found to be 13.6 %, with the majority of infections occurring in male infants (Westenfelder and Beetz 2010).

In infants after newborn age, peaking fever is the most important symptom of pyelonephritis after the age of 1 month. In at least 6 % of febrile infants without a clinically recognizable focus, the source of fever is pyelonephritis (American Academy of Pediatrics 1999; Zorc et al. 2005b).

In young children, lower urinary tract symptoms like frequent voiding or pain at micturition are uncommon before the age of 2 years and are often lacking in acute pyelonephritis (Jodal and Hansson 1994). A first-time UTI classified as acute cystitis occurs especially in girls 2–6 years of age (Jodal and Hansson 1994). In later childhood and youth, frequent voiding, dysuria, and suprapubic, abdominal, or lumbar pain are usually complained of (Shaikh et al. 2007).

> **Take Away**
> Symptoms of UTI in infants and small children are often unspecific and can be misinterpreted.

1.7 Diagnosis

Diagnosis of urinary tract infection depends on the detection of significant bacteriuria and an inflammatory response in the urinary tract (Ma and Shortliffe 2004; Zorc et al. 2005a).

1.7.1 Urine Sampling

Urine sampling by the best method available as well as careful urine investigation and critical interpretation of the results are crucial. In toilet-trained children and adolescents, a *midstream urine* can be obtained (Vaillancourt et al. 2007).

In infancy and in non-toilet-trained children, diagnosing UTI and excluding it both can be challenging and depend not least on the mode of urine sampling (Craig et al. 2010; Tullus 2011).

In these cases, bagged specimen is the most convenient and least traumatic method for obtaining a urine specimen. Unfortunately, the false-positive rate by contamination from outside the bladder is up to 50 %. In daily practice, leukocyturia and bacteriuria from bagged urine samples therefore are often misdiagnosed as signs for UTI due to urine contamination. This can result in unnecessary treatment (radiological), investigations, and even unnecessary operations (like VUR correction). On the other hand, if overlooked, untreated UTI eventually leads to renal damage. For this reason, bagged urine is effective in ruling out the suspicion of urinary tract infection but not useful in documenting it. If the urinalysis suggests an infection, a second urine specimen should be obtained by *bladder puncture* or *catheterization* (American Academy of Pediatrics 2011; Wingerter and Bachur 2011). The success rate regarding sufficient urine sample volumes is best (almost 97 %) if ultrasound is used for the assessment of bladder filling (Kiernan et al. 1993; Buys et al. 1994). Complications of suprapubic bladder aspiration are extremely rare ranging from transient hematuria to bowel perforation (Hildebrand et al. 1981).

1.7.2 Urine Analysis

The diagnosis of UTI is best based upon a leukocyte count of at least 10 per microliter and growth of a single pathogen at a concentration of at least 50.000 colony-forming units/ml (CFU/ml) (Hoberman et al. 1996).

Dipstick Test and Microscopy

Dipstick tests are commonly used for detecting *nitrite* and *leukocyte esterase* as biochemical markers indicative of UTI (Deville et al. 2004). The urine dipstick test alone seems to be useful to exclude the presence of UTI if the results of both nitrite and leukocyte esterase are negative (Deville et al. 2004). If both nitrite and leukocyte esterase test in combination with indicative clinical symptoms are positive, UTI is most likely (Lohr 1991; Deville et al. 2004). However, positive results have to be confirmed by urine culture. It might be useful to add microscopy of uncentrifuged urine within a Neubauer or Fuchs-Rosenthal hemocytometer (Hoberman et al. 1996). Microscopy for bacteria with Gram stain has higher accuracy than all other rapid laboratory tests (Williams et al. 2010), but it is not available in most clinical situations.

Urine Culture

The definitive diagnosis of a UTI is carried out by urine culture, depending on the number of colony-forming units (CFU) per ml. The count can be related to the method of specimen collection, diuresis, time, and temperature of storage until cultivation occurs (Zorc et al. 2005a). Mixed bacterial cultures and low CFU counts are indicative of contamination. Due to its extremely high contamination rates, urine sampled in plastic bags should not be used for urine culture (Schlager et al. 1995).

The classical definition of more than 10^5 colony-forming units per milliliter (cfu/ml) of voided urine representing "significant bacteriuria" is still used in daily practice (Lohr 1991; Piercey et al. 1993; Kass and Finland 2002). In midstream urine (MSU), more than 10^5 cfu/mL is considered to be positive (Cavagnaro 2005). In urine obtained by catheterization or in urine obtained by suprapubic aspiration a number of 10^4 cfu/mL are considered to be significant. Combining bacteriuria and pyuria in febrile children, the finding of >10 WBC/mm^3 and

>50,000 cfu/mL in a specimen collected by catheterization or bladder puncture is significant for a UTI and discriminates between infection and contamination (Hoberman et al. 1993, 1996; Hoberman and Wald 1997).

1.7.3 Differentiation Between Pyelonephritis and Cystitis

The differential diagnosis between upper (pyelonephritis) and lower UTI (cystitis, urethritis) has clinical implications, especially in infants and young children. In this age group, the clinical presentation tends to be nonspecific, and the risk of renal damage caused by pyelonephritis is considered to be higher than in older children. Additionally, concepts of further imaging and treatment are frequently based on the level of UTI (American Academy of Pediatrics 1999).

However, differentiation between pyelonephritis and lower UTI is sometimes difficult. The presence of fever, flank pain, leukocytosis, elevation of C-reactive protein, leukocyte cylinders in the urine, and sonographically documented swelling of the kidney suggest the existence of pyelonephritis; however, specificity and sensitivity of these parameters are quite low (Garin et al. 2007). Today, serum procalcitonin is considered the most reliable serum marker for early prediction of renal parenchymal inflammation in the first febrile UTI (Kotoula et al. 2009).

Cortical scintigraphy ("DMSA scan") has proven to be the most sensitive parameter for the detection of parenchymal involvement; increasingly MRI with diffusion-weighted imaging is seen as an alternative. The commonly used radiopharmaceutical, dimercaptosuccinoc acid, is taken up by the proximal tubular cells directly from the peritubular vessels. Inflammation results in reduced intrarenal blood flow. Areas of decreased cortical uptake of the tracer indicate the presence of an acute pyelonephritis. In a study on piglets, DMSA scan has been shown to have a sensitivity of 91 % and a specificity of 99 % in the diagnosis of acute pyelonephritis (Rushton 1997). Color-coded power doppler sonography is also used for the detection of hypoperfused parenchymal areas but has a lower sensitivity and specificity (Halevy et al. 2004).

> **Take Away**
> An adequate urine sampling technique and urine investigation (including microbiological culture and bacterial resistance testing) are prerequisites for a successful diagnosis and treatment.

1.8 Therapy

The main objectives in the treatment of childhood UTIs are rapid recovery from complaints, prevention of urosepsis and infection-related complications, and the prevention of renal parenchymal damages (Doganis et al. 2007; Coulthard et al. 2009; Doganis and Sinaniotis 2009).

The choice of the appropriate antibiotics, the duration of therapy, and the form of application depend on age, severity of clinical symptoms, and the presence of complicating factors. Additionally, the regional resistance rates of uropathogens have to be considered when calculated antibacterial therapy is initiated.

An acute, symptomatic UTI mostly requires an antibacterial therapy before the pathogen is known and the results of a resistance test are available. Thus, the selection of the antibiotics follows the highest pathogen probability. The pathogen's responsiveness to antibiotics depends on the natural resistance and the actual resistance situation, which can differ largely from region to region. After antibacterial pretreatment and during antibacterial prophylaxis, the risk of resistant uropathogens is particularly high (Lutter et al. 2005). In case of pre-existing abnormalities or dysfunctions of the urinary tract (so-called complicated UTIs), after earlier UTIs, and under antibacterial prophylaxis, non-*E. coli* strains are more often to be reckoned with. This is also true for nosocomial UTIs and in UTI associated with foreign bodies in the urogenital tract or within urolithiasis.

1.8.1 Pyelonephritis in Newborns and Early Infancy

In newborns and young infants, a febrile UTI proceeds considerably more frequent in the form of urosepsis than in older children. In up to approximately 10–15 % positive blood cultures are to be found. Electrolyte disorders with hyponatremia and hyperkalemia can occur, probably because of a temporary pseudo-hypoaldostearonism. For these reasons, newborns and infants in the first two to six months of life initially require a parenteral antibacterial therapy under inpatient conditions. The combination treatment with ampillicin and an aminoglycoside (tobramycin, gentamicin), respectively, a cephalosporin of group 3, achieves a great therapeutic safety (high efficacy of aminoglycosides, respectively, cephalosporins against common uropathogens; enterococcus gap is closed with ampillicin). When applying aminoglycosides, a daily single dose is safe and effective (Contopoulos-Ioannidis et al. 2004; Bloomfield et al. 2005; Hodson et al. 2007). After defervescence, and after the microbiological resistance results are known, a parenteral, calculated therapy can be changed over to a targeted resistance-appropriate medication. The duration of antibiotic therapy is 7–14 days.

1.8.2 Therapy of Pyelonephritis in Late Infancy and Childhood

According to newer studies, an exclusively oral therapy with a cephalosporin of group 3 (i.e., cefixime, ceftibuten) is equal to the usual 2–4 days of intravenous therapy followed by an oral treatment. This is true for the duration of fever, as well as for the development of persistent renal scars (Hoberman et al. 1999; Hodson et al. 2007; Neuhaus et al. 2008). Similar data has been shown for amoxicillin-clavulanate (Montini et al. 2007). However, children with urinary tract abnormalities have been excluded from all randomized studies comparing the equality of an oral therapy to the parental treatment (Hoberman et al. 1999; Montini et al. 2007; Neuhaus et al. 2008). Hence, in case of pyelonephritis in infancy and childhood, the antibacterial treatment with an oral cephalosporin of group three can be carried out after thorough consideration, if a good compliance is to be expected and medical surveillance and therapy are warranted, and if severe urinary tract malformations have been excluded (Bloomfield et al. 2005). Regarding the optimal duration of therapy, a meta-analysis provided an empirical basis for the current practice of treating pediatric UTIs for 7–14 days (Keren and Chan 2002).

1.8.3 Therapy of Complicated Pyelonephritis

In complicated UTI, non-*E. coli* uropathogens, such as *Proteus mirabilis*, *Klebsiella* spp., Indolpos. *Proteus* spp., *Pseudomonas aeruginosa*, *Enterococci*, and *Staphylococci*, are to be anticipated more often. A parenteral treatment with broad-spectrum antibiotics is to be preferred to oral therapy. A temporary urinary diversion (suprapubic cystostomy or percutaneous nephrostomy) might be required in case of therapy failure in obstructive uropathies (i.e., severe pyonephrosis with urethral valves, obstructive megaureter, or ureteropelvic junction obstruction).

1.8.4 Therapy of Acute Focal Bacterial Nephritis, Renal Carbuncle, and Abscess

Acute focal bacterial nephritis ("lobar nephronia") is a localized bacterial infection of the kidney presenting as an inflammatory mass without abscess formation, which may represent a relatively early stage of renal abscess. For the majority of children, the pathogenesis is related to ascending infection due to pre-existing uropathy, especially VUR or urinary obstruction. Prolonged intravenous antibiotic treatment is sufficient in most cases (Klar et al. 1996); 3 weeks of intravenous and oral therapy tailored to the pathogen noted in cultures seem to be superior to shorter treatment (Cheng et al. 2006).

Renal cortical abscesses ("carbuncles") are caused by hematogenous spreading originating from another focus of bacterial infection (e.g., skin infection such as infected wounds, furunculosis, or skin abscess), the most frequent pathogen being *Staphylococcus aureus*. In most of these cases, urine cultures are sterile. Mostly, a prolonged parenteral calculated combination therapy including beta-lactamase-resistant antibiotics targeting *Staphylococcus aureus* is sufficiently effective. More rarely, additional percutaneous drainage, open surgical revision, or nephrectomy is required (Jemni et al. 1992; Steiss et al. 2014).

Renal corticomedullary abscesses are sometimes observed as complications of ascending UTIs with vescicorenal (intrarenal) reflux or in urinary tract obstruction. These abscesses often are preceded by pyelonephritis or by focal bacterial nephritis ("lobar nephronia") caused by gram-negative bacteria, e.g., *E. coli* (Shimizu et al. 2005).

1.8.5 Therapy of Cystitis and Cystourethritis

Symptomatic afebrile UTIs with dysuria, alguria, pollakisuria, lower abdominal pain, and/or onset of secondary urinary incontinence require a treatment which guarantees high urine levels of the antibiotic used. In principle, simple antibiotics should be preferred to highly effective reserve antibiotics in uncomplicated cystitis to avoid further development of resistance in the population. The recommended duration of therapy is 3–5 days (Michael et al. 2003).

1.8.6 Control of Therapeutic Success

Under successful treatment, the urine usually becomes sterile after 24 h, and leukocyturia normally disappears within 3–4 days. Normal body temperature can be expected within 24–48 h after the start of therapy in 90 % of cases. CRP mostly normalizes after 4–5 days (Jodal and Hansson 1994). In cases of prolonged fever and failing recovery, one should consider a resistant uropathogen or the presence of an uropathy or an acute urinary obstruction (e.g., due to a urinary calculus), which urgently demands imaging.

1.8.7 Asymptomatic Bacteriuria

Infants and children with asymptomatic bacteriuria (ABU) have a low risk of developing pyelonephritis. ABU are commonly caused by low virulent uropathogenic bacteria almost leading to a colonization – not, however, to an infection. They can even protect the urinary tract from invasion by bacteria of higher virulence. In most cases, asymptomatic bacteriuria resolves spontaneously after a few weeks or months. It has been shown that the rate of pyelonephritic episodes was higher in girls who were treated for asymptomatic bacteriuria than in those who stayed untreated in spite of bacteriuria (Hansson et al. 1989a, b).

Asymptomatic bacteriuria in patients without accompanying uropathy, bladder dysfunction, or history of pyelonepritic episodes does not call for antibacterial therapy at all. If antibacterial therapy becomes necessary for other reasons, e.g., otitis media or pneumonia, a symptomatic UTI can occur thereafter due to a shift toward more virulent uropathogenic bacteria (Hansson et al. 1989a, b).

> **Take Away**
> The therapeutic strategy for antibacterial treatment depends on the patient's age, the severity of clinical symptoms, as well as underlying complicating factors.

1.9 Diagnostic Work-Up

1.9.1 Diagnostic Imaging

The main aims of diagnostic imaging in symptomatic UTI are the detection of risk factors such as severe congenital anomalies of kidney and urinary tract (CAKUT) and VUR as well as acquired or congenital renal damage. This is especially true after pyelonephritic episodes and at a young age.

Ultrasonography (US) US is available in most pediatric clinics being widely used as first-line imaging in acute UTI. Its relevance has been questioned, especially when prenatal US screening has excluded severe CAKUT (Miron et al. 2007; Montini et al. 2009). However, US is an attractive first-line imaging modality in infants and children with UTI, especially when there is no systematic third-trimester prenatal screening (Preda et al. 2010). Contrast-enhanced sonographic techniques (VUS) have furthermore widened the potential of US for VUR assessment.

DMSA Scan Today, DMSA scan still is considered the most sensitive parameter for the detection of parenchymal involvement in pyelonephritis and has become the gold standard for imaging transient and permanent kidney damages. Areas of decreased cortical uptake of tracer indicate the presence of acute pyelonephritis. As renal scarring then is represented by areas of decreased uptake in association with volume loss, a repeat examination at least 6 months later is necessary to demonstrate if the lesion has resolved or has progressed into a permanent scar.

Voiding Cystourethrogram Current guidelines of the American Association of Pediatrics (AAP) are stating that in infants 2–24 months, "VCUG should not be performed routinely after their first febrile UTI." Rather, VCUG should be performed "if US reveal hydronephrosis, scarring, or other findings that would suggest either high-grade VUR or obstructive uropathy, as well as in other atypical or complex clinical circumstances" (American Academy of Pediatrics 2011). However, normal US does not exclude dilating VUR. Therefore, this statement was criticized by several authors (Friedman et al. 2013; Juliano et al. 2013). Indeed, there is a limitation of VUR assessment to cases with defined risk factors according to the probability of relevant VUR grades and to the risk of renal damage in some other currently published guidelines (Table 2).

If performed more than 1 week after a pyelonephritic episode, the timing of the VCUG does not influence the results (Craig et al. 1997; McDonald et al. 2000; Mahant et al. 2001; Sathapornwajana et al. 2008; Doganis et al. 2009). Commonly, antibacterial therapy or prophylaxis should be continued until the VCUG. For further details, refer to chapter "Vesicoureteric Reflux".

There is no indication for performing an IVU any longer in the setting of UTI. The role for CT and/or MRI is discussed in the respective chapter "Imaging in Urinary Tract Infections").

Imaging Diagnostic Strategies

Today, there exist two principal philosophies regarding the rational usage and sequence of imaging.

"Bottom-Up Strategy" One suggested pathway is to carry out a VCUG (or ce-VUS) and then stop if no VUR is detected. If VUR is seen, then

Table 2 Recommendations for reflux assessment after febrile urinary tract infection in different guidelines

Guideline/approach	Age	Indications for reflux assessment
AAP Guideline (American Academy of Pediatrics 2011) (American Academy of Pediatrics) 2011	Two months–two years	After the second pyelonephritis or In case of sonographically detectable abnormalities of the kidney or/and urinary tract
NICE Guideline (Mori et al. 2007) (England) 2007	Two months–two years <6 months >6 months	Not routinely, but after "atypical UTI" (very severe course of UTI, urosepsis, non-*E. coli* UTI, resistance to adequate therapy after 48 h) or Pathological ultrasonographic findings only with risk factors (urinary tract dilatation, non-*E. coli* UTI, positive family history for reflux)
ISPN (Ammenti et al. 2012) (Italian Society of Pediatric Nephrology) 2014	Two months–three years	Intrauterinely detected sonographic abnormalities, positive family history for reflux, urosepsis, chronic kidney disease, age < 6 months in boys, bladder dysfunction, resistance to adequate therapy after 72 h, non-*E. coli* UTI
"Top-down approach" (Preda et al. 2007, 2011)[6]		Only with signs of renal damage in DMSA scintigram during UTI

a late DMSA scan would probably be required to assess the extent of any renal damage. The goal of this strategy is early detection of VUR and prevention of ascending UTIs. In many European countries, VUR diagnostics is the first-line diagnostics in routine radiological imaging after pyelonephritis, as after UTI, VUR can be detected in 30% of the affected children.

"Top-Down Strategy" The alternative pathway is a DMSA (or US or MRI) scan to identify an abnormal kidney. If abnormal, the child requires VUR assessment. The goal of this strategy is early detection of renal damage.

Today, DMSA scan has become an instrument for the selection of high-risk patients who demand further imaging and prophylaxis. In many studies, DMSA changes in acute UTI indicating pyelonephritis or parenchymal damage, respectively, correlated well with the presence of dilating VUR and the risk of further pyelonephritic episodes, breakthrough infections (Shiraishi et al. 2010), and future renal scarring. Newer strategies therefore support the use of DMSA (if renal involvement is not already detected by US) as first-line diagnostic based on the observation that dilating VUR occurs almost exclusively in children with abnormal DMSA (Hansson et al. 2004; Preda et al. 2007). The new strategies have also influenced current pediatric uroradiological guidelines (Riccabona et al. 2008). However, recent clinical practical guidelines of the American Academy of Pediatrics do not recommend nuclear scans as part of routine evaluation of infants with their first febrile UTI for the findings rarely affect acute clinical management (American Academy of Pediatrics 2011).

1.9.2 Serum and Urine Markers

It is debatable if the current trend toward a "top-down approach" (i.e., indication for VUR assessment dependent on changes in renal imaging) does in fact significantly minimize the overall radiological burden besides sparing VCUGs (Saadeh and Mattoo 2011). Many efforts have been made to find laboratory parameters, which further enable the reduction of evaluation imaging protocols.

Serum procalcitonin and urine markers such as interleukin-8 are also potential noninvasive tools for identifying renal parenchymal involvement and the risk of renal damage (Galanakis et al. 2006; Leroy et al. 2007). Recently, Leroy et al. confirmed that PCT > 0.5 mg/l is a sensitive and validated predictor strongly associated with VUR higher than grade II, regardless of the presence of early renal parenchymal involvement in children with a first UTI (Leroy et al. 2011).

1.9.3 Bladder Function Diagnostics

When voiding dysfunction is clinically suspected (e.g., with incontinence, pollakisuria, urge symptoms, voiding postponement, etc.), a careful history of voiding habits and a urodynamic evaluation, restricted to uroflowmetry with or without pelvic floor electromyography and sonographic measurement of bladder wall thickness and postvoiding residual urine should be performed (see also chapter "Non-neurogenic Bladder-Sphincter Dysfunction ("Voiding Dysfunction")"). Furthermore, fluid intake, voiding frequency, and voiding volumes should be recorded in a two-day protocol. These basic diagnostic parameters enable a clinical functional diagnosis without further invasive measures in most cases (Neveus et al. 2006). Video cystometry should usually be reserved for the evaluation of neuropathic bladders (see chapter "Neurogenic Bladder in Infants and Children").

> **Take Away**
> Diagnostic imaging should follow the "ALARA principle" by opting for the most convenient and informative strategy with the least X-ray burden available.

1.10 Prophylaxis

In infants and children being susceptible to pyelonephritis and UTI recurrences, effective prophylactic measures are eligible. Prophylaxis should always include the efficient management of bladder and/or bowel dysfunction, as well as the treatment of other predisposing factors.

1.10.1 Chemoprophylaxis

A long-term antibacterial prophylaxis is to be considered in cases of high susceptibility to UTIs and risk of acquired renal damage. These are, for instance, patients with dilating VUR (Nuutinen and Uhari 2001), with recurrent pyelonephritic episodes, or with significant urinary tract obstruction (e.g., high-grade megaureters, urethral valves) (Ulman et al. 2000; Herndon 2006; Song et al. 2007; Walsh et al. 2007; Coelho et al. 2008; Lee et al. 2008; Herndon and Kitchens 2009; Gimpel et al. 2010). Whereas several prospective, randomized studies did not support the efficacy of antibacterial prophylaxis in low-grade VUR (Garin et al. 2006; Montini et al. 2008; Pennesi et al. 2008; Roussey-Kesler et al. 2008), currently published data of two elaborate studies showed a clear superiority of prophylaxis over placebo or pure observation strategy in VUR patients after UTI (Brandstrom et al. 2010a, b; RIVUR Trial Investigators 2014).

> **Take Away**
> Antibacterial prophylaxis is recommended in children with the highest risk of recurrence and pyelonephritic scarring.

1.10.2 Treatment of Bladder Dysfunction and Obstipation

Normalization of micturition disorders or bladder overactivity is a paramount measure to lower the recurrence rate of UTIs in a child (Winberg 1990). Often, dysfunctional voiding is associated with constipation. It is well known that treatment of constipation leads to increasing urinary continence and avoidance of UTI recurrences (O'Regan and Yazbeck 1985; O'Regan et al. 1985; Loening-Baucke 1997; De Paepe et al. 2000).

1.10.3 Breast Milk Feeding

Breast milk feeding significantly protects against UTIs at least during the first months of life (Miller and Krieger 2002). In a case control study, the protective effect of breastfeeding was highest soon after birth and declined to zero up to the seventh month of life. It contributed to a diminished rate of UTIs even after ablactation, demonstrating a prolonged effectiveness (Marild et al. 2004).

1.10.4 Circumcision

There is good evidence that circumcision lowers the risk of urinary tract infections, not only in infants but also in toddlers (Wiswell et al. 1988; Herzog 1989; Craig et al. 1996). However, the authors of a recent meta-analysis came to the result that 111 circumcisions would be necessary in the whole male newborn population to avoid one UTI. The number to treat (NTT) is much lower in high-risk patients: a number of 11 for boys with recurrent UTIs and a number of 3 for boys with dilating VUR were calculated in the same study (Singh-Grewal et al. 2005). Some pediatric urologists therefore consider a "prophylactic" circumcision in high-risk male patients, e.g., infants with urethral valves, with high-grade VUR, or with severe neurogenic bladder (Malone 2005).

2 Vesicoureteral Reflux (VUR)

2.1 Introduction

Up to 30–50 % of children presenting with their first UTI are subsequently diagnosed with VUR (Greenfield and Wan 1996; American Academy of Pediatrics 1999).

Scarcely another topic in pediatric urology has been discussed more controversially than VUR. Despite growing knowledge on the interrelations between VUR, UTI, and renal scars, the significance of VUR in the pathogenesis of pyelonephritis and renal damage remains contentious.

2.2 Definition and Classification

The backflow of urine into the ureter or up to the renal pelvis is called vesicoureteral, vesicoureteric, or vesico-renal reflux. Whereas *primary*

VUR relies on an isolated dysfunction of the ureterovesical closing mechanism, *secondary VUR* results among other things from anatomical infravesical obstruction (i.e., urethral valves) or disorders of bladder function (i.e., neurogenic bladder, detrusor-sphincter dyscoordination).

2.3 Etiology and Pathogenesis

Anatomical and functional prerequisites for a normal closing mechanism of the ureterovesical junction are (1) a sufficient anchorage of the distal ureter at the lateral aspect of the trigonum, (2) an angular routing and a sufficient intramural and submucous length of the terminal ureteral segment, (3) a slit-shaped ostium, (4) a regular structure of the trigonal musculature, and (5) an undisturbed bladder function. Failure of one or more of these prerequisites can result in VUR. In extreme cases, the confluence of the ureter becomes widely gaping instead of slit-shaped.

There are several hypotheses regarding the etiology of VUR. One of the mostly accepted is the "bud theory" (Mackie and Stephens 1975) based on the assumption of a dystopic sprouting of the ureteric bud from the Wolff duct, which leads to a lateralized ureteric confluence with a short intramural routing.

One important etiological factor in primary VUR is a genetic disposition caused by polygenic or multifactorial transmission mechanisms (Murawski and Gupta 2006; Murer et al. 2007). About 30% of asymptomatic siblings of an affected child also present with VUR in screening (Redman 1976; Noe 1996, 2002; Hollowell and Greenfield 2002) (Table 3). The risk declines with growing age of the sibling being 10% above the age of 6 years (Connolly et al. 1997).

2.4 "Reflux Nephropathy" and Renal Scarring

Over 30% of children with UTI presenting with a radiologically detected VUR show renal scars in the ipsilateral kidney (Smellie et al. 1975). In contrast, these parenchymal changes rarely exist

Table 3 Percentage of cases with VUR in different risk groups

Risk group	Percentage of children with VUR (approximation) (%)
Unilateral multicystic kidney (contralateral VUR) (Ismaili et al. 2005)	20
Unilateral renal agenesis (contralateral VUR) (Cascio et al. 1999)	28
Ureteropelvic junction obstruction (ipsilateral VUR) (Lebowitz and Blickman 1983)	10
Siblings of reflux patients (Hollowell and Greenfield 2002)	30
Children of parents with VUR (Noe 2002)	66
Children with urinary tract infection	30
Normal population (for comparison) (Bailey 1979)	1

in the non-refluxing contralateral kidney of the same child (Beetz et al. 1989; Polito et al. 2001). Radiologically detectable scars have therefore been classified as "reflux nephropathy" (Smellie and Normand 1979). The proportion of renal units with reflux nephropathy correlates with the VUR grade. Basically, there are two conditions potentially leading to renal damage in association with VUR:

"Congenital Reflux Nephropathy" Approximately one-third of newborns with sonographically presumed and proven VUR present with parenchymal defects in DMSA scans (Yeung et al. 1997; Tsai et al. 1998). Therefore, in many cases of dilating VUR, renal damage is already present at diagnosis and is rather a congenital kidney malformation associated with VUR than an acquired lesion. During the last decade, VUR and reflux nephropathy have been recognized as parts of a multifactorial disturbance of ureterorenal development, "CAKUT" (congenital anomalies of kidneys and urinary tract) (Nakai et al. 2003; Nakanishi and Yoshikawa 2003). This congenital association of VUR and renal damage can

1998; Yeung et al. 2006). These observations support the current trend of a differentiated view of the phenomenon of "VUR": not only are VUR grade or the configuration of ureteral insertion into the bladder crucial prognostic factors in the natural history of VUR, but bladder function is also an important predictive parameter for spontaneous VUR maturation, for susceptibility for pyelonephritic episodes, and for renal damaging. This awareness has implications for conservative therapy, as it must include the treatment of pre-existing bladder dysfunctions to be successful in the long run (Kibar et al. 2007).

VUR Control During Observation Commonly, annual controls of VUR are recommended during conservative treatment. However, the extension of these intervals would have no unacceptable influence on the duration of prophylaxis. Thompson et al. demonstrated by a mathematical model that 2-year intervals with low-grade VURs would decrease the number of VCUGs by 42%, whereas the duration of antibacterial prophylaxis would only be prolonged by 16%. In high-grade VUR, a 3-year interval would decrease the number of VCUGs by 63%, while the duration of prophylaxis would only be prolonged by 10% (Thompson et al. 2005). Therefore, the frequency of repeated VCUGs should be individually based on VUR grade with preference for longer intervals.

2.7.2 Surgical VUR Correction

The surgical concept is based on the assumption that ascension of uropathogens to the kidney leading to pyelonephritis can be avoided by VUR correction, in spite of continuing susceptibility to bacterial growth in the bladder.

Commonly accepted indications for surgical correction are:

- Recurrent pyelonephritis in spite of antibacterial prophylaxis (breakthrough infections)
- Poor compliance with antibacterial prophylaxis
- Progression of pyelonephritic scars
- High-grade VUR (grades IV–V) with low chance of spontaneous resolution
- Persistent high-grade VUR in adolescent girls without tendency to resolve spontaneously
- Refusal of antibacterial prophylaxis by parents and/or patient and desire for surgical correction with high-grade VUR

The principle of all variants in open correction is the prolongation of the submucosal section of the refluxing ureter. There exists a broad spectrum of surgical techniques including ureterocystoneostomy psoas hitch technique (Hertle et al. 1983; Riedmiller et al. 1984), techniques according to Politano-Leadbetter (Politano and Leadbetter 1958), Cohen (Cohen 1975), etc., and anti-reflux plasty, mostly performed according to Lich-Gregoir (Lich et al. 1961; Gregoir 1962).

Endoscopic VUR correction with subureteral injection of bulking substances has become a serious concurrence to open VUR correction due to modern material like NASHA™/Dx (Stabilized, non-animal hyaluronic acid/dextranomer) [Dx/HA, Deflux®]. With exclusive usage of NASHA (Deflux®), experienced surgeons achieved growing success rates similar to open techniques (Puri et al. 2006). Since NASHA (Deflux®) was approved by the FDA (Food and Drug Administration) in 2001, there is a trend toward increasing numbers of surgical VUR corrections in the USA (Lendvay et al. 2006). Interestingly, this is due to the increasing number of endoscopic interventions, whereas the number of open VUR corrections remains stable (Lendvay et al. 2006). Obviously Deflux® injection has not only become an alternative to open procedures but also to conservative VUR management, thereby assuming a position between surgical and conservative strategies.

The success rate of open surgical techniques of VUR grades III–IV is 96–99% in experienced hands (Elder et al. 1997). It is less in VUR grade V (85–90%), mostly due to associated pathologies.

After open ureterocystoneostomy or anti-reflux plasty, routine confirmation of surgical success by a postoperative VCUG is not necessary. However, VUR assessment should be performed in cases of recurrent postoperative pyelonephritis – last but not the least to identify a new VUR into the contralateral ureter. Many authors recommend routine VUR evaluation after (during) VUR correction with bulking agents concerning the possibility of VUR recurrence following endoscopic techniques.

should depend on multiple determinants such as age and sex, bladder function, degree of VUR, recurrences of symptomatic UTIs, pre-existing renal scars, compliance, and the expectations of parents (Tekgul et al. 2012).

2.7.1 Long-Term Observation and Antibacterial Prophylaxis

The proportion of refluxing ureters in the population as well as the degree of VUR in persistently refluxing renal units decreases with growing age. This phenomenon of "reflux maturation" encourages a strategy of "watchful waiting" (Edwards et al. 1977). Conservative strategies today rely on this concept using antibacterial long-term prophylaxis to decrease the risk of UTI recurrences as long as VUR has not been resolved or downgraded.

Today, nitrofurantoin and trimethoprim are the substances of first choice used for antibacterial prophylaxis of UTIs. Cefaclor also has its place in long-term antibacterial prophylaxis (Kaneko et al. 2003).

The indications for antibacterial prophylaxis differ from country to country and from clinic to clinic. The guidelines of the American Urological Association (AUA) recommend antibacterial prophylaxis independent of VUR grade in all cases, if there is no absolute indication for surgical repair (Elder et al. 1997). In a Swedish guideline published in 1999, an antibacterial prophylaxis is exclusively used with VUR grades III–V and continued for 1 year. Thereafter, prophylaxis is continued if the VUR is not downgraded to grades 0–II (Jodal and Lindberg 1999).

In dilating VUR (grades III–IV), the results of randomized prospective studies, especially of the International Reflux Study (IRS), demonstrated that conservative and surgical therapy were equivalent if renal scarring was taken as an endpoint (Jodal et al. 2006). In the IRS, renal growth and recurrence rate of UTIs were almost identical, whereas febrile UTI more frequently occurred with conservative treatment (Jodal et al. 2006).

The optimal duration of long-term antibacterial prophylaxis is as debatable as its indication. Following the rationales for antibacterial prophylaxis, it should be continued until the increased risk of pyelonephritic recurrences is diminished and/or the risk of renal scars is "outgrown."

In girls with VUR, the decision for stopping antibacterial prophylaxis is comparatively more difficult. The cessation of antibacterial prophylaxis is an individual decision which must consider the duration of the previous infection-free period, the degree of reflux, pre-existing parenchymal damage, and the existence of bladder dysfunction. Last but not least, the decision depends on the compliance and reliability of the family. Long-term prophylaxis in boys over 1 year of age with conservatively monitored primary VUR might be dispensable because the risk of recurrence is extremely low in boys at this age (Winberg 1994; Thompson et al. 2001).

Effectiveness of Antibacterial Prophylaxis Current randomized prospective studies from Sweden (Swedish Reflux Study), Australia (PRIVENT Study) and Northern America (RIVUR Study) demonstrated significant superiority of antibacterial prophylaxis compared to surveillance without prophylaxis or placebo regarding the risk of recurrent UTIs (Esbjorner et al. 2004; Greenfield et al. 2008; Keren et al. 2008; Craig et al. 2009; Brandstrom et al. 2010a; RIVUR Trial Investigators 2014). Yet, in the Swedish Reflux Study, prophylaxis was not efficient in boys. In addition, renal scarring could not be avoided in the RIVUR Study, whereas in the Swedish Reflux Study, girls without prophylaxis developed significantly more renal scars with pyelonephritic episodes than girls in the prophylactic group (Brandstrom et al. 2010b).

Importance of Bladder Dysfunction in VUR VUR, UTIs, and bladder dysfunction are frequently associated (Snodgrass 1991; Sillen 1999; Yeung et al. 2006). Bladder dysfunction increases the risk of UTIs and can lead to significant delay in VUR maturation. Its detection by careful history and its efficient treatment are therefore mandatory in all affected children. Overall it is estimated that bladder dysfunction exists in about 50 % of children with VUR (Jodal et al. 2006). Bladder function influences the spontaneous regression rate of VUR (Koff et al.

risk of pyelonephritic renal scarring is highest in early infancy, consensus exists about the indication in this age group. Indications for VUR assessment in different current guidelines after UTI are listed in Table 2. In asymptomatic newborns with unilateral multicystic kidney or renal agenesia, VUR can be found in over 20% of the children in the contralateral uretero-renal unit. Nevertheless, the indication for VCUG should be reluctant. If any abnormalities (i.e., dilatation of urinary tract, sign for renal dysplasia or renal scarring, etc.) are excluded by repeated US in the contralateral uretero-renal unit, a VCUG might be renounced (Ismaili et al. 2005).

Siblings of VUR patients bear a high genetic risk of having VUR. The early diagnosis by screening opens the opportunity of early VUR detection and avoidance of UTIs by prophylaxis (Van den Abbeele et al. 1987; Houle et al. 2004). However, in the overwhelming number of cases, low VUR grades will be found which probably have no pathological relevance (Bonnin et al. 2001; Hollowell and Greenfield 2002). There exists no single study which proves that screening and treatment of asymptomatic siblings of VUR patients reduce the risk of pyelonephritis scarring.

Radiological voiding cystourethrogram (VCUG) remains the gold standard for VUR detection (Riccabona 2002). Several other imaging techniques have been established as promising alternatives to the radiological VCUG. Sophisticated contrast-enhanced sonographic techniques have been proven to reach the same sensitivity and specificity as radiological methods, if appropriate contrast mediums are transurethrally applied (Darge et al. 2005; Darge 2008). Direct radionuclide cystography (e.g., with ^{99m}Tc-MAG3) is also highly sensitive. For further details, refer to chapter "Vesicoureteric Reflux".

> **Take Away**
> The individual indication for VUR diagnostics should consider age, sex, US findings, the number of pyelonephritic episodes, as well as signs of pyelonephritic damage on DMSA renography, if available.

2.7 Therapy

The main goal of any therapy in VUR is the prevention of acquired parenchymal damage by ascending UTIs with their potential sequelae such as hypertension and/or chronic kidney failure. However, in many cases of dilating VUR, renal damage is already present at diagnosis and is rather a congenital kidney malformation associated with VUR than an acquired lesion.

Today, several therapeutic options can be chosen for the therapy of VUR. They include long-term antibacterial prophylaxis, open surgery, endoscopic therapy, and – last but not least – "watchful waiting" without medication.

Due to the fact that low- to medium-grade VURs may spontaneously resolve, the current standard of care for most children, at least initially, is long-term antibacterial prophylaxis to prevent UTI (Peters et al. 2010; Tekgul et al. 2012). Another option, presumably indicated in high-grade VUR, is surgical correction in order to prevent the ascension of bacteria to the kidney. In VUR grades III–IV, surgical correction and long-term antibacterial prophylaxis show no difference regarding the risk of renal damage. However, if dilating VUR persists during long-term antibacterial prophylaxis, the disadvantages of antibiotics such as side effects or the development of bacterial resistance limit its practicability.

Until recently, open surgery was the only option in VUR correction. Currently, endoscopic injection with dextranomer/hyaluronic acid copolymer or other bulking agents is being widely used (Elder et al. 2007). Actually, in lower to mild VUR grades, no treatment at all seems to also be a quite secure strategy if pyelonephritis episodes are promptly treated.

The wide spectrum of treatment options today provides the opportunity of sophisticated therapeutic and prophylactic strategies. However, in spite of several national guidelines published or being in process, no consensus has been found yet regarding the best therapy for different grades of VUR and renal involvement (Peters et al. 2010; Finnell et al. 2011; Tekgul et al. 2012).

The individual, risk-oriented decision for surgical or conservative treatment of dilating VUR

probably be explained by a disorganization of ureteral development in the early embryonic stage (Najmaldin et al. 1990). If the ureteral bud arises aberrantly from its typical origin at the Wolff duct, it can connect to undifferentiated parts of the metanephrogenic blastema, thus inducing dysplastic renal parenchyma. Dilating VUR is predominantly detected in boys, with dilating ureters or renal pelvices being noticed by US (Yeung et al. 1997). As the proportion of renal units with parenchymal damage increases with VUR grade, this might explain why male infants are more often affected by congenital reflux nephropathy than girls.

Acquired Pyelonephritic Renal Damage Associated with VUR The emerging development of renal scars is usually associated with the occurrence of a pyelonephritic episode (Smellie et al. 1985). A VUR is said to favor the ascension of uropathogens up to the kidney. However, there is growing uncertainty on the pathogenic importance of VUR in the development of pyelonephritic scars (Garin et al. 2006; Polito et al. 2006). Systematic studies using DMSA scans demonstrated that pyelonephritic scars can develop in comparable numbers in infants and children with and without VUR (Garin et al. 1998). These results shed a new light on the dignity of VUR: pyelonephritis, not VUR itself, is the crucial mechanism leading to parenchymal damage in acquired "reflux nephropathy" (Gordon et al. 2003; Moorthy et al. 2005).

The following factors increase the risk for acquired renal damage: recurrent pyelonephritis, therapeutic delay of pyelonephritis, and high-grade VUR/intrarenal reflux. Whereas it is well known that infants and young children bear a particular risk for pyelonephritic damage (Vernon et al. 1997), renal scars can also develop during later childhood and adolescence (Smellie et al. 1985; Benador et al. 1997; Jakobsson et al. 1999). In recent years, it has become obvious that the individual risk for pyelonephritic scars might at least be partially genetically determined (Ozen et al. 1999).

Under physiological circumstances, a sterile VUR itself does not lead to renal damage. In the absence of UTIs, acquired refluxive parenchymal damage might only emerge resulting from massive intravesical pressure (by a so-called water hammer effect) like with extremely pronounced detrusor-sphincter dyssynergia or with urethral valves.

In summary, renal scarring associated with VUR might be a partial aspect of a CAKUT or a result of pyelonephritic damage. In boys, connatal reflux nephropathy dominates, whereas in girls pyelonephritis facilitated by VUR is predominantly responsible for renal scarring (Wennerstrom et al. 2000; Swerkersson et al. 2007).

> **Take Away**
> Recurrent pyelonephritic episodes, therapeutic delay, and high-grade VUR increase the risk of acquired renal damage.

2.5 Epidemiology and Symptoms

In a historical study, the prevalence of VUR was 1 % in healthy infants (Bailey 1979). The real percentage might be considerably higher (Sargent 2000; Williams et al. 2008). However, a VUR can be detected in 30 % of children with symptomatic UTI (Sargent 2000). The detection rate in girls is higher than in boys due to the higher cumulative incidence of UTIs in girls beyond the first year of life. VUR is frequently associated with renal anomalies and malformations of the urinary tract (Table 2).

In contrast to UTI, there is no specific symptomatology of VUR. Therefore, VUR is most detected by imaging diagnostics after symptomatic UTIs. Occasionally, micro-hematuria or recurrent flank pain is the only clinical symptoms.

2.6 Diagnosis

The main aim of VUR diagnostics is the detection of VUR before avoidable parenchymal damage arises.

There are some controversies about the indication of VUR diagnostics after UTIs. Since the

2.7.3 Which Therapy for Which Patient?

The individual decision for surgical or conservative treatment depends on multiple factors such as age and sex of the patient, bladder function, degree of VUR, recurrences of symptomatic UTIs, pre-existing renal scars, and the expectations of parents (Tekgul et al. 2012). Last but not least, the availability of a pediatric urologist with experience in surgical correction may play an important role (Smellie et al. 1992). However, in patients with pre-existing reflux nephropathy and dilating VUR, the main factor determining the outcome seems to be the extent of renal parenchymal reduction and the degree of functional impairment at the time of diagnosis.

> **Take Away**
> Today, a multitude of factors informs the decision between surgical (open, minimally invasive, or endoscopic) and conservative (antibacterial prophylaxis or watchful waiting) strategies. These factors include age, sex, severity, as well as frequency of UTIs, VUR grade, congenital or acquired renal damage, and – last but not least – the parents' informed consent.

2.8 Care After Cessation of VUR

Two groups of patients need long-term follow-up even after successful surgical correction or spontaneous cessation of VUR:

2.8.1 Patients with Continuing Susceptibility for UTIs

Many patients who have become conspicuous with UTI before surgical repair or spontaneous cessation of VUR continue suffering recurrences. The infection, however, is mostly restricted to the lower urinary tract (Beetz et al. 2002). Because UTI can lead to risks for mother and fetus, special care is recommended during pregnancy, and urine diagnostics are necessary if symptoms suspicious of UTI appear.

2.8.2 Patients with Reflux Nephropathy

Over 20 % of patients have renal scars at the time of VUR diagnosis. They are at risk of developing renal arterial hypertension (Simoes e Silva et al. 2007). The incidence of renal arterial hypertension is about 12–14 % in young adults with unilateral renal scars and 18 % with bilateral changes (Beetz et al. 1989). With increasing age, the incidence increases up to over 40 % (Kincaid-Smith et al. 1984). Lifelong controls of blood pressure and, if necessary, treatment of arterial hypertension are therefore recommended in patients with reflux nephropathy.

In most cases of unilateral reflux nephropathy, the hypertrophy of non-affected parenchyma compensates the loss of functioning nephrons in scarred areas resulting in normal or only moderately reduced whole kidney function. With bilateral reflux nephropathy, the risk of progressive renal insufficiency demands repeated controls of serum creatinine and calculated glomerular filtration rate. Adequate therapy of hypertension and lowering proteinuria by ACE inhibitors can probably slow down the progress of functional loss.

Reflux nephropathy and increased susceptibility to UTIs seem to be risk factors for EPH-gestosis during pregnancy (Austenfeld and Snow 1988); mild renal insufficiency probably can worsen to higher CKD levels (Becker et al. 1986).

> **Take Away**
> Acquired and congenital renal scarring are risk factors for arterial hypertension, decreased renal function, and complications during pregnancy.

Literature

American Academy of Pediatrics, C. o. Q. I., Subcommittee on Urinary Tract Infection (2011) Urinary Tract Infection: Clinical Practice Guideline for the Diagnosis and Management of the Initial UTI in Febrile Infants and Children 2 to 24 Months. Pediatrics 128(3):595–610

American Academy of Pediatrics. Committee on Quality Improvement. Subcommittee on Urinary Tract Infection (1999) Practice parameter: the diagnosis, treatment, and evaluation of the initial urinary tract infection in febrile infants and young children. Pediatrics 103(4 Pt 1):843–852

Ammenti A, Cataldi L et al (2012) Febrile urinary tract infections in young children: recommendations for the diagnosis, treatment and follow-up. Acta Paediatr 101(5):451–457

Austenfeld MS, Snow BW (1988) Complications of pregnancy in women after reimplantation for vesicoureteral reflux. J Urol 140(5 Pt 2):1103–1106

Austin PF, Bauer SB et al (2014) The Standardization of Terminology of Lower Urinary Tract Function in Children and Adolescents: Update Report from the Standardization Committee of the International Children's Continence Society. J Urol 191(6):1863–1865

Bailey RR (1979) Vesicoureteric Reflux in Healthy Infants and Children. In: Hodson P, Kincaid-Smith P (eds) Reflux Nephropathy. Masson Publishing SA, New York

Becker GJ, Ihle BU et al (1986) Effect of pregnancy on moderate renal failure in reflux nephropathy. Br Med J (Clin Res Ed) 292(6523):796–798

Beetz R, Schulte-Wissermann H et al (1989) Long-term follow-up of children with surgically treated vesicorenal reflux: postoperative incidence of urinary tract infections, renal scars and arterial hypertension. Eur Urol 16(5):366–371

Beetz R, Mannhardt W et al (2002) Long-term followup of 158 young adults surgically treated for vesicoureteral reflux in childhood: the ongoing risk of urinary tract infections. J Urol 168(2):704–707; discussion 707

Benador D, Benador N et al (1997) Are younger children at highest risk of renal sequelae after pyelonephritis? Lancet 349(9044):17–19

Bloomfield P, Hodson EM et al (2005) Antibiotics for acute pyelonephritis in children. Cochrane Database Syst Rev 1, CD003772

Bonnin F, Lottmann H et al (2001) Scintigraphic screening for renal damage in siblings of children with symptomatic primary vesico-ureteric reflux. BJU Int 87(6):463–466

Brandstrom P, Esbjorner E et al (2010a) The Swedish reflux trial in children: III. Urinary tract infection pattern. J Urol 184(1):286–291

Brandstrom P, Neveus T et al (2010b) The Swedish reflux trial in children: IV. Renal damage. J Urol 184(1):292–297

Buys H, Pead L et al (1994) Suprapubic aspiration under ultrasound guidance in children with fever of undiagnosed cause. BMJ 308(6930):690–692

Cascio S, Paran S et al (1999) Associated urological anomalies in children with unilateral renal agenesis. J Urol 162(3 Pt 2):1081–1083

Cavagnaro F (2005) Urinary tract infection in childhood. Rev Chilena Infectol 22(2):161–168

Cheng CH, Tsau YK et al (2006) Effective duration of antimicrobial therapy for the treatment of acute lobar nephronia. Pediatrics 117(1):e84–e89

Coelho GM, Bouzada MC et al (2008) Risk factors for urinary tract infection in children with prenatal renal pelvic dilatation. J Urol 179(1):284–289

Cohen SJ (1975) Ureterozystoneostomie: eine neue Antireflux-Technik. Akt Urol 6(1)

Connolly LP, Treves ST et al (1997) Vesicoureteral reflux in children: incidence and severity in siblings. J Urol 157(6):2287–2290

Contopoulos-Ioannidis DG, Giotis ND et al (2004) Extended-interval aminoglycoside administration for children: a meta-analysis. Pediatrics 114(1):e111–e118

Coulthard MG, Verber I et al (2009) Can prompt treatment of childhood UTI prevent kidney scarring? Pediatr Nephrol 24(10):2059–2063

Craig JC, Knight JF et al (1996) Effect of circumcision on incidence of urinary tract infection in preschool boys. J Pediatr 128(1):23–27

Craig JC, Knight JF et al (1997) Vesicoureteral reflux and timing of micturating cystourethrography after urinary tract infection. Arch Dis Child 76(3):275–277

Craig JC, Simpson JM et al (2009) Antibiotic prophylaxis and recurrent urinary tract infection in children. N Engl J Med 361(18):1748–1759

Craig JC, Williams GJ et al (2010) The accuracy of clinical symptoms and signs for the diagnosis of serious bacterial infection in young febrile children: prospective cohort study of 15 781 febrile illnesses. BMJ 340:c1594

Darge K (2008) Voiding urosonography with US contrast agents for the diagnosis of vesicoureteric reflux in children. II. Comparison with radiological examinations. Pediatr Radiol 38(1):54–63; quiz 126–7

Darge K, Moeller RT et al (2005) Diagnosis of vesicoureteric reflux with low-dose contrast-enhanced harmonic ultrasound imaging. Pediatr Radiol 35(1):73–78

De Paepe H, Renson C et al (2000) Pelvic-floor therapy and toilet training in young children with dysfunctional voiding and obstipation. BJU Int 85(7):889–893

Deville WL, Yzermans JC et al (2004) The urine dipstick test useful to rule out infections. A meta-analysis of the accuracy. BMC Urol 4:4

Doganis D, Sinaniotis K (2009) Early antibiotic treatment of pyelonephritis in children is still mandatory. Pediatrics 123(1):e173–e174; author reply e174

Doganis D, Siafas K et al (2007) Does early treatment of urinary tract infection prevent renal damage? Pediatrics 120(4):e922–e928

Doganis D, Mavrikou M et al (2009) Timing of voiding cystourethrography in infants with first time urinary infection. Pediatr Nephrol 24(2):319–322

Edwards D, Normand IC et al (1977) Disappearance of vesicoureteric reflux during long-term prophylaxis of urinary tract infection in children. Br Med J 2(6082):285–288

Elder JS, Peters CA et al (1997) Pediatric Vesicoureteral Reflux Guidelines Panel summary report on the management of primary vesicoureteral reflux in children. J Urol 157(5):1846–1851

Elder JS, Shah MB et al (2007) Part 3: Endoscopic injection versus antibiotic prophylaxis in the reduction of urinary tract infections in patients with vesicoureteral reflux. Curr Med Res Opin 23(Suppl 4): S15–S20

Esbjorner E, Hansson S et al (2004) Management of children with dilating vesico-ureteric reflux in Sweden. Acta Paediatr 93(1):37–42

Faust WC, Diaz M et al (2009) Incidence of post-pyelonephritic renal scarring: a meta-analysis of the dimercapto-succinic acid literature. J Urol 181(1):290–297; discussion 297–298

Finnell SM, Carroll AE et al (2011) Technical Report--Diagnosis and Management of an Initial UTI in Febrile Infants and Young Children. Pediatrics 128(4):e749–e770

Friedman AA, Wolfe-Christensen C et al (2013) History of recurrent urinary tract infection is not predictive of abnormality on voiding cystourethrogram. Pediatr Surg Int 29(6):639–643

Galanakis E, Bitsori M et al (2006) Urine interleukin-8 as a marker of vesicoureteral reflux in infants. Pediatrics 117(5):e863–e867

Garin EH, Campos A et al (1998) Primary vesicoureteral reflux: review of current concepts. Pediatr Nephrol 12(3):249–256

Garin EH, Olavarria F et al (2006) Clinical significance of primary vesicoureteral reflux and urinary antibiotic prophylaxis after acute pyelonephritis: a multicenter, randomized, controlled study. Pediatrics 117(3):626–632

Garin EH, Olavarria F et al (2007) Diagnostic significance of clinical and laboratory findings to localize site of urinary infection. Pediatr Nephrol 22(7):1002–1006

Gaspari RJ, Dickson E et al (2005) Antibiotic resistance trends in paediatric uropathogens. Int J Antimicrob Agents 26(4):267–271

Ghaemi S, Fesharaki RJ et al (2007) Late onset jaundice and urinary tract infection in neonates. Indian J Pediatr 74(2):139–141

Gimpel C, Masioniene L et al (2010) Complications and long-term outcome of primary obstructive megaureter in childhood. Pediatr Nephrol 25(9):1679–1686

Glauser MP, Meylan P et al (1987) The inflammatory response and tissue damage. The example of renal scars following acute renal infection. Pediatr Nephrol 1(4):615–622

Gordon I, Barkovics M et al (2003) Primary vesicoureteric reflux as a predictor of renal damage in children hospitalized with urinary tract infection: a systematic review and meta-analysis. J Am Soc Nephrol 14(3):739–744

Greenfield SP, Wan J (1996) Vesicoureteral reflux: practical aspects of evaluation and management. Pediatr Nephrol 10(6):789–794

Greenfield SP, Chesney RW et al (2008) Vesicoureteral reflux: the RIVUR study and the way forward. J Urol 179(2):405–407

Gregoir W (1962) Congenital vesico-ureteral reflux. Acta Urol Belg 30:286–300

Halevy R, Smolkin V et al (2004) Power Doppler ultrasonography in the diagnosis of acute childhood pyelonephritis. Pediatr Nephrol 19(9):987–991

Haller M, Brandis M et al (2004) Antibiotic resistance of urinary tract pathogens and rationale for empirical intravenous therapy. Pediatr Nephrol 19(9):982–986

Hansson S, Jodal U et al (1989a) Untreated asymptomatic bacteriuria in girls: II--Effect of phenoxymethylpenicillin and erythromycin given for intercurrent infections. BMJ 298(6677):856–859

Hansson S, Jodal U et al (1989b) Untreated bacteriuria in asymptomatic girls with renal scarring. Pediatrics 84(6):964–968

Hansson S, Dhamey M et al (2004) Dimercapto-succinic acid scintigraphy instead of voiding cystourethrography for infants with urinary tract infection. J Urol 172(3):1071–1073; discussion 1073–1074

Herndon CD (2006) Antenatal hydronephrosis: differential diagnosis, evaluation, and treatment options. ScientificWorldJournal 6:2345–2365

Herndon CD, Kitchens DM (2009) The management of ureteropelvic junction obstruction presenting with prenatal hydronephrosis. ScientificWorldJournal 9:400–403

Hertle L, Becht E et al (1983) Universelle Ureterozystoneostomie nach der Psoas Hitch Technik: Indiaktion - Operationstechnik. Akt Urol 14:167–174

Herzog LW (1989) Urinary tract infections and circumcision. A case–control study. Am J Dis Child 143(3):348–350

Hewitt IK, Zucchetta P et al (2008) Early treatment of acute pyelonephritis in children fails to reduce renal scarring: data from the Italian Renal Infection Study Trials. Pediatrics 122(3):486–490

Hildebrand WL, Schreiner RL et al (1981) Suprapubic bladder aspiration in infants. Am Fam Physician 23(5):115–118

Hiraoka M, Hashimoto G et al (2003) Early treatment of urinary infection prevents renal damage on cortical scintigraphy. Pediatr Nephrol 18(2):115–118

Hoberman A, Wald ER (1997) Urinary tract infections in young febrile children. Pediatr Infect Dis J 16(1):11–17

Hoberman A, Chao HP et al (1993) Prevalence of urinary tract infection in febrile infants. J Pediatr 123(1):17–23

Hoberman A, Wald ER et al (1996) Is urine culture necessary to rule out urinary tract infection in young febrile children? Pediatr Infect Dis J 15(4):304–309

Hoberman A, Wald ER et al (1999) Oral versus initial intravenous therapy for urinary tract infections in young febrile children. Pediatrics 104(1 Pt 1):79–86

Hodson EM, Willis NS et al (2007) Antibiotics for acute pyelonephritis in children. Cochrane Database Syst Rev 4, CD003772

Hollowell JG, Greenfield SP (2002) Screening siblings for vesicoureteral reflux. J Urol 168(5):2138–2141

Houle AM, Cheikhelard A et al (2004) Impact of early screening for reflux in siblings on the detection of renal damage. BJU Int 94(1):123–125

Ismaili K, Avni FE et al (2005) Routine voiding cystourethrography is of no value in neonates with unilateral multicystic dysplastic kidney. J Pediatr 146(6):759–763

Jacobson SH, Eklof O et al (1989) Development of hypertension and uraemia after pyelonephritis in childhood: 27 year follow up. BMJ 299(6701):703–706

Jakobsson B, Jacobson SH et al (1999) Vesico-ureteric reflux and other risk factors for renal damage: identification of high- and low-risk children. Acta Paediatr Suppl 88(431):31–39

Jemni L, Mdimagh L et al (1992) Kidney carbuncle: diagnostic, bacteriological and therapeutic considerations. Apropos of 11 cases. J Urol (Paris) 98(4):228–231

Jodal U, Hansson S (1994) Urinary tract infection. In: Holliday MA, Barratt TM, Avner ED (eds) Pediatric Nephrology. Williams & Wilkins, Baltimore, pp 950–962

Jodal U, Lindberg U (1999) Guidelines for management of children with urinary tract infection and vesicoureteric reflux. Recommendations from a Swedish state-of-the-art conference. Swedish Medical Research Council. Acta Paediatr Suppl 88(431):87–89

Jodal U, Smellie JM et al (2006) Ten-year results of randomized treatment of children with severe vesicoureteral reflux. Final report of the International Reflux Study in Children. Pediatr Nephrol 21(6): 785–792

Juliano TM, Stephany HA et al (2013) Incidence of abnormal imaging and recurrent pyelonephritis after first febrile urinary tract infection in children 2 to 24 months old. J Urol 190(4 Suppl):1505–1510

Kaneko K, Ohtomo Y et al (2003) Antibiotic prophylaxis by low-dose cefaclor in children with vesicoureteral reflux. Pediatr Nephrol 18(5):468–470

Kanellopoulos TA, Salakos C et al (2006) First urinary tract infection in neonates, infants and young children: a comparative study. Pediatr Nephrol 21(8):1131–1137

Kasanen A, Sundquist H et al (1983) Secondary prevention of urinary tract infections. The role of trimethoprim alone. Ann Clin Res 15(Suppl 36):1–36

Kass EH, Finland M (2002) Asymptomatic infections of the urinary tract. J Urol 168(2):420–424

Keren R, Chan E (2002) A meta-analysis of randomized, controlled trials comparing short- and long-course antibiotic therapy for urinary tract infections in children. Pediatrics 109(5), E70

Keren R, Carpenter MA et al (2008) Rationale and design issues of the Randomized Intervention for Children With Vesicoureteral Reflux (RIVUR) study. Pediatrics 122(Suppl 5):S240–S250

Kibar Y, Ors O et al (2007) Results of biofeedback treatment on reflux resolution rates in children with dysfunctional voiding and vesicoureteral reflux. Urology 70(3):563–566; discussion 566–567

Kiernan SC, Pinckert TL et al (1993) Ultrasound guidance of suprapubic bladder aspiration in neonates. J Pediatr 123(5):789–791

Kincaid-Smith PS, Bastos MG et al (1984) Reflux nephropathy in the adult. Contrib Nephrol 39:94–101

Klar A, Hurvitz H et al (1996) Focal bacterial nephritis (lobar nephronia) in children. J Pediatr 128(6):850–853

Koff SA, Wagner TT et al (1998) The relationship among dysfunctional elimination syndromes, primary vesicoureteral reflux and urinary tract infections in children. J Urol 160(3 Pt 2):1019–1022

Kotoula A, Gardikis S et al (2009) Comparative efficacies of procalcitonin and conventional inflammatory markers for prediction of renal parenchymal inflammation in pediatric first urinary tract infection. Urology 73(4):782–786

Lama G, Tedesco MA et al (2003) Reflux nephropathy and hypertension: correlation with the progression of renal damage. Pediatr Nephrol 18(3):241–245

Lebowitz RL, Blickman JG (1983) The coexistence of ureteropelvic junction obstruction and reflux. AJR Am J Roentgenol 140(2):231–238

Lee JH, Choi HS et al (2008) Nonrefluxing neonatal hydronephrosis and the risk of urinary tract infection. J Urol 179(4):1524–1528

Lendvay TS, Sorensen M et al (2006) The evolution of vesicoureteral reflux management in the era of dextranomer/hyaluronic acid copolymer: a pediatric health information system database study. J Urol 176(4 Pt 2):1864–1867

Leroy S, Romanello C et al (2007) Procalcitonin to reduce the number of unnecessary cystographies in children with a urinary tract infection: a European validation study. J Pediatr 150(1):89–95

Leroy S, Romanello C et al (2011) Procalcitonin is a Predictor for High-Grade Vesicoureteral Reflux in Children: Meta-Analysis of Individual Patient Data. J Pediatr 159(4):644–651, e4

Lich R Jr, Howerton LW et al (1961) Childhood urosepsis. J Ky Med Assoc 59:1177–1179

Loening-Baucke V (1997) Urinary incontinence and urinary tract infection and their resolution with treatment of chronic constipation of childhood. Pediatrics 100(2 Pt 1):228–232

Lohr JA (1991) Use of routine urinalysis in making a presumptive diagnosis of urinary tract infection in children. Pediatr Infect Dis J 10(9):646–650

Lutter SA, Currie ML et al (2005) Antibiotic resistance patterns in children hospitalized for urinary tract infections. Arch Pediatr Adolesc Med 159(10):924–928

Ma JF, Shortliffe LM (2004) Urinary tract infection in children: etiology and epidemiology. Urol Clin North Am 31(3):517–526, ix–x

Mackie GG, Stephens FD (1975) Duplex kidneys: a correlation of renal dysplasia with position of the ureteral orifice. J Urol 114(2):274–280

Magin EC, Garcia-Garcia JJ et al (2007) Efficacy of short-term intravenous antibiotic in neonates with urinary tract infection. Pediatr Emerg Care 23(2):83–86

Mahant S, To T et al (2001) Timing of voiding cystourethrogram in the investigation of urinary tract infections in children. J Pediatr 139(4):568–571

Malone PS (2005) Circumcision for preventing urinary tract infection in boys: European view. Arch Dis Child 90(8):773–774

Marchand M, Kuffer F et al (2007) Long-term outcome in women who underwent anti-reflux surgery in childhood. J Pediatr Urol 3(3):178–183

Marild S, Jodal U (1998) Incidence rate of first-time symptomatic urinary tract infection in children under 6 years of age. Acta Paediatr 87(5):549–552

Marild S, Hansson S et al (2004) Protective effect of breastfeeding against urinary tract infection. Acta Paediatr 93(2):164–168

McCracken GH Jr (1984) Recurrent urinary tract infections in children. Pediatr Infect Dis 3(3 Suppl):S28–S30

McDonald A, Scranton M et al (2000) Voiding cystourethrograms and urinary tract infections: how long to wait? Pediatrics 105(4), E50

Merrick MV, Notghi A et al (1995) Long-term follow up to determine the prognostic value of imaging after urinary tract infections. Part 2: Scarring. Arch Dis Child 72(5):393–396

Michael M, Hodson EM et al (2003) Short versus standard duration oral antibiotic therapy for acute urinary tract infection in children. Cochrane Database Syst Rev 1, CD003966

Miller TE, Findon G (1985) Genetic factor(s) influence scar formation in experimental pyelonephritis. Nephron 40(3):374–375

Miller JL, Krieger JN (2002) Urinary tract infections cranberry juice, underwear, and probiotics in the 21st century. Urol Clin North Am 29(3):695–699

Miller T, Phillips S (1981) Pyelonephritis: the relationship between infection, renal scarring, and antimicrobial therapy. Kidney Int 19(5):654–662

Miron D, Daas A et al (2007) Is omitting post urinary-tract-infection renal ultrasound safe after normal antenatal ultrasound? An observational study. Arch Dis Child 92(6):502–504

Montini G, Toffolo A et al (2007) Antibiotic treatment for pyelonephritis in children: multicentre randomised controlled non-inferiority trial. BMJ 335(7616):386

Montini G, Rigon L et al (2008) Prophylaxis after first febrile urinary tract infection in children? A multicenter, randomized, controlled, noninferiority trial. Pediatrics 122(5):1064–1071

Montini G, Zucchetta P et al (2009) Value of imaging studies after a first febrile urinary tract infection in young children: data from Italian renal infection study 1. Pediatrics 123(2):e239–e246

Moorthy I, Easty M et al (2005) The presence of vesicoureteric reflux does not identify a population at risk for renal scarring following a first urinary tract infection. Arch Dis Child 90(7):733–736

Mori R, Lakhanpaul M et al (2007) Diagnosis and management of urinary tract infection in children: summary of NICE guidance. BMJ 335(7616):395–397

Murawski IJ, Gupta IR (2006) Vesicoureteric reflux and renal malformations: a developmental problem. Clin Genet 69(2):105–117

Murer L, Benetti E et al (2007) Embryology and genetics of primary vesico-ureteric reflux and associated renal dysplasia. Pediatr Nephrol 22(6):788–797

Najmaldin A, Burge DM et al (1990) Reflux nephropathy secondary to intrauterine vesicoureteric reflux. J Pediatr Surg 25(4):387–390

Nakai H, Asanuma H et al (2003) Changing concepts in urological management of the congenital anomalies of kidney and urinary tract, CAKUT. Pediatr Int 45(5):634–641

Nakanishi K, Yoshikawa N (2003) Genetic disorders of human congenital anomalies of the kidney and urinary tract (CAKUT). Pediatr Int 45(5):610–616

Neuhaus TJ, Berger C et al (2008) Randomised trial of oral versus sequential intravenous/oral cephalosporins in children with pyelonephritis. Eur J Pediatr 167(9):1037–1047

Neveus T, von Gontard A et al (2006) The standardization of terminology of lower urinary tract function in children and adolescents: report from the Standardisation Committee of the International Children's Continence Society. J Urol 176(1):314–324

Nicholson L, Smith DP (2007) Dysfunctional elimination syndrome. Where constipation, daytime urinary problems and bedwetting merge. Adv Nurse Pract 15(3):26–31; quiz 31–32

Noe HN (1996) Screening for reflux--the current status. J Urol 156(5):1808

Noe HN (2002) Scintigraphic screening for renal damage in siblings of children with asymptomatic primary vesico-ureteric reflux. BJU Int 89(7):792–793; author reply 793

Nuutinen M, Uhari M (2001) Recurrence and follow-up after urinary tract infection under the age of 1 year. Pediatr Nephrol 16(1):69–72

O'Regan S, Yazbeck S (1985) Constipation: a cause of enuresis, urinary tract infection and vesico-ureteral reflux in children. Med Hypotheses 17(4):409–413

O'Regan S, Yazbeck S et al (1985) Constipation, bladder instability, urinary tract infection syndrome. Clin Nephrol 23(3):152–154

Ozen S, Alikasifoglu M et al (1999) Implications of certain genetic polymorphisms in scarring in vesicoureteric reflux: importance of ACE polymorphism. Am J Kidney Dis 34(1):140–145

Pennesi M, Travan L et al (2008) Is antibiotic prophylaxis in children with vesicoureteral reflux effective in preventing pyelonephritis and renal scars? A randomized, controlled trial. Pediatrics 121(6):e1489–e1494

Peters CA, Skoog SJ et al (2010) Summary of the AUA Guideline on Management of Primary Vesicoureteral Reflux in Children. J Urol 184(3):1134–1144

Piercey KR, Khoury AE et al (1993) Diagnosis and management of urinary tract infections. Curr Opin Urol 3:25–29

Politano VA, Leadbetter WF (1958) An operative technique for the correction of vesicoureteral reflux. J Urol 79(6):932–941

Polito C, Rambaldi PF et al (2001) Unilateral vesicoureteric reflux: Low prevalence of contralateral renal damage. J Pediatr 138(6):875–879

Polito C, Rambaldi PF et al (2006) Permanent renal parenchymal defects after febrile UTI are closely associated with vesicoureteric reflux. Pediatr Nephrol 21(4):521–526

Preda I, Jodal U et al (2007) Normal dimercaptosuccinic acid scintigraphy makes voiding cystourethrography unnecessary after urinary tract infection. J Pediatr 151(6):581–584, 584.e1

Preda I, Jodal U et al (2010) Value of ultrasound in evaluation of infants with first urinary tract infection. J Urol 183(5):1984–1988

Preda I, Jodal U et al (2011) Imaging strategy for infants with urinary tract infection: a new algorithm. J Urol 185(3):1046–1052

Puri P, Pirker M et al (2006) Subureteral dextranomer/hyaluronic acid injection as first line treatment in the management of high grade vesicoureteral reflux. J Urol 176(4 Pt 2):1856–1859; discussion 1859–1860

Ransley PG, Risdon RA (1981) Reflux nephropathy: effects of antimicrobial therapy on the evolution of the early pyelonephritic scar. Kidney Int 20(6):733–742

Redman JF (1976) Vesicoureteral reflux in identical twins. J Urol 116(6):792–793

Riccabona M (2002) Cystography in infants and children: a critical appraisal of the many forms with special regard to voiding cystourethrography. Eur Radiol 12(12):2910–2918

Riccabona M, Avni FE et al (2008) Imaging recommendations in paediatric uroradiology: minutes of the ESPR workgroup session on urinary tract infection, fetal hydronephrosis, urinary tract ultrasonography and voiding cystourethrography, Barcelona, Spain, June 2007. Pediatr Radiol 38(2):138–145

Riedmiller H, Becht E et al (1984) Psoas-hitch ureteroneocystostomy: experience with 181 cases. Eur Urol 10(3):145–150

RIVUR Trial Investigators (2014) Antimicrobial Prophylaxis for Children with Vesicoureteral Reflux. N Engl J Med 370(25):2367–2376

Roussey-Kesler G, Gadjos V et al (2008) Antibiotic prophylaxis for the prevention of recurrent urinary tract infection in children with low grade vesicoureteral reflux: results from a prospective randomized study. J Urol 179(2):674–679; discussion 679

Rushton HG (1997) The evaluation of acute pyelonephritis and renal scarring with technetium 99m-dimercaptosuccinic acid renal scintigraphy: evolving concepts and future directions. Pediatr Nephrol 11(1):108–120

Rushton HG, Majd M (1992) Pyelonephritis in male infants: how important is the foreskin? J Urol 148(2 Pt 2):733–736; discussion 737–738

Saadeh SA, Mattoo TK (2011) Managing urinary tract infections. Pediatr Nephrol 26(11):1967–1976

Sargent MA (2000) What is the normal prevalence of vesicoureteral reflux? Pediatr Radiol 30(9):587–593

Sastre JB, Aparicio AR et al (2007) Urinary tract infection in the newborn: clinical and radio imaging studies. Pediatr Nephrol 22(10):1735–1741

Sathapornwajana P, Dissaneewate P et al (2008) Timing of voiding cystourethrogram after urinary tract infection. Arch Dis Child 93(3):229–231

Schlager TA, Hendley JO et al (1995) Explanation for false-positive urine cultures obtained by bag technique. Arch Pediatr Adolesc Med 149(2):170–173

Shaikh N, Hoberman A et al (2003) Dysfunctional elimination syndrome: is it related to urinary tract infection or vesicoureteral reflux diagnosed early in life? Pediatrics 112(5):1134–1137

Shaikh N, Morone NE et al (2007) Does this child have a urinary tract infection? JAMA 298(24):2895–2904

Shaikh N, Morone NE et al (2008) Prevalence of urinary tract infection in childhood: a meta-analysis. Pediatr Infect Dis J 27(4):302–308

Shimizu M, Katayama K et al (2005) Evolution of acute focal bacterial nephritis into a renal abscess. Pediatr Nephrol 20(1):93–95

Shiraishi K, Yoshino K et al (2010) Risk factors for breakthrough infection in children with primary vesicoureteral reflux. J Urol 183(4):1527–1531

Sillen U (1999) Vesicoureteral reflux in infants. Pediatr Nephrol 13(4):355–361

Simoes e Silva AC, Silva JM et al (2007) Risk of hypertension in primary vesicoureteral reflux. Pediatr Nephrol 22(3):459–462

Singh-Grewal D, Macdessi J et al (2005) Circumcision for the prevention of urinary tract infection in boys: a systematic review of randomised trials and observational studies. Arch Dis Child 90(8):853–858

Siomou E, Giapros V et al (2009) Implications of 99mTc-DMSA scintigraphy performed during urinary tract infection in neonates. Pediatrics 124(3):881–887

Slotki IN, Asscher AW (1982) Prevention of scarring in experimental pyelonephritis in the rat by early antibiotic therapy. Nephron 30(3):262–268

Smellie JM, Normand IC (1979) Reflux Nephropathy in Childhood. In: Hodson J, Kincaid-Smith P (eds) Reflux Nephropathy. Masson Publishing USA, New York, pp 14–20

Smellie JM, Edwards D et al (1975) VUR and renal scarring. Kidney Int 8:65–72

Smellie JM, Ransley PG et al (1985) Development of new renal scars: a collaborative study. Br Med J (Clin Res Ed) 290(6486):1957–1960

Smellie JM, Tamminen-Mobius T et al (1992) Five-year study of medical or surgical treatment in children with severe reflux: radiological renal findings. The International Reflux Study in Children. Pediatr Nephrol 6(3):223–230

Snodgrass W (1991) Relationship of voiding dysfunction to urinary tract infection and vesicoureteral reflux in children. Urology 38(4):341–344

Song SH, Lee SB et al (2007) Is antibiotic prophylaxis necessary in infants with obstructive hydronephrosis? J Urol 177(3):1098–1101; discussion 1101

Spencer JD, Schwaderer A et al (2010) Pediatric urinary tract infections: an analysis of hospitalizations, charges, and costs in the USA. Pediatr Nephrol 25(12):2469–2475

Steiss JO, Hamscho N et al (2014) Renal carbuncle and perirenal abscess in children and adolescents. Urologe A

Swerkersson S, Jodal U et al (2007) Relationship among vesicoureteral reflux, urinary tract infection and renal damage in children. J Urol 178(2):647–651; discussion 650–1

Tekgul S, Riedmiller H et al (2012) EAU Guidelines on Vesicoureteral Reflux in Children. Eur Urol 62(3):534–542

Thompson RH, Chen JJ et al (2001) Cessation of prophylactic antibiotics for managing persistent vesicoureteral reflux. J Urol 166(4):1465–1469

Thompson M, Simon SD et al (2005) Timing of follow-up voiding cystourethrogram in children with primary vesicoureteral reflux: development and application of a clinical algorithm. Pediatrics 115(2):426–434

Tokgoz H, Tan MO et al (2007) Assessment of urinary symptoms in children with dysfunctional elimination syndrome. Int Urol Nephrol 39(2):425–436

Tsai JD, Huang FY et al (1998) Asymptomatic vesicoureteral reflux detected by neonatal ultrasonographic screening. Pediatr Nephrol 12(3):206–209

Tullus K (2011) Difficulties in diagnosing urinary tract infections in small children. Pediatr Nephrol 26(11):1923–1926

Ulman I, Jayanthi VR et al (2000) The long-term followup of newborns with severe unilateral hydronephrosis initially treated nonoperatively. J Urol 164(3 Pt 2):1101–1105

Vaillancourt S, McGillivray D et al (2007) To clean or not to clean: effect on contamination rates in midstream urine collections in toilet-trained children. Pediatrics 119(6):e1288–e1293

Van den Abbeele AD, Treves ST et al (1987) Vesicoureteral reflux in asymptomatic siblings of patients with known reflux: radionuclide cystography. Pediatrics 79(1):147–153

Vernon SJ, Coulthard MG et al (1997) New renal scarring in children who at age 3 and 4 years had had normal scans with dimercaptosuccinic acid: follow up study. BMJ 315(7113):905–908

Wallace DM, Rothwell DL et al (1978) The long-term follow-up of surgically treated vesicoureteric reflux. Br J Urol 50(7):479–484

Walsh TJ, Hsieh S et al (2007) Antenatal hydronephrosis and the risk of pyelonephritis hospitalization during the first year of life. Urology 69(5):970–974

Wennerstrom M, Hansson S et al (2000) Primary and acquired renal scarring in boys and girls with urinary tract infection. J Pediatr 136(1):30–34

Westenfelder M, Beetz R (2010) Diagnostic work-up of urinary tract infections in children. In: Naber K, Schaeffer AJ, Hynes CF (eds) Urogenital infections. European Association of Urology

Wettergren B, Fasth A et al (1980) UTI during the first year of life in a Göteborg area 1977–79. Pediatr Res 14:981

Williams G, Fletcher JT et al (2008) Vesicoureteral reflux. J Am Soc Nephrol 19(5):847–862

Williams GJ, Macaskill P et al (2010) Absolute and relative accuracy of rapid urine tests for urinary tract infection in children: a meta-analysis. Lancet Infect Dis 10(4):240–250

Winberg J (1990) What antibiotics should be used for prophylaxis against recurrent urinary tract infections in childhood? Pediatr Nephrol 4:244

Winberg J (1994) Management of primary vesico-ureteric reflux in children--operation ineffective in preventing progressive renal damage. Infection 22(Suppl 1):S4–S7

Winberg J, Andersen HJ et al (1974) Epidemiology of symptomatic urinary tract infection in childhood. Acta Paediatr Scand Suppl (252):1–20

Winberg J, Bergstrom T et al (1975) Morbidity, age and sex distribution, recurrences and renal scarring in symptomatic urinary tract infection in childhood. Kidney Int Suppl 4:S101–S106

Wingerter S, Bachur R (2011) Risk factors for contamination of catheterized urine specimens in febrile children. Pediatr Emerg Care 27(1):1–4

Wiswell TE, Hachey WE (1993) Urinary tract infections and the uncircumcised state: an update. Clin Pediatr (Phila) 32(3):130–134

Wiswell TE, Miller GM et al (1988) Effect of circumcision status on periurethral bacterial flora during the first year of life. J Pediatr 113(3):442–446

Yeung CK, Godley ML et al (1997) The characteristics of primary vesico-ureteric reflux in male and female infants with pre-natal hydronephrosis. Br J Urol 80(2):319–327

Yeung CK, Sreedhar B et al (2006) Renal and bladder functional status at diagnosis as predictive factors for the outcome of primary vesicoureteral reflux in children. J Urol 176(3):1152–1156; discussion 1156–1157

Zorc JJ, Kiddoo DA et al (2005a) Diagnosis and management of pediatric urinary tract infections. Clin Microbiol Rev 18(2):417–422

Zorc JJ, Levine DA et al (2005b) Clinical and demographic factors associated with urinary tract infection in young febrile infants. Pediatrics 116(3):644–648

Congenital Urinary Tract Dilatation and Obstructive Uropathy

Josef Oswald and Bernhard Haid

Contents

1 Epidemiology and Natural Course of Prenatally Detected Urinary Tract Dilatation.................. 243

2 Etiology and Pathophysiology....................... 244
2.1 Pelvic-Ureteric Junction Obstruction............... 246
2.2 Obstruction at the Ureterovesical Junction ("Obstructive Megaureter")........................... 247
2.3 Subvesical Obstruction and UTD (Posterior Urethral Valves)... 247
2.4 Vesicoureteral Reflux (VUR) and UTD............ 248
2.5 Clinical Signs of Obstructive PCD.................. 248

3 Imaging from the Point of View of a Pediatric Urologist: What Is Most Important?... 249
3.1 Use of Grading Systems................................. 249

4 Treatment... 249
4.1 Antibiotic Prophylaxis.................................... 250
4.2 Pyeloplasty and Ureteral Reimplantation......... 250
4.3 Interventional Treatment................................ 251
4.4 Important Aspects for Postoperative Imaging... 251

Conclusion.. 252

References.. 252

1 Epidemiology and Natural Course of Prenatally Detected Urinary Tract Dilatation

The reported incidence of upper urinary tract dilatation (UTD) is 1–5.4% of all pregnancies, dependent on the diagnostic criteria that are being applied, accounting to 60–120,000 children being diagnosed per year in the USA (Mallik and Watson 2008). Of these, around 25% are persistent throughout birth (Barbosa et al. 2012). Sonographically detected intrauterine UTD can be observed in varying degrees in the 18th to 20th week of gestation. A prognostic cutoff level of prenatally diagnosed UTD on the basis of many studies has been determined; the risk of a significant UTDs after birth was linked to its prenatal manifestation (Nguyen et al. 2010): Whereas children with an anteroposterior renal pelvis diameter of ≥15 mm have a risk of 75% of persistence after birth, in children with an anteroposterior renal pelvis diameter of ≤9 mm, it amounts to only 10% (Benfield et al. 2003). The risk for later surgery is connected also with the grade of the prenatal urinary tract dilatation (Fig. 1).

In 2014 a new classification system of pre- and postnatal UTD has been presented as a result of a consensus meeting of members of major mostly American societies in the field in order to unify previously often differing descriptions of UTD (Nguyen et al. 2014). The participating societies included American College of

J. Oswald, FEAPU (✉) • B. Haid, FEAPU
Department of Pediatric Urology, Hospital of the Sisters of Charity, Linz, Austria
e-mail: josef.oswald@bhs.at

Fig. 1 Risk of surgery of antenatal detected urinary tract dilatation (Barbosa et al. 2012)

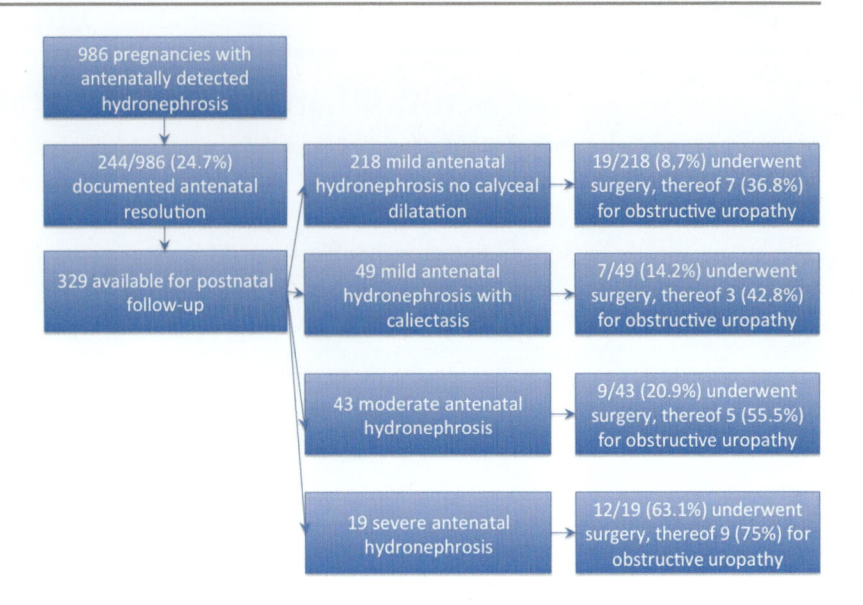

- 986 pregnancies with antenatally detected hydronephrosis
  - 244/986 (24.7%) documented antenatal resolution
  - 329 available for postnatal follow-up
- 218 mild antenatal hydronephrosis no calyceal dilatation → 19/218 (8,7%) underwent surgery, thereof 7 (36.8%) for obstructive uropathy
- 49 mild antenatal hydronephrosis with caliectasis → 7/49 (14.2%) underwent surgery, thereof 3 (42.8%) for obstructive uropathy
- 43 moderate antenatal hydronephrosis → 9/43 (20.9%) underwent surgery, thereof 5 (55.5%) for obstructive uropathy
- 19 severe antenatal hydronephrosis → 12/19 (63.1%) underwent surgery, thereof 9 (75%) for obstructive uropathy

Radiology, the American Institute of Ultrasound in Medicine, the American Society of Pediatric Nephrology, the Society for Fetal Urology, the Society for Maternal-Fetal Medicine, the Society for Pediatric Urology, the Society for Pediatric Radiology, and the Society of Radiologists in Ultrasound. The proposed UTD classification system is based on six categories: (1) anteroposterior renal pelvic diameter, (2) calyceal dilation, (3) renal parenchymal thickness, (4) renal parenchymal appearance, (5) bladder abnormalities, and (6) ureteral abnormalities. The classification system is stratified based on gestational age and whether the UT dilation is detected prenatally or postnatally. The panel also proposed a follow-up scheme based on the UTD classification and its evolution during follow-up examinations (Fig. 2a, b).

In the European ESPT-task force grading scheme, the wording has also been adapted in 2015 and renamed to "pelvicalyceal dilatation/distension (PCD)" instead of "hydronephrosis (HN)," to be consistent with the new standardized terminology, but this scheme intends only to offer a descriptive sonographic grading for postnatal pelvicalyceal appearance not linked with prognostic or therapeutic aspects. The criteria were left unchanged. Obstructive uropathies account for 12.9% of all pediatric kidney transplantations and 23.1% of all pediatric chronic renal failures being the main cause of end-stage renal disease in children (Benfield et al. 2003). Selecting patients with a clear indication for surgical intervention is difficult due to the high variability in the degree of obstruction and the extent of damage as well as the differential function of the affected kidney.

> **Take Away**
> Antenatal diagnosed UTD can be detected after the 18th week of gestation, with an anteroposterior renal pelvis diameter of >15 mm having a 75% risk of persistence after birth. The new American UTD classification system is based on the anteroposterior renal pelvis diameter, calyceal dilatation, renal parenchymal thickness, renal parenchymal appearance, bladder abnormalities, and ureteral abnormalities.

2 Etiology and Pathophysiology

A sonographically dilated renal pelvis and/or calix does not necessarily mean that urinary outflow is impaired; in many patients with UTD, the dilated pelvis needs more time to empty due to a weaker contraction. A clinically significant obstruction should be defined as "any restriction to urinary outflow which, if left untreated, will

a

US parameters		Measurement/findings	Note
Anterior-Posterior Renal Pelvic Diameter (APRPD)		(mm)	Measured on transverse image at the maximal diameter of intrarenal pelvis
Calyceal dilation	Central (major calyces)	Yes/No	
	Peripheral (minor calyces)	Yes/No	
Parenchymal thickness		Normal/Abnormal	Subjective assessment
Parenchymal appearance		Normal/Abnormal	Evaluate echogenicity, corticomedullary differentiation, and for cortical cysts
Ureter		Normal/Abnormal	Dilation of ureter is considered abnormal; however, transient visualization of the ureter is considered normal postnatally
Bladder		Normal/Abnormal	Evaluate wall thickness, for the presence of ureterocele, and for a dilated posterior urethra

b

Ultrasound findings	Time at presentation		
	16–27 weeks	≥28 weeks	Postnatal (>48 h)
Anterior-Posterior Renal Pelvis Diameter (APRPD)	<4 mm	<7 mm	<10 mm
Calyceal dilation			
Central	No	No	No
Peripheral	No	No	No
Parenchymal thickness	Normal	Normal	Normal
Parenchymal appearance	Normal	Normal	Normal
Ureter (s)	Normal	Normal	Normal
Bladder	Normal	Normal	Normal
Unexplained oligohydramnios	No	No	NA

Fig. 2 (**a, b**) Tables to illustrate the UTD classification (Nguyen et al. 2014)

lead to progressive renal deterioration" (Klein et al. 2011).

There are a variety of possible underlying etiologies that possibly manifest as antenatally detected UTD (Fig. 3).

Whereas this figure demonstrates the different etiologies, the percentage of significant pelviureteric junction (PUJ) obstruction remains a matter of definition; in the underlying publications, it is defined as children that ultimately underwent surgery.

PCD is a descriptive sonomorphologic term and is defined as pathological with an anteroposterior renal pelvis diameter of >7 mm at birth and of >10 mm under 1 year of age (Riccabona et al. 2008). However, the definition of normal values for the anteroposterior pelvis remains open to discussion and depends on many factors such as renal function and patient hydration, and in a recent standardization publication by a multidisciplinary consensus board, a normal value of <10 mm at birth has been postulated (Chow and Darge 2015).

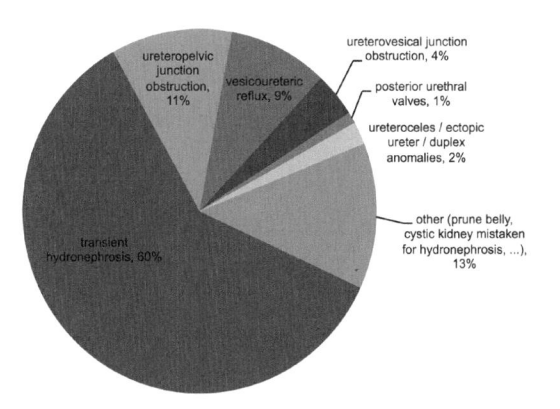

Fig. 3 Etiology of antenatally detected UTD (Sinha et al. 2013)

Both animal models and examinations in humans after pyeloplasty demonstrate that renal damage seems to be caused by complex mechanisms ultimately leading to tubular damage. The main cause, the increased intrapelvic and intrarenal pressure, is compensated first by dilatation and relaxation of the renal pelvis. In the phase of decompensation, inflammatory markers and cytokines lead to structural changes in the ureteric and pelvic wall. Generally, the earlier the onset of obstruction occurs and the longer it persists, the higher the probability of irreversible functional damage gets (Klein et al. 2011). There are, however, reports on recovering renal function also after delayed pyeloplasty in infants, pointing at a possible relevance of renal repair mechanisms and possible postnatal differentiation of nephrons during early life (Chertin et al. 2002).

2.1 Pelvic-Ureteric Junction Obstruction

The most common cause for persistent PCD in children that ultimately undergo surgical treatment is a stenosis at the PUJ reducing the urinary flow from the renal pelvis to the ureter. It is difficult to establish a definite diagnosis of "obstruction" and in particular to indicate a surgical intervention; this additionally may require long-term experience. It is a fact that seemingly relevant obstructions, confirmed by sonographic follow-up and scintigraphic (Tc^{99} MAGIII, mercaptoacetyltriglycine or diuretic renograms) investigations, can resolve spontaneously. In contrast, an apparently mild UTD without signs of significant obstruction can eventually evolve to a relevant situation, endangering kidney function.

2.1.1 Intrinsic Stenosis

Essentially there are two groups of patients: on the one hand, the obstruction is caused by a fibrotic, narrow aperistaltic subpelvic ureteric segment ("intrinsic stenosis"). This hypoplastic adynamic ureteral segment at the PUJ consists of reduced numbers of smooth muscle cells with an increase of collagen and extracellular matrix, respectively (Fig. 4).

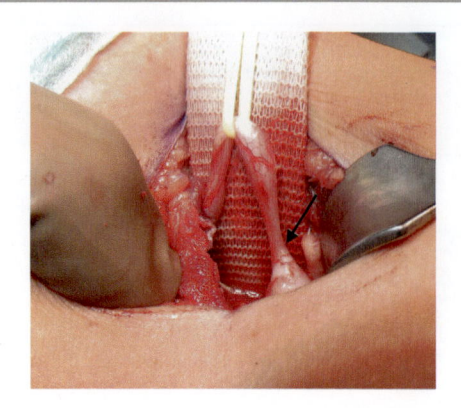

Fig. 4 Adynamic ureteral segment (*arrow*) at the PUJ

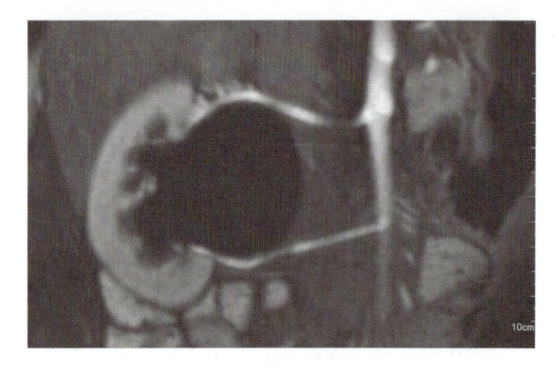

Fig. 5 Extrinsic factor: lower pole vessel of the right kidney (MRI)

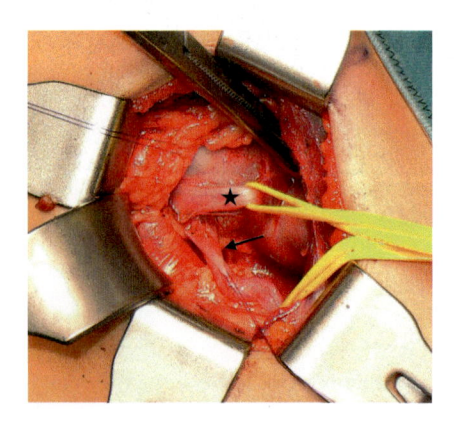

Fig. 6 Extrinsic factor: lower pole vessel (*arrow*), ureter (*asterisk*)

2.1.2 Extrinsic Stenosis

On the other hand, there are extrinsic obstructions: the ureter could be compressed by an aberrant lower pole vessel which supplies the lower pole of the kidney (Figs. 5 and 6). The ureter can also be angulated and distorted, e.g., in high-grade vesicoureteral reflux (VUR) by distinct kinking and tissue adhesions to the pelvis.

An interesting and highly relevant variant is the so-called high inserting ureter, possibly secondarily caused on the basis of the "Brödel effect": An initially orthotropic ureteral insertion into the renal pelvis is transposed upward, by filling a dilated renal pelvis, leading to an often marked obstruction and a long stenotic ureteral segment.

2.2 Obstruction at the Ureterovesical Junction ("Obstructive Megaureter")

Obstruction at the ureterovesical junction (UVJ) is a rarer cause of PCD and – primarily – leads to a ureteral dilatation. Ureters, dilated to more than 7 mm diameter prevesically, are megaureters by definition (Farrugia et al. 2014). The pathophysiology of this condition has been studied extensively leading to insights into the embryological development of the Wolffian ducts, however, not actually explaining why obstruction and/or VUR emerges, sometimes in combination (Oswald et al. 2004). Megaureters can be classified into refluxing, non-refluxing/non-obstructive, obstructive (Fig. 7), and secondary dilated due to an infravesical obstruction or neurogenic bladder (Fig. 8).

Distal ureteral obstruction can be linked as well to the presence of a duplex kidney, where predominantly the upper pole system can present with a relevant UTD. Mainly those obstructed ureters are ectopic or associated with a ureterocele (Meyer-Weigert rule) which correspond to the upper pole moiety (Meyer 1907 and Weigert 1877). In large, ectopic (80%) ureteroceles, the lower pole – lateralized – orifice lies upon the ureteroceles and can present as a refluxing or an obstructed system as well.

2.3 Subvesical Obstruction and UTD (Posterior Urethral Valves)

Subvesical obstruction may lead to secondary ureteral dilatation and UTD, usually in combination with (high grade) VUR. The most common cause of subvesical obstructions in male children is posterior urethral valves (PUV). They are present in one of 8000–25,000 male births and, depending on the severity of obstruction, may eventually lead to renal insufficiency.

The mainly used pathological classification of PUV has been published by Young et al. in 1919.

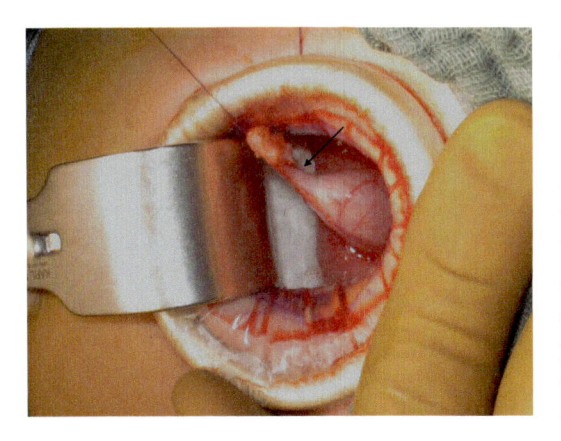

Fig. 7 Obstructive megaureter with narrow distal segment (*arrow*)

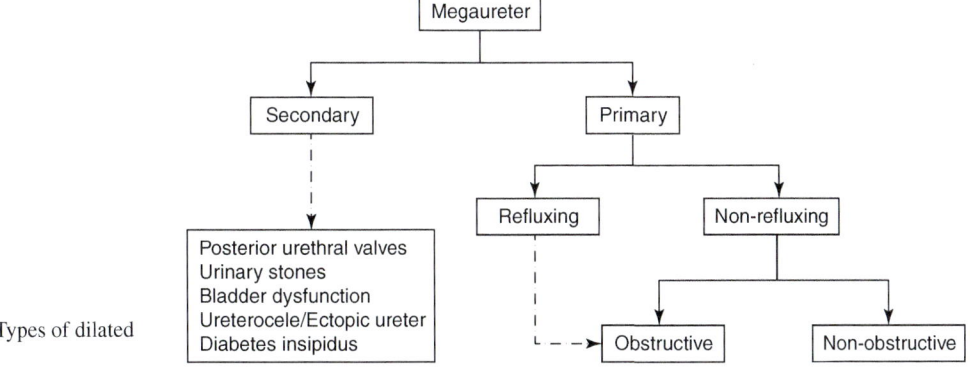

Fig. 8 Types of dilated ureters

Whereas they initially proposed three types of PUV, only type one (bicuspid valves that usually originate on the floor of the urethra arising from the distal lateral aspect of the verumontanum and extend distally and anteriorly to fuse at the midline) and type three are still in use (a membrane, distal to the verumontanum and lying transversely across the urethra, with a small perforation near its center).

The presence of subvesical obstruction often affects the whole urinary tract, with giant HN and renal function impairment as well as pulmonary hypoplasia already before birth. There are, however, also less severe variants, presenting perior postnatally with some grade of UTD or VUR of varying grade. In some boys, valves are only detected at age of 5–8 years in the course of evaluation of bladder emptying disorders. In this context, whereas the concept of so-called mini-valves is heavily discussed, there is no doubt to the fact that later detected and anatomically not/less important valves can have a big functional impact, warranting exact diagnosis and treatment.

The challenge in diagnosis of PUV remains the low sensitivity of VCUG for minor forms and the importance of indirect signs as, for example, hypertrophy of the internal sphincter and alterations of the bladder anatomy as trabeculation or diverticula, as well as secondary VUR.

A subvesical obstruction caused by a PUV that can be presented clinically as VURD syndrome (posterior urethral valve, unilateral vesicoureteral reflux, renal dysplasia) (Hoover and Duckett 1982) is accompanied by high-grade VUR and renal dysplasia (RD) at least on one side and low-grade VUR on the contralateral side in patients with a severely compromised renal function if available (Greenfield et al. 1983). The high-grade VUR serves as pressure pop-off, probably protecting the contralateral kidney.

2.4 Vesicoureteral Reflux (VUR) and UTD

A VCUG (or a contrast-enhanced voiding urosonography = ce-VUS; for details see chapter "Diagnostic Procedures: Excluding MRI, Nuclear Medicine and Video Urodynamics") is required in suspected high-grade VUR as well as in children with (upper, recurrent) urinary tract infections and UTD. The combination of both VUR and real PUJ obstruction, possibly secondary to the VUR, is not uncommon and should be kept in mind. Secondary PUJ obstruction may be caused in these children due to chronic dilatation of the renal pelvis or recurrent inflammatory changes at the PUJ, leading to either anatomical or functional PUJ obstruction (Bomalaski et al. 1997).

2.5 Clinical Signs of Obstructive PCD

The majority of newborns and infants with a significant congenital PUJ narrowing present without any symptoms, neither clinically nor para-clinically. Because of the immaturity of the newborn kidney, it is therefore all the more important to postnatally repeat the ultrasound (US) examination 7–10 days after birth to properly evaluate the extent of the postnatal PCD. Due to the fact that general symptoms, such as poor growth, refusal to feed, vomiting, etc., are usually not observed in these infants with (this asymptomatic) PCD, we recommend a postnatal US around day eight after birth in every newborn with fetal UTD or in every newborn – if no proper fetal US screening is in place – in order to detect any unknown obstruction and to prevent consecutive damage to the affected kidney. An undiagnosed as well as untreated significant PUJ stenosis results in a severely damaged and sometimes even nonfunctional "hydronephrotic" kidney; children with a bilateral PUJ obstruction are particularly at risk of end-stage renal insufficiency.

Take Away
More than 60% of pre- and postnatally diagnosed PCDs are of temporary nature only. The vast majority of clinical significant obstructions are caused by a stenosis at the PUJ. This stricture results from

a congenital dysplastic ureteral segment (intrinsic stenosis) or from an aberrant crossing vessel (extrinsic stenosis). Surgical corrections for stenosis at the UVJ (obstructive megaureters) are rarely indicated; the vast majority of megaureters disappear in time (spontaneous maturation). Other reasons of PCD with dilated ureters are primary (congenital) or secondary VUR. Secondary VUR could be caused by a neurogenic (hypertonic, low compliant bladder, e.g., in myelomeningocele) or by an infravesical obstruction in boys due to posterior PUV.

3 Imaging from the Point of View of a Pediatric Urologist: What Is Most Important?

The main focus in diagnosing persistent UTD in newborns and infants should be detecting significant obstructions requiring surgery. The following examinations are available for evaluating infant UTD:

- US (after birth, e.g., 8 days and 4–6 weeks postnatally)
- Voiding cystourethrography (VCUG) in grade III and IV HN (or ce-VUS)
- Diuretic renography (Tc^{99} MAG III clearance – F+20 protocol)
- (Dynamic functional or anatomic) MR urography (MRU) in selected cases

The essential investigation to evaluate renal split (differential) function as well as drainage from the upper urinary tract is a Tc99 MAG3 diuretic renography with application of furosemide 20mins after injection of the tracer. Essential for an estimation of a significant obstruction are images at 60 and 120 min, also following micturition or after position changes to allow for effects of gravity. Similar information can be retrieved from functional dynamic-diuretic MRU (Gordon et al. 2011; Jones et al. 2011)

3.1 Use of Grading Systems

Grading systems for UTD and PCD are of importance in risk stratification and assessment of the further prognosis. Currently the Society for Fetal Urology (SFU) grading system as well as the adapted grading system from the European Society of Pediatric Radiology (ESPR) Uroradiology Task Force for PCD in childhood is the mainly used classification for UTD; in the USA, the new UTD consensus scheme is being promoted (Fernbach et al. 1993; Riccabona et al. 2008a, b, 2016; Nguyen et al. 2014) (Fig. 9 and Fig. 7 in chapter "Normal Values").

Also, the measurement of the intraparenchymal anteroposterior renal pelvic diameter is of great importance in grading PCD. An AP diameter greater than 7 mm at 8–23 weeks of gestation, greater than 10 mm during the last trimester, and greater than 12 mm at birth should be considered as abnormal. As to its prognostic value, Dhillon followed a great number of children with PCD and found that while virtually all of those with AP diameters greater than 40 mm required surgery, only 11% of those with AP diameters less than 20 mm needed surgical intervention (Dhillon 1998). In between 20 and 30 mm, 40% of children deteriorate with renal function and require a pyeloplasty.

> **Take Away**
> To evaluate infant PCD, the following examinations are recommended: US, VCUG (or ce-VUS), diuretic renography, and in selected patients (functional) MR urography. The most commonly used sonographic classification for PCD is the (adapted) SFU grading system (SFU/ESPR grade 1–4/5), potentially to be partially replaced by the new American UTD classification system if it proves to be workable and beneficial.

4 Treatment

Treatment options for a congenital UTD comprise usually of conservative observation, long-term use of antibiotics, as well as reconstructive surgery

PCD°I (SFU I°)	PCD°II (SFU II°)	PCD°III (SFU III°)	PCD°IV (SFU IV°)
slight splitting of the central renal complex without calyceal involvement, normal parenchyma	splitting of the central renal complex with extenstion to non-dilated calyces	wide splitting of the renal pelvis, dilated outside the renal border, calyces uniformly dilated, normal parenchyma	large dilated calyces, thinning of the parenchyma ≤ 50% of the ipsilateral (normal) kidney

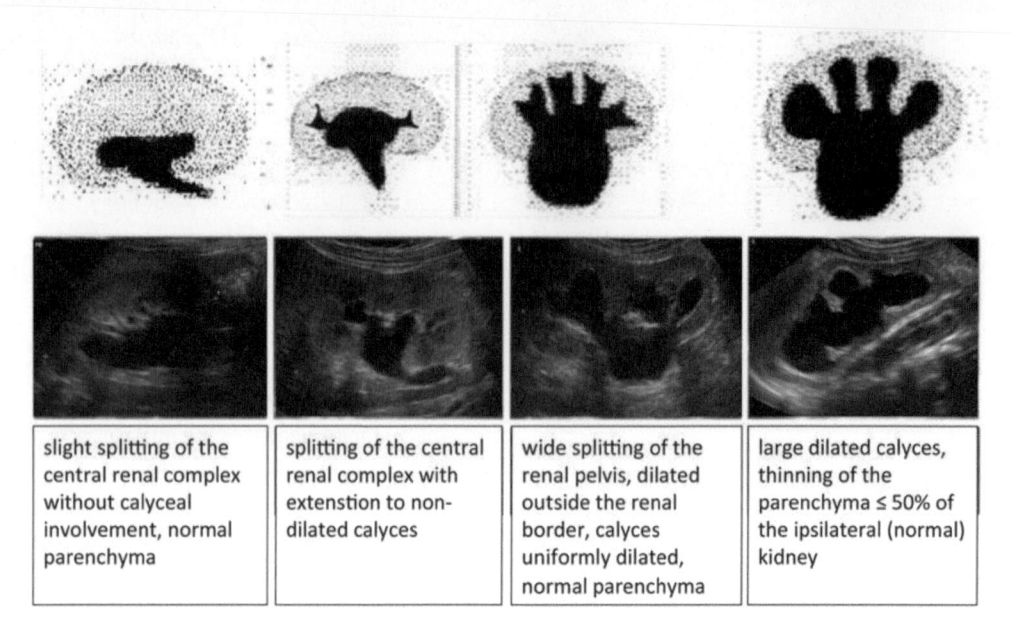

Fig. 9 Adapted SFU grading system (based on the recent ESPR recommendations) for urinary tract dilatation (Modified from Timberlake and Herndon 2013). Note that PCD V° is sometimes used for severe distention (PCD°IV) with only a rim-like residual parenchyma (no corresponding grading in the SFU system)

releasing the subpelvic or prevesical stenotic segment or antireflux surgery in reflexive ureters.

4.1 Antibiotic Prophylaxis

Antibiotic prophylaxis is still partially considered required for UTD associated with ureteral dilatation or known VUR, where it has been shown to diminish the frequency of urinary tract infections significantly (Hoberman et al. 2014). In megaureters, antibiotic prophylaxis reduces the risk for a febrile urinary tract infection during the first 6 months of life for 88% and in the second half of the first year of life for 55% (Gimpel et al. 2010).

4.2 Pyeloplasty and Ureteral Reimplantation (See also Chapter "Surgical Procedures and Indications for Surgery")

The indication for pyeloplasty mainly relies on sequential imaging particularly on deteriorating differential renal function (DRF) in PUJ obstruction and progressive renal scarring as well as recurrent urinary tract infections with a lack of spontaneous maturation in UVJ obstruction and VUR. It is generally accepted that a DRF below 40% or deterioration for more than 5% represents an indication for intervention.

For PUJ obstruction, the dismembered Anderson-Hynes pyeloplasty with – if present – reallocation of crossing vessels to the posterior aspect of the PUJ remains the gold standard, with success rates as high as 98%. In older children laparoscopic of robotic surgery may be an option, while in small children the open retroperitoneal access through a small incision remains the best option.

In UVJ obstruction and VUR, different techniques of antirefluxive ureteral reimplantations are possible. For severely dilated ureters, tailoring (Hendren) or tapering is a necessity in order to assure a non-refluxing implantation. The minimal invasive VUR therapy is defined as the endoscopic injection of bulking agents (usually dextranomer/hyaluronic acid copolymer – Deflux®) and indicated in children with non-dilating VUR.

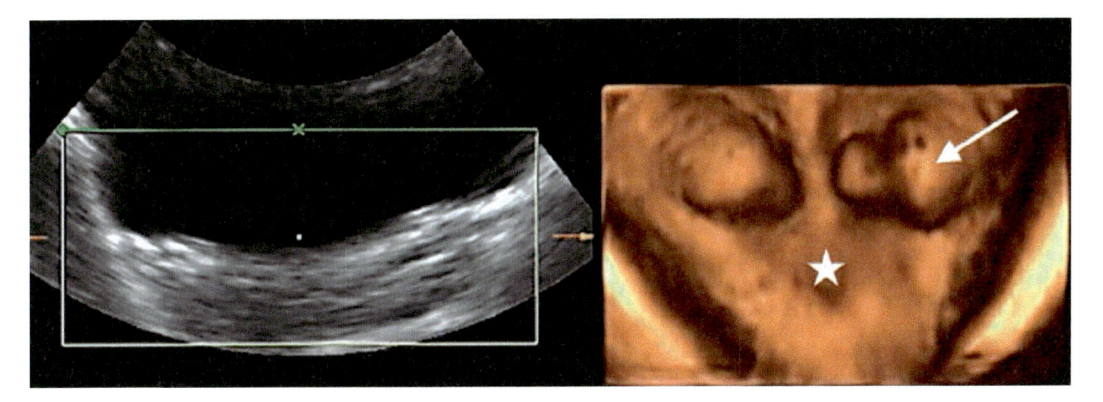

Fig. 10 Postoperative 3D real-time US after endoscopic treatment of VUR. *Arrow*: Beginning lateral shifting of the left Deflux depot. *Asterisk*: Bladder neck

4.3 Interventional Treatment

As well for PUJ obstruction as for UVJ obstruction, interventional treatments have been suggested, mainly comprising balloon dilatation or incision of the narrow segments. These approaches, however, involve a high risk of recurrence and complication (e.g., VUR in UVJ obstruction) and cannot be regarded as standard options.

4.4 Important Aspects for Postoperative Imaging

The role of postoperative imaging is (a) to assess potential complications, (b) to validate the success of the procedure, and (c) to monitor further development. Postoperative US and diuretic renography represent the most important diagnostic tools after pyeloplasty. Despite improvement of drainage a marked dilatation of the renal pelvis, similar to the preoperative finding, may be found for several weeks after a successful pyeloplasty; surgical reduction of the dilated pelvis is rarely indicated – but if performed the reduced pelvic diameter does not necessarily indicate success. An accurate assessment of renal function as well as improved drainage is valid only with diuretic renography (or fMRU) which usually is performed 6 months after operation. Only in severe persistent HN, the isotope evaluation should be preferred at an earlier date. Only if these diagnostic tools technically are not available an intravenous urogram with adapted exposure time and reduced contrast agent could be indicated (ALARA: As Low As Reasonably Achievable; Persliden et al. 2004).

After endoscopic treatment of VUR, a postoperative 3D real-time US demonstrates reliably the exact position of the bulking agent as well as the localization of the orifice – if US is combined with color Doppler (Riccabona et al. 2008a, b; Pichler et al. 2011). Any shifting of the bulking agent can be documented immediately after the operation as well as during follow-up (Fig. 10).

Because of the coaptation of the ureteral wall after injection of the bulking agent especially with the hydrodistention implantation technique, a transient dilatation of the upper urinary tract with megaureter and temporary PCD is common. Later in life bulking agents develop a kind of tissue compression which might be confused with a bladder stone.

For further details, see also chapters "Surgical Procedures and Indications for Surgery", "Upper Urinary Tract Dilatation in Newborns and Infants and the Postnatal Work-Up of Congenital Uro-nephropathies", "Vesicoureteric Reflux", and "Postoperative Imaging and Findings" – as well as "Clinical Management of Common Nephrourologic Disorders (Guidelines and Beyond)".

Take Away

Treatment options for a congenital UTD/PCD consist primarily of a conservative observation strategy. In children with megaureters as well as VUR, long-term use of antibiotics, at least in the first year of life, is still an option. In significant obstruction at the UPJ stenosis and much less at the UVJ (obstructive megaureter), an open – dismembered – pyeloplasty or ureteric reimplantation, respectively, is indicated. In VUR, in most cases an endoscopic minimal invasive therapy is adequate. Postoperative follow-up investigations include US and functional studies as Tc^{99m} MAG3 or fMRU studies. Transient postoperative PCD must be differentiated from significant postoperative obstruction as a complication after surgery.

Conclusion

From a pediatric urologist's point of view, assessment of UTD should be centered at prognostic and practical aspects, involving the use of adequate grading systems (SFU, ESPR, UTD, etc.). The knowledge of indirect signs for subvesical obstruction and on therapeutically implications or functional aspects should lead to a comprehensive assessment of the whole urinary tract.

References

Barbosa JA, Chow JS, Benson CB, Yorioka MA, Bull AS, Retik AB, Nguyen HT (2012) Postnatal longitudinal evaluation of children diagnosed with prenatal hydronephrosis: insights in natural history and referral pattern. Prenat Diagn 32(13):1242–1249

Benfield MR, McDonald RA, Bartosh S, Ho PL, Harmon W (2003) Changing trends in pediatric transplantation: 2001 Annual Report of the North American Pediatric Renal Transplant Cooperative Study. Pediatr Transplant 7(4):321–335

Bomalaski MD, Hirschl RB, Bloom DA (1997) Vesicoureteral reflux and ureteropelvic junction obstruction: association, treatment options and outcome. J Urol 157(3):969–974

Chertin B, Rolle U, Farkas A, Puri P (2002) Does delaying pyeloplasty affect renal function in children with a prenatal diagnosis of pelvi-ureteric junction obstruction? BJU Int 90(1):72–75

Chow JS, Darge K (2015) Multidisciplinary consensus on the classification of antenatal and postnatal urinary tract dilation (UTD classification system). Pediatr Radiol 13

Dhillon HK (1998) Prenatally diagnosed hydronephrosis: the Great Ormond Street experience. Br J Urol 81(Suppl 2):39–44

Farrugia MK, Hitchcock R, Radford A, Burki T, Robb A, Murphy F, British Association of Paediatric Urologists (2014) Urologists consensus statement on the management of the primary obstructive megaureter. J Pediatr Urol 10(1):26–33

Fernbach SK, Maizels M, Conway JJ (1993) Ultrasound grading of hydronephrosis: introduction to the system used by the Society for Fetal Urology. Pediatr Radiol 23:478–480

Gimpel C, Masioniene L, Djakovic N, Schenk JP, Haberkorn U, Tönshoff B, Schaefer F (2010) Complications and long-term outcome of primary obstructive megaureter in childhood. Pediatr Nephrol 25(9):1679–1686

Gordon I, Piepsz A, Sixt R, Auspices of Paediatric Committee of European Association of Nuclear Medicine (2011) Guidelines for standard and diuretic renogram in children. Eur J Nucl Med Mol Imaging 38(6):1175–1188

Greenfield SP, Hensle TW, Berdon WE, Wigger HJ (1983) Unilateral vesicoureteral reflux and unilateral nonfunctioning kidney associated with posterior urethral valves – a syndrome? J Urol 130:733

Hoover DL, Duckett JW Jr (1982) Posterior urethral valves, unilateral reflux and renal dysplasia: a syndrome. J Urol 128:994–997

Jones RA, Grattan-Smith JD, Little S (2011) Pediatric magnetic resonance urography. J Magn Reson Imaging 33(3):510–526

Klein J, Gonzalez J, Miravete M, Caubet C, Chaaya R, Decramer S, Bandin F, Bascands JL, Buffin-Meyer B, Schanstra JP (2011) Congenital ureteropelvic junction obstruction: human disease and animal models. Int J Exp Pathol 92(3):168–192

Mallik M, Watson AR (2008) Antenatally detected urinary tract abnormalities: more detection but less action. Pediatr Nephrol 23(6):897–904

Meyer R (1907) Zur Anatomie und Entwicklungsgeschichte der Ureterverdoppelung. Virchows Arch Pathol Anat Physiol Klin Med 87:408

Nguyen HT, Herndon CD, Cooper C, Gatti J, Kirsch A, Kokorowski P, Lee R, Perez-Brayfield M, Metcalfe P, Yerkes E, Cendron M, Campbell JB (2010) The Society for Fetal Urology consensus statement on the evaluation and management of antenatal hydronephrosis. J Pediatr Urol 6(3):212–231

Nguyen HT, Benson CB, Bromley B, Campbell JB, Chow J, Coleman B, Cooper C, Crino J, Darge K, Herndon CD, Odibo AO, Somers MJ, Stein DR (2014) Multidisciplinary consensus on the classification of prenatal and postnatal urinary tract dilation (UTD classification system). J Pediatr Urol 10(6): 982–998

Oswald J, Schwentner C, Brenner E, Deibl M, Fritsch H, Bartsch G, Radmayr C (2004) Extracellular matrix degradation and reduced nerve supply in refluxing ureteral endings. J Urol 172(3):1099–1102

Persliden J, Helmrot E, Hjort P et al (2004) Dose and image quality in the comparison of analogue and digital techniques in paediatric urology examinations. Eur Radiol 14:638–644

Pichler R, Buttazzoni A, Bektic J, Schlenck B, Radmayr C, Rehder P, Oswald J (2011) Endoscopic treatment of vesicoureteral reflux using dextranomer/hyaluronic acid copolymer in children: results of postoperative follow-up with real-time 3D sonography. Urol Int 87(2):192–198

Riccabona M, Pilhatsch A, Haberlik A, Ring E (2008a) Three-dimensional ultrasonography-based virtual cystoscopy of the pediatric urinary bladder: a preliminary report on feasibility and potential value. J Ultrasound Med 27(10):1453–1459

Riccabona M, Avni FE, Blickman JG, Dacher JN, Darge K, Lobo ML, Willi U (2008b) Imaging recommendations in paediatric uroradiology: minutes of the ESPR workgroup session on urinary tract infection, fetal hydronephrosis, urinary tract ultrasonography and voiding cystourethrography, Barcelona, Spain, June 2007. Pediatr Radiol 38(2):138–145

Riccabona M, Lobo ML, Ording-Muller LS, Augdal TA, Avni FE, Blickman J, Bruno C, Damasio BM, Darge K, Ntoulia A, Papadopoulou F, Vivier PH (2017) ESPR Abdominal (GU and GI) Imaging Task Force – Imaging Recommendations in Paediatric Uroradiology, Part IX: imaging in anorectal and cloacal malformation, imaging in childhood ovarian torsion, and efforts in standardising pediatric uroradiology terminology. Report on the mini-symposium at the ESPR meeting in Graz, June 2015. Pediatr Radiol (in press)

Sinha A, Bagga A, Krishna A, Bajpai M, Srinivas M, Uppal R, Agarwal I, Indian Society of Pediatric Nephrology (2013) Revised guidelines on management of antenatal hydronephrosis. Indian Pediatr 50(2):215–231

Timberlake MD, Herndon CD (2013) Mild to moderate postnatal hydronephrosis – grading systems and management. Nat Rev Urol 10(11):649–656

RIVUR Trial Investigators, Hoberman A, Greenfield SP, Mattoo TK, Keren R, Mathews R, Pohl HG, Kropp BP, Skoog SJ, Nelson CP, Moxey-Mims M, Chesney RW, Carpenter MA (2014) Antimicrobial prophylaxis for children with vesicoureteral reflux. N Engl J Med 370(25):2367–2376

Weigert C (1877) Über einige Bildungsfehler der Ureteren. Virchows Arch Pathol Anat Physiol Klin Med 70:490

Surgical Procedures and Indications for Surgery

Annette Schröder and Wolfgang H. Rösch

Contents

1 Introduction.. 256

2 **Pelvi-ureteric Junction (PUJ) Obstruction**.. 256
2.1 Findings and Indication for Surgery................ 256
2.2 Surgical Procedure... 256
2.3 Postoperative Image... 256
2.4 Possible Complications.................................... 256

3 **Megaureter/Ureterovesical Junction (UVJ) Obstruction**.. 257
3.1 Primary Megaureter... 257

4 **Vesicoureteral Reflux (VUR)**........................ 258
4.1 Findings and Indication for Surgery................ 258
4.2 Surgical Procedures... 258
4.3 Postoperative Imaging..................................... 258
4.4 Possible Complications.................................... 259

5 **Posterior Urethral Valves (PUVs)**................ 259
5.1 Findings and Indication for Surgery................ 259
5.2 Surgical Procedure... 261
5.3 Postoperative Image... 261
5.4 Possible Complications.................................... 261

6 **Ureteroceles**... 261
6.1 Findings and Indication for Surgery................ 261
6.2 Surgical Procedure... 262
6.3 Postoperative Imaging..................................... 262
6.4 Possible Complications.................................... 262

7 **Duplex Systems with Ectopic Ureter**........... 263
7.1 Findings... 263
7.2 Imaging.. 263
7.3 Surgical Approaches.. 263
7.4 Postoperative Imaging..................................... 263

8 **Renal Trauma**.. 263
8.1 Findings and Indications for Imaging............. 263
8.2 Imaging Renal Trauma.................................... 264
8.3 Clinical Management and Surgical Procedures... 264
8.4 Postoperative/Follow-Up Imaging.................. 264
8.5 Possible Complications.................................... 264

9 **Testes**... 265
9.1 Undescended Testes (UDT)............................. 265
9.2 Imaging.. 265
9.3 Surgery... 265
9.4 Postoperative/Follow-Up Imaging.................. 265
9.5 Possible Complications.................................... 265

10 **Urolithiasis**... 266
10.1 Kidney Stones.. 266
10.2 Imaging.. 266
10.3 Indications for Treatment................................ 266
10.4 Possible Complications.................................... 266

Conclusion... 266

References.. 267

A. Schröder • W.H. Rösch (✉)
Department of Pediatric Urology, University Medical Center Regensburg, Steinmetzstraße 1-3, 93049 Regensburg, Germany
e-mail: wolfgang.roesch@barmherzige-regensburg.de

1 Introduction

Often, the decision-making process with regard to indications for surgery is based on clinical findings in combination with the results of radiological imaging. However, sometimes an identical radiological finding will lead to surgery in one patient, and not in another, depending on clinical or other findings. Regardless, in many urological conditions, the results of the radiological tests are indispensable contributions to the decision whether to take the child to the operation room or not. Knowledge of the disease, indications for surgery, and the respective surgical procedure (or conservative management) will help to understand what one is actually looking for and facilitate interpretation and presentation of the radiological findings by the radiologist before and after surgery. This chapter will give an overview of the most commonly seen urological conditions in children that may require surgical correction, the key exams, and findings that lead to an operation, as well as respective surgical procedures and the expected radiological findings during follow-up.

2 Pelvi-ureteric Junction (PUJ) Obstruction

2.1 Findings and Indication for Surgery

The typical ultrasound (US) image of a ballooning extrarenal dilatation of the renal pelvis with caliectasis does not necessarily constitute an indication for surgery. However, increasing dilatation, clinical symptoms, deterioration of renal split function, or decompensation of renal clearance (as assessed by MAG_3 scan or functional MRU) may indicate surgery. On the other hand, the absence of excessive extrarenal dilatation does not necessarily rule out a relevant obstruction, which can be indicated by significant caliectasis; here, it is important to differentiate against nonobstructive megacalycosis (see respective chapters).

2.2 Surgical Procedure

Typically, the operation is performed either in an open fashion or laparoscopically, and most commonly, a dismembered pyeloplasty is performed, during which the ureter and renal pelvis are disconnected and reattached after resection of the narrow segment (Anderson and Hynes 1951). According to the surgeon's preference, a large renal pelvis may be reduced by resecting parts of it. In case of an obstruction by a crossing lower pole vessel, the pelvi-ureteric junction (PUJ) is relocated to the other side of the vessel to avoid recurrence of the (functional) obstruction. According to surgeon's preference, which varies widely, some chose to insert a temporary stent, either an internal double "J" catheter or an externalized drain, which will be removed after a few days or weeks with or without previous imaging.

2.3 Postoperative Image

After surgery, the findings are naturally influenced by whether or not pelvic tissue was resected, which would cause a significant decrease in the size of the renal pelvis diameters immediately after surgery, which – to some extent – may again increase after the removal of the stent without reaching preoperative values. Otherwise, there is usually still a variable degree of dilatation of the renal pelvis as well as the calices, which will decrease over time if the surgery was successful. Residual thickening of the urothelium may be seen.

2.4 Possible Complications

Persistent or recurrent obstruction will be indicated by failure of reduction of or even an increase in dilatation. Hematomas or urine extravasation (urinoma) will be seen as fluid collections near the operative field.

> **Take Away**
> The decision to surgically correct a PUJ obstruction depends on the degree and possible worsening of the Urinary tract dilatation, decrease in renal split function and clinical symptoms (pain). Whether or not a crossing vessel is present does not influence the indication for surgery. Surgical correction is done by open or laparoscopic approach with a high success rate. Mild residual dilatation after surgery is not uncommon.

3 Megaureter/Ureterovesical Junction (UVJ) Obstruction

During routine US, a non-dilated distal ureter is usually not seen. However, after sufficient hydration and with a well-filled bladder, an experienced ultrasonographer can visualize also the normal ureter. A dilated distal ureter can be easily seen.

The possible cause of gross dilatation of the ureter can be obstruction (either at the level of the ureterovesical junction (UVJ) or infravesically), vesicoureteral reflux (VUR), a combination of both (obstruction and reflux), or segmental hypoperistalsis. In the case of an infravesical obstruction, the ureteral dilatation is commonly seen bilaterally; however, bilateral ureteral dilatation does not prove infravesical obstruction. A voiding cystourethrography (VCUG) or a contrast-enhanced voiding urosonography (ce-VUS) will confirm or rule out both VUR and posterior urethral valves (PUVs) (see below).

A grossly dilated tortuous ureter in the absence of VUR or infravesical obstruction can be caused by circular obstruction of the distal ureter, by an ectopic insertion, or by a muscular hypodysplasia of the ureteral wall.

3.1 Primary Megaureter

3.1.1 Findings and Indication for Surgery

A (usually short) obstructing segment of the very distal end of the ureter causes the typical tortuous and dilated image of the primary megaureter (MU). There is a high percentage of spontaneous resolution. The cutoff value of prevesical dilatation that determines the likelihood of spontaneous resolution varies in different publications between 10 and 14 mm (Liu et al. 1994; Chertin et al. 2008). Therefore, among the status of the kidney (degree of dilatation, parenchymal thinning), as well as results of functional tests (MAG3 scan) and clinical symptoms, the width of the distal ureter is one of the key contributors to the decision-making with regard to surgery. Some use the development of the ureteral peristalsis (as documented by M-mode US) as an additional parameter on follow-up (Riccabona 2010).

3.1.2 Surgical Procedure

If surgery is needed during the infant period, primary surgical reconstruction of the UVJ is controversial, and temporary diversion by ureterocutaneostomy may be chosen. For this, the ureter is diverted to the skin for prompt decompression of the respective renal unit. Later in life, after recompensation of the ureter, reimplantation is the therapy of choice. Once the ureter is surgically mobilized far enough to run straight, more proximal segments may be sufficiently narrow for direct reimplantation. Otherwise, tapering of the ureter is necessary by imbrication or resection of surplus tissue (Hendren 1969; Kaliciński et al. 1977; Starr 1979).

Some groups choose to approach the problem in a minimal invasive way by dilating or incising the stenotic segment; however, those methods are not yet widely accepted.

3.1.3 Follow-Up

On postoperative imaging, a residual dilatation of the upper urinary tract is not uncommon, but normally decreases gradually over time.

During the course of spontaneous maturation, the width of the ureter as well as the tortuosity decreases over time until adulthood, and peristalsis may normalize. Often, a short segment of the distal ureter continues to show a mild dilatation with reduced peristalsis, while the upper tract appears entirely normal.

3.1.4 Possible Complications

Persistent or recurrent obstruction will be indicated by failure of reduction or even increase in dilatation of the ureter. Hematomas or urine extravasation (urinoma) will be seen as collections near the operative field.

> **Take Away**
> Primary megaureter does not always require surgical correction, as there is a high rate of spontaneous maturation, the likelihood of which depends on the width of the distal ureter (<10–14 mm). In infants, temporary diversion by means of a ureterocutaneostomy may be necessary; in older children, ureteral reimplantation with or without tapering is the therapy of choice.

4 Vesicoureteral Reflux (VUR)

4.1 Findings and Indication for Surgery

Due to an insufficiency of the anti-reflux mechanism at the ureterovesical junction (UVJ), urine is refluxing up the ureter when the intravesical pressure increases during voiding or even during filling (see chapter "UTI and VUR"). The gold standard to diagnose VUR is the classic fluoroscopic voiding cystourethrogram (VCUG) (see chapter "Diagnostic Procedures: Excluding MRI, Nuclear Medicine and Video Urodynamics"). Some prefer the contrast-enhanced voiding urosonography or radionuclide cystography, which requires less or no radiation, but here visualization of the urethra requires advanced skills (Riccabona 2012). Furthermore, a panoramic overview of the entire ureter and depiction of a possible diverticulum that may pose only late during voiding (and thus is difficult to depict on US) are essential for surgical decision-making; thus, preoperatively, a conventional fluoroscopic VCUG is still deemed necessary.

As there is a known influence by constipation on the occurrence of UTIs and lack of resolution of VUR, it is of interest when signs of fecal loading during ultrasound and fluoroscopy are observed.

4.2 Surgical Procedures

The least invasive surgical approach for treatment of VUR is the endoscopic injection of a bulking agent. This procedure is less successful than the open surgical techniques but often preferred, as it causes less morbidity and can be performed as an outpatient procedure. The higher the degree of VUR is, the lesser is the success rate, and a there is a certain rate of recurrence after initially successful operation (Holmdahl et al. 2010).

Extravesical reimplantation without detaching the ureter, i.e., the Lich-Gregoir procedure (Lich et al. 1962; Gregoir 1964), can be performed when the distal ureter is not grossly dilated (Fig. 1a).

Intravesical reimplantation (i.e., the Cohen procedure) allows operating simultaneously on both ureters by detaching the UVJ and pulling the ureters through a submucosal tunnel to the opposite side of the trigone (cross trigonal) through a midline incision of the bladder (Cohen and Rotner 1969) (Fig. 1b).

Other techniques combine the intra- and extravesical approach, with or without tailoring the ureter or hitching the bladder to the psoas muscle (i.e., Politano-Leadbetter reimplantation).

4.3 Postoperative Imaging

Ultrasound is routinely done after surgery. A transient dilatation of the upper urinary tract is sometimes seen, but will usually disappear over

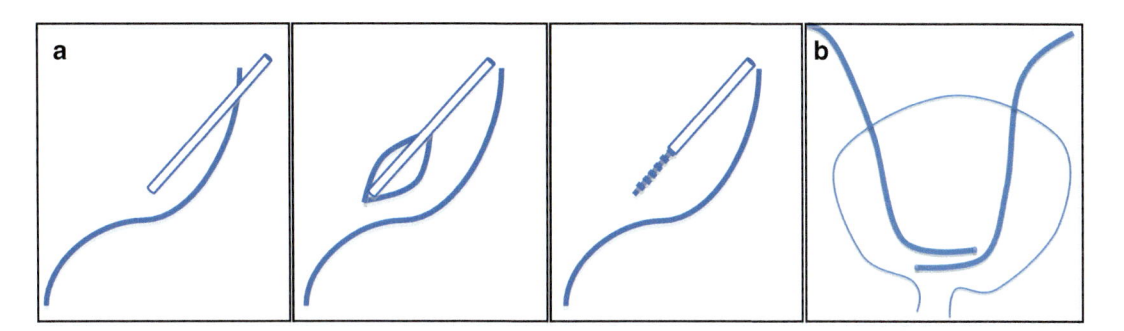

Fig. 1 (a) Cross trigonal position of both ureters after Cohen procedure. Note that the ureteral ostium is now located on the opposite side of each ureter. (b) Extravesical reimplantation without detaching the ureter (Lich-Gregoir)

time. After injection of bulking agent, the submucosal depot is seen as a hyperechoic, round structure at the UVJ, confirming the correct position of the bulking agent. However, not knowing the patient's history, it can be mistaken for a distal ureteral stone (Nelson and Chow 2008).

After surgical correction of VUR, postoperative VCUGs are usually not necessary, unless there is a strong suspicion of recurrence or persistence of VUR, such as recurrence of febrile UTIs.

Depending on the surgical technique, the shape of the bladder may be altered, e.g., the psoas-hitch technique causes a distinct triangular shape at the operated side (Fig. 2). In case of recurrent VUR or when performing an IVU later in adulthood, the ureteral tunnel may be seen (Fig. 3). After Cohen or Politano-Leadbetter reimplantation, the ureter can cross the midline or appear in an unusual angle.

4.4 Possible Complications

De novo obstruction will be indicated by an increase in dilatation of the ureter and renal pelvis. Hematomas or urine extravasation (urinoma) will be seen as collections near the operative field. A hematoma in the ureteral tunnel may cause a fluid collection around the distal, intramural ureter and consecutive dilatation of the upper tract.

> **Take Away**
> The treatment of VUR can be performed conservatively (antibiotic prophylaxis) or surgically. Surgical treatment includes the least invasive endoscopic injection of a bulking agent, as well as open surgical ureteral reimplantation.

5 Posterior Urethral Valves (PUVs)

5.1 Findings and Indication for Surgery

PUVs are often, but not always, diagnosed antenatally. Typical are the "keyhole sign" on fetal US, caused by dilatation of the fetal bladder and posterior urethra, a visibly thickened bladder wall, and bilateral upper tract dilatation (see chapter "Urogenital Fetal Imaging: US and MRI"). The combination of these three findings does not prove, but strongly suggests

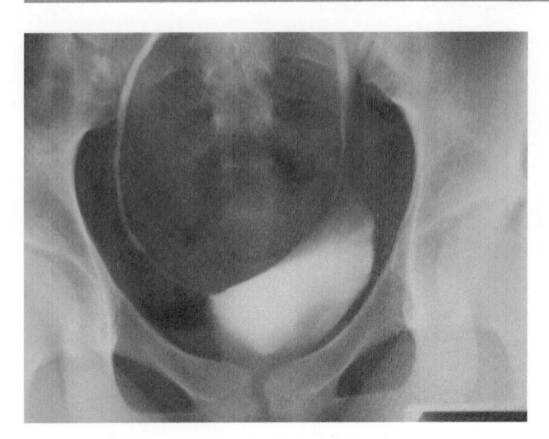

Fig. 2 Intravenous urography in an adult after ureteral reimplantation and psoas-hitch maneuver. Though this imaging technique is not used in pediatric uroradiology for this indication any longer (exceptions for assessing postoperative obstruction using an adapted technique however exist), the image nicely demonstrates the typical postoperative anatomy. Note the typical shape of the bladder, caused by the approximation. The more pronounced is this phenomenon, the lesser is the bladder filled

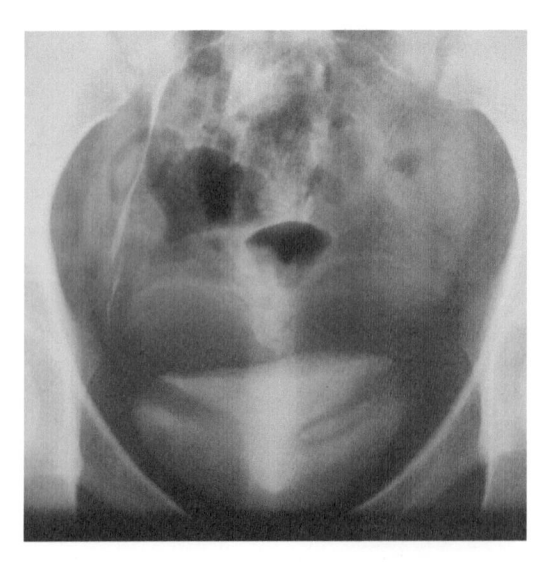

Fig. 3 Intravenous urography in an adult after bilateral ureteral reimplantation (Lich-Gregoir). Though this imaging technique is not used in pediatric uroradiology for this indication any longer (exceptions for assessing postoperative obstruction using an adapted technique however exist), the image nicely demonstrates the typical postoperative anatomy; particularly, the ureteral tunnel is clearly visible on both sides

the presence of PUV. The tiny pieces of soft tissue, blocking the bladder outlet, often have devastating effects (see chapter "Abnormalities of the Lower Urinary Tract and Urachus"). Depending on the severity of the obstruction, oligohydramnios can cause pulmonary hypoplasia, and high mortality rates were described; however, with increased antenatal diagnosis and improved postnatal pulmonary management, the outcome with regard to survival has improved (Thomas 2008). In some cases, prenatal shunting is performed with varying successes. After birth, a catheter is placed immediately for urinary diversion, and after confirming the diagnosis by VCUG (ideally performed without a transurethral catheter), the valves are endoscopically resected (see also chapter "Upper Urinary Tract Dilatation in Newborns and Infants and the Postnatal Work-Up of Congenital Uro-nephropathies").

It is of note that due to the congenital obstruction, irreversible renal damage is often already present at birth, and in up to 50 % of the patients progress to end-stage renal disease sooner or later in life, regardless of early relief of the obstruction. Also, despite early resection of the valves, bladder function is often severely altered, and lifelong treatment and follow-up are required, as the degree and nature of bladder dysfunction can change over time ("valve-bladder syndrome") (Koff et al. 2002). But note that mild PUVs may remain undetected for years and only be diagnosed after presentation of clinical symptoms later during childhood.

VCUG: The VCUG is the most important diagnostic tool to correctly diagnose PUV (see also chapters "Diagnostic Procedures: Excluding MRI, Nuclear Medicine and Video Urodynamics" and "Abnormalities of the Lower Urinary Tract and Urachus"). Differential diagnosis may be difficult, as neuropathic bladder, urethral stricture, and anterior obstruction can appear similarly. To capture the voiding phase from a lateral view is crucial, ideally without the presence of a transurethral catheter, showing the elevated bladder neck. Massive VUR is found in about 50 % of the patients, in case of unilateral VUR mostly on the left side (Hoover and Duckett 1982). Additionally, bladder diverticula are commonly seen.

Ultrasound: Postnatal US will confirm the sometimes massive thickening of the bladder wall, as well as varying degrees of renal (and ureteral) dilatation. In experienced hands, perineal US of the urethra during voiding can reliably demonstrate the valve; US contrast instillation may also depict VUR (e.g., if there is a need for imaging at the bedside in the NICU). Depending on the severity of renal damage, the kidneys can show signs of dysplasia, hyperechogenicity, and parenchymal thinning; sometimes urinary ascites and urinoma are present (see also chapters "Diagnostic Procedures: Excluding MRI, Nuclear Medicine and Video Urodynamics" and "Abnormalities of the Lower Urinary Tract and Urachus").

5.2 Surgical Procedure

The resection of a PUV normally is a straightforward procedure, during which a urethroscope is inserted and the valves are resected or incised with a hook, cold knife, or Bugbee electrode according to surgeon's preference.

5.3 Postoperative Image

After successful destruction/resection of the valves, the bladder wall gradually normalizes and trabeculation decreases; furthermore, a more uniform urethral diameter and improvement or resolution of VUR or obstruction can be seen. However, preexisting renal damage will persist, and monitoring of renal (growth) development is essential.

5.4 Possible Complications

Excessive bleeding can cause a tamponade of the bladder. Incomplete resection of the valve will cause persistent residual urine, although this can also be caused by contractile failure of the detrusor muscle.

> **Take Away**
> Early diagnosis of PUV is crucial, and any suspicion of PUV has to lead to immediate confirmation by VCUG and endoscopy. However, even early treatment cannot prevent a high rate of renal failure in later life.

6 Ureteroceles

6.1 Findings and Indication for Surgery

Ureteroceles are cystiform dilatations of the distal aspect of the ureter, which can be located within the bladder or in ectopic location extravesically (see chapters "Abnormalities of the Lower Urinary Tract and Urachus" and "Upper Urinary Tract Dilatation in Newborns and Infants and the Postnatal Work-Up of Congenital Uro-nephropathies"). Several classifications exist; the clinically most useful one refers to the location of the dilated aspect of the ureter being intra- or extravesical.

Ureteroceles occur more frequently in girls than in boys and are in 85–90 % unilateral. In girls, ureteroceles are associated with a duplex kidney in 95 % of the cases, whereas in boys up to 75 % arise from a single system. Overall 80 % of ureteroceles are associated with a duplex system (Ellerker 1958; Schulman 1976).

A clinically important entity is the cecoureterocele, in which the orifice of the respective ureter is located within the bladder, but the bulk of the ureterocele extends beyond the bladder neck into the urethra and can cause obstruction.

US is regarded as the best study for the examination of a ureterocele (see chapters "Diagnostic Procedures: Excluding MRI, Nuclear Medicine and Video Urodynamics" and "Upper Urinary Tract Dilatation in Newborns and Infants and the Postnatal Work-Up of Congenital Uro-nephropathies"). As the extent of the ureterocele is of clinical relevance, this needs to be properly assessed. Furthermore, different degrees of bladder filling and hydration can influence the diagnosis. A full bladder can compress the ureterocele, whereas an empty bladder can cause the ureterocele to fill out the bladder, thereby effectively hiding it. An insufficient hydration may cause collapse of a then undetectable ureterocele. A pitfall can be a distally dilated ureter that can bulge into the bladder, mimicking a ureterocele ("pseudo-ureterocele"), which can be a tricky differential diagnosis, even for an experienced ultrasonographer. Of help is to pay attention to the thickness of the wall of the intravesical structure, which is much less in a true ureterocele. Also, a dilated ureter will extend more inferiorly beneath the bladder and taper toward the UVJ (Sumfest et al. 1995).

Some surgeons request a VCUG prior to surgery, which shows a filling defect and in cases of a duplex system commonly a VUR into the lower system ureter. It is of note that the ureterocele is often only visible in the early phase of bladder filling. Another pitfall can be the inflated balloon of a Foley catheter, which can be confused for the ureterocele.

6.2 Surgical Procedure

The first step in treating a ureterocele is the endoscopic puncture or incision of the ureterocele, preferably at the base. In case of a cecoureterocele, additional punctures are performed in the extravesical portion of the ureterocele. Some surgeons prefer to create one or a few holes but not to unroof the ureterocele, as – due to the mostly faulty flap valve mechanism at the insertion site – VUR results in many cases. The ideal scenario after surgery is that the punctured ureterocele allows urine to pass through into the bladder without obstruction, but acts as a flap valve, covering the UVJ during voiding and thereby preventing VUR.

6.3 Postoperative Imaging

After a successful procedure, the ureterocele will be deflated, but still be visible as a more or less thick and mobile layer of tissue – sometimes appearing as a pseudo-mass. The upper tract should show decreased or resolved dilatation.

Due to the high incidence of de novo VUR which in duplex systems can affect only the upper or both moieties, a VCUG is usually performed after ureterocele puncture (particularly if not performed previously or if no VUR was present in the initial study).

6.4 Possible Complications

If the puncture of the ureterocele is insufficient, it will fail to collapse. Late recurrent occlusion of the punctured hole is possible and may cause recurrence of the bulging ureterocele. Excessive bleeding can cause a tamponade of the bladder. As mentioned above, de novo VUR is likely.

> **Take Away**
> After diagnosis of a ureterocele and consecutive dilatation of the respective moiety, endoscopic puncture is the first intervention. Persistent dilatation or de novo VUR commonly leads to surgical excision of the ureterocele and ureteral reimplantation.

7 Duplex Systems with Ectopic Ureter

7.1 Findings

Renal duplication per se is quite common (approximately 0.5 % of an unselected population) and in the absence of other abnormalities usually without any consequences. However, particularly in cases of complete duplication, i.e., two ureters that are terminating separately, it can be associated with an ectopic insertion of the upper pole ureter, which can give rise to a number of problems. Following the Weigert-Meyer rule, the ureter of the upper moiety will insert more distally than the one coming from the lower moiety. In girls, in which duplication as well as ectopic insertion is more common, the ectopic ureter can insert above or below the external sphincter, causing continuous loss of urine from the upper moiety despite apparently normal voiding. In boys, the insertion site is always located above the pelvic floor. The other ureter often is refluxing and draining through a more lateral and cranially positioned ostium.

7.2 Imaging

Imaging an ectopic ureteral insertion can be exceedingly challenging, especially when the respective moiety is not dilated and urine excretion is low due to a poor function of the respective renal moiety. Sometimes, MRI may show the ureter (Riccabona et al 2010). However, clinical symptoms and even endoscopic or laparoscopic evaluations may be needed to confirm the suspected diagnosis.

7.3 Surgical Approaches

The most invasive approach to an ectopic ureter with a non- or poorly functioning renal moiety is the heminephrectomy, with or without resection of the distal ureteral stump. However, there is a certain risk for damage of the lower moiety by vascular tear, possibly resulting in loss of the entire kidney (Cabezali et al. 2013). Over the last decade, a tendency toward a less invasive approach emerged, performing a proximal or distal ureteroureterostomy (UU), connecting the distal end of the ectopic ureter to the orthotopic one.

7.4 Postoperative Imaging

US is performed to rule out urine extravasation and will show the missing upper moiety after heminephrectomy. After UU, there can be mild dilatation of the upper moiety. In case of reflux into the ureteral stump, there can be a retrovesical fluid-filled structure; the size is depending on the length of the remaining stump.

7.4.1 Possible Complications

After heminephrectomy, vascular injury can cause ischemia and damage to the remaining moiety. Urinomas can occur around the kidney, in case of UU close to the anastomosis.

When leaving behind a ureteral stump, recurrent infections and empyemas can occur.

Dilatation of the pelvicaliceal system of one or both moieties can occur after UU.

> **Take Away**
> Ectopic ureterocele mostly requires surgical correction. In case of a poorly functioning renal moiety, heminephrectomy used to be the therapy of choice; however, recently there is a tendency to less invasive surgical approaches.

8 Renal Trauma

8.1 Findings and Indications for Imaging

The pediatric kidney is thought to be more susceptible to trauma due to its relatively bigger size and less effective protection by the rib cage, perirenal fat, and abdominal musculature (see also chapter "Urinary Tract Trauma"). It is hypothesized but not proven that renal injury is more common in children than in adults (Brown et al. 1998). Another important difference between children and adults is that hematuria is a less reliable predictor of significant injury, as is hypotension. Therefore, imaging should be performed more aggressively if there is a history of a trauma that may affect the GU tract, even in the absence of hematuria or shock (Brown et al. 1998; Sirlin et al. 2004).

8.2 Imaging Renal Trauma (See Chapter "Urinary Tract Trauma")

Ultrasound has become a major screening tool for trauma (focused assessment with sonography for trauma – FAST) with a specificity range of 95–100 % (i.e., to correctly rule out significant injury). And a detailed US is being increasingly promoted for first-line assessment for mild to moderate blunt abdominal (renal) trauma (Riccabona et al. 2011). However, if the US findings and/or the physical shape of the patient suggests a significant injury, further imaging is needed. The most reliable radiological test is CT, as it allows for assessment of parenchymal and vascular damage as well as urinary extravasation (see chapters "Diagnostic Procedures: Excluding MRI, Nuclear Medicine and Video Urodynamics" and "Urinary Tract Trauma"). Note that a single-phase and single-injection CT as often obtained in an unstable patient or for radiation protection issues and active extravasation will be easily missed (Boone et al. 1993; Al-Qudah and Santucci 2006). Pediatric, age-adapted CT protocols are however essential for optimal diagnostic yield at the lowest possible radiation dose – respective recommendations are available (Riccabona et al. 2010).

8.3 Clinical Management and Surgical Procedures

Nowadays, most and even extensive renal injuries are managed conservatively, as long as the patient is hemodynamically stable or manageable with a limited amount of blood transfusions. Thus, surgery is less often necessary. Urinoma may need drainage (of the collecting system, only sometimes of the urinoma), and large hematoma may pose an indication for interventional or surgical relief. Indications for surgery are based on clinical status (instability and continued need for blood transfusion) and often lead to partial or total nephrectomy. In select cases, selective embolization as well as revascularization can be performed.

8.4 Postoperative/Follow-Up Imaging

Routine follow-up CT scan for high-grade renal injuries, which used to be recommended until recently, is no longer routinely performed in order to reduce radiation exposure. Usually dedicated and detailed US is sufficient to answer all the questions relevant for management decisions. Follow-up CTs are reserved for patients with persistence or new onset of severe symptoms not adequately addressed by US and if MRI is not available or feasible. If available, MRI is increasingly promoted for follow-up, providing excellent imaging without radiation exposure.

8.5 Possible Complications

Renal and vascular injury can cause significant scarring over time, which can be detected by sonography and DMSA scan. Tension caused by a large subcapsular hematoma can cause a page kidney, compressing the vessels and thereby causing ischemia of the previously unaffected regions of the kidney.

> **Take Away**
> Blunt renal trauma in children can be assessed reliably by ultrasound. If CT evaluation is needed, adherence to age-adapted protocols is required.

9 Testes

9.1 Undescended Testes (UDT)

Above the (corrected) age of 6 months, the undescended testis is considered a pathological finding. The clinical evaluation of UDT can be a challenging examination, as the position of the testicle in children and toddlers will be affected by movements, room or hand temperature, and lack of cooperation of the child. A retractile testis, caused by a vivid cremasteric reflex, may be found in the scrotum at the beginning of the examination but can snap up when touching the scrotum or thigh, and the correct diagnosis sometimes requires an experienced examiner.

9.2 Imaging

The primary imaging tool is high-resolution US using a linear high-frequency transducer (see chapter "Imaging in Male Genital Queries"). In some countries, it is still rather common to refer a child with UDT to a radiologist for imaging, although the latest American Urological Association guidelines do not recommend this diagnostic step any longer (Kolon et al. 2014). The main reason for this may be that the referral practice in North America can cause a significant delay in finally sending the child to a surgical specialist, as the often rather lengthy process can take several months. Also, the information gained from imaging will not change the therapeutic pathway, particularly as the physical examination is usually superior to an US study in determining whether or not the UDT is just retractile or requires surgery.

It is of note that a retractile testicle will frequently be found in inguinal position during an US examination, as most children are upset and moving, and the manipulation with the ultrasound probe and the (often not warmed up) gel will elicit the cremasteric reflex leading to the (incorrect) US diagnosis of an inguinally retained testis. In case of an intra-abdominal testis, the radiological diagnosis can be unreliable and will not change the clinical pathway of performing a diagnostic laparoscopy if the testis in not palpable after induction of anesthesia in the OR.

However, in many European countries, (pediatric) urologists or surgeons are performing US themselves and mostly prefer to do the scrotal/inguinal US during the preoperative visit in order to confirm their clinical impression and to plan for the procedural setup.

Any further imaging modalities such as MRI or even CT are not warranted as they will not provide the correct diagnosis with sufficiently high degree of certainty and will not change the surgical management.

9.3 Surgery

A persistently non-palpable testicle has to be evaluated laparoscopically, as no other diagnostic tool can differentiate between a hypoplastic, intra-abdominal, and absent testicle. Furthermore, during laparoscopy, the appropriate treatment is performed in the same procedure, such as orchiectomy, single-stage, or staged orchidopexy.

9.4 Postoperative/Follow-Up Imaging

Postoperative follow-up ultrasounds are routinely performed in order to confirm correct position, sufficient perfusion, and growth of the testicle.

9.5 Possible Complications

After orchidopexy and in particular the Fowler-Stephens maneuver, testicular atrophy can occur. Secondary ascension due to scarring is also possible and requires surgical correction in most cases.

> **Take Away**
> Although ultrasonography is a reliable tool to examine undescended testes, the clinically most relevant criterion is whether or not the testicle is palpable. Also, a retractile testis can only be distinguished from an undescended testis by clinical examination, as the ultrasound examination may trigger the retractile testis to move up into the groin. MRI or CT examinations are not warranted or helpful in this clinical entity.

10 Urolithiasis

10.1 Kidney Stones

Renal concrements in children are considered rather rare; however, due to dietary changes and an increase in childhood obesity, the incidence of urolithiasis has increased significantly over the last decade (VanDervoort et al. 2007). Symptoms in children may differ from those in adults and may occur as abdominal pain, hematuria, UTI, vomiting, and irritability. Hypercalciuria and hypocitraturia are the most common cause for renal stones in children, but metabolic disorders need to be ruled out.

10.2 Imaging

Ultrasonography is a reliable and safe tool to investigate urolithiasis in children, allowing visualization of the entire upper urinary tract. In particular, small stones, which may be missed by IVU or CT, can be detected with adequate hydration (Riccabona et al. 2009). The twinkling artifact has a high positive predictive value for correct diagnosis of a stone (Kielar et al. 2012). Prior to intervention, a plain abdominal radiograph may help to exactly localize a stone. CT scans in children should only be performed in select cases, when other imaging modalities did not suffice to secure the diagnosis.

10.3 Indications for Treatment

Children can pass rather large stones spontaneously; therefore, conservative management is first-line treatment in calculi less than 3 mm (Van Savage et al. 2000). However, in case of pain and/or fever refractory to treatment, emergency placement of an internal or external stent may be necessary. Treatment options for larger calculi include shockwave therapy, endoscopy, percutaneous litholapaxy, and open surgery, depending on location and size of the concrement.

10.4 Possible Complications

Besides UTI and sepsis, all treatment modalities harbor the risk of bleeding, hematoma, and extravasation, which can be visualized by ultrasound and in select cases contrast-enhanced imaging. Residual or passing calculi can cause obstruction and consecutive renal dilatation. Recurrence of urolithiasis is common (40%).

> **Take Away**
> Ultrasonography is the imaging modality of choice in most cases of urolithiasis in children. Plain x-ray and CT or MRI imaging can be performed in select cases.

> **Conclusion**
> In most urological procedures in children, the indication for surgery is based on clinical and imaging findings. For the (pediatric uro-)radiologist, knowledge of the potential impact of specific findings on surgical decision-making is mandatory in order to focus on certain details, such as during "dynamic" investigations by sonography or fluoroscopy. It is important to reassess an imaging finding in context with the clinical symptoms, as the absence or presence of symptoms can make surgery unwarranted in the former, but indicated in the latter scenario.

After surgery, some procedures may lead to altered anatomical findings and can make interpretation difficult. For example, a certain degree of urinary tract dilatation after a procedure does not necessarily mean the measure has failed, as some changes require time to resolve even after successful surgery.

References

Al-Qudah HS, Santucci RA (2006) Complications of renal trauma. Urol Clin North Am 33:41–53, vi. doi:10.1016/j.ucl.2005.10.005

Anderson JC, Hynes W (1951) Plastic operation for hydronephrosis. Proc R Soc Med 44:4–5

Boone TB, Gilling PJ, Husmann DA (1993) Ureteropelvic junction disruption following blunt abdominal trauma. J Urol 150:33–36

Brown SL, Hoffman DM, Spirnak JP (1998) Limitations of routine spiral computerized tomography in the evaluation of blunt renal trauma. J Urol 160:1979–1981

Cabezali D, Maruszewski P, López F et al (2013) Complications and late outcome in transperitoneal laparoscopic heminephrectomy for duplex kidney in children. J Endourol 27:133–138. doi:10.1089/end.2012.0379

Chertin B, Pollack A, Koulikov D et al (2008) Long-term follow up of antenatally diagnosed megaureters. J Pediatr Urol 4:188–191. doi:10.1016/j.jpurol.2007.11.013

Cohen MH, Rotner MB (1969) A new method to create a submucosal ureteral tunnel. J Urol 102(5):567–568

Ellerker AG (1958) The extravesical ectopic ureter. Br J Surg 45:344–353

Gregoir W (1964) The surgical treatment of congenital vesico-ureteral reflux. Acta Chir Belg 63:431–439

Hendren WH (1969) Operative repair of megaureter in children. J Urol 101:491–507

Holmdahl G, Brandström P, Läckgren G et al (2010) The Swedish reflux trial in children: II. Vesicoureteral reflux outcome. J Urol 184:280–285. doi:10.1016/j.juro.2010.01.059

Hoover DL, Duckett JW (1982) Posterior urethral valves, unilateral reflux and renal dysplasia: a syndrome. J Urol 128:994–997

Kaliciński ZH, Kansy J, Kotarbińska B, Joszt W (1977) Surgery of megaureters – modification of Hendren's operation. J Pediatr Surg 12:183–188

Kielar AZ, Shabana W, Vakili M, Rubin J (2012) Prospective evaluation of Doppler sonography to detect the twinkling artifact versus unenhanced computed tomography for identifying urinary tract calculi. J Ultrasound Med 31:1619–1625

Koff SA, Mutabagani KH, Jayanthi VR (2002) The valve bladder syndrome: pathophysiology and treatment with nocturnal bladder emptying. J Urol 167:291–297

Kolon TF, Herndon CDA, Baker LA et al (2014) Evaluation and treatment of cryptorchidism: AUA guideline. J Urol 192:337–345. doi:10.1016/j.juro.2014.05.005

Lich R, Howerton LW, Davis LA (1962) Ureteral reflux, its significance and correction. South Med J 55:633–635

Liu HY, Dhillon HK, Yeung CK et al (1994) Clinical outcome and management of prenatally diagnosed primary megaureters. J Urol 152:614–617

Nelson CP, Chow JS (2008) Dextranomer/hyaluronic acid copolymer (Deflux) implants mimicking distal ureteral calculi on CT. Pediatr Radiol 38:104–106. doi:10.1007/s00247-007-0613-z

Riccabona M (2010) Obstructive diseases of the urinary tract in children: lessons from the last 15 years. Pediatr Radiol 40:947–955. doi:10.1007/s00247-010-1590-1

Riccabona M (2012) Application of a second-generation US contrast agent in infants and children – a European questionnaire-based survey. Pediatr Radiol 42:1471–1480. doi:10.1007/s00247-012-2472-5

Riccabona M, Avni FE, Blickman JG et al (2009) Imaging recommendations in paediatric uroradiology. Minutes of the ESPR uroradiology task force session on childhood obstructive uropathy, high-grade fetal hydronephrosis, childhood haematuria, and urolithiasis in childhood. ESPR Annual Congress, Edinburgh, UK, June 2008. Pediatr Radiol 39:891–898. doi:10.1007/s00247-009-1233-6

Riccabona M, Avni FE, Dacher J-N et al (2010) ESPR uroradiology task force and ESUR paediatric working group: imaging and procedural recommendations in paediatric uroradiology, part III. Minutes of the ESPR uroradiology task force minisymposium on intravenous urography, uro-CT and MR-urography in childhood. Pediatr Radiol 40:1315–1320. doi:10.1007/s00247-010-1686-7

Riccabona M, Lobo ML, Papadopoulou F et al (2011) ESPR uroradiology task force and ESUR paediatric working group: imaging recommendations in paediatric uroradiology, part IV: minutes of the ESPR uroradiology task force mini-symposium on imaging in childhood renal hypertension and imaging of renal trauma in children. Pediatr Radiol 41:939–944. doi:10.1007/s00247-011-2089-0

Schulman CC (1976) The single ectopic ureter. Eur Urol 2:64–69

Sirlin CB, Brown MA, Andrade-Barreto OA et al (2004) Blunt abdominal trauma: clinical value of negative screening US scans. Radiology 230:661–668. doi:10.1148/radiol.2303021707

Starr A (1979) Ureteral plication. A new concept in ureteral tailoring for megaureter. Invest Urol 17:153–158

Sumfest JM, Burns MW, Mitchell ME (1995) Pseudoureterocele: potential for misdiagnosis of an ectopic ureter as a ureterocele. Br J Urol 75:401–405

Thomas DFM (2008) Prenatally diagnosed urinary tract abnormalities: long-term outcome. Semin Fetal Neonatal Med 13:189–195. doi:10.1016/j.siny.2007.10.003

Van Savage JG, Palanca LG, Andersen RD et al (2000) Treatment of distal ureteral stones in children: similarities to the american urological association guidelines in adults. J Urol 164:1089–1093

VanDervoort K, Wiesen J, Frank R et al (2007) Urolithiasis in pediatric patients: a single center study of incidence, clinical presentation and outcome. J Urol 177:2300–2305. doi:10.1016/j.juro.2007.02.002

Urolithiasis and Nephrocalcinosis

Bernd Hoppe

Contents

1 Definition 269
2 Clinical Findings 269
3 Diagnostic Imaging 270
4 Incidence 272
5 Aetiology 272
5.1 Promotors 273
5.2 Inhibitors 277
6 Infectious Stones 277
7 Extrinsic Factors 277
8 General Preventive and Therapeutic Measures 278
8.1 Medication 278
8.2 Surgery 278
Conclusions 278
References 279

1 Definition

Urolithiasis and nephrocalcinosis (NC) are the two types of calcification associated with the urinary tract. *Urolithiasis* is macroscopic calcification in the urinary collecting system. Urinary stones are composed out of crystal agglomerations, sometimes mixed with proteins. Stones are formed on the renal papillae by retention of lithogenic particles (Randall's plaques), either by obstruction or by adherence to damaged renal epithelium (Coe et al. 2010; Evan et al. 2007; Randall 1937). This takes place when urine is supersaturated with regard to stone promoting factors, e.g. increased calcium or oxalate excretion, or because the inhibitor activity is reduced, e.g. low citrate excretion (Karlowicz and Adelman 1995; Verkoelen et al. 1998).

Nephrocalcinosis is microscopic calcification in the tubules, tubular epithelium or interstitial tissue of the kidney. It is classified according to the anatomic area involved. Medullary NC is differentiated from either cortical or diffuse NC. In a variety of diseases urolithiasis and NC occur together (Hoppe et al. 1997; Vervaet et al. 2009; Habbig et al. 2011).

2 Clinical Findings

The most common symptoms of *urolithiasis* are abdominal pain, sometimes clearly identifiable as colicky pain, urinary tract infection, gross or

B. Hoppe
University of Bonn, Department of Pediatrics,
Division of Pediatric Nephrology,
Adenauerallee 119, D-53113 Bonn, Germany
e-mail: bernd.hoppe@ukb.uni-bonn.de

microscopic – non-glomerular – haematuria and, more rarely, flank tenderness or urinary retention. Diagnosis is easily missed if stones are not specifically looked for. Small stones (<2 mm in diameter) may not be detectable even when their presence is strongly suggested. Recurrent urinary tract infections or unexplained sterile pyuria, secondary to noninfectious stones, may provide a clue.

In contrast to patients with urolithiasis, the clinical presentation of *NC* is often asymptomatic especially during infancy. Renal colic has been suspected in some infants with NC and urolithiasis but is difficult to prove. Renal ultrasound screening may detect NC in high-risk infants or as part of the diagnostic evaluation of urinary tract infection. The first symptoms are gross or microscopic haematuria, acute increases in blood pressure and/or sterile leukocyturia. Urinary tract infection may be the first sign of NC too (Hoppe et al. 1997; Karlowicz and Adelman 1995; Habbig et al. 2011) (Table 1).

Take Away
Urolithiasis and nephrocalcinosis are the two types of calcification associated with the urinary tract, the latter often being clinically asymptomatic.

3   Diagnostic Imaging

Urolithiasis and NC are only the symptom of underlying diseases but not the disease itself. Thus, a thorough diagnostic evaluation is required in each child to start specific treatment as early as possible (Hoppe and Kemper 2010; Stapleton 1996a, b). High-resolution ultrasonography (US) is the optimal imaging method for detecting and monitoring NC. The routine use of US in premature infants and in children at risk of developing NC has resulted in a large increase in

Table 1 Nephrocalcinosis grading scale (Dick et al. 1999)

Grade I	Mild increase in echogenicity around the border of the medullary pyramids
Grade II	Mild diffuse increase in echogenicity of the entire medullary pyramid
Grade III	Greater, more homogeneous increase in the echogenicity of the entire medullary pyramid

the number of conditions reported to be associated with NC (Table 4) (Hernanz-Schulman 1991; Jequier and Kaplan 1991; Nayir et al. 1995; Shultz et al. 1991). It has also been increasingly recognised that urolithiasis and NC can coexist in the same patient (Alon 1997; Karlowicz and Adelman 1995).

The bright renal medullary pyramids probably result from interstitial calcium deposition. Patriquin and Robitaille (1986) correlated the sonographic development of medullary NC with four patterns in vivo with the post-mortem pathologic study of Anderson–Carr, which described the progression of intrarenal stone formation (Bruwer 1979). It seems that intratubular calcifications are more common in neonatal NC (Katz et al. 1994).

The varying responses of experimental NC reflect the complex and multifactorial aetiology of NC best. There are two distinct forms of experimental NC in rats: diffuse, but predominantly corticomedullary following sodium phosphate, and predominantly cortical following calcium gluconate (Fourman 1959). Phosphate-induced NC in rabbits occurs maximally at the corticomedullary junction but also frequently in the cortex, seldom in the medulla. NC was not permanent or stable but improved on return to a normal diet (Cramer et al. 1998a, b). Cases of asymmetric NC are described as being due either to renal vein thrombosis or pelvicalyceal dilatation (Navarro et al. 1998).

Diffuse cortical NC by primary hyperoxaluria is most evident both by US and X-ray (Akhan et al. 1995; Hoppe 2012). The correlation of US, CT, pathology and renal function of experimental NC in rabbits demonstrated a better sensitiv-

Table 2 Renal stone analysis in infants and children with infrared spectroscopy (Brühl et al. 1987). Stones are listed in order of decreasing radiopacity

Stones	Girls	Boys
	n = 350	n = 500
Calcium oxalate	*63.4%*	*58.2%*
Weddellite (-monohydrate)	27.7%	29.2%
Whewellite (-dihydrate)	35.7%	29.0%
Infectious	*24.6%*	*29.0%*
Struvite	12.9%	15.0%
Carbonate apatite	9.7%	12.8%
Ammonium hydrogen urate	2.0%	1.2%
Other phosphate stones		
Brushite	1.7%	3.2%
Cystine	0.3%	1.2%
Uric acid	1.4%	2.2%
Uric acid dihydrate	0.3%	0.6%
Proteins	1.4%	1.6%
Artefacts	6.9%	4.0%

ity for US (96–64%) but a better specificity for CT (96–85%), which was later also found in paediatric patients (Cramer et al. 1998a, b; Oner et al. 2004; Palmer et al. 2005; Strouse et al. 2002).

Most urinary tract calculi are visible in X-ray examination as a result of their calcium content (Table 2). *Calcium oxalate stones* may occur in either a pure monohydrate or dihydrate form. Pure *calcium phosphate stones* and calcium oxalate monohydrate stones are the densest calculi for their small size (Jacob et al. 2013). Calcium oxalate dihydrate stones may be spiculated or mamillated and are somewhat less dense than other pure stones of equivalent size (Daudon et al. 2008).

Struvite stones composed of magnesium ammonium phosphate are of low radiopacity in their pure form. This material frequently forms a complex with calcium phosphate, which provides increased radiopacity and which may produce a laminated radiography appearance in the "staghorn" stone.

Cystine stones may develop as small stones or assume a "staghorn" configuration too. Because of their sulphur content, they are less opaque than calcium stones. The density is typically homogeneous, similar to that of "ground glass" (Dyer and Zagoria 1992; Dyer et al. 1998).

Most stones are found in the renal pelvis and/or calyces, the ureter, bladder and rarely in the urethra. The most common ureteral calcification is a stone that has migrated from the kidney. Stones typically become impacted at points of anatomic narrowing in the urinary tract and may be difficult to detect when they overlie bony structures such as the sacrum. To detect a ureteral stone by US may be difficult, but a concomitant dilated ureter or urinary tract dilatation due to a ureteral stone might lead to diagnosis. In general, high-resolution US in combination with colour Doppler twinkling is mostly sufficient for diagnosis. Intravenous urography (IVU) is very rarely necessary, except before extracorporeal shock wave lithotripsy (ESWL).

The comparison between non-contrast-enhanced CT and IVU in adults suspected of a ureteric obstruction by stone demonstrated that non-contrast-enhanced CT is more effective than IVU in precisely identifying ureteric stones, and nearly all stones are visible (Mindell and Cochran 1994; Smith et al. 1995).

It is worth to mention that US detects 90% of kidney stones but only 38% of ureteral stones compared to CT (Palmer et al. 2005). However, in infants and young children, minimisation of exposure to ionising irradiation and the need for sedation to perform a CT favour the use of US over CT.

> **Take Away**
> Urolithiasis and NC are only the symptoms of underlying diseases but not the disease itself! Ultrasound is the primary imaging procedure. It detects 90% of kidney stones but only 38% of ureteral stones compared to CT.

4 Incidence

The incidence of urolithiasis in paediatric patients is considered to be approximately 10% of that in adults; however, it is likely to be underestimated. During past decades, studies reported that 1 in 1000 to 1 in 7500 paediatric hospital admissions were related to urolithiasis (Walther et al. 1980; Milliner and Murphy 1993; Stapleton 1996a, b). However, a recent single-centre study reported a nearly fivefold increase in hospital admissions for paediatric urolithiasis during the last decade (vanDervoort et al. 2007) Another study from the southeast United States, the US "stone belt", observed an increase of children with urolithiasis in an emergency room setting from 7.9 to 18.5 per 100.000 from 1996 to 2007. Interestingly, the number of African-American children remained relatively low (3.2–4.5), whereas the number of Caucasian children in that setting rose from 10.9 to 26.2 per 100.000 in 2007. Hence, Caucasian children are 5.6 times more likely to have kidney stones compared to Afro-American children (Sas et al. 2010).

Children of all ages are affected by urolithiasis and/or NC (Alon 1997). Nephrocalcinosis seems to primarily appear in the first years of life, based on the fact that it is frequently found in tubulopathies or inborn errors of metabolism. Younger children are described to present with a higher proportion of renal calculi, while older children more likely present with ureteral stones (Pietrow et al. 2002; Kalorin et al. 2009; Cameron et al. 2005). A recent study analysed the Kids' Inpatient large-scale paediatric database for sex distribution in more than two million children hospitalised due to urolithiasis and found that the sex distribution changes with age (Novak et al. 2009). Boys were more frequently affected during the first decade (1.2:1 for 0–5 years, 1.3:1 for 6–10 years), while girls were more frequently affected during the second decade of life (0.96:1 for 11–15 years, 0.3:1 for 16–20 years) (Novak et al. 2009). However, other sources even showed more pronounced changes in sex distribution. While in 1996 the reported incidence in boys (8.0/100.000) did not differ from that in girls (7.7/100.000), that in girls showed a faster and stronger increase to 21.9/100.000 in 2007 (boys 15.3/100.000) (Sas et al. 2010).

In contrast to the *infectious stones*, which are mostly found in infants and young children, the incidence of *calcium stones* increases from the age of five. In contrast to adults, *uric acid stones* are very rare in childhood, at least in the Western world: Western Europe 1% and Eastern Europe and the near East 5–10% (Table 2) (Basaklar and Kale 1991; Brühl et al. 1987). *Primary bladder stones* used to be very frequent but have almost disappeared in the Western world (Lopez and Hoppe 2010). There is a family history in more than one third of cases (Danpure 2000).

The incidence of NC is not yet known, but it is very common in metabolic disorders, in which it can be seen as frequently as urolithiasis, e.g. in primary hyperoxaluria (Latta and Brodehl 1990; Habbig et al. 2011), or where it is even the single form of crystal agglomeration and deposition, e.g. in Bartter's syndrome (Buckalew 1989). Preterm infants in particular seem to be prone to NC, which was said to be due to a higher excretion of lithogenic factors (Sonntag and Schaub 1997) but now seems more to be caused by an extremely low urine inhibitory activity by severe hypocitraturia (Sikora et al. 2003; Schell-Feith et al. 2000). The incidence, however, differs drastically between 10 and 65% (Hufnagle et al. 1982; Jacinto et al. 1988; Sikora et al. 2003), with a level of 15% in our premature infants.

> **Take Away**
> Although there are no concrete incidence numbers for paediatric urolithiasis and nephrocalcinosis, incidence seems to increase, like it is the case in the adult population.

5 Aetiology

Urine is a supersaturated solution which may change its concentration very drastically within a short time. It is therefore not surprising that stone formation or the development of NC may take place when the delicate interplay between promotors, e.g. calcium, oxalate and uric acid, and inhibitors – citrate, magnesium and glycosaminoglycans (Ryall 1996) – is disturbed (Karlowicz and Adelman 1995; Evan et al. 2005).

A low urine volume and/or fluctuations in the urinary pH both lead to changes in the solubility product and can therefore predispose to stone formation and stone growth (Coe et al. 1992). A urinary pH of less than 6.0 will increase the risk of uric acid and calcium oxalate stones, whereas a urinary pH >7.4 increases the chances of calcium phosphate precipitation.

An infectious or metabolic cause for stone formation is detected in the majority of paediatric patients (Hoppe et al. 1997). All children with urolithiasis should therefore undergo careful examination (Table 5). Anatomical anomalies are often found to be the reason for stone disease. Renal calculi then develop due to disturbances in urine transport, because of urine stasis or flow changes (Burton et al. 1995).

The stone composition is important for interpretation and for hints of the possible aetiology. The results of stone analysis depend on the origin of the children examined (Table 2).

5.1 Promotors

5.1.1 Hypercalciuria

Hypercalciuria is one of the most frequent conditions in urolithiasis and NC (Table 3,) (Spivacow et al. 2010; Ammenti et al. 2006; Rönnefarth and Misselwitz 2000). There is no sharp limit between normal (up to 0.1 mmol, 4 mg/kg per day) (Ghazali and Barratt 1974; de Santo et al. 1992) and abnormal, except for very high excretions (> 0.2 mmol/kg per day). Whether such children will form stones or develop NC also depends on other factors, e.g. urine volume, pH and the concentration of the other urinary constituents, primarily of oxalate and citrate (Hesse et al. 1986; Hoppe et al. 2008).

Primary/idiopathic hypercalciuria is the most common cause of calcium-containing stones (Coe et al. 1992). It has traditionally been divided into a renal and an absorptive subtype (Stapleton 1983). Theoretically, in patients who have not eaten, urinary calcium excretion is elevated in the former, renal, but normal in the latter, absorptive.

Table 3 Metabolic disturbances associated with urolithiasis/nephrocalcinosis

Metabolic disturbances	
Hypercalciuria	
Normocalcaemic hypercalciuria	Idiopathic hypercalciuria
	dRTA
	Diuretics – furosemide Bartter's syndrome Wilson's disease, Lowe's syndrome Familial hypercalciuria-hypomagnesaemia and nephrocalcinosis syndrome (FHHNC)
Hypercalcaemic, hypercalciuria	Primary hyperparathyroidism
	Immobilisation
	Hyperthyroidism
	Hypothyroidism
	Cushing syndrome – ACTH therapy
	Adrenal insufficiency
	Malignant neoplasm Williams–Beuren syndrome
	Hypervitaminosis D, A CYP24A1 mutation
	Idiopathic hypercalcaemia of childhood
Hyperoxaluria	Primary hyperoxaluria type I, II, III Secondary hyperoxaluria Malabsorption syndromes Lack of intestinal *Oxalobacter formigenes* Short bowel syndrome Dietary
Cystinuria	Type I, II, non-type I/II (3 %)
Hyperuricosuria	Inborn errors of metabolism Lesch–Nyhan syndrome Glycogen storage diseases, type I, III, V, VII
	Overproduction in Leukaemia Non-Hodgkin's lymphoma
	High-protein diet
Hypocitraturia	dRTA Idiopathic Treatment related (e.g. calcineurin inhibitors)

Many paediatric patients, however, cannot easily be classified.

Idiopathic hypercalciuria is considered a multifactorial disease characterised by a complex interaction of environmental and individual factors. Up to 50% of patients have a positive family history (Gambaro et al. 2004; Vezzoli et al. 2010).

Finally, there is a rare but extremely severe form of idiopathic hypercalciuria leading to progressive NC and renal failure: X-linked hypercalciuric nephropathy with tubular proteinuria, also called Dent's disease (Lloyd et al. 1996).

Medullary NC and calcium phosphate stones are common in patients with *distal renal tubular acidosis* (dRTA) (Buckalew 1989; Gückel et al. 1989). A high urinary pH, hypercalciuria and hypocitraturia contribute to these findings (Hamm 1990). In the complete form of dRTA, the urine pH cannot be lowered to less than 6.1 after an acid loading test (Hesse and Vahlensieck 1986).

Medullary NC with hyperechogenic cortex has been described in children with *tyrosinemia*. This rare disease, 1:100.000 live births, is often combined with an impaired renal function: aminoaciduria, hypercalciuria and tubular acidosis (Forget et al. 1999).

There are several clinical entities leading to hypercalcaemia with secondary hypercalciuria (Breslau 1994). *Primary hyperparathyroidism*, although the most frequent cause of hypercalcaemic hypercalciuria in adults, is very rare in children (Damiani et al. 1998). *Hypervitaminosis D* due to administration of multivitamin preparations including vitamin D, or due to vitamin D added to milk preparations, can induce hypercalcaemia and hypercalciuria (Davies 1989; Jacobus et al. 1992; Taylor et al. 1995). Also, mutations in the gene coding for the main enzyme of 1,25-OH dihydroxy-vitamin D3 degradation (CYP24A1) were found to be the culprit for the development of nephrocalcinosis (Schlingmann et al. 2011). CYP24A1 mutations here led to massive hypercalcaemia, suppression of PTH and clinically to dystrophy and muscular hypotonia. An excessive daily intake of *vitamin A*, > 10,000 units, may also lead to hypercalcaemia and can induce hypercalciuria (Ragavan et al. 1982). *Immobilisation* over only 4 weeks will lead to a reduction of bone calcium and bone mass of about 15–20% accompanied by hypercalciuria (Zanchetta et al. 1996).

Long-term administration of furosemide () or dexamethasone and ACTH () can lead to hypercalciuria, NC or stone disease (Downing et al. 1991; Libenson et al. 1999; Myracle et al. 1986; Pope et al. 1996; Rausch et al. 1984; Alon et al. 1994; Hufnagle et al. 1982; Kamitsuka and Peloquin 1991). Hypercalciuria is also found in several syndromes, either linked to the pathogenesis (Bartter's syndrome, William's syndrome) or due to renal tubular damage (Wilson's disease, Lowe's (Dent 2) syndrome) (Gückel et al. 1989; Cote et al. 1989; Hoppe et al. 1993a, b; Sliman et al. 1995). Patients with Bartter's syndrome develop NC but no stones (Table 4). Further conditions include hyper- and hypothyroidism, Cushing syndrome, adrenal insufficiency and metastatic malignant bone disease, long-term assistant ventilation (acid-base changes) and long-term parenteral nutrition, e.g. in very low birth weight infants (Coe et al. 1992; Laufer and Boichis 1989; Campfield and Braden 1989; Hoppe et al. 1993a, b; Pfitzer et al. 1998; Sikora et al. 2003).

5.1.2 Hyperoxaluria

Hyperoxaluria is probably still an underestimated cause of stone formation, although oxalate is a more important risk factor than calcium (Williams and Wandzilak 1989). Therefore, even slightly elevated values are relevant (Leumann et al. 1987). Urinary oxalate is mostly of endogenous origin, only 5–10% derive from the daily nutritional intake (Monico and Milliner 1999; Williams and Wandzilak 1989).

Primary hyperoxaluria type I (PH I) is a rare, autosomal recessive inherited disease caused by a defect in glyoxylate metabolism with low or absent activity of liver-specific peroxisomal alanine:glyoxylate aminotransferase (AGT) (Danpure 1989). The AGXT gene is located on chromosome *2q36-37* (Purdue et al. 1991). The disease prevalence is two patients per million population in Europe (Kopp and Leumann 1995). Around 35–40% of all patients are only diagnosed in end-stage renal disease (Hoppe and Langman 2003).

PH I is characterised by a highly elevated urinary excretion of oxalate and glycolate (> 0.8 mmol/1.73m^{2}body surface area/day, normal <0.5). The urine is saturated with respect

Table 4 Common causes of nephrocalcinosis and differential diagnosis

Nephrocalcinosis	Common causes
Medullary	ACTH therapy
	Adrenal insufficiency
	Bartter's syndrome
	Bone metastases
	Cushing syndrome
	FHHNC
	Hyperoxaluria
	Hyperparathyroidism
	Hyper-, hypothyroidism
	Idiopathic hypercalcaemia
	Lipoid necrosis
	Lesch–Nyhan syndrome
	Lowe syndrome
	Malignant neoplasm
	Medication: furosemide, dexamethasone
	Medullary sponge kidney
	Nutrition: long-time parenteral nutrition, ascorbic acid supplementation
	dRTA
	Tyrosinemia
	Sarcoidosis and other granulomatous diseases
	Sickle cell disease
	Vitamin D, A intoxication
	CYP24A1 mutations
	Williams syndrome, Wilson's disease
Cortical	Chronic hypercalcaemia
	Ethylene glycol intoxication
	Primary hyperoxaluria
	Sickle cell disease
Differential diagnosis	Acute cortical necrosis
	Alport syndrome
	Chronic glomerulonephritis
	Kidney transplant rejection
	Pyelonephritis
	Renal tuberculosis
	Renal vein thrombosis
	Tamm–Horsfall depositions

to calcium oxalate, which causes renal calculi, (medullary) NC or both (Hoppe 2012). With disease progression and declining renal function, calcium oxalate crystals are deposited in the parenchyma of other organs, as well as in the bones and retina (Hoppe 2012).

There is a very large clinical, biochemical and genetic heterogeneity with some patients suffering early renal failure due to NC and others who only have occasional passage of stones in adult life with preserved renal function (Cochat and Rumsby 2013). Renal stones or medullary NC are usually the first signs of PH I (Akhan et al. 1995). However, diagnosis of PH I is often delayed for many years (Kopp and Leumann 1995). Thus, it is important to exclude PH I in all calcium oxalate stone formers (Cochat et al. 2012).

Primary hyperoxaluria type II (PH II), gene on chromosome *9p11*, is less frequently observed than PH I. It is characterised by increased urinary excretion of oxalate and L-glyceric acid due to a defect of both liver-specific D-glycerate dehydrogenase and hydroxypyruvate reductase (Marangella et al. 1992; Cregeen and Rumsby 1999). Urinary glycolate excretion is normal. The clinical course of PH II is much milder than in PH I, although its clinical characteristics are comparable (Hicks et al. 1983). End-stage renal failure is rather the exception (5–10% of patients) (Marangella et al. 1994; Hoppe 2012).

Recently a third PH gene (*HOGA 1*) on chromosome *10q24* was found, which encodes for the mitochondrial 4-hydroxy-2-oxo-glutarate aldolase, and loss of function mutations leads to severe hyperoaxluria but also elevated urinary hydroxy-oxo-glutarate excretion (Belostosky et al. 2010). Very frequently, hyperoxaluria is accompanied by hypercalciuria and hyperuricosuria. It appears as if PH type III is the second most frequent form of PH. Recurrent kidney stones or severe nephrocalcinosis is observed especially in infancy and early childhood. Surprisingly, the clinical symptoms of the disease decrease over time, although hyperoxaluria is ongoing. No case of end-stage renal disease was ever reported (Beck et al. 2013; Monico et al. 2011; Riedel et al. 2012).

Secondary/enteric hyperoxaluria is a typical complication in patients with fat malabsorption, e.g. cystic fibrosis, chronic inflammatory bowel diseases (Crohn's disease) and short bowel syndrome (Hoppe et al. 1998; Sidhu et al. 1998). Normally, oxalate is intestinally bound to calcium to form insoluble calcium oxalate, which is not absorbed. In patients with enteric hyperoxaluria, calcium instead binds to fatty acids; thus, more soluble oxalate is absorbed (Williams and Wandzilak 1989). Secondly, patients with cystic fibrosis lack intestinal oxalate-degrading bacteria, *Oxalobacter formigenes,* which will increase free and absorbable intestinal oxalate (Sidhu et al. 1998). Up to 50 % of our patients with cystic fibrosis have hyperoxaluria and nearly 15 % develop urolithiasis or NC (Hoppe et al. 2005). Enteric hyperoxaluria may also lead to progressive NC and/or recurrent urolithiasis and even end-stage renal disease (Neuhaus et al. 2000; Hueppelshaeuser et al. 2012).

5.1.3 Cystinuria

Cystinuria is one of the most frequent genetic disorders with an overall prevalence of 1:7000 and an autosomal recessive inheritance. It is caused by a defective transport of cystine and the dibasic amino acids lysine, ornithine and arginine through the epithelial cells of the renal tubule and intestinal tract. Two types of cystinuria are now distinguished according to the disease-specific genotype (Font-Llitjos et al. 2005). However, in approximately 3 %, no mutation in these genes is found. In addition, there are differences of the intestinal transport either being disturbed or completely hampered (Horsford et al. 1996; Dello Strologo et al. 2002). Whether stones are formed depend not only on cystine excretion but also on urine volume and pH.

5.1.4 Hyperuricosuria

Uric acid stones are rarely found in children. Hyperuricosuria results from high purine diets, myeloproliferative disorders, tumour lysis syndrome, enzyme defects, etc. (Table 3). Many drugs, e.g. probenecid, high-dose salicylates and contrast media, also increase uric acid excretion. However, low urine pH and low urine volume are far stronger risk factors for stone formation than hyperuricosuria per se.

Some rare inherited deficiencies of the purine salvage enzymes hypoxanthine phosphoribosyltransferase (HPRT) and adenine PRT (APRT) lead to *primary purine overproduction* (Table 3). X-linked Lesch–Nyhan syndrome occurs in complete deficiency of HPRT. It is characterised by mental retardation, automutilation, choreoathetosis, gout and uric acid and NC (Cameron et al. 1993).

Partial deficiency of HPRT results in urolithiasis and renal failure (Choi et al. 1993). Gout and nephrolithiasis have also been reported in glycogen storage disease type I (Restaino et al. 1993) (Table 5).

Deficiency of adenine phosphoribosyltransferase (APRT) results in 2.8-dihydroxyadeninuria (Cebellos-Picot et al. 1992) with autosomal recessive inheritance. Serum uric acid is normal,

Table 5 Diagnostic procedure in urolithiasis/nephrocalcinosis

Patient's history	Familial stone disposition Stone recurrence
Stone localisation	US, (abdominal X-ray), Spiral low enhanced CT
Lab	Electrolytes, uric acid, creatinine, urea, Mg, PO$_4$, plasma oxalate, acid-base status, AP
Urine	Culture, sediment – recurrent infections 24 h urine ≥promotors and inhibitors
Renal function	Clearance
Diet	Daily fluid intake, meat, milk
Drugs	Diuretics, ACTH Vitamin D, A, C overdose Allopurinol chemotherapy
Inherited metabolic disorders	Cystinuria Primary hyperoxalurias Familial hypercalciuria, hypomagnesaemia and nephrocalcinosis syndrome (FHHNC) CYP24A1 (Vit D metabolism) Xanthinuria 2,8 Dihydroxyadeninuria dRTA Dent's disease Lesch–Nyhan syndrome Wilson's disease Bartter's syndrome William's syndrome Lowe's syndrome
Chronic diseases	Malabsorption syndromes (e.g. cystic fibrosis) Steatorrhea Celiac disease Short bowel syndrome
Immobilisation	Hypercalciuria
Stone analyses	Infrared spectroscopy, X-ray diffraction
Differential diagnosis	e.g. appendicitis

and the stones are radiolucent and may be confused with uric acid. The urine contains characteristic brownish round crystals. Diagnosis is confirmed from APRT activity in red blood cells or from excretion of hydroxyadenine in the urine.

In *xanthinuria*, serum uric acid concentration is very low due to deficiency of xanthine oxidase which converts xanthine to uric acid. Characteristic findings of xanthinuria are an orange-brown urinary sediment or orange-stained nappies and later xanthine stones (Arikyants et al. 2007).

5.2 Inhibitors

5.2.1 Hypocitraturia

A low citrate excretion is not always adequately recognised as a risk factor in the pathogenesis of calcium-containing stones (Miller and Stapleton 1985). Low urinary citrate excretion is characteristic for the complete form of dRTA (Preminger et al. 1985). Hypocitraturia is also observed in persistent mild or latent metabolic acidosis, in hypokalaemia and in patients with malabsorption syndromes (Hoppe et al. 2005). Idiopathic hypocitraturia may be secondary to low intestinal alkali absorption (Hoppe et al. 1997).

5.2.2 Further Inhibitors

Glycosaminoglycans (heparin sulphate), Tamm–Horsfall protein (THP) (Hess et al. 1991), nephrocalcin and uropontin are other potent inhibitors of crystallisation processes (Ryall 1996). However, their physiological role, if any, is disputed. The role of THP as inhibitor must be distinguished from the so-called THP kidneys, which can be seen in the first five days of life in neonates (Avni et al. 1983; Berdon et al. 1969; Starinsky et al. 1995).

> **Take Away**
>
> In more than 75% of children with urolithiasis and nephrocalcinosis, a metabolic reason for stone disease can be found. So in all children, diagnostic evaluation is mandatory after the first kidney stone passage or when NC is detected.

6 Infectious Stones

Infectious stones are mainly composed of *struvite* (magnesium ammonium phosphate) but often also contain carbonate apatite. Most struvite stones are found in the kidney, but they may also form in the bladder. Urease-producing bacteria are responsible for the formation of struvite calculi. Ammonia is hydrolysed to ammonium ions which results in a high urinary pH. The high pH also promotes the formation of carbonate ions and the production of trivalent phosphate ions, both components of struvite calculi. Many Gram-positive and Gram-negative bacteria produce urease; however, Proteus species is the predominant organism.

Struvite stones are mainly seen in boys under the age of five. In one third of patients, there is a primary anomaly of the urinary tract, most often a ureteropelvic junction obstruction, or a primary megaureter, or more rarely a ureterocele or urethral valves, etc. (Bruziere and Roubach 1981). Patients with a neurologic bladder, particularly those with meningomyelocele, are particularly prone to struvite stones (Raj et al. 1999). Stones may also occur after renal transplantation (Hess et al. 1994) and during secondary infection on a nidus of different composition, e.g. cystine or calcium oxalate. It is therefore important not to miss an underlying metabolic disorder. Urinary stasis increases the potential for crystallisation to occur. Stones found in patients with ureteropelvic obstruction must therefore not necessarily be of infectious (or metabolic) origin (Oguzkurt et al. 1997).

7 Extrinsic Factors

Urolithiasis may occur from crystallisation of several drugs, e.g. after high-dose sulphonamide therapy (Miller et al. 1993) or after chemotherapy (Hoppe et al. 1997; Cramer et al. 1990). Bladder stones are sometimes found in association with foreign bodies or after surgical procedures, where sutures or metallic staples form the basis of crystal deposition and agglomeration in response to urine exposure.

8 General Preventive and Therapeutic Measures

8.1 Medication

Although stone removal nowadays might be easy to achieve, e.g. via ESWL, prevention of further stone formation is of utmost importance. A large fluid intake at all times, particularly during summer, is the simplest measure. Specific other procedures depend on the underlying condition. In infectious stones, all calculus material should be removed, as it may harbour the organisms. Recurrence of urinary tract infection has to be prevented, e.g. via antibiotic prophylaxis, urine acidification or operation of a vesicoureteral reflux. For all other stones, the underlying metabolic disturbance has to be treated in addition to a high daily fluid intake and to dietary advice. Calcium excretion can be reduced by hydrochlorothiazide medication; in primary hyperoxaluria, therapy with pyridoxine is recommended (Hoppe 2012). Alkaline citrate medication is advisable in both calcium oxalate and uric acid stone disease, as well as in (idiopathic) hypocitraturia, or in patients with dRTA (Leumann et al. 1993). In cystinuria, urine alkalinisation and a high urine volume are extremely helpful, in addition to effective thiol derivatives (D-penicillamine or alpha-mercaptopropionylglycine (Thiola) or ACE inhibitor treatment, which are necessary in recurrent stone formers (Knoll et al. 2005). Allopurinol, an inhibitor of xanthine oxidase, is given in hyperuricosuria that is not amenable to dietary restrictions, particularly in partial or complete HPRT deficiency (Lesch–Nyhan syndrome) (Cameron et al. 1993).

8.2 Surgery

Many pelvic or ureteral stones do not require any intervention and may pass spontaneously, helped by a large urine volume, physical activity and spasmolytics, if needed. An intervention is required in case of persisting or severe obstruction or infection. Small calculi, <5 mm, may be left in situ and observed. Only two kinds of stones can be dissolved chemically: cystine stones by chelating agents and uric acid by alkalisation and administration of allopurinol (Chow and Streem 1996).

Extracorporeal shock wave lithotripsy (ESWL) is now possible even in small children. Ureteral stones may also be treated by ESWL if they are not located very distally or are incrustated in the ureteral wall. Extracorporeal shock waves may damage the renal parenchyma when medullary NC is evident (Boddy et al. 1988). The so-called stone streets in the ureters are very often found after successful ESWL and need specific attention (Dyer et al. 1998).

Other procedures such as percutaneous nephrolithotomy (PNL), ureteroscopy or transureteral lithotripsy (URL), which allow the removal of ureteral stones, are also kidney protective and good alternatives to open surgery (Durkee and Balcom 2006). However, the latter is still required in a considerable proportion of paediatric patients, primarily in those with urinary tract anomalies (El-Damanhoury et al. 1991).

> **Take Away**
> Although stone removal nowadays might be easy to achieve, prevention of further stone formation is of utmost importance. Only symptomatic stones may be removed.

> **Conclusions**
> - Urolithiasis and nephrocalcinosis are not the disease itself; they are only its (first) symptom.
> - High-resolution US is the best method for detecting and monitoring nephrocalcinosis.
> - For detecting urolithiasis – especially ureteral stones – unenhanced low dose spiral CT is the method of choice. However, in children, it is seldom necessary; most relevant stones can be depicted by a meticulous US examination.
> - The most important task in children with urolithiasis and/or nephrocalcinosis is to identify a metabolic reason for stone disease
> - Nephrocalcinosis may persist and even become permanent on US even after eliminating the cause.

References

Akhan O, Özmen MN, Coskun M, Özen S, Akata D, Saatci Ü (1995) Systemic oxalosis: pathognomonic renal and specific extrarenal findings on US and CT. Pediatr Radiol 25:15–16

Alon US (1997) Nephrocalcinosis. Pediatrics 9:160–165

Alon US, Scagliotti D, Garola RE (1994) Nephrocalcinosis and nephrolithiasis in infants with congestive heart failure treated with furosemide. J Pediatr 125:149–151

Ammenti A, Neri E, Agistri R et al (2006) Idiopathic hypercalciuria in infants with renal stones. Pediatr Nephrol 21(12):1901–1903

Arikyants N, Sarkissian A, Hesse A et al (2007) Xanthinuria type I – a rare cause of urolithiasis. Pediatr Nephrol 22(2):310–314

Avni EF, Spehl-Robberecht M, Lebrun D, Gomes H, Garel L (1983) Pathologie Tubulaire Aiguë Transitoire Chez Le Nourrisson: Aspect Échographique Charactéristique. Ann Radiol 26:175–182

Basaklar AC, Kale N (1991) Experiences with childhood urolithiasis (report of 196 cases). Br J Urol 67:203–205

Beck BB, Baasner A, Buescher A et al (2013) Novel findings in patients with primary hyperoxaluria type III and implications for advanced molecular testing strategies. Eur J Hum Genet 21(2):162–172

Belostosky R, Seboun E, Idelson GH, Milliner DS, Becker-Cohen R, Rinat C (2010) Mutations in DHDPSL are responsible for primary hyperoxaluria type III. Am J Hum Genet 87:392–399

Berdon WE, Schwartz RH, Becker J, Baker DH (1969) Tamm-Horsfall proteinuria. Radiology 92:714–722

Boddy SA, Duffy PG, Barratt TM, Whitfield HN (1988) Hyperoxaluria and renal calculi in children. The role of extracorporeal shock wave lithotripsy. Proc R Soc Med 81:604–605

Breslau NA (1994) Pathogenesis and management of hypercalciuric nephrolithiasis. Miner Electrolyte Metab 20(6):328–339

Bruwer A (1979) Primary renal calculi: Anderson-Carr-Randall progression? AJR Am J Roentgenol 132:751–758

Brühl P, Hesse A, Gu KLR (1987) Harnsteinerkrankungen im Kindesalter: ƒtiologie, Diagnostik, Therapie und Metaphylaxe. Wissenschaftliche Verlagsgesellschaft mbH, Stuttgart

Bruziere J, Roubach L (1981) Urinary lithiasis in children. Eur J Urol 7:134–135

Buckalew VM Jr (1989) Nephrolithiasis in renal tubular acidosis. J Urol 141(3 Pt 2):731–737

Burton EM, Hanna JD, Mercado-Deane MG (1995) Nephrocalcinosis in a child with autosomal dominant polycystic kidney disease and a prolapsing ectopic ureterocele. Pediatr Radiol 25:462–465

Cameron JS, Moro F, Simmonds HA (1993) Gout, uric acid and purine metabolism in paediatric nephrology. Pediatr Nephrol 7(1):105–118

Cameron MA, Sakhaee K, Moe OW (2005) Nephrolithiasis in children. Pediatr Nephrol 20(11):1587–1592

Campfield T, Braden G (1989) Urinary oxalate excretion by very low birth weight infants receiving parenteral nutrition. Pediatrics 84(5):860–863

Cebellos-Picot I, Perignon JL, Hamet M, Daudon M, Kamoun P (1992) 2.8 dihydroxyadenine urolithiasis, an underdiagnosed disease. Lancet 339:1050–1051

Choi Y, Koo JW, Ha IS et al (1993) Partial hypoxanthine-guanine phosphoribosyl transferase deficiency in two Korean sisters – a new mutation. Pediatr Nephrol 7:739–740

Chow GK, Streem SB (1996) Medical treatment of cystinuria: results of contemporary clinical practice. J Urol 156:1576–1578

Cochat P, Rumsby G (2013) Primary hyperoxaluria. N Engl J Med 369(7):649–658. doi:10.1056/NEJMra1301564

Cochat P, Hulton SA, Acquaviva C et al (2012) Primary hyperoxaluria type 1: indications for screening and guidance for diagnosis and treatment. Nephrol Dial Transplant 27(5):1729–1736

Coe FL, Parks JH, Asplin JR (1992) The pathogenesis and treatment of kidney stones. N Engl J Med 327:1141–1152

Coe FL, Evan AP, Worcester EM et al (2010) Three pathways for human kidney stone formation. Urol Res 38(3):147–160

Cote G, Jequier S, Kaplan P (1989) Increased renal medullary echogenicity in patients with Williams syndrome. Pediatr Radiol 19:481–483

Cramer B, Husa L, Pushpanathan C (1998a) Nephrocalcinosis in rabbits – correlation of ultrasound, computed tomography, pathology and renal function. Pediatr Radiol 28:9–13

Cramer B, Husa L, Pushpanathan C (1998b) Pattern and permanence of phosphate-induced nephrocalcinosis in rabbits. Pediatr Radiol 28:14–19

Cramer BC, Ozere R, Andrews W (1990) Renal stone formation following medical treatment of renal candidiasis. Pediatr Radiol 21:43–44

Cregeen DP, Rumsby G (1999) Recent developments in our understanding of primary hyperoxaluria type 2. J Am Soc Neprol 10:348–350

Damiani D, Aguiar CH, Bueno VS et al (1998) Primary hyperparathyroidism in children: patient report and review of literature. J Pediatr Endocrinol Metab 11:83–86

Danpure CJ (1989) Recent advances in the understanding, diagnosis and treatment of primary hyperoxaluria type I. J Inherit Metab Dis 12:210–224

Danpure CJ (2000) Genetic disorders and urolithiasis. Urol North Clin Am 27:287–299

Daudon M, Jungers P, Bazin D (2008) Peculiar morphology of stones in primary hyperoxaluria. N Engl J Med 359:100–102

Davies M (1989) High dose vitamin D therapy: indications, benefits and hazards. Int J Vitam Nutr Res Suppl 30:81–86

Dello Strologo L, Pras E, Pontesilli C et al (2002) Comparison between SLC3A1 and SLC7A9 cystinuria patients and carriers: a need for a new classification. J Am Soc Nephrol 13(10):2547–2553

De Santo NG, Iorio BD, Capasso G et al (1992) Population based data on urinary excretion of calcium, magnesium, oxalate, phosphate and uric acid in children from Cimitile (southern Italy). Pediatr Nephrol 6:149–157

Dick PT, Shuckett BM, Tang B, Daneman A, Kooh SW (1999) Observer reliability in grading nephrocalcinosis on ultrasound examinations in children. Pediatr Radiol 29:68–72

Downing GJ, Egelhoff JC, Daily DK, Alon U (1991) Furosemide-related renal calcifications in the premature infant. Pediatr Radiol 21:563–565

Durkee CT, Balcom A (2006) Surgical management of urolithiasis. Pediatr Clin North Am 53:465–477

Dyer RB, Chen MYM, Zagoria RJ (1998) Abnormal calcifications in the urinary tract. Radiographics 18:1405–1424

Dyer RB, Zagoria RJ (1992) Radiological patterns of mineralization as predictor of urinary stone etiology, associated pathology, and therapeutic outcome. J Stone Dis 4:272–282

El-Damanhoury H, Bürger R, Hohenfellner R (1991) Surgical aspects of urolithiasis in children. Pediatr Nephrol 5:339–347

Evan AP, Coe FK, Lingeman JE et al (2005) Insights on the pathology of kidney stone formation. Urol Res 33:383–389

Evan AP, Lingeman J, Coe F et al (2007) Renal histopathology of stone-forming patients with distal renal tubular acidosis. Kidney Int 71(8):795–801

Font-Llitjos M, Jimenez-Vidal M, Bisceglia L et al (2005) New insights into cystinuria: 40 new mutations, genotype-phenotype correlation, and digenic inheritance causing partial phenotype. J Med Genet 42:58–68

Forget S, Patriquin HB, Dubois J, Lafortune M, Merouani A, Paradis K, Russo P (1999) The kidney in children with tyrosinemia: sonographic, CT and biochemical findings. Pediatr Radiol 29:104–108

Fourman J (1959) Two distinct forms of experimental nephrocalcinosis in the rat. Br J Exp Pathol 60:463–464

Gambaro G, Vezzoli G, Casari G et al (2004) Genetics of hypercalciuria and calcium nephrolithiasis: from the rare monogenic to the common polygenic forms. Am J Kidney Dis 44(6):963–986

Gückel C, Benz-Bohm G, Roth B (1989) Die Nephrokalzinose im Kindesalter. Sonographische Befunde und Differentialdiagnostik. Fortschr Röntgenstr 151:301–305

Ghazali S, Barratt TM (1974) Urinary excretion of calcium and magnesium in children. Arch Dis Child 49:97–101

Habbig S, Beck BB, Hoppe B (2011) Nephrocalcinosis and urolithiasis in children. Kidney Int 80(12):1278–1291

Hamm LL (1990) Renal handling of citrate. Kidney Int 38:728–735

Hernanz-Schulman M (1991) Hyperechoic renal medullary pyramids in infants and children. Radiology 181:9–11

Hess B, Nakagawa Y, Parks JH, Coe FL (1991) Molecular abnormality of Tamm-Horsfall glycoprotein in calcium oxalate nephrolithiasis. Am J Physiol 260(4 Part 2):F569–F578

Hess B, Metzger RM, Ackermann D, Montandon A, Jaeger P (1994) Infection-induced stone formation in a renal allograft. Am J Kidney Dis 24(5):868–872

Hesse A, Classen A, Knoll M, Timmerman F, Vahlensieck W (1986) Dependance of urine composition on the age and sex of healthy subjects. Clin Chim Acta 160:79–86

Hesse A, Vahlensieck W (1986) Loading tests for diagnosis of metabolic anomalies in urinary stone formers. Int J Urol Nephrol 18(1):45–53

Hicks NR, Cranston DW, Charlton CAC (1983) Fifteen year follow up of hyperoxaluria type II. N Engl J Med 309:796 (letter)

Hoppe B, Hesse A, Neuhaus T et al (1993a) Urinary saturation and nephrocalcinosis in preterm infants: effect of parenteral nutrition. Arch Dis Child 69:299–303

Hoppe B, Neuhaus T, Superti A, Leumann E (1993b) Hypercalciuria and nephrocalcinosis, a feature of Wilson's disease. Nephron 65:460–462

Hoppe B, Jahnen A, Bach D, Hesse A (1997) Urinary calcium-oxalate saturation in healthy infants and children. J Urol 158:557–559

Hoppe B, Hesse A, Brömme S, Rietschel E, Michalk D (1998) Urinary excretion substances in patients with cystic fibrosis: risk of urolithiasis? Pediatr Nephrol 12:275–279

Hoppe B, von Unruh GE, Blank G et al (2005) Absorptive hyperoxaluria leads to an increased risk of urolithiasis or nephrocalcinosis in cystic fibrosis. Am J Kidney Dis 46(3):440–445

Hoppe B, Langman CB (2003) A United States survey on diagnosis, treatment, and outcome of primary hyperoxaluria. Pediatr Nephrol 18(10):986–991

Hoppe B, Leumann A, Milliner DS (2008) Urolithiasis and nephrocalcinosis in childhood. In: Geary DF, Schaefer F (eds) Comprehensive pediatric nephrology. Elsevier, Philadelphia, pp 499–525

Hoppe B, Kemper M (2010) Diagnostic examination of the child with urolithiasis or nephrocalcinosis. Pediatr Nephrol 25(3):403–413

Hoppe B (2012) An update an primary hyperoxaluria. Nat Rev Nephrol 8(8):467–75

Horsford J, Saadi I, Raelson J, Goodyer PR, Rozen R (1996) Molecular genetics of cystinuria in French Canadians: identification of four novel mutations in type I patients. Kidney Int 49(5):1401–1406

Hufnagle KG, Khan SN, Penn D, Cacciarelli A, Williams P (1982) Renal calcifications: a complication of long term furosemide therapy in preterm infants. Pediatrics 70:360–363

Hueppelshaeuser R, von Unruh GE, Habbig S et al (2012) Enteric hyperoxaluria, recurrent urolithiasis, and systemic oxalosis in patients with Crohn's disease. Pediatr Nephrol 27(7):1103–1109

Jacinto JS, Modanlou HD, Crade MC, Strauss AA, Bosu SK (1988) Renal calcification incidence in very low birth weight infants. Pediatrics 81:31–35

Jacob DE, Grohe B, Geßner M, Beck BB, Hoppe B (2013) Kidney stones in primary hyperoxaluria: new lessons learnt. PLoS One 8(8):e70617

Jacobus CH, Holick MF, Shao Q et al (1992) Hypervitaminosis D associated with drinking milk. N Engl J Med 326(18):1173–1177

Jequier S, Kaplan BS (1991) Echogenic renal pyramids in children. J Clin Ultrasound 19:85–92

Kalorin CM, Zabinski A, Okpareke I et al (2009) Pediatric urinary stone disease does age matter? J Urol 181(5):2267–2271

Kamitsuka MD, Peloquin D (1991) Renal calcification after dexamethasone in infants with bronchopulmonary dysplasia. Lancet 337:626 (letter)

Karlowicz MG, Adelman RD (1995) Renal calcification in the first year of life. Pediatr Clin North Am 42:1397–1413

Katz ME, Karlowicz MG, Adelman RD, Werner AL, Solhaug MJ (1994) Nephrocalcinosis in very low birth weight neonates: sonographic patterns, histologic characteristics, and clinical risk factors. J Ultrasound Med 13:777–782

Knoll T, Zöllner A, Wendt-Nordahl G et al (2005) Cystinuria in childhood and adolescence: recommendations for diagnosis, treatment, and follow-up. Pediatr Nephrol 20(1):19–24

Kopp N, Leumann E (1995) Changing pattern of primary hyperoxaluria in Switzerland. Nephrol Dial Transplant 10:2224–2227

Laufer J, Boichis H (1989) Urolithiasis in children: current medical management. Pediatr Nephrol 3:317–331

Latta K, Brodehl J (1990) Primary hyperoxaluria type I. Eur J Pediatr 149:518–522

Leumann EP, Niederwieser A, Fanconi A (1987) New aspects of infantile oxalosis. Pediatr Nephrol 1:531–535

Leumann E, Hoppe B, Neuhaus T (1993) Management of primary hyperoxaluria: efficacy of oral citrate administration. Pediatr Nephrol 7:207–211

Libenson MH, Kaye EM, Rosman NP, Gilmore HE (1999) Acetazolamide and furosemide for posthemorrhagic hydrocephalus of the newborn. Pediatr Neurol 20:185–191

Lloyd SE, Pearce SH, Fisher SE et al (1996) A common molecular basis for three inherited kidney stone diseases. Nature 379(6564):398–399

Lopez M, Hoppe B (2010) History, epidemiology and regional diversities of urolithiasis. Pediatr Nephrol 25(1):49–59

Marangella M, Petrarulo M, Vitale C, Cosseddu D, Linari F (1992) Plasma and urine glycolate assays for differentiating the hyperoxaluria syndromes. J Urol 148:986–989

Marangella M, Petrarulo M, Cosseddu D (1994) End-stage renal failure in primary hyperoxaluria type II. N Engl J Med 330:1690 (letter)

Miller MA, Gallicano K, Dascal A, Mendelson J (1993) Sulfadiazine urolithiasis during antitoxoplasma therapy. Drug Invest 5:334–337

Miller LA, Stapleton FB (1985) Urinary citrate excretion in children with hypercalciuria. J Pediatr 107(2):263–266

Milliner DS, Murphy ME (1993) Urolithiasis in pediatric patients. Mayo Clin Proc 68:313–315

Mindell HJ, Cochran ST (1994) Current perspectives in the diagnosis and treatment of urinary stone disease. AJR Am J Roentgenol 163:1314–1315

Monico CG, Milliner DS (1999) Hyperoxaluria and urolithiasis in young children: an atypical presentation. J Endourol 13:633–636

Monico CG, Rossetti S, Belostotsky R et al (2011) Primary hyperoxaluria type III gene HOGA1 (formerly DHDPSL) as a possible risk factor for idiopathic calcium oxalate urolithiasis. Clin J Am Soc Nephrol 6(9):2289–2295

Myracle MR, McGahan JP, Goetzman BW, Adelman RD (1986) Ultrasound diagnosis of renal calcification in infants on chronic furosemide therapy. J Clin Ultrasound 14:281–287

Novak TE, Lakshmanan Y, Trock BJ et al (2009) Sex prevalence of pediatric kidney stone disease in the United States: an epidemiologic investigation. Urology 74(1):104–107

Navarro O, Daneman A, Kooh SW (1998) Asymmetric medullary nephrocalcinosis in two children. Pediatr Radiol 28:687–690

Nayir A, Kadioglu A, Sirin A, Emre S, Tonguc E, Bilge I (1995) Causes of increased renal medullary echogenicity in Turkish children. Pediatr Nephrol 9:729–733

Neuhaus T, Belzer T, Blau N, Hoppe B, Sidhu H, Leumann E (2000) Urinary oxalate excretion in urolithiasis and nephrocalcinosis. Arch Dis Child 82:322–326

Oguzkurt L, Karabulut N, Haliloglu M, Ünal B (1997) Medullary nephrocalcinosis associated with vesicoureteral reflux. Br J Radiol 70:850–851

Oner S, Oto A, Tekgul S et al (2004) Comparison of spiral CT and US in the evaluation of pediatric urolithiasis. JBR-BTR 87(5):219–223

Palmer JS, Donaher ER, O'Riordan MA et al (2005) Diagnosis of pediatric urolithiasis: role of ultrasound and computerized tomography. J Urol 174:1413–1416

Patriquin H, Robitaille P (1986) Renal calcium deposition in children: sonographic demonstration of the Anderson-Carr progression. AJR Am J Roentgenol 146:1253–1256

Pfitzer A, Nelle M, Rohrschneider W, Linderkamp O, Tröger J (1998) Inzidenz nephrokalzinosetypischer Sonographiebefunde bei Frühgeborenen während enteraler Kalzium- und Phosphatgabe. Z Geburtsh Neonatol 202:159–163

Pietrow PK, Pope JC, Adams MC et al (2002) Clinical outcome of pediatric stone disease. J Urol 167:670–673

Pope JC, Trusler LA, Klein AM, Walsh WF, Yared A, Brock JW (1996) The natural history of nephrocalcinosis in premature infants treated with loop diuretics. J Urol 156:709–712

Preminger GM, Sakhaee K, Skurla C, Pak CYC (1985) Prevention of recurrent calcium stone formation with potassium citrate therapy in patients with distal renal tubular acidosis. J Urol 134:20–24

Purdue PE, Lumb MJ, Fox M et al (1991) Characterisation and chromosomal mapping of a genomic clone encoding human alanine:glyoxylate aminotransferase. Genomics 10:34–42

Ragavan VV, Smith JE, Bilezikian JP (1982) Vitamin A toxicity and hypercalcemia. Am J Med Sci 283(3):161–164

Raj GV, Bennett RT, Preminger GM, King LR, Wiener JS (1999) The incidence of nephrolithiasis in patients with spinal neural tube defects. J Urol 162:1238–1242

Randall A (1937) The origin and growth of renal calculi. Ann Surg 105(6):1009–1027

Rausch HP, Hanefeld F, Kaufmann HJ (1984) Medullary nephrocalcinosis and pancreatic calcifications demonstrated by ultrasound and CT in infants after treatment with ACTH. Radiology 153:105–107

Restaino I, Kaplan BS, Stanley C, Baker L (1993) Nephrolithiasis, hypocitraturia, and a distal renal tubular acidification defect in type I glycogen storage disease. J Pediatr 122(3):392–396

Riedel TJ, Knight J, Murray MS, Milliner DS, Holmes RP, Lowther WT (2012) 4-hydroxy-2-oxoglutarate aldolase inactivity in primary hyperoxaluria type 3 and glyoxylate reductase inhibition. Biochim Biophys Acta 1822(10):1544–1552

Rönnefarth G, Misselwitz J (2000) Nephrocalcinosis in children: a retrospective survey. Members of the Arbeitsgemeinschaft für pädiatrische Nephrologie. Pediatr Nephrol 14(10-11):1016–1021

Ryall RL (1996) Glycosaminoglycans, proteins, and stone formation: adult themes and child's play. Pediatr Nephrol 10(5):656–666

Sas DJ, Hulsey TC, Shatat IF et al (2010) Increasing incidence of kidney stones in children evaluated in the emergency department. J Pediatr 157(1):132–137

Schell-Feith EA, van Holthe KJE, Conneman N et al (2000) Etiology of nephrocalcinosis in preterm neonates: association of nutritional intake and urinary parameters. Kidney Int 58:2102–2110

Shultz PK, Strife JL, Strife CF, McDaniel JD (1991) Hyperechoic renal medullary pyramids in infants and children. Radiology 181:163–167

Schlingmann KP, Kaufmann M, Weber S et al (2011) Mutations in CYP24A1 and idiopathic infantile hypercalcemia. N Engl J Med 365(5):410–421

Sidhu H, Hoppe B, Hesse A et al (1998) Absence of Oxalobacter formigenes in cystic fibrosis patients: a risk factor for hyperoxaluria. Lancet 352:1026–1029

Sikora P, Roth B, Kribs A et al (2003) Hypocitraturia is one of the major risk factors for nephrocalcinosis in very low birth weight (VLBW) infants. Kidney Int 63:2194–2199

Sliman GA, Winters WD, Shaw DW, Avner ED (1995) Hypercalciuria and nephrocalcinosis in the oculocerebrorenal syndrome. J Urol 153(4):1244–1246

Smith RC, Rosenfield AT, Choe KA et al (1995) Acute flank pain: comparison of non-contrast-enhanced CT and intravenous urography. Radiology 194:789–794

Sonntag J, Schaub J (1997) Oxalate excretion during the first 7 weeks in very-low-birth-weight infants. Biol Neonate 71:277–281

Spivacow FR, Negri AL, del Valle EE et al (2010) Clinical and metabolic risk factor evaluation in young adults with kidney stones. Int Urol Nephrol 42(2):471–475

Stapleton FB (1983) Idiopathic hypercalciuria in children. Semin Nephrol 3(2):116–124

Stapleton FB (1996a) Clinical approach to children with urolithiasis. Semin Nephrol 3:116–124

Stapleton FB (1996b) Clinical approach to children with urolithiasis. Semin Nephrol 16(5):389–397

Starinsky R, Vardi O, Batasch D, Goldberg M (1995) Increased renal medullary echogenicity in neonates. Pediatr Radiol 25:43–45

Strouse PJ, Bates DG, Bloom DA, Goodsitt MM (2002) Non-contrast thin-section helical CT of urinary tract calculi in children. Pediatr Radiol 32(5):326–332

Taylor A, Sherman NH, Norman ME (1995) Nephrocalcinosis in X-linked hypophosphatemia: effect of treatment versus disease. Pediatr Nephrol 9:173–175

Williams HE, Wandzilak TE (1989) Oxalate synthesis, transport and the hyperoxaluric syndromes. J Urol 141:742–747

VanDervoort K, Wiesen J, Frank R et al (2007) Urolithiasis in pediatric patients: a single center study of incidence, clinical presentation and outcome. J Urol 177(6):2300–2305

Verkoelen CF, van der Boom BG, Houtsmuller AB et al (1998) Increased calcium oxalate monohydrate crystal binding to injured renal tubular epithelial cells in culture. Am J Physiol 274:F958–F965

Vervaet BA, Verhulst A, D'Haese PC et al (2009) Nephrocalcinosis: new insights into mechanisms and consequences. Nephrol Dial Transplant 24(7):2030–2035

Vezzoli G, Terranegra A, Arcidiacono T et al (2010) Calcium kidney stones are associated with a haplotype of the calcium-sensing receptor gene regulatory region. Nephrol Dial Transplant 25(7):2245–2252

Walther PC, Lamm D, Kaplan GW (1980) Pediatric urolithiases: a ten-year review. Pediatrics 65(6):1068–1072

Zanchetta JR, Rodriguez G, Negir AL, del Valle E, Spivacow FR (1996) Bone mineral density in patients with hypercalciuric nephrolithiasis. Nephron 73:557–560

Renal Failure and Renal Transplantation

Ekkehard Ring, Holger Hubmann, and Birgit Acham-Roschitz

Contents

1 **Introduction** 283

2 **Acute Renal Failure, Acute Kidney Injury** .. 284
2.1 Definition and Classification 284
2.2 Causes of Acute Kidney Injury 284
2.3 Diagnosis, Treatment, and Prognosis 285

3 **Neonatal Renal Failure** 285
3.1 Fetal and Neonatal Renal Function 285
3.2 Neonatal Acute Kidney Injury 286
3.3 Diagnosis and Treatment 286
3.4 Congenital Renal Disorders 287

4 **Chronic Renal Failure** 287
4.1 Definitions 287
4.2 Epidemiology 287
4.3 Pathophysiology 288
4.4 Diagnosis and Treatment 288
4.5 Planning Dialysis and Transplantation 289

5 **Dialysis** 289
5.1 Basic Considerations 289
5.2 Peritoneal Dialysis 289
5.3 Hemodialysis 290

6 **Renal Transplantation** 290
6.1 Basic Considerations 290
6.2 Acute Problems 291
6.3 Regular Follow-Up 291
6.4 Acute Rejection 291
6.5 Infections 291
6.6 Posttransplant Lymphoproliferative Disorder 292
6.7 Prognosis 292

Conclusion 292

References 293

E. Ring, MD (Retired) (✉) • H. Hubmann, MD
B. Acham-Roschitz, MD
Department of Pediatrics, Division of General Pediatrics, University Hospital Graz, Auenbruggerplatz 34, 8036 Graz, Austria
e-mail: ekkehard.ring@klinikum-graz.at

1 Introduction

Acute renal failure, nowadays called acute kidney injury (AKI), is a sudden-onset disease with the inability of the kidneys to maintain body homeostasis and to excrete creatinine and urea adequately. AKI may be completely reversible but can be the first step to a chronic disease with a diminished number of nephrons, named chronic renal failure (CRF). In addition, AKI may be superimposed on CRF worsening the prognosis significantly. Neonatal AKI (nAKI) has to be seen in the context of switching from fetal situation to postpartal renal function and is discussed separately. Children suffering from congenital, hereditary, or severe acquired renal disease, basically or caused by injury, have a substantially diminished number of nephrons. Loss of nephrons cannot be replaced by new units, and recovery is impossible. Consequently, according to the patient's age, different diseases enter a common pathway of progressive renal dysfunction, CRF. End-stage renal disease (ESRD) is reached when survival is only possible with renal replacement therapy. Aside from all medical and psychosocial care during CRF and ESRD, renal transplantation (RTx) is the ultimate goal to optimize rehabilitation and lifestyle.

2 Acute Renal Failure, Acute Kidney Injury

2.1 Definition and Classification

As indicated above, AKI is a sudden-onset renal compromise with retention of creatinine and urea waste products. The kidneys are unable to maintain electrolyte homeostasis and fluid balance (Lameire et al. 2005). The disease may be slight with just a small increase of creatinine or severe with the need for renal replacement therapy. Urine output may be normal, high, or diminished (oliguria). A uniform definition of AKI was proposed, the *R*isk, *I*njury, *F*ailure, *L*oss, and *E*nd-stage renal disease (RIFLE) classification (Bellomo et al. 2004). Recently, the RIFLE criteria were modified for pediatric AKI, the pRIFLE system, shown in Table 1 (Akcan-Arikan et al. 2007). The KDIGO guidelines (KDIGO 2012) refer to pRIFLE predominantly being in use beyond the neonatal period (Thomas et al. 2014).

2.2 Causes of Acute Kidney Injury

Various diseases can cause AKI traditionally differentiated into prerenal AKI, renal (intrinsic) AKI, and postrenal AKI (Table 2). "Prerenal" implicates a complete reversibility of AKI with restoration of the renal hypoperfusion like in dehydration, acute blood loss, or in heart failure. If impossible during a certain time, prerenal AKI will proceed to intrinsic AKI. *Postrenal* AKI is rare if two functioning kidneys are present and bladder or urethral obstruction is required. It can be found more often in obstructed single kidneys or in renal transplants, e.g., with ureteral necrosis. The majority of children suffer from *renal (intrinsic)* AKI. The disorders can be differentiated into four subgroups. The various types of glomerulonephritis and interstitial nephritis with AKI are discussed in chapter "Renal Parenchymal Disease" as well as the majority of AKI caused by vascular disorders like vasculitis, the renal thrombotic microangiopathies including hemolytic uremic syndrome and antiphospholipid syndrome. Renal venous thrombosis can be found in nephrotic syndrome but mostly is a neonatal renal compromise.

Tubular compromise (acute tubular necrosis, ATN) may be toxin-mediated. Exogenous toxins are bacterial toxins in sepsis or nephrotoxic antibacterial, antifungal, or antineoplastic drugs like aminoglycosides or cisplatin. Contrast agents can cause contrast-induced nephropathy (CIN). Endogenous toxins are hemoglobin, myoglobin (crush syndrome), or uric acid (tumor lysis syndrome). Ischemia/hypoxemia-mediated ATN may be the result of prolonged or irreversible prerenal failure frequently following surgical interventions. Two components have to be considered in the pathophysiology. The microvascular component means vasoconstriction with a decreased oxygen supply and eventually vascular obstruction. The tubular component, in part caused by ischemia, is a cytoskeletal breakdown, desquamation of necrotic cells with tubular obstruction, and backleak of glomerular filtrate (Lameire et al. 2005).

Table 1 Pediatric-modified RIFLE criteria (pRIFLE)

	Estimated GFR	Urine output
Risk	eGFR decrease by 25 %	<0.5 ml/kg/h for 8 h
Injury	eGFR decrease by 50 %	<0.5 ml/kg/h for 16 h
Failure	eGFR decrease by 75 %	<0.3 ml/kg/h for 24 h or
	eGFR <35 ml/min/1,73 m^2	Anuria for 12 h
Loss	Persistent failure >4 weeks	
End stage	End-stage renal disease (persistent failure >3 months)	

Modified from Akcan-Arikan et al. (2007)
eGFR estimated glomerular filtration rate

Table 2 Causes of acute kidney injury. TMA, thrombotic microangiopathy

```
                     Acute kidney injury
                              |
        ┌─────────────────────┼─────────────────────┐
     Prerenal           Renal, intrinsic         Postrenal
                              |
          ┌──────────┬────────┴────────┬──────────┐
      Glomerular  Interstitial      Tubular    Vascular
          |           |                |          |
   Glomerulonephritis Drugs          Toxic     Vasculitis
                     Infections     Ischemic   Thrombosis
                     Autoimmune                Renal TMA
```

2.3 Diagnosis, Treatment, and Prognosis

Diagnosis of AKI is based on an increase of serum creatinine (SCr) or a decrease of GFR. Clinical and laboratory evaluation of these children is urgent to determine the cause and to start appropriate therapy. The volume status and the fractional excretion of sodium (FENa) help to differentiate prerenal AKI from intrinsic AKI; FENa larger than 2 % indicates sodium loss of intrinsic AKI. Hematuria and proteinuria point to glomerular disorders; a normal urinalysis favors tubulointerstitial compromise and ischemic/toxic lesions of ATN. Serum creatinine is a late measure of renal function (Andreoli 2009). Parameters for early detection are warranted enabling early interventions and hopefully leading to an improved prognosis. This is especially true for AKI on the pediatric intensive care unit (PICU) for disorders like sepsis, multiple organ failure, or AKI following cardiac surgery. Different biomarkers have been tested like neutrophil gelatinase-associated lipocalin (NGAL), interleukin-18 (IL18), kidney injury molecule 1 (KIM-1), cystatin C (CysC), etc. (Ho et al. 2014). Yet there is no single biomarker so far to fulfill our expectations. Treatment depends on final diagnosis and is symptomatic in most cases, and continuous hemodiafiltration is the method of choice if renal replacement therapy is needed especially on a PICU (Kellum and Lameire 2013). Prognosis following AKI is questionable and highly dependent on the underlying disease. Mortality is high in AKI as part of multiple organ failure in a PICU in contrast to AKI in isolated renal disorders (Andreoli 2009). In addition, children with AKI directly may proceed to chronic kidney disease (CKD) or have late CKD despite an apparent normalization of renal function. Long-term follow-up is needed in all pediatric AKI patients.

> **Take Away**
> Diagnosis, classification, and therapy of AKI are urgent. Normalization of renal function or CKD may be the outcome.

3 Neonatal Renal Failure

3.1 Fetal and Neonatal Renal Function

Significant fetal urine production starts at approximately 10–12 weeks of gestation. Fetal urine is the major constituent of amniotic fluid, and renal oligohydramnios indicates fetal renal failure. Nephrogenesis has a centrifugal pattern and is completed at 34–36 weeks of gestation. Destroyed nephrons cannot be replaced by new filtering units. Thus, prematurely born infants are the only humans able to harvest new nephrons after birth. Fetal renal blood flow (RBF) and glomerular filtration rate (GFR) are low. Plasma renin activity is high and production of renal prostaglandins is increased. Fetal homeostasis is maintained by the placenta and the maternal renal function, the "fetomaternal unit."

There is a sharp rise in RBF and GFR after birth. Plasma renin activity and production of renal prostaglandins decrease, but remain elevated compared to older children. Maturation of renal function is mostly due to enlargement of the glomerular capillary surface area, a rise in ultrafiltration pressure, and further development of tubular function, but the neonatal kidneys are vulnerable. On the first day of life, serum creatinine roughly equals maternal values even in cases with fetal renal failure. Prematurely born infants have higher levels of creatinine, and their postnatal increase in creatinine clearance is delayed compared to term neonates (see chapter "Normal Values"; Table 4). This is valid especially in very low birthweight infants (Bueva and Guignard 1994; Vieux et al. 2010).

3.2 Neonatal Acute Kidney Injury

Neonatal AKI (nAKI) is common in a neonatal intensive care unit (NICU) and has a significantly negative effect on the outcome. It is best characterized by changes of serum creatinine (SCr) compared to a baseline value. *Stage 1* of nAKI is defined as increase of >0.3 mg/dl within 48 h or up to two times the baseline in 7 days, *stage 2* is an increase up to three times the baseline, and *stage 3* is an increase of more than three times the baseline or SCr >2.5 mg/dl or dialysis (Jetton and Askenazi 2014). Oliguria also can be used for staging of nAKI, but this may be problematic as neonatal AKI frequently is nonoliguric. Special groups with nAKI are severely compromised like very low birthweight infants having a mortality of 42 % compared to 5 % in the non-AKI group (Koralkar et al. 2011). Cases with severe asphyxia and nAKI have mortality rates up to 47 %, and 12 % of neonates with congenital heart disease and AKI die (Gupta et al. 2005; Blinder et al. 2012). Sepsis-associated nAKI is frequent as well as tubular injury by nephrotoxic medications like aminoglycosides. Indomethacin – frequently given for closure of ductus arteriosus – and angiotensin-converting enzyme inhibitors (ACEI) or ATII-receptor blocking drugs (ATII-RB) decrease renal perfusion. ACEI or ATII-RB given during pregnancy can cause oligohydramnios and renal tubular dysgenesis (RTD), a special form of renal dysplasia with lesions of the proximal renal tubule (Spaggiari et al. 2012). Identical lesions are found in the kidneys of the asphyxiated donor twin of twin-to-twin transfusion syndrome, and in genetical forms of RTD where mutations in genes of the ACE system are found (Gubler 2014). These neonates have pulmonary hypoplasia and a nearly intractable arterial hypotension in addition to the kidney injury, and most cannot survive.

3.3 Diagnosis and Treatment

Identification of causes is essential as nAKI is often multifactorial. Due to the immature tubules, urine volume may be high (nonoliguric nAKI) and the ability to conserve sodium is lower. Consequently, determination of fractional excretion of sodium (FENa) is limited to distinguish between prerenal and intrinsic nAKI. Low urine output (<1.5 ml/kg/h) was present in 20 % of NICU patients in a recent study and correlated well with mortality (Bezerra et al. 2013). Additional prognostic factors for non-survival were maximal serum creatinine (nAKI stage 2–3), hyperkalemia, acidosis, thrombocytopenia, long mechanical ventilation, and sepsis. Like in older AKI patients, there is an intensive search for urine biomarkers predicting nAKI early in the course enabling timely interventions and improving prognosis. Urine NGAL, KIM-1, CysC, and other markers were tested with some success, but further research is needed (Krawczeski et al. 2011; Askenazi et al. 2011).

Treatment of nAKI is supportive. Adequate fluid and electrolyte replacement is needed but fluid overload should be avoided. Catecholamines are given as appropriate, and especially theophylline can reduce the AKI incidence significantly (Jetton and Askenazi 2014). Nephrotoxic medications have to be stopped or need proper adjustment for renal function; measurement of drug blood levels are helpful. Neonates with progressive nAKI, severe fluid overload, and intractable electrolyte imbalances need renal replacement therapy mostly performed as continuous hemodiafiltration (Askenazi et al. 2013; Rödl et al. 2012).

3.4 Congenital Renal Disorders

Genetic and nongenetic congenital renal disorders like hypodysplasia, cystic diseases, or urinary tract obstruction already may have caused renal lesions before birth, and renal oligohydramnios indicates fetal renal failure. These "chronic renal lesions" become relevant with birth causing "acute" kidney dysfunction by themselves or lead to superimposed nAKI. This may be intrinsic (prematurity, artificial ventilation, asphyxia, etc.) or postrenal where relief of obstruction is urgently needed. Such cases represent 10–30% of all neonates with nAKI, and avoidance of additional renal lesions is of utmost importance (Klaassen et al. 2007). The pregnancy should be kept intact as long as possible because birth weight below 2000 g is a challenge if neonatal renal replacement therapy is needed; 70% of patients will survive and neonatal end-stage renal disease is exceptional. Follow-up is favorable in many cases with just 50% of patents on dialysis or already being transplanted at the age of 8 years (Kemper and Müller-Wiefel 2007). Yet there are reports indicating much higher mortality rates and a survival of not more than 25% (Grijseels et al. 2011).

> **Take Away**
> Neonatal AKI is frequent with different disorders and a variable prognosis. Neonatal renal replacement therapy may be a challenge in prematurely born neonates.

4 Chronic Renal Failure

4.1 Definitions

Loss of one kidney during life or being born with a single kidney may cause slight renal dysfunction but, in general, does not lead to CRF even in late adulthood (Wikstad et al. 1988). CRF can be defined as a disease state with the loss of more than 50% of nephrons, persistently increased serum creatinine, and a decreased glomerular filtration rate (GFR). CRF implicates a relentless progression to ESRD without the possibility of cure. In the early stages, it is a silent disease defined by biochemical values. When GFR is reduced to 25% of normal, and correspondingly the number of functioning nephrons to 12% of normal, clinical symptoms of uremia appear and dominate in ESRD. To improve the detection and the treatment of children with renal disorders, the term chronic kidney disease (CKD) was established (Hogg et al. 2003). Patients suffer from CKD if kidney damage –with or without a reduced GFR– is present for at least 3 months (not valid for neonatal CKD), characterized by abnormalities in the composition of the blood or urine, abnormalities on imaging tests, or lesions on renal biopsy. The normal values of creatinine, GFR, and the five stages of CKD according to GFR are shown in chapter "Normal Values". The amount of albuminuria (classified A1 to A3) is frequently taken as an additional parameter to the GFR stages for risk evaluation of CRF progression (KDIGO 2013).

4.2 Epidemiology

Approximately one to three children aged up to 18 years per million total population and year will enter ESRD, the figures being similar in Europe and North America. One large survey on CRF with 4666 patients shows that 33% of patients were 6 to 12 years of age and 19% less than 2 years of age (Seikaly et al. 2003). Obstructive uropathy was the most common diagnosis (23%), and 18% suffered from renal aplasia, dysplasia, or hypoplasia. Reflux nephropathy (9%), focal segmental glomerulosclerosis (8%), and polycystic kidney disease (4%) were the next most frequent diagnoses. In general, nearly two-thirds of patients had a structural anomaly. A previous study had shown that 41% had already had urological surgery. Urinary tract malformations and hypodysplasia dominated even more in patients aged less than 2 years, accounting for 67% of cases (Fivush et al. 1998). The largest study from Europe showed similar results with somewhat different groups of diagnoses (Ardissino et al. 2003). Renal hypodysplasia, with or without urological malformations, accounted for 58% of cases. Hypodysplasia with VUR was the most frequent single cause of childhood CRF responsible for 26% of cases. Almost 70% of patients with CRF reached ESRD by 20 years of age with an increasing number of patients with glomerular disorders and a decreasing number of children with hypodysplasia as primary diagnosis. Age and GFR at presentation, the primary disease, and factors like anemia, hypoalbuminemia, blood pressure, and proteinuria influence the progression to ESRD (Seikaly et al. 2003; Gonzales Celedon et al. 2007). Data for patients on dialysis or after renal transplantation are similar. Obstructive uropathy is less frequent and focal glomerulosclerosis more frequent (Neu et al. 2002).

4.3 Pathophysiology

Whatever the underlying disease (e.g., structural anomaly, glomerulopathy, hereditary nephropathy), there is a remarkably similar histological appearance of kidneys with progressive disease, suggesting a common final pathway. Glomerulosclerosis and tubulointerstitial fibrosis are the dominant features (El Nahas and Bello 2005). Various changes seem to perpetuate a vicious cycle with permanent loss of nephrons and ESRD as the endpoint. Extensive nephron loss leads to glomerular hypertrophy (increase in cell size and number). Hyperperfusion and hyperfiltration are the consequence, and glomerular hypertension correlates best with glomerulosclerosis. Renal hemodynamics, the renin-angiotensin system, and factors such as increased glomerular metabolism, mesangial macromolecular deposition, local hypercoagulopathy, and hyperlipidemia are of importance. Glomerular growth promoters like growth hormone, transforming growth factor-β, insulin-like growth factor-I, angiotensin II, or endothelin induce glomerular hypertrophy and mesangial matrix accumulation with glomerular sclerosis as a result. The individual genetic variability may be important as the deletion type of angiotensin-converting enzyme gene seems to be associated with a severe course of disorders like IgA nephropathy and congenital uropathies (Yong et al. 2006). Systemic hypertension, urinary tract infections, and unrecognized or postoperative urinary obstruction perpetuate the damage and enhance progression. Blocking the renin-angiotensin system has the potential for regression or modulation of glomerulosclerosis meaning that we can ameliorate the course of disease (Fogo 2006). Early diagnosis, prevention of infection, close postoperative follow-up, early administration of ACE inhibitors, and proper treatment of systemic hypertension seem to be of utmost importance.

4.4 Diagnosis and Treatment

Diagnosis of CRF is based on laboratory values such as serum creatinine, creatinine clearance, and calculation of the glomerular filtration rate shown in chapter "Normal Values". Urinalysis may show proteinuria, hematuria, or urinary tract infection. Metabolic acidosis, hyperkalemia, renal salt wasting, hypocalcemia, hyperphosphatemia, and anemia are further typical laboratory features. Alkaline phosphatase and parathormone are needed to evaluate renal bone disease (renal osteodystrophy, ROD). Patients with as yet unrecognized CRF may present with a combination of polydipsia, polyuria, secondary enuresis, vomiting, failure to thrive, short stature, systemic hypertension, cardiac failure, and eventually edema as a sign of volume overload. Therapy of patients with known CRF is devoted to preventing such deleterious metabolic derangement.

Treatment intentions are to ameliorating the progressive course of disease, achieving metabolic control, and preventing extrarenal organ diseases. In addition, psychosocial care and planning the future are of importance. Aggressive treatment of severe glomerulopathies with poor outcome such as focal segmental glomerulosclerosis and early administration of ACE inhibitors is mandatory. Blood pressure is best controlled by 24-h measurement, and an intensified blood pressure control with values below the 50th percentile is optimal (Soergel et al. 1997; ESCAPE Trial Group 2009). Dietary measures include adequate caloric and fluid intake; protein is given according to the recommended daily allowances. Salt and potassium requirements depend on renal losses. Strict ROD therapy is mandatory to preventing disabling lesions. It includes dietary phosphate restriction, correction of acidosis, and administration of phosphate-binding agents and calcitriol. Serial determination of phosphate, calcium, acid–base status, alkaline phosphatase, and parathormone is needed (Klaus et al. 2006; Kemper and van Husen 2014). Administration of recombinant human growth hormone can ameliorate growth retardation; correction of renal anemia is achieved by iron and erythropoietin (Warady and Silverstein 2014). Cardiovascular disease is the leading cause of death in children with CRF, and coronary artery calcification is common (Mitsnefes 2012). Adequate therapy can ameliorate severe long-term risk factors.

4.5 Planning Dialysis and Transplantation

Future perspectives must be addressed to families with a child in CRF. The child must be in good physical condition; ABO blood group and HLA system antigens must be known. All necessary vaccinations should be performed during CRF as life vaccines generally are not allowed after RTx. Screening for panel-reactive cytotoxic antibodies and repeated determinations of antibody status against cytomegalovirus, EBV, hepatitis, etc. are mandatory. Urological disorders frequently need nephrectomy or nephrecto–ureterectomy before considering transplantation. Assessment of bladder function is mandatory to prevent bladder problems after transplantation. Children with a small noncompliant bladder may need bladder augmentation, which can be performed before or after renal transplantation. An augmented bladder is no contraindication for transplantation (Fontaine et al. 1998; Rigamonti et al. 2005). The preference of the family for peritoneal dialysis (PD) or hemodialysis (HD), for living-related donor transplantation or a deceased donor, and the option of a preemptive transplantation (before starting dialysis) must be weighed against medical indications. According to the joint decision, vascular access for HD or placement of a PD catheter can be planned. The living-related donor must undergo extensive investigations to ensure that no undue risks are incurred by removal of one kidney.

Take Away
The time of CRF is an active treatment period preventing disabling organ lesions and prolonging the time to end-stage renal failure.

5 Dialysis

5.1 Basic Considerations

If ESRD is reached (CKD 5), survival is possible with only blood purification, performed as PD or HD. It is the steady state from which transplantation is planned and performed in most situations and to which patients return in the case of graft failure. PD or HD can only partially restore metabolic control. As in CRF, proper treatment of hypertension, acidosis, ROD, etc. is mandatory.

5.2 Peritoneal Dialysis

Peritoneal dialysis (PD) is the preferred treatment in children with ESRD. It is the treatment of choice for infants, and 82% of children below

5 years of age are on PD in contrast to 37% of children aged 10–18 years (Watson et al. 2013). A permanent PD catheter is placed surgically into the peritoneal cavity with the tip in the lower abdomen and a long subcutaneous tunnel. Solute clearance and removal of fluid (ultrafiltration) are achieved by changing the dialysate several times per day. PD solutions contain different concentrations of glucose as the osmotic agent (Schmitt et al. 2011). PD can be performed at home during daytime (continuous ambulatory PD, CAPD) or machine-assisted during nighttime (automatic PD, APD, cyclic PD). Thus, a life in the normal surroundings of the family and regular school attendance for older children are possible. Advantages over hemodialysis are the continuous character of treatment with only slow changes in body composition, a relatively free diet and fluid supply, and a stable cardiovascular situation. PD prescription depends on age, body weight or body surface area, and the individual peritoneal membrane solute transport capacity. The latter is determined by a peritoneal equilibration test (PET) (Warady et al. 1996). Determination of creatinine clearance and weekly urea clearance (Kt/V) are of value to check adequacy of PD.

PD complications can be divided into acute or chronic and infectious or noninfectious. Acute catheter dysfunction may be caused by malposition. A too high intraperitoneal pressure may cause inguinal hernias, and herniotomy is frequently needed (Fischbach et al. 2003). Acute respiratory distress should raise suspicion of hydrothorax caused by thoracic leakage of peritoneal fluid (Rose and Conley 1989). Infections of the exit site, the subcutaneous tunnel, and peritonitis are the most common infectious complications. Treatment with intraperitoneal antibiotics is mandatory (Warady et al. 2012). The incidence of peritonitis is estimated to be one infection per 13 treatment months. Recurrent peritonitis may lead to catheter removal. The peritoneal membrane is functionally stable even in children on long-term PD (Warady et al. 1999). However, peritoneal sclerosis can cause ultrafiltration failure and intestinal obstruction. Frequent episodes of peritonitis partially contribute to this severe complication (Shroff et al. 2013).

5.3 Hemodialysis

Hemodialysis is a safe and effective treatment for children with ESRD and is performed in 43% of children aged 10–18 years (Watson et al. 2013). Technical refinements enable HD even in small children and infants (Rees 2013). In this age group, HD is mostly indicated if PD fails or is contraindicated. Vascular access is of utmost importance in pediatric HD. Central venous catheters are preferred in many centers (Neu et al. 2002). Arteriovenous fistulas are an alternative with a lower rate of complications compared to central venous catheters, and sometimes with an improved metabolic control of the patient (Chand et al. 2005; Ramage et al. 2005), but the rapid access to renal transplantation may favor central venous catheters. HD is mostly performed three times per week for 4–6 h per session at the dialysis center. The extracorporeal circuit needs anticoagulation with heparin. Citrate anticoagulation for exclusive anticoagulation of the extracorporeal circuit is a valuable alternative (Fischbach et al. 2005). Like in PD, adequacy of HD is checked by creatinine clearance and weekly urea clearance (Kt/V).

6 Renal Transplantation

6.1 Basic Considerations

Renal transplantation (RTx) is the treatment of choice for children with ESRD and absolute contraindications are few. Patients with HIV disease, malignancies, preexisting metastatic disease, or children with devastating neurological disorders are mostly excluded. Organ-sharing organizations exist for deceased donor Tx, and the allocation criteria mostly give priority to children. There is evidence that giving pediatric donor kidneys to pediatric recipients is the best allocation system, leading to a better prognosis of children with ESRD (Pape et al. 2007). Transplantation from a living-related donor is an alternative and may be performed preemptively (before starting dialysis), and preemptive registration is also accepted by most organizations for Tx. It is performed in about 24% of situations in North America, may prevent dialysis-associated morbidity, and is at least as good as post-dialysis Tx (Cransberg et al. 2006). The graft is placed extraperitoneally into a pelvic site. The vessels of the transplant are anastomosed with the iliac vessels or with the aorta and the inferior vena cava in small children. The ureter is connected to the bladder with an ureterocystoneostomy (Dharnidharka et al. 2014). Immunosuppressive therapy starts with Tx, and most centers use a combination of steroids, calcineurin inhibitor, and mycophenolate mofetil. Tacrolimus is the preferred calcineurin inhibitor as graft survival seems to be superior to cyclosporine A (Filler et al. 2005). New drugs or modifications of established treatment protocols are under investigation for initial and long-term therapy.

6.2 Acute Problems

Acute tubular necrosis (ATN), graft thrombosis, and hyperacute rejection (Rx) are of major concern. ATN is observed in 5.1% of living-related Tx and in 15.6% of deceased donor transplants (NAPRTCS 2010). These patients require dialysis after Tx. Risk factors for ATN are a prolonged cold ischemia, frequent use of blood transfusions, and previous transplantations. Graft thrombosis accounts for 9.6% of graft failure and is more common in young patients. It should be suspected in all cases with primary engraftment and sudden onset of oliguria during the first few days after operation. Hyperacute Rx invariably leads to loss of the graft, but is exceptional nowadays. Tx biopsy is needed in prolonged graft dysfunction. Severe bleeding around the transplant may be caused by anticoagulation or a leak of the vessel anastomoses. Urinary tract obstruction may be the consequence of ureteral kinking, stenosis of ureteral implantation, ureteral necrosis, or large lymphoceles. It is important to note that severe urinary obstruction may present with just minimal or moderate renal pelvic dilatation due to a diminished urinary flow. In addition, these situations are painless as the transplant and the ureter have no nerves.

6.3 Regular Follow-Up

After discharge from hospital, regular visits to the outpatient clinic are necessary. Anthropometric data and the health status are checked. Fluid intake, urine output, and blood pressure are recorded at home. Laboratory investigations include urinalysis, serum creatinine, blood levels of immunosuppressive agents, the antibody status of EBV and cytomegalovirus activity, etc. The dosage of immunosuppressive drugs must be checked and adjusted frequently to avoid the nephrotoxicity of overdosage and the danger for rejection with underdosage.

6.4 Acute Rejection

Various immunological processes are involved in acute rejection. 45.6% of transplants will have at least one rejection (40.9% in living donation and 50.6% in deceased donation). The number of acute rejections has dramatically improved, and just 13.2% had rejection in the years 2007–2010 compared to 31.9% in the years 1999–2002 (NAPRTCS 2010). Clinical symptoms such as graft tenderness and fever are exceptional nowadays. Typical signs are a decrease in urine flow, a rise in serum creatinine, and high blood pressure. Differential diagnosis includes urinary tract obstruction or vascular complications; a transplant biopsy is necessary for definite diagnosis. The type and severity of rejection is classified histologically according to the Banff criteria (Solez and Racusen 2012). As a rule, methylprednisolone pulses are the initial treatment, but this clearly depends on the rejection type. In general, more than 50% of rejections are completely reversible and only 6% lead to graft failure.

6.5 Infections

As a result of immunosuppression, patients are prone to viral and bacterial infections. This is an increasing problem and hospital admissions for infections nowadays exceed admissions for acute rejection. A problematic virus emerging in the last decade is polyoma BK virus (BKV). BKV allograft nephropathy affects 2–8 % of grafts and leads to early graft loss in 50 % of patients, and there is no specific treatment (Acott 2006). Cytomegalovirus infection is a serious complication with a high risk to the patient and the transplant. EBV infections are related to the development of posttransplant lymphoproliferative disease. *Pneumocystis carinii* pneumonia occurs in 3 % of Tx patients. These patients may present acutely with shortness of breath and hypoxemia. Immediate therapy with high-dose cotrimoxazole is frequently effective.

Approximately 50 % of Tx patients have urinary tract infections. Symptomatic infections are found predominantly during the first 3 months after transplantation. Patients with preexisting urological disorders may have recurrent infections, and kidney transplants seem to be prone to scarring in the case of vesicoureteric reflux (Coulthard and Keir 2006).

6.6 Posttransplant Lymphoproliferative Disorder

Posttransplant lymphoproliferative disorder (PTLD) is a serious complication after solid organ transplantation, being related to chronic immunosuppression. The percentage of children with PTLD is increasing and has to be seen in the context of previous EBV infection (Mynarek et al. 2013). Approximately 94 % of PTLD are non-Hodgkin lymphomas. Clinical presentation mostly is not specific and almost every organ including the graft can be affected. Reduction or modification of immunosuppression like switching to mTOR inhibitors like everolimus is mandatory. Treatment with rituximab, an anti-CD20 monoclonal antibody, dramatically could improve the outcome of PTLD. Chemotherapy or radiation is rarely needed, and aside from serologic parameters, imaging has a key role in detecting and long-term monitoring of PTLD (Scarsbrook et al. 2005; Burney et al. 2006).

6.7 Prognosis

The early outcome after renal Tx improves every year. Better care for the patients during CRF and ESRD makes them better candidates for Tx. Improvement of the immunosuppressive regimen and introduction of new drugs eventually will allow a more individual approach. Rehabilitation is optimal, and more than 90 % of patients survive 5 years after Tx. According to the 2010 NAPRTCS report, graft survival rates after 5 years improved to 84.3 % in living donation and to 78.0 % in deceased donation for the years 2003–2010. The rates of chronic kidney loss are unchanged during the last decade and are a cause of major concern. Chronic allograft nephropathy (CAN) is the main cause of kidney loss and is histologically characterized by tubular atrophy and interstitial fibrosis with glomerulopathy and vascular lesions in addition (Alexander et al. 2007). Many immunological and non-immunological factors influence the risk and the rapidity of progression of CAN. Major factors are acute rejections, subclinical rejections, viral infections, nephrotoxicity of CI, and noncompliance with immunosuppression. Protocol biopsies may be helpful to clarify main causes of CAN in the individual patient with hopefully new treatment strategies to reduce the incidence of CAN. In addition, long-term problems such as cardiovascular disease must be addressed early (Oh et al. 2002; Parekh and Gidding 2005). The child and the family need the lifelong support of a multidisciplinary team to optimize therapy.

Take Away
Dialysis is the steady state for children with ESRD, and outcome after RTx is excellent despite various imminent problems.

Conclusion
Various renal and systemic disorders may cause AKI, frequently being reversible but also leading to CKD. Neonatal AKI may be a challenge with a high mortality in special

groups of prematures. Chronic kidney disease is an active treatment time. A preferably short time on dialysis and a successful RTx are warranted. For ESRD, dialysis and preferably RTx are the only long-term options, with a better long-term outcome of RTx after introduction of new immunosuppressive drugs and follow-up regimens. Imaging plays an irreplaceable role during all stages of AKI as discussed in this chapter – from initial diagnosis of AKI up to long-term surveillance including preparation and following RTx.

References

Acott PD (2006) Polyoma virus in pediatric renal transplantation. Pediatr Transplant 10:856–890

Akcan-Arikan A, Zappitelli M, Loftis LL et al (2007) Modified RIFLE criteria in critically ill children with acute kidney injury. Kidney Int 71:1028–1035

Andreoli SP (2009) Acute kidney injury in children. Pediatr Nephrol 24:253–263

Alexander SI, Fletcher JT, Nankivell B (2007) Chronic allograft nephropathy in paediatric renal transplantation. Pediatr Nephrol 22:17–23

Ardissino G, Dacco V, Testa S et al (2003) Epidemiology of chronic renal failure in children: data from the ItalKid project. Pediatrics 111:382–387

Askenazi DJ, Goldstein SL, Koralkar R et al (2013) Continuous renal replacement therapy for children ≤10 kg: a report from the prospective pediatric continuous renal replacement therapy registry. J Pediatr 162:587–592

Askenazi D, Koralkar R, Levitan EB et al (2011) Baseline values of candidate urine acute kidney injury (AKI) biomarkers vary by gestational age in premature infants. Pediatr Res 70:302–306

Bellomo R, Ronco C, Kellum JA et al (2004) Acute renal failure-definition, outcome measures, animal models, fluid therapy and information technology needs: the Second International Consensus Conference of the Acute Dialysis Quality Initiative (ADQI) Group. Crit Care 8:R204–R212

Bezerra CT, Vaz Cunha LC, Liborio AB (2013) Defining reduced urine output in neonatal ICU: importance for mortality and acute kidney injury classification. Nephrol Dial Transplant 28:901–909

Blinder JJ, Goldstein SL, Lee VV et al (2012) Congenital heart surgery in infants: effects of acute kidney injury on outcomes. J Thorac Cardiovasc Surg 143:368–374

Bueva A, Guignard JP (1994) Renal function in preterm neonates. Pediatr Res 36:572–577

Burney K, Bradley M, Buckley A et al (2006) Posttransplant lymphoproliferative disorder: a pictorial review. Australas Radiol 50:412–418

Chand DH, Brier M, Strife CF (2005) Comparison of vascular access type in pediatric hemodialysis patients with respect to urea clearance, anemia management, and serum albumin concentration. Am J Kidney Dis 45:303–308

Coulthard MG, Keir MJ (2006) Reflux nephropathy in kidney transplants, demonstrated by dimercaptosuccinic acid scanning. Transplantation 82:205–210

Cransberg K, Smits JM, Offner G et al (2006) Kidney transplantation without prior dialysis in children: the Eurotransplant experience. Am J Transplant 6:1858–1864

Dharnidharka VR, Fiorina P, Harmon WE (2014) Kidney transplantation in children. N Engl J Med 371:549–558

El Nahas AM, Bello AK (2005) Chronic kidney disease: the global challenge. Lancet 365:331–340

ESCAPE Trial Group, Wühl E, Trivelli A, Picca S et al (2009) Strict blood-pressure control and progression of renal failure in children. N Engl J Med 361:1639–1651

Filler G, Webb NJ, Milford DV et al (2005) Four-year data after pediatric renal transplantation: a randomized trial of tacrolimus vs. cyclosporin microemulsion. Pediatr Transplant 9:498–503

Fischbach M, Edefonti A, Schröder C et al (2005) Hemodialysis in children: general practical guidelines. Pediatr Nephrol 20:1054–1066

Fischbach M, Terzic J, Laugel V et al (2003) Measurement of hydrostatic intraperitoneal pressure: a useful tool for the improvement of dialysis dose prescription. Pediatr Nephrol 18:976–980

Fivush BA, Jabs K, Neu A et al (1998) Chronic renal insufficiency in children and adolescents: the 1996 annual report of NAPRTACS. Pediatr Nephrol 12:328–337

Fogo AB (2006) Progression versus regression of chronic kidney disease. Nephrol Dial Transplant 21:281–284

Fontaine E, Gagnadoux MF, Niaudet P et al (1998) Renal transplantation in children with augmentation cystoplasty: long-term results. J Urol 159:2110–2113

Gonzales Celedon C, Bitsori M, Tullus K (2007) Progression of chronic renal failure in children with dysplastic kidneys. Pediatr Nephrol 22:1014–1020

Grijseels EW, van-Hornstra PT, Govaerts LC et al (2011) Outcome of pregnancies complicated by oligohydramnios or anhydramnios of renal origin. Prenat Diagn 31:1039–1045

Gubler MC (2014) Renal tubular dysgenesis. Pediatr Nephrol 29:51–59

Gupta BD, Sharma P, Bagla J et al (2005) Renal failure in asphyxiated neonates. Indian Pediatr 42:928–934

Ho J, Dart A, Rigatto C (2014) Proteomics in acute kidney injury-current status and future promise. Pediatr Nephrol 29:163–171

Hogg RJ, Furth S, Lemley KV et al (2003) National Kidney Foundation's kidney outcomes quality initiative clinical practice guidelines for chronic kidney disease in children and adolescents: evaluation, classification, and stratification. Pediatrics 111:1416–1421

Jetton JG, Askenazi DJ (2014) Acute kidney injury in the neonate. Clin Perinatol 41:487–502

Kellum JA, Lameire N (2013) Diagnosis, evaluation, and management of acute kidney injury: a KDIGO summary (Part 1). Crit Care 17:204–218

Kemper MJ, Müller-Wiefel DE (2007) Prognosis of antenatally diagnosed oligohydramnios of renal origin. Eur J Pediatr 166:393–398

Kemper MJ, van Husen M (2014) Renal osteodystrophy in children: pathogenesis, diagnosis and treatment. Curr Opin Pediatr 26:180–186

Kidney Disease: Improving Global Outcomes (KDIGO), Acute Kidney Injury Work Group (2012) KDIGO clinical practice guideline for acute kidney injury. Kidney Int 2(Suppl):1–138

KDIGO (2013) Clinical practice guideline for the evaluation and management of chronic kidney disease. Kidney Int 3(Suppl):19–62

Klaassen I, Neuhaus TJ, Mueller-Wiefel DE et al (2007) Antenatal oligohydramnios of renal origin: long-term outcome. Nephrol Dial Transplant 22:432–439

Klaus G, Watson A, Edefonti A et al (2006) Prevention and treatment of renal osteodystrophy in children on chronic renal failure: European guidelines. Pediatr Nephrol 21:151–159

Koralkar R, Ambalavanan N, Lwvitan EB et al (2011) Acute kidney injury reduces survival in very low birth weight infants. Pediatr Res 69:354–358

Krawczeski CD, Woo JG, Wang Y et al (2011) Neutrophil gelatinase-assiciated lipocalin concentrations predict development of acute kidney injury in neonates and children after cardiopulmonary bypass. J Pediatr 158:1009–1015;e1

Lameire N, Van Biesen W, Vanholder R (2005) Acute renal failure. Lancet 365:417–430

Mitsnefes MM (2012) Cardiovascular disease in children with chronic kidney disease. J Am Soc Nephrol 23:578–585

Mynarek M, Schober T, Behrends U et al. Posttransplant lymphoproliferative disease after pediatric solid organ transplantation. Clin Dev Immunol. 2013; Article ID 814974.

North American Pediatric Renal Trials and Collaborative Studies. 2010 annual transplant report. https://web.emmes.com/study/ped/annlrept/2010_Report.pdf.

Neu AM, Ho PL, McDonald RA et al (2002) Chronic dialysis in children and adolescents. The 2001 NAPRTCS annual report. Pediatr Nephrol 17:656–663

Oh J, Wunsch R, Turzer M et al (2002) Advanced coronary and carotid arteriopathy in young adults with childhood onset chronic renal failure. Circulation 106:100–105

Pape L, Ehrich JH, Offner G (2007) Young for young! Mandatory age-matched exchange of paediatric kidneys. Pediatr Nephrol 22:477–479

Parekh RS, Gidding SS (2005) Cardiovascular complications in pediatric end-stage renal disease. Pediatr Nephrol 20:125–131

Ramage IJ, Bailie A, Tyerman KS et al (2005) Vascular access survival in children and young adults receiving long-term hemodialysis. Am J Kidney Dis 45:708–714

Rees L (2013) Infant dialysis-what makes is special? Nat Rev Nephrol 9:15–17

Rigamonti W, Capizzi A, Zacchello G et al (2005) Kidney transplantation into bladder augmentation or urinary diversion: long-term results. Transplantation 80:1435–1440

Rödl S, Marschitz I, Mache CJ et al (2012) Hemodiafiltration in infants with complications during peritoneal dialysis. Artif Organs 96:590–593

Rose GM, Conley SB (1989) Unilateral hydrothorax in small children on chronic continuous peritoneal dialysis. Pediatr Nephrol 3:89–91

Scarsbrook AF, Warakaulle DR, Dattani M et al (2005) Posttransplantation lymphoproliferative disorder: the spectrum of imaging appearances. Clin Radiol 60:47–55

Schmitt CP, Bakkaloglu SA, Klaus G et al (2011) Solutions for peritoneal dialysis in children: recommendations by the European Pediatric Dialysis Working Group. Pediatr Nephrol 26:1137–1147

Seikaly MG, Ho PL, Emmett L et al (2003) Chronic renal insufficiency in children: the 2001 annual report on the NAPRTCS. Pediatr Nephrol 18:796–804

Shroff R, Stefanidis CJ, Askiti V et al (2013) Encapsulating peritoneal sclerosis in children on chronic PD: a survey from the European Paediatric Dialysis Working Group. Nephrol Dial Transplant 28:1908–1914

Soergel M, Kirschstein M, Busch C et al (1997) Oscillometric 24-hour ambulatory blood pressure values in healthy children and adolescents. A multicenter trial including 1,141 subjects. J Pediatr 129:178–184

Solez K, Racusen LC (2012) The Banff classification revisited. Kidney Int 83:201–206

Spaggiari E, Heidet L, Grange G et al (2012) Prognosis and outcome of pregnancies exposed to renin-angiotensin system blockers. Prenat Diagn 32:1071–1076

Thomas ME, Blaine C, Dawnay A et al (2014) The definition of acute kidney injury and its use in practice. Kidney Int 87(1):62–73

Vieux R, Hascoet J-M, Merdariu D et al (2010) Glomerular filtration rate reference values in very preterm infants. Pediatrics 125:e1186–e1192

Warady BA, Alexander SR, Hossli S et al (1996) Peritoneal membrane transport function in children receiving long-term dialysis. J Am Soc Nephrol 7:2385–2391

Warady BA, Fivush B, Andreoli SP et al (1999) Longitudinal evaluation of transport kinetics in children receiving peritoneal dialysis. Pediatr Nephrol 13:571–576

Warady BA, Bakkaloglu S, Newland J (2012) Consensus guidelines for the prevention and treatment of catheter-related infections and peritonitis in pediatric patients receiving peritoneal dialysis: 2012 update. Perit Dial Int 32:529–586

Warady BA, Silverstein DM (2014) Management of anemia with erythropoietic-stimulating agents in children with chronic kidney disease. Pediatr Nephrol 29:1498–1505

Watson AR, Hayes WN, Vondrak K et al (2013) Factors influencing choice of renal replacement therapy in European Pediatric Nephrology Units. Pediatr Nephrol 28:2361–2368

Wikstad I, Celsi G, Larsson L et al (1988) Kidney function in adults born with unilateral renal agenesis or nephrectomized in childhood. Pediatr Nephrol 2:177–182

Yong D, Qing WQ, Hua L et al (2006) Association of angiotensin I-converting enzyme gene insertion/deletion polymorphism and IgA nephropathy: a meta-analysis. Am J Nephrol 26:511–518

Part IV

Lower Urinary Tract Anomalies, Malformations and Dysfunctions

Abnormalities of the Lower Urinary Tract and Urachus

Samuel Stafrace, Marie Brasseur-Daudruy, and Jean-Nicolas Dacher

Contents

1	**Prenatal Diagnosis**..................................	299
1.1	Absence of Normal Bladder.......................	300
1.2	Megacystis..	301
1.3	Management Concepts and Options Available......................................	301
2	**Posterior Urethral Valves**......................	302
2.1	Posterior Urethral Valves in Neonates: Imaging and Follow-Up.............................	302
2.2	Diagnosis of Posterior Urethral Valves in Older Boys...	307
3	**Other Causes of Bladder Outlet Obstruction**.................................	308
3.1	Urethral Polyp..	308
3.2	Ureterocele Prolapse..................................	308
3.3	Cobb's Collar, Urethral Diverticula, and Cowper's Gland Cysts.........................	308
3.4	Tumor..	309
4	**Other Urethral Congenital Abnormalities**...	310
5	**Bladder Diverticula**................................	311
6	**Congenital Cystic Disease of the Seminal Vesicle**..	311
7	**Bladder Stones**...	312
8	**Infection**..	312
9	**Urachus**...	313
	Conclusion...	314
	References...	314

S. Stafrace, MD, MRCP (UK), FRCR, FRCP Edin
Sidra Medical and Research Center, Doha, Qatar
e-mail: sstafrace@sidra.org

M. Brasseur-Daudruy • J.-N. Dacher (✉)
Department of Radiology,
University Hospital of Rouen, 1, Rue de Germont, F-76031 Rouen, France
e-mail: Marie.Brasseur-Daudruy@chu-rouen.fr; Jean-Nicolas.Dacher@chu-rouen.fr

1 Prenatal Diagnosis

Nowadays, maternal-fetal sonography is able to diagnose most congenital abnormalities of the lower urinary tract (Eurin et al. 1999). Production of urine begins around the tenth week of gestation when the bladder becomes theoretically visible (McHugo J 2001). By 12 weeks of gestation a normal bladder is visible in the fetal abdomen in 87% of cases and should be seen in all during the second trimester (Clayton and Brock 2012). Its identification can be facilitated by color Doppler encoding of blood flow in the umbilical arteries present alongside. Later during pregnancy, the bladder should be examined on several occasions during fetal sonography to ensure that the bladder fills and empties; cycles last 30–45 min (Patten et al. 1990). The normal ureters are not usually visible. The normal bladder appears as a thin-walled fluid-filled cavity. Any bladder abnormality (size, wall thickening) should lead to an

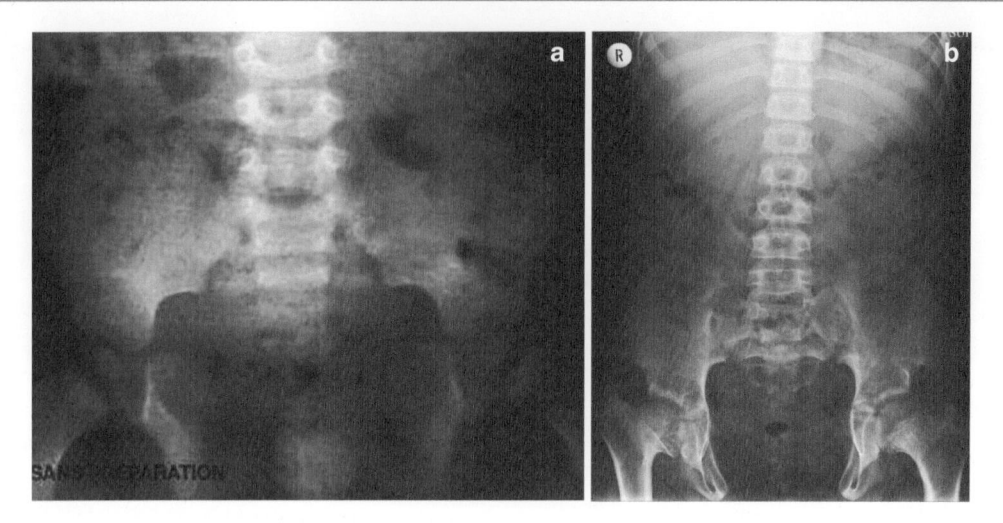

Fig. 1 (**a**) AP radiograph of the pelvic cavity showing widening of the pubic symphysis in an infant girl with vesical exstrophy. (**b**) Similar appearances in an older child—note the associated dysplastic appearances in the right hip

intense analysis of the kidneys (calyces, pelvis, and parenchyma), fetal gender, volume of amniotic fluid, and the fetal lungs.

1.1 Absence of Normal Bladder

The absence of any visible bladder should alert for an abnormality on the exstrophy-epispadias complex. This is a spectrum with epispadias being the mildest manifestation followed by classic bladder exstrophy (intermediate) and cloacal exstrophy (most severe manifestation on the spectrum). The bladder is normally still identified in epispadias. In the two more severe malformations, there is an open defect of the abdominal or perineal wall. Classic bladder exstrophy and cloacal exstrophy can also present with an omphalocele (Grignon and Dubois 1999). The spectrum of abnormalities normally involves the bladder, abdominal wall, pelvic floor, and bony pelvis (Tekes et al. 2013). Widening of the distance between the pubic bone echoes can be shown by prenatal ultrasound (US) (see also chapter "Epispadias-Exstrophy Complex"). This finding, also appreciated on plain film post delivery, can also be seen in epispadias (Fig. 1). Postnatal abdominal and pelvic MRI may be helpful for decision-making and surgery planning in assessing all the anatomical structures involved in the epispadias-exstrophy complex, if plain film and US cannot answer all relevant questions.

Cloacal malformation exclusively occurs in the female phenotype and should not be confused with cloacal exstrophy (see above and chapter "Urinary Problems Associated with Imperforate Anus") (Lebowitz 1997). A cloacal malformation represents the most severe degree of an imperforate anus on the anorectal malformation complex spectrum (Hendren 1998). Prenatal diagnosis is difficult because a septated fluid-filled cavity can be mistaken for a normal bladder. However, echogenic debris can substantiate such a suspected diagnosis because it has been shown to result from a mixture of urine and meconium (Bear and Gilsanz 1981). At birth, there is only one perineal opening, and communication between the urethra, the vagina, and the rectum is seen. Widening of the pubic bones may also be associated to the cloacal malformation as well as many other associated malformations (involving the axial skeleton, spinal cord, heart, and urinary tract). The prognosis of this severe malformation improved dramatically with the contribution of Hardy Hendren who developed novel surgical techniques to deal with these complex anomalies (Miller 1993).

1.2 Megacystis

Megacystis (which has differing criteria dependent on the trimester) has been described as a physiological finding in two scenarios. Firstly, transient megacystis has been reported during the first trimester of pregnancy (Sebire et al. 1996). Secondly, megacystis can be observed in normal female fetuses by the end of pregnancy (Eurin et al. 1999). Establishing a physiological cause requires the presence of normal kidneys, nondilated upper tracts, and the visualization of normal fetal micturition. In female fetuses, megacystis should not be confused with a distended vagina due to an imperforate hymen or the presence of a duplicated uterus.

Transient megacystis may be a sign of obstruction and/or vesicoureteric reflux (VUR). In boys, it could be the consequence of transient bladder outlet obstruction and the starting point of a series of abnormalities. Notably, it could explain the male predominance in neonatal VUR. This hypothesis was raised after the observation of children presenting with VUR, a dilated posterior urethra, and no posterior urethral valves (PUV) (Avni et al. 1992; Avni and Schulman 1996) (see also chapter "Vesicoureteric Reflux"). Another hypothesis has come from experimental surgery. Premature urachal closure could induce hydroureteronephrosis in male fetuses (Gobet et al. 1998). Such a transient obstruction has also been suspected as being responsible for the prune-belly syndrome which associates megacystis, ureterohydronephrosis, undescended testis, and hypoplasia of muscles of the abdominal wall (Pagon et al. 1979) (see chapter "Imaging in Prune Belly Syndrome and Other Syndromes Affecting the Urogenital Tract").

Table 1 Prenatal diagnosis of megacystis

Pathology	Physiology (see text)
Lower urinary tract obstruction	Transient megacystis (10–14 weeks)
Posterior urethral valves	
Urethral atresia (mostly fatal)	Isolated megacystis by the end of pregnancy in girls
Prolapsed ectopic ureterocele	
Vesicoureteric reflux (Megacystis-megaureter association in high-grade reflux)	
Megacystis microcolon intestinal Hypoperistalsis syndrome (MMIHS)	
Neurologic disorders	
Prune-belly syndrome	
Caudal regression syndrome	
Anorectal anomalies and cloaca	

The differential diagnosis for megacystis includes other pathological conditions (Abbott et al. 1998; Fievet et al. 2014), and postnatal radiological investigations are still useful to assess the anatomy of the lower urinary tract (Table 1). When assessing fetal megacystis, the gestational age at diagnosis is helpful in stratifying the potential cause. The most common diagnosis for megacystis diagnosed in the first 6 months of gestation is bladder outflow obstruction, topped by posterior urethral valves. Beyond the 6 months of gestation, the most common cause for megacystis is VUR (Fievet et al. 2014).

1.3 Management Concepts and Options Available

Many factors have to be taken into account in the management of megacystis diagnosed antenatally. In the cases caused by severe obstruction, poor outcome factors include early diagnosis, oligohydramnios, lung hypoplasia, sonographic signs of renal dysplasia, the presence of any other fetal malformation, elevated urinary sodium, and urinary beta$_2$-microglobulin. Assessment for other anomalies and karyotyping should be done first and, if normal, serial urinary testing for electrolytes and protein profiles. Fetal intervention is offered in specialized centers in cases of confirmed severe lower urinary tract obstruction, the absence of other anomalies, normal karyotyping, and favorable urinary analysis. Intervention can involve fetal cystoscopy (and laser fulguration for posterior urethral valves) and/or the insertion of a vesicoamniotic shunt. Alternatives to therapeutic intervention include expectant pregnancy management or termination (depending on local legislation) (Ruano et al. 2014).

> **Take Away**
> Bladder examination is part of any maternal-fetal sonography. An abnormality can reveal either transient or constituted obstruction of the lower urinary tract requiring intense monitoring and further assessment.

2 Posterior Urethral Valves

Posterior urethral valves (PUV) consist of abnormal mucosal folds between the urethral wall and the distal end of the verumontanum. The classification established by Young at the beginning of the twentieth century appears questionable from an endoscopic perspective (Dewan et al. 1992). Young had identified three types of valves. Type I was described as a bicuspid valve radiating distally from the posterior edge of the verumontanum to the anterior aspect of the proximal membranous urethra. Type I valves are by far the most frequent, representing 95% of all cases. Type III posterior urethral valves are more circumferential (diaphragm-like) and have been thought to be a remnant of the urogenital membrane.

Young type II valves were first described as "mucosal folds extending cranially from the verumontanum to the bladder neck" (Dewan et al. 1992); they could be a different disease and the consequence of dysfunctional voiding with bladder-sphincter dyscoordination.

Membranous obstruction is more likely than the "valvular mechanism" that gave its name to the malformation (Dewan and Goh 1995). This concept is referred to as congenital obstructive posterior urethral membrane (COPUM). As a matter of fact, most children seem to present with the same membranous abnormality more or less modified by the passage of indwelling catheters or a Whitaker diathermy hook (Whitaker and Sherwood 1986).

On endoscopy, valves are described as a membranous obstruction with a posterior pinhole orifice adjacent to the verumontanum. Disposition of valves is oblique, the distal attachment being anterior. Valves usually balloon distally so that they can traverse the external sphincter (see also Chap. 15).

There is great variability in clinical presentation. The most obstructive forms are usually detected by prenatal US, and the child's management starts before or at birth. Less severe forms can be detected during early infancy or even during later childhood. Renal consequences are extremely variable—from no alteration in forms revealed in older children to severe renal impairment and bladder dysfunction in infantile/neonatal cases.

2.1 Posterior Urethral Valves in Neonates: Imaging and Follow-Up

Management of fetuses and neonates with prenatal diagnosis of PUV should be performed in a fetal medicine and pediatric surgery/urology reference center. In each new case, the great variability of presentation makes different specialists' participation necessary in the difficult decision-making process (Fig. 2). Fetal specialists, surgeons, neonatologists, nephrologists or urologists, and radiologists should be involved in the discussions before birth. The quality of management is frequently improved when the surgeon/urologist and the nephrologist can

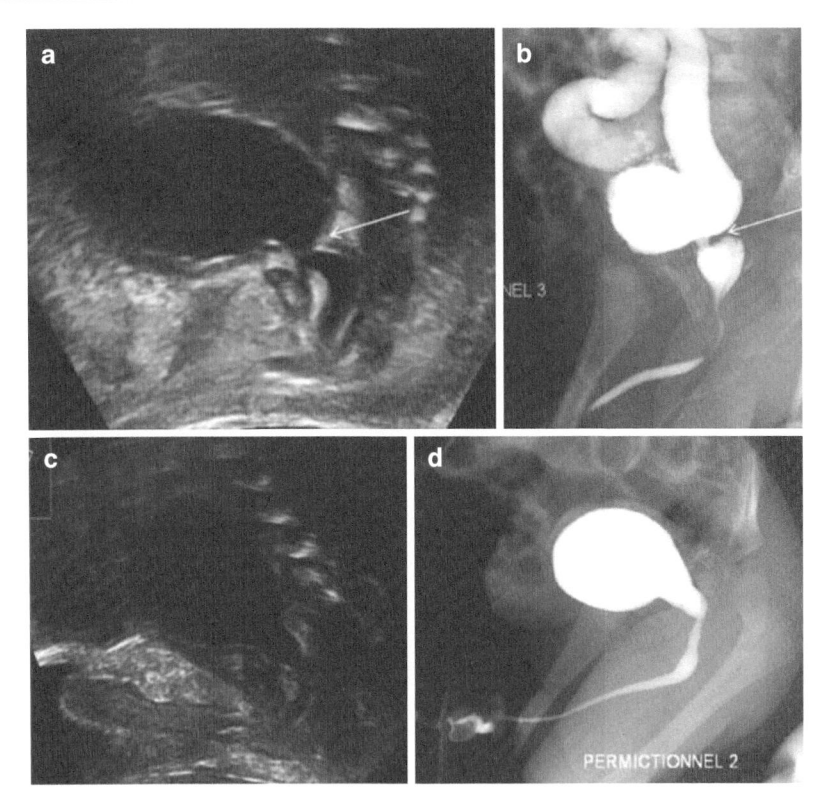

Fig. 2 Antenatal US images of PUV with postnatal MCUG in two separate cases. (**a**) Sagittal US image of the fetal bladder and urethra during micturition; the dilated posterior urethra is seen accompanied by bladder and bladder neck hypertrophy (*arrow*). (**b**) Sagittal selected image during MCUG. Appearances on US are confirmed on the MCUG obtained soon after birth. (Note also the significant associate VUR) (**c**) Similar case with dilated posterior urethra demonstrated on the sagittal prenatal US during micturition. (**d**) Reciprocal sagittal MCUG obtained soon after birth with correlation of the expected findings. Both cases above had confirmed PUV

explain the principles of postnatal treatment and perspectives to the parents during pregnancy. In order to plan postnatal management, prenatal findings including images, US measurements, and biological findings should be communicated to the pediatric radiologist.

After birth, radiological evaluation is routinely performed during the first 24 h of life. Prenatal US findings are confirmed, and precise assessment is facilitated by usage of a high-frequency transducer and perineal scans. The huge bladder with a thickened and trabeculated wall and the dilated posterior urethra are shown and measured. Bilateral dilatation fo teh ureters and the pelvicaliceal system are frequent. Analysis of the renal parenchyma (echogenicity, cysts, thickness) is important even if US cannot quantify renal function (Fig. 3). Renal dysplasia seems to depend on the timing in gestation and the presence of individual factors such as VUR or urinoma (Blane et al. 1994; Peters et al. 1992).

Perirenal urinoma (ascites or even hydrothorax) may be present (Fig. 4). Such fluid collections are the consequence of the rupture of calyceal fornices due to increased pressure. This has been described as the "pop-off" mechanism (Rittenberg et al. 1988). However, the presence or absence of urinoma does not clearly correlate with renal function impairment.

At birth, a voiding cystourethrogram (VCUG) is performed either through a feeding tube or more commonly after suprapubic puncture (Fig. 5). Aspiration of any stagnant urine is first performed. All precautions must be taken to ensure sterility given the increased risk of post-procedural infection (Dacher et al. 1992). Infection could be life threat-

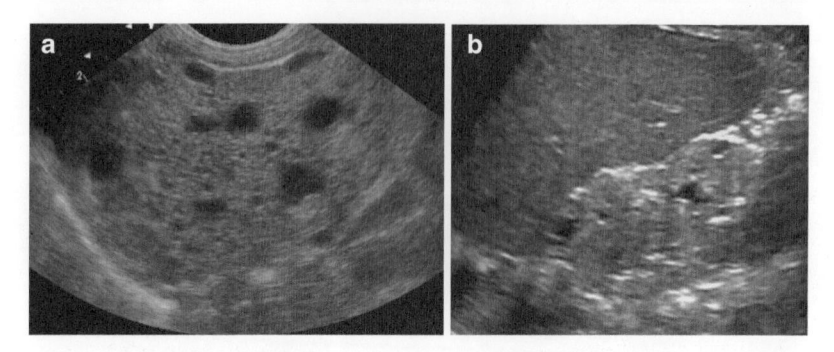

Fig. 3 Cystic dysplastic appearance of the kidneys in a case of posterior urethral valves. The left kidney demonstrates loss of corticomedullary differentiation, irregularity of the outline, and numerous cysts. (**a**) At birth when the kidneys also appeared enlarged. (**b**) At 6 months of age, the kidneys are now small and the cysts still discernable

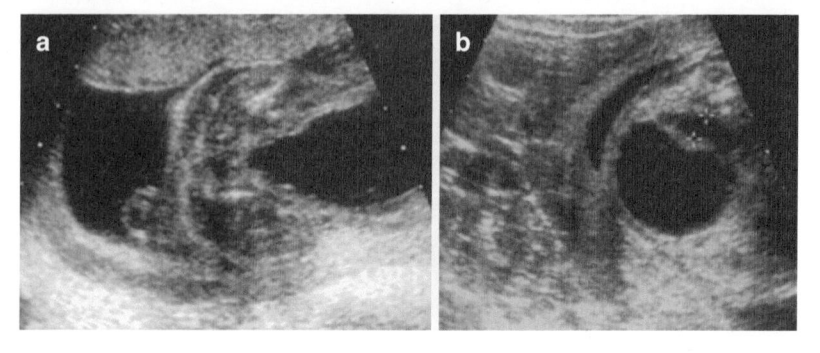

Fig. 4 Prenatal sonography in a 22-week gestational age male fetus. (**a**) Megacystis with dilated posterior urethra. Moderately dilated left kidney (not shown). (**b**) Huge dilatation of the right kidney with perirenal urinoma (Courtesy of D. Eurin)

ening for the baby and devastating for the already challenged renal function. Retrograde opacification is technically possible since valves produce only one-way obstruction. However, it can be difficult to pass through the bladder neck due to the dilated posterior urethra, which can retain the tip of the tube. Retrograde catheterization yields a higher risk of infection, and it could probably modify the endoscopic appraisal of the anatomy.

When the initial study is performed percutaneously, leakage into the prevesical space can occur. This should not interrupt the examination since it resolves spontaneously. The bladder appears thick-walled with marked sacculations and trabeculations. Diverticula may be present.

VUR (often only unilateral) is a frequent finding (Fig. 6). Oblique views can be taken to analyze the lower segment of the refluxing ureter. Delayed films should be taken to analyze reflux clearance and to grade the obstructive component. Voiding time is often long and patience is required when performing these studies. This is, however, an essential diagnostic step since it shows the discrepancy between the anterior and posterior segments of the urethra with a posteriorly located orifice. In classical descriptions, VCUG demonstrates the "sail in the wind" sign in Young type I posterior urethral valves and the "wind in sock" sign in Young type III posterior urethral valves (Figs. 5 and 7). Again, these different patterns are more likely to be the consequence of endourethral procedures rather than different diseases.

The main differential diagnosis is the megacystis-megaureter association, which is due to massive VUR and the phenomenon of aberrant micturition. (Willi and Lebowitz 1979; Reuter and Lebowitz 1985). Prenatal diagnosis is relatively straightforward in female fetuses, but more subtle in males (in the absence of a dilated posterior urethra). Prune-belly syndrome is another important consideration with similar dynamics but more extensive multisystemic pathological

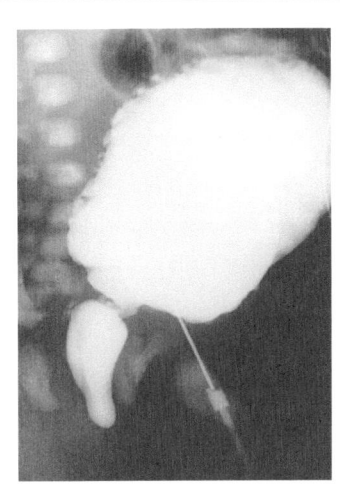

Fig. 5 Suprapubic micturating cystourethrography in a neonate with posterior urethral valves. A high-capacity heavily trabeculated bladder was opacified. Distended posterior urethra. Valves are ballooned by contrast medium ("sail in the wind" sign)

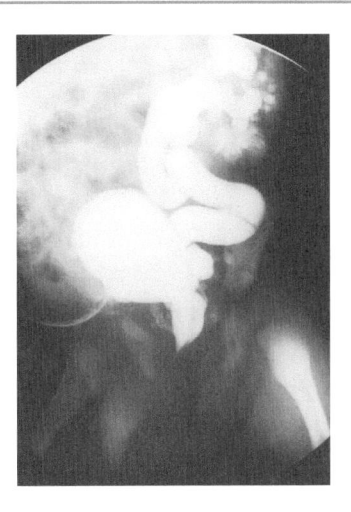

Fig. 6 Suprapubic voiding cystourethrography (VCUG) in a neonate with posterior urethral valves (PUV). Contrast reflux into the seminal vesicles. High-grade left VUR into a very dilated upper urinary tract. Note intrarenal reflux

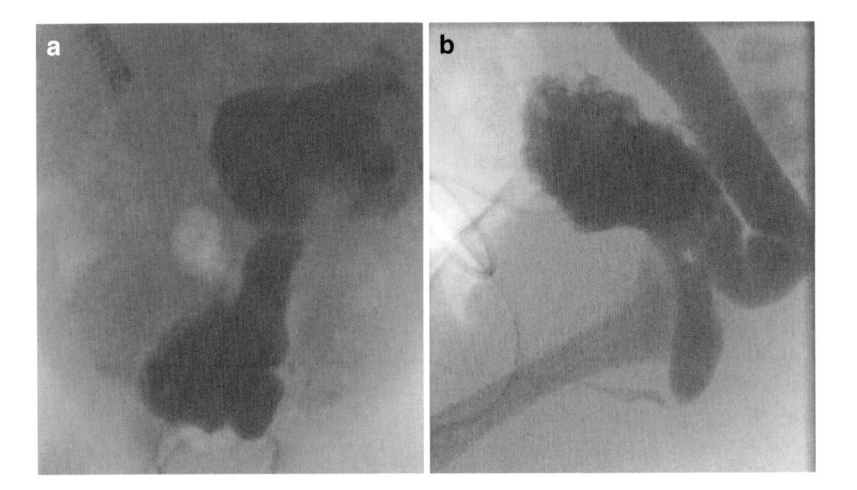

Fig. 7 VCUG through a suprapubic catheter in a neonate with PUV. AP (**a**) and lateral (**b**) projections. PUV with change in caliber in the posterior urethra, trabeculated bladder, and gross VUR into tortuous dilated left ureter

associations (Fig. 8). In prune-belly syndrome, the bladder is often three to four times the expected size with dilated bilateral refluxing elongated ureters. Urachal anomalies are common. The bladder neck is wide and an associated utricle is often seen. The detrusor musculature is thickened. There is commonly renal dysplasia further affecting renal function. Other characteristic anomalies include the absence or deficiency of the abdominal wall musculature, cryptorchidism (in boys who represent 95 % of the cases), gastrointestinal, cardiac, and orthopedic abnormalities (Zugor et al. 2012). Alternative diagnosis could include a neuropathic cause with dysfunctional voiding. Appearances can be very similar to PUV and presentation is typically in the neonate (Fig. 9).

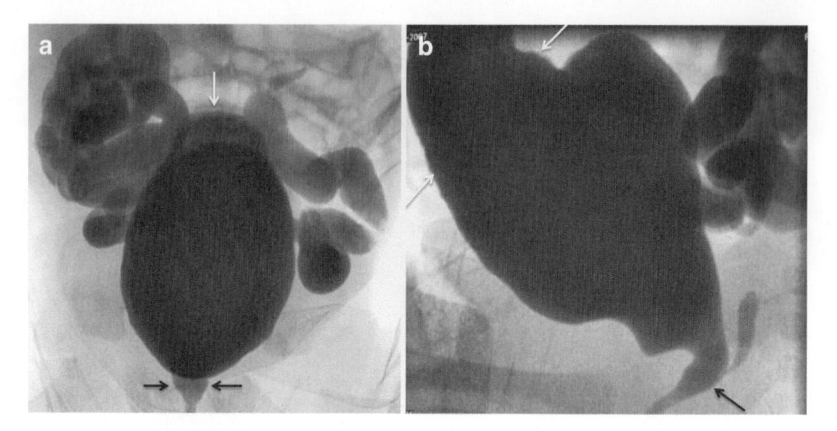

Fig. 8 VCUG in a neonate with diagnosis of prune-belly syndrome. (**a**) AP view. The bladder is enlarged (megacystis) with bilateral dilated tortuous ureters. There is malrotation of the kidneys with gross right intrarenal reflux. (**b**) Lateral projection. A large urachal remnant is present (*white arrows*). The bladder neck is widened (*black arrow*), and the posterior urethra demonstrates a prominent utricle posterior to the dilated bladder neck

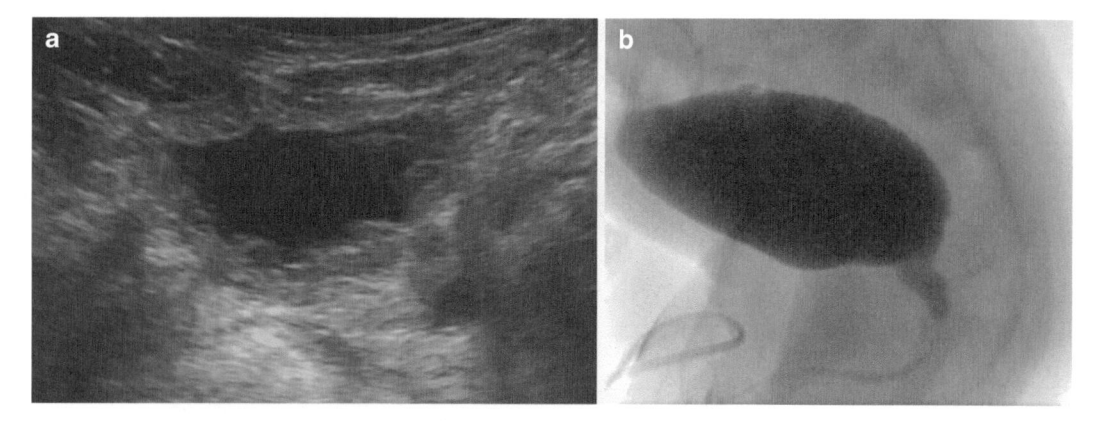

Fig. 9 Ultrasound and VCUG in a neonate with suspected PUV. (**a**) Transverse US image of the thickened bladder. (**b**) Lateral projection from VCUG study. This demonstrates clear change in caliber in the posterior urethra with some trabeculations of the bladder. The initial diagnosis was PUV. However, cystoscopy did not identify any anatomical abnormality in the posterior urethra. The lower sacral elements are missing (difficult diagnosis on a VCUG) with the abnormality presumed to be neurological (see also Fig. 11)

After VCUG, iodinated contrast medium is aspirated, and the bladder is slowly drained by the catheter. Fulguration of the valves is performed during the following hours or days. Because the bladder catheter cannot be left inside the bladder for an extended period, and because there is severe alteration of the bladder contractility, renal diversion is frequently required during the first few months of life, particularly if there is a significant upper obstruction component at the ureterovesical junction or the pelvi-ureteric junction (bilateral nephrostomy or ureterostomy). Imaging follow-up is based on US, nuclear medicine studies, MR urography, and contrast studies as required based on the individual findings.

Continence is often a problem in children and adolescents with a history of an obstructive PUV. Urodynamic studies are sometimes helpful to evaluate vesical and sphincteral function. Growth of the prostate gland during puberty often yields transient or definite improvement (Pfister et al. 1996).

In spite of extensive and precocious surgical treatment following prenatal diagnosis, many patients with a perinatal history of PUV have subsequent deterioration of their renal function. Usually, if renal function quickly improves immediately after relief of the anatomical obstruction, then deterioration will only develop slowly over the years sometimes only after puberty (Drozdz et al. 1998; Pereira et al. 2013).

End-stage renal disease occurs in most patients with a history of severe obstruction during the first 20 years of life.

2.2 Diagnosis of Posterior Urethral Valves in Older Boys

The clinical presentation is completely different in older children. The main complaint is usually dysuria or urinary tract infection (Fig. 10).

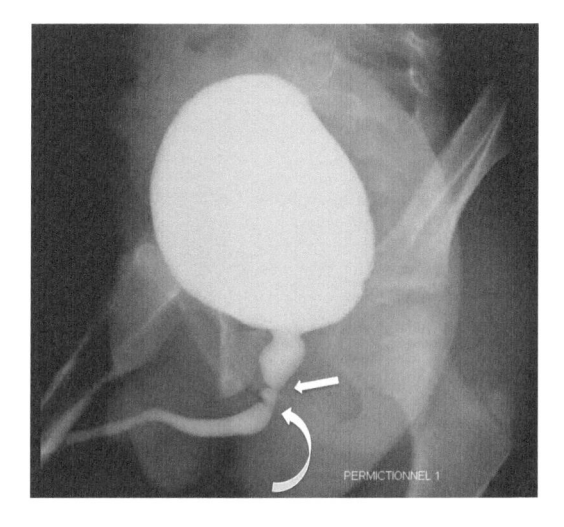

Fig. 10 A 6-year-old boy with dysuria and sensation of incomplete voiding. No prenatal history. No history of urinary tract infection. VCUG shows moderately obstructive PUV (*straight arrow*). Fulguration was performed with success. Note the imprinting of the external sphincter (*curved arrow*)

Megacystis and thickening of the bladder wall are less frequent. The kidneys are usually normal, as is the measured renal function. The differential diagnosis should include the other causes of bladder outlet obstruction and functional disorders such as dysfunctional voiding with severe bladder-sphincter dyscoordination (Fig. 11) (see chapters "Non-neurogenic Bladder-Sphincter Dysfunction ("Voiding Dysfunction")" and "Neurogenic Bladder in Infants and Children"). Both VCUG and urodynamic studies can be diagnostic; US may sometimes show indirect findings.

There is a broad spectrum in PUV. It should be remembered that some boys may have marked folds with no obstruction at all (Dewan and Goh 1995). This frequent radiological or endoscopic finding should be correlated with clinical complaints in order to ensure proper management of patients.

> **Take Away**
> Optimal neonatal management of boys with a prenatal diagnosis of PUV necessitates excellent cooperation among fetal specialists, obstetricians, neonatologists, surgeons/urologists, nephrologists, and radiologists. Early and comprehensive imaging by US and VCUG is essential. Unfortunately, end-stage renal disease is still a frequent outcome.

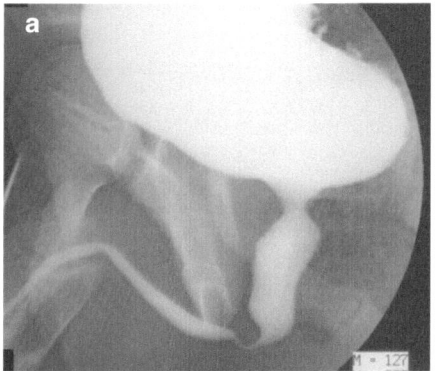

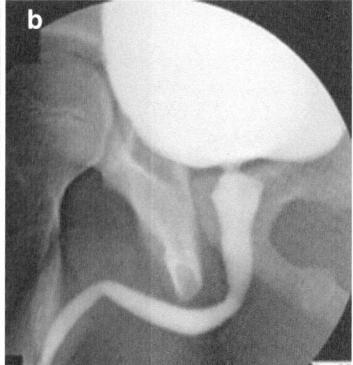

Fig. 11 (a) VCUG in a 7-year-old boy with dysuria showing extrinsic compression of the urethra due to abnormal sphincter contraction during micturition. This functional anomaly should not be mistaken for a PUV. Urodynamic studies favor dysfunctional voiding with bladder-sphincter dyscoordination during voiding. Biofeedback physiotherapy was carried out. Clinical outcome was favorable. (b) Follow-up VCUG shows normalization of urethral anatomy during micturition

3 Other Causes of Bladder Outlet Obstruction

3.1 Urethral Polyp

Extremely rare in childhood, the urethral polyp is usually solitary and consists of a pedunculated structure, originating from the posterior urethra, developing in the bladder neck, which can prolapse in the urethra during micturition (Foster and Garrett 1986). The abnormality can present with hematuria, nonneurogenic bladder-sphincter dysfunction, or urinary tract infection. On US it appears as an echogenic area. The main differential diagnosis of a urethral polyp is an ectopic ureterocele that has ruptured either spontaneously or after endoscopic incision (Fig. 12). VCUG is helpful, showing a mobile filling defect in the projection of the base of the bladder. Bladder trabeculations and diverticula can be associated. Surgical removal is the treatment of choice. An association has been described with hepatoblastoma in the Beckwith-Wiedemann syndrome (Bockrath et al. 1982).

3.2 Ureterocele Prolapse

An ectopic ureterocele typically develops at the lower end of the upper pole ureter of a duplicated kidney (see also Chap. 15). It is a cyst-like thin-walled structure that is known to be mobile and variable in shape. During fetal or later life, the ureterocele can prolapse into the posterior urethra and create obstruction. Usually the respective ureter is dilated; bilateral dilated urinary tract and megacystis can subsequently develop. Clinical diagnosis can be made at birth in girls with a perineal soft tissue mass, megacystis, and bilateral urinary tract obstruction. US diagnosis can be difficult when the ectopic ureterocele has spontaneously ruptured or with poor hydration or reduced renal function within insufficient urine production to fill and distend the urethrocele. In this case, the differential diagnosis with a urethral polyp is challenging (see above). The phenomenon has also been described in boys with a single ureterocele (Diard et al. 1981).

3.3 Cobb's Collar, Urethral Diverticula, and Cowper's Gland Cysts

Cobb's collar is a congenital narrowing of the bulbar urethra with no connection to the verumontanum (Cobb et al. 1968; Dewan et al. 1994). This entity is frequently associated with tubular or cystic dilatation of Cowper's gland ducts (also called syringocele) (Dewan 1996). Both structures arise embryologically from the urogenital membrane area.

In most cases, narrowing of the bulbar urethra with or without retrograde opacification of Cowper's gland ducts has no pathological significance (Beluffi et al. 2006) (Fig. 13). However, retention cysts may occur and induce urinary flow obstruction. Fetal infravesical obstruction

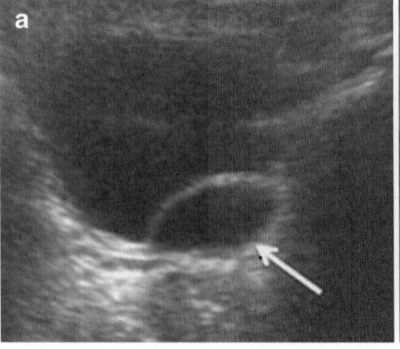

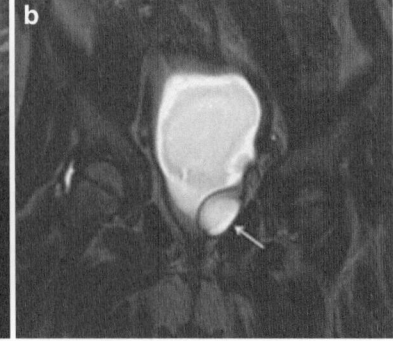

Fig. 12 A 5-year-old girl with a left ureterocele (*arrows*). (a) Transverse US image demonstrating the thin-walled ureterocele indenting the left aspect of the bladder base. (b) Corresponding coronal T2 MRI image

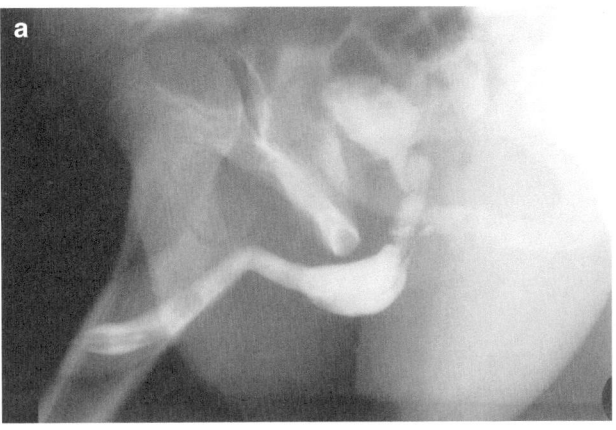

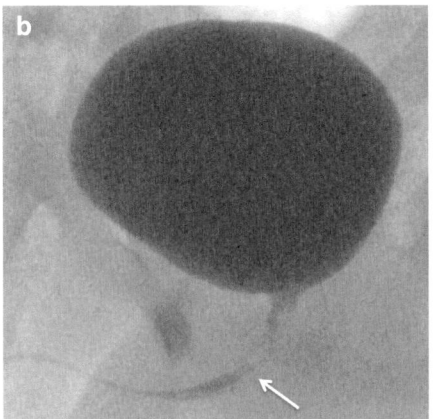

Fig. 13 (a, b) Normal appearances of Cowper's gland ducts on MCUG in two adolescent males (*arrows*)

may complicate Cowper's gland cysts as well (Dhillon et al. 1993). Urethral diverticulum can be either acquired or congenital (Fig. 14). Congenital diverticula can be found anywhere in the urethra, but largely predominate on the ventral surface of the penile urethra (Rimon et al. 1992). It is hypothesized that anterior urethral valves and diverticula could be the consequence of a ruptured Cowper's gland cyst (McLellan et al. 2004).

Secondary urethral diverticula seem to be more frequent than a primary etiology. These can be related to previous trauma from catheterization (in patients with neurogenic bladder), previous surgery (e.g., in cases of anorectal malformation), or to periurethral infection (bacterial or parasitic). A stone may develop in any kind of urethral diverticulum.

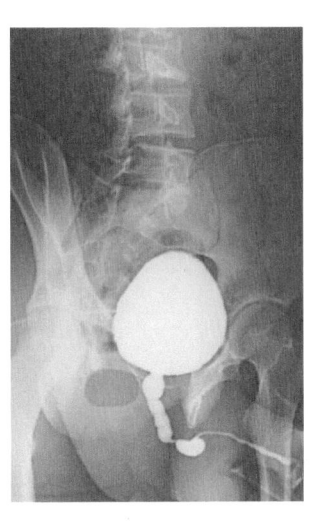

Fig. 14 VCUG in a 7-year-old boy with history of dysuria; no history of trauma. During micturition, a distended posterior urethra was identified as well as a diverticulum associated with stenosis

3.4 Tumor

Rhabdomyosarcoma is the most frequent malignant tumor of the lower urinary tract (Bisset et al. 1991). Peak incidence is during the first 3 years of life, and cases have been reported in neonates. The bladder, the prostate gland, and the vagina are the most commonly involved sites. Urinary frequency, hematuria, a palpable abdominal mass, fever, and constipation may all be the presenting symptoms of the disease. Passage of the tumor is most common in vaginal lesions. The site of origin is often difficult to detect, and conclusions should not be based on ultrasound findings alone.

Imaging helps determine the extent of the lesion. Ultrasound usually shows an irregular polypoid mass (grape-like) infiltrating the base of the bladder (Fig. 15). Thickening of the bladder wall can be associated, as well as dilatation of one or both ureters. A periurethral tumor causing lower obstruction may also be depicted by US particularly when using a perineal approach. On VCUG, an irregular filling defect of the base of the bladder is shown, and the floor of the bladder appears elevated. There may be

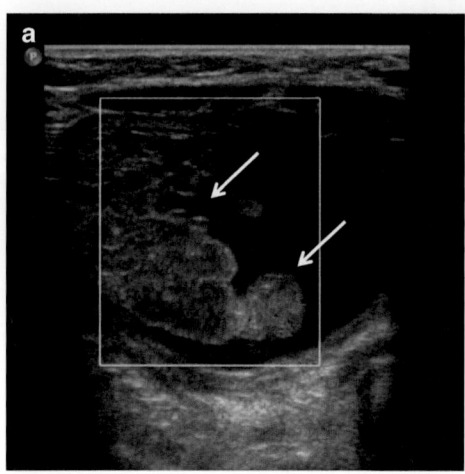

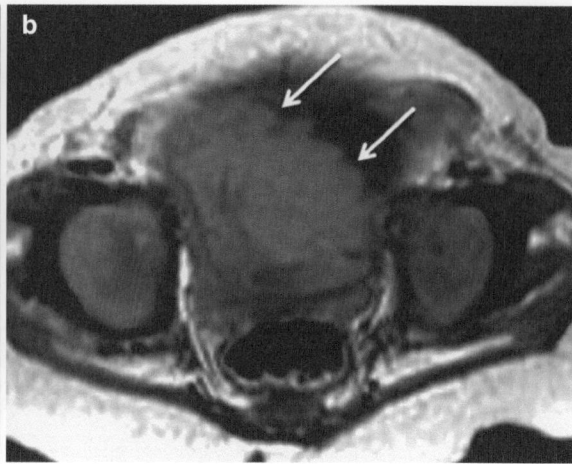

Fig. 15 Rhabdomyosarcoma of the bladder. (**a**) Longitudinal image of the bladder demonstrating an intraluminal lobulated polypoid mass (*arrows*) arising from the dorsal superior wall. (**b**) Transverse axial T1 image of the same solid lesion (*arrows*). The lesion was demonstrated to represent a rhabdomyosarcoma on biopsy (Courtesy of Dr. Gurdeep S Mann; Alder Hey Children's Hospital, Liverpool, UK)

irregular thinning of the posterior urethra in boys. Residual urine is frequent. Nowadays, the reference imaging modality is multiplanar MRI with fat-suppression sequences and gadolinium enhancement.

> **Take Away**
> The combination of US, VCUG, and cystoscopy helps establish a proper differential diagnosis among the causes of congenital or acquired bladder outlet obstruction.

4 Other Urethral Congenital Abnormalities

A great variety of urethral abnormalities may be found, most of them in boys. Evaluation is based on VCUG or retrograde urethrography (Riccabona et al. 2015). Cystourethroscopy is often useful to confirm findings. Normal variants should be kept in mind in order to avoid misinterpretation. For example, compression of the pendulous urethra by a nonopaque urinal and proximal dilatation is a frequent misinterpretation (Rink and Mitchell 1990).

Hypospadias is a frequent anomaly of the urinary meatus that can be associated with significant stenosis and dilatation of the male urethra. Though possible in most cases, catheterization of the urethra can be difficult and painful. In general, however, particularly low-grade hypospadias does not require extensive imaging; if at all, a US of the urinary tract will suffice except for postoperative complications such as strictures.

Epispadias is part of the heterogeneous exstrophy-epispadias complex (see chapter "Epispadias-Exstrophy Complex"). It may occur in males and females. Widening of the pubic symphysis is usually associated (see above). Continence is variable in these patients, so imaging and urodynamic studies should be directed toward this issue and the detection of associated anomalies.

Duplication of the bulbous urethra is extremely rare. It may be complete or blind-ended, ventral or dorsal (Barbagli et al. 1996) (Fig. 16).

Finally, megalourethra is an enlargement of the pendulous urethra with no evidence of distal obstruction (Stephens and Fortune 1993). It could be the consequence of late canalization of the epithelial core in the glans. It may also be a part of the prune-belly syndrome.

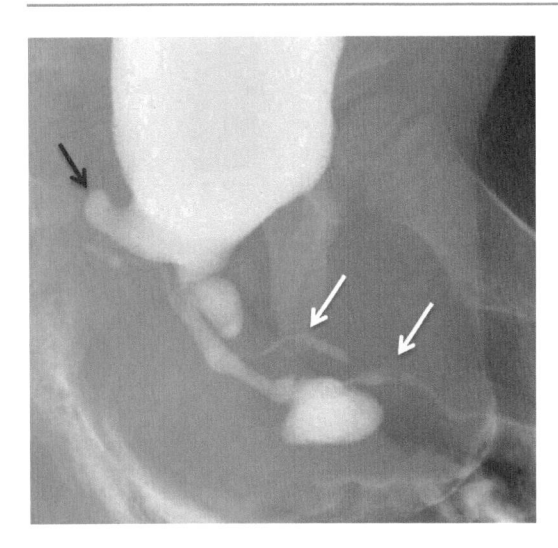

Fig. 16 MCUG demonstrating near-complete duplication of the urethra (*white arrows*). A bladder diverticulum is also noted arising from the right side of the bladder base (*black arrow*) (Courtesy of Dr. Gurdeep S Mann; Alder Hey Children's Hospital, Liverpool, UK)

> **Take Away**
> Diagnosis of urethral congenital abnormalities is based on clinical examination, the voiding phase of the VCUG study, retrograde urethrography, perineal (ce-)US during voiding, and cystoscopy.

5 Bladder Diverticula

A bladder diverticulum consists of herniation of the vesical mucosa through a defect in the muscular wall of the bladder. This entity was first described in paraplegic patients with neurogenic bladder. In rare cases, a dilated upper urinary tract has been described in association with bladder diverticula associated with compression or disturbance of ureteric emptying (Lebowitz 1997). More commonly, (paraostial) diverticula are associated with ipsilateral VUR. There is an association with the absence of spontaneous resolution of VUR (Blane et al. 1994). US is often negative particularly if performed without sufficient bladder filling or without post-void evaluation. VCUG usually yields the accurate diagnosis dependent on the performance of left and right oblique views of the full bladder, as diverticula may be hidden behind the opacified bladder on AP views and missed. Diverticula may only pose during voiding, while some even evert during voiding to an extent that an initially non-refluxing ureter may become refluxive. A bladder diverticulum may be an incidental finding, and it does not require any treatment when no association with either VUR, urinary tract infection, or obstruction is identified. The main differential diagnosis consists of an everted ectopic ureterocele (Bellah et al. 1995).

> **Take Away**
> Oblique films on VCUG (during voiding) are the best imaging approach to demonstrate bladder diverticula that can cause obstruction and VUR or represent a normal variant.

6 Congenital Cystic Disease of the Seminal Vesicle

This uncommon disorder (King et al. 1991) can be acquired or congenital. When congenital, the cyst is usually associated with anomalies of the ipsilateral mesonephric duct such as a multicystic dysplastic kidney. A cyst can be discovered on a pelvic US. On an axial plane, it can be confused with a dilated ureter. An orthogonal scan helps to make the differential diagnosis (the structure remains rounded in case of a congenital cyst). Associated renal and/or ureteral anomalies (multicystic dysplastic kidney, renal agenesis, duplication of collecting system, and ectopic ureter) and urethral or bladder anomalies (PUV, VUR into the cyst and/or the ipsilateral ureter) can be detected on US, cystography, MR, and/or CT (Hernanz-Schulman et al. 1989). Cystoscopy is a useful complementary examination to look for trigonal abnormalities and an ectopic ureteral orifice.

> **Take Away**
> Congenital cystic disease of the seminal vesicle is often associated with anomalies of the ipsilateral kidney and ureter.

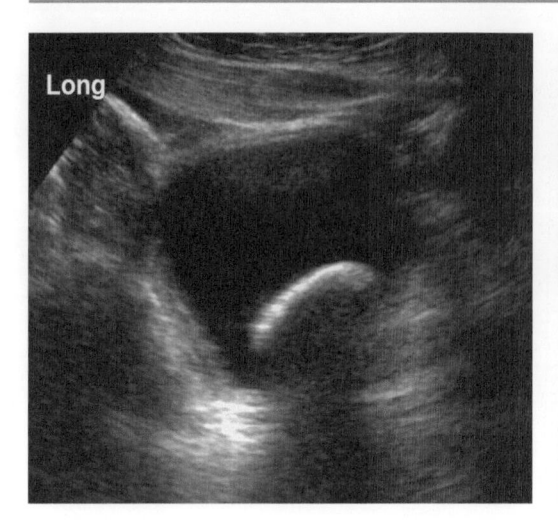

Fig. 17 US of the bladder demonstrating a large single stone in the bladder (Courtesy of Dr. Gurdeep S Mann; Alder Hey Children's Hospital Liverpool, UK)

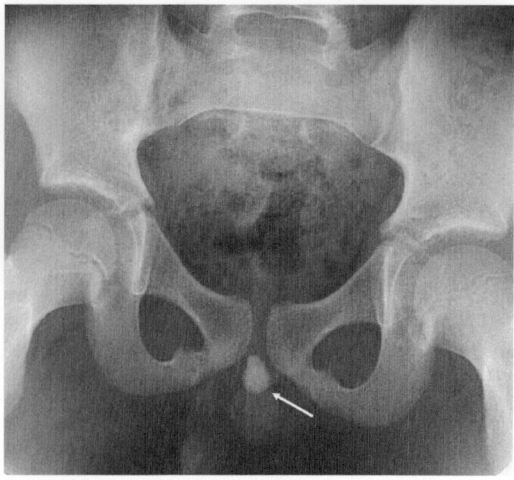

Fig. 18 Plain film showing a calcified stone in the posterior urethra (*arrow*) in a boy complaining of dysuria

7 Bladder Stones

Endemic bladder stones are mostly observed in boys in Africa and in the Indian subcontinent. These primary calculi are likely related to nutritional deficiencies. In contrast, the bladder stone has become very uncommon in children in western countries. The recognized lithogenic factors are infection (*Proteus mirabilis*), stasis, hypercalciuria (which can be associated with nephrocalcinosis), bladder scars, intestinal tissue in the bladder mucosa (in exstrophy or after surgical augmentation of the bladder), cystinuria, ileal dysfunction (inflammatory bowel disease, intestine inserted into the urinary tract), and long-standing intravesical foreign bodies (catheter) (see also chapters "Urolithiasis and Nephrocalcinosis" and "Imaging of Urolithiasis and Nephrocalcinosis"). Diagnosis is obvious on US and plain film when the stone is located in the bladder (Fig. 17). It should be remembered that a stone can be located in the posterior urethra and thus only is depictable sonographically by a perineal access; a calcified stone can be hidden behind a lead shielding of the gonads (Fig. 18).

> **Take Away**
> If a diagnosis of a bladder stone is obvious as seen in most cases on plain film and US, finding its explanation can be more challenging.

8 Infection

The spectrum of urinary tract infection includes cystitis in children (see also chapters "UTI and VUR" and "Imaging in Urinary Tract Infections"). Imaging is not relevant in common cystitis in an adolescent girl. However, in some patients, children with cystitis may present with dysuria, gross hematuria, and moderate fever. If US is performed, irregular thickening of the bladder wall can be shown. Such thickening can be tricky to interpret when the bladder is not filled, which is common in these children with frequent voiding.

In some patients, inflammatory changes can be so intense that infravesical obstruction with bilateral hydronephrosis is created. Differentiating pseudotumoral cystitis and a tumor can be difficult and occasionally may require sophisticated imaging (MRI), cystoscopy, and biopsy (Hoeffel et al. 1993) (Fig. 19). This applies to another rare inflammatory

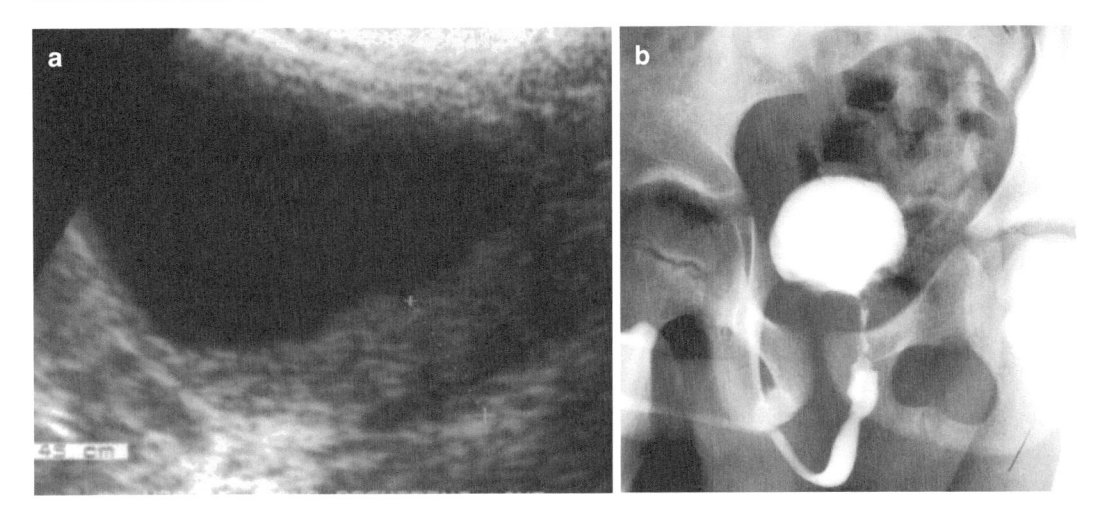

Fig. 19 US and VCUG in a 7-year-old boy with gross hematuria and painful dysuria. (**a**) Irregular thickening of the base of the bladder on US. (**b**) Elevation of the bladder, irregular stenosis of the bladder neck, and proximal posterior urethra. Prostatic rhabdomyosarcoma was suspected. Cystoscopy and biopsies were negative. Urinary culture was positive. Final diagnosis was *E. coli* pseudotumoral cystitis

condition of the urinary bladder of unknown origin, the eosinophilic cystitis. This inflammatory process is characterized by eosinophilic infiltration of the bladder wall. MR findings of this condition are specific; there is a smooth and nearly circumferential thickening of the bladder wall showing prominent low intensity on T2-weighted images (as also seen on US), which may histologically represent high cellularity due to massive eosinophilic infiltration (Tamai et al. 2007).

In children living in Africa, parasitic infection should be included in the differential diagnosis of cystitis. In schistosomiasis, nodular infiltrates of the bladder wall are commonly shown with US as well as calcification of the wall (also seen on plain films in later stages) (Fig. 20).

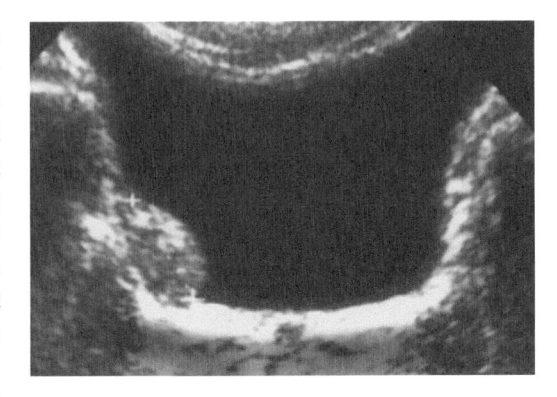

Fig. 20 Bladder US in an 8-year-old girl returning from Western Africa. Nodular echogenic lesion is protruding into the bladder lumen. Diagnosis was urinary schistosomiasis

> **Take Away**
> Bacterial, viral, or fungal infection of the bladder can be associated with a pseudotumoral appearance causing difficulties in imaging diagnostics.

9 Urachus

The urachus is the remnant of an embryonic connection coursing from the dome of the fetal bladder to the umbilicus. After birth in normal children, it is limited to a thin cord-like structure. Rarely, a patent urachus is present at birth. More commonly, urachal diverticulum is present at the dome of the bladder. It is more commonly associated with bladder outflow obstruction such as posterior urethral valves and prune-belly syndrome (Fig. 21). Diagnosis can be made on VCUG on lateral views or on US. Note that a pseudotumoral irregularity of the anterior upper aspect of the bladder wall is a normal remnant of the urachus and often seen on US in children which should not be mistaken for bladder wall tumor. A urachal cyst is another pathogenic remnant of a urachus when communication to the bladder or skin surface has sealed. It may be isolated or multiple, and infection can occur within this (Newman et al. 1986). Diagnosis is based on the association of clinical findings and US, which shows a superficial midline abscess-like structure. Urachal carcinoma does not occur in childhood, but this possible complication in adulthood may justify prophylactic surgical excision of urachal cysts in children (Thomas et al. 1986).

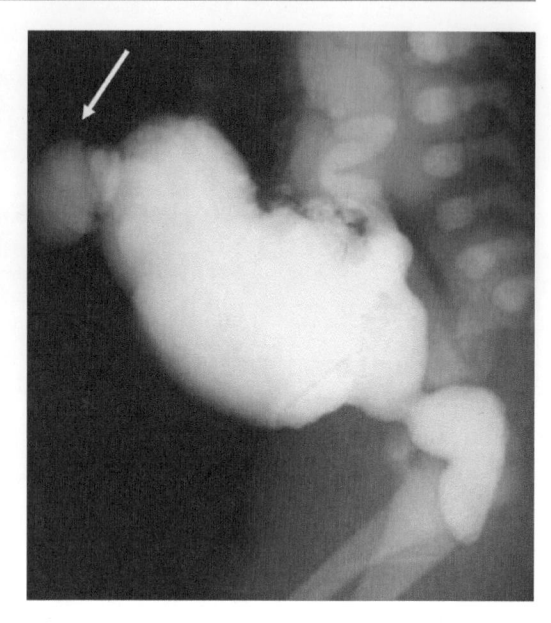

Fig. 21 VCUG in a neonate with PUV. Huge diverticulum of the urachus is visible on this lateral view (*arrow*)

Conclusion

Abnormalities of the lower urinary tract are relatively common conditions. A significant number of these are diagnosed antenatally. Post delivery of the imaging should be performed by experienced radiologists and rests mainly with US and VCUG.

References

Abbott JF, Levine D, Wapner R (1998) Posterior urethral valves: inaccuracy of prenatal diagnosis. Fetal Diagn Ther 13:179–183

Avni EF, Schulman CC (1996) The origin of vesico-ureteric reflux in male newborns: further evidence in favour of a transient fetal urethral obstruction. Br J Radiol 78:454–459

Avni EF, Gallety E, Rypens F et al (1992) A hypothesis for the higher incidence of vesico-ureteral reflux and primary megaureters in male babies. Pediatr Radiol 22:1–4

Barbagli G, Selli C, Palminteri E et al (1996) Duplications of the bulbous urethra: clinicoradiologic findings and therapeutic options. Eur Urol 29:67–71

Bear JW, Gilsanz V (1981) Calcified meconium and persistent cloaca. AJR Am J Roentgenol 137:867–868

Beluffi G, Fiori P, Pietrobono L, Romano P (2006) Cowper's glands and ducts: radiological findings in children. Radiol Med (Torino) 111:855–862

Bellah RD, Long FR, Canning DA (1995) Ureterocele eversion with vesicoureteral reflux in duplex kidneys: findings at voiding cystourethrography. AJR Am J Roentgenol 165:409–413

Bisset GS, Strife JL, Kirks DR (1991) In: Kirks D (ed) Genitourinary tract in practical pediatric imaging. Little, Brown, Boston, pp 905–1056

Blane CE, Zerin JM, Bloom DA (1994) Bladder diverticula in children. Radiology 190:695–697

Bockrath JM, Maizels M, Firlit CF (1982) Benign bladder neck polyp causing tandem obstruction of the urinary tract in a patient with Beckwith-Wiedemann syndrome. J Urol 128:1309–1312

Cobb BG, Wolf JA, Ansell JS (1968) Congenital stricture of the proximal urethral bulb. J Urol 99:629–631

Clayton DB, Brock JW (2012) Prenatal ultrasound and urological anomalies. Pediatr Clin N Am 59:739–756. doi:10.1016/j.pcl.2012.05.003

Dacher JN, Mandell J, Lebowitz RL (1992) Urinary tract infection in infants in spite of prenatal diagnosis of hydronephrosis. Pediatr Radiol 22(6):401–404; discussion 404–5

Dewan PA, Zappala SM, Ransley PG et al (1992) Endoscopic reappraisal of the morphology of congenital obstruction of the posterior urethra. Br J Urol 70:439–444

Dewan PA, Keenan RJ, Morris LL et al (1994) Congenital urethral obstruction: Cobb's collar or prolapsed congenital obstructive posterior urethral membrane (COPUM). Br J Urol 73:91–95

Dewan PA, Goh DG (1995) Variable expression of the congenital obstructive posterior urethral membrane. Urology 45:507–509

Dewan PA (1996) A study of the relationship between syringoceles and Cobb's collar. Eur Urol 30:119–124

Dhillon HK, Yeung CK, Duffy PG et al (1993) Cowper's glands cysts-a cause of transient intra-uterine bladder outflow obstruction. Fetal Diagn Ther 8:51–55

Diard F, Eklöf O, Lebowitz RL et al (1981) Urethral obstruction in boys caused by prolapse of simple ureterocele. Pediatr Radiol 11:139–142

Drozdz D, Drozdz M, Gretz N et al (1998) Progression to endstage renal disease in children with posterior urethral valves. Pediatr Nephrol 12:630–636

Eurin D, Vaast P, Robert Y (1999) Voies urinaires et rétropéritonie. In: Avni F, Robert Y (eds) Imagerie du foetus. Société Française de Radiologie, Paris, pp 85–95

Fievet L, Faure A, Coze S et al (2014) Fetal megacystis. Etiologies, management and outcome according to the trimester. Pediatr Urol 84:185–190

Foster RS, Garrett RA (1986) Congenital posterior urethral polyps. J Urol 136:670–672

Gobet R, Bleakley J, Peters CA (1998) Premature urachal closure induces hydroureteronephrosis in male fetuses. J Urol 160:1463–1467

Grignon A, Dubois J (1999) Malformations de la paroi antérieure du foetus. In: Avni F, Robert Y (eds) Imagerie du foetus. Société Française de Radiologie, Paris, pp 75–83

Hendren H (1998) Cloaca, the most severe degree of imperforate anus. Ann Surg 228:331–346

Hernanz-Schulman M, Genieser N, Ambrosino M et al (1989) Bilateral duplex ectopic ureters terminating in the seminal vesicles: sonographic and CT diagnosis. Urol Radiol 11:49–52

Hoeffel JC, Drews K, Gassner I et al (1993) Pseudotumoral cystitis. Pediatr Radiol 23:510–514

King BF, Hattery RR, Lieber MM et al (1991) Congenital cystic disease of the seminal vesicle. Radiology 178:207–211

Lebowitz RL (1997) Trying to understand the cloacal malformation: a systematic approach in difficulties in imaging and understanding of children's disease. In: Willi U (ed) European Society of Pediatric Radiology, 20th postgraduate course. Springer, Heidelberg/Berlin/New York, pp 47–50

McHugo J, Whittle M (2001) Enlarged fetal bladders: aetiology, management and outcome. Prenat Diagn 21(11):958–63

McLellan DL, Gaston MV, Diamond DA et al (2004) Anterior urethral valves and diverticula in children: a result of ruptured Cowper's duct cyst? BJU Int 94:375–378

Miller GW (1993) The work of human hands. Hardy Hendren and surgical wonder at Children's Hospital. Random House, New York

Newman BM, Karp MP, Jewett TC et al (1986) Advances in the management of infected urachal cysts. J Pediatr Surg 21:1051–1054

Pagon RA, Smith DW, Shepard TW (1979) Urethral obstruction malformation complex: a cause of abdominal muscle deficiency and the "prune belly". J Pediatr 94:900–906

Patten RM, Mack LA, Wang KY et al (1990) The fetal genitourinary tract. Radiol Clin North Am 28:115–130

Peters CA, Carr MC, Lais A et al (1992) The response of the fetal kidney to obstruction. J Urol 148:503–509

Pereira PL, Martinez Urrutia MJ et al (2013) Long term consequences of posterior urethral valves. J Pediatr Urol 9:590–596

Pfister C, Wagner L, Dacher JN et al (1996) Long-term bladder dysfunction in boys with posterior urethral valves. Eur J Pediatr Surg 6(4):222–224

Reuter KL, Lebowitz RL (1985) Massive vesicoureteral reflux mimicking posterior urethral valves in a fetus. J Clin Ultrasound 13:584–587

Riccabona M, Darge K, Lobo ML, et al (2015) ESPR uroradiology task force – imaging recommendations in paediatric uroradiology – Part VIII: Rethrograde urethrography, imaging in intersex queries, and imaging in childhood testicular torsion. Report on the minisymposium at the ESPR meeting in Amsterdam, June 2014, Pediatr Radiol in review

Rimon U, Hertz M, Jonas P (1992) Diverticula of the male urethra: a review of 61 cases. Urol Radiol 14:49–55

Rink RC, Mitchell ME (1990) Physiology of lower urinary tract obstruction. Radiol Clin North Am 17:329–334

Rittenberg MH, Hulbert WC, Snyder HM et al (1988) Protective factors in posterior urethral valves. J Urol 140:993–996

Ruano R, Sananes N, Sangi-Haghpeykar H et al (2014) Fetal intervention for severe lower urinary tract obstruction: a multicenter case–control study comparing fetal cystoscopy with vesico-amniotic shunting. Ultrasound Obstet Gynecol 45(4):452–458. doi:10.1002/uog.14652

Sebire NJ, Von Kaisenberg C, Rubio C et al (1996) Fetal megacystis at 10–14 weeks of gestation. Ultrasound Obstet Gynecol 8:387–390

Stephens FD, Fortune DW (1993) Pathogenesis of megalourethra. J Urol 149:1512–1516

Tamai K, Koyama T, Saida S et al (2007) MR imaging findings of eosinophilic cystitis in an 8-year-old girl. Pediatr Radiol 37:836–839

Tekes A, Ertan G, Solaiyappan M et al (2013) 2D and 3D MRI features of classic bladder exstrophy. Clin Radiol 69(2014):e223–e229

Thomas AJ, Pollack MS, Libshitz HI (1986) Urachal carcinoma: evaluation with computed tomography. Urol Radiol 8:194–198

Whitaker RH, Sherwood T (1986) An improved hook for destroying posterior urethral valves. J Urol 135:531–532

Willi UV, Lebowitz RL (1979) The so-called megauretermegacystis syndrome. AJR Am J Roentgenol 133:409–416

Zugor V, Schott GE, Labanaris AP (2012) The prune belly syndrome: urological aspects and long term outcomes of a rare disease. Pediatr Rep 4:e20

Female Genital Anomalies and Important Ovarian Conditions

Gisela Schweigmann, Theresa E. Geley, and Ingmar Gassner

Contents

1	**Introduction**..	317
2	**Embryology of the Female Genitalia**............	318
3	**Müllerian Duct Anomalies**............................	320
3.1	Müllerian Agenesis..	321
3.2	Disorders of Vertical Fusion.............................	323
3.3	Disorders of Lateral Fusion..............................	324
3.4	Vaginal Anomalies With or Without Obstruction..	324
3.5	Diagnostic Imaging of Müllerian Duct Anomalies...	326
4	**Lower Urinary Tract Anomalies of Urogenital Sinus**..	332
4.1	Female Hypospadias..	333
4.2	Urogenital Sinus in Disorders of Sexual Development...	334
4.3	Cloacal Malformation..	338
5	**Important Ovarian Conditions**......................	343
5.1	Characteristics of the Normal Ovary................	343
5.2	Ovarian Cysts..	344
5.3	Ovarian Torsion...	347
	References..	349

1 Introduction

Congenital anomalies of the female genital tract result from Müllerian duct anomalies and/or abnormalities of the urogenital sinus or cloaca. Failure of fusion of the Müllerian ducts results in a wide variety of fusion abnormalities of the uterus, cervix, and vagina (Gruenwald 1941). Müllerian duct abnormalities may occur alone or in association with urogenital sinus or cloacal malformations. Persistence of the cloaca is believed to be caused by an abnormal development of the dorsal part of the cloaca and the urorectal septum (Stephens 1983b; Nievelstein et al. 1998). Urogenital sinus malformations occur after the cloaca has been organized into the urogenital sinus and the anus (Williams and Bloomberg 1976). Early and complete assessment of these patients, including radiological and biochemical examinations, is mandatory to provide an optimal basis for treatment that will have a great influence on the quality of the patient's later life. Due to the close embryologic relationship between the urinary and the genital tract, malformations involving both organ systems are very common. Understanding the development of the urogenital system is necessary to comprehend the full spectrum of congenital anomalies of the female genitalia.

Ovarian cysts are frequently seen on ultrasound, and ovarian torsion is an important differential diagnosis in lower abdominal pain or ovarian mass and has therefore been included in

G. Schweigmann, MD (✉) • T.E. Geley
I. Gassner (Retired)
Section of Pediatric Radiology, Medical University of Innsbruck, Anichstrasse 35, 6020 Innsbruck, Austria
e-mail: gisela.schweigmann@i-med.ac.at

© Springer International Publishing AG, part of Springer Nature 2018
M. Riccabona (ed.), *Pediatric Urogenital Radiology*, Medical Radiology,
https://doi.org/10.1007/978-3-319-39202-8_19

this chapter, although they are not closely related etiologically to the abovementioned malformations and organ systems.

2 Embryology of the Female Genitalia

Sex determination at the chromosome level is related to the presence or absence of a Y chromosome. Those individuals with a Y chromosome (including XXY, XXXY, etc.) will develop into males, and those without one will become females. Some individuals, however, will undergo what is referred to as 46,XX testicular disorder of sex development (DSD) or 46,XY complete gonadal dysgenesis, also called primary sex reversal, whereby the X and Y chromosomes cross over and exchange the sex determination SRY gene (Hughes et al. 2006; Koopman 1995; Marrakchi et al. 2005). This relatively rare occurrence (approximately 1 in 20,000 births) can lead to males with two X chromosomes and females with a Y chromosome.

Historically the development of the female phenotype was thought to occur by default, when SRY gene was not activated. Recently female sex determination genes (WNT4, RSP01, FOXL2) whose expression is required for normal female genital differentiation have been identified (Hersmus et al. 2008; Barbaro et al. 2011). While gonad development is a result of the presence of the sex determination gene, sex differentiation is determined by the hormonal products of the gonads including the Müllerian-inhibiting substance (MIS) produced by Sertoli cells.

The two factors produced by the testes, androgen and MIS, are essential for the formation of the external and internal male genitalia as well as for the suppression of further development of the Müllerian duct into female genital structures. In the absence of a Y chromosome, zygotes with two or more X chromosomes will develop ovaries and female internal and external genitalia. Whereas the X chromosome is essential for development, zygotes lacking a Y chromosome (45,X) are viable but are unable to develop differentiated gonads (streak gonads) (Wilson and Goldstein 1975).

Both the internal and the external genital organs develop in coordination with the urinary and anorectal system at an early stage of gestation (Fig. 1). The internal genital organs as well as the lower urinary system originate from two paired urogenital structures that develop in both sexes: the mesonephric ducts (Wolffian ducts) and the paramesonephric ducts (Müllerian ducts) (Moore et al. 2011). At 5 weeks of gestation, the ureteral bud arises from the distal segment of the Wolffian duct to grow dorsally and soon becomes connected with the primordium of the permanent kidney or metanephric blastema. The ureteral bud forms the ureter, the renal pelvis, the calyces, and the intrarenal collecting ducts and acts as an inducer of differentiation of the renal

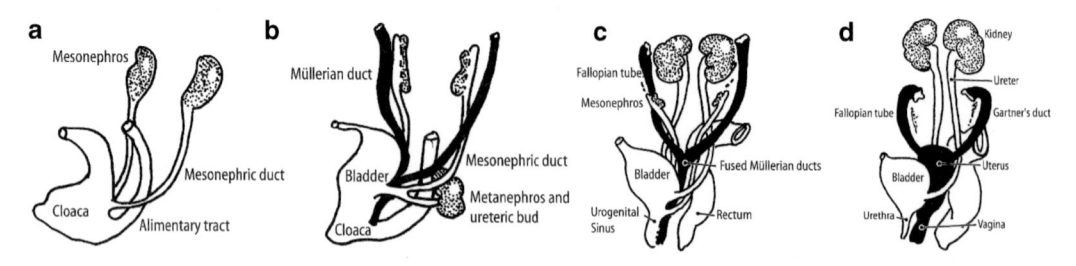

Fig. 1 Schematic representation of the embryology of the female genitourinary tract. (**a**) The mesonephric ducts (Wolffian ducts) connect the mesonephros to the cloaca. (**b**) At approximately 5 weeks of gestation, the ureteric bud originates from the Wolffian duct, reaches the metanephros, and induces its differentiation into the kidney while the mesonephros degenerates. The Müllerian ducts fuse at about 7–9 weeks in the midline to form the uterovaginal canal. (**c**) At 8 weeks the uterovaginal canal reaches the urogenital sinus at the Müllerian tubercle. The urogenital sinus results from the separation of the cloaca into the urogenital sinus and rectum. (**d**) The vagina becomes patent at approximately 22 weeks. The Wolffian ducts are resorbed and remnants are referred to as Gartner's duct

blastema into the adult kidney. Between the sixth and the eighth week, the segment of the Wolffian duct distal to the origin of the ureteral bud dilates and is incorporated into the wall of the vesicourethral canal. The ureter undergoes a craniolateral shift relative to the Wolffian duct to open into the bladder. With further growth of the surrounding structures, the ureteral opening migrates to the lateral corners of the bladder trigone, while the Wolffian ducts descend with the urogenital sinus. In the female, the Wolffian duct epithelium forms the posterior wall of the entire urethra (Stephens 1983a).

During the sixth week of gestation, the Müllerian ducts develop alongside the Wolffian ducts (Gruenwald 1941). The Müllerian ducts are divided into two segments demarcated by the insertion of the ligamentum inguinale, which eventually becomes the round ligament. The distal segments of the Müllerian ducts induced by the mesonephric ducts move toward the midline and soon fuse into a single tube, the uterovaginal canal (Acién and Acién 2011). The septum that divides the uterovaginal canal disappears at 11 weeks. The uterovaginal canal elongates to join the urogenital sinus at the Müllerian tubercle between the two openings of the Wolffian ducts. Further differentiation and canalization result in the formation of the uterus and the cervix. At 12 weeks the vagina forms. Induced by the fusion of the uterovaginal canal with the urogenital sinus, bilateral endodermal evaginations, the sinovaginal bulbs, form in the area of the Müllerian tubercle (Moore et al. 2011). The sinovaginal bulbs proliferate into the primitive vaginal plate. Canalization of this plate starts at the urogenital sinus forming the vaginal epithelium and the entire wall of the distal third of the vagina. The nonepithelial components of the proximal two-thirds of the vagina, however, are of uterovaginal canal origin. However in literature embryology of the vagina is very controversial. In contrast to the classical embryological concept, various studies have proved the participation of the mesonephric ducts in the formation of the vagina. Bok and Drews (1983) demonstrated that the "sinovaginal bulbs" are in fact the caudal segments of the Wolffian ducts. Drews (2007) considered that the Wolffian ducts do not contribute to the vagina itself but have a helper function during downward movement of the vaginal bud. In contrast according to Acién and Acién (2011), the mesonephric ducts form the vagina together with the Müllerian tubercle.

The proximal segments of the Müllerian ducts remain ununited to form the fallopian tubes. In females the Wolffian duct is finally resorbed, leaving only scattered remnants forming an interrupted channel alongside the fallopian tubes, the proximal uterus, within the cervix, and the anterolateral wall of the vagina, ending at or just above the level of the hymen. These remnants are then referred to as Gartner's duct.

Development of the external genital organs, the urethra, and the anus involve transformation processes of the internal and external cloaca, which are separated by the cloacal membrane in a transverse plane (Stephens 1983a; Nievelstein et al. 1998). At 4 weeks the internal cloaca is a single chamber, into which lead the large intestine, the hindgut, the allantois, and the Wolffian ducts.

Between the fourth and sixth weeks, the complex process of partitioning the internal and the external cloaca into separate urinary and anorectal systems takes place. The theories formulated by Rathke (1882), Retterer (1890), and Tourneux (1888) dominated the understanding of the development of the cloaca for decades. More recently, however, a new model of cloacal development has been put forward by Van der Putte (1986), Hartwig (1992), and Kluth et al. (1995). According to their theory, the distance between the caudal tip of the urorectal septum and the cloacal membrane decreases due to the unfolding process of the embryo and does not involve an active proliferation process of the urogenital septum as suggested earlier. According to this model, the urorectal septum is formed by fusion of the surrounding extraembryonic mesoderm of the yolk sac and allantois. The tip of this septum marks the cranial border of the cloaca and subdivides the internal cloaca into the urogenital sinus and the anorectal canal. However, fusion between the cloacal membrane and the urorectal septum, as suggested by the previous theories, never occurs (Nievelstein et al. 1998). The cloacal membrane eventually ruptures to allow communication between the internal and the external cloaca.

The process of partitioning then spreads caudally into the external cloaca. The perineal mound (i.e., the tip of the urorectal septum) separates the urogenital sinus from the anus. The inner genital folds proliferate to form the perineum and the labia minora, whereas the outer genital folds develop into the labia majora.

3 Müllerian Duct Anomalies

Based on the embryological development of the female genital system, uterovaginal malformations are classified as Müllerian agenesis in cases of a developmental defect of the caudal portion of the Müllerian ducts (Mayer-Rokitansky-Küster-Hauser syndrome), disorders of lateral fusion resulting from failure of the two Müllerian ducts to fuse, and disorders of vertical fusion that are caused by faults in the union between the Müllerian tubercle and derivatives of the urogenital sinus (transverse vaginal septum, cervical agenesis, disorders of the hymen). Disorders of lateral fusion are very heterogeneous but are best classified according to Buttram and Gibbons who proposed a classification of Müllerian anomalies in 1979, which was subsequently modified by the American Society of Reproductive Medicine in 1988 (formerly American Fertility Society). According to this classification, Müllerian duct anomalies are classified into seven groups. A particular patient, however, may not necessarily fit neatly into a single category. Then an exact description of each anomaly in detail is needed. Class I to class VI are shown in Figs 2, 3, and 4; class VII (not shown) refers to a uterus with luminal changes secondary to in utero exposure to diethylstilbestrol (DES), used to prevent miscarriage between the late 1940s and the 1970s.

Due to the frequent association of vertical and lateral fusion disorders, vaginal anomalies are best considered according to the presence or absence of an obstruction.

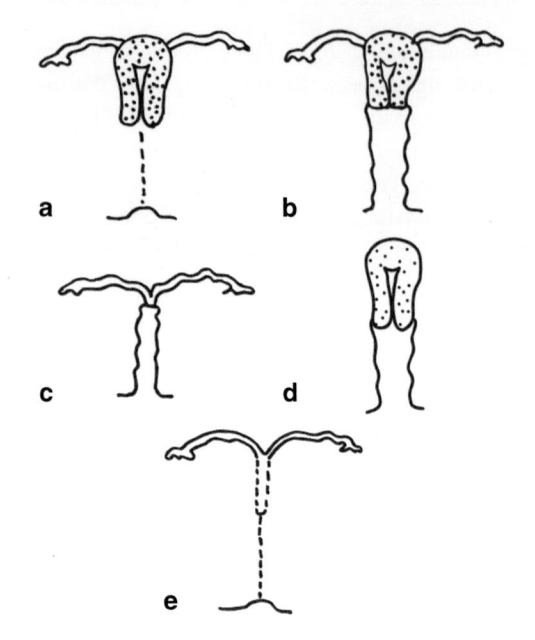

Fig. 2 Schematic representation of class I: Müllerian agenesis or hypoplasia. (**a**) Vaginal. (**b**) Cervical. (**c**) Fundal. (**d**) Tubal. (**e**) Combined vaginal and fundal

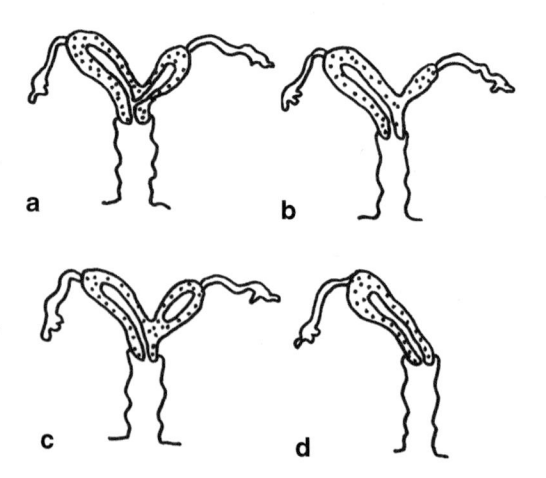

Fig. 3 Schematic representation of class II: unicornuate uterus. (**a**) With a rudimentary, communicating horn. (**b**) The rudimentary horn has no cavity, no endometrium. (**c**) The rudimentary horn is noncommunicating with active endometrium. (**d**) No rudimentary horn

Syndromes reported to be associated with genital anomalies in the female encompass Mayer-Rokitansky-Küster-Hauser syndrome (Müllerian agenesis); MURCS association (*Mü*llerian duct aplasia, *r*enal agenesis/ectopia, *c*ervical *s*omite dysplasia) (Duncan et al. 1979);

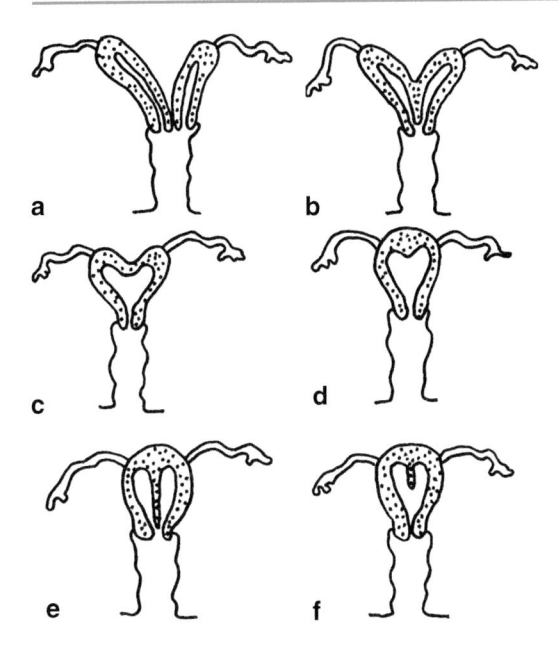

Fig. 4 Schematic representation of classes III, IV, and V. (**a**) Uterus didelphys (class III); (**b–d**). bicornuate uterus (class IV): (**b**) complete, (**c**) partial; (**d**) arcuate (class VI); (**e, f**) septate uterus (class V): (**e**) complete, (**f**) partial

hand-foot-genital syndrome (bifid uterus, double uterus, septate vagina); VATER, VACTEL, VACTERL, and VACTER association (*v*ertebral, *v*ascular, and *a*nal *a*nomalies, *a*uricular defects, *c*ardiovascular anomalies, *t*racheoesophageal fistula, esophageal atresia, renal anomalies, *r*adial defects, *r*ib and *l*imb anomalies); Beckwith-Wiedemann syndrome (bicornuate uterus); EEC syndrome (transverse vaginal septum); Fraser syndrome (bicornuate uterus, vaginal atresia, rudimentary uterus); Roberts syndrome (septate vagina); renal-genital-ear anomalies (vaginal atresia); Schinzel-Giedion syndrome (hymenal atresia); Jarcho-Levin syndrome (uterus didelphys) (Taybi and Lachman 2007); and finally Pallister-Hall syndrome (vaginal atresia) (Unsinn et al. 1995).

3.1 Müllerian Agenesis

Mayer-Rokitansky-Küster-Hauser syndrome is characterized by the absence of the entire vagina or, more commonly, the proximal two-thirds of the vagina, absence or abnormalities of the uterus, and malformations of the upper urinary tract (Fig. 5). It affects 1 in 4000–5000 otherwise normal (46 XX) girls and is regarded as resulting from the cessation of development of the Müllerian duct due to a deficiency of the estrogen and gestagen receptors (Ludwig 1998). Mayer-Rokitansky-Küster-Hauser syndrome type A (typical form) shows normal-appearing external genitalia, absence of the vagina and uterus, normal fallopian tubes, normal ovaries, and no renal anomalies. In type B (atypical form), the uterus may be normal except for the lack of a conduit to the introitus or may be rudimentary, commonly showing disorders of the lateral fusion with aplasia of one or both uterine horns, or asymmetry of the horns if both are present. However, any of the lateral or vertical fusion abnormalities with or without obstruction may be seen. The fallopian tubes are abnormally developed (hypoplasia and aplasia of one or both tubes), and ovarian anomalies such as inguinal hernia containing an ovary, no descent of the ovary, absence of the ovary, or streak ovaries have been reported (Taybi and Lachman 2007; Bazi et al. 2006).

Malformations of the upper urinary tract occur in up to 50 % (Rosenberg et al. 1986) of all affected females and include renal hydronephrosis, agenesis, fusion, dysplasia, and unilateral ectopia. Associated anomalies of the ureters such as ectopia and vesicoureteral reflux have also been reported. Skeletal anomalies are seen in approximately 10 % (Taybi and Lachman 2007) of patients who have malformations of the spine, such as wedge vertebrae, fusions, rudimentary vertebral bodies, and supernumerary vertebrae. The absence or underdevelopment of one lower sacral segment and coccyx as well as tethered spinal cord have been reported. Other skeletal anomalies include syndactyly, absence of a digit, long proximal phalanx of digits three and four, long metacarpals of digits one to four, carpal abnormalities, hypoplasia of the thenar eminence, and bilateral femoral hypoplasia.

The typical patient seeks medical advice at the expected time of onset of puberty because of primary amenorrhea. Upon physical examination the external genitalia are those of a normal

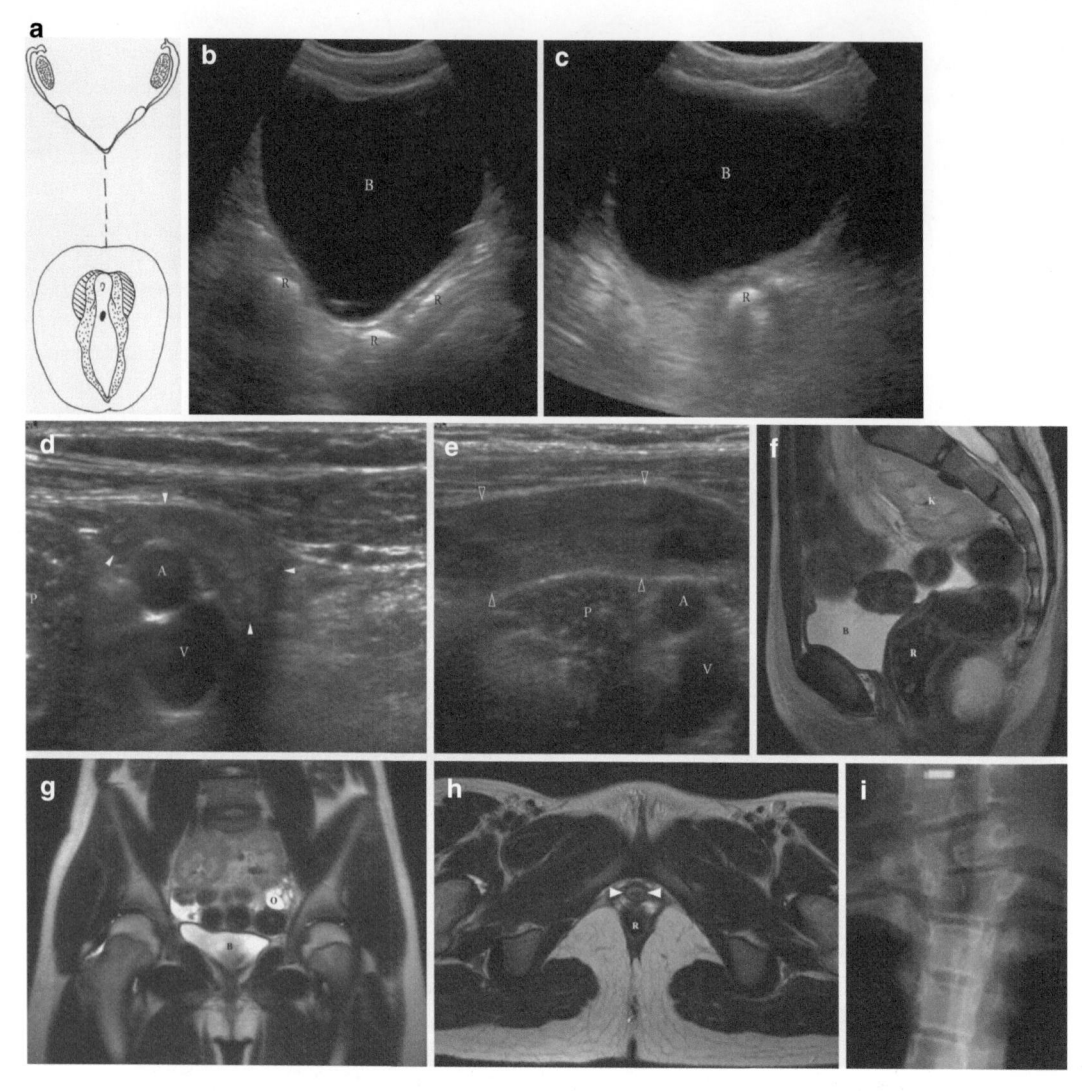

Fig. 5 Mayer-Rokitansky-Küster-Hauser syndrome (MRKHS): (**a**) schematic representation of genital anomalies encountered in Mayer-Rokitansky-Küster-Hauser syndrome. The rudimentary uterine horn consists of muscle bundles and some endometrial tissue. The tubes and ovaries are normally displayed. The perineal anatomy shows a female phenotype, but no vaginal opening or a blind vaginal pouch. (**b–e**) A 17-year-old girl with normal external genitalia and normal female karyotype. (**b**) Longitudinal, (**c**) transverse pelvic sonogram: behind the fluid-filled bladder (*B*), neither the vagina nor uterus, but only the rectum (*R*) is visualized. (**d, e**) Transverse scans through the right iliac fossa: (**d**) fallopian tube (*closed arrowheads*) in front of the iliac vessels. (**e**) More laterally the normal ovary with follicles (*open arrowheads*) is in front of the psoas muscle. The iliac artery (*A*) and vein (*V*), psoas muscle (*P*). (**f–h**) A 13-year-old girl with MURCS association (*Mü*llerian duct aplasia, *R*enal agenesis/ectopia, *C*ervivcal *S*omite dysplasia). (**f**) Sagittal, (**g**) coronal, (**h**) axial T2-weighted MR images show complete absence of the vagina, cervix, and uterus. The patient has two normal ovaries (right not shown) and a pelvic kidney. *K* kidney, *B* bladder, *R* rectum, *O* ovary. Urethra: *arrowheads*. (**i**) Anteroposterior radiograph of the cervicothoracic spine: fused cervicothoracic vertebrae (spine anomaly of the Klippel-Feil variety)

female, although the introitus may end in a shallow blind pouch. Depending on whether there is a functional endometrium, cyclic or intermittent abdominal pain may be present due to hematocolpos or hematometrocolpos. Mayer-Rokitansky-Küster-Hauser syndrome is the second most frequent cause of primary amenorrhea after the classic Turner syndrome.

The classic Turner syndrome (55 % of 45 XO patients) shows ovarian dysgenesis, primary amenorrhea, and infantile uterus, vagina, and breasts (Fig. 6). Less commonly, a mosaicism (X/XX, X/XY, X/XX/XY), isochromosome X, ring X, or partial deletion of the X chromosome is found. In chromosomal mosaic patients, the whole spectrum from absent to infantile to normal-sized ovaries, uterus, and vagina can be seen, explaining why 5 % of all Turner syndrome patients have spontaneous menstruation. Patients carrying a Y chromosome in their karyotype have a higher risk for developing gonadoblastoma (Siegel 2011).

3.2 Disorders of Vertical Fusion

The disorders of the vertical fusion of the Müllerian ducts consist of transverse vaginal septa, imperforate cervix, and cervical agenesis and result from faults in the junction between the descending Müllerian ducts and the ascending urogenital sinus. In transverse septa the interruption may be complete or incomplete and occur at any level of the vagina, sometimes at multiple levels. The vagina is obliterated by fibrous connective tissue with vascular and muscular elements lined by squamous epithelium. The septum may be a thin membrane but more commonly involves a whole segment of the vagina (segmental vaginal atresia). An increased incidence of associated proximal Müllerian duct anomalies is found, such as lateral fusion abnormalities of the uterus, stenosis, hypoplasia, or the absence of the uterus and the fallopian tubes (Silverman and Kuhn 2013).

Although of different embryological origin, the imperforate hymen is commonly listed together with defects of the vertical fusion of the Müllerian ducts. The hymen membrane separates the vaginal lumen from the urogenital sinus and is entirely of urogenital sinus origin. The hymen membrane usually ruptures in the perinatal period and remains as a thin fold around the vaginal orifice. As with all vaginal obstructions found in association with a normal uterus, imperforate hymen may either be symptomatic in the newborn period or after onset of puberty due to the development of hydrocolpos/

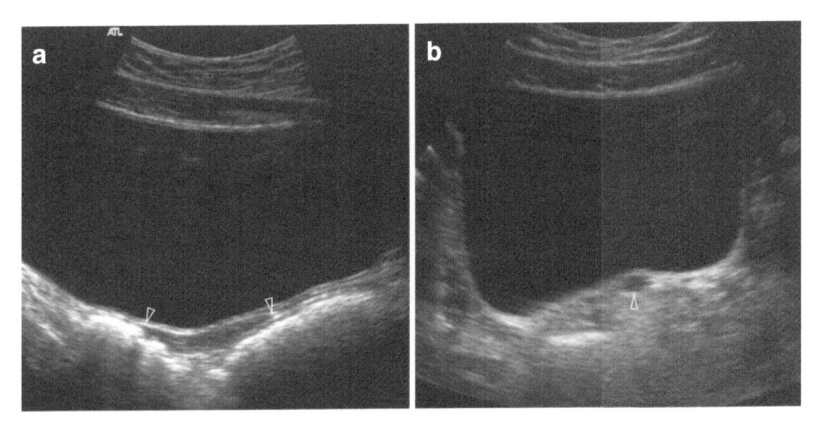

Fig. 6 Turner Syndrome. A 13-year-old girl with 45 XO karyotype. (**a**) Longitudinal and (**b**) transverse pelvic sonogram show a small-sized uterus (*open arrowheads*). The ovaries could not be identified

hydrometrocolpos or hematocolpos/hematometrocolpos, respectively. A protruding interlabial mass in association with a midline pelvic mass is found upon physical examination. Imperforate hymen is the simplest and most easily correctable of all vaginal obliterations. It is not associated with an increased incidence of Müllerian duct or renal anomalies (Silverman and Kuhn 2013).

3.3 Disorders of Lateral Fusion

Incomplete fusion of the distal segments of the two Müllerian ducts results in various degrees of bifidity of the uterus and/or vagina (Jarcho 1946) (Fig. 8). Disorders of the lateral fusion are rare in the general population and, in the absence of obstruction, are asymptomatic during childhood or at puberty. However, these anomalies are more frequently encountered in infertile women. This group of uterine malformations includes septate, bicornuate, didelphic, and unicornuate uterus (Figs. 2, 3, and 4) (Buttram and Gibbons 1979; American Fertility Society 1988).

To differentiate bicornuate from septate uterus in adults, a line drawn between the uterine ostia is used. In septate uterus the apex of the external fundal contour in adults is more than 5 mm above the interosteal line. When it is below or less than 5 mm, above the uterus is bicornuate (Fig. 9) (Behr et al. 2012; Homer et al. 2000; Fedele et al. 1988). In prepubescent girls, however, the entire uterus is so small that these criteria may not be applied for differentiation. Hence the approach is to describe anatomy exactly (number of cervices, number of uterine horns, communication of atrophic horn).

A minor and relatively common form of fusion defects is simple septate vagina, in which the vagina is divided in two lateral compartments by a midline sagittal septum without uterine anomalies (Figs. 7, 8, and 9).

3.4 Vaginal Anomalies With or Without Obstruction

Because of the frequent association of vertical with lateral fusion anomalies, it is useful to consider vaginal anomalies according to the presence or the absence of obstruction (Fig. 10). Nonobstructive vaginal anomalies encompass bifid vagina, longitudinal vaginal septum, and incomplete transverse septum. Among the obstructive vaginal anomalies are imperforate hymen, complete transverse vaginal septum (Fig. 14), and atresia of the uterine cervix and vagina, as mentioned above, as well as unilateral obstructive vaginal septum and obstruction of a unilateral rudimentary horn.

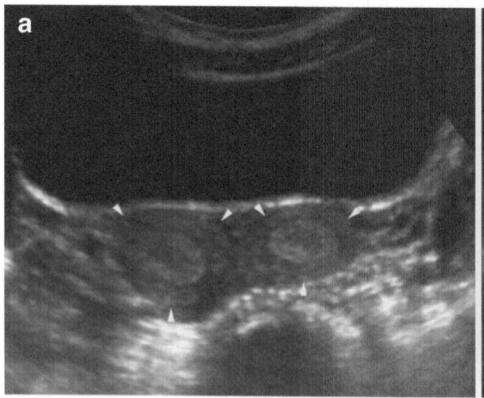

Fig. 7 Bicornuate uterus (uterus duplex unicollis). A 13 ½-year-old girl. (**a, b**) Transverse pelvic sonograms shows (**a**) two uterine bodies (*closed arrowheads*) and two endometrial cavities and (**b**) the cervix (*open arrowheads*) with a single endometrial cavity

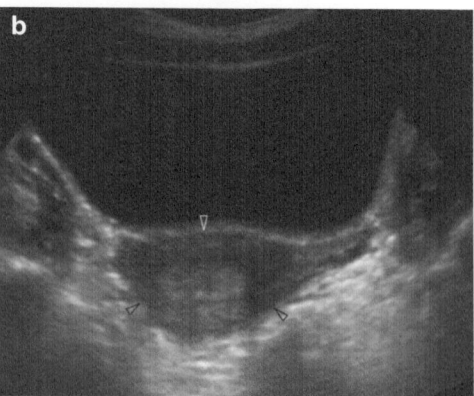

Fig. 8 Uterus didelphys with double vagina in a 16-year-old girl. (**a**) Filling of the vagina with plain sodium solution. Transverse sonogram shows two uteri (*closed arrowheads*) with thickened, echogenic endometrium (*asterisks*) and two fluid-filled vaginas (*V*) behind the empty bladder. (**b**) With a slightly angulated transducer position, no sonographic dropout occurs and allows clear demonstration of the two separate vaginas (*V*). *B* bladder. (**c**) Contrast filling of the vagina. Anterior posterior view of the double vagina after retrograde filling. The septum is clearly visible

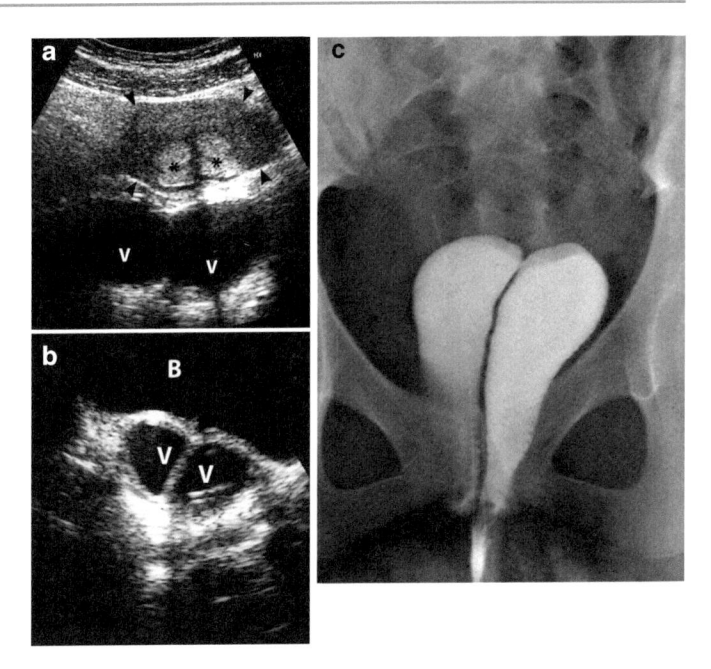

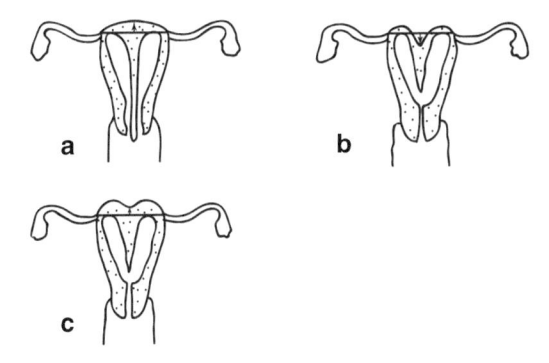

Fig. 9 Classification criteria for differentiation of septate from bicornuate uteri (measurements valid for adults). After Behr et al. 2012, (**a**) septate uterus: The apex of the fundal contour is more than 5 mm (*arrow*) above the interosteal line. (**b**, **c**) Bicornuate uteri: The apex of the fundal contour is below (*arrow* in **b**), or less than 5 mm above (*arrow* in **c**) the interosteal line

Unilateral obstructive vaginal septum In some cases of duplicated uterus with a midline vaginal septum, the caudal end of one hemivagina, more often the left, is obstructed (uterus didelphys with septate vagina and uterovaginal obstruction) (Fig. 11). No hymen tissue is found on the obstructed side. The disorder may present at birth with a pelvic mass due to accumulated genital secretion. The ipsilateral fallopian tube may also be enlarged. More commonly, however, the patient presents at puberty with a pelvic mass and cyclic abdominal pain despite a normal menstrual blood flow. The obstructed vaginal compartment may protrude as a cystic mass from the introitus. An obstructed hemivagina and double uterus are almost always associated with severe ipsilateral renal anomalies (renal agenesis, renal dysplasia, ectopia, ipsilateral ectopic ureter, and urinary tract dilatation) due to the close developmental association between the genital system (originating from the Müllerian ducts) and the urinary system (originating from the Wolffian ducts) (Silverman and Kuhn 2013). Uterus didelphys, blind hemivagina, and ipsilateral renal agenesis are referred as Herlyn-Werner-Wunderlich syndrome (Orazi et al. 2007). In this context a multicystic dysplastic kidney develops in consequence of ureteric obstruction due to an ectopic opening of the ureter into the ipsilateral obstructed half of the double vagina. The cysts of MCDK may involute in the course of time – in rare cases prenatally, commonly postnatally – resulting in a small dysplastic kidney or even its complete disappearance, thus mimicking renal

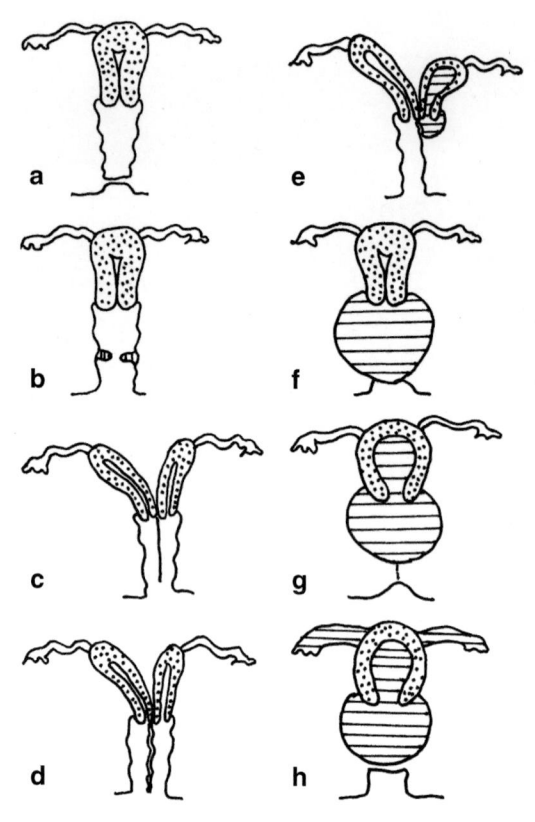

Fig. 10 Schematic representation of vaginal anomalies with and without obstruction. (**a**) Imperforate hymen. (**b**) Incomplete transverse vaginal septum. (**c**) Longitudinal vaginal septum, uterus didelphys. (**d**) Bifid vagina, uterus didelphys. (**e**) Obstruction of a hemivagina, hematometrocolpos, uterus didelphys. (**f**) Imperforate hymen, hematocolpos; a protruding vestibular mass is found. (**g**) Partial vaginal agenesis, hematometrocolpos. (**h**) Transverse vaginal septum, hematometrocolpos, spilling of menstrual blood via the fallopian tubes

agenesis later in life (Kiechl-Kohlendorfer et al. 2011).

Therefore, it is advisable to look for an uterus didelphys with obstructed hemivagina whenever a multicystic dysplastic kidney or renal agenesis in a girl is discovered. This is important for correct management at the onset of puberty to prevent patients from becoming symptomatic with acute abdominal pain and dysmenorrhea (Fig. 12).

Obstruction of an unilateral rudimentary horn This condition is found at the extreme end of the spectrum of Müllerian duct anomalies (Fig. 3). One of the two Müllerian ducts fails to develop or is partially or completely (unicornuate uterus) resorbed. The ipsilateral fallopian tube is, therefore, absent or rudimentary, whereas both ovaries are present and functional. If a rudimentary hemiuterus contains functioning endometrium, the patient may develop an accumulation of mucus within this structure, during the neonatal period, or blood, at the time of puberty. Renal agenesis or severe renal dysplasia on the side of the missing or malformed hemiuterus is the rule (Gilsanz et al. 1982; Woolf and Allen 1953).

> **Take Away**
> Due to the close developmental relationship of the urinary and the genital tract, malformations frequently occur in both of these systems. Major renal anomalies are common in patients presenting with unilateral obstruction or agenesis of duplicated structures derived from the Müllerian duct.

3.5 Diagnostic Imaging of Müllerian Duct Anomalies

Pediatric radiologists will commonly come across Müllerian duct anomalies at two different stages of a girl's life. In neonates diagnostic requests encompass evaluation of a palpable abdominal mass and delineation of associated genital malformation in urogenital sinus anomalies. In adolescent girls delay in puberty or primary amenorrhea and pelvic abdominal pain after the onset of puberty are the most common reasons for consultation.

Ultrasound (US) is the most common first-step imaging technique in the evaluation of patients of both age groups. Subsequent tests such as MR imaging and fluoroscopic studies provide additional information (Fielding 1996; Wagner and Woodward 1994). In particular, patients with Müllerian agenesis may need MR imaging to clearly document their ovaries and the rudimentary uterus (Rosenberg et al. 1986; Rosenblatt et al. 1991; Lang et al. 1999).

On MR imaging T2-weighted images are best to characterize anatomy of the female

Fig. 11 Uterus didelphys with left multicystic dysplastic kidney (*MCDK*) and ipsilateral vaginal obstruction. (**a**) Longitudinal scan (coronal plane) of the left flank. *MCDK*: multiple anechoic cysts of variable size and shape that do not communicate with each other. The dilated ureter (*arrows*) could be traced from the MCDK to the obstructed ipsilateral left vagina. (**b**) Transverse pelvic sonogram shows two uterine fundi: right fundus (*closed arrowheads*), left fundus (*open arrowheads*). (**c**) Transverse scan at lower level than b shows a left-sided cyst representing obstructed left vagina (*LV*). (**d, e**) Longitudinal sonograms obtained after instilling saline solution in the vagina demonstrated (**d**) fluid-filled patent right vagina (*RV*) with right uterus (*arrowheads*); (**e**) atretic left vagina (*LV*) with left uterus (*arrowheads*). Obstructing membrane (*arrow*). (**f**) Transverse scan shows the atretic left ureter (*closed arrowheads*) bulging into the atretic left vagina (*asterisk*). Functional right vagina (*open arrowheads*). (**g**) Schematic representation

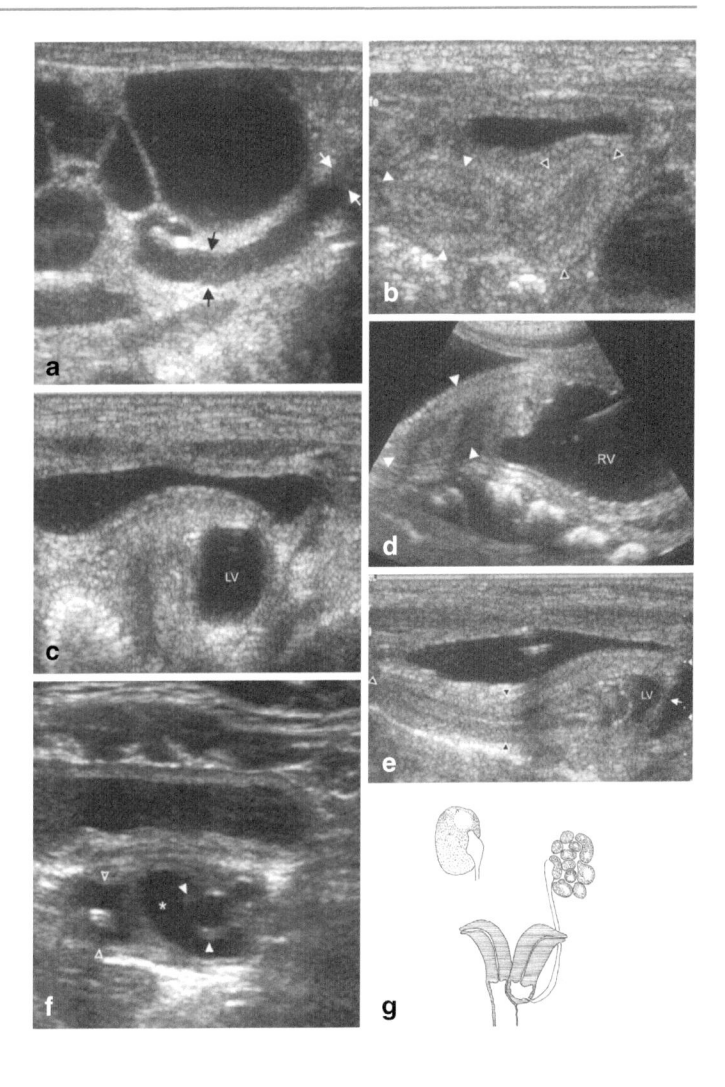

reproductive tract. Multiplanar reformatting of 3D T2-weighted images, done retrospectively at the workstation, avoids the need for exact prescription of the imaging plane and therefore reduces imaging time (Fig. 16e). For small pelvic lower UGT pathology, additional (isotropic) HR-MR 3D-CISS-sequence can help to establish the correct anatomic diagnosis by offering increased contrast and spatial resolution at little additional examination time (Ehammer et al. 2011). T1-weighted images help to identify high-signal-intensity blood products.

In US and MR imaging sagittal plane is helpful to determine a diagnosis of uterine or vaginal agenesis or hypoplasia. Oblique coronal images in the long axis of the uterus are necessary for proper assessment of the external uterine fundal contour to differentiate bicornuate from septate and didelphic uterus (Fig. 9). Axial planes best characterize vaginal agenesis (Fig. 5h).

Due to the high association of Müllerian duct anomalies with anomalies of the urinary tract, every patient diagnosed with genital malformations, whether newborn or adolescent, needs a careful investigation of the urinary tract. Renal US and voiding cystourethrography should be performed on all patients diagnosed with a duplicated uterine system. Pelvic sonography, on the other hand, is mandatory in patients with unilateral renal agenesis, ectopia, multicystic dysplastic, or horseshoe kidney (Gilsanz et al. 1982; Woolf and Allen 1953; Gilsanz and Cleveland 1982; Kiechl-Kohlendorfer et al. 2011). In cases of Müllerian agenesis, spinal ultrasound in newborns and MR imaging in older girls as well as plain X-rays are required to rule out spinal cord anomalies and skeletal anomalies, respectively (Fig. 13).

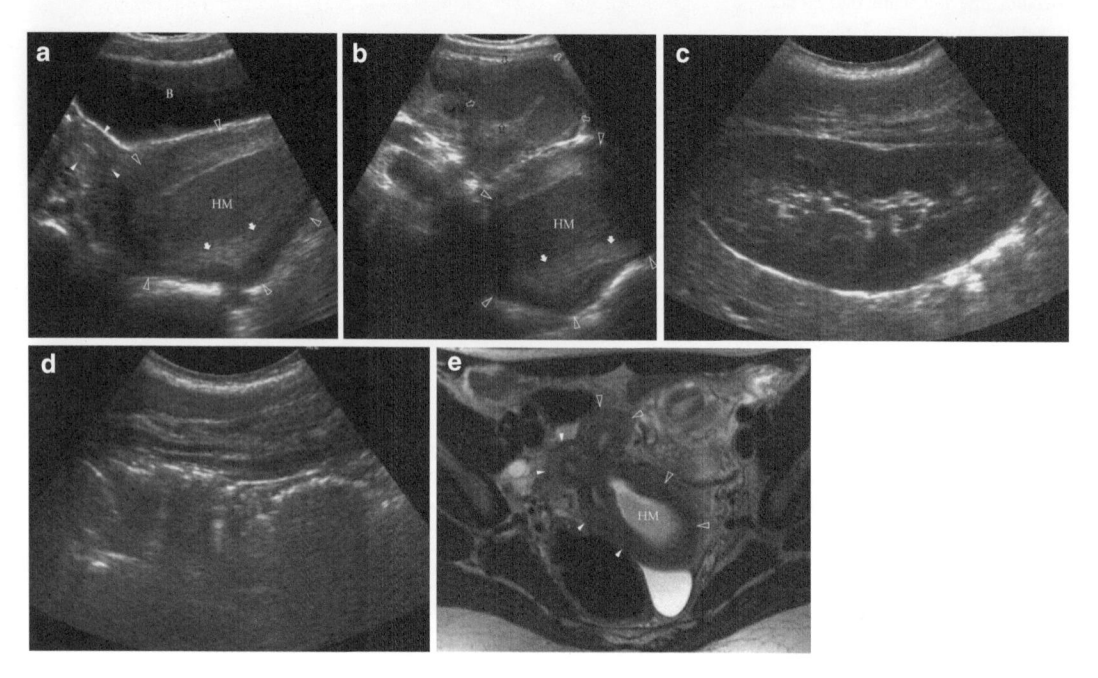

Fig. 12 Uterus didelphys with left-sided vaginal atresia and the absent left kidney. A 14-year-old girl with cyclic and progressive abdominal pain and a pelvic mass. (**a**) Transverse and (**b**) left coronal pelvic sonogram show a normal right uterus (*closed arrowheads*) and a left-sided enormous dilated blood-filled uterus (*open arrowheads*) with a sedimentation level (*closed arrows*) in the hematometra (*HM*). Bladder (*B*). (**b**) On left coronal sonogram, both the left-sided hematometra and the hematosalpinx (*open arrows*) are seen. (**c**) Right and (**d**) left longitudinal dorsal sonogram show a normal right and the absent left kidney (key to the diagnosis!). (**e**) Axial T2-weighted image shows the normal right uterus (*closed arrowheads*) and the left uterus (*open arrowheads*) with the dilated blood-filled cervix, representing the hematometra (*HM*)

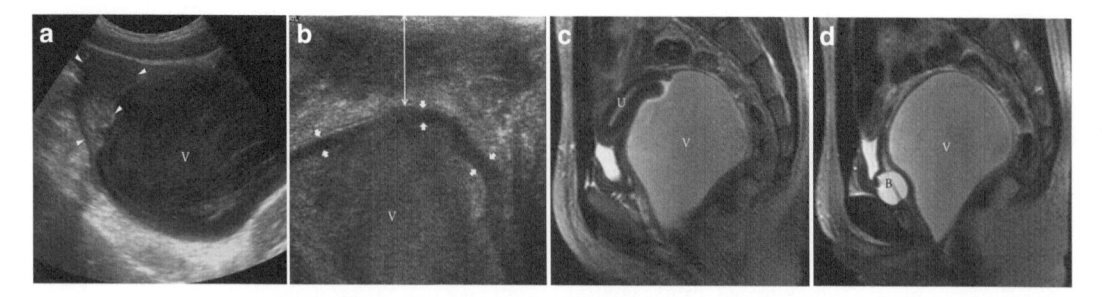

Fig. 13 Distal vaginal atresia with hematocolpos. A 14-year-old girl. (**a**) Longitudinal pelvic sonogram: huge distension of the vagina (*V*). Internal echos reflect cellular debris or blood. Normal-sized pubertal uterus (*arrowheads*). (**b**) Transperineal sagittal sonogram shows clearly the thick vaginal septum (*arrows*) and the distance (*double arrow*) from the perineum to the caudal aspect of the distended vagina (*V*) corresponding to the short zone of vaginal atresia. (**c**, **d**) T2-weighted magnetic resonance images of the pelvis in the midsagittal plane show the markedly distended vagina (*V*) filled with material consistent with subacute blood. The uterus (*U*) is not enlarged. Balloon catheter (*B*) in the empty bladder

Morphologic features of the uterus in neonate, prepubertal, and pubertal girls Under the influence of maternal and placental hormones, the neonatal uterus is more prominent and measures between 2.3 and 4.6 cm (mean 3.4 cm) in length, the fundal width ranges from 0.8 to 2.1 cm (mean 1.2 cm), and cervical width ranges from 0.8 to 2.2 cm (mean 1.4 cm), with a definable endometrial stripe (Fig. 14) (Siegel 2011).

The prominent neonatal uterus provides a unique opportunity for early and accurate diagnosis of these anomalies by sonography, and every US investigation in a neonate girl should include its assessment. A uterus didelphys or bicornuate uterus can, therefore, readily be demonstrated. The prepubertal uterus is smaller, has a tube shape, and a non-apparent endometrium, making it almost impossible to evaluate uterine anomalies (Fig. 15).

Estrogen stimulation at the onset of puberty results in fundal swelling and apparent endometrium (Fig. 16). The postpubertal uterus has the

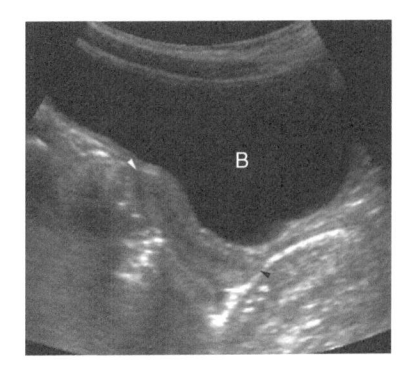

Fig. 15 Normal prepubertal uterus of a 2 ½ -year-old girl. Longitudinal sonogram shows a tubular uterus (*arrowheads*) with no differentiation between the fundus and cervix. The inner layer of myometrium is hypoechoic (subendometrial halo). *B* bladder

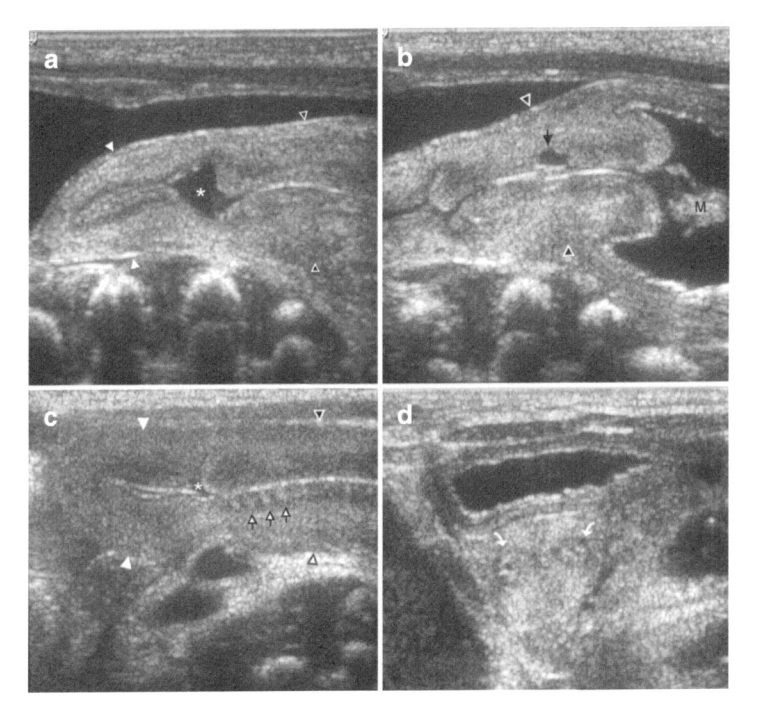

Fig. 14 Normal neonatal uterus. (**a–c**) Longitudinal sonograms: The cervix and fundus are clearly discernible. The cervix (*open arrowheads*) has a greater diameter and length than fundus (*closed arrowheads*). There is a small amount of fluid within the endometrial canal at the junction of the fundus and cervix (*asterisk*). Single nabothian cyst in the cervix (*closed arrow*). The inner layer of myometrium is hypoechoic (subendometrial halo). Echogenic endometrial glands (*open arrows*). In the fluid-distended vagina, cervical mucus adherent to the vaginal part of cervix is visible (M). (**d**) Transverse scan at the level of the fundus shows the uterine horns (area where the tubes enter the uterus; *curved arrows*)

adult pear-shaped appearance and measures 5–8 × 1.5 × 3 cm (Teele and Share 1992; Ziereisen et al. 2005) (Fig. 16).

Sonographic features of hydro-/hematocolpos and hydrometro-/hematometrocolpos Sonographic evaluation of a newborn or adolescent girl with a palpable abdominal mass may reveal a midline cystic mass reflecting congenital hydrocolpos or hydrometrocolpos in the former and hematocolpos or hematometrocolpos in the latter (Figs. 17 and 18).

In some cases the cystic dilatation of the vagina may be very impressive with the less

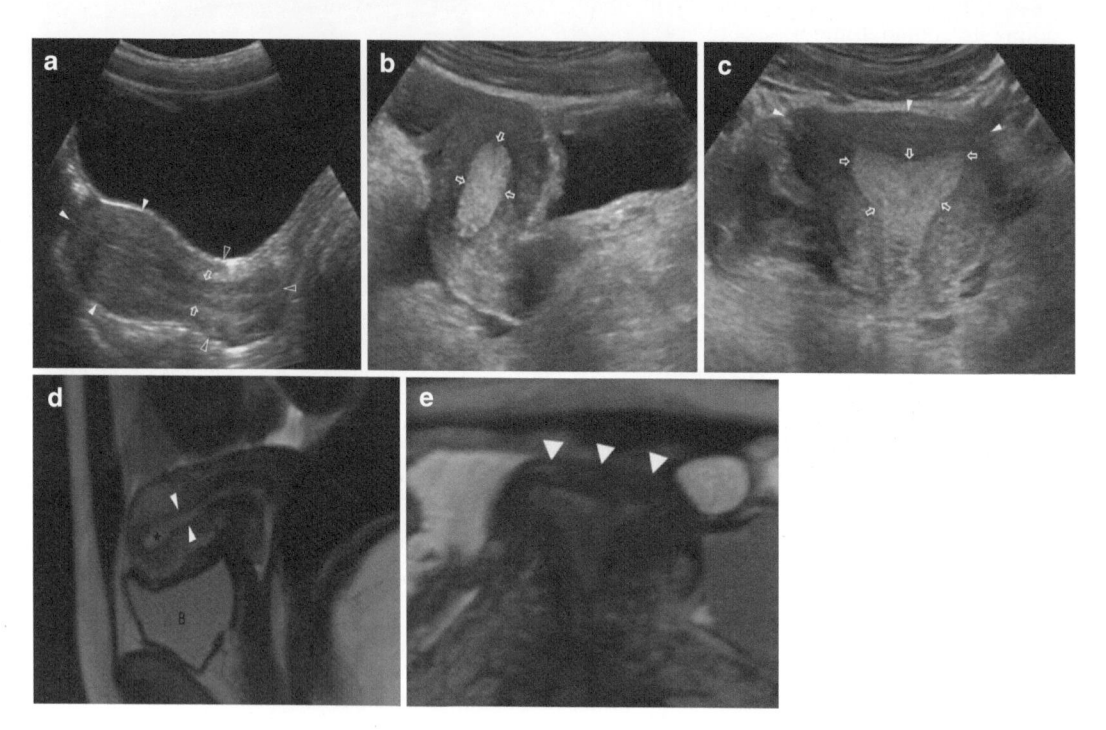

Fig. 16 Normal postmenarchal pear-shaped uterus and the phases of endometrial development. (**a**) A 13 ½ -year-old girl. Longitudinal sonogram: Diameter and length of the fundus (*closed arrowheads*) are greater than those of the cervix (*open arrows*). Proliferative phase: The central canal is echogenic and surrounded by the hypoechoic functionalis layer (*open arrows*). (**b**, **c**) A 14-year-old girl. Secretory phase. (**b**) Longitudinal, (**c**) coronal sonogram: thickened echogenic endometrium (*open arrows*). The internal (*open arrows*) and external (*closed arrowheads*) fundal contour is clearly visible. (**d**) A 17-year-old girl. Sagittal T2-weighted image of a normal zonal anatomy of the uterus: high-signal endometrium (*asterisks*), low-signal junctional zone (*arrowheads*), intermediate-signal myometrium. *B* bladder. (**e**) Coronal oblique T2-weighted reformatted image: normal external fundal contour (*arrowheads*)

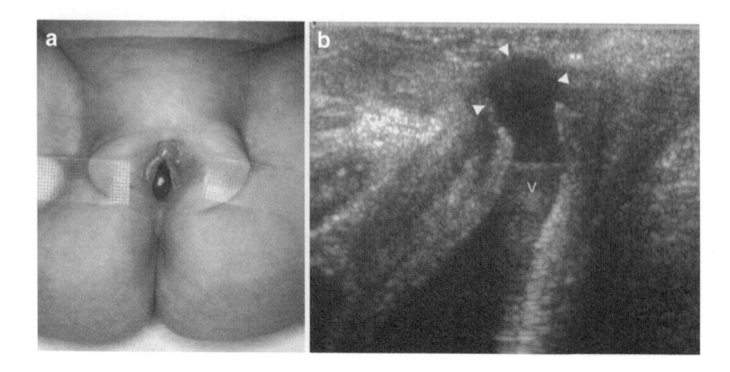

Fig. 17 Imperforate hymen with moderate hydrocolpos. (**a**) The imperforate hymen protrudes between the labia. (**b**) Translabial sagittal scan: The vagina (*V*) is moderately dilated and the fluid protrudes the hymen (*arrowheads*) spherically

easily distensible uterus attached to it as a small cap-like structure. The fluid-filled vagina and/or uterus may be seen as a cystic structure homogeneously and completely filled appearing as a solid mass, cystic with scattered internal echoes, or completely anechoic. A fluid-debris level might be found and is a crucial finding in congenital hydrocolpos/hydrometrocolpos that differentiates the vagina from the bladder (Blask et al. 1991a, b). Association of hydro-/hematocolpos and hydrometro-/hematometrocolpos with an obliterate introitus or a shallow blindly ending vaginal pouch is strongly suggestive of Müllerian agenesis or transverse vaginal septum but has to be distinguished from pelvic masses caused by an imperforate hymen or unilateral occlusion of a duplicated vagina (Blask et al. 1991b).

In addition, fluid may be found in the peritoneal cavity due to spillage of genital secretion/menstrual blood via the fallopian tubes. Repeated backflow of menstrual blood results in endometriosis and chronic epithelial tubal changes that jeopardize fertility (Fig. 19).

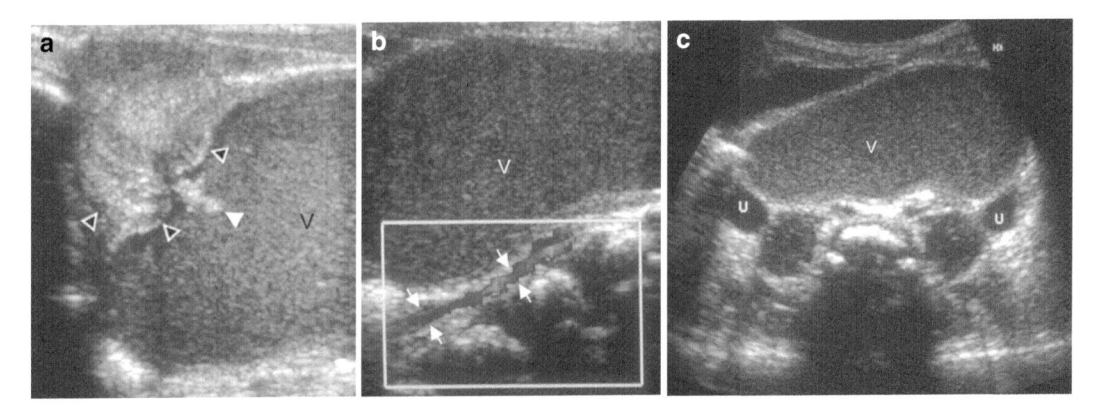

Fig. 18 Imperforate hymen with excessive hydrocolpos. (**a, b**) Longitudinal scans: The low-level echoes within the markedly dilated vagina (*V*) represent mucous secretions. (**a**) The uterus with cervix (*open arrowheads*) projects into the dilated vagina (*V*). Mucus plug (*closed arrowhead*) adherent to the cervical ostium. (**b**) The hydrocolpos (*V*) compresses the inferior vena cava (*blue color*). (**c**) Transverse pelvic scan: The ureters (*U*) are dilated due to distal ureteral compression. *V* hydrocolpos

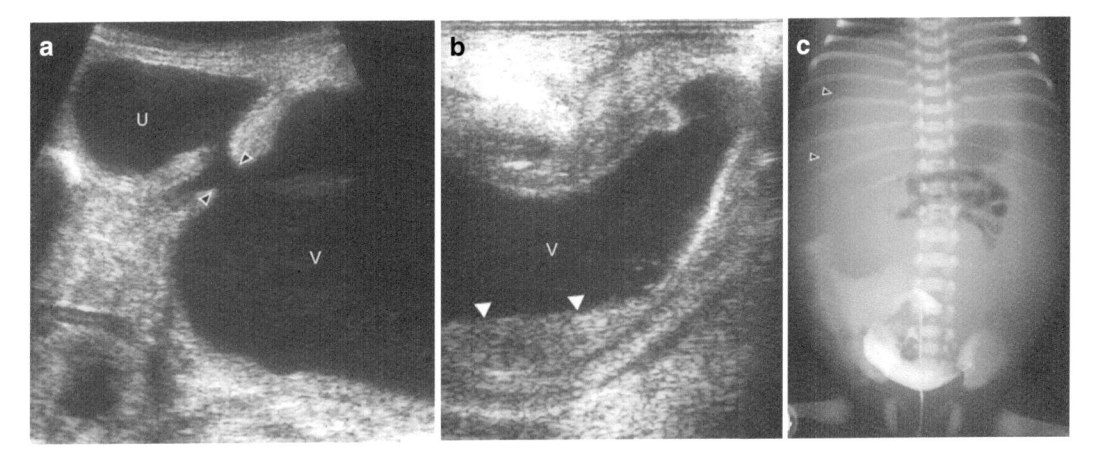

Fig. 19 Imperforate hymen with hydrometrocolpos and ascites due to spillage of genital secretions via the fallopian tubes into the peritoneal cavity. (**a, b**) Sagittal scans: The vagina (*V*) and the uterus (*U*) are dilated with broad communication through the cervical ostium (*open arrowheads*). The vagina shows a fluid-debris level (*closed arrowheads*). (**c**) Distended, fluid-filled abdomen. The air-filled loops of bowel cluster in the center of the abdomen. The lateral edge of the liver (*arrowheads*) is visible

Diagnostic imaging of vaginal anomalies. Vaginal anomalies without obstruction are usually asymptomatic unless they represent a mechanical obstacle during intercourse or delivery. Either fluid filling of the vagina under sonographic guidance or traditional vaginography with contrast material is effective in delineating these malformations (Pellerito et al. 1992; Rosenberg et al. 1986). In our experience traditional vaginography is restricted in value by only demonstrating the inner contour of the vagina (Gassner and Geley 2004). Frequently the uterus does not opacify, and the proximal impression of the cervix/cervices or the lateral impression caused by an obstructed hemivagina may at times be difficult and confusing. Filling the vagina with either ultrasound contrast agents or plain salt solution combined with ultrasound, however, overcomes these problems. In our experience, fluid instillation into either the bladder or the rectum or both significantly increases the performance of ultrasound by generating "sonographic windows" surrounding the uterus and vagina (Kiechl-Kohlendorfer et al. 2001).

Filling the vagina in a newborn is performed via an 8-F feeding tube (Riccabona et al. 2014). A catheter of adjusted size is used in older girls. Simultaneously performed transabdominal or perineal ultrasound delineates the internal anatomy and patency of the vagina, the presence of one or two cervices, and allows the differentiation of a cystic mass being related to an obstructed vagina, a ureterocele, renal cysts (multicystic dysplastic kidney) (Fig. 11), or a dilated Gartner's duct or a Gartner's duct cyst. Gartner's duct cysts are usually asymptomatic, do not exceed 2 cm in size, and typically exhibit a hypoechoic, sharply delineated cystic structure in close proximity to the anterolateral wall of the cervix (Rosenfeld and Lis 1993). In the rare cases of the ureteral bud failing to separate from the Wolffian ducts, a single ectopic ureter may terminate directly or via Gartner's duct or a Gartner's duct cyst into the bladder neck, the urethra, the vaginal vestibule, or the vagina itself (Currarino 1982). A single ectopic ureter is always accompanied by ipsilateral renal hypoplasia, dysplasia, or agenesis (Gharagozloo and Lebowitz 1994).

> **Take Away**
> In the evaluation of Müllerian duct anomalies in neonates and adolescent girls, sonography is the most useful first-step examination technique. In all patients with congenital malformations of the inner genitalia, the urinary tract needs to be evaluated and vice versa.

4 Lower Urinary Tract Anomalies of Urogenital Sinus

The most common urogenital sinus malformations a radiologist will come across are patients suffering from female hypospadias (simple urogenital sinus), intersexual conditions, and cloacal malformation (urogenital sinus associated with anorectal malformation) (Fig. 20).

Urogenital sinus is suspected during physical examination of a newborn with a normally placed anus in association with either ambiguous genitalia or a normal external genitalia, but only a single perineal opening within the vestibulum.

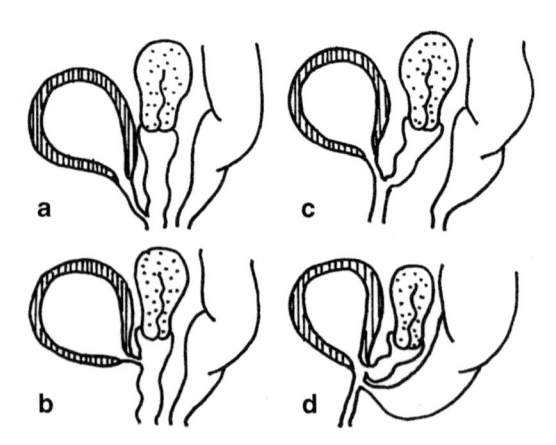

Fig. 20 Schematic representation of lower urinary tract anomalies of the urogenital sinus. (**a**) Distal female hypospadia: The urethral meatus lies in the roof of the vagina. (**b**) Proximal female hypospadia. (**c**) Urogenital sinus. (**d**) Persistent cloaca. The most common anatomy of persistent cloaca is shown. There is a urogenital sinus; the vagina enters just below the bladder neck, and the rectum enters just below the vagina. The confluence level can be high, intermediate, or low

It is either isolated or found in association with chromosomal and hormonal abnormalities or as a cloacal variant. Neonates with urogenital sinus frequently have ambiguous genitalia, since a main cause of this malformation stems from virilization of a female fetus or an intersex anomaly. However, urogenital sinus may also result from incomplete development of the lower vagina, and the external genitalia may appear completely normal (Marshall et al. 1979).

In patients with ambiguous genitalia, determination of the sex has to be performed using biochemical, genetic, and radiological studies in order to exclude the life-threatening salt-losing form of adrenogenital syndrome and to provide adequate information to the parents.

4.1 Female Hypospadias

In female hypospadias the urethral meatus is positioned in the anterior wall of the vagina (Figs. 20 and 21). Merguerian and McLorie (1992) regard female hypospadias as a mild form of urogenital sinus. Currarino (1986) and Knight et al. (1995) describe female hypospadias as an abnormality of the urethra itself caused by a defect in the differentiation of either the Wolffian ducts, which form the dorsal part of the urethra, or the urogenital sinus, which develops into the distal third of the vagina. Differentiation defects of the Wolffian duct lead to the development of the more severe proximal hypospadias, whereas developmental anomalies of the urogenital sinus result in the less severe distal hypospadias.

Distal hypospadia is more likely to have a urethra of normal diameter with no meatal stenosis and may, therefore, be asymptomatic or cause symptoms such as postmicturition incontinence and imperfect control, recurrent urinary tract infections, and urethral syndrome (referring to isolated urethritis with symptoms of increased frequency, pain during micturition, urgency, and dyspareunia) once sexual intercourse has commenced (Van Bogaert 1992).

The more severe cases of proximal hypospadias often show a narrowing of the urethra with signs of urinary outflow obstruction and are commonly associated with cloacal anomalies and female pseudohermaphroditism (46,XX DSD) (Knight et al. 1995).

4.1.1 Diagnostic Imaging of Female Hypospadias

In mild forms of female hypospadias, the urethral meatus is on the roof of the vagina just inside the introitus and might be entirely overlooked unless attempts to catheterize the urethra, usually for radiologic evaluation of the urinary tract, are frustrated by the inability to locate the meatus (Balk et al. 1982). In these patients the urethra must be catheterized blindly using a catheter with a curved tip (coudé catheter). To rule out associated malformations, both the kidneys, the uterus, and the vagina of these patients should be examined. The more severe cases of female hypospadias are usually part of a complex urogenital malformation, and diagnostic evaluation will, therefore, be discussed below.

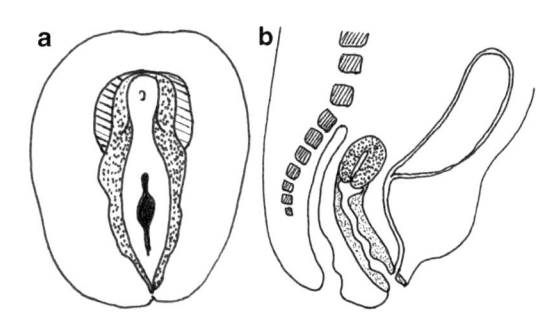

Fig. 21 Schematic representation of female hypospadia. (**a**) The perineal anatomy shows a female phenotype but no urethral opening. (**b**) The urethral meatus is in the roof of the vagina

> **Take Away**
>
> Inability to locate the urethral meatus in a little girl may be due to the presence of female hypospadias. In these patients the urethral meatus is positioned in the anterior wall of the vagina, and catheterization has to be attempted blindly.

4.2 Urogenital Sinus in Disorders of Sexual Development

Disorders of the external genitalia are especially troubling for parents because of the unconscious emotional significance of these reproductive structures. The role of the radiologist is to assist in assigning the correct gender of the neonate and to anticipate and diagnose any life-threatening conditions related to intersexual states. According to the consensus statement on management of intersex 2006, the three major types of disorders of sexual development (DSD) with ambiguous genitalia are referred to as 46,XX DSD, 46,XY DSD and sex chromosome DSD. There is some overlap between these three subgroups (Hughes et al. 2006). Table 1 presents the adapted classification according to the European Society for Pediatric Endocrinology (Riccabona 2013). Recommendations on imaging in "intersex" queries are given by the ESPR uroradiology task force part VIII (Riccabona et al. 2015).

4.2.1 46,XX Disorders of Sexual Development

In most instances 46,XX disorders with ambiguous genitalia (former female pseudohermaphroditism) result from exposure of a female fetus to excessive androgens.

The most common causes of androgen excess are *congenital adrenal hyperplasia*, followed by *placental aromatase deficiency, masculinizing maternal hormones*, and *administration of androgenic drugs to women during pregnancy*. The increased level of androgens within the fetal

Table 1 Classification of disorders of sexual development (DSD), according to the Lawson Wilkins Pediatric Endocrine Society and European Society for Pediatric Endocrinology

Numerical sex chromosome anomalies	46,XY	46,XX

47,XXY Klinefelter syndrome and variants	Disorders of gonadal (testicular) development
	    Complete or partial gonadal dysgenesis
	    Ovotestiscular DSD (true hermaphroditism)
	    Testis regression syndrome
		Disorders of gonadal (ovarian) development
		    Gonadal dysgenesis
		    Ovotesticular DSD (true hermaphroditism)
		    Testicular DSD

45,XO Turner syndrome and variants		

45,XO/46,XY MGD ovotesticular DSD (true hermaphroditism)	Disorders in androgen synthesis or action
	    Leydig cell failure
	    LH receptor mutations
	    Androgen biosynthesis defects
	    Defects in androgen metabolism
	    Defects in androgen action
	    Androgen insensitivity syndrome
	    Drugs and environmental modulators
		Androgen excess

46,XX/46,XY chimeric ovotesticular DSD	Disorders of AMH gene/persistent Müllerian duct syndrome	

	Others
	    Syndromic associations of male genital development cloacal anomalies, etc.
	    Vanishing "testes" syndrome
	    Maternal excessive exogenous estroprogestins
	    Congenital hypogonadotropic hypogonadism
	    Isolated hypospadias
	    Cryptorchidism
	    Environmental influences
		Others
		    Syndromic associations (and cloacal anomalies)
		    Müllerian agenesis/hypoplasia
		    Uterine anomalies
		    Vaginal atresia
		    McKusick-Kaufman syndrome
		    Mayer-Rokitansky-Kuster-Hauser syndrome
		    Labial adhesions

Adapted according to presentation of Orazi et al. (2012)

bloodstream causes virilization of the external genitalia, which may vary from minimal phallic enlargement of the clitoris to almost complete masculinization (Fig. 22). The degree of masculinization of the fetus is thought to be related to the time and amount of androgen exposure. If the androgen stimulus is received after 12 weeks of gestation, only clitoral hypertrophy will occur (Merguerian and McLorie 1992). Earlier androgen exposure results in urogenital sinus and a higher degree of ambiguity of the external genitalia. At birth these patients present with marked clitoral enlargement and variable degree of labioscrotal fold fusion and rugation. The opening of the urogenital sinus at the clitoral base may mimic penile hypospadias.

Congenital adrenal hyperplasia. This is caused by a family of autosomal recessive disorders of adrenal steroidogenesis leading to a deficiency of cortisol. Lack of glucocorticoid hormone causes an increase in corticotropin, hyperstimulation of the fetal adrenal gland, and excessive androgen synthesis. One out of three adrenal enzymes involved in the pathway on which glucocorticoids are synthesized is affected. The condition 21-hydroxylase deficiency counts for 90–95%, and a defect of 11β-hydroxylase is found in 5–8% of cases (New 2003). The remaining patients show defects of other enzymes involved in steroidogenesis. Due to impaired aldosterone biosynthesis, salt-losing symptoms are common in 21- and 3β-hydroxysteroid dehydrogenase deficiencies and usually present soon after birth. Owing to allelic variants, severe and mild forms are described for each defect (Chan-Cua et al. 1989).

Placental aromatase deficiency This results from a very low aromatizing activity of the placenta and thus failure to convert androgens derived

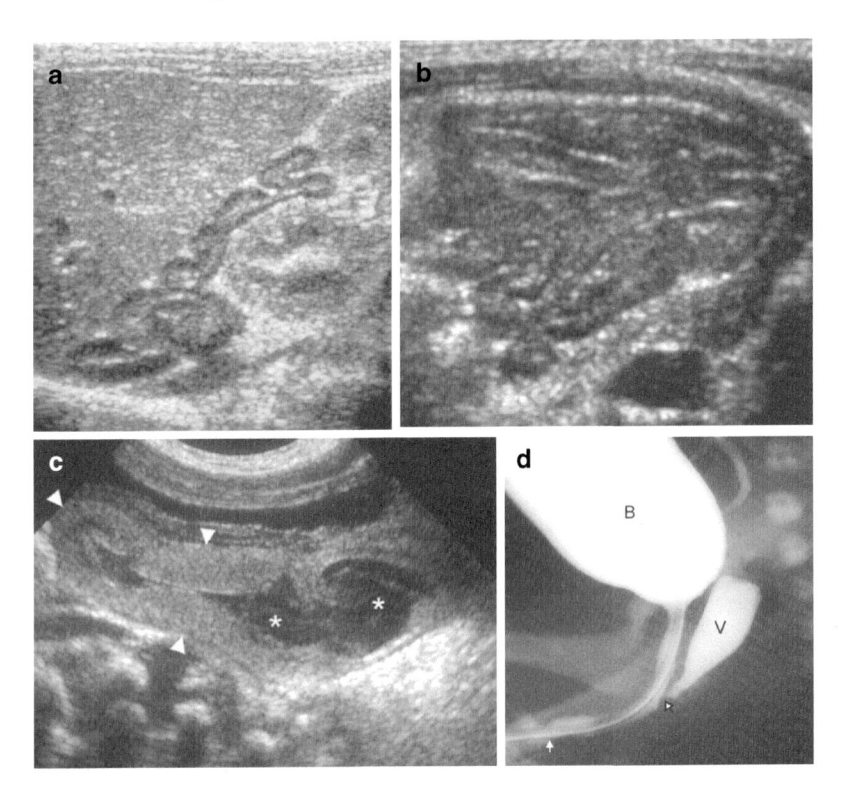

Fig. 22 Congenital adrenal hyperplasia with virilization of the external genitalia and urogenital sinus with vaginal stenosis in a 1-day-old female. (**a**) Right longitudinal sonogram; (**b**) left axial sonogram. The adrenal gland is enlarged with the so-called cerebriform pattern (resembling the cerebral cortex). (**c**) Longitudinal pelvic scan confirms the presence of the uterus (*arrowheads*). There is moderate hydrometrocolpos (*asterisks*) due to urogenital sinus with vaginal stenosis. (**d**) The bladder is catheterized. Contrast material fills the bladder (*B*) and during micturition in the vagina (*V*). Stenotic vaginal communication (*open arrow*). Urogenital sinus opening (*closed arrow*)

from fetal dehydroepiandrosterone into estrogens (Shozu et al. 1991; MacGillivary et al. 1998).

Virilizing maternal tumors These include adrenal adenoma, androblastoma, luteomas, and Krukenberg tumors and are reported to cause fetal virilization. In cases of unclear hermaphroditism, evaluation of the mother should always include measurement of her plasma androgen levels.

Administration of androgenic drugs to pregnant women Over the past couple of years, this mainly iatrogenic problem has been significantly reduced by replacing virilizing progestational compounds with nonvirilizing analogs in the treatment of threatening abortion.

4.2.2 46,XY Disorder of Sexual Development

46,XY DSD with ambiguous genitalia (former male pseudohermaphroditism) is most frequently caused by an abnormal plasma testosterone level or an abnormal testosterone response. The most common causes are disorders in androgen synthesis or action.

A *5-alpha reductase deficiency* is an androgen biosynthesis defect that blocks the transformation of testosterone into the more potent 5-alpha dihydrotestosterone (DHT). The affected 46,XY individuals have high normal to elevated plasma testosterone levels with decreased DHT levels and elevated testosterone/DHT ratios. DHT is necessary to exert androgenic effects farther from the site of testosterone production. A 5-alpha reductase deficiency results in a disorder characterized by female phenotype or severely undervirilized male phenotype with development of the epididymis, vas deferens, seminal vesicle, and ejaculatory duct, but also a pseudovagina (Imperato-McGinley and Zhu 2002).

Androgen insensitivity syndrome (AIS) is also called testicular feminization and results from a complete or partial absence of cytoplasmic receptors for testosterone in target tissues (Holterhus et al. 2005). The feminization is a consequence of increased testicular secretion of estradiol, peripheral conversion of androgens to estradiol, and a lack of testosterone function during fetal development. Serum LH and FSH are elevated as testosterone is ineffective at the hypothalamus. The syndrome is characterized by a 46,XY karyotype and negative sex chromatin. It is divided into two main categories: complete (CAIS) and partial (PAIS). CAIS results in bilateral testes, absent or hypoplastic Wolffian ducts, and female-appearing external genitalia with diminished axillary and pubic hair development (Collins et al. 1993). In PAIS the degree of sexual ambiguity varies widely from individual to individual.

CAIS is rarely discovered during childhood, unless a mass is felt in the abdomen or groin that turns out to be a testicle. Most with this condition are not diagnosed until they fail to menstruate or they try to become pregnant. PAIS, however, is often discovered during childhood because the affected child has both male and female physical characteristics and/or ambiguous genitalia such as partial fusion of the outer vaginal lips, an enlarged clitoris, or a short, blind-ending vagina.

4.2.3 Sex Chromosome DSD

The frequent cause of ambiguous genitalia in sex chromosome DSD is mixed gonadal dysgenesis. A very rare form is ovotesticular disorder of sex development.

Mixed gonadal dysgenesis is a condition of abnormal and asymmetrical gonadal development and/or sex chromosomal mosaicism, as well as retained Müllerian ducts. A number of abnormalities have been reported in the karyotype, most commonly a mosaicism 45,X/46,XY. The phenotypical expression may be ambiguous, or male or female depending on the extent of the mosaicism. The gonads may not be symmetrical; thus, the development of the Müllerian duct and Wolffian duct may be asymmetrical, too (Donahoe et al. 1979). In the presence of dysgenetic gonadal tissue and Y chromosome material, there is a high risk of the development of tumors such as gonadoblastomas and seminoma-dysgerminomas with the risk exceeding 50% as the third decade is approached. Removal of the gonads is usually indicated.

Chimeric, ovotesticular (46,XX/46,XY) DSD (former true hermaphroditism) is a very rare form of intersex disorder characterized by the presence of both ovarian and testicular tissue in the same individual. There may be an ovary on one side and a testis on the other, but more commonly one or both gonads are an ovotestis containing both types of tissue. External genitalia are often ambiguous, the degree depending mainly on the amount of testosterone produced by the testicular tissue between 8 and 16 weeks of gestation. It is rare for both types of gonadal tissue to function.

> **Take Away**
> Phenotypic sex differentiation is determined by hormonal products of the gonads. Anomalous hormone production during fetal development frequently results in ambiguous genitalia.

4.2.4 Diagnostic Imaging of Urogenital Sinus Anomalies

In *congenital adrenal hyperplasia* (Willi 1991; Chertin et al. 2000), the primary task of the radiologist is to demonstrate the level of communication between the vagina and the urethra and the anatomy of the internal genitalia or to rule out kidney anomalies and adrenal gland hyperplasia. Sonographic evaluation of the patient is usually the first-step imaging technique to provide detailed information on the urogenital system. Transabdominal US demonstrates the internal genitalia, delineates Müllerian duct anomalies, rules out any obstructions such as hydrocolpos and hydrometrocolpos (Blask et al. 1991a), and allows for investigation of the kidneys and adrenal glands at the same time. Urinary tract anomalies are common and include renal agenesis, ectopia, and cystic dysplasia as well as uni- and bilateral hydronephrosis, vesicoureteral reflux, and signs of urinary outflow obstruction (Woolf and Allen 1953). Enlargement of the adrenal cortex occurs in many, but not all babies with congenital adrenal hyperplasia. Demonstration of enlarged adrenal glands with a wavy configuration of their limbs, however, is highly suspicious of congenital adrenal hyperplasia even before biochemical or genetic data can be obtained (Fig. 22) (Teele and Share 1991; Hernanz-Schulman et al. 2002; Barwick et al. 2005).

In *androgen insensitivity syndrome*, US will demonstrate an absent uterus, no or a blind-ending vagina, and testes located in the inguinal canal, labia, or intra-abdominal. Coexistence with urologic abnormalities has to be is expected such as unilateral renal agenesis (Tokgoz et al. 2006). The patient is at increased risk of undergoing malignant transformation of the undescended gonad. The gonads should not be removed until puberty and growth are complete but closely monitored sonographically during childhood.

Procedural recommendations on imaging of the neonatal and infant genital tract are given by the *ESPR uroradiology task force* (Riccabona et al. 2014). A systematic transabdominal and transperineal US approach of the pelvic cavity with full-filled bladder is fundamental. Whenever genital US is insufficient for adequate characterization, a specific sonographic genitography is recommended. It consists of prewarmed saline instillation into the vagina through a small flexible feeding tube (8-F, thinner if urogenital sinus tract) that improves visualization. If the bladder fails to fill via urogenital sinus, blind bladder catheterization with second (curved tip) catheter is done. Additional rectal saline filling may also be useful.

For depiction of complex malformations or surgical planning, subsequent complementary imaging may include fluoroscopic genitography. Water-soluble iodinized contrast material (100 mg I/ml, or less) is required (Fig. 22). Barium paste or another opaque material is useful for marking the external orifice on the perineum. If done in the same session as US genitography, catheters are reused. Otherwise the urethra and/or the urogenital sinus is catheterized. If the catheter enters the bladder, voiding cystourethrography should be performed in the lateral position to demonstrate the urethra as well as the vagina during micturition and to rule out vesicoureteral reflux. If only the vagina is filled, however, the catheter should be left in place and a second curved-tip catheter passed anteriorly into the urogenital sinus in an attempt to catheterize the urethra. The relative position of the vaginal orifice both to the urethra and to the vestibulum can then be demonstrated. Using US and contrast studies, a definitive diagnosis of anatomical features and associated genitourinary tract malformations can be made.

Although US is the examination of choice, some authors recommend MRI to be performed before surgery (Lang et al. 1999). Unlike in adults or in older children, MRI evaluation of the genital tract is limited in neonates due to resolution issues and may be therefore less useful. A high-resolution 3D sequence after saline instillation into the vagina and bladder as well as rectal filling with diluted contrast material may yield more differentiated anatomical information (Riccabona et al. 2014).

In DSD, MR imaging reliably identifies the presence and size of ovaries, testes, uterus, vagina, and penis (Moshiri et al. 2012). Ectopic gonads, testes, and immature ovaries without cysts have intermediate signal on T1-weighted images and high-signal-intensity with an intermediate-signal-intensity outer rim on T2-weighted images (Chavhan et al. 2008). To detect and characterize streak gonads is much more challenging with any imaging modality. On T2-weighted images, low-signal-intensity stripes can be seen. High-signal-intensity foci in streak gonads could represent neoplastic changes (Gambino et al. 1992). The presence or absence of bulbospongiosus muscle and location of the transverse perinei muscles are helpful to differentiate clitoric hypertrophy from penile structures. The examination has to be completed by additional assessment of the kidneys and adrenal glands.

> **Take Away**
> Narrowing differential diagnosis of the possible cause of a urogenital sinus as well as demonstration of its anatomical features can be achieved at a high confidence level using contrast studies and US to assess pelvic structures and the adrenal glands.

4.3 Cloacal Malformation

The cloacal malformation is the most complex type of imperforate anus with confluence of the rectum, vagina, and bladder into a single common channel. Cloaca is exclusively seen in phenotypic females and occurs in 1 of every 40,000–50,000 newborns. Cloaca should not be confused with cloacal exstrophy, a malformation due to a failed closure of the lower abdominal wall seen in boys and girls. The diagnosis of cloacal malformation includes a wide spectrum of pelvic and perineal anomalies (Jaramillo et al. 1990; Hendren 1998). At the mild end of the spectrum is a persistent urogenital sinus opening with an anteriorly placed anus adjacent to it (incomplete cloaca), while in more severe malformations, all three tracts converge inside the pelvis (see also chapter "Urinary Problems Associated with Imperforate Anus"). Variants of the cloacal malformations include the presence of an accessory filiform channel or sinus that connects the bladder or urethra to the perineum, anomalies of the vagina, and the so-called posterior cloaca, where the urogenital sinus is posteriorly placed and found to open either into the orthotopic rectum or perineally close to the normal anus (Pena and Kessler 1998) (Fig. 23). Jaramillo et al. (1990) characterize the anatomy of persistent cloaca according to its urinary-cloacal or urinary-rectal communication pattern. Urinary-cloacal communication is called either urethrocloacal or vesicocloacal.

Vaginal anomalies include bifid vagina, unilateral obstruction of one hemivagina, distal vaginal stenosis or atresia, the absence of the vagina, a mislocalized retrorectal vagina, and a bifid vagina communicating widely with the trigonal area of the bladder (Fig. 24) (Jaramillo et al. 1990; Tolete-Velcek et al. 1989).

Apart from the incomplete cloaca with two perineal openings, most patients present with a single perineal opening. The perineal anatomy varies from an almost normal female phenotype (Fig. 25) to a rudimentary phallic structure with poorly formed labia (Hendren 1998). Additional pelvic anomalies include fusion defects of the Müllerian ducts, with a duplication of the uterus in

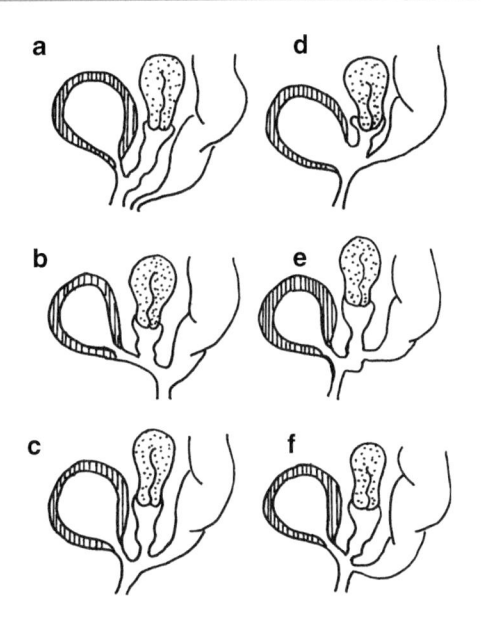

Fig. 23 (Schematic representation of cloacal malformation variants. (**a**) Incomplete cloacal malformation: A persistent urogenital sinus opening is found adjacent to an anteriorly placed anus. (**b**) Posterior cloaca: The urogenital sinus derives posteriorly and opens in the anterior rectal wall at the anus or immediately anterior to it. (**c**) Urethrocloacal communication: The urethra empties into the proximal end of the cloaca and is well formed. (**d**) Vesicocloacal communication: The urethra is rudimentary or absent. Rectal communication is called either vaginal or cloacal. (**e**) Vaginal communication of the rectum: The rectum usually joins the vagina low on its posterior wall. (**f**) Cloacal communication of the rectum: The rectum joins the cloaca

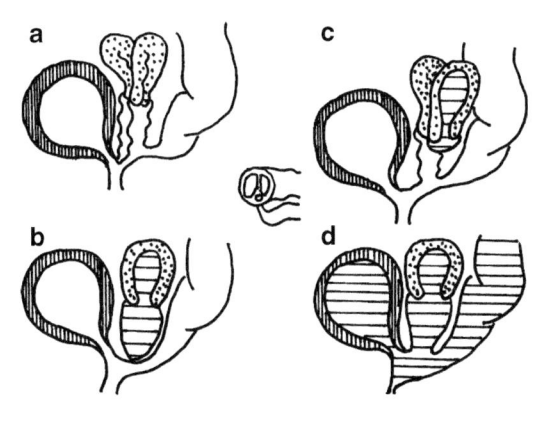

Fig. 24 Schematic representation of cloacal variants and genital anomalies. (**a**) Bifid vagina and uterus, the rectal fistula enters at the base of the septum dividing the vagina. (**b**) Distal vaginal stenosis or atresia leading to hydrometrocolpos. (**c**) Bifid uterus and vagina, unilateral obstruction, and hydrometrocolpos. (**d**) Obstruction of the urogenital sinus resulting in distention of the vagina by a combination of genital secretion, meconium, and urine

55 % of patients and obstruction of the genital tract in 25 % (Jaramillo et al. 1990; Blask et al. 1991a, b; Tolete-Velcek et al. 1989). Major renal anomalies such as renal agenesis, multicystic dysplasia, or renal ectopia are frequently associated with cloacal malformation. Vesicoureteral reflux usually occurs bilaterally and is sometimes associated with bladder diverticula and ectopia of the ureter (Jaramillo et al. 1990; McLorie et al. 1987). The ureteral ostium might then be found in a lateral or inferior location in the bladder, the vagina, or the cloaca. In cases of functional bladder outlet obstruction, hydronephrosis is common (Rich et al. 1988; Hassink et al. 1996). Furthermore, cloacal malformation can be associated with anomalies of the pelvic osseous structures such as sacral agenesis or hypoplasia, dysraphism, and pubic diastasis. Pubic diastasis, if wider than 4 cm, is frequently associated with either duplication of the bladder or a common vesicovaginal or vesicocloacal chamber. In addition, lower spinal cord abnormalities such as lipomyelomeningocele, high cord, and most frequently (affecting one-third of all patients with cloacal malformation) tethered cord (Karrer et al. 1988; Metts et al. 1997; Barkovich 2012) are found.

Except for the rare instances of incomplete cloaca, immediate colostomy is required to prevent fecal contamination of the urinary tract and renal damage, which is the most significant potential cause of morbidity and mortality in these patients. Obstruction of the cloaca may occur at any level and determines whether the proximal distended urinary and/or genital system is filled solely with genital secretions or contains urine and/or meconium as well (Fig. 24). In patients with urinary tract dilatation usually due to hydrocolpos placement of a vaginostomy, tube is required. Vesicostomy is rarely also needed (Levitt and Peña 2010). Immediate correction of high-grade vesicoureteral reflux or another potentially life-threatening uropathy is essential. In cases with a tethered cord, neurosurgical release may sometimes prevent neuronal deficits during growth but usually fails to alleviate already established neurological deficits.

Definitive correction of the cloaca can now be performed between the ages of 6 and 24 months

(Hendren 1998). The prognosis of infants with cloacal malformations has improved significantly due to surgical repair techniques pioneered by Hendren and depends on the length of the common channel on endoscopy. Children with a common channel less than 3 cm length have a good prognosis and can usually undergo posterior sagittal anorectoplasty with total urogenital mobilization. Children with a common channel longer than 3 cm usually require additional laparotomy to provide extra colon length for pull-through. They are more likely to have long-term sequelae (Levitt and Peña 2010).

> **Take Away**
> The diagnosis of cloacal malformation includes a wide spectrum of pelvic and perineal anomalies. Associated malformations of the inner genitalia and urinary tract need to be considered. Operative management and prognosis depend on the length of the common cannel.

4.3.1 Diagnostic Imaging of Cloacal Malformation

Prenatal US often fails to provide an early diagnosis, and the large, sometimes septated, fluid-filled pelviabdominal mass is often mistaken for the urinary bladder. Fetal MRI may provide additional information about the presence or absence of a cloacal anomaly in a fetus with hydrometrocolpos, which is diagnosed by location, image morphology, and fluid signal intensity of the lesion (Servaes et al. 2010) (see also chapter "Urogenital Fetal Imaging: US and MRI").

After delivery the diagnosis of cloacal malformation is suspected when, in addition to an absent anus, only one perineal orifice is found between the labia (Fig. 25). These patients need urgent referral to the pediatric radiology department for early definition of the abnormal anatomy and detection of associated malformations to adequately address potentially life-threatening complications.

US is the most efficient first-step imaging technique in the diagnostic work-up of these patients.

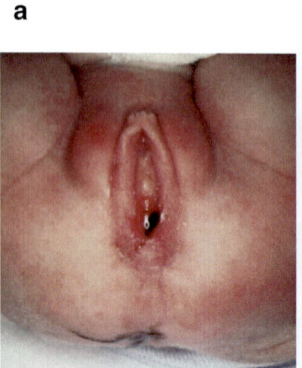

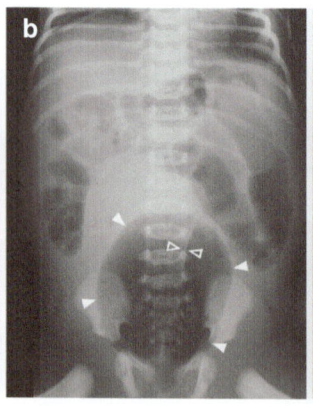

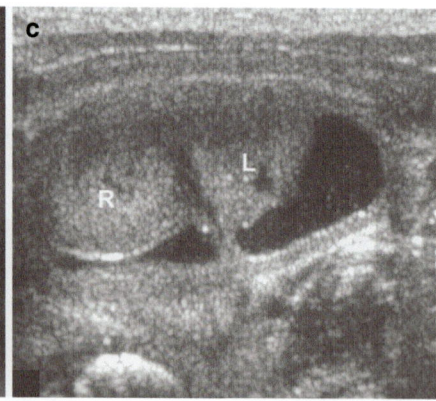

Fig. 25 Cloacal malformation with uterus didelphys. (**a**) The perineal anatomy shows a female phenotype, but only a single perineal opening. Meconium is seen within the ostium of the cloaca. (**b**) Plain X-ray. The vagina is dilated (*closed arrowheads*) and contains air. A sagittal vaginal septum is visible (*open arrowheads*). (**c**) Transverse pelvic scan: right (*R*) and left (*L*) cervix uteri behind the empty bladder. (**d**) Transverse pelvic scan at lower level than c shows the right and left vagina (*V*), urethra (*open arrowheads*), and the rectocloacal fistula (*arrowhead*). (**e**) Axial MR view (T2 weighted) of the fluid-filled vagina shows the sagittal vaginal septum with the rectocloacal fistula (*closed arrowhead*) and the dilated vagina halves with air-fluid levels. The *open arrowhead* marks the catheter. (**f**) Longitudinal pelvic scan shows the cloacal fistula (*asterisk*), rectum (*R*), and vagina (*V*). (**g, h**) Frontal and lateral view after contrast filling of the colon via colostomy demonstrates the rectum (*R*), the right and left vagina (*V*), and the rectocloacal fistula (*arrowheads*). (**i**) Transperineal sagittal scan: the urethra (*U*), vagina (*V*), and rectum (*R*) converge to a short common cloacal channel (*arrows*). (**j**) Lateral view after contrast filling: the bladder (*B*), vagina (*V*), and rectum (*R*). Three separate catheters are inserted through the single perineal opening. (**k**) Lateral view during voiding after removal of the catheters in the rectum and vagina. The short common cloacal channel is clearly demonstrated (*arrows*). The bladder (*B*), vagina (*V*), and rectum (*R*)

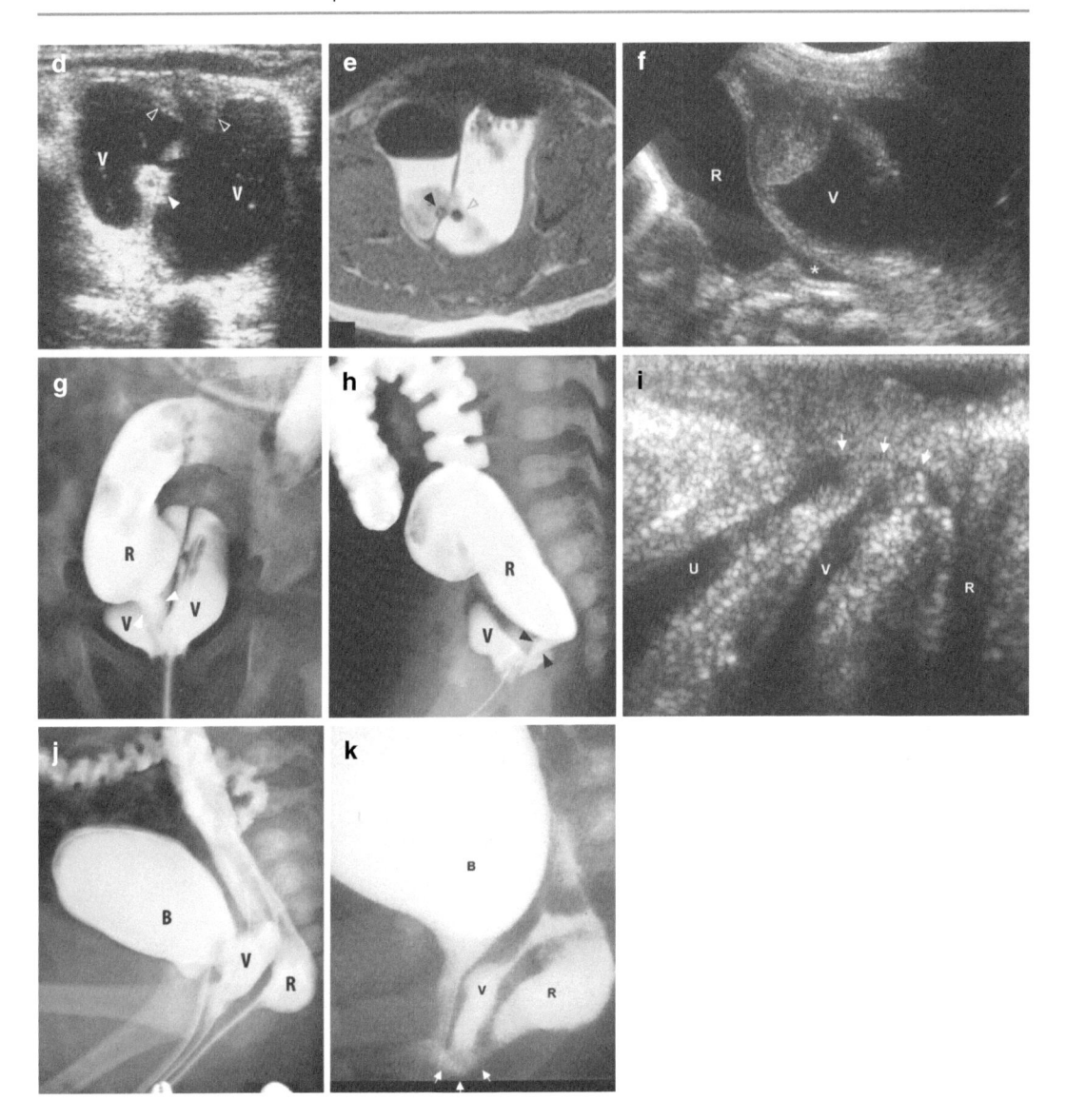

Female Genital Anomalies and Important Ovarian Conditions

Fig. 25 (continued)

Early after birth, no or only a small amount of intestinal gas will be present, and a clearer documentation of the intrapelvic structures can be obtained (Fig. 25). A pelvic mass, which is almost always a distended vagina and/or uterus, can readily be visualized (Blask et al. 1991a). A fluid-debris level is frequently seen and the level of obstruction can be determined. If there is obstruction of the common outlet, retrograde flow via the fallopian tubes may result in accumulation of intra-abdominal fluid. Depending on the level of obstruction, this fluid may consist of genital secretion only (obstruction lies above the communication between the bladder, rectum, and vagina) or contains urine and/or meconium as well. Vaginal and bladder duplication as well as malformations of the uterus can be visualized. In cases of duplicated genital structures, care should be taken to

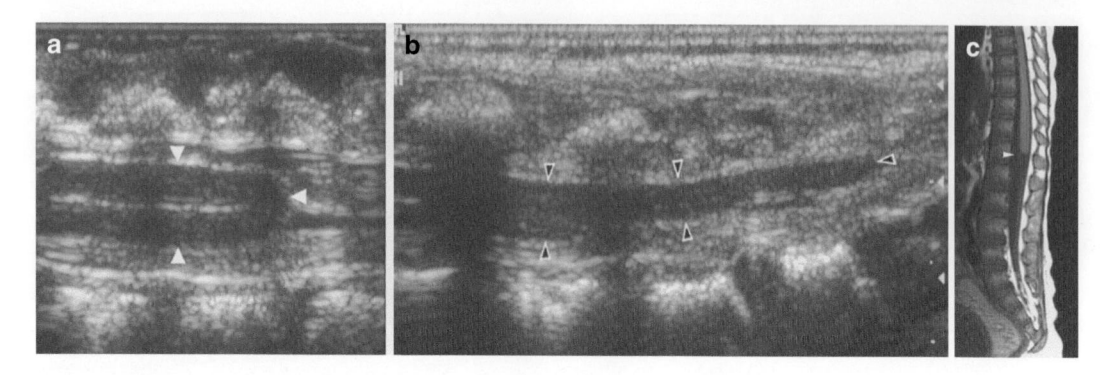

Fig. 26 Spinal cord anomalies in cloacal malformation. Newborn with (**a**) high-lying stubby conus (*arrowheads*). (**b**) With a tethered cord that extends into the sacral canal (*open arrowheads*). (**c**) A 16 ½ -year-old girl after cloacal malformation repair. T1-weighted image shows the cord terminus opposite L1 vertebral body (*arrowhead*). The terminus of the spinal cord has a characteristic blunted or chisel-shaped appearance with greater preservation of the dorsal sensory portion of the conus

document any obstruction (Tolete-Velcek et al. 1989; Blask et al. 1991a). The distance between the blind end of the rectum and the perineum can accurately be measured by transperineal US (Teele and Share 1997). The US evaluation of the newborn is completed by analysis of the abdomen including the kidney and the spinal cord. The result of the US examination of the upper urinary tract is used to choose further diagnostic tests, such as MR urography or scintigraphy.

In every patient with cloacal malformation, the spinal cord needs to be evaluated, since anomalies of the lower spinal cord occur with an incidence of up to 43%. The spinal cord can either be examined by means of spinal US during the neonatal period or, if necessary, using MR preferably imaging later in life.

Sonographic features of spinal anomalies in patients with cloacal malformations are either a high-lying plump conus or a tethered cord with a thickened filum terminale (greater than 2 mm at L5-S1), a low-lying conus medullaris (the tip of the conus lies below the level of L2), a posterior position, and a restricted motion of the conus and filum terminale within the thecal sac. In some cases of tethered cord, no distinct filum can be seen, but the spinal cord is markedly elongated, extending downward to the lower end of the dural sac (Fig. 26). This feature is particularly common in caudal regression syndrome, frequently associated with anal atresia and cloacal malformation (Barkovich 2012).

After having obtained a good sonographic overview of the pelvic anatomy, radiological examination should then be continued with plain radiographs performed a couple of hours after birth to provide evidence of any distal bowel obstruction due to the accumulation of air (Fig. 25). Gas seen in the bladder indicates urinary-intestinal communication. A pelvic mass is usually a distended vagina and/or uterus, secondary to obstruction. If this mass contains gas, it is a sign of a rectovaginal communication. Linear calcifications in the abdomen along the peritoneal surface are signs of calcifying peritonitis, which is not necessarily a result of congenital intestinal perforation, but can occur whenever either meconium (Jaramillo et al. 1990) or genital secretion (Nidecker and Humphry 1978; Ceballos and Hicks 1979) spills into the peritoneal cavity via the fallopian tubes. Granular abdominal calcifications suggest calcified intraluminal meconium (enteroliths) due to mixing of urine and meconium that are commonly associated with vaginal atresia or stenosis and rectovesical or rectourethral communication.

The next step in the imaging process is fluoroscopic studies using water-soluble contrast material to visualize the often unpredictable and erratic courses of the communication between the multiple structures and to provide functional information about reflux and competence of the urinary sphincter (Fig. 25). Contrast material is injected into the cloaca using an 8-F feeding tube if the perineal opening is small. A wider opening may need partial sealing using the balloon of a Foley catheter or a nipple (the

Poznanski technique). Accessory perineal openings should be sought. A second rudimentary urethra (phallic urethra) is expected in cases where an additional small opening is found at the base or the tip of the clitoris (Jaramillo et al. 1990). Imaging during injection should begin in the lateral projection to display the various communications. Frontal projections are useful to delineate vaginal or bladder duplications. A competent urethral sphincter can be expected when the bladder fails to opacify, and vaginal obstruction or atresia is documented if contrast material fails to visualize the vagina. It might sometimes be difficult to distinguish between the bladder and the vagina. Contrast reflux into a ureter or a urachal remnant helps to identify the bladder; a cervical impression or a septum identifies the vagina. However, in our experience this cervical impression is often difficult to observe.

Following the injection into the cloaca, an attempt to catheterize the bladder should be made to perform a voiding cystourethrogram, the only way to rule out vesicoureteral reflux. In some cases catheterization of the bladder may be difficult and needs to be supported by the use of a coudé catheter, cystoscopy, or suprapubic puncture.

The rectum frequently fails to opacify after the injection of contrast material into the cloaca. In patients who have already had a colostomy, contrast material can be directly injected into the distal limb of the colostomy prior to retrograde cloacal injection. This technique regularly demonstrates the level of rectal occlusion and the presence of communication between other pelvic structures, making further cloacal injections unnecessary (Fig. 25). Most commonly, a balloon catheter is used to inject contrast material under moderate pressure to demonstrate the narrow communication between the organ systems.

Even though not available at all pediatric institutions, rotational fluoroscopy and 3D reconstruction also have been shown to provide precise anatomical information to facilitate accurate surgical planning of a cloacal malformation and to define prognosis regarding long-term bowel, bladder, and sexual function (Patel et al. 2011). Accurate 3D representation of all urogenital and hindgut components and connections is also possible with simultaneous performance of micturating cystogram, excretory urogram, and thin-section MDCT as demonstrated by Adams et al. 2006.

Some authors recommend using MR imaging to delineate the anatomy of the inner genitalia prior to definitive surgical repair of the cloacal malformation (Metts et al. 1997; Tolete-Velcek et al. 1989). In selected cases MR imaging in combination with fluoroscopic imaging and ultrasound may be helpful to unravel the anatomy. An orienting imaging algorithm on how to proceed with suspected anorectal malformations as well as procedural recommendations on the fluoroscopic and sonographic technique has been recently issued by the ESPR uroradiology task force (Lobo 2015; Riccabona et al. 2017).

Take Away

To assess pelvic structures in cloacal malformation, US should be performed as soon as possible after birth since no or only a small amount of intestinal gas will be present. Fluoroscopic studies are mandatory to demonstrate the complex anatomy, to evaluate the urinary tract and the details of the inner genitalia, and to delineate connections and fistulas as well as the level of a possible obstruction.

5 Important Ovarian Conditions

5.1 Characteristics of the Normal Ovary

During fetal life the ovaries descend from the upper abdomen into the pelvis. At birth they usually are located within the mesovarium of the broad ligaments. On occasion descent is arrested and the ovaries may be found anywhere from the inferior edge of the kidney down to the broad ligament. Rarely, the ovaries descend below the broad ligaments and lie in the inguinal canal (Goske et al. 1984; Jedrzejewski et al. 2008) (Fig. 27).

The shape of the ovaries is variable, although the majority of ovaries are ovoid. The presence of small follicles (maximal diameter 10 mm) is a common and normal finding in children of all ages.

In the neonate ovarian size is around 1 cm³. The ovaries contain frequently one or more follicles, which measure usually less than 1 cm (Fig. 28). Between 6 and 12 months, when maternal hormonal influence subsides, size of the ovaries decreases progressively, averaging 0.7 cm³ (Cohen et al. 1993). The ovaries are relatively stable in volume before puberty, between the ages of two and nine (volume < 2 cm³, small follicles <9 mm). From the age of nine onward, there is progressive increase in the size of the ovaries. In response to gonadotropin stimulation, the ovaries migrate deeper into the pelvis, and the ovarian volume ranges between 2 and 4 cm³. After menarche the ovarian volume is more than 4 cm³ (Ziereisen et al. 2005). Multiple cortical cysts representing stimulated and unstimulated follicles can be seen during each menstrual cycle (antral follicle 5–10 mm, Graafian follicle 15–30 mm, mature corpus luteum follicle 15–30 mm) (Siegel 2011).

5.2 Ovarian Cysts

Ovarian cysts in neonates are thought to be caused by follicular stimulation due to maternal hormones and have been found to be associated with hypersecretion of placental hCG or increased placental permeability to hCG. Congenital ovarian cysts have also been reported in infants of diabetic mothers, in infants of mothers who had toxemia, a large placenta complicating Rh sensitization, or in infants suffering from adrenogenital syndrome (Silverman and Kuhn 2013; Topaloglu et al. 1997). Great variations exist in size of ovarian cysts, and cases where they occupy nearly the whole abdomen are seen (Fig. 29).

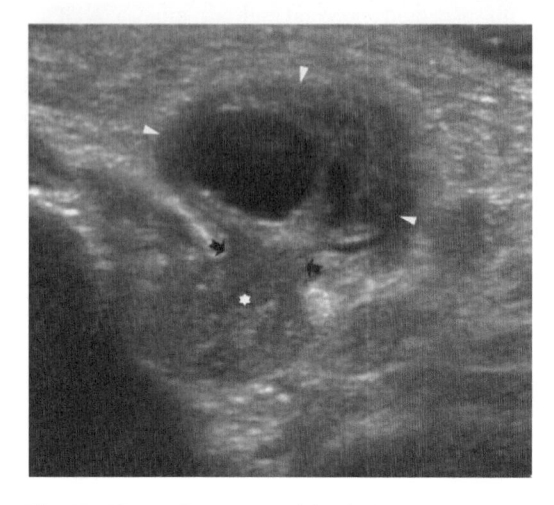

Fig. 27 Neonatal ovary-containing indirect inguinal hernia of the canal of Nuck. Longitudinal scan in the left inguinal area shows a subcutaneous oval mass containing small cysts (*arrowheads*). The appearance suggests that this mass is a neonatal ovary. The ovarian ligament (*asterisk*) extends to the abdominal cavity through the neck of the canal of Nuck (*arrows*)

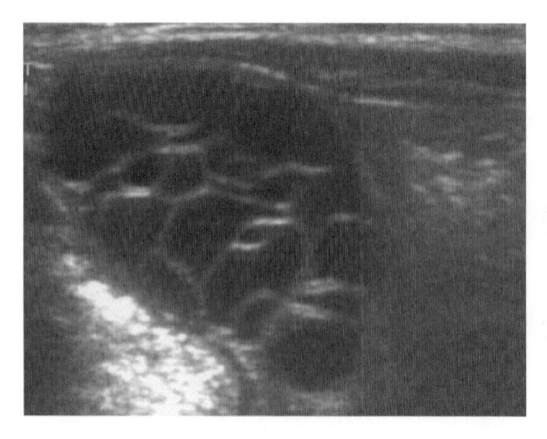

Fig. 28 Normal ovarian appearance in the neonate. Transverse scan: The ovary contains multiple follicular cysts

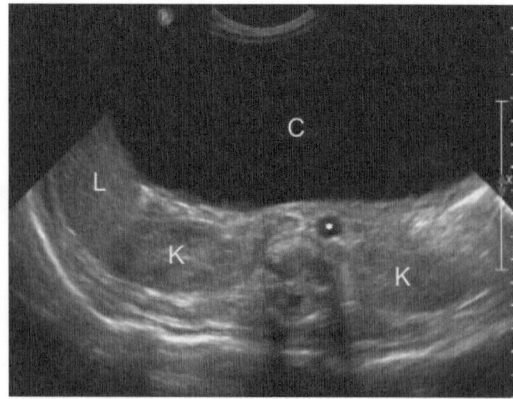

Fig. 29 Huge neonatal ovarian cyst. The cyst (*C*) is anechoic and extends to the upper abdomen. Liver (*L*), kidney (*K*), aorta (*asterisk*)

In childhood the incidence of ovarian cysts is lower than in neonates and postmenarchal girls according to low levels of gonadotropin and estradiol production. Nonetheless follicular maturation and involution is going on throughout childhood. Unilateral or bilateral ovarian follicular cysts of various sizes are frequently observed in girls with precocious puberty (onset of secondary sexual characteristics before 8 years of age). These cysts may either be secondary to ovarian stimulation by an increased level of circulating pituitary gonadotropins (central precocious puberty) or functional cysts similar to those seen in normal girls (partial precocious development). However, in some cases a large ovarian cyst may assume an autonomous function and be responsible for precocious puberty due to excessive estrogen production. In these instances, imaging of uterus length and quality of the endometrium helps to assess estrogenization.

Bilateral ovarian cysts in older girls are often found in association with cystic fibrosis, untreated hypothyroidism (Lindsay et al. 1983), Cushing syndrome, and other endocrinopathies with increased circulating androgen levels. Bilateral ovarian enlargement with discrete cysts has been seen in children with McCune-Albright syndrome (fibrous dysplasia, patchy cutaneous pigmentation, sexual precocity) (Rieth et al. 1981) and in patients suffering from polycystic ovarian disease.

In polycystic ovarian disease, both of the generally enlarged ovaries contain many small follicular cysts (2–6 mm), but larger cysts may also be present. Polycystic ovarian syndrome (Stein-Leventhal syndrome) is characterized by the association of polycystic ovaries with irregular menses, prolonged uterine bleeding, amenorrhea, anovulation, and often hirsutism and obesity. The clinical manifestation of this syndrome begins at or shortly after puberty.

According to their sonographic appearance, a simple and a complex cyst have been described. Simple cysts have a thin wall, an anechoic content, and no calcifications or associated mass. A daughter cyst is a specific sonographic finding for an ovarian cyst and should not be considered as complex (Lee et al. 2000) (Fig. 30).

Complex cysts show a fluid-debris level, a retracting clot, or thick septae as a result of salpingo torsion and subsequent ovarian infarction or hemorrhage into a simple cyst (Fig. 31 and 32).

To differentiate between a hemorrhagic ovarian cyst and a complex ovarian mass, like a tumor or dermoid cyst, may not be possible on imaging. Follow-up imaging of hemorrhagic cysts demonstrates decrease in size over the next menstrual cycle and resolves over two to three menstrual cycles. Lesions, which do not resolve or grow, need further surgical evaluation.

Controversy still exists about the management of ovarian cysts as to whether conservative (close observation), intermediate (percutaneous needle aspiration of large simple cyst under sonographic guidance, percutaneous drainage of complex cysts), or aggressive (surgical removal) therapy of ovarian cysts is more appropriate.

In general, most ovarian cysts are functional in nature and usually will resolve spontaneously (Brandt and Helmrath 2005). Müller-Leisse et al. (1992) demonstrated considerable regression of the ovarian cysts in conservatively treated neonates, regardless of the sonographic appearance of the cyst and, therefore, recommend conservative treatment in asymptomatic

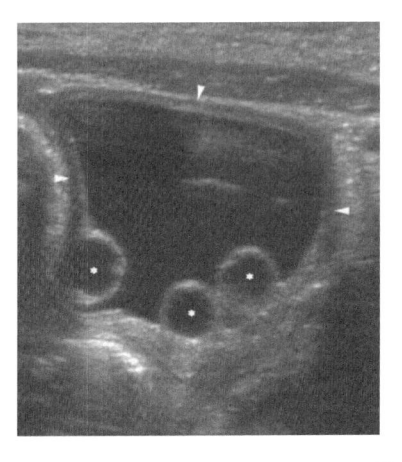

Fig. 30 Neonatal ovarian cyst. Transverse scan. The cyst (*arrowheads*) contains small "daughter cysts" (*asterisks*), representing follicles

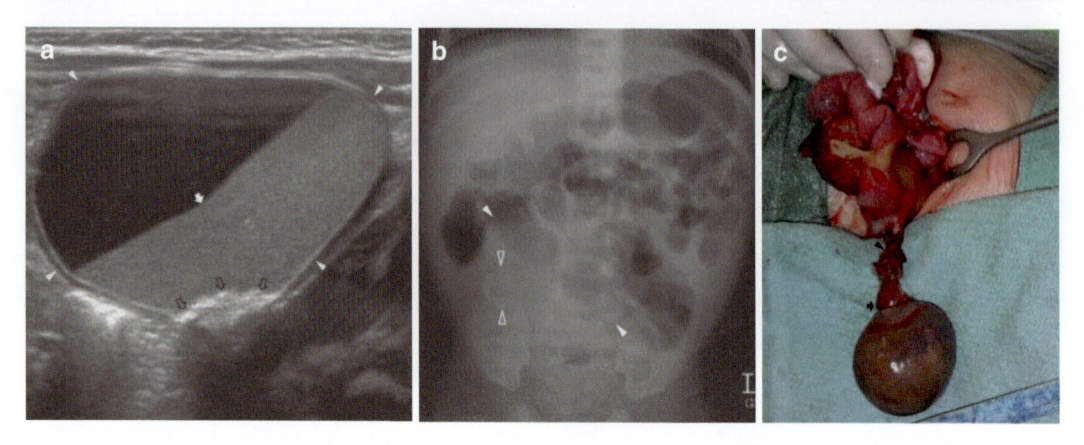

Fig. 31 Congenital ovarian cyst complicated by intrauterine adnexal torsion. (**a**) Longitudinal sonogram of the right hemiabdomen at the age of 2 months shows a large cyst (*arrowheads*) with a fluid-debris (blood) level (*arrow*). The necrotic ovary (*open arrows*) is highly echogenic (calcified). (**b**) Plain abdominal radiograph shows a soft tissue mass in the right lower quadrant (*arrowheads*) with the calcified ovary (*open arrowheads*). (**c**) Photograph taken at time of surgery shows the hemorrhagic ovarian cyst, the necrotic ovary (*arrow*), and the torsed fallopian tube (*arrowhead*)

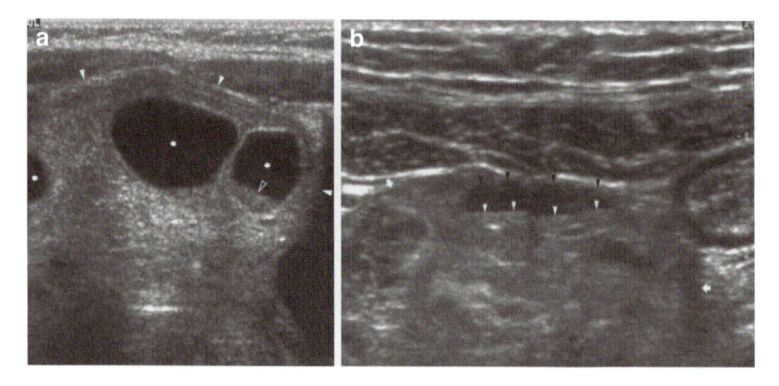

Fig. 32 (**a**) Ovarian torsion. High-resolution oblique sonogram through the left lower abdomen in a 4-month-old girl demonstrates an enlarged left ovary (*arrows*) with fluid-debris level in follicular cysts (*open arrowhead*) indicative of hemorrhagic infarction (**b**). A 17-year-old girl with left ovarian torsion. Transabdominal axial high-resolution US reveals fluid-debris levels (*white arrowheads*) in peripheral follicles (*black arrowheads*) of the enlarged ovary (*arrows*) indicative of hemorrhagic infarction

patients and percutaneous puncture of space-occupying cysts.

Surgical evaluation is indicated if the diagnosis is in question; the cyst persists or is symptomatic.

Most pediatric surgeons for the treatment of ovarian cysts favor laparoscopy. If surgical exploration is performed, every attempt to salvage the gonad should be made. Simple cysts should be fenestrated. Complex or functional cysts should be excised, with preservation of the remaining ovary. Viable ovarian tissue may still be present, even if macroscopically invisible (Brandt et al. 1991; Brandt and Helmrath 2005).

Take Away
The presence of small follicles (maximal diameter 10 mm) is a common and normal finding in children of all ages. A daughter cyst is a specific sonographic finding for an ovarian cyst. Most ovarian cysts are functional in nature and will usually resolve spontaneously. Surgical evaluation is indicated if the diagnosis is in question; the cyst persists or is symptomatic. If surgical exploration is performed, every attempt to salvage the gonad should be made.

5.3 Ovarian Torsion

Ovarian torsion results from partial or complete twisting of the ovarian pedicle on its axis. With progressive torsion, there is initial compromise of lymphatic drainage, which causes enlargement of the ovary due to lymphatic edema. This is followed by venous obstruction and hemorrhagic infarction. The final step is interruption of the arterial blood supply, which can result in gangrene, infection, peritonitis, and its sequelae (Graif and Itzchak 1988).

Torsion occurs in normal ovaries, but more frequently in ovarian masses that increase the risk of torsion.

Torsion may also occur antenatally and may not be always symptomatic (Nussbaum et al. 1988) (Fig. 31). In the neonate it may cause fever, irritability, vomiting, leukocytosis, and abdominal tenderness. In all age groups, clinical presentation is nonspecific and includes pelvic pain, nausea, and vomiting (Meyer et al. 1995) and may mimic appendicitis. The possibility of ovarian torsion should, therefore, be considered in every female patient with pelvic pain. Symptoms often occur repeatedly, suggesting recurrent torsion and detorsion. Undiagnosed and untreated ovarian torsion commonly results in loss of the ovary and may lead to infertility. Timely diagnosis is mandatory to avoid these complications. Management of suspected ovarian torsion should have the same priority as the surgical emergency management of testicular torsion.

Sonography is the imaging modality of choice to evaluate girls with suspected torsion because it involves no ionizing radiation to the patient, is immediately available, and provides good visualization of pelvic organs. Several characteristic sonographic features of ovarian torsion in children have been described:

Enlargement of the ovary is one of these signs. The mean volume of the torsed ovary is, on average, 12 times that of the normal contralateral side (Servaes et al. 2007). However, this diagnostic sign is nonspecific and can also be seen in other ovarian mass lesions, such as benign or malignant tumor, hemorrhagic or simple ovarian cyst, endometrioma or tubo-ovarian abscess, which are more common in postmenarchal adolescents.

Multiple cortical follicles (8–15 mm in size) in the periphery of a unilaterally enlarged ovary have been reported in up to 74% of patients with ovarian torsion (Graif et al. 1984). Multifollicular enlargement has been attributed to transudation of fluid into the follicles as part of congestion of the ovary from circulatory impairment and should be considered presumptive evidence of torsion.

Color and spectral Doppler sonography can provide important information regarding ovarian vascularity. Studies have shown that while the absence of blood flow does indeed indicate torsion (provided Doppler is sensitive enough to depict ovarian blood flow), maintenance of blood flow does not exclude the diagnosis (Hurh et al. 2002). Possible explanations for this are (1) a dual blood supply from the ovarian and uterine arteries that provides persistent arterial flow even when the ovary is torsed, (2) intermittent torsion with the Doppler findings being dependent on whether torsion is present at the time of examination (Peña et al. 2000), or (3) partial torsion that compromises venous flow with limited or no effect on arterial flow (Hurh et al. 2002).

Circulatory impairment in the torsed ovary leads to transudation of fluid and hemorrhage in the follicles of the ovary. *Using high-resolution US*, transudation can be seen as *fluid-debris levels* in these peripheral follicles at least in advanced stages of the disease (Fig. 32). This should be considered as a highly specific finding that may facilitate the immediate and correct diagnosis of ovarian torsion and is indicative of hemorrhagic infarction (Kiechl-Kohlendorfer et al. 2006).

A *twisted vascular pedicle and the whirlpool sign are also promising findings*. At gray-scale US the twisted vascular pedicle appears as a round hyperechoic structure with multiple concentric hypoechoic stripes (target appearance), as a beaked structure with concentric low echoic stripes, or as an ellipsoid or tubular structure with internal heterogeneous echoes (Lee et al. 1998). At color Doppler sonography (CDS) of the twisted vascular pedicle, visualization of circular or coiled vessels is the whirlpool sign. The ovaries without flow in the vascular pedicle at CDS were necrotic or infarcted at surgery (Lee et al. 1998; Vijayaraghavan 2004). Thus, the whirlpool sign may also be helpful in determination of preoperative ovarian viability (Chang et al. 2008). However, this depends on accessibility and also to a certain extent on patient age.

As additional, nonspecific finding free pelvic fluid in the cul-de-sac has been detected with US in one- to two-thirds of the reported cases of ovarian torsion (Graif et al. 1984), and *medial displacement of the torsed ovary to the midline* may be a helpful sign (Siegel 2011) (Fig. 33).

The role of CT has expanded, and it is increasingly used in evaluation of abdominal pain. Common CT features of ovarian torsion include an enlarged ovary, uterine deviation to the twisted side, smooth wall thickening of the twisted adnexal cystic mass, fallopian tube thickening, peripheral cystic structures, and ascites (Chang et al. 2008). Although CT shows features suggestive of torsion, the study of Chiou et al. (2007) demonstrated that the diagnostic value of initial CT was less than that of initial US; furthermore CT is not recommended as the first-step imaging in infants and children with lower abdominal pain or suspicion of ovarian torsion (Ording-Müller 2015; Riccabona et al. 2017).

An MRI study can be helpful in selected cases, when the symptoms of torsion are subacute/chronic or recurrent in nature, but it should not delay emergency management.

Similar to US in MRI a twisted vascular pedicle between the enlarged ovary and uterus may be shown. Enlargement of the ovary and multiple follicles separated by edematous stroma characterize early stages of torsion (Togashi 2003). Hyperintense signal of enlarged ovarian stroma on T2-weighted images indicates edema (Ghossain et al. 2004; Haque et al. 2000) (Fig. 33). With hemorrhagic necrosis, the lesion may exhibit high intensity on T1-weighted images (Rha et al. 2002; Minutoli et al. 2001). Enhancement on postcontrast MR images identifies viable tissues in the affected ovary (Haque et al. 2000) (Fig. 33). Lack of enhancement in the torsed ovary is consequence of complete interruption of blood flow and is a delayed sign suggesting hemorrhagic infarction of the lesion (Rha et al. 2002). Diffusion-weighted sequences may show diffusion restriction – some advocate to use low ADC values as an indicator of hemorrhagic infarction (Kato et al. 2014).

When ovarian torsion is suspected, urgent surgical intervention is indicated and is usually performed by laparoscopy. Despite macroscopic appearance of early necrosis, the twisted ischemic ovary may be successfully reperfused by detorsion. Adnexectomy should be avoided as ovarian function is preserved in 88–100% of cases (Oelsner and Shashar 2006).

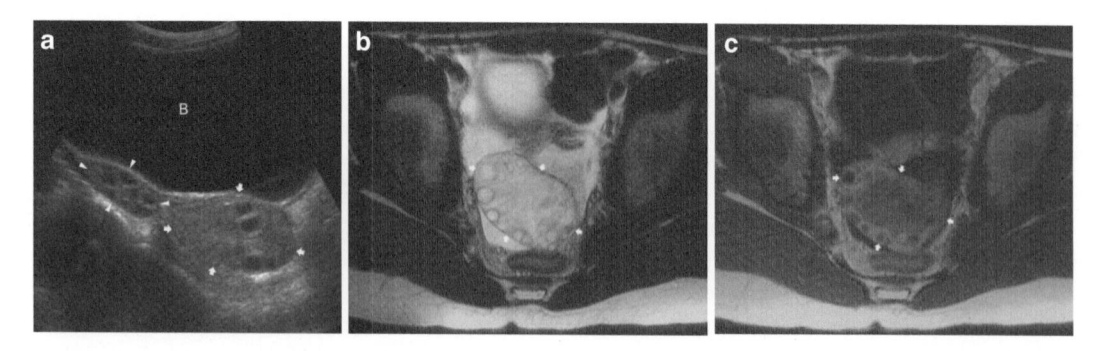

Fig. 33 An 11 ½-year-old girl with adnexal torsion. (**a**) Left oblique sonogram, (**b**) axial T2-weighted MR image, and (**c**) axial postcontrast T1-weighted MR image. Enlarged medially displaced left ovary (*arrows*) with increased stromal echogenicity (**a**) hyperintense stroma (**b**) reflecting edema and containing peripheral follicles. Postcontrast T1-weighted image (**c**) shows heterogeneous enhancement in the ovarian stroma and the wall of the follicles. The right ovary (*arrowheads*) is normal. Bladder (*B*)

> **Take Away**
> Imaging characteristics of ovarian torsion are unilaterally enlargement and medial displacement of the torsed ovary, multiple cortical follicles in the periphery of the ovary, whirlpool sign of the vascular pedicle, fluid-debris levels in peripheral follicles indicating hemorrhagic infarction, and free fluid in the cul-de-sac (nonspecific).

References

Acién P, Acién MI (2011) The history of female genital tract malformation classifications and proposal of an updated system. Hum Reprod Update 17(5):693–705

Adams ME, Hiorns MP, Wilcox DT (2006) Combining MDCT, micturating cystography, and excretory urography for 3D imaging of cloacal malformation. AJR Am J Roentgenol 187:1034–1035

American Fertility Society (1988) The American Fertility Society classifications of adnexal adhesions, distal tubal occlusion, tubal occlusion secondary to tubal ligation, tubal pregnancies, müllerian anomalies and intrauterine adhesions. Fertil Steril 49:944–955

Balk SJ, Dreyfus NG, Harris P (1982) Examination of genitalia in children: the remaining taboo. Pediatrics 70:751–753

Barbaro M, Wedell A, Nordenström A (2011) Disorders of sex development. Semin Fetal Neonatal Med 16(2):119–127

Barkovich AJ (2012) Pediatric neuroimaging, vol 862, 3rd edn. Lippincott Williams & Wilkins, Philadelphia, pp 887–888

Barwick TD, Malhotra A, Webb JA, Savage MO, Reznek RH (2005) Embryology of the adrenal glands and its relevance to diagnostic imaging. Clin Radiol 60:953–959

Bazi T, Berjawi G, Seoud M (2006) Inguinal ovaries associated with Mullerian agenesis: case report and review. Fertil Steril 85:1510–1518

Behr SC, Courtier JL, Qayyum A (2012) Imaging of Müllerian duct anomalies. Radiographics 32:E233–E250

Blask AR, Sanders RC, Gearhart JP (1991a) Obstructed uterovaginal anomalies: demonstration with sonography. I. Neonates and infants. Radiology 179:79–83

Blask AR, Sanders RC, Rock JA (1991b) Obstructed uterovaginal anomalies: demonstration with sonography. II. Teenagers. Radiology 179:84–88

Bok G, Drews U (1983) The role of the Wolffian ducts in the formation of the sinus vagina: an organ culture study. J Embryol Exp Morphol 73:275–295

Brandt ML, Helmrath MA (2005) Ovarian cysts in infants and children. Semin Pediatr Surg 14:78–85

Brandt ML, Luks FI, Filiatrault D et al (1991) Surgical indications in antenatally diagnosed ovarian cysts. J Pediatr Surg 26:276–282

Buttram VC, Gibbons WE (1979) Müllerian anomalies: a proposed classification (an analysis of 144 cases). Fertil Steril 32:40–46

Ceballos R, Hicks GM (1979) Plastic peritonitis due to neonatal hydrometrocolpos: radiologic and pathologic observations. J Pediatr Surg 5:63–70

Chan-Cua S, Freidenberg G, Jones KL (1989) Occurrence of male phenotype in genotypic females with congenital virilizing adrenal hyperplasia. Am J Med Genet 34:406–410

Chang HC, Bhatt S, Dogra VS (2008) Pearls and pitfalls in diagnosis of ovarian torsion. Radiographics 28:1355–1368

Chavhan GB, Parra DA, Oudjhane K, Miller SF, Babyn PS, Pippi Salle JL (2008) Imaging of ambiguous genitalia: classification and diagnostic approach. Radiographics 28:1891–1904

Chertin B, Hadas-Halpern I, Fridmans A, Kniznik M, Abu-Arafeh W, Zilberman M, Farkas A (2000) Transabdominal pelvic sonography in the preoperative evaluation of patients with congenital adrenal hyperplasia. J Clin Ultrasound 28:122–124

Chiou SY, Lev Toaff AS, Masuda E et al (2007) Adnexal torsion new clinical and imaging observations by sonography, computed tomography, and magnetic resonance imaging. J Ultrasound Med 26:1289–1301

Cohen HL, Shapiro MA, Mandel FS et al (1993) Normal ovaries in neonates and infants: a sonographic study of 77 patients 1 day to 24 months old. AJR Am J Roentgenol 160:583–586

Collins GM, Kim DU, Logrono R, Rickert RR, Zablow A, Breen JL (1993) Pure seminoma arising in androgen insensitivity syndrome (testicular feminization syndrome): a case report and review of the literature. Mod Pathol 6:89–93

Currarino G (1982) Single vaginal ectopic ureter and Gartner's duct cyst with ipsilateral renal hypoplasia and dysplasia (or agenesis). J Urol 128:988–993

Currarino G (1986) Large prostatic utricles and related structures, urogenital sinus and other forms of urethrovaginal confluence. J Urol 136:1270–1279

Donahoe PK, Crawford JD, Hendren WH (1979) Mixed gonadal dysgenesis, pathogenesis, and management. J Pediatr Surg 14:287–300

Drews U (2007) Helper function of the Wolffian ducts and role of androgens in the development of the vagina. Sex Dev 1:100–110

Duncan PA, Shapiro LR, Stangel JJ, Klein RM, Addonizio JC (1979) The MURCS association: Müllerian duct aplasia, renal aplasia, and cervicothoracic somite dysplasia. J Pediatr 95(3):399–402

Ehammer T, Riccabona M, Maier E (2011) High resolution MR for evaluation of lower urogenital tract malformations in infants and children: feasibility and preliminary experiences. Eur Radiol 78:388–393

Fielding JR (1996) MR imaging of Müllerian anomalies: impact on therapy. AJR Am J Roentgenol 167:1491–1495

Fedele L, Ferrazzi E, Dorta M, Vercellini P, Candiani GB (1988) Ultrasonography in the differential diagnosis of "double" uteri. Fertil Steril 50(2):361–364

Gambino J, Caldwell B, Dietrich R, Walot I, Kangarloo H (1992) Congenital disorders of sexual differentiation: MR findings. AJR Am J Roentgenol 158:363–367

Gassner I, Geley TE (2004) Ultrasound of female genital anomalies. Eur Radiol 14(Suppl 4):L107–L122

Gharagozloo AM, Lebowitz RL (1994) Detection of poorly functioning malpositioned kidney with single ectopic ureter in girls with urinary dribbling. AJR Am J Roentgenol 164:957–961

Ghossain MA, Hachem K, Buy JN, Hourany-Rizk RG, Aoun NJ, Haddad-Zebouni S, Mansour F, Attieh E, Abboud J (2004) Adnexal torsion: magnetic resonance findings in the viable adnexa with emphasis on stromal ovarian appearance. J Magn Reson Imaging 20:451–462

Gilsanz V, Cleveland RH (1982) Duplication of the Müllerian ducts and genitourinary malformations. Part I: the value of excretory urography. Radiology 144:793–796

Gilsanz V, Cleveland RH, Reid BS (1982) Duplication of the Müllerian ducts and genitourinary malformations. Part II: analysis of malformations. Radiology 144:797–801

Goske MJ, Emmens RW, Rabinowitz R (1984) Inguinal ovaries in children demonstrated by high resolution real-time ultrasound. Radiology 151:635–636

Graif M, Itzchak Y (1988) Sonographic evaluation of ovarian torsion in childhood and adolescence. AJR Am J Roentgenol 150:647–649

Graif M, Shalev J, Strauss S et al (1984) Torsion of the ovary: sonographic features. AJR Am J Roentgenol 143:1331–1334

Gruenwald P (1941) The relation of the growing Müllerian ducts to the Wolffian duct and its importance for the genesis of malformations. Anat Rec 81:1–19

Hartwig NG (1992) Pathoembryology: developmental processes and congenital malformations. Thesis, State University Leiden, Leiden

Haque TL, Togashi K, Kobayashi H, Fujii S, Konishi J (2000) Adnexal torsion: MR imaging findings of viable ovary. Eur Radiol 10:1954–1957

Hassink EAM, Rieu PNMA, Hamel BCJ, Severijnen RSVM, vd Staak FHJ, Festen C (1996) Additional congenital defects in anorectal malformations. Eur J Pediatr 155:477–482

Hendren H (1998) Cloaca, the most severe degree of imperforate anus. Ann Surg 228:331–346

Hernanz-Schulman M, Brock JW III, Russell W (2002) Sonographic findings in infants with congenital adrenal hyperplasia. Pediatr Radiol 32:130–137

Hersmus R, Kalfa N, de Leeuw B, Stoop H, Oosterhuis JW, de Krijger R, Wolffenbuttel KP, Drop SL, Veitia RA, Fellous M, Jaubert F, Looijenga LH (2008) FOXL2 and SOX9 as parameters of female and male gonadal differentiation in patients with various forms of disorders of sex development (DSD). J Pathol 215(1):31–38

Holterhus PM, Werner R, Hoppe U, Bassler J, Korsch E, Ranke MB, Dorr HG, Hiort O (2005) Molecular features and clinical phenotypes in androgen insensitivity syndrome in the absence and presence of androgen receptor gene mutations. J Mol Med 83:1005–1013

Homer HA, Li TC, Cooke ID (2000) The septate uterus: a review of management and reproductive outcome. Fertil Steril 73(1):1–14

Hughes IA, Houk C, Ahmed SF, Lee PA, LWPES/ESPE Consensus Group (2006) Consensus statement on management of intersex disorders. Arch Dis Child 91:554–563

Hurh PJ, Meyer JS, Shaaban A (2002) Ultrasound of a torsed ovary: characteristic gray-scale appearance despite normal arterial and venous flow on Doppler. Pediatr Radiol 32:586–588

Imperato-McGinley J, Zhu YS (2002) Androgens and male physiology: the syndrome of 5alpha-reductase-2 deficiency. Mol Cell Endocrinol 198:51–59

Jaramillo D, Lebowitz RL, Hendren WH (1990) The cloacal malformation: radiologic findings and imaging recommendation. Radiology 177:441–448

Jarcho J (1946) Malformation of the uterus: review of the subject, including embryology, comparative anatomy, diagnosis and report of cases. Am J Surg 71:106–166

Jedrzejewski G, Stankiewicz A, Wieczorek AP (2008) Uterus and ovary hernia of the canal of Nuck. Pediatr Radiol 38:1257–1258

Karrer FM, Flannery AM, Nelson MD, McLone DG, Raffensperger JG (1988) Anorectal malformations: evaluation of associated spinal dysraphic syndromes. J Pediatr Surg 3:45–48

Kato H, Kanematsu M, Uchiyama M, Yano R, Furui T, Morishige K (2014) Diffusion-weighted imaging of ovarian torsion: usefulness of Apparent Diffusion Coefficient (ADC) values for the detection of hemorrhagic infarction. Magn Reson Med Sci 13:39–44

Kiechl-Kohlendorfer U, Geley TE, Unsinn KM, Gassner I (2001) Diagnosing neonatal female genital anomalies using saline-enhanced sonography. AJR Am J Roentgenol 177:1041–1044

Kiechl-Kohlendorfer U, Maurer K, Unsinn KM, Gassner I (2006) Fluid debris level in follicular cysts: a pathognomonic sign of ovarian torsion. Pediatr Radiol 36:421–425

Kiechl-Kohlendorfer U, Geley T, Maurer K, Gassner I (2011) Uterus didelphys with unilateral vaginal atresia: multicystic dysplastic kidney is the precursor of "renal agenesis" and the key to early diagnosis of this genital anomaly. Pediatr Radiol 41:1112–1116

Kluth D, Hillen M, Lambrecht W (1995) The principles of normal and abnormal hindgut development. J Pediatr Surg 30:1143–1147

Knight HML, Phillips NJ, Mouriquand PDE (1995) Female hypospadias: a case report. J Pediatr Surg 30:1738–1740

Koopman P (1995) The molecular biology of SRY and its role in sex determination in mammals. Reprod Fertil Dev 7:713–722

Lang IM, Babyn P, Oliver GD (1999) MR imaging of paediatric uterovaginal anomalies. Pediatr Radiol 29:163–170

Lee EJ, Kwon HC, Joo HJ, Suh JH, Fleischer AC (1998) Diagnosis of ovarian torsion with color Doppler sonography: depiction of twisted vascular pedicle. J Ultrasound Med 17(2):83–89

Lee HJ, Woo SK, Kim JS, Suh SJ (2000) "Daughter Cyst" sign: a sonographic finding of ovarian cyst in neonates, infants and young children. AJR Am J Roentgenol 174:1013–1015

Levitt MA, Peña A (2010) Cloacal malformations: lessons learned from 490 cases. Semin Pediatr Surg 19:128–138

Lindsay AN, Voorhess ML, MacGillivary MH (1983) Multicystic ovaries in primary hypothyroidism. Obstet Gynecol 61:433–437

Lobo L (2015) Recommendation for an imaging algorithm in neonatal and childhood ano-rectal/cloacal malformation. Pediatr Radiol 45(S2):S310

Ludwig KS (1998) The Mayer-Rokitansky-Küster syndrome. An analysis of its morphology and embryology. Part I: morphology. Part II: embryology. Arch Gynecol Obstet 262:1–42

MacGillivary MH, Morishimo A, Conte F, Grumbach M, Smith EP (1998) Pediatric endocrinology update: an overview. The essential roles of estrogens in pubertal growth, epiphyseal fusion and bone turnover: lessons from mutations in the gene for aromatase and the estrogen receptor. Horm Res 49:2–8

Marrakchi A, Belhaj L, Boussouf H, Chraibi A, Kadiri A (2005) Pure gonadal dysgenesis XX and XY: observations in 15 patients. Ann Endocrinol (Paris) 66:553–556

Marshall FF, Jeffs RD, Sarafyan WK (1979) Urogenital sinus abnormalities in the female patient. J Urol 122:568–572

McLorie GA, Sheldon CA, Fleisher M, Churchill BM (1987) The genitourinary system in patients with imperforate anus. J Pediatr Surg 22:1100–1104

Merguerian PA, McLorie GA (1992) Disorders of the female genitalia. In: Kelalis PP, King LR, Belman AB (eds) Clinical pediatric urology, 3rd edn. Saunders, Philadelphia, pp 1084–1105

Metts JC, Kotkin L, Kasper S, Shyr Y, Adams MC, Brock JW (1997) Genital malformations and coexistent urinary tract or spinal anomalies in patients with imperforate anus. J Urol 158:1298–1300

Meyer JS, Harmon CM, Harty MP et al (1995) Ovarian torsion: clinical and imaging presentation in children. J Pediatr Surg 30:1433–1436

Minutoli F, Blandino A, Gaeta M, Lentini M, Pandolfo I (2001) Twisted ovarian fibroma with high signal intensity on T1-weighted MR image: a new sign of torsion of ovarian tumors? Eur Radiol 11:1151–1154

Moore KL, Persaud TVN, Mark GT (2011) The developing human: clinically oriented embryology, 9th edn. W.B. Saunders Company, Philadelphia

Moshiri M, Chapman T, Fechner PY, Dubinsky TJ, Shnorhavorian M, Osman S, Bhargava P, Katz DS (2012) Evaluation and management of disorders of sex development: multidisciplinary approach to a complex diagnosis. Radiographics 32:1599–1618

Müller-Leisse C, Bick U, Paulussen K et al (1992) Ovarian cysts in the fetus and neonate: changes in sonographic pattern in the follow-up and their management. Pediatr Radiol 22:395–400

New MI (2003) Inborn errors of adrenal steroidogenesis. Mol Cell Endocrinol 211:75–83

Nidecker AC, Humphry A (1978) Peritoneal calcification in a neonate with imperforate hymen. J Can Assoc Radiol 29:277–279

Nievelstein RAJ, Van der Werff JFA, Verbeek FJ, Valk J, Vermeij-Keers C (1998) Normal and abnormal embryonic development of the anorectum in human embryos. Teratology 57:70–78

Nussbaum AR, Sanders RC, Hartman DS, Dudgeon DL, Parmley TH (1988) Neonatal ovarian cysts: sonographic-pathologic correlation. Radiology 168:817–821

Oelsner G, Shashar D (2006) Adnexal torsion. Clin Obstet Gynecol 49(3):459–463

Orazi C, Lucchetti MC, Schingo PMS, Marchetti P, Ferro F (2007) Herlyn-Werner-Wunderlich syndrome: uterus didelphys, blind hemivagina and ipsilateral renal agenesis. Sonographic and MR findings in 11 cases. Pediatr Radiol 37:657–665

Orazi C, Silveri M, Cappa M, Bizarri C, Schingo PMS, Toma P (2012) Disorders of sexual development: role of imaging. Oral presentation at the 49th meeting of the European Society of Pediatric Radiology, Athens, 2012 May

Ording-Müller LS (2015) Paediatric urogenital radiology – ovarian torsion. Pediatr Radiol 45(S2):S309–S310

Patel M, Racadio JM, Levitt MA, Bischoff A, Racadio JM, Peña A (2011) Complex cloacal malformations: use of rotational fluoroscopy and 3-D reconstruction in diagnosis and surgical planning. Pediatr Radiol 42:355–363

Pellerito JS, McCarthy SM, Doyle MB, Glickman MG, DeCherney AH (1992) Diagnosis of uterine anomalies: relative accuracy of MR imaging, endovaginal sonography, and hysterosalpingography. Radiology 183:795–800

Pena A, Kessler O (1998) Posterior cloaca: a unique defect. J Pediatr Surg 33:407–412

Peña JE, Ufberg D, Cooney N et al (2000) Usefulness of Doppler sonography in the diagnosis of ovarian torsion. Fertil Steril 73:1047–1050

Rathke H (1882) Abhandlung zur Bildungsgeschichte der Tiere. Leipzig

Retterer E (1890) Sur l'origine et l'évolution de la région anogénitale des mammifères. J Anat Physiol 26:126–216

Rha SE, Byun JY, Jung SE, Jung JI, Choi BG, Kim BS, Kim H, Lee JM (2002) CT and MR imaging features of adnexal torsion. Radiographics 22:283–294

Riccabona M (2013) Imaging of the neonatal female pelvis. Pediatr Radiol 43(Suppl3):S496

Riccabona M, Lobo ML, Willi U, Avni F, Damasio B, Ording-Mueller LS, Blickman J, Darge K, Papadopoulou F, Vivier PH (2014) ESPR uroradiology task force and ESUR Paediatric Work Group—Imaging recommendations in paediatric uroradiology, part VI: childhood renal biopsy and imaging of neonatal and infant genital tract. Pediatr Radiol 44:496–502

Riccabona M, Darge K, Lobo ML, Ording-Muller LS, Augdal TA, Avni FE, Blickman J, Damasio BM, Ntoulia A, Papadopoulou F, Vivier PH, Willi U (2015) ESPR Uroradiology Task Force – Imaging Recommendations in Paediatric Uroradiology – Part VIII: Rethrograde urethrography, imaging in disorders of sexual development, and imaging in childhood testicular torsion. Report on the mini-symposium at the ESPR meeting in Amsterdam, June 2014. Pediatr Radiol 45:2023–8

Riccabona M, Lobo ML, Ording-Muller LS, Augdal ThA, Vivier PH, Avni FE, Blickman J, Damasio BM, Darge K, Ntoulia A, Papadopoulou F, Willi U (2017) ESPR abdominal (GU and GI) imaging Task Force – Imaging Recommendations in Paediatric Uroradiology – Part IX: imaging in anorectal and cloacal malformation, imaging in childhood ovarian torsion, and efforts in standardising pediatric uroradiology terminology. Report on the mini-symposium at the ESPR meeting in Graz, June 2015. Pediatr Radiol 47:1369-1380. doi: 10.1007/s00247-017-3837-6. Epub 2017 Aug 29

Rich MA, Brock WA, Pena A (1988) Spectrum of genitourinary malformations in patients with imperforate anus. Pediatr Surg Int 3:110–113

Rieth KG, Comite F, Shawker TH, Cutler GB (1981) Pituitary and ovarian abnormalities demonstrated by CT and ultrasound in children with features of McCune-Albright syndrome. Radiology 153:389–393

Rosenberg HK, Sherman NH, Tarry WF, Duckett JW, McCrum Snyder H (1986) Mayer-Rokitansky-Kuster-Hauser syndrome: US aid to diagnosis. Radiology 161:815–819

Rosenblatt M, Rosenblatt R, Kutcher R, Coupey SM, Kleinhaus S (1991) Utero-vaginal hypoplasia. Pediatr Radiol 21:536–537

Rosenfeld DL, Lis E (1993) Gartner's duct cyst with single vaginal ectopic ureter and associated renal dysplasia or agenesis. J Ultrasound Med 12:775–778

Shozu M, Akasofu K, Harda T, Kubota Y (1991) A new cause of female pseudohermaphrodism: placental aromatase deficiency. J Clin Endocrinol Metab 72:560–566

Servaes S, Victoria T, Lovrenski J, Epelman M (2010) Contemporary pediatric gynecologic imaging. Semin Ultrasound CT MR 31:116–140

Servaes S, Zurakowski D, Laufer MR, Feins N, Chow JS (2007) Sonographic findings of ovarian torsion in children. Pediatr Radiol 37:446–451

Siegel MJ (2011) Pediatric sonography, 4th edn. Wolters Kluwer/Lippincott Williams & Wilkins, Philadelphia

Silverman FN, Kuhn JP (2013) Caffey's pediatric X-ray diagnosis: an integrated imaging approach, 12th edn. Elsevier Saunders, Philadelphia

Stephens FD (1983a) Normal embryology of the cloaca. In: Stephens FD (ed) Congenital malformation of the urinary tract. Praeger, New York, pp 1–14

Stephens FD (1983b) Abnormal embryology-cloacal dysgenesis. In: Stephens FD (ed) Congenital malformation of the urinary tract. Praeger, New York, pp 15–52

Taybi H, Lachman RS (2007) Radiology of syndromes, metabolic disorders, and skeletal dysplasias, 5th edn. Mosby, St. Louis

Teele RL, Share JC (1991) Ultrasonography of infants and children. Saunders, Philadelphia, pp 240–244

Teele RL, Share JC (1992) Ultrasonography of the female pelvis in childhood and adolescence. Radiol Clin North Am 30:743–758

Teele RL, Share JC (1997) Transperineal sonography in children. AJR Am J Roentgenol 168:1263–1267

Togashi K (2003) MR imaging of the ovaries: normal appearance and benign disease. Radiol Clin North Am 41:799–811

Tokgoz H, Turksoy O, Boyacigil S, Sakman B, Yuksel E (2006) Complete androgen insensitivity syndrome: report of a case with solitary pelvic kidney. Acta Radiol 47:222–225

Topaloglu AK, Vade A, Zeller WP (1997) Congenital adrenal hyperplasia and bilateral ovarian cysts in a neonate. Clin Pediatr (Phila) 36:719–720

Tolete-Velcek F, Hansbrough F, Kugaczewski J, Coren CV, Klotz DH, Price AF, Laungani G, Kottmeier PK (1989) Uterovaginal malformations: a trap for the unsuspecting surgeon. J Pediatr Surg 24:736–740

Tourneux F (1888) Sur les premiers développements du cloaques du tubercule génital et de l'anus chez l'embryon de mouton. J Anat 24:503–517

Unsinn KM, Neu N, Krejci A, Posch A, Menardi G, Gassner I (1995) Pallister-Hall syndrome and McKusick-Kaufmann syndrome: one entity? J Med Genet 32:125–128

Van Bogaert LJ (1992) Surgical repair of hypospadias in women with symptoms of urethral syndrome. J Urol 147:1263–1264

Van der Putte SCJ (1986) Normal and abnormal development of the anorectum. J Pediatr Surg 24: 434–440

Vijayaraghavan SB (2004) Sonographic whirlpool sign in ovarian torsion. J Ultrasound Med 23:1643–1649

Wagner BJ, Woodward P (1994) Magnetic resonance evaluation of congenital uterine anomalies. Semin Ultrasound CT MR 15:4–17

Willi UV (1991) Pediatric genitourinary imaging. Curr Opin Radiol 3:936–945

Williams DJ, Bloomberg S (1976) Urogenital sinus in the female child. J Pediatr Surg 11:51–56

Wilson JD, Goldstein JL (1975) Classification of hereditary disorders of sexual development. Birth Defects Orig Artic Ser 11:1–16

Woolf RB, Allen WM (1953) Concomitant malformations: the frequent simultaneous occurrence of congenital malformations of the reproductive and urinary tracts. Obstet Gynecol 2:236–265

Ziereisen F, Guissard G, Damry N, Avni EF (2005) Sonographic imaging of the paediatric female pelvis. Eur Radiol 15:1296–1309

Imaging in Male Genital Queries

Thomas A. Augdal, Lil-Sofie Ording-Müller, and Michael Riccabona

Contents

1	Introduction	353
2	Imaging Technique and Normal Imaging Anatomy	354
3	Embryology of the Male Genital Tract	355
4	Congenital Anomalies	356
4.1	Hypospadias	356
4.2	Penile Anomalies	356
4.3	Scrotal Anomalies	357
5	The Inguinal Canal, Hernias and Hydroceles	357
6	Cryptorchidism	358
7	Acute Scrotum	358
7.1	Torsion of the Spermatic Cord in Children and Adolescents	359
7.2	Perinatal Torsion of the Spermatic Cord	360
8	Other Causes of Acute Scrotum	360
8.1	Torsion of the Intrascrotal Appendages	360
8.2	Epididymitis and Epididymoorchitis	361
8.3	Acute Idiopathic Scrotal Oedema	361
8.4	Henoch-Schönlein Purpura	361
9	Haemorrhage and Trauma	362
9.1	Testicular Trauma	362
9.2	Scrotal Haematoma	363
10	Testicular and Paratesticular Tumours and Pseudotumours	363
10.1	Germ Cell Tumours	364
10.2	Sex Cord-Stromal Tumours	364
10.3	Miscellaneous Conditions	364
11	Vascular Conditions	367
11.1	Vascular Lesions of the Genitalia	367
11.2	Priapism	367
11.3	Varicocele	368
12	Superficial Genital Lesions	368
Conclusion		368
References		368

T.A. Augdal, MD (✉)
Department of Radiology, University Hospital of North Norway, Tromsø, Norway
e-mail: Thomas.Angell.Augdal@unn.no

L.-S. Ording-Müller, MD, PhD
Department of Radiology and Nuclear Medicine, Unit for Paediatric Radiology, Oslo University Hospital, Oslo, Norway

M. Riccabona, MD
Department of Radiology, Division of Pediatric Radiology, University Hospital Graz, Graz, Austria

1 Introduction

A great variety of congenital and acquired conditions may affect the male genital tract, many of them rarely encountered by radiologists, as a thorough history and clinical examination will reveal their nature and guide treatment. Most often the indication for imaging of congenital anomalies is to establish the extent of disease and detect associated anomalies to inform decision-making with regard to management, whereas in conditions like vascular malformations, imaging is necessary to guide treatment before the malformation becomes potentially debilitating. The true emergency of spermatic cord torsion is discussed in more detail, as correct management can be challenging. Malignancy is thankfully rare in children, but must always be kept in mind by the vigilant radiologist.

The intention of this chapter is to provide an overview the conditions where imaging has a role in the diagnosis and follow-up of the disease.

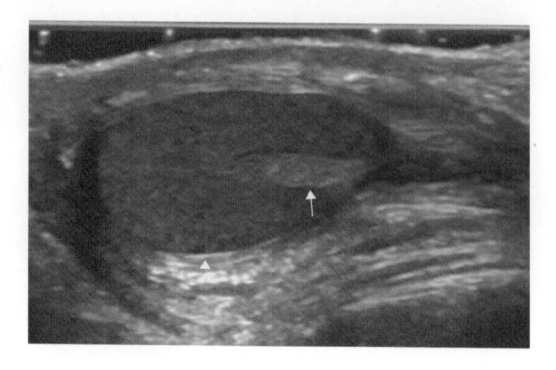

Fig. 1 Normal prepubertal testicle. The testicle is oval, of homogeneous structure and of intermediate echogenicity. In this boy the mediastinum (*arrow*) is highly reflective, whereas the tunica vaginalis (*arrowhead*) is barely visible

2 Imaging Technique and Normal Imaging Anatomy

Ultrasonography (US) is the modality of choice in most queries of the male genital tract. It is dynamic, readily available, offers assessment of circulation and has excellent resolution, particularly in superficial tissues. The role of elastography (for instance, in suspected malignancy) and intravenous contrast enhancement (for instance, in testicular torsion) is yet to be defined, particularly in children. Modern equipment offers improved reproducibility with the option of video storage. The examination should take place in a comfortable environment with the patient supine and the scrotum supported by a towel. Remember to respect the privacy of even a young patient. The inguinal canal, scrotum and penis are examined with a high-frequency linear transducer in a systematic matter including greyscale and colour and spectral Doppler assessment of the relevant structures. The latter can be challenging in prepubertal boys; thus it may be helpful to first calibrate the Doppler settings on the asymptomatic side.

Normal scrotal layers are thin and not discernible at US. The prepubertal testicle (ss) is smaller (typical volume of 1–2 ml) and has a lower reflectivity than in adults (Hamm and Fobbe 1995). The thin, echogenic surface of the testicle is the tunica albuginea (Figs. 1 and 6). Projections from the tunica albuginea form

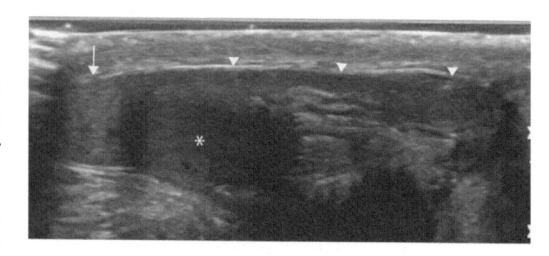

Fig. 2 Oblique longitudinal plane of most of a normal epididymis (*arrow* and *arrowheads*) in a 12 y.o. The epididymal head (*arrow*) is seen as a triangular structure expected to be in close proximity to the upper pole of the testicle (*asterisk*)

septa (sometimes visible) and the echogenic mediastinum where the rete testis drains into the epididymis (Fig. 1). The epididymis is seen posterior to the testicle as a tubular structure of equal or slightly higher echogenicity (Fig. 2). The intrascrotal appendages are five small, oval and often pedunculated structures potentially seen at their respective locations, particularly in the presence of a hydrocele.

Three main arteries and their interconnecting anastomoses supply the scrotum and its contents: the testicular artery (testicle and epididymis), cremasteric artery (paratesticular tissue) and deferential artery (vas deferens). Of particular interest is the low-resistance spectral Doppler tracing of a normal testicular artery, the normal resistive index is in the area of 0.54, and is independent of

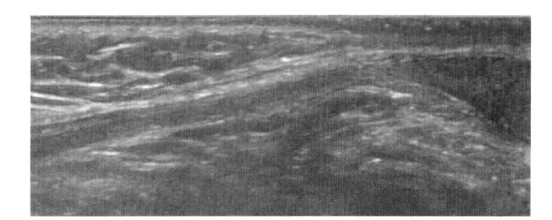

Fig. 3 Normal width and course of the inguinal canal and spermatic cord in a prepubertal boy. The spermatic cord and its vessels has a straight (as here) or slightly tortuous course to the testicle

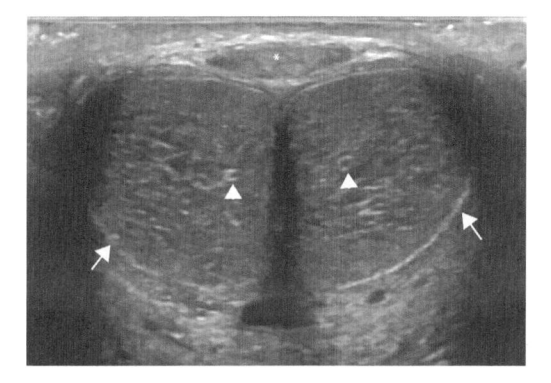

Fig. 4 Ventral, transverse view of a normal penis in a teenager. The corpus spongiosum (*asterisk*) is easily compressed (as here) and then becomes more echogenic than the paired cavernous bodies. Note the cavernosal arteries (*arrowheads*), the highly echogenic tunica albuginea (*arrows*) and the shadowing by the tunica albuginea not to be misinterpreted as a pathological finding

age and volume (Schneble et al. 2011). The main venous drainage of the testicle and epididymis is through the pampiniform plexus to the testicular veins.

The spermatic cord contains the vessels and the vas deferens (Fig. 3). It is surrounded by a thin echogenic sheath and courses the inguinal canal as a straight, tubular structure of no more than 10 mm thickness (Baud et al. 1998).

The penile shaft consists of the ventral corpus spongiosum surrounding the urethra and the paired dorsal cavernous bodies enveloped by the tunica albuginea and connective tissue (Fig. 4). The influx of blood decreases the echogenicity of the cavernous bodies during tumescence. The main arterial supply is from the internal pudendal artery via its branches. The cavernosal artery supplies the erectile tissue of the cavernous bodies.

The main role of magnetic resonance imaging (MRI) is to provide detailed (usually intrapelvic) information about complex congenital anomalies, to reveal metastatic disease and to unravel complicated scrotal disease. MRI may also show the extent of vascular lesions, and if available, both MRI (using DWI and contrast enhancement) and scintigraphy can reliably diagnose testicular torsion (Paltiel et al. 1998; Watanabe et al. 2007; Maki et al. 2011), but is rarely used for this purpose due to the potential treatment delay. Computed tomography is irrelevant except in detection of pulmonary metastatic disease and in staging of malignant conditions if MRI is unavailable.

> **Take Away**
> Ultrasonography is the primary choice for imaging male genital queries.

3 Embryology of the Male Genital Tract

Development of the male gender begins in gestational week seven when somatic support cells in the genital ridges differentiate into Sertoli cells. Sertoli cells then recruit Leydig cells and secrete the Müllerian-inhibiting substance necessary to induce regression of the female genital precursors. Leydig cells secrete the testosterone needed to stabilise the mesonephric duct and promote its differentiation into the epididymis, vas deferens, seminal vesicles and ejaculatory ducts, and they also convert testosterone to dihydrotestosterone – essential for the development of the male urethra, penis, scrotum and prostate gland.

From the eighth week the inguinal canal and the vaginal process develop in conjunction as caudal evaginations of the abdominal wall and peritoneum, respectively. During its elongation to the scrotum, the vaginal process precedes the testicle and becomes ensheathed by the layers of the abdominal wall (Biasutto et al. 2009). The testicle moves towards the future inguinal canal by the regression of the cranial suspensory ligament and the swelling and shortening of the gubernaculum (Hutson 2013). The gubernaculum widens the internal inguinal ring, where it keeps the testicle positioned until its descent into the scrotum. The influence of the gubernaculum, hormonal factors and abdominal pressure on the testicular descent through the inguinal canal to the scrotum is not well understood.

> **Take Away**
> Knowledge and understanding of the embryological development of the male genital tract is essential to understand congenital anomalies and to properly read imaging studies.

4 Congenital Anomalies

4.1 Hypospadias

With an annual incidence of 1–4 per 1000, hypospadias is one of the most common congenital anomalies of the male genital tract. It is caused by incomplete formation of the urethra resulting in an ectopic urethral meatus seen anywhere along the ventral penis, scrotum or perineum, and the meatus' position is commonly used for classification (Tekgul et al. 2015).

Imaging rarely influences surgical management, but occasionally the surgeon may request a retrograde urethrography (RUG) (Riccabona et al. 2015) and subsequent voiding cystourethrography (VCUG) (Riccabona et al. 2008) to assess the urethra, bladder function and vesicoureteral reflux (VUR). Contrary to previous statements, a recent review concluded that there is no relationship between the severity of hypospadias and the prevalence of associated urogenital anomalies, and the authors also disputed the need for screening of the renal tract (Chariatte et al. 2013). However, in the setting of severe hypospadias and non-palpable testicles or ambiguous genitalia, thorough assessment for disorders of sexual development is recommended, in particular exclusion of the potential life-threatening bilateral adrenal hyperplasia.

Up to 25% of patients experience surgical complications, in which imaging may help detect conditions such as anastomotic leakage (resulting in urethrocutaneous fistulas), strictures, aneurysmal dilatation of the neourethra or stone formation (Milla et al. 2008; Tekgul et al. 2015).

4.2 Penile Anomalies

A thorough clinical examination reveals the nature of penile anomalies such as phimosis, paraphimosis and penile curvature (dorsal, lateral or ventral) and the webbed and concealed forms of inconspicuous penis. Micropenis is a subtype of inconspicuous penis most commonly caused by insufficient secretion or action of testosterone, where cerebral MRI to assess the hypothalamic-pituitary axis is part of the endocrinological workup (Wiygul and Palmer 2011). In congenital megaprepuce (a subtype of concealed penis) and trapped penis, symptoms of obstruction and infection may call for exclusion of other causes of lower urinary tract infection. Aphallia is a rare anomaly in which the penis is absent or rudimentary. MRI will demonstrate the absence of the corpora cavernosa and corpus spongiosum, which is of clinical importance because, unlike in micropenis, testosterone treatment has no effect due to the lack of growth potential. More than 50% of the patients have associated anomalies, in particular genitourinary, which MRI may be helpful to delineate (Goenka et al. 2008).

In the rare instance of duplication of the penis, US or preferably MRI helps classify the anomaly

4.3 Scrotal Anomalies

Penoscrotal transposition, ectopic or accessory scrotum, bifid scrotum, scrotal hypoplasia and scrotal agenesis are all rare conditions seen in conjunction with, but not restricted to, anomalies of the urogenital tract. A detailed outline of these associations is beyond the scope of this text. US may detect the cryptorchid testicle in ectopic scrotum and scrotal agenesis or hemiagenesis, as well as the upper urinary tract anomalies of penoscrotal transposition and ectopic scrotum, whereas MRI is necessary to outline the VACTERL pattern of anomalies in an accessory scrotum.

and delineate the associated anomalies such as bladder duplication, imperforate anus, rectosigmoid duplication, bifid scrotum and vertebral anomalies (Gyftopoulos et al. 2002).

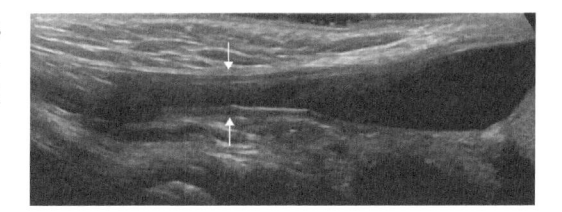

Fig. 5 Right-sided hydrocele communicating with the peritoneal cavity through a patent vaginal process (*arrows*) in a 6 y.o. The fluid was easily compressed

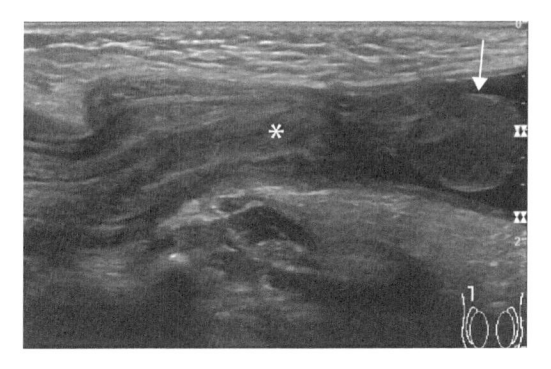

Fig. 6 Widened inguinal canal containing a bowel loop (*asterisk*) in manifest inguinal hernia. The echogenic tunica albuginea (*arrow*) at the testicular surface is easily appreciated in the presence of a hydrocele (Image courtesy of Dr. T. Köhler)

> **Take Away**
> Imaging is usually redundant for diagnosing anomalies of the male genital tract, but may be necessary to delineate the extent of pathology and to assess surgical complications.

5 The Inguinal Canal, Hernias and Hydroceles

Hydroceles and hernias are the most common causes of swelling of the groin in children. The primary variants are communicating, funicular and encysted *hydrocele* and result from a failed closure of the vaginal process. On US, uncomplicated hydroceles are anechoic masses with a striking through transmission. Communicating hydroceles (Fig. 5) are more common on the right side in infants and premature boys. Prognosis is excellent with up to 90% spontaneous regression within the first year of life (Naji et al. 2012).

The presence of omental fat, bowel wall signature or peristalsis defines an *inguinal hernia* (Fig. 6). Hernias are important to detect because they require prompt elective surgery due to the risk of incarceration (Zamakhshary et al. 2008). Meticulous scanning of the inguinal canal including Valsalva's manoeuvre is indicated to increase sensitivity, because the intra-abdominal content may retract with the child lying supine.

Complications include haemorrhage (haematocele), infection (pyocele) or obstructive symptoms from large hydroceles like the rare abdominoscrotal hydrocele – a condition where the ipsilateral testicle is typically elongated or fusiform (Vaos et al. 2014). It is important to assess intratesticular Doppler in large hydroceles as increased intrascrotal pressure may develop and compromise testicular circulation (Dagrosa et al. 2015).

Simple hydroceles presuppose a confined vaginal process to allow a collection of fluid within the parietal and visceral layer of the tunica vaginalis. The aetiology often remains unknown, though it can be associated with infection, trauma or tumour which is more commonly seen in adolescence and adulthood (Cimador et al. 2010).

> **Take Away**
> Because of the risk of incarceration, it is most important do discern hernias from hydroceles.

6 Cryptorchidism

Cryptorchidism is present in 1 % of boys aged 1 year and particularly common in low-birth-weight individuals (Sijstermans et al. 2008). The development is not well understood but involves both genetic and environmental factors. The testicles are expected to be in the scrotal position from 6 months of age. Relocation is indicated within 18 months of age due to the increased risk of malignancy, reduced fertility, testicular torsion and inguinal hernia. Prepubertal orchiopexy reduces, but does not eliminate, the risk of testicular malignancy (Walsh et al. 2007).

According to guidelines experienced examiners (i.e. surgeons) are expected to identify all extra-abdominal testicles by palpation (Kolon et al. 2014). Hence, in most cases imaging is regarded unnecessary and has also been found to cause significant delay to definite treatment (Kanaroglou et al. 2015). However, if US is undertaken, the typically small and hypoechoic testicle is often identified in the inguinal, femoral, paravesical, penile or perineal region (Fig. 7). If a testicle is not found and suspected to be intra-abdominal, no further imaging is advocated for two reasons: US and MRI cannot reliably confirm the presence or absence of the testicle, and laparoscopy is indicated to identify, relocate or resect the testicle or its remnant in any way (Tasian and Copp 2011; Krishnaswami et al. 2013). If an abdominal survey is done, an assessment of the renal tract is often included.

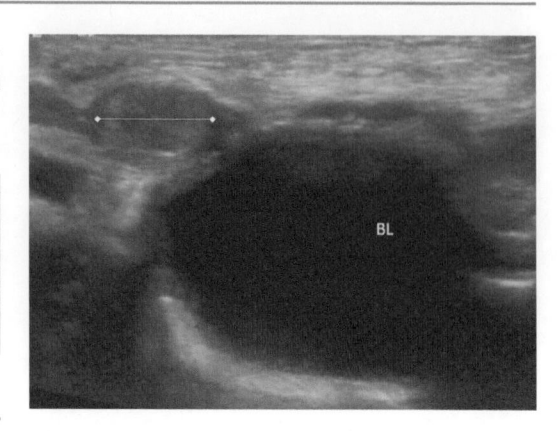

Fig 7 Cryptorchidism. The right testicle (+...+) located next to the urinary bladder (BL)

> **Take Away**
> Thorough clinical examination is regarded sufficient for the diagnosis of cryptorchidism.

7 Acute Scrotum

The three most common causes of acute scrotal pain in children and adolescents are torsion of one of the testicular appendages, testicular torsion and acute epididymitis. The main cause of scrotal swellings in the neonate is hydroceles; the important differentials are testicular torsion and tumours. A detailed description of all possible differential diagnoses is beyond the scope of this text.

The clinical history, symptoms and signs of an acute scrotum are variable and do not clearly differentiate between the causes, making correct management challenging. Due to the early onset of irreversible injury, immediate surgical treatment is indicated when spermatic cord torsion is the most likely diagnosis. In equivocal cases, non-delayed inguinoscrotal US is the preferred examination, as it is fast, available, non-invasive and reliable when adequately performed. Scintigraphy and MRI both perform well, but are hampered by availability, duration, cost, need for venous access and radiation (scintigraphy only). Imaging algorithms for suspected testicular torsion in neonates and children, respectively, have recently been suggested (Riccabona et al. 2015).

7.1 Torsion of the Spermatic Cord in Children and Adolescents

Testicular torsion is most commonly seen in early adolescence, after the age of ten. There is also a peak in neonates and young infants, but it may occur at all ages. About 90% of torsions are intravaginal due to the 'bell-clapper' appearance in which the distal spermatic cord, epididymis and testicle are encircled by the tunica vaginalis. No single symptom or sign is able to confirm or rule out testicular torsion, and attempts to predict testicular torsion from the history and clinical findings trade a high sensitivity for a low specificity (Srinivasan et al. 2011; Boettcher et al. 2012). Because sole reliance on colour Doppler sonography (CDS) is associated with false-negative examinations, the preferred US technique includes meticulous inguinoscrotal greyscale and a complete Doppler examination (i.e. including the assessment of intraparenchymal spectral Doppler flow pattern) in combination (Kalfa et al. 2007).

All testicular findings are indirect signs of the underlying pathology, i.e. the twisted vascular pedicle. The typical US finding in a twisted spermatic cord is a snail-shaped mass displacing the epididymis away from the upper pole of the testicle (Fig. 8). However, any focal or general thickening or loss of the straight or slightly tortuous course of the spermatic cord and its vessels (whirl pool or spiral sign) is suspicious of a spermatic cord torsion in acute scrotal pain (Baud et al. 1998). The ipsilateral epididymis is usually enlarged with circulation equal to that of the testicle. Additional extratesticular findings in spermatic cord torsion are thickened scrotal skin and hydrocele.

The affected testicle is typically enlarged and rounded with a coarse echostructure, and its echogenicity changes in association with the duration and severity of the torsion from hyperechoic to hypoechoic or heterogeneous (Figs. 8

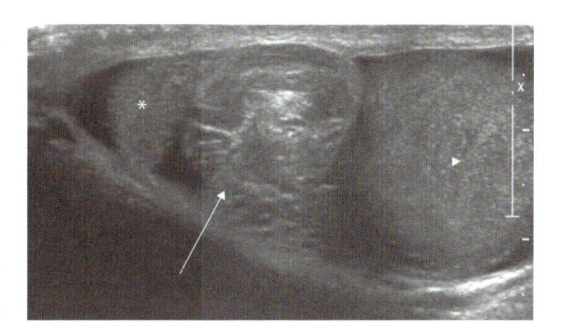

Fig. 8 Acute testicular torsion. The typical snail-shaped appearance of the twisted spermatic cord seen as a pseudomass (*arrow*) between the epididymis (*asterisk*) and the testicle (*arrowhead*). The testicle is enlarged with a coarse structure, and there is an accompanying hydrocele (Image courtesy of Dr. C. Baud)

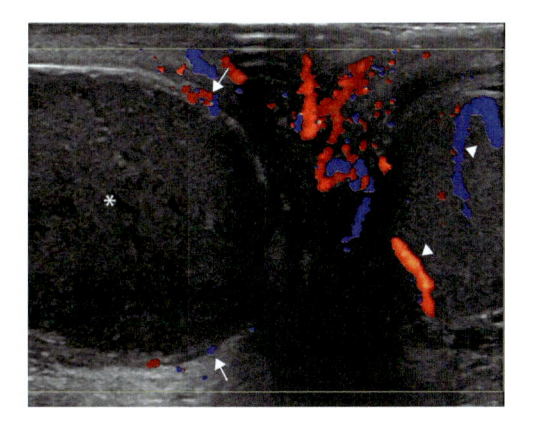

Fig. 9 Right-sided testicular torsion. The right testicle (*asterisk*) displays signs of spermatic cord torsion with enlargement, a coarser structure and lack of internal Doppler, as opposed to the contralateral normally perfused testicle (*arrowheads*). It is important to not interpret capsular Doppler (*arrows*) as proof of internal perfusion

and 9). Intratesticular blood flow assessed with CDS or power Doppler may be absent (complete torsion) (Fig. 9), reduced (incomplete or partial torsion) or increased (intermittent torsion). Assessment of intratesticular blood flow in young boys can be challenging, but is often possible with modern equipment. The Doppler examination should include spectral analysis of the intratesticular parenchymal arterial circulation, which may be the only finding that differentiates intermittent torsion from acute epididymitis. In the right clinical setting, any Doppler asymmetry raises suspicion of testicular torsion.

7.2 Perinatal Torsion of the Spermatic Cord

The more rare perinatal testicular torsion is extravaginal and has a poorer salvage rate. The findings at clinical examination and US are time dependent. In an intrauterine event, the expected finding at birth would be a firm, non-tender scrotal mass, lack of the cremasteric reflex and a corresponding size-reduced, non-perfused, hypoechoic testicle with calcifications at US (Fig. 10). Such a testicle is necrotic and cannot be salvaged. In a perinatal (or neonatal) event, the more likely clinical findings are a non-translucent scrotal swelling, skin discoloration and varying degrees of tenderness and retraction of the testicle. At US, the testicle is enlarged with any echogenicity and altered perfusion (Fig. 11) (Ricci et al. 2001). Prediction of viability is uncertain.

The management of these boys is controversial due to historically low salvage rates and the

> **Take Away**
> Immediate surgical exploration is indicated if there is any doubt whether the testicular circulation is compromised. Imaging should be reserved to equivocal cases and must not delay surgical treatment.

risk, albeit small, of general anaesthesia in neonates. A recent systematic review found an overall salvage rate of 9% for the entire group, but noteworthy, 23 out of the 24 testicles that were salvaged had undergone immediate surgery, and the overall salvage rate in the emergency group was 21% (Nandi and Murphy 2011). Also in favour of emergency exploration and bilateral orchiopexy is the risk of (asynchronous) bilateral disease. For these reasons the European Association of Urology considers perinatal testicular torsion an emergency (Tekgul et al. 2015).

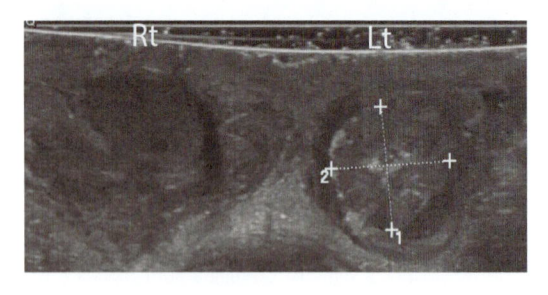

Fig. 10 Long-standing perinatal testicular torsion. The left (Lt) testicle is size reduced and inhomogeneous with hyperechoic areas suggestive of calcification

8 Other Causes of Acute Scrotum

8.1 Torsion of the Intrascrotal Appendages

The testicular appendages are remnants of the mesonephric and paramesonephric ducts. Torsion of a testicular appendage typically occurs in prepubertal boys and is indicated by insidious onset

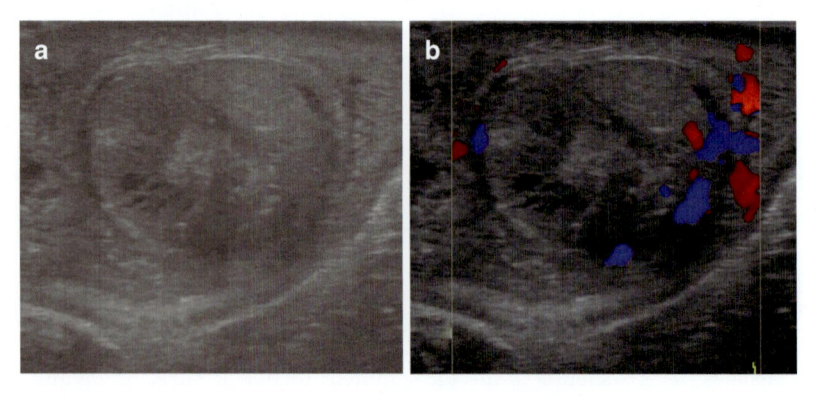

Fig. 11 Acute perinatal testicular torsion in a neonate. The testicle is enlarged with a coarse and inhomogeneous texture (**a**) and altered perfusion (**b**)

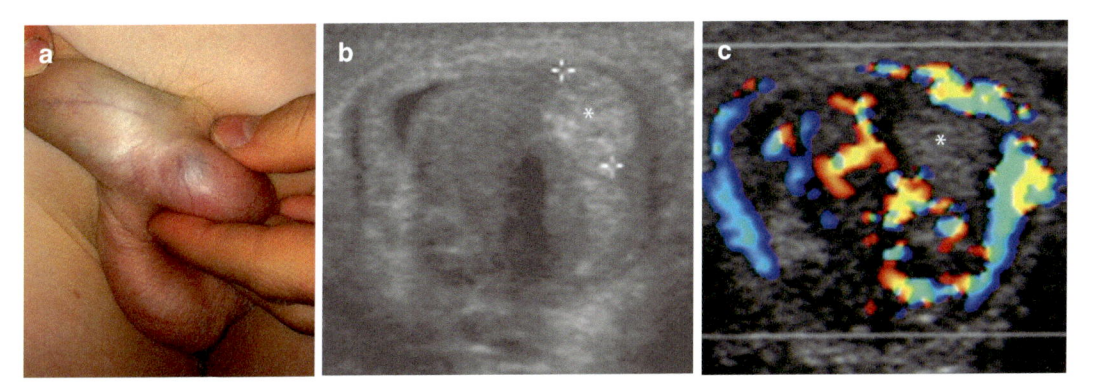

Fig. 12 Torsion of the appendix testis. Photograph (**a**) of the '*blue dot*' sign. On US, an enlarged, rounded and hyperechoic (**b**) appendix testis (*asterisk*) without internal Doppler (**c**). Note subtle hydrocele and hyperaemia of the testicle and epididymis ((**a**) Courtesy of Dr. S. Müller (**a**) with permission from Riccabona (2014a) (**b, c**))

and a positive 'blue dot sign' on the overlaying skin (Boettcher et al. 2013). Torsed testicular appendages (Fig. 12) are rounder and larger than the normal 1–7 mm, lack circulation and may have any echogenicity (Yang et al. 2005). They evoke an inflammatory response with an accompanying ipsilateral hydrocele (80–90 %), enlarged and hyperechoic epididymis (50–100 %) and hyperaemia in the nearby testis (50–90 %). Unlike testicular torsion, the spermatic cord is linear without focal irregularities.

Direct visualisation of the torsed appendage strengthens this diagnosis versus that of acute epididymitis.

8.2 Epididymitis and Epididymoorchitis

The cause of acute epididymitis with or without orchitis usually remains unknown. Whereas infection is exceedingly rare in prepubescent boys, it occurs in adolescents – not always related to sexual activity. Up to 40 % of boys with epididymitis have associated urogenital anomalies, though not all of these conditions are considered causative (Karmazyn et al. 2009). Many accept proven infection, recurrent infection or young age as indications for further imaging (urinary tract US and VCUG).

Acute epididymitis presents with insidious onset scrotal pain, a tender epididymis and dysuria, sometimes accompanied by fever, abdominal pain or nausea (Boettcher et al. 2013). US shows an enlarged (focal or general) and hyperaemic epididymis of any echogenicity with associated hydrocele and often augmented testicular perfusion and swelling (Fig. 13). Complications include abscess formation and testicular ischemia, primarily reported in adults (Yusuf et al. 2013).

8.3 Acute Idiopathic Scrotal Oedema

Acute idiopathic scrotal oedema is a self-limiting rare cause of acute scrotal pain, diagnosed clinically by the characteristic (bilateral) discomfort, swelling and erythema of the scrotum, and sometimes extending to the perineum, lower abdomen or penis. US is done to exclude other causes and shows a thickened, hypoechoic scrotal wall with a typical appearance of the increased vascularity ('fountain sign') (Geiger et al. 2010). Some patients also have inguinal lymphadenopathy and a mild hydrocele (Klin et al. 2002).

8.4 Henoch-Schönlein Purpura

Henoch-Schönlein purpura is the most common vasculitis of childhood. Scrotal symptoms are accounted in 13 % of affected boys,

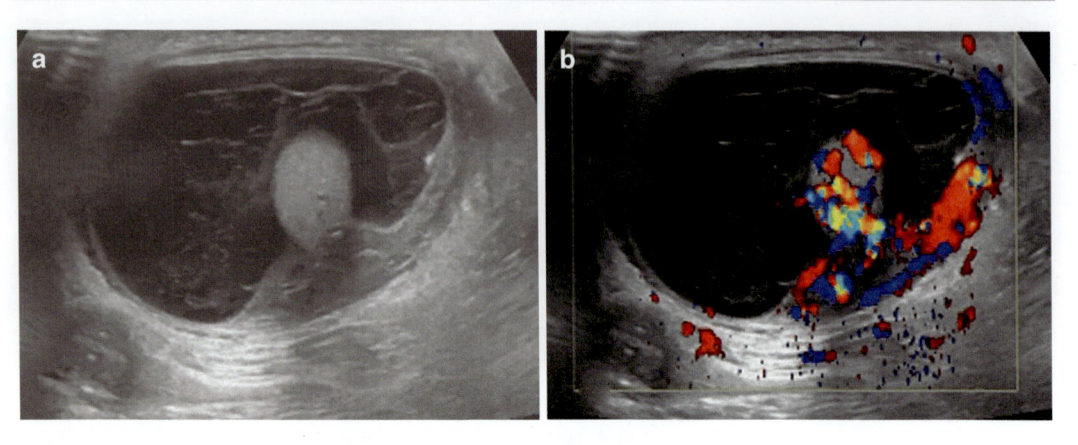

Fig. 13 Enlarged, hyperaemic epididymis in acute epididymitis. Associated augmented testicular perfusion and a fibrinous hydrocele

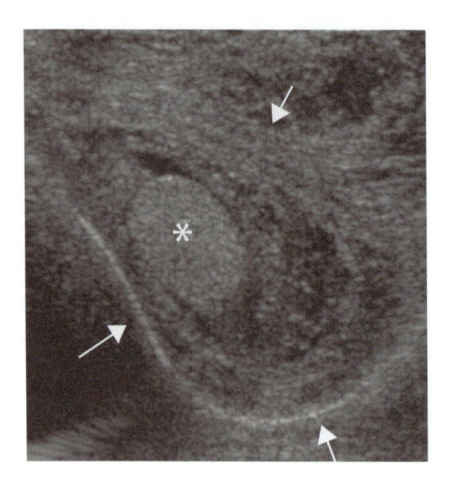

Fig. 14 Severe scrotal oedema (*arrows*) and a normal testicle (*asterisk*) in Henoch-Schönlein purpura involving the scrotum

> **Take Away**
> Torsion of one of the intrascrotal appendages and acute epididymitis are by far the most common differential diagnoses to spermatic cord torsion in acute scrotal pain after the neonatal period.

the commonest being swelling and pain, which may include the penis (Soreide 2005; Balevic et al. 2013). Despite testicular torsion being uncommon in the typical 3–6-year-old boy with purpura, it should be kept in mind as a potential differential diagnosis. US (Fig. 14) reveals oedema of the scrotal wall, hydrocele and enlarged and hyperaemic epididymides (Ben-Sira and Laor 2000). The spermatic cords and testicles are expected to be normal, but rare complications include haemorrhage of the spermatic cord and thrombosis of the spermatic vein (Diana et al. 2000).

9 Haemorrhage and Trauma

9.1 Testicular Trauma

Testicular contusions are seen as solitary or multiple hypoechoic areas on US. The appearance of *intratesticular haematomas* varies with time; hyperacute haematomas are isoechoic, acute haematomas are hyperechoic and chronic haematomas appear more hypoechoic. All haematomas should be followed until resolution. *Testicular fracture* is a discontinuity of the normal parenchyma seen as a straight, hypoechoic and avascular area with or without associated rupture of the tunica albuginea. In *testicular rupture* the tunica albuginea is disrupted with extrusion of testicular parenchyma (Fig. 15). The loss of testicular contour and a heterogeneous parenchyma at US detects most ruptures, however, with a rather poor specificity of 65 % (Guichard et al. 2008). Surgical exploration and treatment is indicated

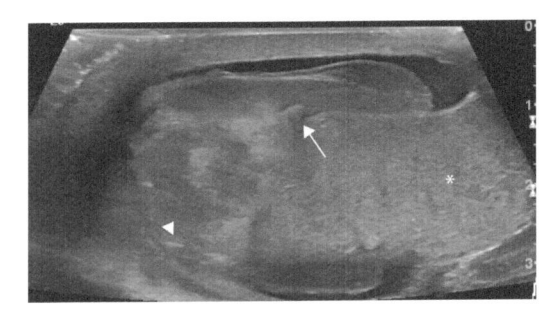

Fig. 15 Traumatic testicular rupture. The disrupted tunica albuginea is easily appreciated (*arrow*). The upper pole appeared heterogeneous with a mixture of haemorrhage and necrosis (*arrowhead*) and was devascularised (not shown). The rest of the testicle appeared homogenous (*asterisk*) and was well perfused. The parietal layer of the tunica vaginalis contained the homogeneous haematoma separated from a small surrounding hydrocele (Image courtesy of Dr. T. Sakinis)

if testicular rupture is suspected. Extratesticular injury includes haematoma of the epididymis and scrotal wall. In equivocal cases MRI may clarify the pattern of injury including disruption of the tunica albuginea (Kim et al. 2009).

9.2 Scrotal Haematoma

Haematoma of the scrotal wall can be caused by direct trauma or indirectly by the dissection of blood along the fascial planes to the scrotum. US detects a scrotal wall haematoma and normal scrotal content usually accompanied by a simple hydrocele. In neonates a scrotal haematoma may be secondary to an adrenal haemorrhage, which is why the adrenals should be examined for the presence of masses. Such secondary scrotal haematomas may present in the scrotal wall, in the space between the two tunica vaginalis layers or both.

> **Take Away**
> Scrotal/testicular imaging after trauma is performed in clinically equivocal cases, as surgical exploration is indicated if a rupture of the tunica albuginea is demonstrated or suspected.

10 Testicular and Paratesticular Tumours and Pseudotumours

The annual incidence of testicular neoplasms is 0.5–2 per 100,000 (Agarwal and Palmer 2006) with a peak before 3 years of age and after puberty. In prepubertal boys, most tumours are benign (Taskinen et al. 2008). Tumours usually present as a painless scrotal mass, but pain is sometimes caused by haemorrhage, necrosis or associated infection. The role of US is to determine the location as intra- or extratesticular and to assess the potential for testis-sparing surgery. A survey of inguinal and retroperitoneal lymph nodes and the abdominal organs is recommended in the presence of a tumour. If histology reveals malignancy, then depending on the diagnosis, subsequent pelvic and abdominal MRI and thoracic CT is done to evaluate for metastatic disease (Fig. 16). Scrotal US is excellent for follow-up, as is pelvic and abdominal MRI. In general, histology is required for diagnosis as most tumours are inconsistent or nonspecific at US and MRI, and many tumours have cystic components. The exception is the virtually diagnostic concentric rings of alternating hypo- and hyperechoic strands in epidermoid cysts.

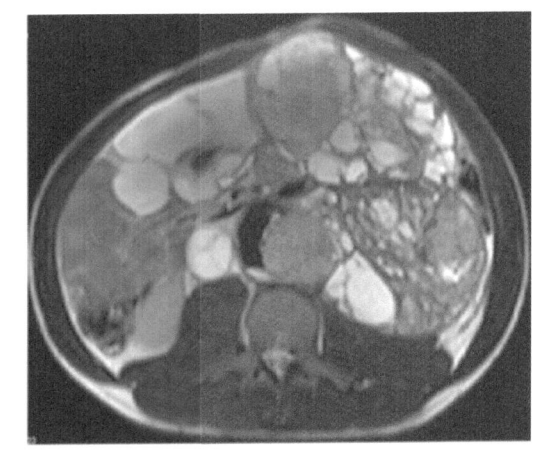

Fig. 16 Axial T2w section of the mid-abdomen demonstrating the multicystic nature of all involved compartments in a huge germ cell tumour of the testis

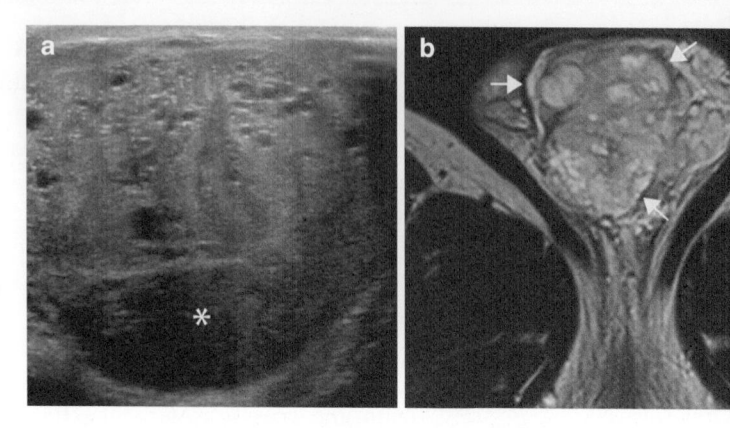

Fig. 17 Ultrasound (**a**) and axial T2w tSE (**b**) images of a mixed germinal cell tumour (*arrows*) in a 14 y.o. On US, the large tumour is hyperechoic relative to normal testicular tissue (*asterisk*). It consisted of multiple small and some larger cysts also appreciated on MRI

10.1 Germ Cell Tumours

The most common primary testicular neoplasms are the germ cell tumours (Fig. 17). *Teratomas* (Fig. 18) are heterogeneous lesions with a mixture of solid and cystic areas, often fat or calcifications and usually well circumscribed (Epifanio et al. 2014). Prepubertal teratomas show a benign clinical course contrary to their adult counterpart (Grady et al. 1997). *Yolk sac tumour* is the most common malignant testicular tumour in children and is suggested by a palpable tumour and raised alpha-foetoprotein in a prepubertal boy (Fig. 19). The prognosis is generally good, particularly if the disease is restricted to the testicle. The imaging findings are nonspecific. The most common testicular tumour in adult life, *seminoma*, is irrelevant before puberty except in boys with cryptorchidism.

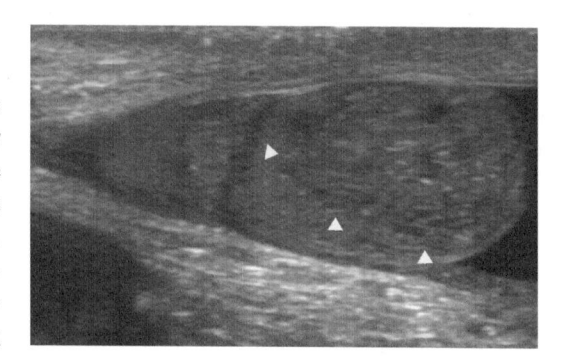

Fig. 18 Immature teratoma of the testicle in an infant. On US the solid and cystic lesion appeared fairly well circumscribed (*arrowheads*) despite taking up most of the space of the right testicle

10.2 Sex Cord-Stromal Tumours

Sex cord-stromal tumours in children are all rare with scarce reports of inconsistent imaging findings. All *juvenile granulosa cell tumours* and most *Sertoli and Leydig cell tumours* in children are benign. Leydig cell tumours are endocrinological active and typically present with precocious puberty. Hormonal disturbance is also found in a smaller percentage of Sertoli cell tumours (Ahmed et al. 2010). *Gonadoblastoma* occurs almost exclusively in individuals with disorder of sex development.

10.3 Miscellaneous Conditions

Secondary testicular malignancy is rare, but typically seen in lymphoma or leukaemia as bilaterally enlarged, hypoechoic and hyperaemic testicles; the testis may even be a hiding place for residual tumour. *Ectopic adrenal remnants* are seen as multiple hypoechoic nodules near the hilus in both testicles in conditions associated with increased circulating corticotropin (Avila et al. 1999). Other multifocal lesions include granulomatous processes.

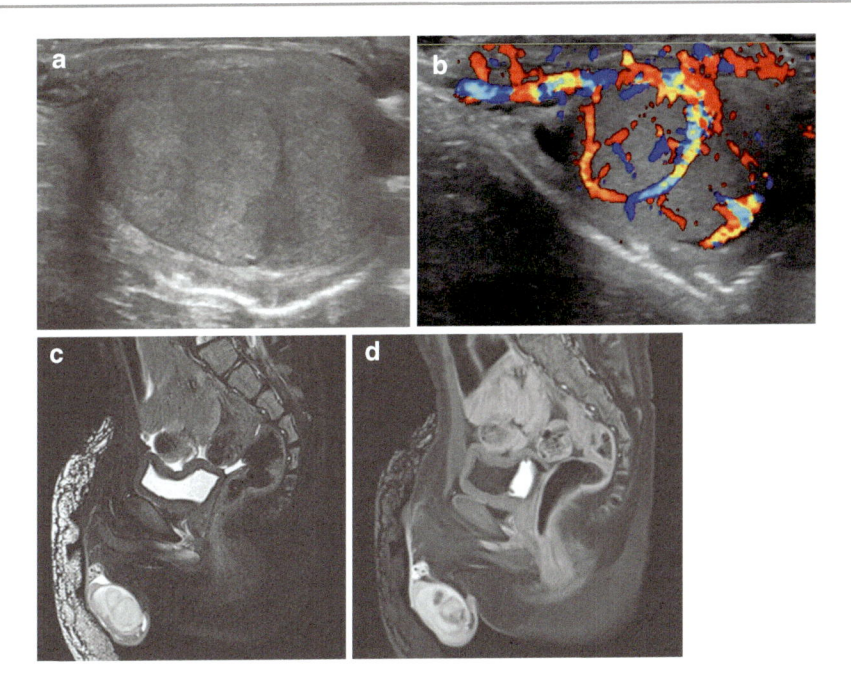

Fig. 19 Yolk sac tumour in a 2 y.o. presenting an enlarged left testicle. Ultrasound (**a**, **b**) shows inhomogeneous, lobulated architecture and hyperaemia with enlarged pathological vessels. Sagittal T2 with Dixon fat suppression (**c**) shows an inhomogeneous testicular mass with inhomogeneous enhancement on T1 fs sequence (**d**). Note that MRI is mainly performed for the assessment of metastasis (see Fig. 16), less for identification of the tumour itself which is usually sufficiently imaged by US

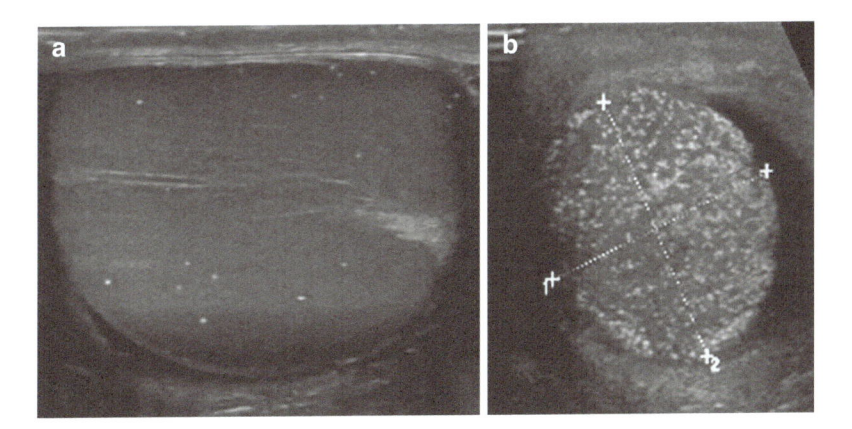

Fig. 20 Testicular microlithiasis. Punctuated hyperechoic foci without shadowing seen scattered in otherwise normal testicular tissue (**a**). Note the transmediastinal artery, a normal variant (**b**) (Reprinted with permission from Riccabona (2014b))

Testicular microlithiasis occurs in about 2 % of boys undergoing scrotal US and is typically seen bilaterally as scattered, punctuated, non-shadowing echogenic foci (Fig. 20). It is rare in infants and young boys. In general, and particularly in the adult population, there appears to be an association between microlithiasis and malignant testicular tumours (Wang et al. 2015), but whether or not this holds true for children is still under discussion (Cooper et al. 2014; Volokhina et al. 2014; Suominen et al. 2015). Thus no strong recommendations for regular US follow-up of these patients can be given, though often performed annually, as there obviously is some association between microlithiasis and testicular tumors (Trout et al. 2017).

Malignant paratesticular tumours are exceedingly rare, but suspected in all rapidly growing paratesticular masses. They often appear ill defined, solid or mixed solid and cystic, heterogeneous and hypoechoic with increased blood flow. The most common lesion is rhabdomyosarcoma of the embryonal subtype which has a better prognosis with early onset (Agarwal and Palmer 2006). MRI may help delineate the involvement of the scrotal content, as well as the presence of metastatic disease.

Benign cysts, like intratesticular (Fig. 21), tunica albuginea or epididymal cysts, should have the classic appearance of simple cysts – any solid component should raise suspicion of a cystic tumour. MRI may help to differentiate cystic tumours from cysts by their contrast enhancement pattern. *Spermatoceles* have a discrete echogenicity due to spermatozoa and proteinaceous fluid. *Cystic dysplasia of the rete testis* is a rare congenital condition due to failed connection between the efferent ducts and the rete testis, strongly associated with renal malformations (Jeyaratnam and Bakalinova 2010). The affected testicle is typically enlarged and asymptomatic (Fig. 22).

Lipomas are frequently seen in the spermatic cord, whereas the *adenomatoid tumour* is found in the epididymis or testicular tunica.

Meconium periorchitis results from meconium passage through a patent vaginal process to the scrotum following bowel wall rupture in late foetal or early postnatal life. Meconium incites a sterile inflammation and development of a soft paratesticular mass that calcifies later on and is accompanied by a hydrocele. The rest of the scrotal content is normal and scattered peritoneal calcifications support the diagnosis. Conservative treatment is sufficient in most cases, but surgery is undertaken if the lesion is indistinguishable from a tumour (Alanbuki et al. 2013).

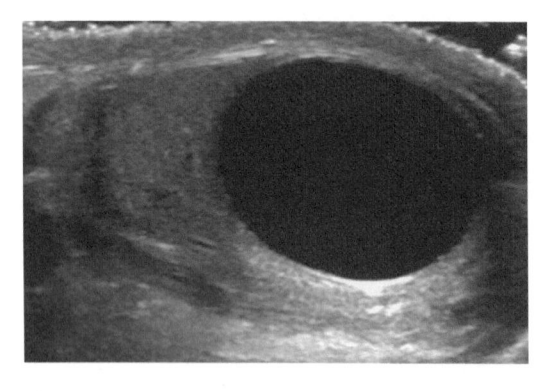

Fig. 21 The findings of a simple intratesticular cyst. Simple cysts are anechoic, show strong posterior acoustic enhancement and are well demarcated without evidence of solid parts

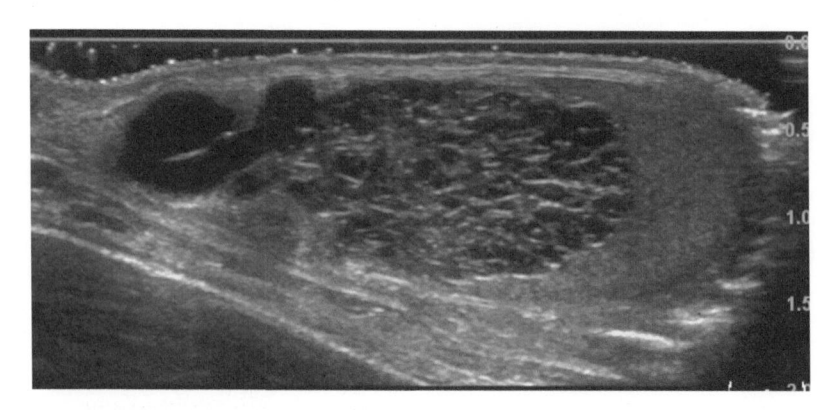

Fig. 22 Enlargement of the testicle caused by a large cystic dysplasia of the rete testis. The countless small tubular, cystic structures may become large and compress and displace the normal-appearing testicular tissue towards the periphery. May have atypical US appearance due to mucoid material

> **Take Away**
> Cautious interpretation of imaging is advocated, as benign and malignant lesions may be indiscernible based on imaging findings, rendering histology necessary for correct diagnosis.

11 Vascular Conditions

11.1 Vascular Lesions of the Genitalia

US is the initial examination when a vascular lesion is suspected. The most common *vascular tumour* is infantile haemangioma, seen as a well-circumscribed, uniformly enhancing soft tissue mass with increased arterial flow at Doppler and dilated feeding and draining vessels (Kulungowski et al. 2011). They often present with ulceration or bleeding, and in particular perineal lesions are associated with urogenital, anorectal and spinal malformations.

Vascular malformations account for 90 % of genital vascular lesions in boys, and usually present early with swelling, pain, bleeding (haematuria), infection or altered urinary mechanism. Vascular malformations grow with the child and can become debilitating. The findings depend upon the type of malformation present (venous, arterial, lymphatic or any combination) (Kulungowski et al. 2011). US is helpful to differentiate between slow-flow (appr. 90 %) and high-flow (appr. 10 %) vascular malformations and for follow-up, whereas MRI delineates the lesion and its associated anomalies (Leavitt et al. 2012). Subtraction angiography may be needed for diagnosis, and also has the option of treatment. While lymphoedema is seen secondary to tumour and infection in adults, in children it usually is a primary anomalous development of the lymphatic vessels that presents during infancy. The genitals are affected in approximately 20 %. History and clinical examination are usually sufficient for diagnosis, but in equivocal cases lymphoscintigraphy confirms lymphoedema (Gloviczki et al. 1989; Bellini et al. 2008). US and/or MRI may be used to detect the cause of secondary lymphoedema (Warren et al. 2007; White et al. 2014).

11.2 Priapism

Prolonged erection is uncommon in children. The ischaemic subtype is the most common, typically due to sickle cell disease. It presents with painful and rigid cavernous bodies. A hypoxic, hypercapnic and acidotic blood gas confirms the diagnosis and renders imaging unnecessary. Immediate treatment is recommended to avoid necrosis (Donaldson et al. 2014).

Non-ischaemic priapism is caused by a loss of inflow regulatory mechanisms, typically due to a fistula from the cavernosal artery. US usually identifies the fistula and its low-resistance, high-flow Doppler tracing (Fig. 23) in the boy presenting a non-tender, not fully erect penis and a history of trauma to the perineal region (Halls et al. 2012). In children, imaging is recommended before blood gas sampling (Donaldson et al. 2014).

Neonatal priapism usually occurs during the first few days of life and persists for 2–12 days, rendering laboratory workup, US and careful observation as the appropriate level of care (Donaldson et al. 2014).

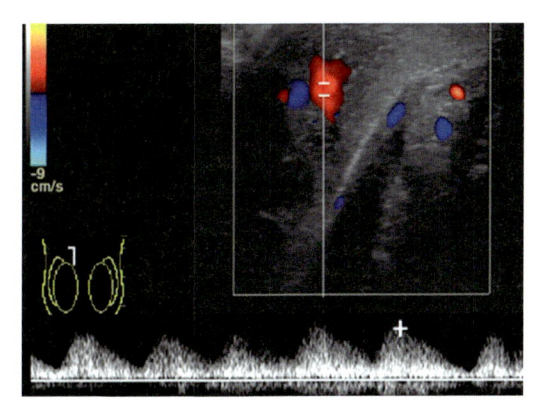

Fig. 23 Posttraumatic arteriosinusoidal fistula causing non-ischaemic priapism (Image courtesy of Dr. J. Westvik)

11.3 Varicocele

Varicocele usually manifests in adolescence as a left-sided scrotal swelling and dull discomfort. The associated decreased ipsilateral testicular volume is correlated to poorer semen quality (Diamond et al. 2007) and is one indication for treatment, in addition to pain (Pastuszak et al. 2014). The role of US is to confirm the tortuous, ectatic veins of the pampiniform plexus (Fig. 24) and to assess testicular structure and volume. Up to 15% volume asymmetry is a normal finding in adolescent boys, which is why follow-up for at least 12 months should be encouraged (Kolon et al. 2008). Doppler examination including compulsory Valsalva's manoeuvre will demonstrate increased flow and is often used for classification. However, none of the proposed classification systems correlate with impairment of spermatogenesis (Valentino et al. 2014). US should be done to assess for potential causes of vessel compression in atypical age groups, right-sided varicocele and recurrence after treatment and should always include at least the complete urinary tract, better also the entire pelvis and abdomen.

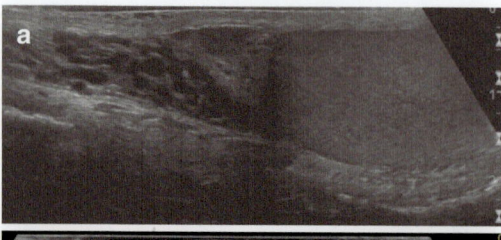

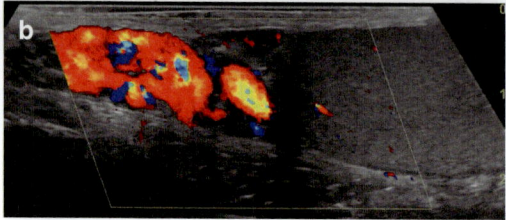

Fig. 24 Varicocele. The typical ectatic, tortuous veins of pampiniform plexus (**a**) are further dilated and show extensive reversed blood flow during Valsalva's manoeuvre (**b**)

Conclusion
Ultrasonography is the primary imaging choice for all male genital queries, though in some instances MRI provides necessary additional information. Detailed knowledge of imaging anatomy and pathology is as essential as proper technique and meticulous scanning. It is most important that the radiologist engages in and contributes to adequate patient care, which also includes correct use and utilisation of imaging studies.

Take Away
US and MRI provide complementary information in the workup of vascular lesions.

12 Superficial Genital Lesions

The many causes of superficial lesions of the male genitals can be classified as cystic, vascular, dermatological, infectious or neurogenic. Most of them are diagnosed and treated without imaging. If encountered on US or MRI, cysts of the median raphe have the features of cysts, and lesions such as epidermoid and dermoid cysts, neurinomas and Schwannomas have their usual appearance. In juvenile xanthogranuloma, imaging detects systemic involvement, which is important as it is associated with increased morbidity and mortality (Patel et al. 2010).

References

Agarwal PK, Palmer JS (2006) Testicular and paratesticular neoplasms in prepubertal males. J Urol 176(3):875–881. doi:10.1016/j.juro.2006.04.021

Ahmed HU, Arya M, Muneer A, Mushtaq I, Sebire NJ (2010) Testicular and paratesticular tumours in the prepubertal population. Lancet Oncol 11(5):476–483. doi:10.1016/s1470-2045(10)70012-7

Alanbuki AH, Bandi A, Blackford N (2013) Meconium periorchitis: a case report and literature review. Can Urol Assoc J 7(7–8):E495–E498. doi:10.5489/cuaj.316

Avila NA, Premkumar A, Merke DP (1999) Testicular adrenal rest tissue in congenital adrenal hyperplasia: comparison of MR imaging and sonographic findings. AJR Am J Roentgenol 172(4):1003–1006. doi:10.2214/ajr.172.4.10587136

Balevic S, Taylor M, Amaya M (2013) Penile and scrotal swelling mimicking child abuse. Clin Pediatr 52(10):988–990. doi:10.1177/0009922813497826

Baud C, Veyrac C, Couture A, Ferran JL (1998) Spiral twist of the spermatic cord: a reliable sign of testicular torsion. Pediatr Radiol 28(12):950–954. doi:10.1007/s002470050507

Bellini C, Boccardo F, Campisi C, Villa G, Taddei G, Traggiai C et al (2008) Lymphatic dysplasias in newborns and children: the role of lymphoscintigraphy. J Pediatr 152(4):587–589. doi:10.1016/j.jpeds.2007.12.018, 9.e1-3

Ben-Sira L, Laor T (2000) Severe scrotal pain in boys with Henoch-Schonlein purpura: incidence and sonography. Pediatr Radiol 30(2):125–128

Biasutto SN, Repetto E, Aliendo MM, Borghino VN (2009) Inguinal canal development: the muscular wall and the role of the gubernaculum. Clin Anat 22(5):614–618. doi:10.1002/ca.20820

Boettcher M, Bergholz R, Krebs TF, Wenke K, Aronson DC (2012) Clinical predictors of testicular torsion in children. Urology 79(3):670–674. doi:10.1016/j.urology.2011.10.041

Boettcher M, Bergholz R, Krebs TF, Wenke K, Treszl A, Aronson DC et al (2013) Differentiation of epididymitis and appendix testis torsion by clinical and ultrasound signs in children. Urology 82(4):899–904. doi:10.1016/j.urology.2013.04.004

Chariatte V, Ramseyer P, Cachat F (2013) Uroradiological screening for upper and lower urinary tract anomalies in patients with hypospadias: a systematic literature review. Evid Based Med 18(1):11–20. doi:10.1136/eb-2012-100520

Cimador M, Castagnetti M, De Grazia E (2010) Management of hydrocele in adolescent patients. Nat Rev Urol 7(7):379–385. doi:10.1038/nrurol.2010.80

Cooper ML, Kaefer M, Fan R, Rink RC, Jennings SG, Karmazyn B (2014) Testicular microlithiasis in children and associated testicular cancer. Radiology 270(3):857–863. doi:10.1148/radiol.13130394

Dagrosa LM, McMenaman KS, Pais VM Jr (2015) Tension hydrocele: an unusual cause of acute scrotal pain. Pediatr Emerg Care 31(8):584–585. doi:10.1097/pec.0000000000000283

Diamond DA, Zurakowski D, Bauer SB, Borer JG, Peters CA, Cilento BG Jr et al (2007) Relationship of varicocele grade and testicular hypotrophy to semen parameters in adolescents. J Urol 178(4 Pt 2):1584–1588. doi:10.1016/j.juro.2007.03.169

Diana A, Gaze H, Laubscher B, De Meuron G, Tschantz P (2000) A case of pediatric Henoch-Schonlein purpura and thrombosis of spermatic veins. J Pediatr Surg 35(12):1843. doi:10.1053/jpsu.2000.9293

Donaldson JF, Rees RW, Steinbrecher HA (2014) Priapism in children: a comprehensive review and clinical guideline. J Pediatr Urol 10(1):11–24. doi:10.1016/j.jpurol.2013.07.024

Epifanio M, Baldissera M, Esteban FG, Baldisserotto M (2014) Mature testicular teratoma in children: multifaceted tumors on ultrasound. Urology 83(1):195–197. doi:10.1016/j.urology.2013.07.046

Geiger J, Epelman M, Darge K (2010) The fountain sign: a novel color Doppler sonographic finding for the diagnosis of acute idiopathic scrotal edema. J Ultrasound Med 29(8):1233–1237

Gloviczki P, Calcagno D, Schirger A, Pairolero PC, Cherry KJ, Hallett JW et al (1989) Noninvasive evaluation of the swollen extremity: experiences with 190 lymphoscintigraphic examinations. J Vasc Surg 9(5): 683–689; discussion 90

Goenka A, Jain V, Sharma R, Gupta AK, Bajpai M (2008) MR diagnosis of penile agenesis: is it just absence of a phallus? Pediatr Radiol 38(10):1109–1112. doi:10.1007/s00247-008-0910-1

Grady RW, Ross JH, Kay R (1997) Epidemiological features of testicular teratoma in a prepubertal population. J Urol 158(3 Pt 2):1191–1192

Guichard G, El Ammari J, Del Coro C, Cellarier D, Loock PY, Chabannes E et al (2008) Accuracy of ultrasonography in diagnosis of testicular rupture after blunt scrotal trauma. Urology 71(1):52–56. doi:10.1016/j.urology.2007.09.014

Gyftopoulos K, Wolffenbuttel KP, Nijman RJ (2002) Clinical and embryologic aspects of penile duplication and associated anomalies. Urology 60(4):675–679

Halls JE, Patel DV, Walkden M, Patel U (2012) Priapism: pathophysiology and the role of the radiologist. Br J Radiol 85(Spec No 1):S79–S85. doi:10.1259/bjr/62360925

Hamm B, Fobbe F (1995) Maturation of the testis: ultrasound evaluation. Ultrasound Med Biol 21(2): 143–147

Hutson JM (2013) Journal of Pediatric Surgery-Sponsored Fred McLoed Lecture. Undescended testis: the underlying mechanisms and the effects on germ cells that cause infertility and cancer. J Pediatr Surg 48(5):903–908. doi:10.1016/j.jpedsurg.2013.02.001

Jeyaratnam R, Bakalinova D (2010) Cystic dysplasia of the rete testis: a case of spontaneous regression and review of published reports. Urology 75(3):687–690. doi:10.1016/j.urology.2009.05.067

Kalfa N, Veyrac C, Lopez M, Lopez C, Maurel A, Kaselas C et al (2007) Multicenter assessment of ultrasound of the spermatic cord in children with acute scrotum. J Urol 177(1):297–301. doi:10.1016/j.juro.2006.08.128; discussion

Kanaroglou N, To T, Zhu J, Braga LH, Wehbi E, Hajiha M et al (2015) Inappropriate use of ultrasound in management of pediatric cryptorchidism. Pediatrics 136(3):479–486. doi:10.1542/peds.2015-0222

Karmazyn B, Kaefer M, Kauffman S, Jennings SG (2009) Ultrasonography and clinical findings in children with epididymitis, with and without associated lower urinary tract abnormalities. Pediatr Radiol 39(10):1054–1058. doi:10.1007/s00247-009-1326-2

Kim SH, Park S, Choi SH, Jeong WK, Choi JH (2009) The efficacy of magnetic resonance imaging for the diagnosis of testicular rupture: a prospective preliminary study. J Trauma 66(1):239–242. doi:10.1097/TA.0b013e318156867f

Klin B, Lotan G, Efrati Y, Zlotkevich L, Strauss S (2002) Acute idiopathic scrotal edema in children – revisited. J Pediatr Surg 37(8):1200–1202

Kolon TF, Clement MR, Cartwright L, Bellah R, Carr MC, Canning DA et al (2008) Transient asynchronous testicular growth in adolescent males with a varicocele. J Urol 180(3):1111–1114. doi:10.1016/j.juro.2008.05.061; discussion 4–5

Kolon TF, Herndon CD, Baker LA, Baskin LS, Baxter CG, Cheng EY et al (2014) Evaluation and treatment of cryptorchidism: AUA guideline. J Urol 192(2):337–345. doi:10.1016/j.juro.2014.05.005

Krishnaswami S, Fonnesbeck C, Penson D, McPheeters ML (2013) Magnetic resonance imaging for locating nonpalpable undescended testicles: a meta-analysis. Pediatrics 131(6):e1908–e1916. doi:10.1542/peds.2013-0073

Kulungowski AM, Schook CC, Alomari AI, Vogel AM, Mulliken JB, Fishman SJ (2011) Vascular anomalies of the male genitalia. J Pediatr Surg 46(6):1214–1221. doi:10.1016/j.jpedsurg.2011.03.056

Leavitt DA, Hottinger DG, Reed RC, Shukla AR (2012) A case series of genital vascular anomalies in children and their management: lessons learned. Urology 80(4):914–918. doi:10.1016/j.urology.2012.06.011

Maki D, Watanabe Y, Nagayama M, Ishimori T, Okumura A, Amoh Y et al (2011) Diffusion-weighted magnetic resonance imaging in the detection of testicular torsion: feasibility study. J Magn Reson Imaging 34(5):1137–1142. doi:10.1002/jmri.22698

Milla SS, Chow JS, Lebowitz RL (2008) Imaging of hypospadias: pre- and postoperative appearances. Pediatr Radiol 38(2):202–208. doi:10.1007/s00247-007-0697-5

Naji H, Ingolfsson I, Isacson D, Svensson JF (2012) Decision making in the management of hydroceles in infants and children. Eur J Pediatr 171(5):807–810. doi:10.1007/s00431-011-1628-x

Nandi B, Murphy FL (2011) Neonatal testicular torsion: a systematic literature review. Pediatr Surg Int 27(10):1037–1040. doi:10.1007/s00383-011-2945-x

Paltiel HJ, Connolly LP, Atala A, Paltiel AD, Zurakowski D, Treves ST (1998) Acute scrotal symptoms in boys with an indeterminate clinical presentation: comparison of color Doppler sonography and scintigraphy. Radiology 207(1):223–231. doi:10.1148/radiology.207.1.9530319

Pastuszak AW, Kumar V, Shah A, Roth DR (2014) Diagnostic and management approaches to pediatric and adolescent varicocele: a survey of pediatric urologists. Urology 84(2):450–456. doi:10.1016/j.urology.2014.04.022

Patel P, Vyas R, Blickman J, Katzman P (2010) Multimodality imaging findings of disseminated juvenile xanthogranuloma with renal involvement in an infant. Pediatr Radiol 40(Suppl 1):S6–S10. doi:10.1007/s00247-010-1798-0

Riccabona M (2014a) Ultrasound of the urogenital tract. In: Riccabona M (ed) Pediatric ultrasound, requisites and applications. Springer, Berlin/Heidelberg, p 384

Riccabona M (2014b) Ultrasound of the urogenital tract. In: Riccabona M (ed) Pediatric ultrasound, requisites and applications. Springer, Berlin/Heidelberg, p 382

Riccabona M, Avni FE, Blickman JG, Dacher JN, Darge K, Lobo ML et al (2008) Imaging recommendations in paediatric uroradiology: minutes of the ESPR workgroup session on urinary tract infection, fetal hydronephrosis, urinary tract ultrasonography and voiding cystourethrography, Barcelona, Spain, June 2007. Pediatr Radiol 38(2):138–145. doi:10.1007/s00247-007-0695-7

Riccabona M, Darge K, Lobo ML, Ording-Muller LS, Augdal TA, Avni FE et al (2015) ESPR uroradiology Taskforce-imaging recommendations in paediatric uroradiology, part VIII: retrograde urethrography, imaging disorder of sexual development and imaging childhood testicular torsion. Pediatr Radiol 45(13):2023–2028. doi:10.1007/s00247-015-3452-3

Ricci P, Cantisani V, Drudi FM, Carbone I, Coniglio M, Bosco S et al (2001) Prenatal testicular torsion: sonographic appearance in the newborn infant. Eur Radiol 11(12):2589–2592. doi:10.1007/s003300100868

Schneble F, Pohlmann T, Segerer H, Melter M (2011) Scrotal ultrasound in children and adolescents with duplex Doppler analysis of intratesticular arteries. Ultraschall Med 32(Suppl 2):E51–E56. doi:10.1055/s-0031-1273377

Sijstermans K, Hack WW, Meijer RW, van der Voort-Doedens LM (2008) The frequency of undescended testis from birth to adulthood: a review. Int J Androl 31(1):1–11. doi:10.1111/j.1365-2605.2007.00770.x

Soreide K (2005) Surgical management of nonrenal genitourinary manifestations in children with Henoch-Schonlein purpura. J Pediatr Surg 40(8):1243–1247. doi:10.1016/j.jpedsurg.2005.05.005

Srinivasan A, Cinman N, Feber KM, Gitlin J, Palmer LS (2011) History and physical examination findings predictive of testicular torsion: an attempt to promote clinical diagnosis by house staff. J Pediatr Urol 7(4):470–474. doi:10.1016/j.jpurol.2010.12.010

Suominen JS, Jawaid WB, Losty PD (2015) Testicular microlithiasis and associated testicular malignancies in childhood: a systematic review. Pediatr Blood Cancer 62(3):385–388. doi:10.1002/pbc.25343

Tasian GE, Copp HL (2011) Diagnostic performance of ultrasound in nonpalpable cryptorchidism: a systematic review and meta-analysis. Pediatrics 127(1):119–128. doi:10.1542/peds.2010-1800

Taskinen S, Fagerholm R, Aronniemi J, Rintala R, Taskinen M (2008) Testicular tumors in children and adolescents. J Pediatr Urol 4(2):134–137. doi:10.1016/j.jpurol.2007.10.002

Tekgul S, Dogan H, Erdem E, Hoebeke P, Kocvara R, Nijman J et al (2015) Guidelines on Paediatric urology. European Association of Urology. European Society for Paediatric Urology. http://uroweb.org/guideline/paediatric-urology/. Accessed 10 Nov 2015

Trout AT, Chow J, McNamara ER, Darge K et al. (2017) Association between Testicular Microlithiasis and Testicular Neoplasia: Large Multicenter Study in a Pediatric Population. Radiology 285:576–583.

Valentino M, Bertolotto M, Derchi L, Pavlica P (2014) Children and adults varicocele: diagnostic issues and therapeutical strategies. J Ultrasound 17(3):185–193. doi:10.1007/s40477-014-0088-3

Vaos G, Zavras N, Eirekat K (2014) Testicular dysmorphism in infantile abdominoscrotal hydrocele: insights into etiology. Int Urol Nephrol 46(7):1257–1261. doi:10.1007/s11255-014-0665-6

Volokhina YV, Oyoyo UE, Miller JH (2014) Ultrasound demonstration of testicular microlithiasis in pediatric patients: is there an association with testicular germ cell tumors? Pediatr Radiol 44(1):50–55. doi:10.1007/s00247-013-2778-y

Walsh TJ, Dall'Era MA, Croughan MS, Carroll PR, Turek PJ (2007) Prepubertal orchiopexy for cryptorchidism may be associated with lower risk of testicular cancer. J Urol 178(4 Pt 1):1440–1446. doi:10.1016/j.juro.2007.05.166; discussion 6

Wang T, Liu L, Luo J, Liu T, Wei A (2015) A meta-analysis of the relationship between testicular microlithiasis and incidence of testicular cancer. Urol J 12(2):2057–2064

Warren AG, Brorson H, Borud LJ, Slavin SA (2007) Lymphedema: a comprehensive review. Ann Plast Surg 59(4):464–472. doi:10.1097/01.sap.0000257149.42922.7e

Watanabe Y, Nagayama M, Okumura A, Amoh Y, Suga T, Terai A et al (2007) MR imaging of testicular torsion: features of testicular hemorrhagic necrosis and clinical outcomes. J Magn Reson Imaging 26(1):100–108. doi:10.1002/jmri.20946

White RD, Weir-McCall JR, Budak MJ, Waugh SA, Munnoch DA, Sudarshan TA (2014) Contrast-enhanced magnetic resonance lymphography in the assessment of lower limb lymphoedema. Clin Radiol 69(11):e435–44. doi:10.1016/j.crad.2014.06.007

Wiygul J, Palmer LS (2011) Micropenis. ScientificWorldJournal 11:1462–1469. doi:10.1100/tsw.2011.135

Yang DM, Lim JW, Kim JE, Kim JH, Cho H (2005) Torsed appendix testis: grayscale and color Doppler sonographic findings compared with normal appendix testis. J Ultrasound Med 24(1):87–91

Yusuf G, Sellars ME, Kooiman GG, Diaz-Cano S, Sidhu PS (2013) Global testicular infarction in the presence of epididymitis: clinical features, appearances on grayscale, color Doppler, and contrast-enhanced sonography, and histologic correlation. J Ultrasound Med 32(1):175–180

Zamakhshary M, To T, Guan J, Langer JC (2008) Risk of incarceration of inguinal hernia among infants and young children awaiting elective surgery. Can Med Assoc J 179(10):1001–1005. doi:10.1503/cmaj.070923

Urinary Problems Associated with Imperforate Anus

Erich Sorantin, Michael E. Höllwarth, and Sandra Abou Samaan

Contents

1 Introduction 373
2 **Anorectal Malformations (ARMs)** 374
2.1 Embryology of Imperforate Anus 374
2.2 Associated Malformations 375
3 **Urologic Problems** 377
3.1 Incidence 378
3.2 Structural Anomalies 378
3.3 Functional Anomalies 379
4 **Imaging** 380
5 **Therapy** 382
Conclusion 382
References 382

1 Introduction

The term "imperforate anus" includes all kinds of anorectal malformations: from covering of the anus by a thin skin membrane to high anorectal atresia – with or without a fistula into the urethra or the bladder – to cloacal anomalies in females. Overall incidence is 1 in 5000 live births with a slight male predominance (Alamo et al. 2013).

It is well known that in a high proportion of imperforate anus patients, this maldevelopment will be in association with anomalies of one or several other organ systems (e.g., spinal cord and spine, cardiovascular, gastrointestinal, musculoskeletal, as well as urogenital system – see below). Among those, urinary tract anomalies with or without infections, as well as functional disorders of the urinary system, are common and may cause serious complications. Thus the overall morbidity and mortality of patients with anorectal malformations are considerably influenced by those potentially genitourinary tract anomalies. To facilitate the understanding of the problem, we briefly describe the different types of imperforate anus and the incidence of associated anomalies before we focus on the related urinary tract problems (see also chap. 19).

E. Sorantin, MD (✉)
Department of Radiology, Division of Pediatric Radiology, Medical University Graz,
Auenbruggerplatz 34, A-8036 Graz, Austria
e-mail: Erich.Sorantin@medunigraz.at

M.E. Höllwarth, MD (Retired)
Department of Pediatric and Adolescent Surgery,
Medical University Graz,
Auenbruggerplatz 34, A-8036 Graz, Austria

S. Abou Saaman, MD
Department of Radiology, Hamad General Hospital,
P.O. Box 3050, Doha, Qatar

2 Anorectal Malformations (ARMs)

In earlier years anorectal malformations were classified into two subtypes: a high and low form, depending on whether the distal rectal pouch ended above or below the levator muscle level. On the occasion of the international Wingspread workshop meeting in 1984, the different types of imperforate anus were classified into three major groups and into the male and female patterns of the malformation (Stephens and Smith 1986). Briefly, a high-intermediate-low classification was agreed upon, and minor and rare subtypes were omitted. "High" anomalies are characterized by anorectal agenesis or rectal atresia with or without a rectovesical or rectoprostatic fistula in males or a rectovaginal fistula in females. The blind rectal pouch ends definitely above a hypotrophic puborectalis muscle sling. In "intermediate" malformations, the rectal pouch enters that sling; there may be a rectobulbar fistula in males and a rectovestibular or rectovaginal fistula in females. In the "low" forms the rectum passes through a well-developed puborectalis muscle and may end in an anocutaneous fistula in males and an anovestibular or anocutaneous fistula in females. The consensus conference placed the female cloaca in a separate group classifying the malformation in a high, an intermediate, or a low form depending on the length of the common channel (see below and also chapter "Female Genital Anomalies and Important Ovarian Conditions"). With regard to anal function and continence, it is evident that the high forms of imperforate anus have clearly less satisfying results than the low forms. Beyond that, the high and intermediate forms have a higher incidence of associated malformations and urinary tract function disorders. In 2005 an international group of experts elaborated the so-called "Krickenbeck" classification which is not based on anatomical or embryological features but on the frequency of occurrence into "major clinical groups" and "rare/regional variants." Furthermore, an additional grouping of the surgical procedures has been published, with the intention to make them comparable with each other, and uniform methods of assessment of outcome have been agreed by the participants (Murphy et al. 2006).

2.1 Embryology of Imperforate Anus

A complete overview of embryology is given within chapters "Urinary Tract Embryology, Anatomy, and Anatomical Variants" and "Female Genital Anomalies and Important Ovarian Conditions".

Briefly, in the 4-week-old embryo, the hindgut expands to form the internal cloaca, into which issues the large intestine, the allantois, and the Wolffian or mesonephric ducts. The internal cloaca is separated from the external cloaca by the cloacal membrane. The partitioning of the internal cloaca by a craniocaudally growing septum begins at the 4 mm stage and is completed at the 16 mm stage, when the septum reaches the cloacal membrane. Once the septum is completed, the cloaca is divided into a ventral urogenital sinus and the dorsal rectum. The Wolffian ducts become organized into the vasa deferentia and the vesicae seminales in the male, while in the female they are the leading structures for the proceeding of the Müllerian ducts into the vestibule. The external cloaca is a depression of tissue formed by the bilateral genital folds and the genital tubercle on the ventral aspect. When the septum reaches the cloacal membrane, the latter atrophies and both systems enter the common external cloaca. The process of partitioning now extends caudally by the Uroanal septum. The high and intermediate groups of anorectal malformation can be seen as the result of a disturbed development of the partitioning of the internal cloaca with the gut ending in a fistula to the verumontanum or higher in males, and into the vagina or fossa navicularis of the vestibule in females. The low forms refer to developmental errors affecting the partitioning of the external cloaca, resulting in a fistula to the perineum or to the female vestibule or a completely or partially persisting anal membrane (Stephens and Smith 1971).

Duhamel (1961) reported that the most frequent malformations associated with imperforate anus are just those that one finds constantly in the siren anomaly, and he concluded that the whole pattern of anorectal malformations belongs to the syndrome of caudal regression. This hypothesis is in agreement with the work of Berdon et al. (1966) and Elliott et al. (1970)), who explained the common association of lumbosacral vertebral anomalies and hindgut malformations by a disturbed development of the notochordal organizer at a very early stage of embryogenesis (Fig. 1).

2.2 Associated Malformations

As mentioned above, there is an agreement in the literature that ARMs are highly associated with anomalies of other organ systems – a complete list can be found in Table 1. The overall reported incidence varies from 20 to 70 %, a range that depends largely on a careful and systematic search for additional anomalies (Stephens and Smith 1971; Alamo et al 2013). In a series of 75 patients, an overall incidence of 72 % additional anomalies was found, reaching nearly 100 % in the subgroup of deceased patients (Höllwarth and Menardi 1983) (Table 2). These findings confirm the conclusion from a necropsy study of babies dying with AMRs that there is a nearly 100 % association with other malformations (Moore and Lawrence 1952).

Moreover, frequently more than one organ system is involved, and therefore several syndromes including imperforate anus are known – a list of the most frequent ones can be found in Table 3.

Stephens and Smith (1971) and others have demonstrated that the incidence of additional anomalies is twice as high in the high and intermediate groups of anorectal malformations (85 %) as in the low group (46 %). These findings

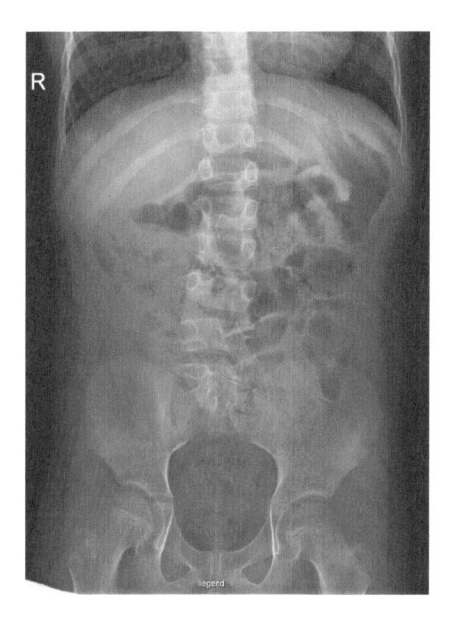

Fig. 1 A 12-year-old boy with imperforate anus and sacral agenesis; plain abdominal film: sacral agenesis can be noted. Additionally, right convex lumbar scoliosis due to left sided malformation of the articular process in LV and SI is seen

Table 1 Associated malformations in ARMs (after Alamo et al. 2013)

Affected system	Anomalies
Cardio-vascular	Tetralogy of Fallot, atrial septal defect, ventricular septal defect, dextrocardia, coarctation of the aorta
Gastrointestinal	Esophageal atresia; duodenal, jejunal, or ileal atresia; absent colon; intestinal malrotation; volvulus; Meckel diverticulum
Musculoskeletal	Hip dislocation or dysplasia, fusion of iliac bones, Madelung deformity, arthrogryposis, clubfoot, polydactyly, syndactyly, limb deficiency, sacral agenesis, vertebral dysplasia, spina bifida, tethered cord
Spinal cord and spine	Sacral agenesis, vertebral dysplasia, spina bifida, tethered cord, myelomeningocele
Urogenital	Vesicoureteral reflux, hydronephrosis, bilateral or unilateral renal agenesis, renal dysplasia, renal ectopia, horseshoe kidney, polycystic kidney, renal duplication, megaureter, bladder exstrophy, micropenis, hypospadias, uterine duplications or double vagina, vulvo-vaginal atresia, ambiguous genitalia

Table 2 Associated malformations in 75 patients with anorectal malformations

Anatomical system	Total ($n=75$) (%)	Survivors ($n=59$) (%)	Deceased ($n=16$) (%)
Urinary tract	41.3	35.5	62.5
Genitalia	12.0	10.1	18.7
Skeletal system	46.6	37.2	37.5
Cardiac system	18.6	11.8	37.5
Intestinal tract	18.6	8.4	62.5
Cerebral	13.3	8.4	25.0
Others	22.6	20.3	31.2
Total	*72.0*	*65.5*	*100*

Table 3 Most common syndromes with ARM association (after Alamo et al. 2013)

Associated entity	Syndromes or multisystemic involvement
Associations of congenital anomalies	VACTERL (Vertebral anomalies, Anal atresia, Cardiac malformations, Tracheo-Esophageal fistula, Renal and Limb anomalies), OEIS (Omphalocele, Exstrophy, Imperforate anus, Spinal defects), MURCS (Müllerian duct aplasia, Renal aplasia, Cervicothoracic Somite dysplasia)
Chromosomopathies	Trisomy 13, 18, and 21; parental unidisomy 16; deletion of 22q11.2 and 13q; heterotaxia
Syndromes	Baller-Gerold, cat-eye, caudal regression, Christian, Currarino triad, Down, facio-auriculo-vertebral, Feingold, fetal alcohol, FG (Opitz-Kaveggia), Fraser, Ivemark, Johanson-Blizzard, Kabuki, Klippel-Feil, Lowe, MIDAS, Okihiro, Opitz, Pallister-Hall, Pallister-Killian, Rieger, Townes-Brock, ulnar-mammary, Walker-Warburg

Table 4 Associated malformations in relation to the atresia level

	Total	Urogenital	Skeletal	Intestinal	Cardiac	Cerebral	Others
High and intermediate ($n=34$) (%)	85.0	76.4	52.9	29.4	23.5	11.7	32.3
Low ($n=41$) (%)	61.0	34.0	41.4	9.7	14.6	24.6	17.0

have been confirmed by the analysis of 75 patients with anorectal malformations which has shown an incidence of 85 % in the high and intermediate forms versus 61 % in the low forms (Höllwarth and Menardi 1983) (Table 4).

Although almost every known malformation has been reported in association with anorectal malformations, the analysis of anatomical localization shows that organ systems within the lower part of the body, e.g., the urogenital tract, are significantly more affected than those in the upper part. Similarly, detailed studies of the associated skeletal malformations of our patients showed that vertebral anomalies are significantly more common in the lumbar and sacrococcygeal spine in patients with imperforate anus (Figs. 2 and 3) – confirming the findings of an earlier study carried out by Pellerin and Bertin (1967).

As mentioned above, partial or complete sacral agenesis can be seen as a part of the caudal regression syndrome and may strongly imply additional neurogenic disorders of the bladder. For the radiologist it is important to analyze lumbosacral plain radiographs of patients with imperforate anus carefully, since the presence of lumbosacral anomaly malformations gives rise to strong suspicion of additional urogenital malformations and dysfunctions. Moreover, it was reported that about one-third of ARM patients suffered from a tethered cord with a male predominance in the low ARMs (Golonka et al. 2002). Additionally, 45 % of patients with low ARMs and tethered

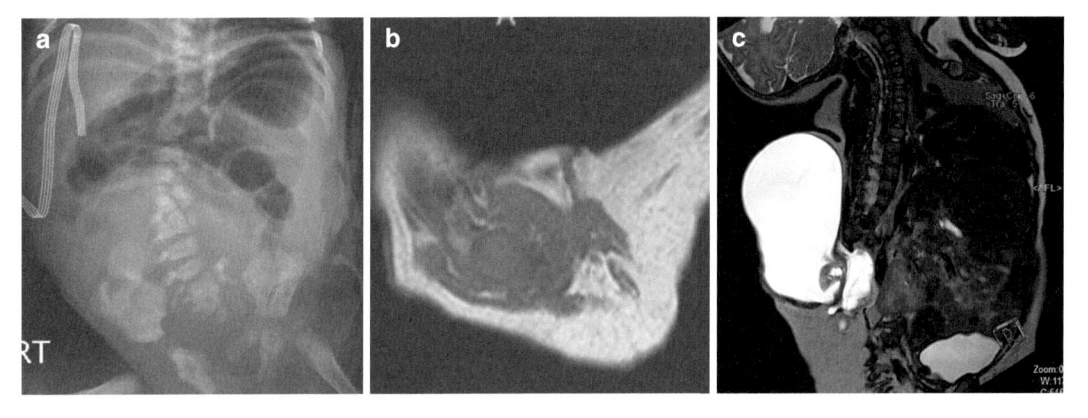

Fig. 2 Baby with imperforate anus and multiple malformations: (**a**) plain film of the abdomen: malformed lumbar spine with multiple hemivertebra and sacral dysplasia. (**b**) MRI, transversal plane: left thigh and gluteal muscles are missing. (**c**) MRI, sagittal plane: a high meningomyelocele is depicted. It is obvious that a neurogenic bladder must exist

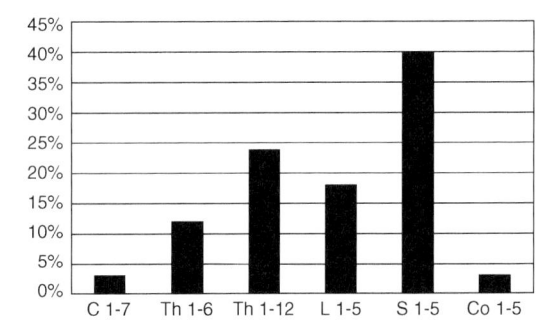

Fig. 3 Distribution of associated vertebral anomalies in patients with imperforate anus ($n=33$)

cord did not reveal any other lumbosacral anomalies as reported by the last cited authors.

> **Take away**
> Anorectal anomalies are classified into three subtypes of malformations: high, intermediate, and low. Associated anomalies occur twice as often in the high and intermediate groups as in the low group.

3 Urologic Problems

Structural anomalies of the urinary tract as well as functional disorders and – in a minority of patients – complications after surgical correction of the imperforate anus contribute to a significant degree to the final outcome of those patients

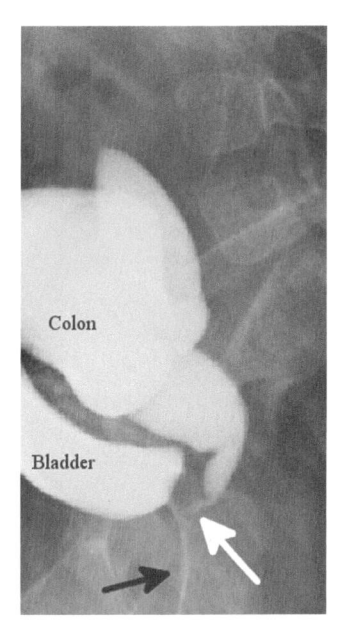

Fig. 4 Male baby boy with a rectourethral fistula at VCUG → *white arrow* marks the fistula, *black arrow* urethral catheter

(McLorie et al. 1987; Wilcox and Warne 2006). Furthermore, the overall morbidity may be influenced by urinary tract infections, which occur either as a consequence of the recto-urinary fistula (Fig. 4) in males or on the basis of anatomic or neurogenic disorders. A high or intermediate form of imperforate anus and the association of vertebral anomalies have already been emphasized as an important hint that a careful

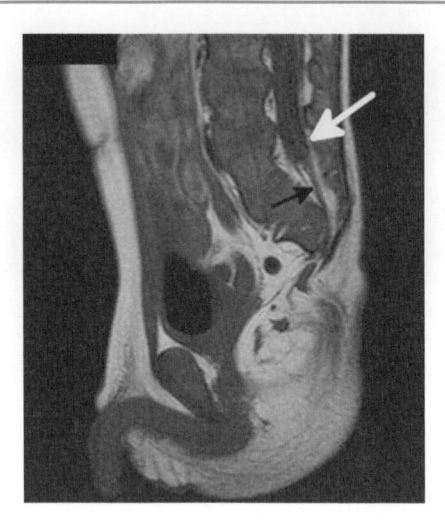

Fig. 5 Same baby boy as Fig. 3, T1 weighted MRI, sagittal plane, tethered chord: *white arrow* points to the low positioned and malformed medullary cone, whereas the *black arrow* indicates the thickened terminal filum

and thorough radiological/urologic evaluation is required in order to establish the proper management plan. However, even in patients with low forms of atresia and no additional vertebral malformations, the incidence of associated urologic anomalies, including vesicoureteric reflux (VUR), is significantly higher when compared to the normal population (Yeung and Kiely 1991). Therefore, it is advisable to perform a careful evaluation of the urinary system in all patients with imperforate anus. As already mentioned, the situation can be further complicated by tethered cord (Fig. 5) and consecutively a neurogenic bladder dysfunction.

3.1 Incidence

Several studies with large numbers of patients have been performed in the past to assess the incidence and type of associated urogenital tract anomalies. The numbers differ from author to author and over the years, depending on how carefully a search has been performed as well as imaging modalities and technology used. All authors agree that supralevator anorectal lesions have not only a higher incidence of urologic malformations but also the more serious forms, especially in males.

Out of 200 consecutive patients with imperforate anus, Wiener and Kiesewetter (1973) found a 64% rate of urologic anomalies among the high forms (including the intermediate forms) and 18% in the low forms. According to Hoekstra et al. (1983), 71% of the supralevator atresias are associated with urogenital malformations, but also the infralevator malformations have a remarkably high association rate of 34%. McLorie et al. (1987) encountered non-fistula genitourinary abnormalities in 60% of the high and in 20% of the low lesions. All these authors found no gender differences with regard to the incidence of associated urogenital malformations, while Wiener and Kiesewetter (1973) as well as Ralph et al. (1992) described a significantly higher incidence in males. Eighty-four percent of the anomalies in the former authors' series were major, with a potential for serious problems; 18% were incompatible with life.

3.2 Structural Anomalies

Fistulas to the urinary tract in patients with imperforate anus can be seen as a part of the malformation itself. In male patients with a high or intermediate ARM, 80% have a rectourethral fistula and 8% a rectovesical fistula (Stephens and Smith 1971). Additionally, a number of other malformations of the urinary tract can be found in these patients (Table 1). In the upper urinary tract, the most common anomalies are renal dysplasia or renal agenesis, hydronephrosis, duplications, and renal ectopia. Furthermore, 47% of the supralevator group and 35% of the low group showed a VUR, which might be caused in one-third of the cases by a malformation of the ureterovesical junction, but more commonly by a functional disorder due to a neurogenic bladder (Fig. 6) (Ralph et al. 1992). Associated malformations of the lower urinary tract are hypospadias, epispadias and exstrophy, urethral diverticula, valves, strictures, or duplications. While some of these anomalies do not require immediate treatment, others require surgical repair in the newborn period, e.g., exstrophy, or at an appropriate time later on, e.g., obstructions or VUR.

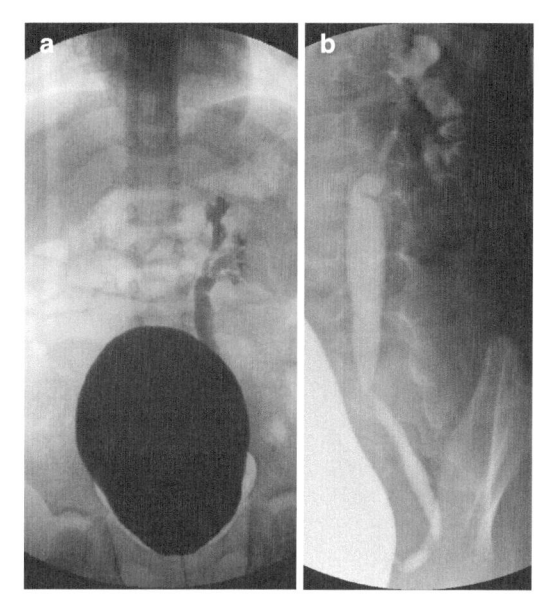

Fig. 6 A 3-year-old girl, Currarina trias, neurogenic bladder with hypotone detrusor mixed type (see chapter "Neurogenic Bladder in Infants and Children") under anticholinergic therapy. VCUG: (**a**) "last image hold" during filling phase – a huge bladder with VUR on the left side is depicted. (**b**) Same study, full exposed shot – the refluxing left ureter inserts into the bladder with a pathologic angelhook deformity

Obviously, agenesis of both kidneys is not compatible with postpartal life, but nearly as important are dysplastic or hypoplastic kidneys on both sides. Hoekstra et al. (1983) found that 75 % of cases of early death were related to urogenital tract anomalies. The overall incidence of death from renal failure out of a series of 484 infants with imperforate anus was 6.4 % with high and intermediate lesions and 1.1 % with low lesions, and in each the incidence was higher in male infants (McLorie et al. 1987).

3.3 Functional Anomalies

Holschneider et al. (1982) described a urinary incontinence rate of 19 % in patients 11 years after the correction of an anorectal atresia which has been explained by the position of the rectourethral fistula close to the external sphincter region and the surgical trauma of the abdominoperineal pull-through procedure, as well as by additional malformations of the spine. The latter argument is supported by the fact that two-thirds of the urologic anomalies in patients with imperforate anus are associated with spinal deformities, mainly with sacral anomalies. Among them, occult spinal dysraphism including lipomeningocele, ventral meningocele (Currarino syndrome – Fig. 6), and tethered cord is associated with lower urinary tract dysfunction. Boemers et al. (1996a) described a normal urinary tract function in 98 % of the children with a normal sacrum, sacral dysplasia only, or sacral agenesis affecting only smaller parts of the segments S4 and S5. Severe dysfunction was observed in all but one patient with a more extended sacral agenesis, indicating that this subgroup of patients needs careful urologic assessment. In contrast, Parrott (1985) found a neurogenic bladder in 7–18 % of the cases of imperforate anus, but not all of them had abnormalities of the lumbosacral spine, indicating that excessive dissection and rectal mobilization may cause denervation. Similarly, Greenfield and Fera (1991) and Kakizaki et al. (1994) point to the fact that a significant association of voiding dysfunctions in patients with anorectal malformations can be observed even in the absence of vertebral anomalies. It can be concluded that these children should not be excluded from a urological evaluation including urodynamic studies, video urodynamics if available, or modified voiding cystourethrography (VCUG) (see chapters "Video Urodynamics" and "Neurogenic Bladder in Infants and Children").

To answer the question of whether the surgical trauma imposes a major insult to the pelvic nerves, pre- and postoperative investigations of bladder function have been performed. Urodynamic studies before any pull-through surgery showed a sphincter-detrusor dyssynergia in 4 out of 14 patients with bladder trabeculation and VUR or hydronephrosis (Greenfield and Fera 1991). Kakizaki et al. (1994) found a voiding dysfunction in 9 (38 %) out of 24 children before anorectoplasty, and partial sacral agenesis was present in only 4 of those 9 babies. Out of 27 patients studied pre- and postoperatively, the urodynamic studies showed minor changes in only 4 patients when compared with the preoperative results

(Boemers et al. 1995). Another three boys had an atonic bladder with loss of the detrusor contractility consistent with autonomic denervation; two of them had a standard posterior sagittal anorectoplasty combined with a transabdominal procedure with dissection of the distal rectum.

In comparison to earlier studies, one has to consider that the surgical strategies have changed considerably over the years. Today, the preferred procedure consists of a close rectal dissection by the posterior sagittal anorectoplasty, according to Pena (1967)) or using laparoscopy (Georgeson et al. 2000). Boemers et al. (1995) conclude from their study that a posterior sagittal anorectoplasty is only rarely followed by an additional bladder dysfunction in a few patients when special attention is given to the surgical details and a significant rectovesical dissection can be avoided. Furthermore, a hyperreflexive bladder cannot be caused by an iatrogenic injury, because a surgical trauma results mostly in a lower motor lesion with an atonic sphincter followed by incontinence, as three patients in the Boemers et al. (1995) study have shown. A preexisting deficient nerve supply in cases of sacral agenesis might increase the vulnerability to iatrogenic nerve damage. In conclusion, the most common cause of a postoperative bladder dysfunction is not the surgical damage, but a hyperreflexic neuropathic bladder which is present in up to 55 % of the patients, namely, in 61 % of those with a high anomaly and 36 % of those with low malformations (Ralph et al. 1992).

Thus, the high incidence of VUR in patients with imperforate anus may partly be caused by a malformation of the ureterovesical junction but more often results from a neurogenic disorder. Boemers et al. (1996b) showed that 60 % of the patients with a neurogenic dysfunction had VUR; additionally 32 % had reflux nephropathy. All children with impaired renal function had a neurogenic bladder-sphincter dysfunction.

In adulthood ARM patients may present with difficulties of stool evacuation or anal incontinence. An MRI study demonstrated that thinned pelvic floor muscles can be detected in the vast majority of patients, most commonly of the external sphincter and less frequently of the levator plate (Gartner et al. 2013).

> **Take away**
> Structural as well as functional anomalies are reported commonly in babies with anorectal malformations. Therefore, a careful evaluation of the urogenital tract is essential in these cases.

4 Imaging

Boemers et al. (1999) have published detailed guidelines for the diagnostic screening and initial management of babies with imperforate anus. These recommendations are based on the complexity of the malformation and malfunction pattern in patients with imperforate anus and their impact on morbidity and mortality, which calls for a pre- and postoperative evaluation of the vertebral spine and the urogenital tract. Furthermoe the ESPR Abdominal Imaging Task Force has also recently iproposed updated recommendations for imaging and imaging procedures of patients with anorectal malformations (Riccabona et al. 2017).

The first issue is to evaluate whether there are skeletal malformations by performing of chest as well as spine radiographs immediately after birth. Thus the number and the qualitative anomalies of the vertebral bodies within the different sections and the number and asymmetry of ribs can be counted. A careful screening for sacral anomalies is mandatory, since they can be associated with a tethered chord (Carson et al. 1984). In neonates and young babies, spinal US can depict a tethered chord (Boemers et al. 1996A; Gartner et al. 2013; Pang 1993). Moreover, movements of the cauda equina fibers can be observed in real time. In older children with restricted US access to the spinal canal, MRI can depict a tethered chord and other associated anomalies. Rivosecchi et al. (1995) studied 50 patients with anorectal malformations by MRI and found 25 patients with spinal cord abnormalities such as fibrolipoma with or without tethered cord ($n=19$), syringomyelia ($n=4$), tethered cord ($n=2$), and meningocele ($n=1$). Abdominal

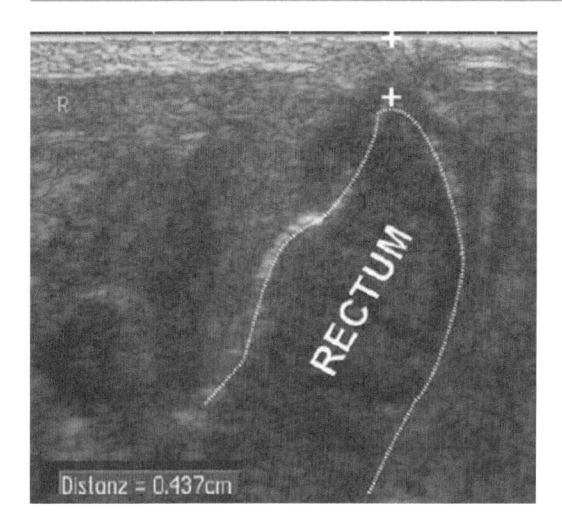

Fig. 7 Male newborn, low ARM, transperineal sonography in coronal plane: the two + markers indicate the atretic segment, whereas the *dashed line* depicts the inner contours of the pre-atretic, meconium filled rectum

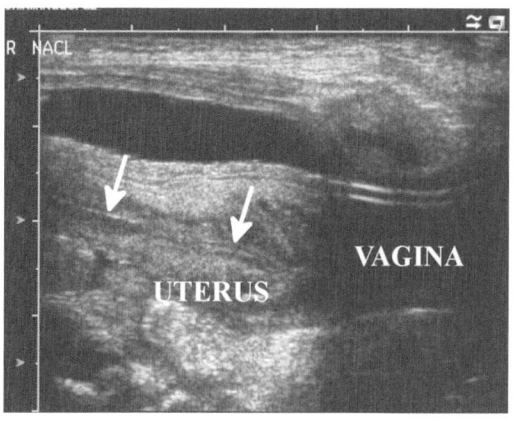

Fig. 8 Female neonate, sonographic genitography, midline sagittal plane – normal findings: vagina and the urinary bladder were filled with physiologic saline via thin catheters, thus the uterus including the cervix is easily visualized. Even the mucosal line can be demonstrated (*white arrows*). Genitosonography represents an excellent method for evaluation of the female genitourinary tract, especially within the first week of life (due to prenatal maternal hormonal stimulation of the fetus)

plain films in bottom-up position were used for length assessment of the atretic rectal segment. The anal dimple was indicated by a metallic marker. Today, perineal US can deliver the same information in a much more comfortable way but should be performed as early as possible after birth (Fig. 7) (Haber et al. 2007).

With regard to the urogenital tract, US is highly accurate in the newborn period and has been shown to be of great advantage for these patients (Karrer et al. 1988). Except for the first days of life, when urinary output is low and a dilatation of the collecting system can be missed, US is the primary screening method for detecting structural urinary tract anomalies. Repeated opening of the bladder neck and the posterior urethra may indicate a neurogenic bladder disorder. Any anomaly or dilatation of the upper urinary tract should prompt for VCUG (or contrast-enhanced voiding urosonography, ce-VUS). Some authors recommend VUR assessment in all male patients with no perineal opening even without upper tract dilatation on US (Boemers et al. 1999). Yeung and Kiely (1991) point at the high incidence of VUR even in babies with low anorectal malformations and recommend performing VCUG in all these patients. Backflow through the fistula into the rectum or reflux into the ductuli can be detected in some male patients. Transperineal US after retrograde filling the vagina with physiologic saline ("Genitosonography") represents an excellent modality to study the female genitourinary tract (Fig. 8). In girls with a persistent cloaca, Genitosonography and/or fluoroscopic genitography (with water-soluble contrast medium) should be performed (Riccabona et al 2014; Lobo 2015).

If a VCUG is performed, the modified technique should be used for orienting function assessment (see chapters "Video Urodynamics" and "Neurogenic Bladder in Infants and Children"); if available, a video-urodynamic (VUD) study is the method of choice. In boys with a rectourethral fistula, abdominal pressure can be recorded either through an existing colostomy or – if no colostomy is needed – through a microtip catheter placed in the stomach. If VUD is not available, an additional urodynamic study is recommended during the first 3 months of life in patients with concomitant sacral agenesis. Depending on the type of bladder dysfunction, a follow-up urodynamic study has to be performed after conservative – anticholinergic – therapy or surgical interventions (Lobo 2015). Imaging should be completed by echocardiography for detection of associated cardiac malformations.

> **Take away**
> The entire spectrum of imaging investigations and functional studies is necessary to detect urogenital anomalies in anorectal malformations.

5 Therapy

In general the clinical condition of the baby, the existence of other severe malformations (e.g., esophageal atresia or cardiac failure), the type of the anorectal malformation, and the severity of associated urinary tract malformation govern the timing and the order of the surgical interventions. Low atresia forms can be immediately treated in the male with a cutback procedure or in females with primary bouginage or modified translocation of the fistula. High forms may require primary colostomy with postponement of an abdominoperineal pull-through procedure in order to allow the treatment of associated anomalies. Intermediate forms can be treated by a simple posterior anorectoplasty using a perineal approach without laparotomy. In most cases this procedure may require no time delay.

The treatment of the anatomical urinary tract abnormalities is the same as it would be for similar abnormalities occurring in isolation. The treatment of functional disorders was neglected for many years. Since Boemers et al. (1996b) and other authors showed that a severe hyperreflexive bladder dysfunction may exist even before the operation, early clean intermittent catheterization, either alone or combined with parasympathetic medications or surgical measures, has been recommended for these babies from the beginning in order to avoid later deterioration of the upper urinary tract due to the voiding dysfunction. A paralytic bladder strongly suggests pelvic nerve injury secondary to a surgical pull-through procedure.

Urinary tract infection may be caused by a long rectourethral fistula remnant, as a consequence of urinary stasis with associated anomalies, a neurogenic bladder dysfunction, and/or VUR, respectively. Regular monitoring of urine specimens is necessary, with appropriate antibiotic therapy in the case of infection.

> **Take away**
> The treatment of functional or anatomical urinary tract abnormalities in patients with anorectal malformations does not differ from the treatment of those with isolated malformations.

> **Conclusion**
> Anorectal malformations have a high incidence of associated malformations. Among these, the functional and/or anatomical abnormalities of the genitourinary tract are of primary importance because of their impact on the overall morbidity and mortality of these patients. Although urogenital tract malformations can be associated in all patients with imperforate anus, there is a significantly higher incidence in the high forms of atresia and/or when lumbosacral vertebral malformations exist. Careful radiological and urodynamic investigation, including lumbosacral plain radiographs, US (of the perineum, the bladder and kidneys, and the spinal cord), and a VUD study (if available, or an urodynamic study complemented by a modified VCUG), should be performed before and/or after the pull-through procedure according to published guidelines (Boemers et al. 1999). Additionally, an MRI may become necessary in selected cases to plan a neurosurgical procedure and its appropriate timing.

References

Alamo L, Meyrat BJ, Meuwly JY, Meuli RA, Gudinchet F (2013) Anorectal malformations: finding the pathway out of the labyrinth. Radiographics 33:491–512

Berdon WE, Hochberg B, Baker DH, Grossman H, Santulli TV (1966) The association of lumbosacral spine and genitourinary anomalies with imperforate anus. Am J Radiol 98:181–191

Boemers TML, Bax KMA, Rövekamp MH, van Gool JD (1995) The effect of posterior sagittal anorectoplasty and its variants on lower urinary tract function in children with anorectal malformations. J Urol 153:191–193

Boemers TML, de Jong TPVM, van Gool JD, Bax KMA (1996a) Urologic problems in anorectal malformations. 1. Urodynamic findings and significance of sacral anomalies. J Pediatr Surg 31:407–410

Boemers TML, de Jong TPVM, van Gool JD, Bax KMA (1996b) Urologic problems in anorectal malformations. 2. Functional urologic sequelae. J Pediatr Surg 31:634–637

Boemers TML, Beek FJA, Bax NMA (1999) Guidelines for urological screening and initial management of lower urinary tract dysfunction in children with anorectal malformations – the ARGUS protocol. BJU Int 83:662–671

Carson JA, Barnes PD, Tunell WP (1984) Imperforate anus: the neurologic implication of sacral abnormalities. J Pediatr Surg 19:838–842

Duhamel B (1961) From the mermaid to anal imperforation: the syndrome of caudal regression. Arch Dis Child 36:152–155

Elliott GB, Tredwell SJ, Elliott KA (1970) The notochord as an abnormal organizer in production of congenital intestinal defect. Am J Radiol 110:628–634

Gartner L, Peiris C, Marshall M, Taylor SA, Halligan S (2013) Congenital anorectal atresia: MR imaging of late post-operative appearances in adult patients with anal incontinence. Eur Radiol 23:3318–3324

Georgeson KE, Inge TH, Albanese CT (2000) Laparoscopically assisted anorectal pull-through for high imperforate anus – a new technique. J Pediatr Surg 35:927–930

Greenfield SP, Fera M (1991) Urodynamic evaluation of the patient with an imperforate anus: a prospective study. J Urol 146:539–541

Golonka NR, Haga LJ, Keating RP, Eichelberger MR, Gilbert JC, Hartman GE, Newman KD et al (2002) Routine MRI evaluation of low imperforate anus reveals unexpected high incidence of tethered spinal cord. J Pediatr Surg 37:966–969; discussion 999

Haber HP, Seitz G, Warmann SW, Fuchs J (2007) Transperineal sonography for determination of the type of imperforate anus. AJR Am J Roentgenol 189:1525–1529

Hoekstra WJ, Scholtmeijer RJ, Molenaar JC (1983) Urogenital tract abnormalities associated with congenital anorectal anomalies. J Urol 130:962–963

Holschneider AM, Kraeft H, Scholtissek C (1982) Urodynamische Untersuchungen von Blasenentleerungsstörungen bei Analatresie und Morbus Hirschsprung. Z Kinderchir 35:64–68

Höllwarth M, Menardi G (1983) Begleitmißbildungen bei anorektalen Anomalien. In: von Kapherr H (ed) Anorektale Fehlbildungen. Fischer, Stuttgart, pp 63–67

Kakizaki H, Nonomura K, Asano Y (1994) Preexisting neurogenic voiding dysfunction in children with imperforate anus: problems in management. J Urol 151:1041–1044

Karrer FM, Flannery AM, Nelson MD (1988) Anorectal malformations: evaluation of associated spinal dysraphic syndromes. J Pediatr Surg 23:45–48

Lobo LM (2015) Recommendation for an imaging algorithm in neonatal and childhood ano-rectal/cloacal malformation. Pediatr Radiol 45:310

McLorie GA, Sheldon CA, Fleisher M (1987) The genitourinary system in patients with imperforate anus. J Pediatr Surg 22:1100–1104

Moore TC, Lawrence EA (1952) Congenital malformations of the rectum and anus: associated anomalies encountered in a series of 120 cases. Surg Gynecol Obstet 95:281–284

Murphy F, Puri P, Hutson JM (2006) Incidence and frequency of different types, and classification of anorectal malformations. In: Holschneider AM, Hutson JM (eds) Anorectal malformation in children. Springer, Heidelberg, pp 163–184

Pang D (1993) Sacral agenesis and caudal spinal cord malformations. Neurosurgery 32:755–758

Parrott TS (1985) Urologic implications of anorectal malformations. Urol Clin North Am 12:13–21

Pellerin D, Bertin P (1967) Genito-urinary malformations and vertebral anomalies in ano-rectal malformations. Z Kinderchir 4:375–383

Pena A (1967) Posterior sagittal anorectoplasty: results in management of 332 cases of anorectal malformations. Pediatr Surg Int 3:94–104

Ralph DJ, Woodhouse CRJ, Ransley PG (1992) The management of the neuropathic bladder in adolescents with imperforate anus. J Urol 148:366–368

Riccabona M, Lobo ML, Willi U, Avni F, Damasio B, Ording-Mueller LS, Blickman J, Darge K, Papadopoulou F, Vivier PH et al (2014) ESPR uroradiology task force and ESUR Paediatric Work Group – Imaging recommendations in paediatric uroradiology, part VI: childhood renal biopsy and imaging of neonatal and infant genital tract. Minutes from the task force session at the annual ESPR Meeting 2012 in Athens on childhood renal biopsy and imaging neonatal genitalia. Pediatr Radiol 44:496–502

Riccabona M, Lobo ML, Ording-Muller LS, Augdal TA, Avni FE, Blickman J, Bruno C, Damasio B, Darge K, Ntoulia A, Papadopoulou F, Vivier PH (2017) ESPR abdominal (GU and GI) imaging task force – imaging recommendations in paediatric uroradiology, part IX: imaging in anorectal and cloacal malformation, imaging in childhood ovarian torsion, and efforts in standardising pediatric uroradiology terminology. Report on the mini-symposium at the ESPR meeting in Graz, June 2015. Pediatr Radiol 47:1369–1380. https://doi.org/10.1007/s00247-017-3837-6. Epub 2017 Aug 29

Rivosecchi M, Lucchetti MC, Zaccara A (1995) Spinal dysraphism detected by magnetic resonance imaging in patients with anorectal anomalies: incidence and clinical significance. J Pediatr Surg 30:488–490

Stephens FD, Smith ED (1971) Ano-rectal malformations in children. Year Book, Chicago

Stephens FD, Smith ED (1986) Classification, identification, and assessment of surgical treatment of anorectal anomalies. Pediatr Surg Int 1:200–205

Wiener ES, Kiesewetter WB (1973) Urologic abnormalities associated with imperforate anus. J Pediatr Surg 8:151–157

Wilcox DT, Warne SA (2006) Urological problems in children with anorectal malformations. In: Holschneider AM, Hutson JM (eds) Anorectal malformations in children. Springer, Heidelberg, pp 269–279

Yeung CK, Kiely EM (1991) Low anorectal anomalies: a critical appraisal. Pediatr Surg Int 6:333–335

Epispadias-Exstrophy Complex

Erich Sorantin and Sandra Abou Samaan

Contents

1 Introduction 385
2 Incidence 386
3 Prenatal Diagnosis 386
4 Embryology 386
5 Anatomy of the Epispadias-Exstrophy Complex 387
   5.1 Epispadias 387
   5.2 Classical Bladder Exstrophy 388
   5.3 Variants 389
   5.4 Cloacal Exstrophy (Vesicointestinal Fissure) 390
6 Surgical Repair 390
   6.1 Initial Bladder Closure 391
   6.2 Epispadias Repair 392
   6.3 Bladder Neck Reconstruction 392
7 Outcome of Bladder Exstrophy 392
   7.1 Vesicoureteral Reflux 392
   7.2 Bladder Function 392
   7.3 Continence 392
   7.4 Psychosexual Function and Fertility 393
8 Imaging in Epispadias-Exstrophy Complex ... 393
Conclusion 395
References 395

E. Sorantin, MD (✉)
Department of Radiology, Division of Pediatric Radiology, Medical University Graz, Auenbruggerplatz 34, 8036 Graz, Austria
e-mail: Erich.Sorantin@medunigraz.at

S. Abou Samaan, MD
Department of Radiology, Hamad General Hospital, P.O. Box 3050, Doha, Qatar

1 Introduction

The epispadias-exstrophy complex represents a spectrum of malformations ranging from epispadias to cloacal exstrophy (Wood 1990). The most common entities of this complex and their frequencies are listed in Table 1 (Duckett and Cladamone 1985).

Historically, bladder exstrophy was first mentioned in 2000 BC. The earliest description was given in 1597 by Scheuke and Grafenberg, a complete one about 150 years later by Mowat in 1747. The term "exstrophy" was coined by Chaussier in 1780 (Kelly 1998).

Today multistage surgical repair is favored over other treatment alternatives. Due to the complexity of the problem, management of the affected patients requires close interdisciplinary teamwork involving pediatric surgery, pediatric urology, pediatric orthopedics, pediatric radiology, as well as psychological support. During all the different stages, the pediatric radiologist is responsible for the rational use of imaging modalities in order to facilitate treatment planning, to assess therapeutic success, and to detect and monitor complications.

Table 1 Types and frequencies of epispadias-exstrophy complex

Types	Frequency (%)
Classical bladder exstrophy	60
Epispadias (balanitic, penile, subsymphyseal, penopubic)	30
Cloacal exstrophy, superior vesical fissure, duplicate exstrophy, pseudoexstrophy	10

2 Incidence

Epispadias occurs in 1 in 117,000 of the population, with a 5:1 male predominance. The incidence of classical bladder exstrophy is reported to be between 1 in 10,000 and 1 in 50,000 births (Duffy 1995). There is a 3:1 male predominance. Variants of bladder exstrophy tend to occur more often in females than in males (Duckett and Cladamone 1985; Inouye et al. 2013).

The risk of occurrence is 400–500 times higher if one parent suffers from bladder exstrophy (Ben-Chaim et al. 1996; Duffy 1995). There is evidence that a slightly increased risk for bladder exstrophy or epispadias exists in children whose mothers are less than 20 years old and after in vitro fertilization (Ben-Chaim et al. 1996; Inouye et al. 2013). In addition, a possible concordance of intrauterine exposure to diazepam and occurrence of omphalocele-exstrophy-imperforate anus-spina bifida (OEIS) complex has been published (Lizscano-Gil et al. 1995). Cloacal exstrophy has an incidence of about 1:200,000 births. For this malformation no sex predominance is reported (Duckett and Cladamone 1985). Epispadias-exstrophy complex seems to be more frequent in Caucasian children than in non-Caucasian (Inouye et al. 2013).

Take Away
Bladder exstrophy is an underdiagnosed condition on prenatal US. The absence of the urinary bladder on those scans is the hallmark of bladder exstrophy.

3 Prenatal Diagnosis

Bladder exstrophy is diagnosed prenatally in only 13% of cases (Ben-Chaim et al. 1996; Dickson 2014). In a retrospective study on 43 prenatal ultrasound (US) examinations, they identified five criteria that were related to bladder exstrophy (the number in parentheses represents the estimated frequency of each symptom):

- Bladder never identified (71%)
- Lower abdominal bulge representing the exstrophied bladder (47%)
- Diminutive penis and anterior displaced scrotum (57% of males)
- Low set of the umbilicus (29%)
- Abnormal widening of iliac crests (18%)

Normally, the urinary bladder can be visualized on prenatal US after 14 weeks of gestation (Ben-Chaim et al. 1996). Therefore, in the absence of the urinary bladder on prenatal US or if any of the other abovementioned symptoms are present, the diagnosis of bladder exstrophy should be raised.

Take Away
Bladder exstrophy is more common in boys. Variants of bladder exstrophy are more common in girls. There is no sex predominance in cloacal exstrophy.

4 Embryology

The defect has to be dated within the first 8 weeks of gestation (Duffy 1995). It is believed to originate from an abnormal mesodermal migration during the development of the lower abdominal wall as well as the urogenital and anorectal canals (Duffy 1995). This mesoderm will later transform to the muscles of the abdominal wall and the urinary bladder, to the penis or clitoris, to the scrotum or labia, as well as to the bones, joints, and ligaments of the anterior pelvic girdle.

Muecke (1964) postulated that an overdevelopment of the cloacal membrane causes the abnormal mesodermal migration. After the rupture of the cloacal membrane to produce the urogenital and anal orifices, the entire urogenital tract is exposed, thus producing the exstrophic bladder and the associated epispadias (Sponseller et al. 1995). This theory is supported by the experimental findings in chicks, in which exstrophied bladders could be produced by replacing the cloacal membrane with a foreign body (Muecke 1964).

A recently published immunohistochemical study revealed that specimens of exstrophied bladders reveal fewer myelinated nerve fibers than normal individuals (Mathews et al. 1999). Normally, the innervation of the detrusor determines its ability to contract. Since the exstrophied bladder does not store any urine during intrauterine development, there is no need for contractions and innervation, which may explain the abovementioned difference in innervation (Mathews et al. 1999). Up to now it is unclear whether this finding can predict contractility of the former exstrophied bladder.

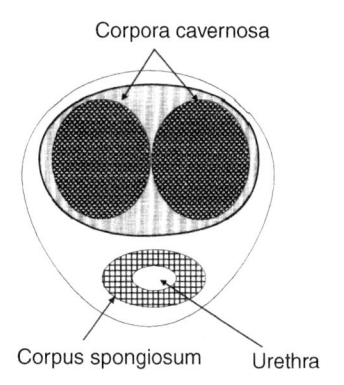

Fig. 1 Cross-sectional anatomy of a normal penis: the corpora cavernosa share a common fibrous wall (tunica albuginea corporis spongiosum)

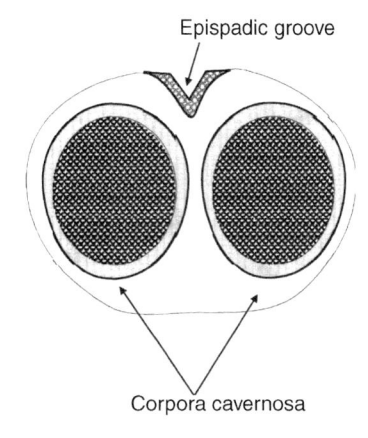

Fig. 2 Cross-sectional anatomy of an epispadiac penis: the corpora cavernosa are separated, and there is a urethral groove on the dorsal side of the penis

> **Take Away**
>
> The embryological defect producing the epispadias-exstrophy complex occurs about 8 weeks of gestation. Immunohistochemical differences between exstrophied and normal bladders exist.

5 Anatomy of the Epispadias-Exstrophy Complex

5.1 Epispadias

5.1.1 Male Epispadias

Normally, the urethra is located on the ventral side of the penis. Both corpora cavernosa are located on the dorsal side of the penis and share a common fibrous wall (Fig. 1). In male epispadiac patients, however, instead of the urethra, there is a continuous groove extending from the internal urethral orifice to the glans penis, and the corpora cavernosa are separated (Fig. 2).

Three different types can be differentiated: balanitic, penile, and penopubic (or complete) epispadias. In balanitic and penile epispadias, continence is present, and musculoskeletal deformities of bladder exstrophy are mild or absent. On the other hand, in penopubic or complete epispadias, the whole length of the penis is involved, and these patients are always incontinent to a certain degree. Usually the penis is short and stubby.

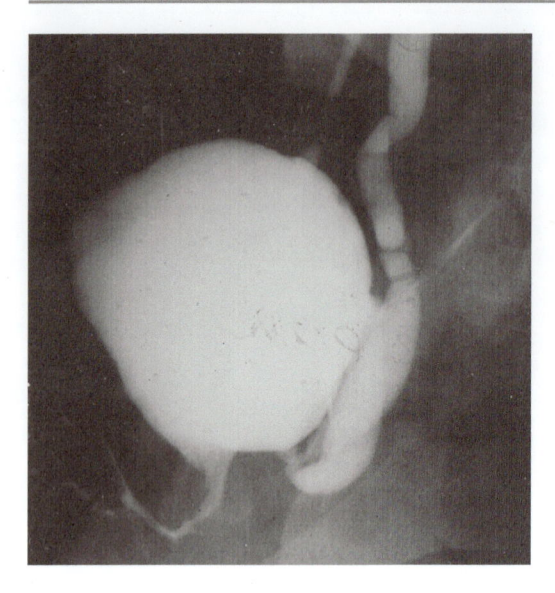

Fig. 3 Spot film of a VCUG in a baby with patient with epispadias: bilateral VUR is present as well as a hook deformity of the ureterovesical junction. The urethra is short and irregular after surgery

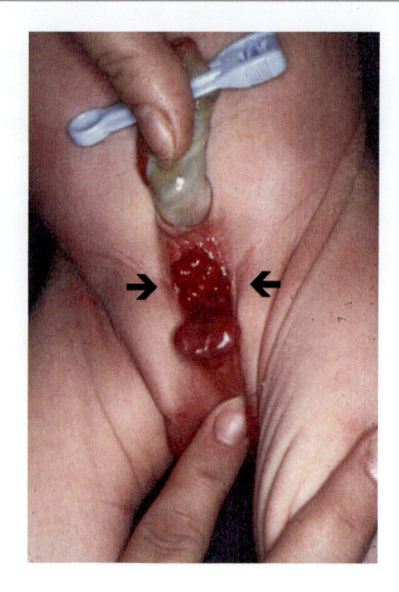

Fig. 4 Photograph of a baby boy with classic exstrophy: the umbilicus is low set, and the bladder is exstrophied (*solid arrows*). The penis is short, and the corpora cavernosa are separated by the epispadiac groove

In addition, this subtype reveals the musculoskeletal deformities of bladder exstrophy, but to a minor degree (Currarino et al. 1993).

5.1.2 Female Epispadias

Most frequently the complete or subsymphyseal type can be observed (Currarino et al. 1993). In addition, a bifid clitoris exists and the labia are abnormally separated (Currarino et al. 1993). These patients are always incontinent, and the musculoskeletal deformities of bladder exstrophy are present (Currarino et al. 1993). Minor continent forms, exhibiting an absence of the distal urethra or a short patulous urethra, eventually are accompanied by a bifid clitoris and may occasionally be seen (Currarino et al. 1993).

In 90 % of all patients with epispadias, vesicoureteral reflux (VUR) will be present. This is due to an abnormal trigone and laterally displaced ureterovesical junctions (Duckett and Cladamone 1985) (Fig. 3).

5.2 Classical Bladder Exstrophy

An excellent overview and a detailed anatomical description are given by Kelly (1998) and Wood (1990), respectively (Fig. 4).

5.2.1 Urogenital Features

The anterior wall of the abdomen is widely open over the entire dorsal surface of the penis as well as the bladder neck and the anterior bladder wall (Wood 1990). The mucosa of the exstrophied bladder is irritable and becomes hyperemic and polypoid. On histologic examination the mucosa shows cystitis cystica, cystitis glandularis, and polypoid changes (Crankscon and Ahmed 1997). If no surgical repair is undertaken, acute and chronic inflammatory changes will lead to squamous metaplasia, and malignancy may occur (Crankscon and Ahmed 1997). In addition, disorganization of the detrusor muscle bundles will occur in this situation, causing bladder dysfunction even after successful anatomical repair (Crankscon and Ahmed 1997). In affected male babies, the penis is short, and a posterior chordee causes it to curve upward to the area of the exstrophied bladder (Currarino et al. 1993). In normal individuals the corpora cavernosa fuse at the penile shaft and share a common fibrous wall with the urethra located at the anterior side of the penis. In contrast the corpora cavernosa remain separated up to the glans penis in patients with the epispadias-exstrophy complex because of the split symphysis. The epispadiac groove lies between the separated

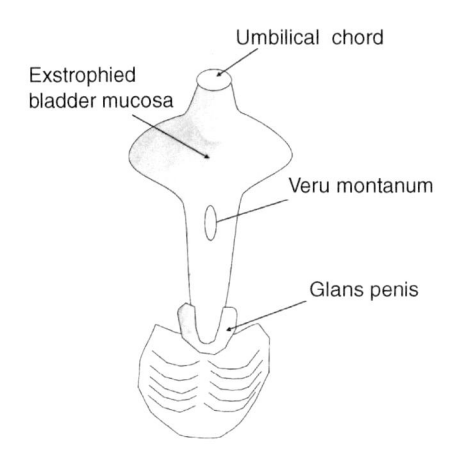

Fig. 5 Schematic urogenital findings in a male patient suffering from bladder exstrophy

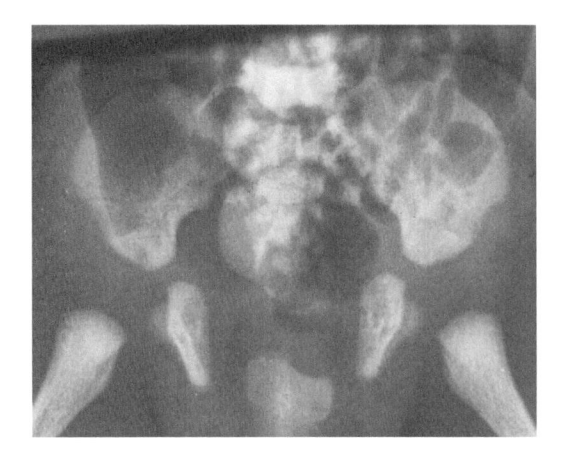

Fig. 6 Pelvic X-ray of a male baby with classic exstrophy: a split symphysis is present. The pubic and iliac bones are rotated outward with an increase in the intertriradiate distance

corpora cavernosa at the dorsum of the penis (Kelly 1998) (Fig. 5). Unilateral or bilateral cryptorchidism may be present (Currarino et al. 1993).

In females there is a short epispadiac urethra; the clitoris is bifid and may consist of two widely separated parts. The vaginal introitus is tilted upward (Crankscon and Ahmed 1997).

In patients with bladder exstrophy, associated anomalies of the upper urinary tract are infrequent (Currarino et al. 1993). However, after surgical correction VUR will be present in almost all cases of bladder exstrophy (Ben-Chaim et al. 1996 and Dickson 2014).

5.2.2 Musculoskeletal Features

The rectus abdominis muscle is deficient and widely separated. The umbilicus is low set, and an omphalocele can frequently be observed (Currarino et al. 1993). Inguinal hernias are present in up to 20% of patients, boys being more affected than girls (Connolly et al. 1995). In the later course, an incidence of inguinal hernias between 65 and 82% can be expected for males, with rates between 11 and 15% for females (Connolly et al. 1995; Husmann et al. 1990).

One of the hallmarks in bladder exstrophy is the split symphysis, where the width of the split increases with the size of the exstrophy (Currarino et al. 1993). Therefore, in bladder exstrophy the pelvic girdle appears rather C shaped instead of forming a ring. In detail, the iliac bones are rotated about 12° externally (increasing the iliac wing angle) and the pubic bones about 18° (increasing the ischiopubic angle) (Sponseller et al. 1995). Compared to normal individuals, the pubic bones tend to be shortened by 30%, and the transverse diameter of the pelvis, measured at the level of the intertriradiate cartilage, is increased by 31% (Sponseller et al. 1995). Since the corporal bodies of the penis diverge laterally to the pubic rami, the osseous malformation contributes to the short penis appearance (Sponseller et al. 1995). Figure 6 exhibits a pelvic X-ray of a patient suffering from bladder exstrophy. Vertebral malformations can be found in up to 7% (Cadeddu et al. 1997) of cases.

5.3 Variants

Pseudoexstrophy of the Bladder

This malformation is a rare variant of classical bladder exstrophy. It is characterized by the presence of the musculoskeletal defects of classic bladder exstrophy without the urinary tract defects. There is a deficient abdominal wall, and the bladder has a subcutaneous position and is only covered by a thin epithelial membrane. The umbilicus is low set, and the pubic symphysis is widened. At operation the bladder and urethra appear intact (Swana et al. 1997; Ahmed and Abu Daia 1998).

Covered Exstrophy of the Bladder
Similar to pseudoexstrophy of the bladder, the same musculoskeletal defects exist, and the closed bladder is protruding through the deficient rectus muscles. In contrast to pseudoexstrophy, the anterior bladder wall is covered by a varying degree of subcutaneous tissue and skin (Borwankar et al. 1998; Sahoo et al. 1997). A female predominance and a high incidence of genital anomalies (e.g., bifid clitoris, hypoplastic vagina, stenosed duplicated vagina) have been reported (Sahoo et al. 1997). Anorectal malformations are more common than in classical bladder exstrophy (Sahoo et al. 1997).

Superior Vesical Fissure
The musculoskeletal features of classic bladder exstrophy can be observed as well as a minimal bladder eventration below an abnormally low-set umbilicus (Borwankar et al. 1998; Sahoo et al. 1997).

Inferior Vesical Fissure
To date only a few cases have been reported (Johnson et al. 1995). Bladder exstrophy is limited to the bladder neck, whereas the penis and urethra are normal. Split symphysis is present too.

Duplicate Exstrophy
Duplicate exstrophy is comprised of a normal bladder and an additional exstrophied bladder. Complete and incomplete entities have been reported (Perren and Frey 1998).

Bladder Exstrophy with Normal Umbilicus and Normal Infraumbilical Wall
There was a case that was reported revealing the abovementioned features (Sripathi et al. 1997).

OEIS Complex
Bladder exstrophy can be part of the omphalocele-exstrophy-imperforate anus-spinal defects (OEIS) complex. The OEIS complex is rare and affects only 1 in 200,000 to 1 in 400,000 pregnancies (Smith et al. 1992).

5.4 Cloacal Exstrophy (Vesicointestinal Fissure)

5.4.1 Urogenital and Intestinal Features

There are two halves of the exstrophied bladder separated by an exstrophied ileocecal bowel area. On the rostral side of the bowel exstrophy, the ileum prolapses. In addition there is an imperforate anus, and the colon may be duplicated. Usually a duplicated appendix is found. In males a small and duplicated penis can be seen. In females the vagina is septet, and uterine abnormalities are likely. A high proportion of these patients will also present a small to giant omphalocele (Duckett and Cladamone 1985).

5.4.2 Musculoskeletal Features

The same skeletal features as in classic bladder exstrophy can be observed. Myelomeningoceles are present in 50% of these patients. Spinal abnormalities are common.

> **Take Away**
> All subtypes of the epispadias-exstrophy complex exhibit a split symphysis to a certain degree. Incontinent epispadias is more common than continent epispadias. In addition to classic bladder exstrophy, covered variants exist. Cloacal exstrophy represents the most severe part of the spectrum, comprising urogenital, intestinal, and musculoskeletal malformations.

6 Surgical Repair

The overall goal of treatment in patients with the epispadias-exstrophy complex is the well, dry, fertile, and happy (both cosmetically and functionally) adult (Kelly 1998).

Today staged surgical repair is favored, consisting of the steps described in Sects. 6.1, 6.2, and 6.3 (Wood 1990; Kelly 1998; Ben-Chaim et al. 1996; Ben-Chaim and Gearhart 1996;

Canning 1996). Recently an excellent overview, the "Modern Staged Repair of Bladder Exstrophy," was published (Dickson 2014).

Urinary diversion using bowel segments is no longer the first treatment choice due to its inherent disadvantages such as the need for intermittent catheterization through a reconstructed urethra, mucus plugs, bladder infection, electrolyte disturbances, stones, disruption of the anastomosis, long-term potential for renal deterioration, and bladder or bowel cancer (Kelly 1998; Canning 1996). Bladder augmentation can be regarded as an alternative approach for patients where the staged repair has failed (Kelly 1998). In these patients bladder augmentation can improve the quality of life significantly.

6.1 Initial Bladder Closure

Due to improvements in anesthesia and postoperative care, surgical correction of the exstrophied bladder and osteotomies can be done safely within the neonatal period. Newborns are under the influence of the maternal hormone (relaxin). Therefore if bladder closure is performed within 72 h of life, there is a good chance of achieving pelvic closure without osteotomies. Of course the size of the symphyseal split represents a prognostic factor (Kelly 1998; Ben-Chaim and Gearhart 1996). In addition, the swelling of the exstrophied bladder mucosa is less severe within the time frame of 72 h. If closure is delayed, osteotomies will become necessary more frequently (Inouye et al. 2013). If the male urethral plate is too short, it can be elongated by paraexstrophy flaps using the paraexstrophy tissue as described by Duckett and Cladamone (1985; see also Kelly 1998; Ben-Chaim et al. 1996). It is mandatory to follow the principles of plastic surgery to maintain good blood supply to the flaps. The urethra is closed proximally in order to stimulate bladder growth, and ureteral stents are placed to prevent obstruction and hypertension (Ben-Chaim et al. 1996). Coexisting omphaloceles and inguinal hernias should also be repaired (Kelly 1998; Connolly et al. 1995; Husmann et al. 1990).

Postoperative complications include ischemia of paraexstrophy flaps, thus leading to urethral strictures (Kelly 1998; Ben-Chaim et al. 1996; Ben-Chaim and Gearhart 1996). Suprapubic leakage is another problem, but usually there is spontaneous closure within several months. VUR is present in almost all cases postoperatively (Currarino et al. 1993; Dickson 2014). Two children were reported who developed significant hypertension postoperatively after primary bladder closure and pelvic osteotomies followed by immobilization using skin traction (Husmann et al. 1993). In both children hypertension subsided spontaneously after removal of the immobilization.

Failed bladder exstrophy closure is defined by wound dehiscence, bladder prolapse, bladder outlet obstruction, or formation of fistulas (Fig. 7, Inouye et al. 2013). Pelvic osteotomies and postoperative immobilization were reported

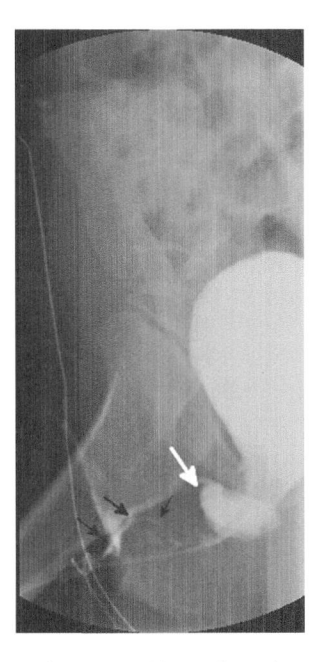

Fig. 7 Screenshot from videourodynamics of a 5-year-old boy. There is bag-like dilatation of the proximal posterior urethra (*white arrow*) due to surgery as well as a system of multiple penile fistulas (*black arrows*)

to decrease the rate of failure (Inouye et al. 2013).

6.2 Epispadias Repair

Epispadias repair is performed at the age of one up to 3 years (Dickson 2014).

Testosterone can be given 2 weeks preoperatively in order to stimulate penile skin growth, thus making the surgical repair easier.

For epispadias repair several procedures are available like the Cantwell-Ranswell and variants (Kelly 1998; Ben-Chaim et al. 1996; Canning 1996; Husmann et al. 1993). Briefly, the urethra is tubularized over a catheter. The corporal bodies are freed completely from the glans and the proximal urethra, then rotated inward, and sutured together. The procedure is finished by reconstruction of the glans and moving the distal end of the urethra to the ventral side of the penis. Penile ischemia can lead to an asymmetric appearance of the penis afterward.

6.3 Bladder Neck Reconstruction

Bladder neck reconstruction is undertaken at the age of 4–5 years, where it can be expected that the child can cooperate actively with toilet training. A prerequisite for bladder neck repair is a bladder capacity of more than 60 ml (Ben-Chaim et al. 1996) or 100 ml, respectively (Dickson 2014). Today the Young-Dees-Leadbetter procedure is recommended (Inouye et al. 2013).

Since nearly all patients suffer from VUR, new ureteral implantation must also be performed too. Afterward muscle flaps are created from the mid-trigone to the prostatic urethra, and these flaps are closed over a catheter in order to produce a bladder neck. In cases where the bladder neck is wide open or continence is inadequate, submucosal injection of Teflon, collagen, or silicone microspheres can be an alternative treatment choice (Kelly 1998).

> **Take Away**
> Management of bladder exstrophy aims to result in a well, dry, fertile, and happy (both cosmetically and functionally) adult. Therapy of bladder exstrophy consists of staged surgical repair. Factors for successful outcome of bladder closure have been identified. VUR is common after bladder closure.

7 Outcome of Bladder Exstrophy

7.1 Vesicoureteral Reflux

Vesicoureteral reflux will be present in nearly all patients after bladder closure, thus making antireflux surgery necessary. Pyelonephritis and renal scarring are reported to occur in 25–50 % of patients (Hollowell et al. 1992).

7.2 Bladder Function

Generally, besides bladder capacity, urodynamic parameters decline after bladder neck reconstruction, thus leading to the search for alternative surgical strategies (Canning 1996). After bladder closure, up to 80 % of patients will have normal filling urodynamics before bladder neck reconstruction (Canning 1996; Diamond et al. 1999). Following bladder neck reconstruction, only 25 % of patients will exhibit normal detrusor function (Canning 1996; Diamond et al. 1999; Stein et al. 1994). Bladder capacity is about one-third of the expected age-matched bladder capacity before bladder neck repair and will be about half of the expected bladder capacity afterward (Diamond et al. 1999).

7.3 Continence

Kelly evaluated achieved continence in a series of 26 patients older than 6 years who underwent sphincter reconstruction at the Royal Children's Hospital Melbourne (Kelly 1998). Patients were classified as being physiologically continent (voluntary urinary control, only sporadic nighttime wetting), socially continent (imperfect bladder control, adjustments for daily life such as pads necessary), or incontinent (urine leakage cannot be prevented). Of these 26 patients, 40 % belonged to the physiologically continent group, 30 % to the socially continent group, and 30 % were incontinent. Therefore, it can be expected that about two-thirds of the patients will achieve some kind of continence after surgical repair of bladder exstrophy. In recent publications, these figures were reported to be improved (Dickson 2014). About 70 % of patients are dry during day and night, and 15–20% being incontinent with no significant sex difference.

7.4 Psychosexual Function and Fertility

It has been reported that about 70 % of adolescents and 33 % of younger school-aged children will have behavioral, social, and school competency problems (Ben-Chaim et al. 1996). The beginning of sexual activity seemed to be delayed. Following staged repair of bladder exstrophy, males will be able to have erections, but about one-third will describe the erections as unsatisfactory due to the small penis appearance. Only a minority will father children, mainly because of obstruction of the ejaculatory ducts and associated infections. Retrograde ejaculation seems to be an additional problem (Ben-Chaim and Gearhart 1996). Similar findings were reported by Stein et al. (1994), who investigated 101 patients after urinary diversion with and without genital reconstruction. No male with genital reconstruction could ejaculate normally and had fathered children, whereas all patients without genital reconstruction could ejaculate normally, and 40 % had fathered children (Stein et al. 1994). Therefore, genital reconstruction and closure of the urethra in males are burdened with the risk of infertility.

Recently Salem et al. reported a long-term evaluation in male patients with bladder exstrophy (Salem and Eisa 2012). One-third of those patients were married, 40 % of those having fathered children, 75 % of them after normal conception, and 25 % using assisted reproductive techniques.

However, 92 % of women are satisfied with the cosmetic outcome. Nearly all woman can engage in sexual intercourse, but a quarter consider it as unpleasant or painful (Stein et al. 1994). Pregnancies have been reported to occur (Ben-Chaim et al. 1996; Stein et al. 1994).

> **Take Away**
> In up to three-quarters of patients, behavioral, social, and school competency problems can be expected. The majority of patients will be sexually active. In males, genital reconstruction seems to be burdened by the risk of infertility. The majority of women will be satisfied with the cosmetic outcome, and pregnancies occur.

8 Imaging in Epispadias-Exstrophy Complex

Various imaging modalities are involved during the tortuous course of patients suffering from the epispadias-exstrophy complex (Wood 1990). In newborns with bladder exstrophy, *chest films* are taken as a part of the preoperative workup within the first days of life. *Pelvic X-rays* depict the skeletal deformity. *Plain films of the lumbar spine* should be evaluated with the chest film for vertebral anomalies.

Ultrasound examinations of the entire abdomen (including kidneys) and the spinal canal should be performed to assess coexisting malformations. In the case of premature babies, the US study should be completed by a cranial US for the evaluation of intraventricular hemorrhage. After bladder closure, *voiding cystourethrography* (VCUG) is the method of choice for demonstration and grading of VUR. Using Fotter's modified VCUG technique, functional information regarding detrusor contractions can be obtained during the same investigation (Fotter et al. 1986; Fotter 1992, 1994, 1996) (see chapters "Video Urodynamics" and "Neurogenic Bladder in Infants and Children").

Complete workup of the lower urinary tract regarding the simultaneous assessment of morphology and functional disorders can be achieved by videourodynamics, if available (see chapter "Video Urodynamics"). Since the bladder outlet and urethral morphology are of particular interest in these patients, at any time of the staged surgical correction, there is no role for a direct radionuclide cystogram and ce-VUS.

Renal US, potentially including 3D US and volumetry, will allow noninvasive monitoring of kidney growth. Furthermore, dilatation of the pelvico-caliceal system can be detected. In cases of suspected reflux nephropathy, isotope studies (DMSA scans) or MR urography should be performed (Riccabona 2007). Added Doppler sonography assesses renal perfusion in the long term. Serial US examinations of the urinary bladder, including the estimation of the residual urine, give information about bladder filling capacity and the voiding function. There is a role for 3D US, which provides the generation of 3D anatomic images and allows more accurate estimations of bladder volume than those derived from two orthogonal sections using the ellipsoid formula (Riccabona et al. 1996).

For long times intravenous urography (IVU) was the standard method for the evaluation of the upper urinary tract in terms of morphology, semi-quantitative estimation of kidney function, and dynamics of urinary drainage. This has been replaced by MR urography which is now the method of choice (Riccabona 2007); IVU is reserved to a limited number of patients with special questions especially after surgery or if MRI is not available.

After antireflux surgery serial US examinations including color Doppler sonography (CDS) are mandatory. It has to be mentioned that a decreasing size of pelvico-caliceal dilatation, after an initial increase, can be also caused by a decrease in renal urine production, i.e., kidney function. Dynamic scintigraphy can be helpful in this situation; technique of and indication for other imaging modalities should follow the (procedural) recommendations of the ESPR "Abdominal (GI & GU) Imaging Task Force" (Riccabona et al. 2008, 2009, 2010).

For the standardized and reproducible assessment of the split renal function and urine drainage, isotope studies are performed. Nowadays MR urography may represent an alternative, thus avoiding the hazards of radiation (Riccabona 2007).

For imaging of the skeletal features in the epispadias-exstrophy complex, especially in patients who did not undergo pelvic osteotomies, multislice computed tomography or musculoskeletal MR with subsequent 3D reconstructions provides a valuable tool. The underlying skeletal deformities can be assessed and the necessary parameters obtained, as needed for orthopedic correction (Yazici et al. 1998; Gargollo et al. 2005).

Magnetic resonance imaging is the best choice for imaging of spinal problems beyond the neonatal period. Patients suffering from cloacal exstrophy and coexisting myelomeningoceles can be evaluated for postoperative complications such as the tethered cord syndrome. In addition, in these patients MRI can be used for assessment of the pelvic floor, the urinary bladder, the gonads, the uterus, and the rectum.

Take Away

Still plain films of the chest, the pelvis and the spine are mandatory. In the neonatal period, US can be used for assessment of coexisting renal and spinal malformations. Modified VCUG assesses both lower urinary tract function and morphology.

Videourodynamics, if available, allows complete workup of the lower urinary tract. After antireflux surgery serial US examinations and an abbreviated IVU can be helpful in troublesome cases of evaluation of urine drainage.

MR urography is increasingly becoming the noninvasive alternative for isotope studies.

Conclusion

The epispadias-exstrophy complex represents a spectrum of malformations ranging from epispadias to cloacal exstrophy, with classical bladder exstrophy being the most common form occurring more frequently in boys. Several variants exist which are more frequent in girls. Concomitant malformations are present. Today treatment consists of a staged surgical repair. VUR is one of the most frequent complications. Imaging must be directed to detect associated malformations as well as to monitor surgical success. Moreover imaging should follow international established guidelines such as those from the ESPR Abdominal (GI & GU) Imaging Task Force.

References

Ahmed S, Abu Daia J (1998) Exstrophic abdominal wall defect without bladder exstrophy (pseudo-exstrophy). Br J Urol 81:762–763

Ben-Chaim J, Gearhart JP (1996) Current management of bladder exstrophy. Tech Urol 2:22–33

Ben-Chaim J, Docimo S, Jeffs RD (1996) Bladder exstrophy from childhood into adult life. J R Soc Med 89:39–46

Borwankar SS, Kasat LS, Naregal A (1998) Covered exstrophy: a rare variant. Pediatr Surg Int 14:129–130

Cadeddu JA, Benson JE, Silver RI (1997) Spinal abnormalities in classic bladder exstrophy. Br J Urol 79:975–978

Canning DA (1996) Bladder exstrophy: the case for primary bladder reconstruction. J Urol 48:831–834

Connolly JA, Peppas DS, Jeffs RD (1995) Prevalence and repair of inguinal hernias in children with bladder exstrophy. J Urol 154:1900–1901

Crankscon SJ, Ahmed S (1997) Female bladder exstrophy. Int Urogynecol J Pelvic Floor Dysfunct 8:98–104

Currarino G, Wood B, Majd M (1993) The genitourinary tract and retroperitoneum–epispadias-exstrophy complex. In: Silverman F, Kuhn J (eds) Caffey's pediatric X-ray diagnosis. An integrated imaging approach. Mosby, St. Louis, pp 1298–1301

Dickson AP (2014) The management of bladder exstrophy: the Manchester experience. J Pediatr Surg 49(2):244–250

Diamond DA, Bauer SB, Dinlenc C (1999) Normal urodynamics in patients with bladder exstrophy: are they achievable? J Urol 162:841–845

Duckett JW, Cladamone AA (1985) Bladder and urachus. In: Kelalis PP, King LR, Belman AB (eds) Clinical pediatric urology. Saunders, Philadelphia, pp 726–742

Duffy PG (1995) Bladder exstrophy. Semin Pediatr Surg 5:129–132

Fotter R (1992) Functional disorders of the lower urinary tract: urodynamic and radiological diagnosis. In: Thomsen HS (ed) European uroradiology 1992. FADL, Copenhagen, pp 127–132

Fotter R (1994) Children. In: Dalla Palma L, Thomsen HS (eds) European uroradiology 1994. FADL, Copenhagen, pp 120–127

Fotter R (1996) Neurogenic bladder in infants and children–a new challenge for the radiologist. Abdom Imaging 21:534–540

Fotter R, Kopp W, Klein E, Höllwarth M, Uray E (1986) Unstable bladder in children: functional evaluation by modified voiding cystourethrography. Radiology 161:811–813

Gargollo PC, Borer JG, Retik AB (2005) Magnetic resonance imaging of pelvic musculoskeletal and genitourinary anatomy in patients before and after complete repair of bladder exstrophy. J Urol 174:1559–1566

Hollowell JG, Hill PD, Duffy PG (1992) Lower urinary tract function after exstrophy closure. Pediatr Nephrol 6:428–432

Husmann DA, McLorie GA, Churchill BM, Ein SH (1990) Inguinal pathology and is association with classical bladder exstrophy. J Pediatr Surg 25:332–334

Husmann DA, McLorie GA, Churchill BM (1993) Hypertension following primary bladder closure for vesical exstrophy. J Pediatr Surg 28:239–241

Inouye BM, Massanyi EZ, Di Carlo H, Shah BB, Gearhart JP (2013) Modern management of bladder exstrophy repair. Curr Urol Rep 14(4):359–365

Johnson P, Sarin YK, Kapoor R (1995) Inferior vesical fissure. J Urol 154:1478

Kelly CH (1998) Exstrophy and epispadias: Kelly's method of repair. In: O'Neill JA (ed) Pediatric surgery, 5th edn. Mosby, St. Louis, pp 1732–1759

Lizscano-Gil LA, Garcia-Cruz D, Sanchez-Corona J (1995) Omphalocele–exstrophy–imperforate anus–spina bifida complex in a male prenatally exposed to diazepam. Arch Med Res 26:95–96

Mathews R, Wills M, Perlman E (1999) Neural innervation of the newborn exstrophic bladder: an immunohistochemical study. J Urol 162:506–508

Muecke EC (1964) The role of the cloacal membrane in exstrophy: the first successful experimental study. J Urol 92:659

Perren F, Frey P (1998) The exstrophy-epispadias complex in the duplicated lower urinary tract. J Urol 159:1681–1683

Riccabona M (2004) Pediatric MRU – its potential and its role in the diagnostic work-up of upper urinary tract dilatation in infants and children. World J Urol 22;79–87

Riccabona M, Avni FE, Blickman JG (2008) Imaging recommendations in paediatric uroradiology: minutes of the ESPR workgroup session on urinary tract infection, fetal hydronephrosis, urinary tract ultrasonography and voiding cystourethrography, Barcelona, Spain, June 2007. Pediatr Radiol 38(2):138–145

Riccabona M, Avni FE, Blickman JG (2009) Imaging recommendations in paediatric uroradiology. Minutes of the ESPR uroradiology task force session on childhood obstructive uropathy, high-grade fetal hydronephrosis, childhood haematuria, and urolithiasis in childhood. ESPR Annual Congress, Edinburgh, UK, June 2008. Pediatr Radiol 39(8):891–898

Riccabona M, Avni FE, Dacher JN (2010) ESPR uroradiology task force and ESUR paediatric working group: imaging and procedural recommendations in paediatric uroradiology, part III. Minutes of the ESPR uroradiology task force minisymposium on intravenous urography, uro-CT and MR-urography in childhood. Pediatr Radiol 40: 1315–1320

Riccabona M, Nelson TR, Pretorius DH, Davidson TE (1996) In vivo three–dimensional sonographic measurement of organ volume: validation in the urinary bladder. J Ultrasound Med 15: 627–632

Sahoo SP, Gangopadhyay AN, Sinha CK (1997) Covered exstrophy: a rare variant of classical bladder exstrophy. Scand J Urol Nephrol 31:103–106

Salem HK, Eisa M (2012) Long-term follow-up (18–35 years) of male patients with history of bladder exstrophy (BE) repair in childhood: erectile function and fertility potential outcome. J Sex Med 9(5):1466–1472. doi:10.1111/j1743-6109-2011-02536.x

Smith NM, Chambers HM, Furness ME (1992) The OEIS complex (omphalocele-exstrophy–imperforate anus–spinal defects): recurrence in sibs. J Med Genet 29: 730–732

Sponseller BD, Bisson LJ, Gearhart JP (1995) The anatomy of the pelvis in the exstrophy complex. J Bone Joint Surg Am 77:177–189

Sripathi V, Sen S, Ahmed S (1997) Normal umbilicus and infra-umbilical abdominal wall in bladder exstrophy. Br J Urol 80:672

Stein R, Stockle M, Fisch M (1994) The fate of the adult exstrophy patient. J Urol 152:1413–1416

Swana HS, Gallagher PG, Weiss RM (1997) Pseudoexstrophy of the bladder: case report and literature review. J Pediatr Surg 32:1480–1481

Wood BP (1990) Cloacal malformations and exstrophy syndromes. Radiology 177:326–327

Yazici M, Sözübir S, Kilicoglu G (1998) Three-dimensional anatomy of the pelvis in bladder exstrophy: description of bone pathology by using three-dimensional computed tomography and its clinical relevance. J Pediatr Orthop 18:132–135

Non-neurogenic Bladder-Sphincter Dysfunction ("Voiding Dysfunction")

Michael Riccabona and Richard Fotter

Contents

1 Introduction.. 397
2 Terminology: Categorization.......................... 398
3 Incidence.. 400
4 Physiology.. 401
5 Toilet Training (Bladder Control)................... 402
6 Pathophysiology.. 402
7 Constipation... 404
8 Urinary Tract Infection (UTI) and Uretero-vesical Reflux (VUR) in Voiding Dysfunction...................................... 405
9 Enuresis and Incontinence............................. 407
10 Non-neurogenic Bladder-Sphincter Dysfunction in Neonates and Infants........... 410
11 Modified Voiding Cystourethrography (VCUG)... 413
12 Evaluation.. 415
Conclusion.. 417
References.. 418

M. Riccabona, MD (✉)
Department of Radiology, Division of Pediatric Radiology, University Hospital Graz, Auenbruggerplatz 34, 8036 Graz, Austria
e-mail: michael.riccabona@meduni-graz.at

R. Fotter, MD (Retired)
Department of Radiology, Formerly Division of Pediatric Radiology, Medical University Graz, Auenbruggerplatz 34, 8036 Graz, Austria

1 Introduction

Non-neurogenic bladder-sphincter dysfunction ("voiding dysfunction") is a very common childhood disorder that all pediatric urologists, pediatricians, and (pediatric) radiologists encounter in their daily practice (Farhat et al. 2000). The most common clinical presentations are recurrent urinary tract infections (UTI), vesicoureteral reflux (VUR), and daytime and/or nighttime wetting. If constipation and/or encopresis are associated with non-neurogenic bladder-sphincter dysfunction ("voiding dysfunction"), it is called dysfunctional elimination syndrome (Koff et al. 1998; Austin et al. 2014). One or more of the clinical symptoms of voiding dysfunctions were reported in 26% of 7-year-old Swedish children; most had moderate urgency as a sign of incomplete voluntary bladder control (Hellström et al. 1990).

The prevalence of daytime wetting has been reported to be 0.2–9% in children aged 6–12 years, with daytime wetting more common in girls than in boys (Bakker et al. 2002; Lee et al. 2000; Swithinbank et al. 1994). Combined daytime and nighttime wetting occurs in 1.5–2.8% (Lee et al. 2000; Gür et al. 2004; Järvelin et al. 1988). Therefore, voiding dysfunction in children should not be seen as an isolated phenomenon. It should always be seen in the context of the pertinent clinical symptoms, in particular frequency, urge, and (urge) incontinence, and it should be seen as one among other risks or predisposing factors such as VUR of the disease complex urinary tract infection-permanent renal damage (Yeung et al. 2006a, b; Batisky 1996), which in addition are very closely associated (Chen et al. 2004). Furthermore, "voiding dysfunction" probably is also a causal factor for the development of VUR (Barroso et al. 2001; Koff et al. 1979; Nasrallah and Simon 1984; Homsy et al. 1985; Scholtmeijer and Nijman 1994; Koff 1992).

However, in textbooks and scientific publications, VUR and non-neurogenic bladder-sphincter dysfunction are commonly dealt with separately; furthermore, only little new knowledge has been published over the last decade, whereas increasingly nice overview articles are available (Nepple and Cooper 2014). As a clinical consequence, regular management often consists of ad hoc treatment for every UTI with only minor attention to an underlying bladder dysfunction. This monosymptomatic approach may cause undue morbidity from non-neurogenic bladder-sphincter dysfunction and UTIs in a group of patients with a prevalence as high as 40 % for VUR and 30 % for reflux nephropathy (Van Gool 1995; Koff et al. 1979; Griffith and Scholtmeijer 1987; Van Gool et al. 1992a). This problem is further enhanced by a mislabeling: The nighttime component of wetting is often misinterpreted as enuresis nocturna, although the wetting is not exclusively at nighttime (Van Gool 1995).

In addition, numerous definitions and categories are in use for non-neurogenic bladder-sphincter dysfunction, blaming either the bladder or the urethral sphincter for the various clinical expressions. In this chapter not only the spectrum of voiding dysfunction will be described but how dysfunction is embedded into a disease; complex UTI and renal damage will be shown. Furthermore, the associations and the causal relationship to VUR, UTI, renal damage, and constipation will be discussed, and the various clinical manifestations will be elucidated.

In the past imaging and research predominantly were focused on VUR, and pediatric radiologists mostly were not adequately aware of the important role that non-neurogenic bladder-sphincter dysfunction plays in this common nephrourologic disease complex. Though voiding dysfunction is one of the most underestimated topics in pediatric uroradiological daily work, education, and research, still pediatric radiologists are often the first and only experts who get in touch with those children. Missing recognition of dysfunction may lead to treatment delay or failure; it may also increase treatment costs (Benoit et al. 2002). Furthermore, it may lead to reimplantation surgery failure, and last but not least, it may lead to renal damage.

2 Terminology: Categorization

Different terminologies and categorizations have been used for children who present with varying degrees of "functional" urinary symptoms. Some are based on the urodynamic pattern (reflecting the underlying pathophysiology and the diagnosis), others on clinical presentation. The term "urge syndrome" has been used to describe both the clinical symptoms and the overactivity of the detrusor muscle (unstable bladder). As uninhibited detrusor contractions – the underlying pathology of unstable bladder – cannot be demonstrated in all children during a urodynamic study, although the symptoms are indicative of an overactive detrusor, it would be better to use the term unstable bladder or overactive bladder for these patients presenting with frequency and urge – with or without incontinence. Over the last years, numerous articles dealing with all aspects of non-neurogenic bladder-sphincter dysfunction in infants and children have been published, though little new insight has been presented in the last 15 years.

A broad spectrum of terms is still in use for sometimes overlapping patterns of pediatric non-neurogenic bladder-sphincter dysfunction, such as non-neuropathic vesicourethral dysfunction (Koff 1984), overactivity of the bladder and striated urethral muscle (Van Gool et al. 1984), non-neuropathic or non-neurogenic bladder-sphincter dysfunction (Hoebecke et al. 1999), dysfunctional bladder (Hinman 1986), unstable bladder (Koff 1982), non-neurogenic neurogenic bladder (Allen 1977), and Hinman syndrome (Hinman 1986).

Non-neurogenic neurogenic bladder or the so-called *Hinman syndrome* is the extreme end of the spectrum of non-neurogenic bladder-sphincter dysfunction. This syndrome shows severe clinical manifestations including urinary retention, severe bladder-sphincter dysfunction, VUR, hydronephrosis and hydroureter, as well as renal scarring (see respective other chapters in this book).

Voiding dysfunction is a rather vague, today commonly used overall term in the literature for urinary symptoms resulting from non-neurogenic bladder-sphincter dysfunction. It presents with a mixture of lower urinary tract symptoms – in particular urge, urge incontinence, frequency, infrequency, and UTI. Furthermore, voiding dysfunction is used as a misnomer for *dysfunctional voiding*. This term describes a sign and is now used in an imprecise way as well, because it is indiscriminately applied to two pathophysiologically different disturbances that may overlap and coincide but may require different treatment. One is overactivity of the detrusor during bladder filling, which is represented by uninhibited detrusor contractions (*unstable or overactive bladder*). The other is overactivity of the external urethral sphincter during voiding (*dysfunctional voiding* in particular) (Koff 1982). These children may also demonstrate uninhibited detrusor contractions indicative for unstable bladder on urodynamic studies and clinically often present with urge and frequency, with or without incontinence.

There are at least three theories on how those two patterns of dysfunction are seen in terms of categorization and treatment. In the first, there are two distinct entities that can manifest in isolation or in combination. The second theory states that there is a spectrum ranging from minor unstable detrusor contractions during higher filling volumes of the bladder to the full-blown type, the so-called Hinman syndrome at the far end of the spectrum. The third theory claims that the two entities are closely related and are two components of the dysfunctional voiding complex with different expression. Referring to the latter theory, there is disagreement about whether the primary abnormality is overactivity of the detrusor during bladder filling or overactivity of the external urethral sphincter during voiding.

Bauer (1992) grouped into primarily unstable bladder (small capacity, hypertonic bladders, and detrusor hyperreflexia), infrequent voiding associated with large-capacity bladders (lazy bladder syndrome), and psychogenic non-neuropathic bladder.

Others such as Van Gool et al. (1992a, b) and Hjälmas (1992) published other urodynamic classifications. Hjälmas (1992) described unstable bladder, sphincter dyscoordination, lazy bladder, and occult neurogenic bladder. Van Gool et al. (1992a) divided conditions into two main groups, urge syndrome and dysfunctional voiding; the latter is subdivided into staccato voiding, fractionated voiding, and lazy bladder syndrome.

Mayo and Burns (1990) confirmed the hypothesis that children with bladder instability and dysfunctional voiding represent two separate groups. They described one group with instability alone and a second group with dysfunctional voiding with or without instability. They found infection and/or VUR to be common in the former, the more devastating urinary tract changes to occur in the latter group, particularly heavy trabeculation of the bladder.

This confusing use of different terms in original articles, editorials, and review articles makes it not only difficult for the reader to understand this important topic but inhibits comparative research on diagnosis, treatment, outcome, and costs. Therefore, a standardization of lower urinary tract dysfunction in children has been published by the International Children's Continence Society (Nørgaard et al. 1998, Nijman 2000). Two main dysfunctions are classified: unstable bladder (urge syndrome) and dysfunctional voiding (Table 1). The authors state that those disorders might not be the completely separate entities they seem, as transitional phases between urge syndrome and dysfunctional voiding do occur. Also, the associated complex of functional incontinence and recurrent urinary tract infection (UTI) may start with detrusor overactivity and hold maneuvers with a gradual progression to fractioned and incomplete voiding (dysfunctional voiding).

All these rather divergent discussions on terminology and categories can be reduced to one common pathophysiological denominator: impaired coordination between the smooth muscle of the

Table 1 Voiding disorders – definition and symptoms

Normal voiding (toilet-trained children = as in healthy adults)
Definition:
No involuntary/uninhibited detrusor contractions during bladder filling,
No contractions at full bladder even with physiologic urge
Coordinated relaxation of external urethral sphincter when voiding = low intravesical pressure during emptying
Detrusor-sphincter dysfunction during bladder filling (unstable bladder):
Primary abnormality = failure to voluntarily suppress involuntary detrusor contractions
Includes all stages
From minor unstable detrusor contractions at large filling volume to high-amplitude unstable detrusor contractions at less filling, potentially combined with urge
Compensation by voluntary constriction of external urethral sphincter to stay dry, causing increased intravesical pressure
Leads to (urge) incontinence (clinically daytime wetting) or "hidden instability" with less specific voiding symptoms (clinically frequency and urge, UTI with/without VUR, constipation and/or fecal soiling)
Detrusor-sphincter dysfunction during micturition (dysfunctional voiding):
Overactivity of urethral closure mechanism during voiding
Most severe form in childhood = Hinman syndrome, non-neurogenic neurogenic bladder
Less common – clinically fecal retention/soiling, emotional disturbance, psychosocial problems
Bladder trabeculation, diverticula, VUR, and upper tract dilatation, large post-void residual urine volume
Three main forms:
Staccato voiding – caused by bursts of pelvic floor activity during voiding, resulting in bladder pressure peaks with interrupted urinary flow
Fractioned voiding – caused by detrusor muscle hypoactivity, voiding = several unsustained detrusor contractions, low voiding frequency, large bladder capacity
Lazy bladder syndrome – long-standing dysfunctional voiding and resulting detrusor decompensation, voiding achieved by abdominal pressure; leads to large residual urine volume

Adapted from Riccabona (2012)

urinary bladder (the detrusor muscle) and the striated muscle of the external urethral sphincter (pelvic floor muscles) which leads to repeated pathologically high intravesical pressure during bladder filling and/or voiding with all its negative consequences for the bladder, the ureterovesical junction, the ureteric orifices, the ureters, and the kidneys.

> **Take Away**
> The classification of the International Children's Continence Society should be used to eliminate confusion, to facilitate and enable comparative research and meta-analyses. This classification recognizes two main dysfunctions: overactive bladder or unstable bladder (urge syndrome) and dysfunctional voiding. The common denominator of lower urinary tract dysfunction is bladder-sphincter dyscoordination leading to chronic high intravesical pressure with resulting negative consequences for the urinary tract.

3 Incidence

Bauer et al. (1980) found that the majority of children with urinary tract dysfunction had an unstable bladder, and only a small number had the severest type of dysfunction, which is called non-neurogenic neurogenic bladder (Allen 1977). Schulman et al. (1999) described an unstable bladder or urge syndrome in 52 % of cases of non-neurogenic bladder-sphincter dysfunction followed by dysfunctional voiding in 25%. Himsl and Hurwitz (1991) state as well that the underlying problem in the great majority of children with functional disorders of the lower urinary tract is an unstable bladder.

The study by Mayo and Burns (1990) and the publication of Hoebeke et al. (1999) show that the number of cases with unstable bladder is around 60%. Passerini-Glazel et al. (1992) describe a rate of unstable bladder of 90% in children with non-neurogenic bladder-sphincter dysfunction. In 156 children with daytime incontinence, Van Gool et al. (1992a) found an unstable bladder in 53% and dysfunctional voiding in 59%. Weerasinghe and Malone (1993) reported an unstable bladder in 54% and dysfunctional voiding in 3.5%. In a study on the utility of videourodynamics in children with UTI and non-neurogenic bladder-sphincter dysfunction, Glazier et al. (1997) also found a majority of cases with unstable bladder and only 30% of patients with dysfunctional voiding. Hoebeke et al. (2001) – in a publication about 1,000 videourodynamic studies in children with non-neurogenic bladder dysfunction – found urge syndrome (overactive bladder or unstable bladder) in 58% (male:female ratio 58:42), dysfunctional voiding (overactivity of the external urethral sphincter) in 32% (male:female ratio 49:51), and lazy bladder in 4% (male:female ratio 20:80). Furthermore, he found that the age distribution provided evidence against a dysfunction sequence as mentioned above. Furthermore, urinary incontinence decreases with a similar rate in boys and girls – in spite of a higher prevalence of daytime incontinence in girls than in boys (Swithinbank et al. 2010).

> **Take Away**
> The prevalence of non-neurogenic bladder-sphincter dysfunction ("voiding dysfunction") in children is high. One or more symptoms of disturbed bladder function were reported in up to 26% of children. Overactive bladder (unstable bladder) turned out to be the most common dysfunction.

4 Physiology

For many years uninhibited detrusor contractions have been considered a normal phenomenon in neonates. In several publications a normal functioning infant bladder has been described as unstable (Hjälmas 1988; Lapides and Diokno 1970; Couillard and Webster 1995). A possible explanation was a lack of cortical inhibition of the micturition reflex (Muellner 1960; de Groat 1993). But recently, the hypothesis that uninhibited detrusor contractions are physiological in neonates was challenged by Yeung et al. (1995), who observed detrusor instability in only 1 out of 21 normal infants using natural filling cystometry. Therefore, it was concluded that the function of the infant bladder is under control of higher centers, and uninhibited detrusor contractions are an abnormal phenomenon resulting from a lack of inhibition through the central nervous system.

Yeung et al. (1995) suggested that "incomplete coordination between detrusor contraction and urinary sphincter relaxation could be normal." In a further study by Yeung et al. (1998), two separate patterns of micturition could be distinguished: a normal pattern typified by a continuous urinary stream coordinating with a detrusor contraction and an immature pattern typified by an interrupted stream and apparently dyscoordinated micturition. This is in agreement with our own observations.

By the age of 4–5 years, many children have been toilet trained successfully and have adopted an adult pattern of urinary control. This is also characterized by the absence of involuntary or uninhibited detrusor contractions during bladder filling. Even if the bladder is full and there is a strong desire to void, no bladder contractions will occur. With micturition, coordinated relaxation of the external urethral sphincter takes place. Therefore, bladder emptying is under low intravesical pressure in children and adults.

> **Take Away**
> From the immature bladder with a yet incomplete coordination between detrusor contraction and urinary sphincter relaxation, a complex maturation process takes

years to eventually achieve the adult pattern of urinary control. Nevertheless, uninhibited detrusor contractions probably are an abnormal phenomenon even in neonates resulting from a lack of inhibition through the central nervous system.

5 Toilet Training (Bladder Control)

Toilet training is a highly complex process that is normally completed during the first 4–6 years of life; much of it is not completely understood. In addition to a normal anatomy of the lower urinary tract, a diffuse neuronal network must be present, centrally connected, and controlled. Bladder emptying of the young infant is reflexive; it undergoes a gradual change to the voluntary control of micturition as the central nervous system gains control of the micturition process during the first 4–5 years of life. Daytime control mostly precedes nighttime continence. The development of continence and voluntary micturition needs maturation of the nervous system and behavioral learning. Cognitive perception of the maturing urinary tract is a prerequisite for toilet training. This implies a high susceptibility to the development of non-neurogenic bladder-sphincter dysfunctions.

Feeding typically stimulates micturition in infants, which is under control of the pontine-mesencephalic micturition center in the brain stem – with only minimal cortical influence. To gain normal bladder function, there are specific developments while the child is maturing. The bladder capacity has to increase, which takes place by about 30 ml per year until puberty. The cortical inhibitory pathways to and from the pontine micturition center develop between 1 and 3 years of age, allowing the child to gain voluntary control over the reflexes that control the detrusor and sphincter muscles. This development gives the child the possibility to feel bladder fullness and initiate or inhibit a detrusor contraction voluntarily, thus suppressing voiding at socially inappropriate places and times. Normal urinary bladder control is mostly achieved by the age of 4 years. At this age the urethral sphincter reflexively constricts during bladder filling and relaxes during a voluntary detrusor contraction, allowing micturition to occur.

Non-neurogenic bladder-sphincter dysfunction is thought to originate from behavioral factors that affect toilet training and inhibit the maturation of normal urinary control. Since the gastrointestinal tract plays a prominent role in lower urinary tract dysfunction, the term dysfunctional elimination syndromes (Koff et al. 1998) is applied, if functional bowel disturbances are associated in terms of chronic constipation and encopresis.

Take Away

Toilet training is a highly complex process that is normally completed during the first 4–6 years of life. The development of continence and voluntary micturition needs maturation of the nervous system and behavioral learning. Cognitive perception of the maturing urinary tract is a prerequisite for toilet training. This implies a high susceptibility to the development of non-neurogenic bladder-sphincter dysfunctions, which are thought to originate from behavioral factors that affect toilet training and inhibit the maturation of normal urinary control.

6 Pathophysiology

If abnormalities of toilet training and aberrations in the development of normal urinary control persist, pathologic significance increases as the child becomes older.

For purposes of a better understanding of the pathophysiology and enabling comparative research on the impact on therapeutic efficacy, on outcome, on cost effectiveness, and on life quality, and referring to the abovementioned discussion on categorization, two main types of dysfunction can be subdivided – according to whether the dysfunction occurs during bladder filling or during bladder emptying (or both).

Detrusor-Sphincter Dysfunction During Bladder Filling (Unstable Bladder or Overactive Bladder) The primary abnormality is the failure to suppress involuntary detrusor contractions due to the inability to exert complete voluntary control over the micturition reflex. This dysfunction ranges from minor unstable detrusor contractions at high filling volumes to the severe type with high-amplitude unstable detrusor contractions at lesser bladder-filling volumes, frequently but not always combined with an urge to void.

The child, attempting to maintain continence during such contractions, must voluntarily and tightly constrict the external urethral sphincter to stay dry. This results in simultaneous and unphysiological contraction of both the bladder and external urethral sphincter. During this event functional urinary obstruction and high intravesical pressure develop and persist until the bladder either relaxes or empties.

In about 70% of cases, this dysfunction leads to (urge) incontinence, which is clinically manifested as wetting (mostly daytime but nighttime as well). But even in severe cases, the obligatory voluntary contraction of the striated urethral sphincter against the contracting detrusor can prevent leakage in up to 30% of cases.

The clinical symptoms of an unstable bladder are frequency, urge, and urge incontinence. Uninhibited detrusor contractions leading to symptoms such as urgency, frequency, and urge incontinence can be called overactive bladder syndrome (Staskin and Dmochowski 2002).

Unstable bladder (overactive bladder) is the most common non-neurogenic bladder-sphincter dysfunction, accounting for 175 cases out of 226 children in a study by Hellerstein and Linebarger (2003). Children with this dysfunction use various posturing maneuvers (e.g., Vincent's curtsy) to avoid urinary incontinence. Children who are able to avoid incontinence showed a significantly higher incidence of UTIs than those who did not attempt to obstruct urine outflow (Hellerstein and Linebarger 2003). This means that the lack of wetting does not exclude unstable bladder. These children may present with irritating voiding symptoms such as frequency and urge with UTI, with and without VUR, reflux nephropathy, constipation, and/or fecal soiling. Especially in primary nocturnal enuresis not responding to treatment, an unstable bladder not only during sleep but also during daytime may be detected.

Detrusor-Sphincter Dysfunction During Micturition (Dysfunctional Voiding) The primary abnormality of this dysfunction is overactivity of the urethral closure mechanism during voiding. The most severe form of dysfunctional voiding in childhood is the Hinman syndrome (Hinman 1986) or the so-called non-neurogenic neurogenic bladder (Allen 1977). This syndrome includes fecal retention and soiling, emotional disturbances with family psychosocial problems, bladder trabeculation, diverticula, VUR, and upper tract dilatation. In addition, there is a large post-void residual urine volume. Unstable bladder is mostly associated. This severe type of dysfunction is uncommon; more commonly seen are children with less severe symptoms of dysfunctional voiding. Dysfunctional voiding can be subdivided into the following three types:

Staccato voiding is caused by bursts of pelvic floor activity during micturition resulting in peaks in bladder pressure together with interruption in urinary flow.

Fractionated voiding is caused by hypoactivity of the detrusor muscle, and voiding consists of several unsustained detrusor contractions each with its own flow. Voiding frequency tends to be low, and bladder capacity is large.

Lazy bladder syndrome is the consequence of long-standing dysfunctional voiding. It results from detrusor decompensation. Abdominal pressure is mostly responsible for voiding, and large residual urine volume can be observed (Nørgaard et al. 1998).

It is important to consider that with any type of bladder-sphincter dysfunction, an obstruction of the lower urinary tract is associated. In the case of unstable bladder, this occurs during bladder filling; in the case of dysfunctional voiding, this happens during bladder emptying. Resulting high intravesical pressure is the main mediator that leads to morphologic changes of the urinary bladder in terms of trabeculation and formation of diverticula with negative consequences for the ureteric orifices. The development of VUR probably has its main cause in the anatomical distortion of the uretero-vesical junction as a consequence of chronic high pressure; high pressure itself does not cause VUR (Koff 1992). In cases of borderline competent ureteric orifices, chronic high pressure itself may directly induce and perpetuate VUR.

Especially in cases of dysfunctional voiding with upper tract dilatation and even reflux nephropathy, high intravesical pressure and morphologic distortion of the bladder are associated (Naseer and Steinhardt 1997). It has to be underlined that the clinical expression of dysfunctional voiding is not only staccato voiding or fractionated incomplete voiding but also clinical symptoms such as frequency and urgency with and without incontinence as well and recurrent UTIs. Wetting in fractionated voiding is probably intrinsically a form of overflow incontinence.

Take Away
Functional obstruction is the central problem in non-neurogenic bladder-sphincter dysfunction. Bladder distortion, VUR, upper urinary tract dilatation, UTI, and reflux nephropathy are potential consequences.

7 Constipation

Worldwide constipation is a common problem in children. Estimated prevalence rates have varied from 4 to 37% (Yong and Beattie 1998; Van der wal et al. 2005; De Araújo Sant'Anna and Calcado 1999; Zaslavsky et al. 1988; Maffei et al. 1997). Constipation may vary from mild and short lived to severe and chronic and is sometimes associated with fecal and urinary incontinence, UTI, and abdominal pain. The prevalence of fecal incontinence ranges in children from about 0.3% to 8% (Van der Wal et al. 2005; Bellman 1966; Howe and Walker 1992). In a study by Loening-Baucke (2007), a prevalence rate of 22.6% for constipation, 4.4% for fecal incontinence, and 10.5% for urinary incontinence in a US primary care clinic was found. In this study on 482 children, the fecal incontinence was coupled with constipation in 95% of their children. From the 10.5% prevalence rate for urinary incontinence, 3.3% were found for daytime only, 1.8% for daytime with nighttime, and 5.4% for nighttime urinary incontinence. And it was concluded that fecal and urinary incontinence was significantly more commonly observed in constipated than non-constipated children.

Koff et al. (1998) termed functional bowel and bladder disorders – including unstable bladder, constipation, and infrequent voiding – dysfunctional elimination syndromes. He considers non-neurogenic bladder-sphincter dysfunction as only one part of the spectrum of functional disturbances that affect VUR and UTI. In his study on 153 children with primary VUR, he showed that 56% had dysfunctional elimination syndromes. The phenomenon of an association of overactive bladder, infrequent voiding, recurrent UTI, anatomic bladder distortion, upper urinary tract dilatation, VUR, residual urine, and a negative effect upon the reimplanted ureter with constipation remains incompletely understood (Blethyn et al. 1995; Dohil et al. 1994; O'Regan et al. 1986; Savage 1973; Loening-Baucke 1997; Shopfner 1968). It is postulated that a mechanical effect of the full rectum displacing the bladder, distorting the bladder base, and elongating the urethra might be responsible (Shopfner 1968; Dohil et al. 1994). Another explanation might be the similar spinal innervation of the urethral and anal sphincters. Although the precise causal relationship remains unknown, a study by Loening-Baucke (1997) showed that the treatment of constipation played an important role in successful treatment of daytime and nighttime urinary incontinence and recurrent UTI in children without urologic anatomic abnormalities. Therefore, for evaluating and treating UTI and primary VUR, the assessment of bladder and bowel function disturbances is essential (Burgers et al. 2013). In addition dysfunctional elimination syndromes might lead to idiopathic urethritis which is a common childhood problem characterized by blood spotting in the underwear between voiding (Herz et al. 2005). The authors showed a higher cure rate when children with idiopathic urethritis were treated according to dysfunctional elimination syndrome guidelines.

Dysfunctional elimination syndromes in childhood may have a negative impact on bladder and bowel function later in life. Women with urogynecological symptoms had significantly higher childhood dysfunctional elimination syndrome scores than normal women.

> **Take Away**
> Fecal and urinary incontinence are more commonly observed in constipated than non-constipated children. Constipation and/or encopresis is commonly associated with non-neurogenic bladder-sphincter dysfunction; comprehensive treatment is mandatory for successful management of affected children. Idiopathic urethritis might be a manifestation of an underlying dysfunctional elimination syndrome.

8 Urinary Tract Infection (UTI) and Uretero-vesical Reflux (VUR) in Voiding Dysfunction

As mentioned above non-neurogenic bladder-sphincter dysfunction is one important risk factor among others in the disease complex UTI-renal damage (Van Gool 1995). It has a strong correlation with recurrent UTI and breakthrough infections and may also delay the spontaneous resolution of VUR (Allen 1977; Bachelard et al. 1998; David et al. 1998; Hellström et al. 1987; Hinman and Baumann 1973; Koff 1982; Koff and Murtagh 1983; Koff et al. 1979; Lapides and Diokno 1970; Naseer and Steinhardt 1997; Smellie et al. 1988; Snodgrass 1998; van Gool et al. 1984; Wan et al. 1995; Mazzola et al. 2003; Feldman and Bauer 2006; Chen et al. 2004; Schulman et al. 1999; Chiozza 2002; Hoebeke et al. 2001; Chandra 1995). The well-known combination of primary VUR and UTI predisposing to pyelonephritis, renal scarring, hypertension, and chronic renal damage has formed the basis for diagnostic and therapeutic concepts over the last 25 years (Fanos and Cataldi 2004).

Girls evaluated for UTI after toilet training have in 50–60% of cases typical symptoms of unstable bladder. Koff and Murtagh (1983) reported that unstable bladder was present in 54% of children with VUR. Snodgrass (1998) reported an incidence of 33%. These authors concluded that unstable bladder might be the most common non-neurogenic bladder-sphincter dysfunction associated with VUR. Similarly, Homsy et al. (1985) demonstrated a doubled VUR resolution rate in children treated with anticholinergics compared to that in a historical control.

In a study by Penido Silva et al. (2006), non-neurogenic bladder-sphincter dysfunction was identified in 94 (19.1%) girls and in 20 boys (11%) with VUR. The main clinical implication of this multivariate analysis was that gender as an isolated variable is a poor predictor of clinical outcome in an unselected series of primary VUR. Although boys in this study had a more severe VUR pattern at baseline, girls had a greater risk of recurrent UTI and non-neurogenic bladder-sphincter dysfunction during follow-up.

Koff (1992) described two patterns of dysfunction that have important implications on patients with VUR: the non-neurogenic neurogenic bladder (Allen 1977; Hinman 1986) and the unstable bladder (Bauer et al. 1980; Koff and Murtagh 1983). The greatest degrees of VUR and the severest changes of the upper urinary tract including reflux nephropathy were found at the lowest bladder pressure. This can be explained by the sustained effect of chronically increased bladder pressure that produces anatomical changes, including bladder wall thickening, bladder diverticula, and alterations of the ureterovesical junction. It is the chronic effect of high pressure on the bladder that produces bladder decompensation, leading to the lazy bladder syndrome with infrequent voiding, now lower intravesical pressure and high residual urine volume. There are many studies dealing with the close association between VUR and non-neurogenic bladder-sphincter dysfunction (Van Gool et al. 1984; Hellström et al. 1987; Seruca 1989; Van Gool and Dejonge 1989; Griffith and Scholtmeijer 1987; Fotter 1992; Pfister et al. 1996). An interesting study in this context was presented by Noé (1988), who showed the relationship between siblings' VUR and dysfunctional voiding. He concluded that VUR is indeed polygenetic in its inheritance and significantly influenced by environmental factors such as dysfunctional voiding.

Koff et al. (1998) suggested that there is a relationship among dysfunctional elimination syndromes and that all children with VUR need to be carefully and specifically evaluated for unstable bladder, constipation, and infrequent voiding, because successful management may significantly improve the outcome of VUR and prevent breakthrough UTIs, thereby reducing the need for reimplantation surgery and ultimately better ensuring kidney health. But children with VUR, non-neurogenic bladder-sphincter dysfunction, and dysfunctional elimination syndromes remain at significant risk for a breakthrough UTI despite antibiotic prophylaxis, anticholinergic therapy, timed voiding, and regular bowel evacuation (Koff et al. 1998).

Of greatest importance is the observation by Naseer and Steinhardt (1997) who, in their study on 538 patients with a history of daytime urinary incontinence, identified 51 children with VUR, UTI, and dysfunctional voiding in whom new renal scars had developed while they were under care. They concluded that voiding dysfunction is a significant risk factor not only for UTI and VUR development and perpetuation but also for the development of new renal scars when associated with UTI and VUR. An association between urinary tract dysfunction and reflux nephropathy was also demonstrated by Nielsen et al. (1984).

In their 1987 publication, Griffith and Scholtmeijer described two different VUR/dysfunction complexes. One type included unstable bladder and VUR that frequently occurred on one side only; reflux nephropathy or upper urinary tract abnormalities were rare in this group. The other group included poorly contracting bladders during voiding and overactivity of the external urethral sphincter. The bladder was usually stable and VUR occurred frequently on both sides; reflux nephropathy and upper urinary tract abnormalities were relatively common. VUR in an unstable bladder occurred as a direct consequence of abnormally high detrusor pressure occurring during unstable bladder contractions. In the second group with a poorly contracting bladder (lazy bladder syndrome), VUR occurred at low detrusor pressure and often was bilateral.

In the multivariate large-scale analysis of the relationship between dysfunctional elimination syndromes, UTI and VUR by Chen et al. (2004), the authors believe that both VUR and UTI are not independently associated with non-neurogenic bladder-sphincter dysfunction. The authors conclude that only together UTI and VUR are associated with non-neurogenic bladder-sphincter dysfunction. This is in agreement with the concept that non-neurogenic bladder-sphincter dysfunction together with chronic constipation and/or encopresis (dysfunctional elimination syndromes) causes UTI, and abnormal voiding pressures cause VUR to develop which would result in the observed association (Chen et al. 2004).

In a study by Yeung et al. (2004), it could be shown that the resolution of VUR significantly correlated with renal and bladder functional status at diagnosis. Normal renal and bladder functions at diagnosis were highly predictive of complete resolution of VUR, whereas abnormal renal and bladder functions were prognostic for persistence of VUR.

Non-neurogenic bladder-sphincter dysfunction in patients with renal transplantation may have a negative effect on the transplanted kidney (Van der Weide et al. 2006; Luke et al. 2003; Adams et al. 2004). In a study by Luke et al. (2003) comparing the long-term outcomes of graft survival between children with dysfunctional lower urinary tract and children with a normal lower urinary tract, it was found that lower urinary tract pressure plays an important role in graft survival. The role of VUR into the renal allograft with chronic/recurrent, potentially subclinical infection is being increasingly recognized as a risk factor for transplant survival, and thus antirefluxive surgery techniques are being promoted (see chapter "Imaging in Renal Failure, Neonatal Oligoanuria, and Renal Transplantation")

> **Take Away**
> Non-neurogenic bladder-sphincter dysfunction has a strong correlation with UTI and breakthrough infections, as well as with VUR and renal scarring. Successful management of voiding and bowel dysfunction significantly improves the outcome of VUR, allows VUR resolution, and prevents breakthrough infections, thereby reducing the need for reimplantation surgery and ultimately better ensuring kidney health.

9 Enuresis and Incontinence

For therapeutic and prognostic reasons, it is important to distinguish between enuresis and incontinence. Enuresis is defined as normal voiding occurring at an inappropriate time or place. Primary nocturnal enuresis is defined as bedwetting that is lifelong and that does not have an intervening dry period of at least 6 months. If there was a dry period of 6 months before recurrence of nighttime wetting, it is called secondary nocturnal enuresis. Monosymptomatic nocturnal enuresis is bedwetting with normal daytime voiding; in polysymptomatic nocturnal enuresis, bedwetting is associated with daytime symptoms of frequency and urgency – with or without incontinence. Incontinence is the involuntary loss of urine together with non-neurogenic bladder-sphincter dysfunction – often in combination with UTI, constipation, and fecal incontinence.

The causes of enuresis are always functional; the causes of incontinence may be organic or functional but are mostly functional (Kelleher 1997). Functional causes can be divided as mentioned above in this chapter into overactive bladder (unstable bladder) and dysfunctional voiding in particular.

At least one nocturnal enuresis event per month has been reported in over 10% of children 6 years of age (Lackgren et al. 1999), in 2–5% of 10 year olds (Nørgaard et al. 1998; Chiozza et al. 1998; Lackgren et al. 1999) and 0.5–3.0% of adolescents (Spee-van der Wekke et al. 1998). The incidence of nocturnal enuresis is 1.5–2%-fold more frequent among boys than among girls (Hellström et al. 1990).

Only monosymptomatic bedwetting without urge and UTI should be termed monosymptomatic (or isolated) enuresis nocturna. Chandra (1998) states that children with isolated nocturnal enuresis have a lower prevalence of constipation and/or encopresis. Urge incontinence, mostly as a daytime symptom of bladder instability, may be combined with nighttime wetting. In this case bedwetting should not be categorized as enuresis but as incontinence.

Several causal mechanisms in nocturnal enuresis have been described. Nørgaard et al. (1995) describe insufficient nocturnal production of arginine vasopressin and impaired renal sensitivity to this substance and to desmopressin. This leads to nocturnal polyuria, which might be one of the most important etiologic factors in nocturnal enuresis. Koff (1995) describes an afferent and efferent developmental delay in terms of a failure of the central nervous system to recognize bladder fullness or contraction and to suppress the micturition reflex arc during sleep. He underlines that this developmental delay is not responsible for all cases of nocturnal enuresis; etiology is indeed multifactorial.

Chandra (1998) underscores that nocturnal enuresis results from an interaction of unstable detrusor contractions, delayed arousal from sleep, and nocturnal polyuria. Some children with nocturnal enuresis can hold urine well for several hours during the day and have isolated nocturnal enuresis, while others manifest diurnal voiding symptoms as well, including urinary frequency, urgency, urge incontinence, and pelvic withholding. Pathogenesis of isolated nocturnal enuresis may be different in comparison to children with daytime and nighttime wetting. In the latter, unstable detrusor contractions of overactive bladder may play a major role, whereas delayed arousal from sleep at bladder fullness may be the cause in patients with isolated nocturnal enuresis. In children with isolated nocturnal enuresis, sleep cystometry has also disclosed unstable bladder (overactive bladder) in 50% of cases (Nørgaard et al. 1989). Therefore, among several pathological factors that have been described in association with isolated enuresis nocturna, there may be a significant underlying non-neurogenic bladder-sphincter dysfunction, especially in children in whom treatment has failed (Medel et al. 1998; Yeung et al. 1999, 2004, 2006b; Kajiwara et al. 2006).

Chandra (1996) and Hellström et al. (1990) reported that 60% of girls and 50% of boys with nighttime wetting manifested daytime wetting symptoms as well. In bedwetting the bladder may get full because of large production of nighttime urine or because of reduced bladder capacity. This reduced capacity could be the result of incomplete bladder relaxation or from uninhibited detrusor contractions while sleeping. If the child is a deep sleeper or manifests delayed sleep arousal, the full bladder may empty itself during sleep (Hjälmas 1995, 1997; Wille 1994; Nevéus et al. 1999). In normal children contraction of the detrusor during sleep leads to a change from deep to light sleep followed by arousal for urination (Watanabe et al. 1994).

Another causal factor in enuresis nocturna might be rapid bladder filling (Nørgaard et al. 1989). In this context the rare anatomic abnormality of a completely duplicated ureteral system in which an ectopic ureter empties directly outside the bladder has to be kept in mind. In this case the upper renal moiety drains through a ureter that empties below the urethral sphincter or at some other ectopic site such as the vagina, uterus, or even the perineum. Hence, these children are wet all of the time. This condition occurs exclusively in girls.

Altogether, it can be concluded that for therapeutic and diagnostic reasons, it is essential to focus on the distinction between enuresis and incontinence. The term enuresis should be reduced to the symptom of isolated (monosymptomatic) primary nocturnal enuresis. These children void in bed while asleep and generally are not aroused by the wetting. The problem is that occult daytime wetting of bladder instability or dysfunctional voiding may coexist. The polyetiologic mechanism may include daytime unstable bladder, nocturnal bladder contractions, failure of antidiuretic hormone nocturnal increase, and disturbances in arousal mechanisms. All could be related to a developmental delay of the central nervous system control of micturition, partly genetic and partly due to environmental factors (Koff 1995).

Most cases of daytime and nighttime wetting are functional forms of urinary incontinence resulting from non-neurogenic bladder-sphincter dysfunction, clinically manifested by frequency, urgency, and urge incontinence. UTIs, covered bacteriuria, VUR, constipation, encopresis, and structural abnormalities of the urinary tract are often associated, and vaginal voiding should be differentiated as another cause of daytime wetting in girls (Bernasconi et al. 2009).

It is accepted that evaluation of the child with wetting with a history of infection is indicated because some 30–50% of children who present with UTI will have VUR demonstrated on voiding cystourethrography (VCUG). However, no clear guidelines have been established for the evaluation of wetting children with sterile urine demonstrated at the time of admission or without a history of UTI. In a study on children with enuresis, Sujka et al. (1991) demonstrated that no one symptom or combination of symptoms segregated these patients likely to have VUR: 16% of their 83 patients with sterile urine and no history of infection had VUR; out of those, 16 showed reflux nephropathy as well. They concluded that one of six children who present with enuresis and sterile urine will have VUR. And therefore screening these children with VCUG should be considered. This corresponds to our results and roughly to our policy of performing a comprehensive urinary tract ultrasound (US) (including a post-void assessment) in children of more than 6 years of age with persistent severe enuresis nocturna despite treatment and performing VCUG with a history of UTI. Assessment of stool retention by US measurement of the rectal diameter should be included (Klijn et al. 2004). The authors found a mean diameter of the rectum of 4.9 cm (95% CI 4.4–5.3) in constipated children; in the control group, they found a mean diameter of the rectum of 2.1 cm (95 % CI 1.8–2.4). Therefore, the transverse diameter of the rectum measured by pelvic US provides an additional accurate parameter with which to diagnose constipation in patients with non-neurogenic bladder-sphincter dysfunction.

Any attempt to make the important distinction between monosymptomatic nocturnal enuresis and incontinence based on the patient's history and clinical symptoms alone may fail, and occult underlying functional disorders of the lower urinary tract may be overlooked. This may contribute to the different rates of success for a heterogeneous spectrum of therapeutic measures in different studies and may contribute to different statements regarding prognosis and associated disorders of enuresis.

Incontinence and clinical symptoms of non-neurogenic bladder-sphincter dysfunction can be found in children after *sexual abuse*. Ellsworth et al. (1995) found a 6 % rate of sexual abuse in 300 children with non-neurogenic bladder-sphincter dysfunction. Abidari and Shortliffe (2002) mentioned that sexual abuse of children is not limited to penetration but may include fondling, exhibitionism, or pornography. Davila et al. (2003) report that sexual abuse survivors have a significantly higher incidence of genitourinary dysfunction symptoms, including urge incontinence and voluntary urinary retention.

Giggle incontinence is another type of incontinence in girls. Those girls wet with a coordinated full or partial void during laughter. According to a study by Chandra et al. (2002), giggle incontinence results from unstable detrusor contractions induced by laughter, and it improves with effective treatment of unstable bladder by methylphenidate or biofeedback (Berry et al. 2009; Richardson and Palmer 2009). In this study diurnal voiding symptoms were noted in 95 % of patients with giggle incontinence, while giggle incontinence was noted in 23 % of those presenting with predominantly diurnal voiding symptoms.

It was reported that incontinence and clinical symptoms of non-neurogenic bladder-sphincter dysfunction occur in some genetic syndromes. In *William's syndrome* deletions on the long arm of chromosome 7 are associated with mild cognitive deficits, a highly social personality, and vascular and visceral defects (Abidari and Shortliffe 2002). A 32 % prevalence of genitourinary symptoms, predominantly daytime wetting and increased frequency, was reported in a series of 41 patients (Schulman et al. 1996).

Ochoa syndrome has an autosomal dominant pattern of inheritance. Children who have this syndrome exhibit all the clinical features of Hinman syndrome, and in addition they have an unusual inversion of facial expression when smiling is attempted. The face becomes contorted into a grimace that makes it appear that the child is crying. Therefore, this syndrome is also known as the urofacial syndrome. Treatment is the same as for the Hinman syndrome. Despite the concern of children and parents regarding urinary incontinence, there is little research into the *psychological problems* associated with daytime wetting. In a study by Joinson et al. (2006), it was reported that there is increased vulnerability to psychological problems in children as young as 7 years of age with daytime wetting. There should be awareness of the increased risk of disorders such as *attention-deficit/hyperactivity disorder in children* with daytime wetting because this is likely to interfere with treatment.

Take Away

Distinction should be made between monosymptomatic enuresis nocturna and incontinence. Patients with persistent and severe monosymptomatic enuresis nocturna despite treatment should undergo urinary tract US and VCUG as well, if there are positive US findings and/or a history of UTI. In wetting children (daytime with or without nighttime urinary incontinence) with UTI with or without urge, urinary tract US and a VCUG have to be performed; here, the assessment of signs for potential stool retention has to be part of the imaging studies.

10 Non-neurogenic Bladder-Sphincter Dysfunction in Neonates and Infants

In a study by Yeung et al. (1995), a considerably greater rise in detrusor pressure with micturition was found, especially in male neonates and infants than in older children. Sillen et al. (1992) described pronounced detrusor hypercontractility in male infants with gross bilateral VUR, and in a follow-up study, they described a gradual decrease in this initial detrusor hypercontractility until the age of 38 months (Sillen et al. 1996). Bachelard et al. (1998) described low bladder capacity, high-frequency bladder instability, high voiding pressure, and increased activity of the pelvic floor during voiding in male infants with UTI. Hiraoka et al. (1999) found that male neonates had larger residual urine volumes and smaller urinary flow rates than female neonates.

One potential explanation for the increased voiding pressure in male newborns and infants as described by Yeung et al. (1999), Sillen et al. (1992), and Bachelard et al. (1998) could be the change in the configuration of the external urinary sphincter after birth, which starts as a complete ringlike structure and changes its configuration into an omega-shaped or horseshoe-like posteriorly open muscle structure by splitting, which occurs during the first year of life. This sex-linked developmental anatomy seems to coincide in time with the observation of high voiding pressure reported predominantly in male newborns and infants (Kokoua et al. 1993).

Unstable detrusor contractions combined with trabeculated thickened bladder wall, reduced capacity, and somewhat dilated posterior urethra in male newborns with high-grade dilating (bilateral) VUR can be detected on routine VCUG performed for prenatally dilated upper urinary tracts. In these male newborns and young infants, a highly dyscoordinated voiding pattern was observed (Fotter 1994; Allen and Bright 1978; Hjälmas 1988; Wen and Tong 1998) (Figs. 1 and 2).

In a study by Godley et al. (2001), it was reported that VUR outcome in infants had a strong correlation with the initial renal functional status at diagnosis with a high incidence of early resolution of even high-grade VUR in infants. Bilateral abnormal kidneys associated with high-grade VUR turned out to be a poor prognostic sign for VUR resolution. And Yeung et al. (1997) reported that resolution of VUR correlated with bladder function. A high VUR resolution rate was observed in infants with normal bladder function, and children with non-neurogenic bladder-sphincter dysfunction seem to have more

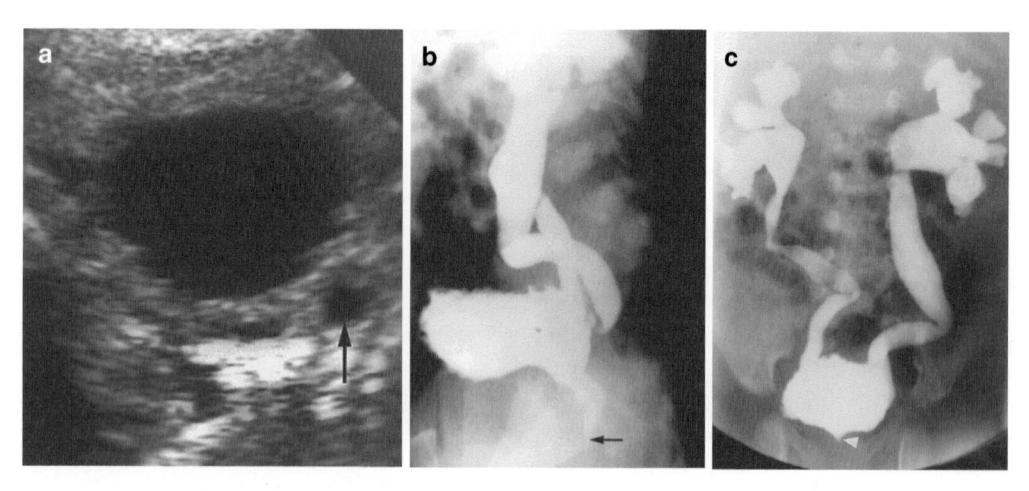

Fig. 1 Bilateral high-grade fetal dilatation of upper urinary tract in the neonate. (**a**) Transverse US scan of the bladder: bladder wall thickening, trabeculation, dilatation of the left pelvic ureter (*arrow*), filling volume immediately before voiding 10 ml. (**b, c**) VCUG: bladder trabeculation, diverticula, bilateral VUR grade 5, wide bladder neck anomaly (*arrowhead*), unstable detrusor contractions, transformed into premature micturition, dyscoordinated voiding, contrast-filled posterior urethra up to contracted external sphincter (*arrow*), residual urine

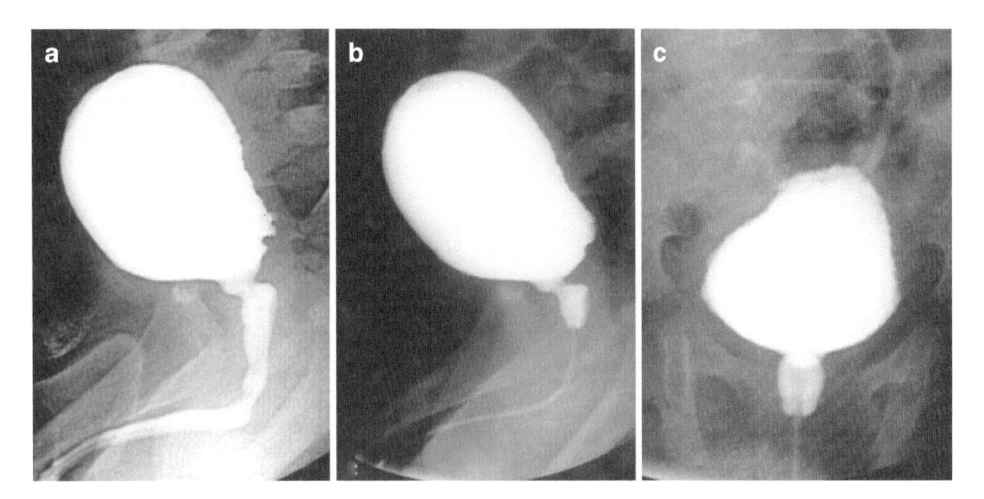

Fig. 2 Male, 2 months old: moderate bilateral fetal hydronephrosis, VCUG. Reduced bladder filling volume (20 ml), residual urine, early uninhibited detrusor contractions transformed into premature micturition. (**a**) Minor bladder trabeculation, short phase of normal micturition. (**b**, **c**) Dyscoordinated voiding, contraction of external urethral sphincter, dilated posterior urethra, male spinning top urethra

breakthrough infections, which may have a role in new renal scar formation.

The coexistence of non-neurogenic bladder-sphincter dysfunction with VUR in infants and with kidney abnormalities could all arise from a single primary maldevelopment during differentiation of the ureteral bud and bladder trigone (Yeung et al. 2006a). Therefore, normal renal and bladder functions seem to be highly predictive of complete resolution of VUR; on the other hand, abnormal renal and bladder function would be associated with poor prognosis and persistence of VUR. This could be proved in a study by Yeung et al. (2006a).

Special attention must be paid to the critical assessment of adequate functional bladder capacity, since so-called covert instability manifests as significantly reduced bladder capacity. This means that after a short stable filling phase, the first unstable detrusor contraction is immediately transformed into a premature and forceful micturition contraction (Sillen et al. 1992). In this context it has to be taken into account that development of bladder volume in relation to age is not linear. There is a massive increase in bladder capacity after the 12th to 18th month of life with a gain in perception and unconscious as well as conscious inhibition of detrusor contraction (Zerin et al. 1993).

Jayanthi et al. (1997) reported on seven patients (5 males and 2 females), newborn to 2 months old, obviously with the severest form of neonatal bladder-sphincter dysfunction and called this pattern the *non-neurogenic neurogenic bladder of early infancy*. None of the infants had neurologic pathology or anatomical outflow obstruction. Five of the seven patients presented with thick-walled poorly compliant bladders and incomplete bladder emptying. Significant upper tract pathology was found in all cases. Although the primary pathophysiological problem – low bladder capacity combined with detrusor hypercontractility during the filling as well as the voiding phase and abnormal contraction or perhaps non-relaxation of the external urinary sphincter – is similar to the disorders encountered in older children, the clinical presentation is certainly more severe in infants. And since dysfunction has started during development of the nephrons prenatally, the risks for the upper urinary tract are much greater than in other forms of non-neurogenic bladder-sphincter dysfunction.

In 15 out of 25 baby boys with VUR, Avni and Schulman (1996) found a spectrum of bladder and urethral anomalies; they drew the conclusion that these findings may support the theory that a significant number of cases of VUR in baby boys results from a transient fetal urethral obstruction. But one central question remains in this context, if we consider a transient urethral obstruction between the ninth and thirteenth week of gestation as the cause of prenatal VUR and upper tract dilatation: how does the postnatally detected bladder-sphincter dysfunction fit into this hypothesis, how does it start, and why does it persist after birth? These questions can only be answered speculatively. It is well known that subvesical obstruction leads to bladder hypertrophy, reduced bladder compliance and capacity, high detrusor pressure during bladder filling and voiding, and unstable detrusor contractions. Based on this well-known pathophysiological mechanism, the speculative conclusion could be drawn that after a transient early fetal urethral obstruction, functional disturbances (bladder dysfunctions) could be induced and persist obviously at least until early infancy (Fotter 1994; Avni and Schulman 1996) and longer. According to the results of the study by Sillen et al. (1996), either a delay in maturation of the coordination between the detrusor and the external sphincter with lacking sphincteric relaxation or reflexive contraction of the external sphincter could explain the high-pressure waves without leakage of urine during unstable detrusor contractions in these newborn males. The hypercontractile detrusor with altered tension of the bladder wall and/or longer-lasting elevated detrusor pressures during the remainder of pregnancy might be an important contributory factor for the development of VUR and megaureters in these children (Herndon et al. 1999; Kokoua et al. 1993). In this context it is interesting that Risdon et al. (1993) found that in children with gross VUR submitted to unilateral nephrectomy, evidence of dysplastic renal development was confined to male patients. This corresponds to other studies that indicate a marked male preponderance among patients with reflux nephropathy diagnosed early in life, particularly those detected by antenatal ultrasound. Studies by Glick et al. (1993) and Beck (1971) have shown that upper tract obstruction can cause dysplastic kidneys. Therefore, it seems likely that early fetal transient urethral obstruction in males followed by bladder-sphincter dysfunction with anatomic bladder distortion and persistent intrauterine high-pressure VUR may result in dysplastic kidneys.

Similar dysfunctional states can also be found in preschool children. This suggests that there may be a subgroup of children in whom non-neurogenic bladder-sphincter dysfunction may be congenital rather than acquired, as is postulated for the classical Hinman syndrome (Hinman 1986).

Summarizing these studies and observations, it can be concluded that non-neurogenic bladder-sphincter dysfunction is not limited only to later childhood after toilet training; it can be observed more often in males with (bilateral) high-grade VUR neonatally, as well as in infancy and early childhood. VUR resolution depends on renal status and bladder function. Unstable contractions of a hypercontractile detrusor with high filling and voiding pressure in utero may be an important contributory factor for the development of (bilateral) VUR and megaureters in these children. Another explanation could be that VUR, congenital kidney damage, and bladder-sphincter dysfunction could all arise from a single primary maldevelopment during differentiation of the ureteral bud and bladder trigon. Male preponderance of bilateral high-grade VUR and of reflux nephropathy in early life and the high percentage of dysplastic elements in damaged kidneys in males may be explained by a causal relationship to a sex-linked in utero bladder dysfunction that persists after birth. Potential causes could be a transient fetal urethral obstruction (Avni and Schulman 1996) and/or the specific anatomical configuration of the striated external sphincter and its change with postnatal life in male infants (Kokoua et al. 1993).

Take Away
Non-neurogenic bladder-sphincter dysfunction can be found more often in male neonates and infants with (bilateral) high-grade VUR and megaureters. Abnormal renal and bladder function is associated with poor prognosis and persistence of VUR. Reduced bladder capacity, trabeculation, dilated posterior urethra, and a highly disturbed voiding pattern are characteristic VCUG signs.

11 Modified Voiding Cystourethrography (VCUG)

A slightly modified VCUG technique allows the diagnosis of (uninhibited) unstable detrusor contractions and therefore the diagnosis of unstable bladder with accuracy similar to that of urodynamic techniques (sensitivity 93%, specificity 90.7%) (Fotter et al. 1986).

For this technique the bladder has to be catheterized with a 6–10-French feeding tube, and the diluted contrast agent is dripped into the bladder from a constant height of 30 cm above the level of the bladder, at a rate of 5% of expected age-matched volume per minute (Fotter 1996). The radiologist has to maintain visual contact with the child and with the infusion bottle at all times. Bladder filling has to be carried out under brief intermittent fluoroscopic observation with the patient in a supine position. Additional fluoroscopic observations have to be carried out during slowing or spontaneous cessation of the infusion flow. Normally the bladder will fill to the expected age-matched capacity without significant slowing or cessation of the drip infusion flow. The drip infusion acts as a manometer of sorts.

If a first desire to void is announced, the point of bladder filling should be noted (normally greater than 20% of expected capacity). The drip infusion is stopped and the catheter removed if a strong urge to void is announced or when expected age-matched capacity is reached.

The combination of a transient opening of the bladder neck with a flow of contrast agent into the posterior urethra up to the voluntarily contracted striated urethral sphincter together with cessation and/or backup of contrast agent drip flow suggests the presence of an uninhibited detrusor contraction (Fotter et al. 1986; Passerini-Glazel et al. 1992) (Fig. 3). These findings are valid; they can stand alone without urodynamic results. Modified VCUG allows detection of the majority of these dysfunctions in neonates, infants, and small children with the same reliability and in the same way as in older age groups.

Assessing dyscoordination between bladder and external sphincter during voiding without interrupted flow by VCUG is a weak point of this technique. However, it is well known that electromyographic assessment of pelvic floor muscles assessment also is not reliable, with many artifacts noted (e.g., leg movements) (Hoebecke et al. 1999).

Two specific cystographic signs have been found to be closely associated with unstable bladder (Saxton et al. 1988; Hausegger et al. 1991; Saxton and Robinson 1992; Naseer and Steinhardt 1997). The first is the so-called spinning top urethra (STU) (Combs et al. 1998; Van Gool et al. 1992a) (Fig. 4). In a retrospective VCUG study on 102 girls, Hausegger et al. (1991) found 28 to have STU, 16 of whom had an unstable bladder as well (57%). There was a statistically positive correlation between STU and unstable bladder; similar results were published

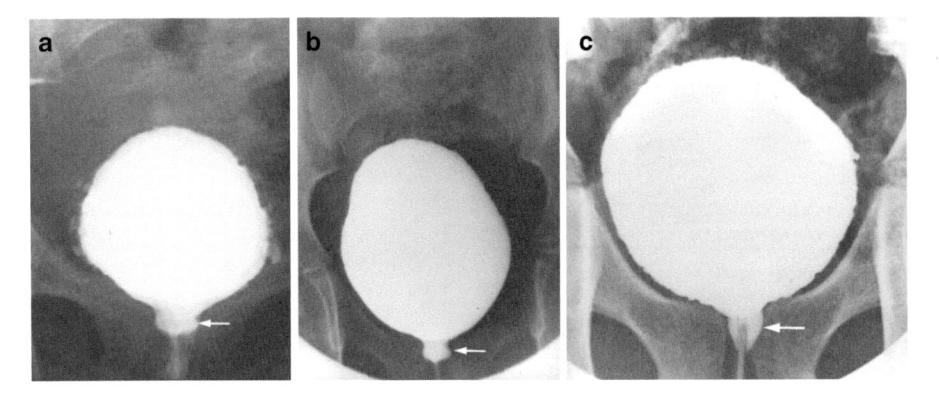

Fig. 3 Different appearances of bladder neck opening (*arrow*) with unstable detrusor contractions on VCUG. (**a**) Male, 4 years old: urge incontinence, bladder trabeculation and sacculation, leakage around the catheter, high-grade unstable bladder. (**b**) Female, 6 years old: daytime and nighttime wetting, minor bladder trabeculation, unstable bladder. (**c**) Female, 7.5 years old: daytime incontinence, bladder trabeculation, unstable bladder

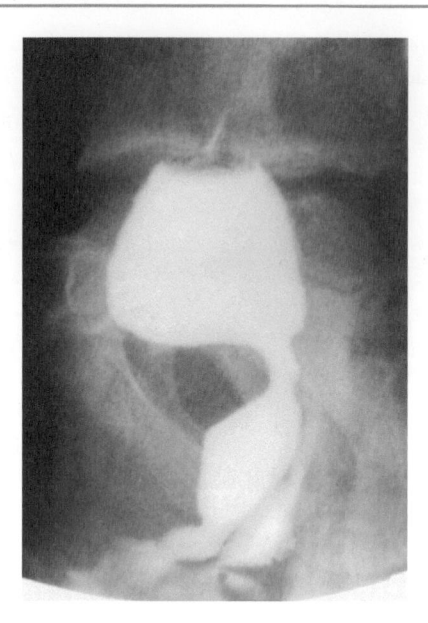

Fig. 4 Female, 6 years old: daytime wetting, VCU. High-grade spinning top urethra, marked widening of the muscular segment of the urethra during voiding

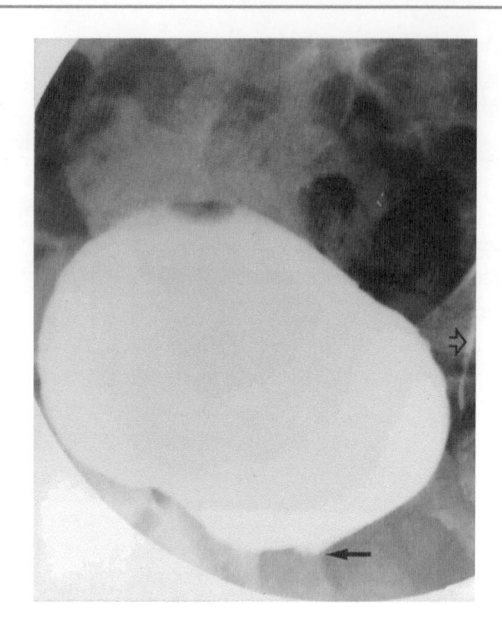

Fig. 5 Female, 6 years old: daytime and nighttime wetting, VCU. Wide bladder neck anomaly (*arrow*), uretero-vesical reflux grade 1 (*open arrow*)

by Saxton et al. (1988). These studies confirmed the close association between unstable bladder and STU. Spinning top urethra was described in boys as well; this dilatation of the posterior urethra was found in male infants with high-grade VUR (Avni and Schulman 1996; Sillen et al. 1992; Fotter 1994) (Figs. 1 and 2) and boys with unstable bladder (Saxton and Robinson 1992).

Second, the so-called wide bladder neck anomaly (WBNA) (Saxton et al. 1988; Hoebecke et al. 1999) is a permanent passive bladder neck opening in the filling phase of the VCU independent of uninhibited detrusor contractions (Fig. 5). Wide bladder neck anomaly might be an acquired phenomenon and unstable bladder an important etiologic factor contributing to WBNA. This is in contrast to the opinion of Saxton et al. (1988), who see in WBNA a congenital disorder. Both cystographic signs should alert the observer's attention to possible non-neurogenic bladder-sphincter dysfunctions, even in the absence of unstable detrusor contractions.

Careful attention must always be given to precise assessment of the urethral morphology in order to detect narrowing of the bulbar urethra (Cobb's collar) (Dewan et al. 1995; Nonomura et al. 1999) and congenital obstructing posterior urethral membranes (COPUM) (Dewan 1993; Dewan et al. 1997).

Altogether, assessment of lower urinary tract by VCUG should include bladder and urethra morphology, detection and grading of VUR, bladder function during filling (unstable bladder?), age-matched bladder-filling capacity (Zerin et al. 1993), residual urine, urinary flow (if smooth or interrupted), and sphincter behavior during voiding (voiding dysfunction?). In addition, an assessment of the fullness with stool of the entire colon and rectum (fecal retention?) and an evaluation for spinal defects must always be done.

Take Away
A slightly modified VCUG technique allows the diagnosis of unstable detrusor contractions with similar accuracy to urodynamic techniques. Spinning top urethra and wide bladder neck anomaly, even in the absence of unstable bladder, should alert the attention to occult or healed dysfunction.

12 Evaluation

The evaluation process begins with a good history. A standardized questionnaire using a scoring system for the quantitative evaluation of incontinence symptoms in children should be used to improve pretest probability, in particular, if we consider that routine urodynamics in children with non-neurogenic bladder-sphincter dysfunction in many cases do not change therapy or influence outcome (Akbal et al. 2005; Bartkowski and Doubrava 2004; Sureshkumar et al. 2006; Parekh et al. 2001). Equally important is the physical examination, which includes a careful inspection of the lower spine to look for a cutaneous manifestation of an occult spinal dysraphism and/or sacral agenesis and an examination of the external genitalia.

The radiological assessment of children with non-neurogenic bladder-sphincter dysfunction includes a comprehensive urinary tract US and a modified VCUG in children with persistent and severe dysfunction – in particular if associated with UTI and breakthrough infections (Parekh et al. 2001). In girls, radionuclide cystography or echo-enhanced sonography may replace VCUG – when only VUR is searched for – and other means of functional assessment such as uroflowmetry are performed.

For the evaluation of children with symptoms of non-neurogenic bladder-sphincter dysfunction by US, a careful examination of the urinary bladder has to be performed in particular. Not only structural abnormalities have to be searched for; bladder wall thickness, bladder volume, and residual urine volume after voiding have to be assessed (Käfer et al. 1997). Similar as described before for the modified VCUG technique, the bladder base and bladder neck, respectively, have to be observed carefully as well. A transient opening of the bladder neck together with uninhibited detrusor contractions with filling of the posterior urethra up to the contracted external sphincter can be seen sometimes with continuous observation of the bladder base by US as well (Fig. 6).

To overcome the weaknesses of urodynamics in children and the invasiveness and the radiation burden of VCUG, several articles have been published recently describing various measurements and calculations in an attempt to detect non-neurogenic bladder-sphincter dysfunction by bladder US: According to Leung et al. (2007), nomograms of total renal volume, urinary bladder volume index, and bladder volume wall thickness index are described as useful indicators of bladder dysfunction in children with enuresis and UTI (Yeung et al. 2007). In 1997, Kaefer et al. published that the bladder thickness index (bladder wall thickness was indexed to inner wall diameter) is a sensitive US predictor of infravesical obstruction; application of this index could be

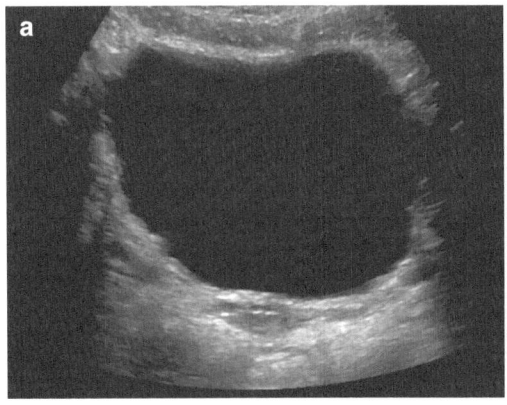

Fig. 6 (**a**, **b**) School age girl: urge incontinence, UTI, unstable bladder, bladder US. (**a**) Full bladder, minor bladder trabeculation, bladder neck closed. (**b**) Uninhibited detrusor contractions with bladder neck opening and filling the posterior urethra up to contracted external sphincter with urine (*arrow*)

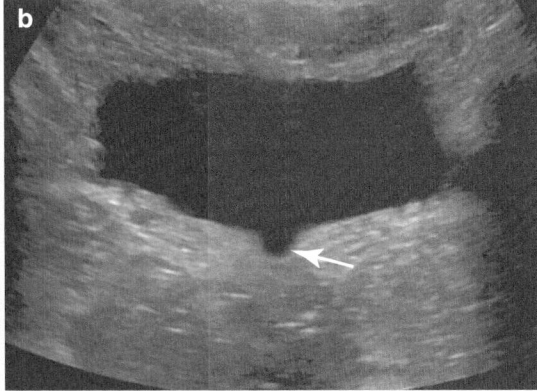

a noninvasive screening tool for the patient with persistent non-neurogenic bladder-sphincter dysfunction. Ukimura et al. (1998) described in 1998 that US-estimated bladder weight might be used to evaluate bladder compliance in children and concluded that this might be a suitable noninvasive urodynamic test in children with suspected urodynamic abnormalities.

Another interesting feature of bladder US seems to be the assessment of the ureteric jet Doppler patterns (Leung et al. 2002a, b, 2006). The authors conclude that the persistence of an immature pattern was highly associated with UTI and VUR. Furthermore, the authors found that there was significant increase in the incidence of immature patterns in enuretic children when compared with controls. Enuretic children with bilateral immature ureteric jet wave forms and markedly thickened bladder wall showed multiple significant urodynamic abnormalities, which could be accounted for by immaturity of both uretero-vesical junction and detrusor muscle.

Pediatric radiologists performing US studies in children with clinical symptoms of non-neurogenic bladder-sphincter dysfunction and in enuretic children should not only evaluate for structural abnormalities but should search for signs of unstable bladder (open bladder neck?) and should measure residual volume after voiding and bladder wall thickness according to published standards (bladder wall thickness varies minimally with age, with a mean of 3 mm, when the bladder is full and 5 mm when empty) (Leung et al. 2007). Calculating urinary bladder volume index and bladder volume wall thickness index and assessing the ureteric jet Doppler patterns seem to be useful adjuncts.

Important aspects in the evaluation process are the indications for VCUG: Children with persistent and severe symptoms of non-neurogenic bladder-sphincter dysfunction including urgency, urge incontinence, and infrequent voiding (lazy bladder syndrome) and positive findings in the urinary tract US study, in particular with (recurrent) UTI, should undergo VCUG (Greenfield et al. 1997; Opsomer et al. 1998; Fotter 1994). A pelvic floor electromyography and uroflowmetry should be an obligatory part of the evaluation in those children. The role of urodynamics regarding sensitivity and specificity and impact on therapeutic efficacy and outcome is under debate.

Neonates and young infants with prenatally detected upper urinary tract dilatation or other uropathology who undergo urinary tract US and VCUG must be carefully evaluated for signs of non-neurogenic bladder-sphincter dysfunction as well. Special attention to non-neurogenic bladder-sphincter dysfunction must also be given for infants and children with UTI who are referred for VCUG because 30% of children with voiding dysfunction do not have urgency and/or incontinence.

Detection of non-neurogenic bladder-sphincter dysfunction is an important contribution for adequate management of these children. The radiologist must be aware of the important responsibility she/he has for these patients and must take charge in detecting non-neurogenic bladder-sphincter dysfunction, which otherwise could be overlooked. Since dysfunctional voiding and unstable bladder are often associated or coincide with the detection of unstable detrusor contractions on VCUG, they can be a first and indirect sign indicating the need for further detailed examination (even videourodynamics which allows the most detailed assessment of the underlying, often complex, pattern of dysfunction) for planning tailored and individualized treatment.

The close relationship between dysfunctional voiding and unstable bladder and urge with or without incontinence, recurrent UTI, breakthrough infections, VUR, and constipation makes urinary tract US and VCUG (and possibly videourodynamics) an important part of the evaluation algorithm in these children. Successful treatment of these dysfunctions has a positive effect on the resolution rate and resolution time of VUR, of UTI, of (urge) incontinence, and on costs (Benoit et al. 2002) and prevents kidney damage.

Videourodynamics remains the gold standard if a combination of a detailed functional assessment combined with a morphologic assessment of the urinary tract is desired (Glazier et al. 1997). But videourodynamic studies are seldom needed in children with non-neurogenic bladder-sphincter dysfunction. These studies are reserved for a selected group of patients with severe and/or persistent symptoms despite treatment. Videourodynamics is not available in many institutions where children have to be assessed uroradiologically, and it is an expensive and time-consuming method. Therefore, the radiologist has to know a great deal about pediatric urology and urinary tract pathophysiology to exhaust all the possibilities that an adequate VCUG technique provides. Severe and persistent urgency and urge incontinence together with UTI suggest severe urinary tract pathology. In these patients imaging with US and a VCUG should be performed (Himsl and Hurwitz 1991). However, we have to keep in mind that VCUG and videourodynamics are invasive methods and should not be used as screening tests in children.

We do not perform VCUG for monosymptomatic, primary nocturnal enuresis or initially in children with daytime and nighttime wetting in the absence of severe urge, urge incontinence, or UTI.

Altogether, it should be underlined that a slightly modified VCUG technique allows the diagnosis of unstable bladder (overactive bladder) to be made in centers without urodynamic facilities with similar accuracy. Therefore, modified VCUG is recommended in all children for the evaluation of symptoms of persistent and severe non-neurogenic bladder-sphincter dysfunction, in particular with (febrile) UTI and breakthrough infections, and in all neonates and infants for the evaluation of upper urinary tract dilatation and extended US signs indicative of VUR.

> **Take Away**
> Evaluation of non-neurogenic bladder-sphincter dysfunction begins with a careful history and a physical examination followed by urine analysis. The radiological investigation starts with a comprehensive urinary tract US. A VCUG is performed in persistent and severe cases of non-neurogenic bladder-sphincter dysfunction and in children with associated UTI or breakthrough infections.

There is still low general awareness of the problem of non-neurogenic bladder-sphincter dysfunction, especially among radiologists. There are still many children with non-neurogenic bladder-sphincter dysfunction, whose real problem has not been understood and who therefore receive delayed treatment or no treatment at all.

In primary monosymptomatic enuresis nocturna and in children with minor wetting before treatment, without irritative voiding symptoms and without UTI, VCUG should not be performed.

Conclusion

The common pathophysiological denominator of all subtypes of non-neurogenic bladder-sphincter dysfunction ("voiding dysfunction") is functional urinary obstruction caused by detrusor-sphincter dyscoordination during bladder filling and/or micturition, leading to high intravesical pressure. Clinical manifestation in terms of irritative voiding symptoms and/or incontinence and urinary tract pathology in terms of anatomical distortion, VUR, and dilatation of the upper urinary tract are the consequences. Constipation, encopresis, UTI, and breakthrough infections are part of a syndrome. To find a single common etiological denominator seems to be unrealistic; a complex polyetiologic concept has to be considered, and etiology may differ by age and gender.

Pediatricians, pediatric urologists, and pediatric radiologists must learn to differentiate between symptoms such as enuresis nocturna and (urge) incontinence and signs such as unstable bladder or dysfunctional voiding. Unstable bladder is often the cause of (urge) incontinence in children, but it may be an associated sign of the symptom nighttime bedwetting (enuresis nocturna). The underlying etiology for both, the symptom and the sign, might be a disturbance of higher central nervous centers. The enormous complexity of this problem and rather divergent results of several treatment studies make treatment decisions still difficult. Even today, there is a major research deficit in this context due to the lack of systematic and large studies on the impact of various diagnostic tools and signs on the diagnostic and therapeutic efficacy, and there is still a lack of large comparable prospective and randomized treatment studies measuring outcome and life quality. The (pediatric) radiologist performing VCUG and US studies of the urinary tract in neonates, infants, and children has to know which functional and morphological findings are indicators of non-neurogenic bladder-sphincter dysfunction to bring out the crucial clues for further patient management.

References

Abidari JM, Shortliffe L (2002) Urinary incontinence in girls. Urol Coin N Am 29:661–675

Adams J, Mehls O, Wiesel M (2004) Pediatric renal transplantation and the dysfunctional bladder. Transpl Int 17:596–602

Akbal C, Genc Y, Burgu B et al (2005) Dysfunctional voiding and incontinence scoring system: quantitative evaluation of incontinence symptoms in pediatric population. J Urol 173:969–973

Allen T (1977) The non-neurogenic neurogenic bladder. J Urol 117:232

Allen T, Bright T (1978) Urodynamic patterns in children with dysfunctional voiding problems. J Urol 119:247–252

Austin PF, Bauer SB, Bower W et al (2014) The standardization of terminology of lower urinary tract function in children and adolescents: update report from the Standardization Committee of the International Children's Continence Society. J Urol 191:1863

Avni EF, Schulman CC (1996) The origin of vesico-ureteric reflux in male newborns: further evidence in favour of a transient fetal urethral obstruction. Br J Urol 78:454–459

Bachelard M, Sillen U, Hansson S et al (1998) Urodynamic pattern in infants with urinary tract infection. J Urol 160:522–526

Bakker E, Van Sprundel M, Van der Auwera JC et al (2002) Voiding habits and wetting in a population of 4,332 Belgian schoolchildren aged between 10 and 14 years. Scand J Urol Nephrol 36:354–362

Barroso U, Jednak R, Barthold JS et al (2001) Outcome of ureteral reimplantation in children with the urge syndrome. J Urol 166:1031–1035

Bartkowski DP, Doubrava RG (2004) Ability of a normal dysfunctional voiding symptom score to predict uroflowmetry and external urinary sphincter electromyography patterns in children. J Urol 172:1980–1985

Batisky D (1996) Pediatric urinary tract infections. Pediatr Ann 25(266):269–276

Bauer SB (1992) Neuropathology of the lower urinary tract. In: Kelalis PP, King LR, Belman AB (eds) Clinical pediatric urology, 3rd edn. Saunders, Philadelphia

Bauer SB, Retik AB, Colodney AH et al (1980) The unstable bladder of childhood. Urol Clin North Am 7:321–336

Beck AD (1971) Effect of intra-uterine obstruction upon the development of the fetal kidney. J Urol 105:784–789

Bellman M (1966) Studies on encopresis. Acta Paediatr Scand 170:1–151

Benoit RM, Wise BV, Naslund MJ et al (2002) The effect of dysfunctional voiding on the costs of treating vesicoureteral reflux: a computer model. J Urol 168:2173–2176

Bernasconi M, Borsari A, Garzoni L et al (2009) Vaginal voiding: a common cause of daytime urinary leakage in girls. J Pediatr Adolesc Gynecol 22:347

Berry AK, Zderic S, Carr M (2009) Methylphenidate for giggle incontinence. J Urol 182:2028

Blethyn AJ, Jenkins HR, Roberts R et al (1995) Radiological evidence of constipation in urinary tract infection. Arch Dis Child 73:534–535

Burgers RE, Mugie SM, Chase J et al (2013) Management of functional constipation in children with lower urinary tract symptoms: report from the Standardization Committee of the International Children's Continence Society. J Urol 190:29

Chandra M (1995) Reflux nephropathy, urinary tract infection, and voiding disorders. Curr Opin Pediatr 7:164–170

Chandra M (1996) Incidence of voiding dysfunction in elementary school children. Pediatr Res 39:359A

Chandra M (1998) Nocturnal enuresis in children. Curr Opin Pediatr 10:167–173

Chandra M, Saharia R, Shi Q et al (2002) Giggle incontinence in children: a manifestation of detrusor instability. J Urol 168:2184–2187

Chen JJ, Mao W, Homayoon K et al (2004) A multivariate analysis of dysfunctional elimination syndrome and its relationships with gender, urinary tract infection and vesicoureteral reflux in children. J Urol 171:1907–1910

Chiozza ML (2002) Dysfunctional voiding. Ped Med Chir 24:137–140

Chiozza ML, Bernardinelli L, Caione P et al (1998) An Italian epidemiological multicentre study of nocturnal enuresis. Br J Urol 81(Suppl):86–89

Combs AJ, Glassberg AD, Gerdes D et al (1998) Biofeedback therapy for children with dysfunctional voiding. Urology 52:312–315

Couillard DR, Webster GD (1995) Detrusor instability. Urol Clin North Am 22:593–612

David C, Dacher JN, Monroc M et al (1998) Retrograde cystography after a first episode of acute pyelonephritis in the child. J Radiol 79:133–137

Davila GW, Bernier F, Franco J et al (2003) Bladder dysfunction in sexual abuse survivors. J Urol 170:476–479

De Araújo Sant'Anna AM, Calcado AC (1999) Constipation in school-aged children at public schools in Rio de Janeiro, Brazil. J Pediatr Gastroenterol Nutr 29:190–193

De Groat WC (1993) Anatomy and physiology of the lower urinary tract. Urol Clin North Am 20:383–401

Dewan PA (1993) Congenital obstructing posterior urethral membranes (COPUM): further evidence for a common morphological diagnosis. Pediatr Surg Int 8:45–50

Dewan PA, Goh DG, Crameri J (1995) Cobb's collar. Pediatr Surg Int 10:243–246

Dewan PA, Pillay S, Kaye K (1997) Correlation of the endoscopic and radiological anatomy of congenital obstruction of the posterior urethra and the external sphincter. Br J Urol 79:790–796

Dohil R, Roberts E, Verrier-Jones K et al (1994) Constipation and reversible urinary tract abnormalities. Arch Dis Child 70:56–57

Ellsworth PI, Merguerian PA, Copening ME (1995) Sexual abuse: another causative factor in dysfunctional voiding. J Urol 153:773–776

Fanos V, Cataldi L (2004) Antibiotics or surgery for vesicoureteric reflux in children. Lancet 364:1720–1722

Farhat W, Bägli DJ, Capolicchio G et al (2000) The dysfunctional voiding scoring system: quantitative standardization of dysfunctional voiding symptoms in children. J Urol 164:1011

Feldman AS, Bauer SB (2006) Diagnosis and management of dysfunctional voiding. Curr Opin Pediatr 18:139–147

Fotter R (1992) Functional disorders of the lower urinary tract: urodynamic and radiological diagnosis. In: Thomsen HS (ed) European uroradiology 1992. FADL Publishers, Copenhagen, pp 127–132

Fotter R (1994) Children. In: Dalla Palma L, Thomsen HS (eds) European uroradiology 1994. FADL Publishers, Copenhagen, pp 120–127

Fotter R (1996) Neurogenic bladder in infants and children – a new challenge for the radiologist. Abdom Imaging 21:534–540

Fotter R, Kopp W, Klein E et al (1986) Unstable bladder in children: functional evaluation by modified VCU. Radiology 161:811–813

Glazier DB, Murphy DP, Fleisher MH et al (1997) Evaluation of the utility of video-urodynamics in children with urinary tract infections and voiding dysfunction. Br J Urol 80:806–808

Glick PL, Harrison MR, Neall RA (1993) Correction of congenital hydronephrosis in utero III. Early midtrimester ureteral obstruction produces renal dysplasia. J Pediatr Surg 18:681–687

Godley ML, Desai D, Yeung CK et al (2001) The relationship between early renal status and the resolution of vesicoureteric reflux and bladder function at 16 months. BJU Int 87:457–462

Greenfield SP, Ng M, Wan J (1997) Experience with vesicoureteral reflux in children: clinical characteristics. J Urol 158:574–577

Griffith DJ, Scholtmeijer RJ (1987) Vesico-ureteral reflux and lower urinary tract dysfunction: evidence for two different reflux-dysfunction complexes. J Urol 137:240–244

Gür E, Turhan P, Can G et al (2004) Enuresis: prevalence, risk factors and urinary pathology among school children in Istanbul, Turkey. Pediatr Int 46:58–63

Hausegger KA, Fotter R, Sorantin E et al (1991) Urethral morphology and bladder instability. Pediatr Radiol 21:278–280

Hellerstein S, Linebarger JS (2003) Voiding dysfunction in pediatric patients. Clin Pediatr (Phila) 42:43–49

Hellström AL, Hjälmas K, Jodal U (1987) Rehabilitation of the dysfunctional bladder in children: method and 3-year follow-up. J Urol 138:847–849

Hellström AL, Hanson E, Hansson S et al (1990) Micturition habits and incontinence in 7-year-old Swedish school entrants. Eur J Pediatr 149:434–437

Herndon CDA, McKenna P, Kolon TF (1999) A multicenter outcome analysis of patients with neonatal reflux presenting with prenatal hydronephrosis. J Urol 162:1203–1208

Herz D, Weiser A, Collette T et al (2005) Dysfunctional elimination syndrome as an etiology of idiopathic urethritis in childhood. J Urol 173:2132–2137

Himsl KK, Hurwitz RS (1991) Pediatric urinary incontinence. Urol Clin North Am 18:283–293

Hinman F (1986) Nonneurogenic neurogenic bladder (the Hinman syndrome)-15 years later. J Urol 136:769–777

Hinman F, Baumann FW (1973) Vesical and ureteral damage from voiding dysfuncion in boys without neurologic or obstructive disease. J Urol 109:727–732

Hiraoka M, Hori C, Tsukahara H et al (1999) Voiding function study with ultrasound in male and female neonates. Kidney Int 55:1920–1926

Hjälmas K (1988) Urodynamics in normal infants and children. Scand J Urol Nephrol Suppl 114:20–27

Hjälmas K (1992) Urinary incontinence in children: suggestions for definitions and terminology. Scand J Urol Nephrol Suppl 141:1–6

Hjälmas K (1995) SWEET, the Swedish enuresis trial. Scand J Urol Nephrol Suppl 173:89–93

Hjälmas K (1997) Pathophysiology and impact of nocturnal enuresis. Acta Paediatr 86:919–922

Hoebecke P, Vande Walle J, Everaert K et al (1999) Assessment of lower urinary tract dysfunction in children with non-neuropathic bladder sphincter dysfunction. Eur Urol 35:57–69

Hoebeke P, Van Laecke E, Van Camp C et al (2001) One thousand video-urodynamic studies in children with non-neurogenic bladder sphincter dysfunction. BJU Int 87:575–580

Homsy YL, Nsouli I, Hamburger B et al (1985) Effects of oxybutynin on vesicoureteral reflux in children. J Urol 134:1168–1171

Howe AC, Walker CE (1992) Behavioral management of toilet training, enuresis and encopresis. Pediatr Clin North Am 39:413–432

Järvelin MR, Vikevainen-Tervonen L, Moilanen J et al (1988) Enuresis in 7-year-old children. Acta Paediatr 77:148–153

Jayanthi VR, Khoury AE, McLorie GA et al (1997) The nonneurogenic neurogenic bladder of early infancy. J Urol 158:1281–1285

Joinson C, Heron J, Von Gontard A et al (2006) Psychological problems in children with daytime wetting. Pediatrics 118:1985–1993

Käfer M, Barnewolt C, Retik AB et al (1997) The sonographic diagnosis of intravesical obstruction in children: evaluation of bladder wall thickness indexed to bladder filling. J Urol 157:989–991

Kajiwara M, Inoue K, Kato M et al (2006) Nocturnal enuresis and overactive bladder in children: an epidemiological study. Int J Urol 13:36–41

Kelleher RE (1997) Daytime and nighttime wetting in children: a review of management. J Soc Pediatr Nurs 2:73–82

Klijn AJ, Asselman M, Vijverberg MAW et al (2004) The diameter of the rectum on ultrasonography as a diagnostic tool for constipation in children with dysfunctional voiding. J Urol 172:1986–1988

Koff SA (1982) Bladder-sphincter dysfunction in childhood. Urology 14:457–461

Koff SA (1984) Non-neuropathic vesico-urethral dysfunction in children. In: Urodynamics, principles, practice and application. Churchill Livingstone, New York, pp 311–325

Koff SA (1992) Relationship between dysfunctional voiding and reflux. J Urol 148:1703–1705

Koff SA (1995) Why is desmopressin sometimes ineffective at curing bedwetting? Scand J Urol Nephrol Suppl 173:103–108

Koff SA, Murtagh DS (1983) The uninhibited bladder in children: effect of treatment on recurrence of urinary tract infection and on vesico-ureteral reflux resolution. J Urol 130:1138–1141

Koff SA, Lapides J, Piazza DH (1979) Association of urinary tract infection and reflux with uninhibited bladder contractions and voluntary sphincteric obstruction. J Urol 122:373–376

Koff SA, Wagner TT, Jayanthi VR (1998) The relationship among dysfunctional elimination syndromes, primary vesicoureteral reflux and urinary tract infections in children. J Urol 160:1019–1022

Kokoua A, Homsy Y, Lavigne JF (1993) Maturation of the external urinary sphincter: a comparative histotopographic study in humans. J Urol 150:617–622

Lackgren G, Hjalmas K, Van Gool J et al (1999) Nocturnal enuresis: a suggestion for a European treatment strategy. Acta Paediatr 88:679–690

Lapides J, Diokno AC (1970) Persistence of the infant bladder as cause for urinary tract infection in girls. J Urol 103:243–248

Lee SD, Sohn DW, Lee JZ et al (2000) An epidemiological study of enuresis in Korean children. BJU Int 85:869–873

Leung VY, Metreweli C, Yeung CK (2002a) Immature ureteric jet Doppler patterns and urinary tract infection and vesicoureteric reflux in children. Ultrasound Med Biol 28:873–878

Leung VY, Metreweli C, Yeung CK (2002b) The ureteric jet Doppler waveform as an indicator of vesicoureteric sphincter function in adults and children. An observational study. Ultrasound Med Biol 28:865–872

Leung VY, Chu WC, Yeung CK et al (2006) Ureteric jet Doppler waveform and bladder wall thickness in children with nocturnal enuresis. Pediatr Res 60:582–586

Leung VY, Chu WC, Yeung CK (2007) Nomograms of total renal volume, urinary bladder volume and bladder wall thickness index in 3,376 children with a normal urinary tract. Pediatr Radiol 37:181–188

Loening-Baucke VA (1997) Urinary incontinence and urinary tract infection and their resolution with treatment of chronic constipation of childhood. Pediatrics 100:228–232

Loening-Baucke VA (2007) Prevalence rates for constipation and faecal and urinary incontinence. Arch Dis Child 92(6):486–489

Luke PPW, Herz DB, Bellinger MF et al (2003) Long-term results of pediatric renal transplantation into a dysfunctional lower urinary tract. Transplantation 76:1578–1582

Maffei HV, Moreira FL, Oliveira WM et al (1997) Constipacao intestinal em escolare. J Pediatr 73:340–344

Mayo ME, Burns MW (1990) Urodynamic studies in children who wet. Br J Urol 65:641–645

Mazzola BL, Von Vigier RO, Marchand S et al (2003) Behavioral and functional abnormalities linked with recurrent urinary tract infections in girls. J Nephrol 16:133–138

Medel R, Dieguez S, Brindo M et al (1998) Monosymptomatic primary enuresis: differences between patients responding or not responding to oral desmopressin. Br J Urol 81(Suppl 3):46–49

Muellner SR (1960) Development of urinary control in children. JAMA 172:1256–1261

Naseer SR, Steinhardt GF (1997) New renal scars in children with urinary tract infections, vesicoureteral reflux and voiding dysfunction: a prospective evaluation. J Urol 158:566–568

Nasrallah PF, Simon JW (1984) Reflux and voiding abnormalities in children. Urology 24:243–245

Nepple KG, Cooper CS (2014) Etiology and clinical features of bladder dysfunction in children. UpToDate 2014; Wolters Kluwer Health. www.uptodate.com. Last updated 26 Jun 2014

Nevéus T, Hetta J, Cnattingius S et al (1999) Depth of sleep and sleep habits among enuretic and incontinent children. Acta Paediatr 88:748–752

Nielsen JB, Djurhuus JC, Jørgensen TM (1984) Lower urinary tract dysfunction in vesicoureteral reflux. Urol Int 39:29–31

Nijman RJ (2000) Classification and treatment of functional incontinence in children. BJU Int 85(Suppl 3): 574–577

Noé HN (1988) The relationship of sibling reflux to index patient dysfunctional voiding. J Urol 130:1138–1141

Nonomura K, Kanno T, Kakizaki H et al (1999) Impact of congenital narrowing of the bulbar urethra (Cobb's collar) and its transurethral incision in children. Eur Urol 36:144–149

Nørgaard JP, Hansen JH, Wildschiodlz G et al (1989) Sleep cystometrics in children with nocturnal enuresis. J Urol 141:1156–1159

Nørgaard JP, Jønler M, Rittig S et al (1995) A pharmacodynamic study of desmopressin in patients with nocturnal enuresis. J Urol 153:1984–1986

Nørgaard JP, van Gool JD, Hjälmas K et al (1998) Standardization and definitions in lower urinary tract dysfunction in children. Br J Urol 81(Suppl 3):1–16

O'Regan S, Schick E, Hamburger B et al (1986) Constipation associated with vesicoureteral reflux. Urology 27:394–396

Opsomer RJ, Clapuyt P, De Groote P et al (1998) Urodynamic and elecotrophysiological testing in pediatric neurourology. Acta Urol Belg 66:31–34

Parekh DJ, Pope JC, Adams MC et al (2001) The use of radiography, urodynamic studies and cystoscopy in the evaluation of voiding dysfunction. J Urol 165:215–218

Passerini-Glazel G, Cisternino A, Camuffo MC et al (1992) Video-urodynamic studies of minor voiding dysfunctions in children: an overview of 13 years' experience. Scand J Urol Nephrol Suppl 141:70–84

Penido Silva JM, Araujo Oliveira E, Santos Diniz JS et al (2006) Gender and vesico-ureteral reflux: a multivariate analysis. Pediatr Nephrol 21:510–516

Pfister C, Wagner L, Caher JN et al (1996) Long-term bladder dysfunction in boys with posterior urethral valves. Eur J Pediatr Surg 6:222–224

Riccabona M (2012) Functional disorders of the lower urinary tract in childhood: an update. Pediatr Radiol 42(S3):S433–S434

Richardson I, Palmer LS (2009) Successful treatment for giggle incontinence with biofeedback. J Urol 182:2062

Risdon RA, Yeung CK, Ransley PG (1993) Reflux nephropathy in children submitted to unilateral nephrectomy: a clinicopathological study. Clin Nephrol 6:308–314

Savage JP (1973) The deleterious effect of constipation upon the reimplanted ureter. J Urol 109:501–503

Saxton HM, Robinson LB (1992) Nonobstructive posterior urethral widening (spinning top urethra) in boys with bladder instability. Radiology 182:81–85

Saxton HM, Borzyskowski M, Mundy AR et al (1988) Spinning top urethra: not a normal variant. Radiology 168:147–150

Scholtmeijer RJ, Nijman R (1994) Vesicoureteric reflux and videourodynamic studies: results of a prospective study after three years follow-up. Urology 43:714–718

Schulman SL, Zderic S, Kaplan P (1996) Increased prevalence of urinary symptoms and voiding dysfunction in Williams' syndrome. J Pediatr 129:446–469

Schulman SL, Quinn CK, Plachter N et al (1999) Comprehensive management of dysfunctional voiding. Pediatrics 103:658

Seruca H (1989) Vesico-ureteral reflux and voiding dysfunction: a prospective study. J Urol 142:494–498

Shopfner CE (1968) Urinary tract pathology associated with constipation. Radiology 90:865–877

Sillen U, Hjalmas K, Aili M et al (1992) Pronounced detrusor hypercontractility in infants with gross bilateral reflux. J Urol 148:598–599

Sillen U, Bachelard M, Hermanson G et al (1996) Gross bilateral reflux in infants: gradual decrease of initial detrusor hypercontractility. J Urol 155:668–672

Smellie JM, Grüneberg RN, Bantock HM et al (1988) Prophylactic co-trimoxazole and trimethoprim in the management of urinary tract infection in children. Pediatr Nephrol 2:12–17

Snodgrass W (1998) The impact of treated dysfunctional voiding on the nonsurgical management of vesicoureteral reflux. J Urol 160:1823–1825

Spee-van der Wekke J, Hirasing RA, Meulmeester JF et al (1998) Childhood nocturnal enuresis in the Netherlands. Urology 51:1022–1026

Staskin DR, Dmochowski RR (2002) Future studies of overactive bladder: the need for standardization. Urology 60(5 Suppl 1):90–93

Sujka SK, Piedmonte MR, Greenfield SP (1991) Enuresis and the voiding cystourethrogram: a re-evaluation. Urology 38:139–142

Sureshkumar P, Cumming RG, Craig CJ (2006) Validity and reliability of parental report of frequency, severity and risk factors of urinary tract infection and urinary incontinence in children. J Urol 175:2254–2262

Swithinbank LV, Carr JC, Abrams PH (1994) Longitudinal study of urinary symptoms and incontinence in local schoolchildren. Scand J Urol Nephrol 163(Suppl):67–73

Swithinbank LV, Heron J, von Gontard A, Abrams P (2010) The natural history of daytime urinary incontinence in children: a large British cohort. Acta Paediatr 99:1031

Ukimura O, Kojima M, Inui E et al (1998) Noninvasive evaluation of bladder compliance in children using ultrasound estimated bladder weight. J Urol 160:1459–1462

Van der Wal MF, Benninga MA, Hirasing RA (2005) The prevalence of encopresis in a multicultural population. J Pediatr Gastroenterol Nutr 40:345–348

Van der Weide MJA, Cornelissen EAM, Van Achterberg T et al (2006) Dysfunction of lower urinary tract in renal transplant children with nephrologic disease. Urology 67:1060–1065

Van Gool JD (1995) Dysfunctional voiding: a complex of bladder/sphincter dysfunction, urinary tract infections and vesicoureteral reflux. Acta Urol Belg 63:27–33

Van Gool JD, Dejonge GA (1989) Urge syndrome and urge incontinence. Arch Dis Child 64:1629–1634

Van Gool JD, Kuijten RH, Donckerwolcke RA et al (1984) Bladder-sphincter dysfunction, urinary infection and vesicoureteral reflux, with special reference to cognitive bladder training. Contrib Nephrol 39:190–210

Van Gool JD, Vijverberg MA, de Jong TPVM (1992a) Functional daytime incontinence: clinical and

urodynamic assessment. Scand J Urol Nephrol Suppl 141:58–69
Van Gool JD, Vijverberg MA, Messer AP et al (1992b) Functional daytime incontinence: non-pharmacological treatment. Scand J Urol Nephrol Suppl 141:93–103
Wan J, Kaplinsky R, Greenfield S (1995) Toilet habits of children evaluated for urinary tract infection. J Urol 154:797–799
Watanabe H, Kawauchi A, Kitamori T et al (1994) Treatment for nocturnal enuresis according to an original classification system. Eur Urol 25:43–50
Weerasinghe N, Malone PS (1993) The value of videourodynamics in the investigation of neurologically normal children who wet. Br J Urol 71:539–542
Wen JG, Tong EC (1998) Cystometry in infants and children with no apparent voiding symptoms. Br J Urol 81:468–473
Wille S (1994) Nocturnal enuresis: sleep disturbance and behavioral patterns. Acta Paediatr 83:772–774
Yeung CK, Godley ML, Ho CKW et al (1995) Some new insights into bladder function in infancy. Br J Urol 76:235–240
Yeung CK, Godley ML, Ransley PG (1997) The evolution of bladder function as an important indicator for the natural outcome of vesicoureteric reflux during the first 2-years of life. In: Proceedings of the American Academy of Pediatrics, New Orleans, p 112
Yeung CK, Godley ML, Dhillon HK et al (1998) Urodynamic patterns in infants with normal lower urinary tracts or primary vesico-ureteric reflux. Br J Urol 81:461–467
Yeung CK, Chiu HN, Sit FKY (1999) Bladder dysfunction in children with refractory monosymptomatic primary nocturnal enuresis. J Urol 162:1049–1055
Yeung CK, Sreedhar B, Leung VT et al (2004) Ultrasound bladder measurements in patients with primary nocturnal enuresis: a urodynamic and treatment outcome correlation. J Urol 171:2589–2594
Yeung CK, Sreedhar B, Sihoe JDY et al (2006a) Renal and bladder functional status at diagnosis as predictive factors for the outcome of primary vesicoureteral reflux in children. J Urol 176:1152–1157
Yeung CK, Sreedhar B, Sihoe JDY et al (2006b) Differences in characteristics of nocturnal enuresis between children and adolescents: a critical appraisal from a large epidemiological study. BJU Int 97:1069–1073
Yeung CK, Sreedhar B, Leung YFV et al (2007) Correlation between ultrasonographic bladder measurements and urodynamic findings in children with recurrent urinary tract infection. BJU Int 99: 651–655
Yong D, Beattie RM (1998) Normal bowel habit and prevalence of constipation in primary-school children. Amb Child Health 4:277–282
Zaslavsky C, Ávila EL, Araújo MA et al (1988) Constipacao intestinal da infancia-um estudo de prevalencia. Rev AMRIGS 32:100–102
Zerin JM, Chen E, Ritchey ML et al (1993) Bladder capacity as measured at voiding cystourethrography in children: relationship to toilet training and frequency of micturition. Radiology 187:803–806

Neurogenic Bladder in Infants and Children

Erich Sorantin, R. Fotter, and K. Braun

Contents

1 **Anatomy and Physiology** 423
2 **Etiology of Neurogenic Bladders** 424
3 **Classification of Neurogenic Bladder** 424
4 **Diagnostic Imaging in Neurogenic Bladder** 425
4.1 Radiological, Functional Assessment and Classification of Neurogenic Bladder Based on mVCUG 427

Conclusion 428

References 428

1 Anatomy and Physiology

The bladder can be divided into three parts: apex, body, and fundus. The detrusor muscle corresponds to the smooth muscle component of the bladder and forms a complex mesh of muscle bundles extending into the bladder neck as well as surrounding of the proximal urethra – thus forming the internal urethral sphincter. The striated external sphincter covers only the distal part of the internal urethral sphincter and extends than downwards to the level of the urogenital diaphragm. In the normal case, a single ureter, on each body side, enters the bladder on the lateral circumference at an angle of less than 45°. The trigone represents the area between the two ureteric orifices and the internal urethral meatus.

Somatic and autonomous nervous systems control the lower urinary tract. The somatic nerves originate from the dural sac within the sacral chord and innervate the external sphincter via pudendal nerve, whereas for autonomic innervation, sympathetic nerves leave the spinal cord at T10 to L1. Parasympathetic counterpart originates from the dural sac at S2 to S4.

Regarding function the urinary bladder acts as a reservoir for urine and is responsible for evacuation of the collected urine. There are three features, which characterize a normal, mature bladder function: sensation about bladder filling and voiding that can be induced and interrupted voluntarily. If any of those features is missing, a neurogenic bladder will be present.

E. Sorantin, MD (✉) • R. Fotter, MD (Retired)
Department of Radiology, Division of Pediatric Radiology, Medical University Graz,
Auenbruggerplatz 34, A-8036 Graz, Austria
e-mail: Erich.Sorantin@medunigraz.at

K. Braun, MD
Department of Pediatric and Adolescent Surgery,
Medical University Graz,
Auenbruggerplatz 34, A-8036 Graz, Austria
e-mail: karin.braun@medunigraz.at

Storage is achieved at almost the same intraluminal pressure (10 bis 15 cm H_2O – isobaric state). The are several formulas available to calculate the normal, age-dependent bladder capacity (see also chapter "Normal Values"):

- Normal expected bladder capacity (ml) = (age in years + 2) × 30 = 30 × (age in years) + 60 (Koff 1983)
- Normal expected bladder capacity (ml = 16 × age in years) + 70 (Houle et al. 1993)

In the first 6 months of life, the bladder volume does not show a linear increase due to the increased fluid load caused by breastfeeding. There are already published normograms of normal bladder capacity (Zerin et al. 1993). In children with myelodysplasia, the bladder capacity will be usually reduced by 20–25% and can be calculated by the following formula:

- Bladder capacity in myelodysplasia (ml) = (24.5 × age in years) + 62 (Palmer et al. 1997)

Continence is maintained by the resistance of the bladder neck as well as by the voluntary controlled, striated external sphincter.

Voiding is achieved by detrusor muscles contraction and simultaneous opening of the bladder neck as well as relaxation of the external, striated sphincter. It has to be considered that voiding in unfamiliar surrounding a partially filled bladder or overfilled bladder may promote residual volume. Residual void of more than 20 ml or more than 10% of the total bladder capacity, on repeated occasions, may be regarded as abnormal.

2 Etiology of Neurogenic Bladders

Myelodysplasia, cerebral palsy, teratoma, and imperforate anus with sacral dysplasia (e.g., Currarino triad) represent frequent causes of neurogenic bladder in childhood (Goepel et al. 1999; Ozkan et al. 2006). In particular the outcome of patients with myelodysplasia does not anymore depend on the underlying neurological pathology but from the urological course. In children with myelodysplasia, pyelonephritis and renal failure are the most common causes for morbidity and mortality within the first 3 years. It is not worthy to mention that 50% of these patients will end up with urinary tract deterioration within the first years without any intervention (Bauer and Joseph 1990). The pressure volume characteristics of the neurogenic bladder determine the fate of the upper urinary tract. Intermittent or continuous elevated bladder pressure is related to urinary tract infections, upper urinary tract deterioration, and renal failure. Predicted factors for upper urinary tract deterioration are sphincter detrusor dyssynergia, high bladder-filling pressure (more than 40 cm H_2O – see chapter "Video-Urodynamics"), and poor bladder compliance (Bauer and Joseph 1990; Galloway et al. 1991; Ghoniem et al. 1989, 1990; Kurzrock and Polse 1998; McGuire et al. 1981). Furthermore, high leak point pressure and vesicoureteral reflux (VUR) (Seki et al. 2004) as well as detrusor fibrosis are related to poor prognosis (Özkan et al. 2005).

Therefore the therapeutic goal is to preserve the renal function and to avoid urinary tract infection as well as achievement of social continence. Several strategies like clean, intermittent catheterization, appropriate medication (e.g., anticholinergic drugs, antibiotics), as well as urological procedures (e.g., continence operations, bladder augmentations) facilitate the achievement of the abovementioned goals (Bauer and Joseph 1990; Kasabian et al. 1992; Rickwood et al. 1982; Stein et al. 2005; Hayashi et al. 2006; Morrisroe et al. 2005).

3 Classification of Neurogenic Bladder

Classification can be made on anatomical (in relation to the anatomic level of the underlying neurological disorders) or on functional aspects. A functional classification of the bladder property can be derived from features like compliance (hyper-/normo-/hypotonic), urine storage, and voiding:

(a) Inability to void (normal bladder capacity, high residual volume),

Table 1 Classification of detrusor activity

Type	Detrusor contractions	SWI*	Passive bladder neck opening
Acontractile	−	+++	+++
Contractile	++	−	−
Mixed	+	+	+

*Sphincter Weakness Incontinence

(b) Inability to store (low bladder capacity, no residual volume)
(c) Balanced function (bladder capacity acceptable, residual volume tolerable)
(d) Combined dysfunction (inadequate bladder capacity, unacceptable high residual volume)

Furthermore the reflexive activity of the detrusor can be classified in three types (Rickwood et al. 1982):

(a) Contractile detrusor (detrusor hyperreflexia)
(b) Acontractile detrusor (detrusor areflexia)
(c) Mixed type – especially when an underlying neurologic pathology affects different portions of the micturition control centers and pathways – most frequently in myelodysplasia.

On voiding cystourethrography (VCUG), a contractile detrusors present always with closed bladder neck and unstable detrusor contractions. As opposed, acontractile detrusors show a passive open neck during the VCUG filling phase and are lacking detrusor contractions. Mixed types share features of other types to a varying extent; thus sometimes further subtypes like mixed acontractile or mixed contractile are differentiated.

Putting all these features together, classification of the detrusor activity can be achieved as demonstrated in Table 1.

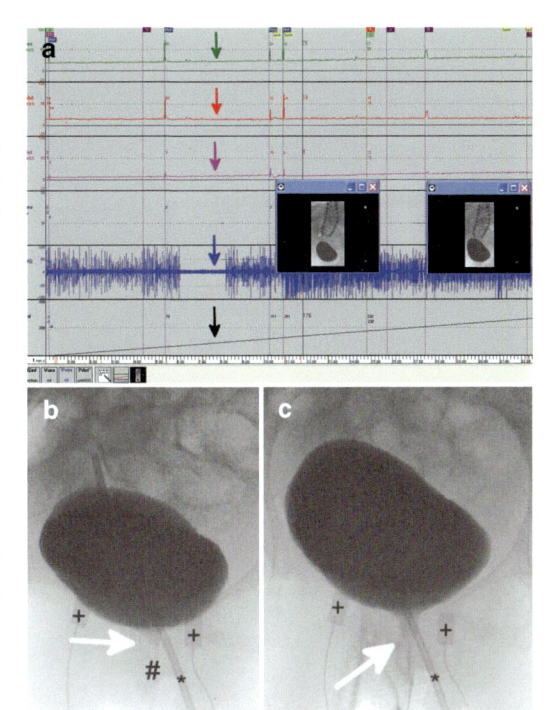

Fig. 1 (a) VUD, 14-year-old girl, operated for a meningomyelocele and underwent later spine surgery. VUD pressure tracings with the following *arrows*: *green* → intravesical pressure, *red* → intra-abdominal pressure, *pink* → detrusor pressure (intravesical – intra-abdominal pressure), *blue* → pelvic floor EMG, *black* → instilled volume. Secondary capture screenshots from fluoroscopy are superimposed – detailed views in (b, c). There is no significant change of detrusor pressure during the examination – indicating an acontractile detrusor type. The minimal steady increase of detrusor pressure indicates that the bladder tone increases with filling, which does not occur in normal bladders. (**b, c**) Secondary screen capture shots from VUD. Rectal (*) and urethral catheters (#) in place as well as perineal electrodes (+). (**b**) VUD filling phase, an open bladder neck can be seen (*white arrow*), (**c**) end of filling, bladder catheter was removed; there is leakage of urine due to straining (*white arrow*). Final combined findings (VUD and fluoroscopy report): normtonic, acontractile detrusor, inability to void

4 Diagnostic Imaging in Neurogenic Bladder

Imaging of neurogenic bladder must depict all details necessary for clinical management. Video urodynamics represents the imaging modality of choice and allows the determination of parameters as listed in chapter "Video-Urodynamics". A recent overview can be found at Drzewiecki and Bauer (Drzewiecki and Bauer 2011). Figures 1 and 2 demonstrate examples of VUD findings in acontractile and contractile detrusor types.

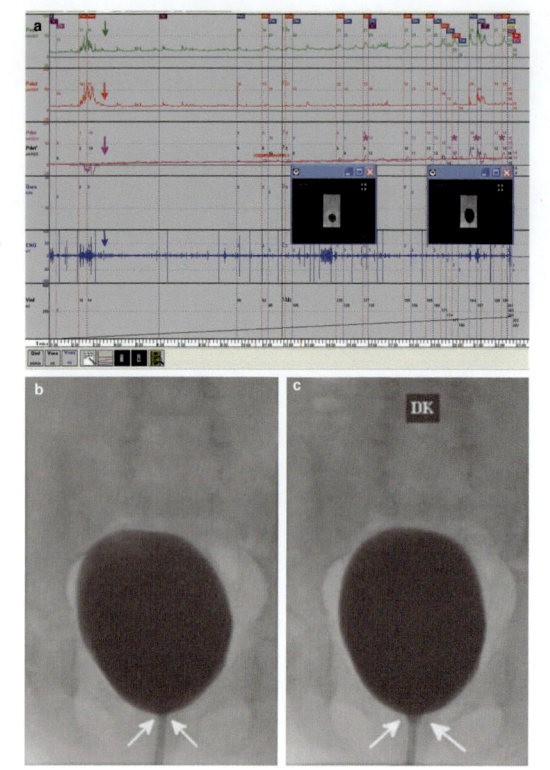

Fig. 2 (a) VUD, 5-year-old boy, operated for a meningomyelocele. VUD pressure tracings marked with *arrows* – colors the same as in Fig. 1a. Secondary capture screenshots from fluoroscopy are superimposed – detailed view in (b, c). In the later part of the examination, several detrusor contractions are depicted and marked by*. (b, c) Secondary screen capture shots from VUD (a). Rectal and urethral catheters are superimposed due to straight a-p view. (b) VUD filling phase bladder neck closed, (c) Detrusor contraction on VUD tracings → bladder neck opened. Final combined findings (VUD and fluoroscopy report): normtonic, contractile detrusor, inability to void

However, VUD demands dedicated equipment, which is, unfortunately, not ubiquitously available. Therefore the question remains: which of the necessary parameters can be obtained by performing VCUG in a modified fashion? In children with myelodysplasia, it is not enough to fill the bladder and describe only morphology. A modified VCUG technique (mVCUG) in combination with an expertise in pathophysiology of neurogenic bladders provides nearly all this information needed for functional assessment (Fotter et al. 1986; Fotter 1996).

In mVCUG there is just a minor change in the setting of standard VCUG: the bottle with contrast medium is just put 30 cm above the patient. The placement of the contrast bottle 30 cm above the patient is done since the critical intervesical pressure is 40 cm H_2O. Values above this limit lead to upper urinary tract dilatation, especially if there are intermittent pressure values of more than 90–100 cm H_2O – consequences are bladder wall thickening, trabeculation, subsequent diverticular formation, and VUR.

The drip infusion dropping speed serves as a manometer. This means that if the dropping speed is normal, the intravesical pressure will be below 30 cm of water → so well below the critical intravesical pressure value of 40 cm H_2O. Stopped dropping of the drip infusion indicates that there is a rise in the intravesical pressure to more than 30 cm. At this moment a short intermittent fluoroscopy with a last image hold shot is taken to demonstrate if the bladder neck is open or closed – an opened bladder neck indicates detrusor contraction (Fig. 3) (Fotter et al. 1986; Fotter 1996). In case of straining of the patient or movement, the intervesical pressure will rise, but due to the lacking detrusor contraction, the bladder neck will be kept closed. Therefore, mVCUG allows semiquantitative assessment of the intravesical pressure changes.

The filling phase of mVCUG ends if there is an urge to void, if there is abdominal discomfort claimed by the patient, if the expected age-related bladder capacity is reached, or if the drip infusion has completely stopped due to constantly increasing intravesical pressure or as a consequence of uninhibited detrusor contractions. The catheter removal is done under fluoroscopic control with the child in lateral position. Furthermore it is documented how the child tries to empty the bladder. Spontaneous micturations can be achieved by triggering the infraumbilical belly in order to provoke detrusor contractions or by raising intra-abdominal pressure (e.g., straining).

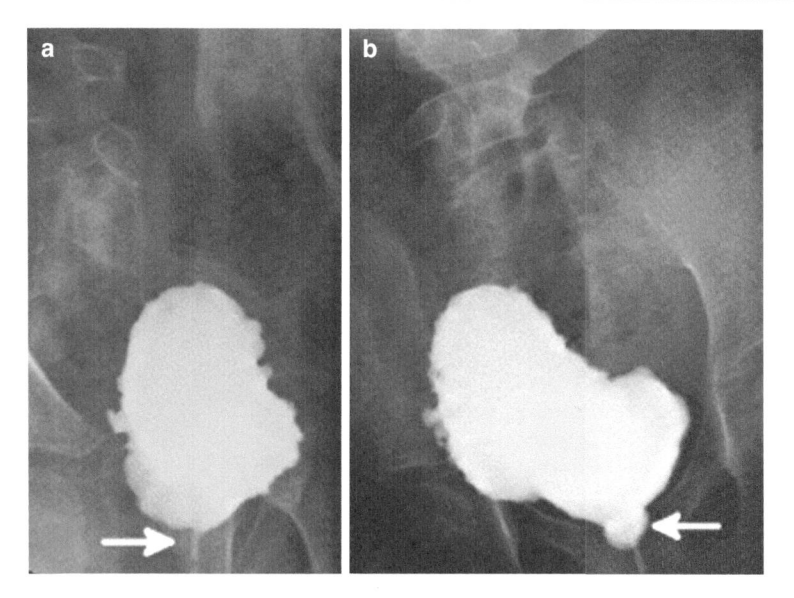

Fig. 3 Patient with neurogenic bladder at mVCUG (**a**) depicts the resting state, where the contrast medium is dropping at constant speed and the bladder neck is closed (*arrow*). (**b**) Drip infusion stops with simultaneous bladder neck opening (*arrow*) → both findings indicate inhibited detrusor contractions. A few seconds later, dropping will start and the bladder neck will close again

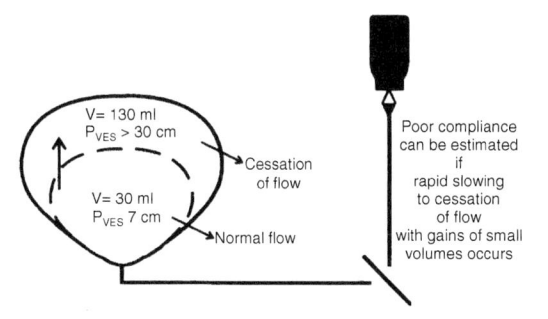

Fig. 4 Estimation of poor bladder compliance by modified VCUG (*V* bladder-filling volume, P_{VES} vesical pressure)

4.1 Radiological, Functional Assessment and Classification of Neurogenic Bladder Based on mVCUG

In correspondence to VUD, the following parameters can be defined by mVCUG.

4.1.1 Bladder Compliance

As already mentioned the speed of the drip infusion represents the manometer – thus a noncompliant bladder can be assumed if there is a constant decrease of drip infusion speed until sensation at inadequate low filling volumes (Fig. 4).

4.1.2 Unstable Detrusor Contraction

In mVCUG these are defined by a stop of the drip infusion with simultaneous opening of the bladder neck. The frequency and time period of those unstable detrusor contractions is noted.

4.1.3 Safe Storage Volume

The amount of instilled contrast medium before-gradual slowing down of drip infusion speed or detrusor contractions occurs represents "safe storage volume". The intravesical pressure doesn't reach 30 cm of H_2O, and therefore the speed of the drip infusion doesn't slow down until leakage occurs or age-related bladder capacity is reached (Fig. 5).

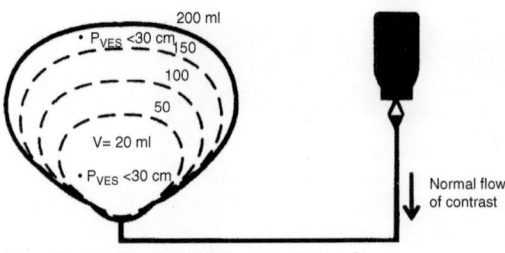

Fig. 5 Estimation of the safe storage period (the bladder volume at which vesical pressure remains well below 40 cm H$_2$O, the safe storage pressure) by modified VCUG (P_{VES} vesical pressure, V bladder-filling volume)

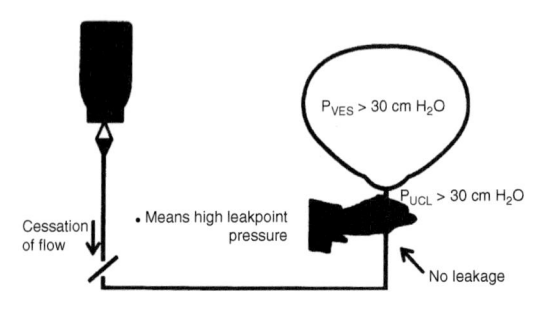

Fig. 6 Leak point pressure estimation by modified VCUG (P_{VES} vesical pressure, P_{UCL} urethral closure pressure)

4.1.4 Leak Point Pressure

In patients with no leakage at continuous slowing down or cessation of the drip infusion a high leak point pressure can be assumed (more than 30 cm absolute – Fig. 6).

4.1.5 Sphincter Detrusor Dyssynergia

An intermittent closing external sphincter during voiding indicates sphincter detrusor dyssynergia.

4.1.6 Detrusor Function

A classification of the detrusor function can be done using Table 1.

By putting the abovementioned features together, a classification of bladder function can be achieved.

Conclusion

Comprehensive assessment of lower urinary tract function and morphology is essential in neurogenic bladders. VUD represents the modality of choice and allows full workup. In institutions with no VUD, mVCUG represents a valuable alternative and allows, in addition of morphology, semiquantitative estimation of relevant factors with only minor setting modification. For mVCUG no special hardware is necessary.

References

Bauer SB, Joseph D (1990) Management of the obstructed urinary tract associated with neurogenic bladder dysfunction. Urol Clin North Am 17:395–405

Drzewiecki B, Bauer S (2011) Urodynamic testing in children: indications, technique, interpretation and significance. J Urol 186(4):1190–1197

Fotter R (1996) Neurogenic bladder in infants and children – a new challenge for the radiologist. Abdom Imaging 21:534–540

Fotter R, Kopp W, Klein E (1986) Unstable bladder in children: functional evaluation by modified voiding cystourethrography. Radiology 161:812–813

Galloway NTM, Mekras JA, Helms M (1991) An objective score to predict upper tract deterioration in myelodysplasia. J Urol 145:535–539

Ghoniem GM, Bloom DA, McGuire EJ (1989) Bladder compliance in meningomyelocele children. J Urol 141:1404–1406

Ghoniem GM, Roach MB, Lewis VH, Harmon EP (1990) The value of leak pressure and bladder compliance in the urodynamic evaluation of meningomyelocele patients. J Urol. 144(6):1440–2.

Goepel M, Krege S, Portgys P (1999) Urologische Diagnostik bei Kindern mit Myelomeningozele. Urologe 38:10–13

Houle A, Gilmour R, Churchill B (1993) What a volume can child normally store in the bladder at a safe pressure? J Urol 149:561–564

Hayashi Y, Yamataka A, Kaneyama K (2006) Review of 86 patients with myelodysplasia and neurogenic bladder who underwent sigmoidocolocystoplasty and were followed more than 10 years. J Urol 176:1806–1809

Kasabian NG, Bauer SB, Dyro FM (1992) The prophylactic value of clean intermittent catheterization and anticholinergic medication in newborns and infants with myelodysplasia at risk and developing urinary tract deterioration. Am J Dis Child 146:840–843

Koff S (1983) Estimating bladder capacity in children. Urology 21:248

Kurzrock EA, Polse S (1998) Renal deterioration in myelodysplastic children: urodynamic evaluation and clinical correlates. J Urol 159:1657–1661

McGuire EJ, Woodside JR, Bordin TA (1981) Prognostic value of urodynamic testing in myelodysplastic children. J Urol 126:205–209

Ozkan KU, Bauer SB, Khoshbin S (2006) Neurogenic bladder dysfunction after sacrococcygeal teratoma resection. J Urol 175:292–296

Özkan B, Demirkesen O, Durak H (2005) Which factors predict upper urinary tract deterioration in overactive neurogenic bladder dysfunction? Urology 66:99–104

Morrisroe SN, O'Connor RC, Nanigian DK (2005) Vesicostomy revisited: the best treatment for the hostile bladder in myelodysplastic children? BJU Int 97:397–400

Palmer L, Richards I, Kaplan W (1997) Age-related bladder capacity and bladder capacity growth in children with myelomeningocele. J Urol 158:1261–1264

Rickwood AMK, Thomas DG, Philip NH (1982) A system of management of the congenital neuropathic bladder based upon combined urodynamic and radiological assessment. Br J Urol 54:507–511

Seki N, Masuda K, Kinukawa N (2004) Risk factors for febrile urinary tract infection in children with myelodysplasia treated by clean intermittent catheterization. Int J Urol 11:973–977

Stein R, Wiesner C, Beetz R (2005) Urinary diversion in children and adolescents with neurogenic bladder: the Mainz experience – Part II: continent cutaneous diversion using the Mainz pouch I. Pediatr Nephrol 20:926–931

Zerin JM, Chen E, Ritchey ML, Bloom DA (1993) Bladder capacity as measured at voiding cystourethrography in children: relationship to toilet training and frequency of micturition. Radiology 187(3):803–806

Part V

Congenital Malformations, Vesico-Ureteric Reflux, and Postoperative Imaging

Congenital Anomalies of the Renal Pelvis and Ureter

Freddy Avni, Elisa Amzallag-Bellenger, Marianne Tondeur, and Pierre-Hugues Vivier

Contents

1	**Introduction**...	434
2	**Imaging the Pelvis and Ureter**.................	434
3	**Anomalies of the Pelvis and Ureter in Single and Bifid Collecting Systems**........	435
3.1	Calyceal Diverticulum................................	435
3.2	Hydrocalyx, Fraley's Syndrome, and Infundibular Stenosis........................	436
3.3	Megacalicosis..	437
3.4	Ureteropelvic Obstruction...........................	438
3.5	Megaureter and Hydroureter.......................	445
3.6	Ureteral Wall Lesions and Look-Alike........	448
3.7	Ectopic Ureter..	449
3.8	Ureterocele and Single Collecting System...	450
3.9	Bifid Collecting Systems.............................	450
4	**Duplex Collecting Systems**........................	451
4.1	Etiology and Epidemiology.........................	451
4.2	Presentation and Circumstances of Diagnosis..	451
4.3	The Work-Up of Duplex Kidneys: General Considerations...............................	452
4.4	Duplication and VUR..................................	452
4.5	Ureteral Ectopia...	454
4.6	Ureterocele..	458
4.7	(Cystic) Dysplasia of the Upper Pole..........	458
4.8	Other Types of Obstruction in Duplex Kidney..	460
5	**Triplication and Quadruplication of the Ureter**...	461
	Conclusion...	461
	References...	461

F. Avni, MD, PhD (✉)
Department of Pediatric Radiology, Jeanne de Flandre Hospital, Lille University Hospital, 59037 Lille, France
e-mail: favni@skynet.be

E. Amzallag-Bellenger, MD
Department of Pediatric Imaging, Jeanne de Flandre Mother and child hospital, Lille University Hospitals, Lille, France

M. Tondeur, MD
Department of Radio-Isotopes, CHU Saint-Pierre, Rue Haute 322, 1000 Brussels, Belgium

P.-H. Vivier, MD, PhD
Service de radiologie, CHU Charles-Nicolle, 1, rue de Germont, 76031 Rouen Cedex, France

X-Ray Expert, Maison médicale, Hôpital Privé de l'Estuaire, 505, rue Irène-Joliot-Curie, 76620 Le Havre, France

1 Introduction

Congenital anomalies may involve any level of the collecting system; the most usual presentation is urinary tract dilatation that may already be detected during fetal life. The role of imaging is to determine the origin of the dilatation, i.e., obstructive versus nonobstructive (Table 1 lists the causes of urinary tract dilatation). Other useful information includes the level of the impairment to drainage (so-called obstruction) and its impact on renal function. All these data are important in order to determine the best therapeutic approach.

Two imaging techniques have been classically used in order to demonstrate the morphology of the collecting system: ultrasound (US) and intravenous urography (IVU). The latter has been almost completely abandoned and replaced by MR urography as well as, in selected conditions, by computed tomography (CT). The work-up of most anomalies has to be completed by voiding cystourethrography (VCUG) and isotopic studies for the evaluation of renal function and drainage studies.

2 Imaging the Pelvis and Ureter

In pediatric uro-nephrology, US has a central position; whatever the anomaly, it will be performed first and will determine the subsequent work-up. US is very efficient for the demonstration of dilatation of the urinary tract and the level of "obstruction"; yet, the method can hardly differentiate between obstructive and nonobstructive dilatation. Also, the degree of dilatation is influenced by the state of hydration of the patient; therefore, some teams advocate the use of furosemide and measurement of the resistive index in order to diagnose obstruction. Another interest of US is that the technique also provides information on the renal parenchyma (Patriquin 1991; Peerboccus et al. 2012; Bude et al. 1992; Palmer 2006).

Intravenous urography used to be performed frequently for the work-up of uro-nephropathies. Its indications have progressively faded, and the technique is replaced by CT, scintigraphy, and mainly MR imaging.

Table 1 Causes of urinary tract dilatation

Congenital etiologies
Ureteropelvic junction obstruction
Ureterovesical junction obstruction
Nonobstructive and nonrefluxing dilatation
Vesicoureteric reflux (grades III–V)
Nonobstructive nonrefluxing megaureter
Duplex collecting system
Posterior urethral valves
Megacalycosis
Pelvi-infundibular stenosis
Secondary etiologies
Tumoral involvement
Extrinsic compression
Retroperitoneal fibrosis
Constipation
Megabladder
Lithiasis

CT has proved informative in many pathological or doubtful situations involving the pyelocalyceal and ureteral system; it may demonstrate the connections of atypical cystic parenchymal lesions with the collecting system, and it may determine the primitive or secondary origin of an "obstruction." CT completes the information given by US; if necessary 2D or 3D reconstructions or urographic images post-contrast injection may also be obtained. The technique is irradiating, and therefore, its use must be well-thought-out and cautious (Palmer 2006; Renjen et al. 2012; Darge et al. 2013).

These last years, the use of MR urography has been gaining popularity for the visualization of the urinary tract, both the parenchyma and collecting system. Its best indications are the morphological assessment of a very dilated urinary tract, ectopic ureteral insertion, and assessment of renal parenchymal damage. The combination of hydrographic sequences and gadolinium-enhanced sequences provides information on both morphology and (indirect) function. In the near future, further studies will determine whether MR imaging can be considered as an "all-in-one" examination and will replace both IVU and isotope studies (Wille et al. 2002; Jones et al. 2004; Rohrschneider et al. 2003; Nolte-Ernstig et al. 1998).

Till then, the best evaluation of separate renal functions and of the degree of renal drainage impairment is obtained by isotope studies with furosemide injection (Roarke and Sandler 1998; Piepsz and Ham 2006; Palmer 2006; Gordon et al. 2001, 2011; Vivier et al. 2010a, b; Riccabona et al. 2010). Other techniques such as retrograde pyelography have almost completely been abandoned.

> **Take Away**
>
> US is the central imaging technique for the visualization of a dilated collecting system. Morphology of the urinary tract is best assessed by MR imaging or CT. Function is best assessed by isotope studies.

3 Anomalies of the Pelvis and Ureter in Single and Bifid Collecting Systems

3.1 Calyceal Diverticulum

A calyceal diverticulum is an eventration of a calyx into the renal parenchyma that is filled with urine. Most of the diverticula are small and asymptomatic. Complications include the development of milk of calcium and urolithiasis and rarely hematuria; infection is unusual. The relation between diverticulum and isolated renal cyst is unclear. The diverticulum is usually detected by US as an isolated cystic structure. However, the connection with the pyelocalyceal system may be missed on US; it can be more easily demonstrated on MRU or on CT (Fig. 1). Treatment is necessary only when complications such as hemorrhage or lithiasis occur.

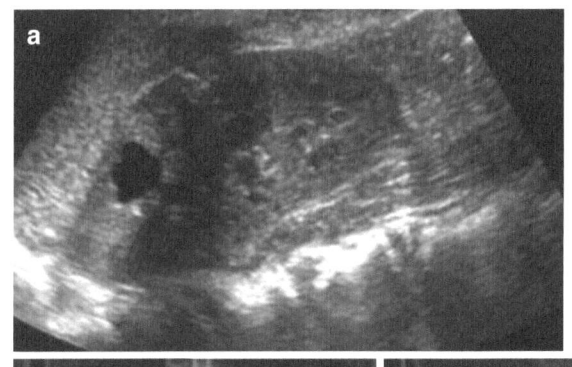

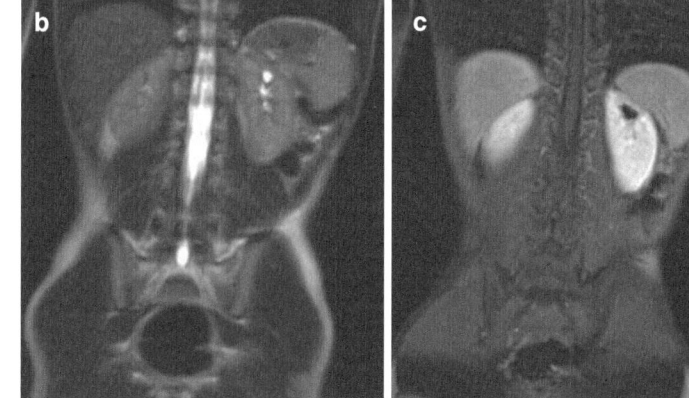

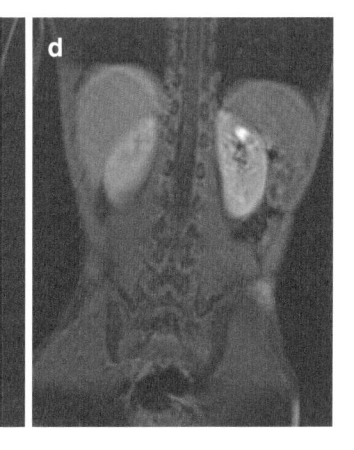

Fig. 1 Calyceal diverticulum 7-year-old girl. Incidental finding. (**a**) Ultrasound: sagittal scan of the left kidney – a cystic mass is visible at the upper pole of the kidney. (**b**) MRI of the kidneys. HASTE T2 sequence; a cystic structure is visible close to the collecting system. (**c**) (early) and (**d**) (delayed) MRI scan T1 sequence after Gd enhancement: The signal of the cystic structure seen in the left kidney increases confirming a connection with the pyelocalyceal system

3.2 Hydrocalyx, Fraley's Syndrome, and Infundibular Stenosis

Hydrocalyx refers to a dilatation limited to one or more calyces in the absence of renal pelvis dilatation. The condition may be congenital or acquired. Congenital hydrocalyx results from a stenosis of the infundibulum draining the calyx into the renal pelvis. The narrowing induces a (cystiform) dilatation of one of the calyces (Fig. 2). When more than one calyx is involved, the condition is also referred to as infundibular stenosis. MR urography is able to demonstrate the anomaly. The most extensive form of the disease is infundo-pelvic stenosis, in which a small pelvis may also be associated (Figs. 3 and 4). The condition may also be acquired secondarily to infection (tuberculosis) or urolithiasis (Uhlenhuth et al. 1990).

The dilatation of the calyx may be secondary to extrinsic compression by a vessel (the so-called Fraley's syndrome), to scarring following inflammatory or infectious processes (tuberculosis), and to obstruction by a lithiasis or a blood clot.

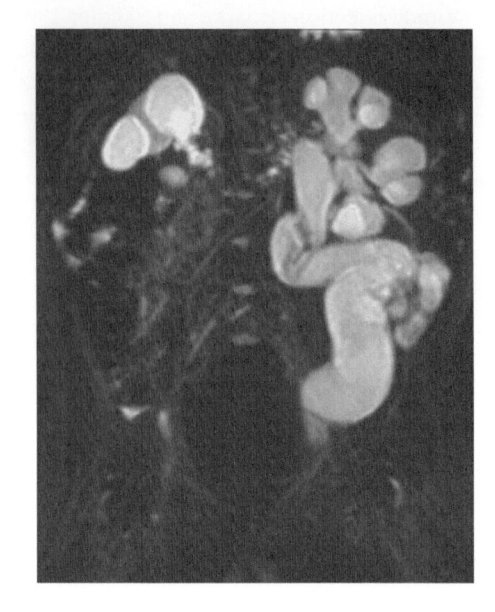

Fig. 3 Pelvi-infundibular stenosis – MR urography T2W sequence. Right MCDK + left infundibular stenosis and megaureter

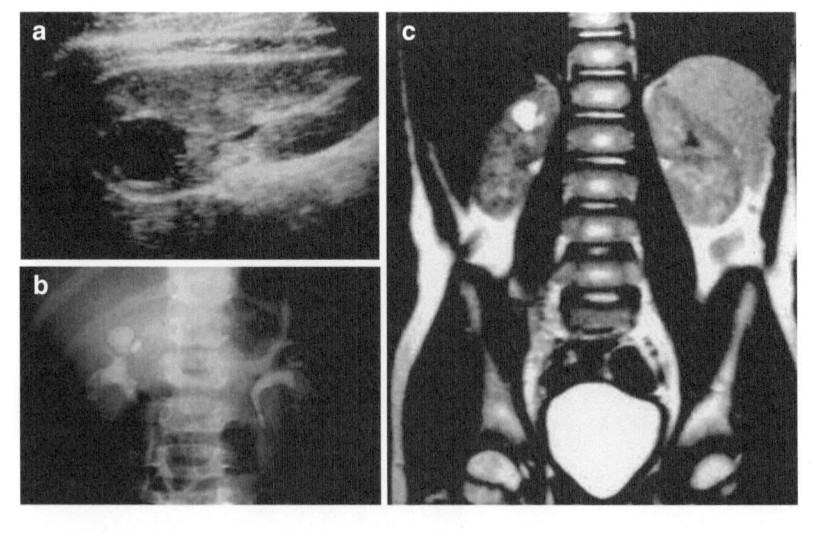

Fig. 2 Hydrocalyx. (**a**) US: cystic mass (between crosses) at the upper pole of the right kidney. (**b**) IVU: typical appearance of the right hydrocalyx. (**c**) MR: T2W coronal view demonstrating the right hydrocalyx

3.3 Megacalicosis

Mega(poly)calicosis is characterized by the presence of 12–20 dilated dysplastic calyces in the absence of obstruction and is probably related to or associated with a developmental hypoplasia of the medullary pyramids. The condition may be difficult to diagnose on classical US and better evaluated on 3D US (see chapter "Imaging in Renal Agenesis, Dysplasia, Hypoplasia and Cystic Diseases of the Kidney") or on MR urography (Figs. 5 and 6). The small renal pelvis is easier to demonstrate, and the dilated numerous calyces are easier to count by it. Megacalycosis may typically also be associated with a primary megaureter (MU) (Vargas and Lebowitz 1986; Mandell et al. 1986). Complications include the development of urolithiasis (Figs. 5 and 6).

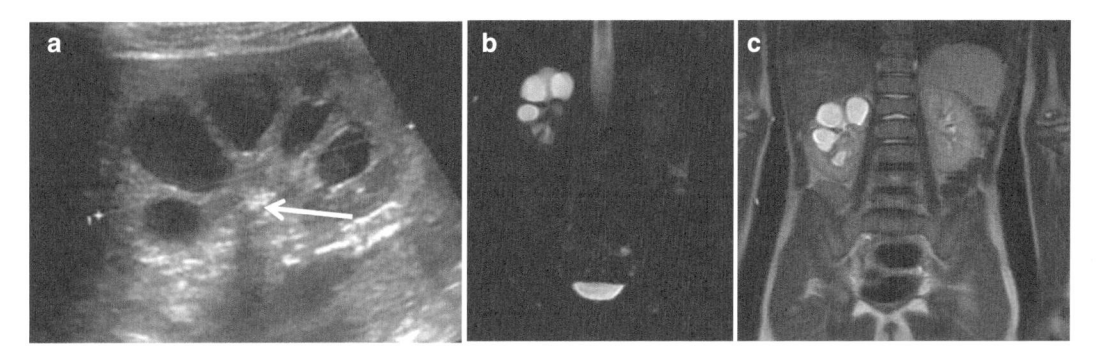

Fig. 4 Infundibular stenosis with pelvic urolithiasis: (**a**) Ultrasound: sagittal scan of the right kidney; all the calyces appear dilated, the renal pelvis is not dilated; a lithiasis is present within the pelvis (*arrow*). (**b**) MR urography. Coronal T2 (MRCP) sequence. (**c**) Coronal T2 SSFE sequence demonstrating a small renal pelvis in comparison with the dilated calyces

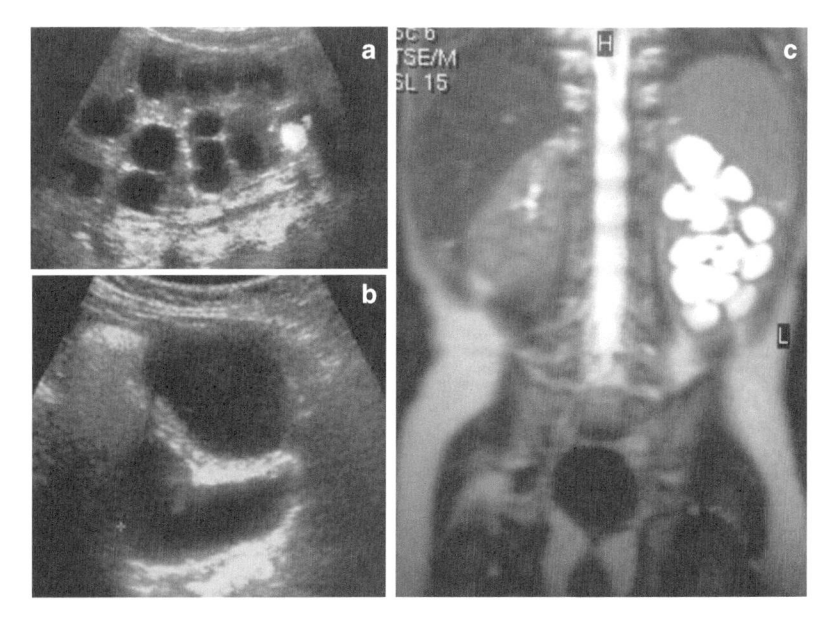

Fig. 5 Megacalycosis and megaureter. (**a**) US: sagittal scan of the left kidney. Unusual cystic dilatation of all the calyces. A lithiasis is visible at the lower pole. (**b**) US of the pelvis showing an associated dilated ureter (1.8 cm between crosses). (**c**) MR urography: typical megacalycosis of the left kidney

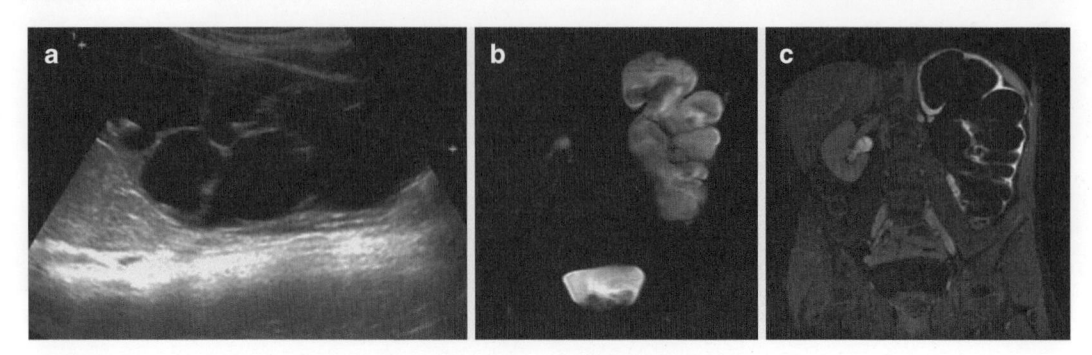

Fig. 6 Megacalycosis. (**a**) US sagittal scan of the left kidney. Numerous dilated renal calyces. (**b**) MR urography: Coronal T2W sequence and (**c**). T1 FS post-Gd enhancement showing highly dilated numerous calyces with poor enhancement

3.4 Ureteropelvic Obstruction

3.4.1 Diagnosis of "Obstruction"

Dilatation of the urinary tract may occur secondary to obstruction and/or vesicoureteric reflux (VUR) or as a primary process (like nonobstructive megaureter). The main objective of all the imaging techniques will be to diagnose among all the cases those that might require surgical correction in order to preserve or improve function. Noteworthy, the definition of obstruction lacks consensus, and the terminology such as impairment of urinary tract drainage should be the preferred wording. Still, obstruction is the common denomination used.

The antenatal diagnosis and postnatal follow-up of fetal uropathies have brought lots of new information on the natural history of obstructive or pseudo-obstructive uropathies. Unfortunately, no clear-cut conclusions can be drawn from these many examples. There are still controversies concerning the diagnosis of obstruction and the yield of early surgery (Prigent et al. 1999; Eskild-Jensen et al. 2004; Piepsz et al. 2009; Riccabona et al. 2009; Gordon et al. 2011; Piepsz 2011; Ismaili 2013).

The first step toward the detection of obstruction is US (Fig. 7a), the main landmark being the demonstration of dilatation of the urinary tract. Dilatation is best evaluated on an anteroposterior measurement of the renal pelvis on a transverse scan of the kidney. In the newborn, a pelvic diameter greater than 7 mm is considered abnormal; dilatation of the calyces (and of the ureter) indicates the need for further work-up. In older children, a diameter higher than 10 mm should be considered abnormal. The following step in the work-up of a uropathy is VCUG. Once VUR is excluded, it becomes more probable that the urinary tract dilatation is secondary to obstruction. It is noteworthy that VUR and obstruction may coexist in the same collecting system (Maizels et al. 1992; Stocks et al. 1996; Riccabona et al. 2010).

Many hopes were placed on US for the diagnosis of obstruction. Various grading systems have been described in order to categorize the urinary tract dilatation (Maizels et al. 1992). However, besides diagnosing urinary tract dilatation, conventional US alone does not provide direct information on renal function or the degree of obstruction. Therefore, several authors have proposed Doppler analysis of the renal arteries with calculation of the resistive index after furosemide injection. In case of obstruction, the resistive index tends to be greater than 85 % and takes longer to return to baseline values after a diuretic stress test. The first results are promising, but the use of the technique in newborns and small infants is more difficult and less reproducible (Yagci et al. 1999; Patti et al. 2000). Infants and neonates tend to have a physiologically higher resistive index.

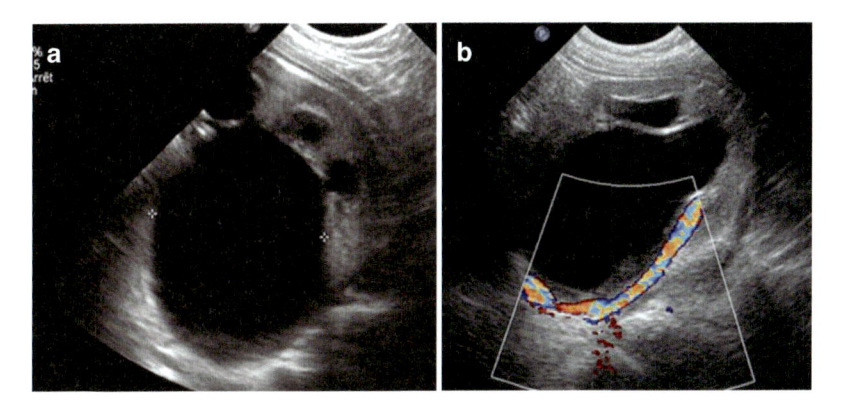

Fig. 7 PUJ obstruction: ultrasound – transverse scans of the left kidney. (**a**) Standard US: marked dilatation of the renal pelvis. (**b**) Color Doppler ultrasound demonstrating a crossing vessel

The best method to evaluate and to quantify renal function and drainage is the radioisotope study with furosemide injection ("diuretic radionuclide renogram"). Radiation dose delivered from the radionuclide renogram is low, about 0.2–0.4 mSv, depending essentially on the age and the level of renal function (Stabin et al. 1992; Ismaili 2013). Calculation of separate clearances requires both the measurements of GFR and of differential renal functions (DRF) from the isotopic renogram. GFR is determined by injection of chromium isotope-ethylnediamine-tetraacetic acid (51Cr-EDTA) using a simple plasma sample technique (Piepsz et al. 2001).

The renograms are best performed using tubular tracers with a high extraction rate such as 99mTc-mercaptoacétyltriglycine (99mTc-MAG3) or 99mTc ECD (ethyl cysteinate dimer) (Piepsz et al. 2009; Gordon et al. 2011; Piepsz 2011; Ismaili 2013). The same radiopharmaceutical should be used on follow-up studies (Piepsz et al. 2009). The renogram allows to evaluate both DRF (input) and renal excretion (output) of the tracer.

The differential renal function (DRF) is calculated from the early phase of the renograms. Two different methods (area under the curve and Rutland-Patlak plot) are available; using both allows a quality control (Piepsz et al. 2009; Gordon et al. 2011; Piepsz 2011; Ismaili 2013). Normal values are between 45 and 55 % (Prigent et al. 1999; Eskild-Jensen et al. 2004; Gordon et al. 2011).

The second part of the renogram provides information about tracer excretion, the renal drainage. As far as dilatation is concerned, drainage stimulation using furosemide is the procedure of choice. In young patients furosemide is often injected simultaneously with the radiopharmaceutical (F0), reducing the duration of the examination and the number of venous punctures (Piepsz 2011). Other schemes are available, the diuretic being injected 15 min prior to the radiotracer (F-15) or at the end of the dynamic phase of the renogram (F+20). As kidney drainage may be artificially delayed in the presence of a full bladder at the end of the renogram, post-micturition post-erect images are mandatory (Piepsz et al. 2009; Gordon et al. 2011; Piepsz 2011). The erect position allows taking into account the effect of gravity (Fig. 8).

Interpretation of renal drainage is approached by visual analysis of the images and curves. Two quantitative parameters, output efficiency (OE) and normalized residual activity (NORA), are currently available, allowing an accurate analysis of the drainage. They replace the previously used T1/2 which depended on the level of renal function and which cannot be calculated on the late post-micturition images (Piepsz et al. 2009; Piepsz 2011; Gordon et al. 2011; Ismaili 2013).

OE is the fraction of tracer that has left the kidney at a given time and NORA is defined as

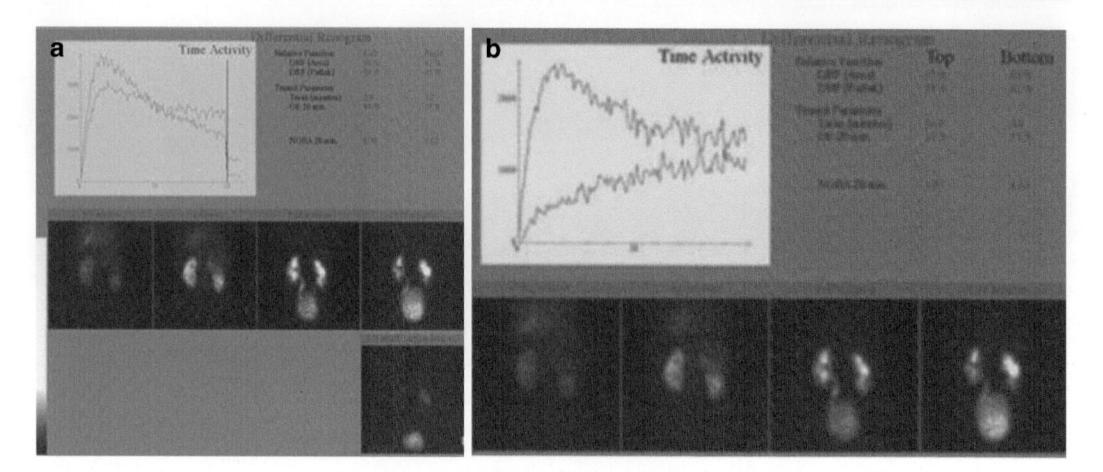

Fig. 8 Diuretic renogram (Tc99MAG3) in a case of R duplex kidney (upper pole atrophy). (**a**) Classical calculation: impaired right kidney DRF and poor function of the upper part of the right kidney. Important bilateral retention of the tracer at the end of the first part of the renogram. Complete emptying of the left kidney and quasi-complete emptying of the right kidney after micturition. (**b**) Upper and lower poles calculated separately. The upper part contributes to 15–20 % of right kidney function

the ratio of retained renal activities at two different time points. Both parameters may be calculated at the end of the renogram and after post-micturition post-erect images. OE and NORA do not depend on the individual input function and on the overall clearance. The determination of OE and NORA is highly intra- and interobserver reproducible (Tondeur et al. 2013); values of both parameters in normal and dilated kidneys have been determined in children (Piepsz et al. 2002; Nogarède et al. 2010). Several authors (Piepsz 2009; Piepsz 2011; Ismaili 2013) and the guidelines from the European Association of Nuclear Medicine recommend the use of both OE and NORA in daily practice (Gordon et al. 2011) (Fig. 9).

The definition of risk factors for functional deterioration in the absence of surgical treatment upon the basis of the renogram remains a matter of debate (Piepsz et al. 2001; Gordon et al. 2001; Piepsz 2009; Ismaili 2013). There is a consensus that there is no risk for a further deterioration in the presence of good renal drainage (Piepsz 2009) (Fig. 10).

Unfortunately poor renal drainage does not allow predicting functional deterioration in case of conservative treatment. In such cases surgical treatment is sometimes proposed. In the last years the predictive role of a delayed "cortical transit time" has been suggested. Cortical transit time is the duration the tracer is present only in the cortical rim from the beginning of the renogram. It has been shown that a delayed cortical transit time, more than 3 min, predicts functional deterioration in the absence of surgical treatment and also predicts improvement after pyeloplasty (Fig. 11) (Schlotmann et al. 2009; Piepsz et al. 2011; Duong et al. 2013). However, a normal cortical transit does not exclude the risk of DRF deterioration.

The Whitaker test or pressure measurements after urinary tract nephrostomy are used with some success in selected cases (Peters 1995). It necessitates sedation and the placement of a nephrostomy tube. It can therefore not be used in every case.

MR urography is increasingly used in patients with obstructive uropathy (Figs. 12 and 13a). After contrast injection, early angiographic phases can be obtained and curves of gadolinium uptake can be drawn in a similar way to isotopes (Fig. 13b). The results seem promising, although there is a need to standardize the conditions of

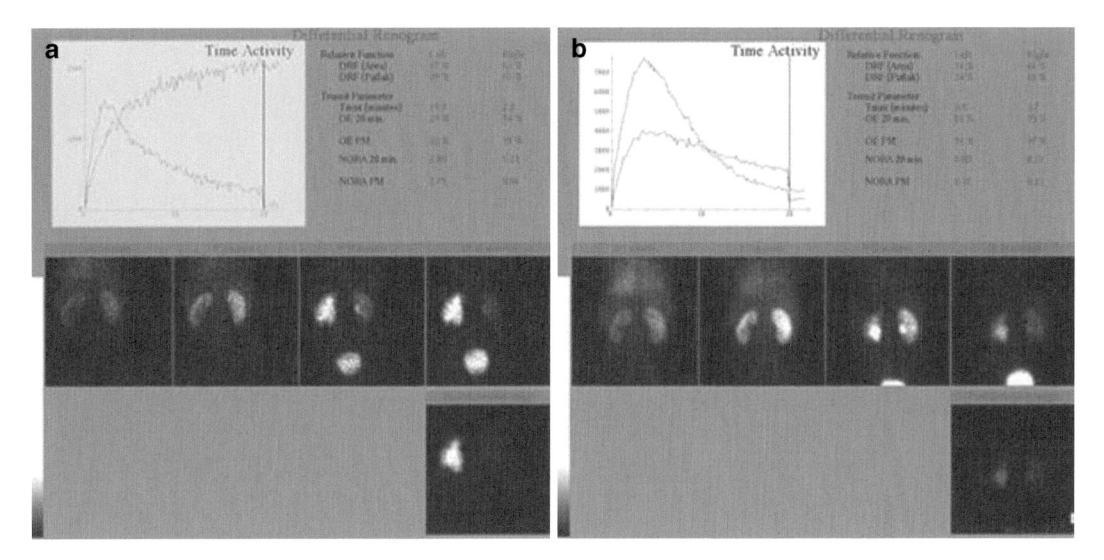

Fig. 9 F0 diuretic renogram (Tc^{99m}-MAG3) – left PUJ obstruction. (**a**) Abnormal left DRF (<45%) and severely impaired drainage of left kidney with no emptying after micturition. (**b**) 6 months after surgery. Improvement of left kidney drainage but no improvement of left DRF

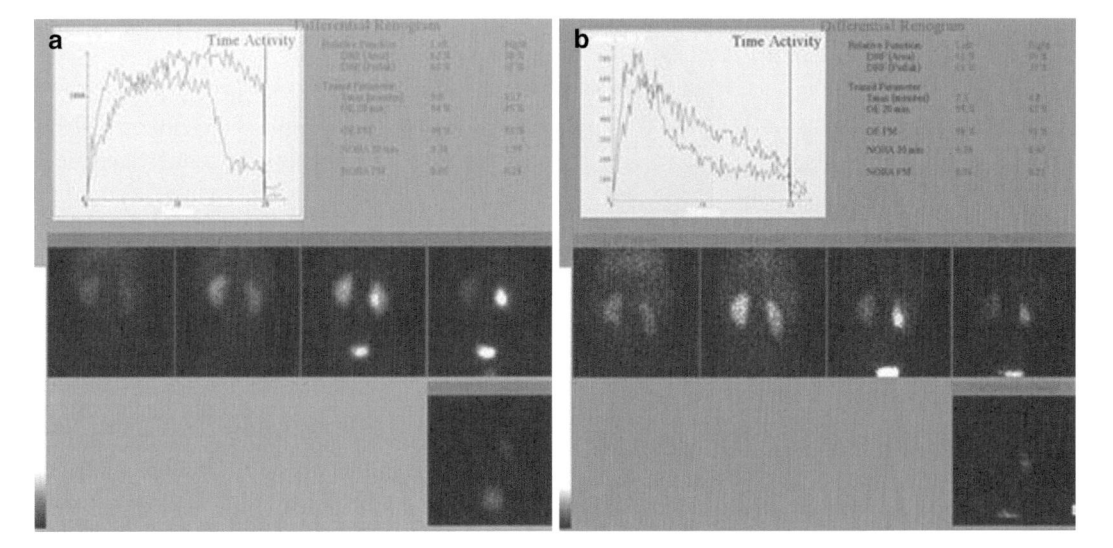

Fig. 10 F0 diuretic renogram (Tc^{99m}-MAG3). Right PUJ obstruction 3-month-old baby girl. At 3 months. Increasing size of the right pelvis. Impaired right kidney DRF; nearly complete emptying after micturition. 18-month-old. Conservative treatment. Improvement of renal drainage with the right kidney emptying at the end of the first part of the renogram

the examination. Also, correlation between renal function and parenchymal enhancement after gadolinium injection has still to be demonstrated (Regan et al. 1996; Nolte-Ernstig et al. 1998; Vivier et al. 2011; Claudon 2014).

3.4.2 Etiology of Pelviureteric Junction Obstruction (PUJO)

PUJO represents the leading cause of dilatation of the urinary tract (about 35–40% of the cases). Its origin is not always understood or can be

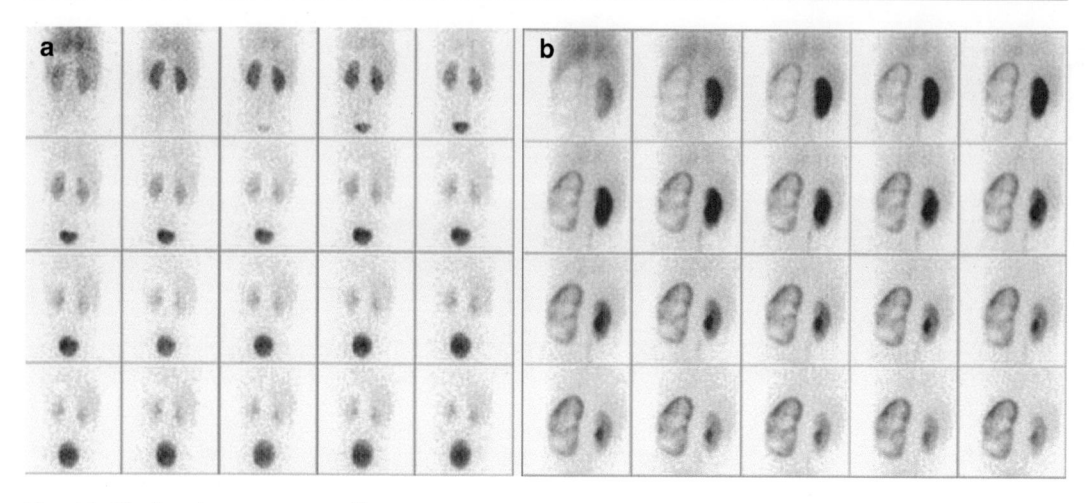

Fig. 11 F0 diuretic renogram (Tc^{99m}-MAG3), 1 min frames: (**a**) example of normal cortical transit time. The entire renal parenchyma of both kidneys is visualized early. (**b**) Example of delayed cortical transit time. Severely delayed left kidney cortical transit: no parenchymal activity appearing during the 20 min of the renogram

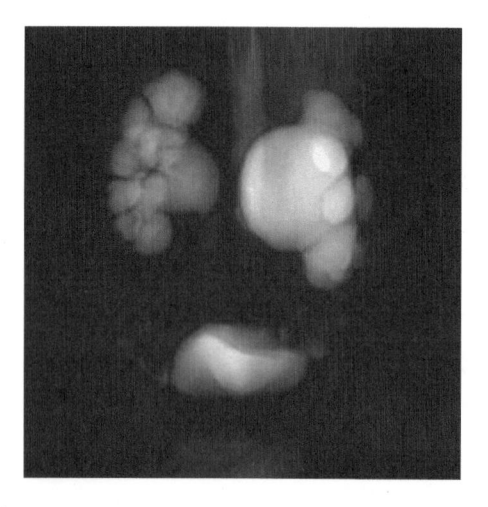

Fig. 12 MR urography T2W sequence showing bilateral PUJO

interpreted as multifactorial. PUJO can result from anatomic anomalies or abnormal peristalsis. At surgery, muscular discontinuity or extrinsic compression of the PUJ due to vessels or ureteral kinks can be found. US and MR imaging can very nicely display the crossing vessel (Figs. 7b and 14) (Calder et al. 2007; Frauschner et al. 1999; Veyrac et al. 2003).

Nowadays, since the widespread use of obstetrical US, most cases of PUJ obstruction are detected in utero or in the direct neonatal period in asymptomatic patients. Rarely, the condition is revealed after the palpation of an abdominal mass, hematuria, or urinary tract infection. Interestingly, despite antenatal diagnosis, cases of PUJ obstruction are still detected later in childhood. In older children, symptoms leading to the diagnosis include, among others, hematuria following an abdominal trauma, nausea, failure to thrive, and flank pain (Cendron et al. 1994; Coplen et al. 2006).

3.4.3 Particular Forms of PUJO

Giant PUJO

Giant PUJO is usually detected in the newborn after an antenatal diagnosis (Fig. 15). A flank mass is often palpated, and gastrointestinal discomfort is present. Pelvic dilatation is huge, extending from the diaphragm up to the bladder and across the midline. Besides MR imaging, it is difficult for imaging procedures to identify the type of uropathy. The kidney functions poorly and the condition usually necessitates nephrectomy. The condition may mimic a giant multicystic dysplastic kidney (MCDK).

UPJ Obstruction and VUR

See chapter "Vesicoureteric Reflux" (Bomalski et al. 1997).

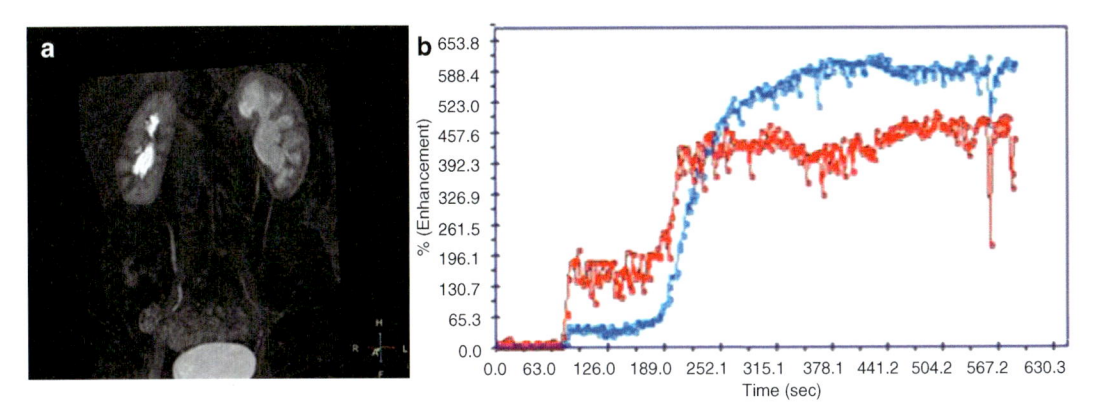

Fig. 13 MR urography bilateral (apparently) moderate PUJO. (**a**) Delayed view after Gd enhancement. (**b**) Bilateral enchancement curves of delayed excretion

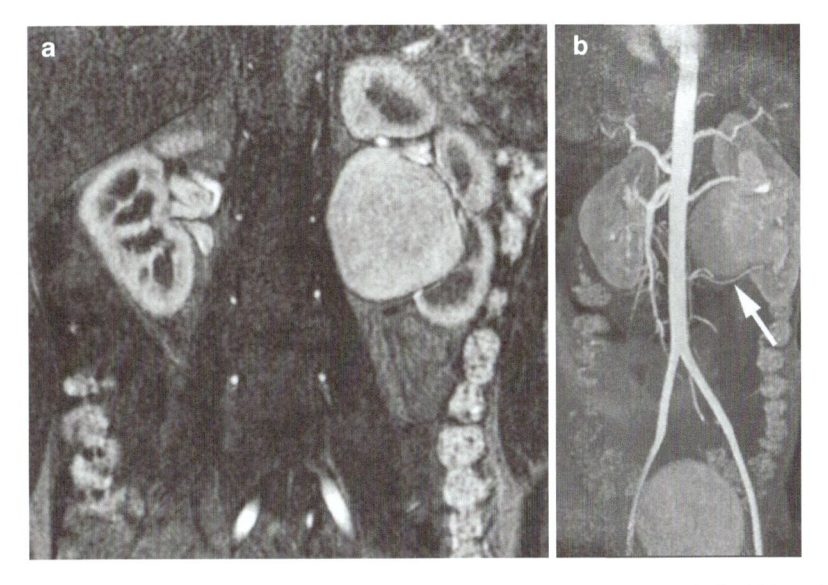

Fig. 14 UPJ obstruction. (**a**) T1-weighted sequence + Gd enhancement. Typical left PUJO. (**b**) MR angiography displays the crossing vessel (*arrow*) (Courtesy of JN Dacher, MD, PhD)

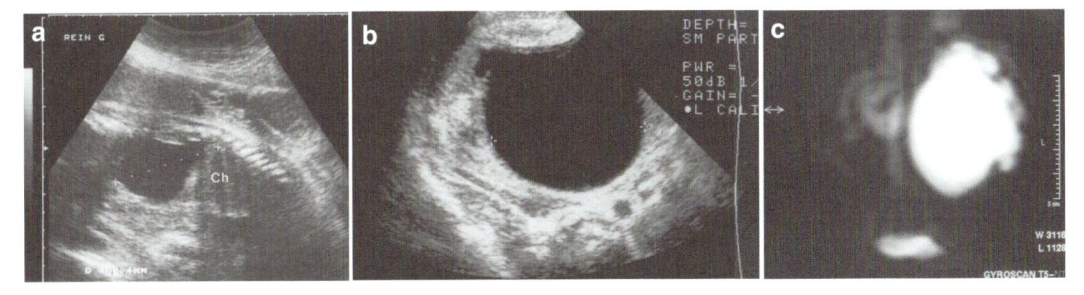

Fig. 15 Giant PUJO. (**a**) In utero 32 weeks LMP. Sagittal scan of the left kidney displays a huge dilatation (6 cm between crosses). Ch, fetal chest. (**b**) US at birth: transverse scan of the kidney, the renal pelvis (between crosses) measures 5.5 cm. (**c**) MR urography, T2W coronal image displays a typical PUJO

PUJ and Ureterovesical Junction (UVJ) Obstruction

Both PUJ and UVJ obstruction may coexist. UVJ obstruction may evolve unrecognized, especially on IVU, up to the surgical correction of the PUJ obstruction (Fig. 16); only thereafter will the lower obstruction be detected and eventually corrected. The condition might be easier to diagnose on MR urography (McGrath et al. 1987).

PUJ Obstruction and Urolithiasis

Any condition favoring urinary stasis may induce the development of urolithiasis (Fig. 17) (Kraus et al. 1999) (see chapters "Urolithiasis and Nephrocalcinosis" and "Imaging in Renal Agenesis, Dysplasia, Hypoplasia and Cystic Diseases of the Kidney").

PUJ Obstruction and Horseshoe Kidney

Horseshoe kidney may present PUJ obstruction due to the crossing between the vessels and the ureters. This usually involves one of the collecting systems (Fig. 18).

PUJ Obstruction and Urinoma

A urinoma may complicate a PUJO. This type of complication may occur already in utero. It is more common with posterior urethral valves and acts like a protecting mechanism against obstruction (Silveri et al. 2002).

Intermittent PUJO

Intermittent PUJ obstruction is a condition where stable conditions alternate with acute dilatation of the collecting system. During an acute phenomenon, the patient experiences pain, nausea, and vomiting (Dietl's crisis). The clue to the diagnosis is thickening of the pelvic wall on US during convalescence (Tsai et al. 2006).

3.4.4 Differential Diagnosis of PUJO

Differential diagnosis of PUJO should include multicystic dysplastic kidney (MCDK), infundibular stenosis, and UVJ obstruction. This differential diagnosis is easy in most cases. In MCDK, no or little amount of renal parenchyma is seen, there are cysts of variable sizes, and there are no connections between the cysts. In infundibular stenosis, the calyces are dilated, more than the renal pelvis. Finally, in UVJ obstruction, the ureter is dilated.

3.4.5 The Natural History and Treatment of Neonatal PUJO

The postnatal follow-up of fetal hydronephrosis has shown that more than half of the cases of hydronephrosis resolve spontaneously in utero or after birth (see chapter "Upper Urinary Tract Dilatation in Newborns and Infants and the Postnatal Work Up of Congenital Uro-nephropathies"). This evidence has led to a more conservative approach toward all uropathies and among them PUJO. On the other hand, many urologists stress the fact that early surgery would improve renal function, while others publish opposite conclusions, although they agree that pyeloplasty is safe in early life.

It seems reasonable to follow these patients during their first year of life with US and isotope studies and to propose surgery if any complication occurs, if renal function diminishes, or if there is evidence of contralateral renal hypertrophy (Koff et al. 1994; Koff and Campbell 1994).

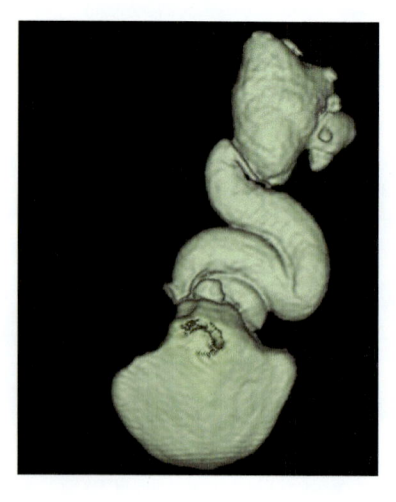

Fig. 16 PUJ and UVJ obstruction. 3D – T2W MR urography. Obstruction is seen at the PUJ and at the UVJ

3.4.6 Progression of Obstruction

It has rarely been shown that patients with normal kidneys in early life present a true UPJ obstruction later in childhood, necessitating surgical correction (Rickwood and Godiwalla 1997; Flaschner et al. 1993).

> **Take Away**
> PUJO is the leading cause of a urinary tract dilatation. More and more cases are diagnosed with antenatal diagnosis. The confirmation of the obstruction and the best timing for surgery remain controversial.

3.5 Megaureter and Hydroureter

Ureteral dilatation, or hydroureter, is a frequent cause of a dilatation of the fetal urinary tract. Under normal conditions, on fetal or postnatal US, the normal ureter is not visualized. Once it is visible (Fig. 19), a urinary tract dilatation is present and must be investigated (Keller et al. 1993).

The presence of a dilated ureter may correspond to primary megaureter (MU), to refluxing MU (see chapter "Congenital Anomalies of the Renal Pelvis and Ureter" and "Vesicoureteric Reflux"), to nonobstructive nonrefluxing MU, or to secondary MU. The various imaging techniques will be necessary in order to differentiate between these entities.

3.5.1 Primary Megaureter

Primary MU corresponds to a dilatation of the ureter above an adynamic ureteral segment at the ureterovesical junction. The degree of dilatation is variable. On US, the dilated ureter is especially visualized behind the bladder; due to peristalsis, the caliber of the ureter varies and the dilatation may "disappear" during a few seconds; therefore, the examiner should remain focused on the area in order to not underestimate the dilatation. MR urography displays easily the dilated ureter up to the UVJ (Fig. 20). The adynamic segment may or may not be visible. There may also be a ballooning of the distal ureter. The degree of associated pelvicalyceal dilatation varies, and it may even sometimes be absent. As mentioned, more and

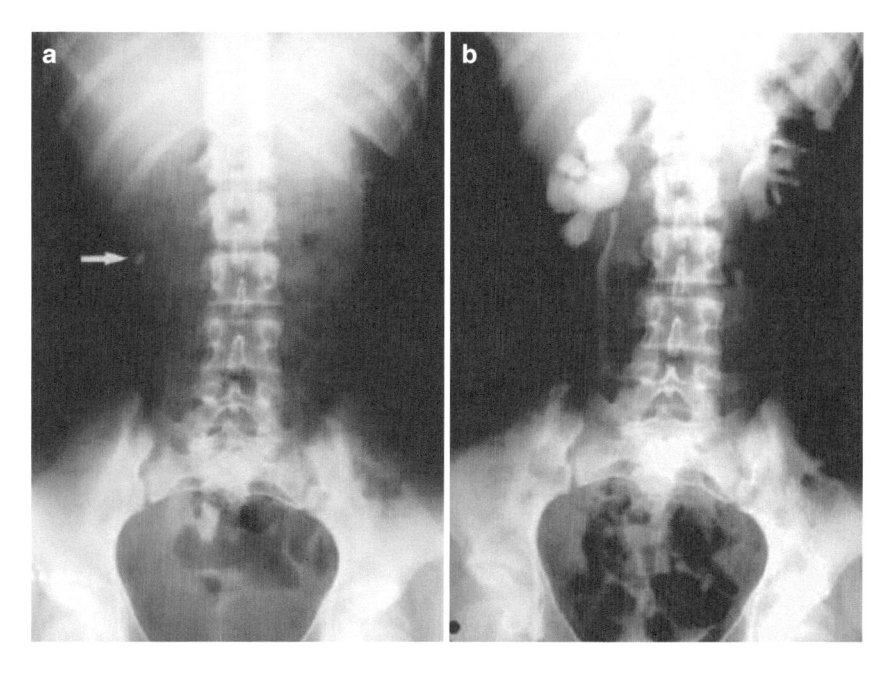

Fig. 17 PUJ obstruction and lithiasis. (**a**) Plain film of the abdomen; right calcified lithiasis (*arrow*). (**b**) IVU: UPJ obstruction; the lithiasis is in the inferior calyx

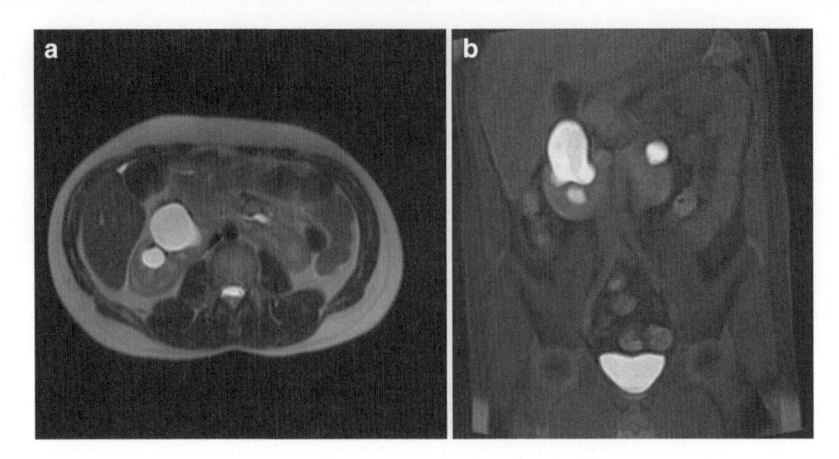

Fig. 18 Right PUJ in a horseshoe kidney–MR urography. (**a**) Axial T2 HASTE sequence. (**b**) Coronal T1 Vibe FS Gd enhanced

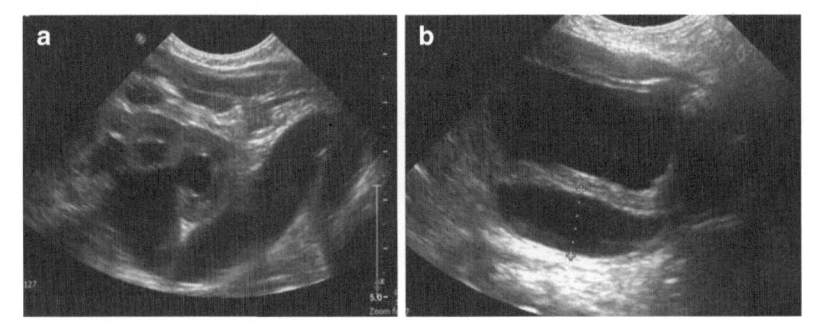

Fig. 19 Megaureter on US. (**a**) Sagittal scan of the left kidney showing a dilated pyelocalyceal system as well as proximal and lumbar ureter. (**b**) Left parasagittal scan of the bladder, a dilated ureter is visible behind the bladder

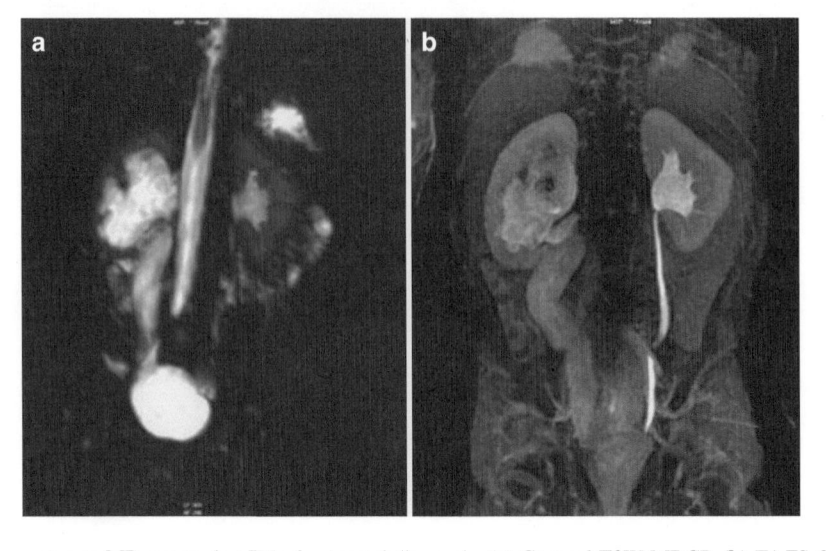

Fig. 20 Megaureter on MR urography: FU of antenatal diagnosis. (**a**) Coronal T2W MRCP. (**b**) T1 FS Gd enhanced sequences confirming the right ureteral dilatation

more cases are diagnosed during fetal life and evaluated after birth. MU tends to resolve spontaneously in a large percentage, and therefore, a conservative attitude has been proposed. The patients are put under prophylactic antibiotic therapy and followed clinically and by US for several years. Surgery is elected if any complication occurs or if renal function deteriorates (Wilcox and Mouriquand 1998; Baskin et al. 1994; Liu et al. 1994).

3.5.2 Refluxing Megaureter

High-grade VUR should be preferred to refluxing megaureter to avoid misunderstanding. However, primary MU and VUR can rarely coexist (Fig. 21) (see chapters "Congenital Anomalies of the Renal Pelvis and Ureter" and "Vesicoureteric Reflux"). Treatment should include both ureteral modeling and antireflux reimplantation.

3.5.3 Secondary Megaureter

Intrinsic Causes

Ureteral dilatation may occur secondarily to ureteral valves and midureteral (Fig. 22) or distal stenosis or due to ureteral diverticula (Cope and Snow 1991; Pinter et al. 1997). Valves should be differentiated from pseudo-valves corresponding to the persistence of a fetal pattern that is transitory and nonobstructive (Fig. 23).

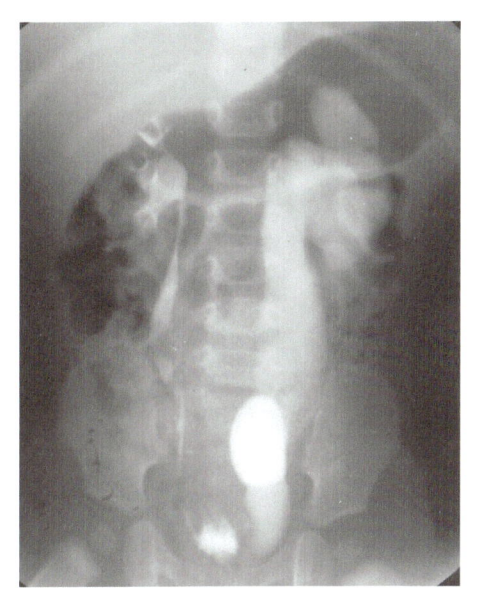

Fig. 21 Coexisting UVJ obstruction and VUR: post-void film of a VCU; there is bilateral VUR. On the left, VUR has occurred in a dilated collecting system

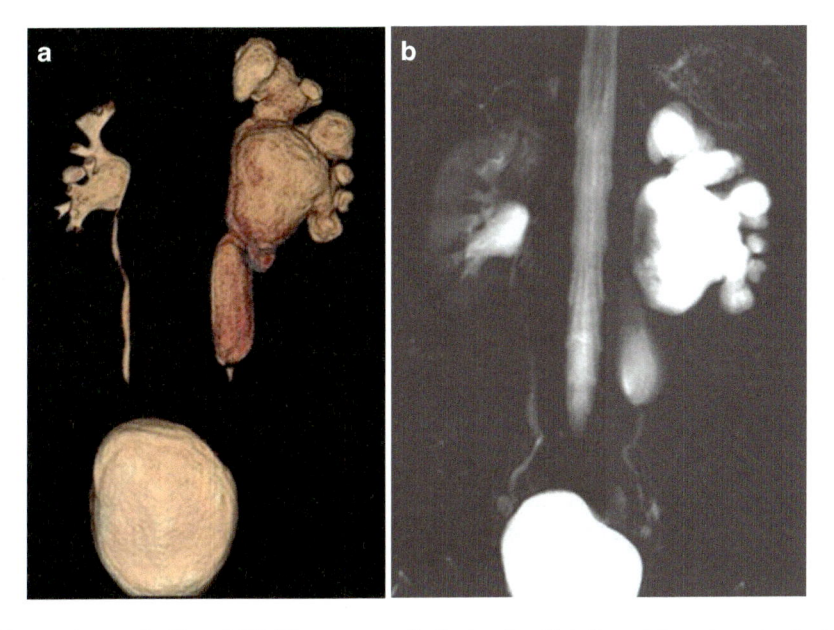

Fig. 22 Midureteral stenosis 3D and 2D T2 sequences displaying the dilatation of the urinary tract up to the midlumbar ureter

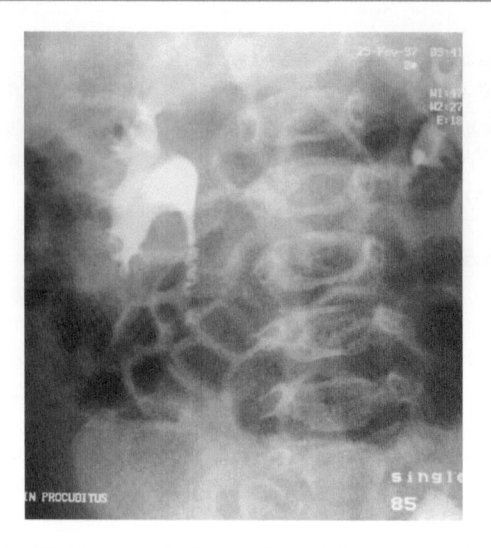

Fig. 23 Persisting fetal ureter determining pseudo-valves on the proximal ureter (30-s view of an IVU)

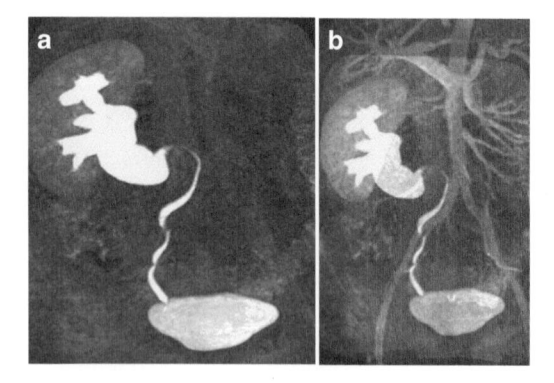

Fig. 24 Retrocaval ureter. (a) MIP T1 EG3D and (b) fusion views (Courtesy L Lemaître MD (Lille))

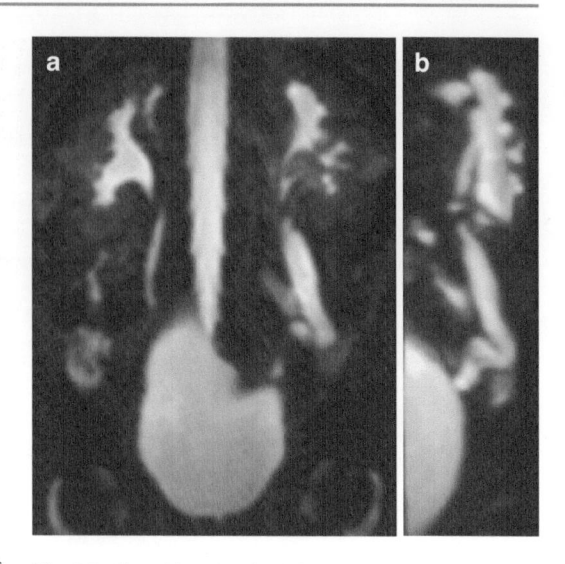

Fig. 25 Crural hernia of a left megaureter. MR imaging T2W sequence. (a) Upright AP view. (b) Lateral view showing the anterior course of the ureter

Extrinsic Causes

Retrocaval ureter causes a typical medial displacement of the right lumbar ureter that is (Fig. 24) best demonstrated on CT or MR urography. Ischiatic or crural herniation of the ureter may also occur; the ureter will display an unusual lateral and anterior course (Fig. 25). Retroperitoneal tumor processes and genitourinary pelvic tumors may determine displacement and secondary obstruction of the ureters (Fig. 26). A distended bladder also induces ureteral and pyelocalyceal dilatation, and, therefore, the size of the collecting system must be controlled after micturition. In severe cases constipation may displace and distend the ureters (Fig. 27). Urolithiasis and hematoma may induce ureteral dilatation, and the work-up must be adapted according to the potential diagnosis (Lautin et al. 1988; Herbetko and Hyde 1990; Oyen et al. 1987; Sherman et al. 1988).

3.5.4 The Natural History of Primary Megaureter

See chapter "UTI and VUR".

3.6 Ureteral Wall Lesions and Look-Alike

Ureteral wall lesions most often correspond to inflammatory and infectious lesions. They are best visualized on CT (IVU like views) where they appear as filling defects (cystic ureteritis) or striations (ureteritis) (see chapters "Surgical Procedures and Indications for Surgery" and "Congenital Anomalies of the Renal Pelvis and Ureter"). Differential diagnosis should include hematoma and varices (Matsumoto 1986).

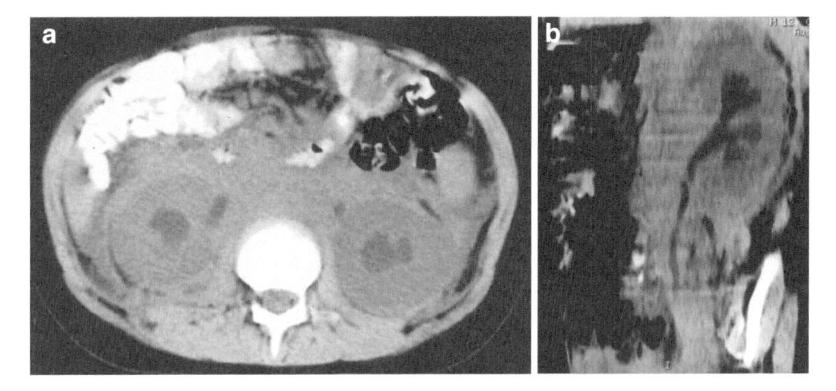

Fig. 26 Retroperitoneal malignant fibrosis (leukemic infiltration) determining bilateral ureterohydronephrosis visualized on a CT scan without contrast injection. (**a**) Transverse scan. (**b**) Oblique 2D reconstruction showing the ureteral entrapment

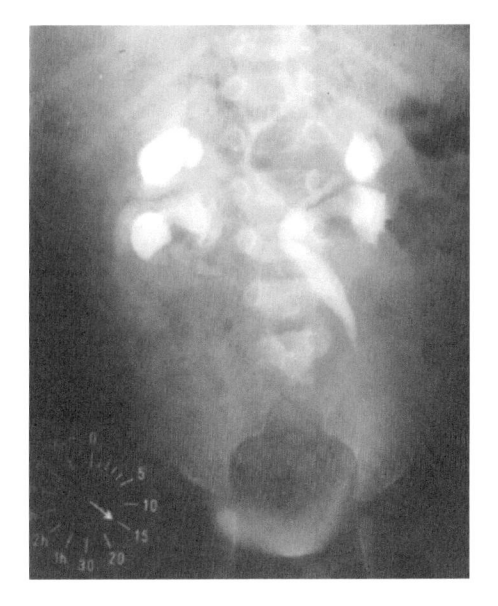

Fig. 27 Ureterohydronephrosis induced by fecaloma (patient with caudal regression syndrome and dysplastic kidneys)

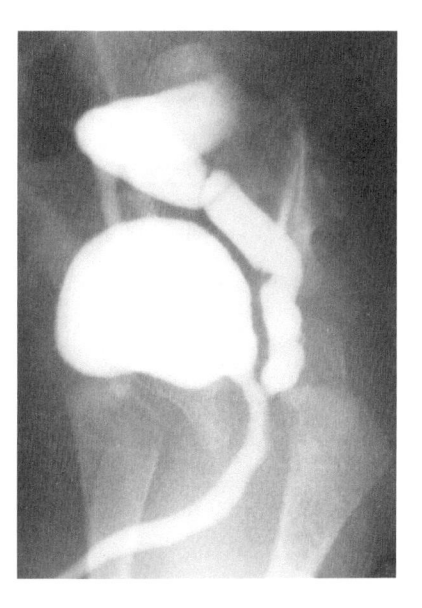

Fig. 28 VUR into an ectopic ureter inserting into the posterior urethra (patient with pelvic horseshoe kidneys)

3.7 Ectopic Ureter

Ureteral ectopia may be associated with single or duplex collecting systems (see below). Ureteral ectopia with a single system is much rarer than in the duplex kidney. Unilateral ectopia is more common in boys, whereas bilateral ectopia is more frequent in girls. It is usually associated with poorly functioning dysplastic kidney(s); the kidney may even correspond to a MCDK. The ectopic ureter may drain into the bladder neck, the posterior urethra, or the vas deferens in boys (Fig. 28). It drains into the bladder neck (Fig. 29), the urethra, the vagina, or the uterus in girls; it may also drain into the rectum or a Gartner duct cyst (Sheih et al. 1996). VUR into the ectopic ureter may appear during cycling VCU.

The anomaly is best demonstrated on MR urography or on contrast-enhanced CT (Borer et al. 1998; Pantuck et al. 1996; Gharagoloo and Lebowitz 1995; Braveman and Lebowitz 1991).

3.8 Ureterocele and Single Collecting System

Ureterocele (U-cele) represents cystic dilatation of the intravesical segment of the ureter. It is more common with duplex kidneys. When it is associated with a single system, the U-cele is commonly intravesical. On US, the U-cele appears as a cystic structure within the bladder that is connected with the ureter (Fig. 30); the upper urinary tract is somewhat obstructed or dilated. On VCUG, the U-cele appears as a filling defect within the bladder, especially on early films. The exact anatomy is assessed by MR urography (Fig. 31). The treatment is similar to that for U-cele in duplex kidneys depending on the degree of secondary obstruction. It is worth noting that a U-cele may be associated with a MCDK.

3.9 Bifid Collecting Systems

Bifid collecting systems correspond to incomplete duplication of the ureter; the ureters may meet at any level between the PUJ and the UVJ. US can only rarely differentiate the complete from the incomplete duplex kidney. Nowadays it is best evaluated by MR urography. An obstruction may occur at the lower pole collecting system or at the meeting point of the two ureters. Uretero-ureteral or pyelo-pyelic reflux (yo-yo reflux) is also typical for this condition (Fig. 32) (see chapter "Renal Agenesis, Dysplasia, Hypoplasia and Cystic Diseases of the Kidney").

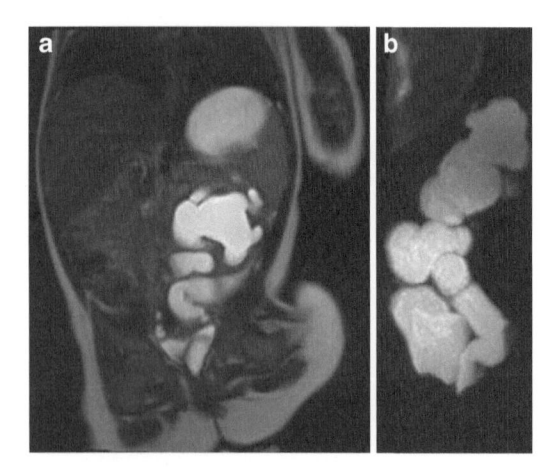

Fig. 29 Ectopic insertion of a ureter from a left markedly dilated and dysplastic kidney – MR urography. (**a**) Coronal T2W sequence, (**b**) sagittal MIP T2W sequence. The dilated left ureter inserts at the level of the bladder neck

> **Take Way**
> Primary MU has a typical appearance best demonstrated on MR urography, though often US is sufficient. An MU may or may not be secondary to obstruction and associated with VUR.

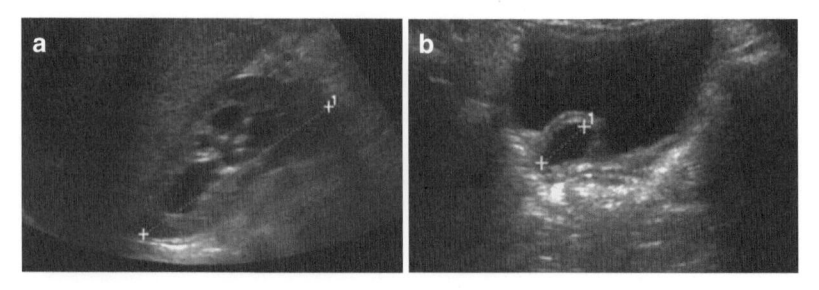

Fig. 30 Single U-cele on US. (**a**) Sagittal scan of the right kidney, displaying a slight dilatation of a single system. (**b**) Transverse scan of the bladder, typical U-cele

Fig. 31 Single U-cele on MR urography. (**a**) Frontal T2W sequence shows the mildly dilated right system. (**b**) Frontal T2W sequence, demonstrating the U-cele within the bladder

and lateral than the ureter draining the upper part of the kidney (Weigert-Meyers law). When both orifices open close to each other at a normal location, no complications occur. On the contrary, when they open apart from each other and away from the normal location, complications occur: the lower pole is usually associated with VUR and the upper pole with ureteral ectopia or U-cele with secondary obstruction. Dysplasia of the upper pole is also very common and seems to be related to an abnormal position of the ureteral bud on the renal blastema (Mckie and Stephens 1975). Complete ureteral duplication occurs in 1 out of 500 patients, most often with no complications.

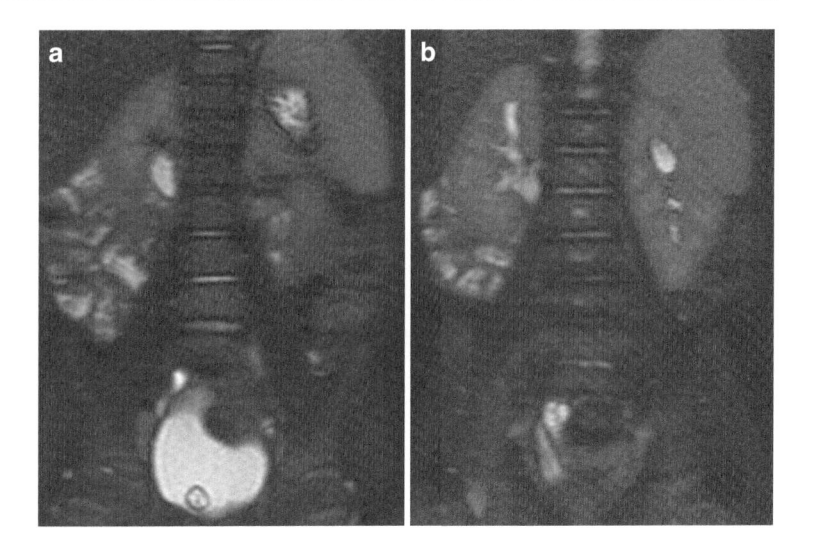

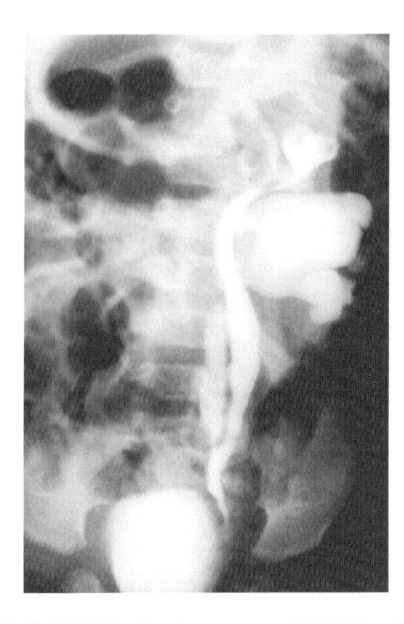

Fig. 32 Left bifid collecting system with VUR on VCUG

4 Duplex Collecting Systems

4.1 Etiology and Epidemiology

Complete duplication is thought to result from two separate ureteral buds presenting on the mesonephric duct (Glassberg et al. 1984). The orifice of the ureter draining the lower segment of the kidney migrates more cephalad

4.2 Presentation and Circumstances of Diagnosis

An uncomplicated duplex kidney is usually detected during a US examination that demonstrates two distinct renal hila separated by a bridge of normal parenchyma (Fig. 33). Unless there is a clinical indication, no further examination is necessary.

Still, many complications may occur and involve any of the poles of the duplex kidney, sometimes both, such as dilatation of the upper or lower pole, VUR, MCDK ectopic ureter, or U-cele.

Abnormal duplex kidneys used to be and are still detected during the work-up of urinary tract infection or urinary dribbling in girls. They are more and more often demonstrated during fetal life. In utero, it is possible to differentiate between the two collecting systems particularly if one is dilated. It is even possible to differentiate between ectopic ureteral insertion and U-cele in utero (Vergani et al. 1999). Other forms of presentation include interlabial mass in girls or bladder outlet obstruction. Both conditions are related to urethral prolapse of the U-cele (Nussbaum and Lebowitz 1983).

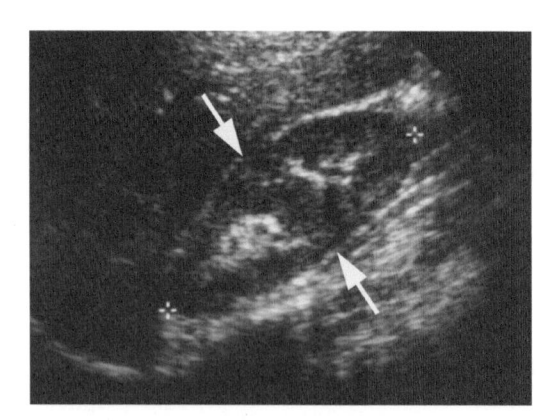

Fig. 33 US of renal duplication: sagittal scan of the right kidney. The two hyperechoic sinusal entities are separated by a parenchymal bridge (*arrows*)

4.3 The Work-Up of Duplex Kidneys: General Considerations

The findings of obstetrical US have to be confirmed after birth by US first. US usually demonstrates the two renal poles and the ureterohydronephrosis involving one or both moieties (Fig. 34a). It displays easily intravesical U-celes (Fig. 34b); however, the technique cannot always demonstrate ectopic ureters. VCUG is performed thereafter in order to detect VUR, including reflux into an ectopic ureter, and to evaluate the U-cele (Fig. 35). MR urography is performed whenever anatomical information is needed on the morphology of the duplex system. The technique is able to provide all the anatomical (Fig. 36a) details as well as some functional information after gadolinium enhancement (Fig. 36b–d). Isotope studies are mandatory to determine renal function particularly of the dilated and dysplastic upper moiety (Fig. 8). This complete work-up is mandatory in order to orient the best therapeutic approach.

4.4 Duplication and VUR

VUR is much more likely to occur into the lower than in the upper moiety of a duplex kidney. Lower-pole VUR is the most common abnormality that is associated with a duplex kidney

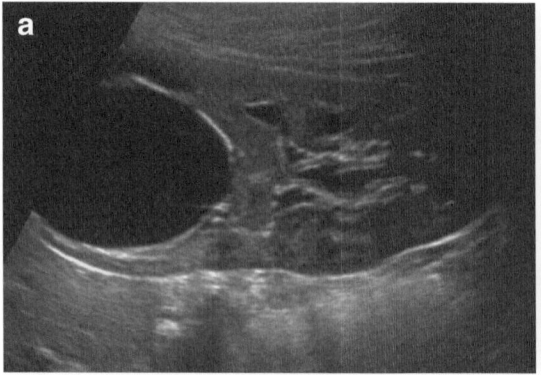

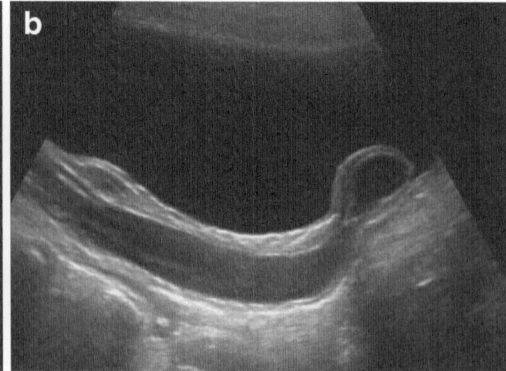

Fig. 34 US of a (classical) complicated left duplex kidney. (**a**) US of the kidney showing a dilated upper pole. (**b**) US of the bladder (left parasagittal scan, a dilated ureter ends into a typical U-cele)

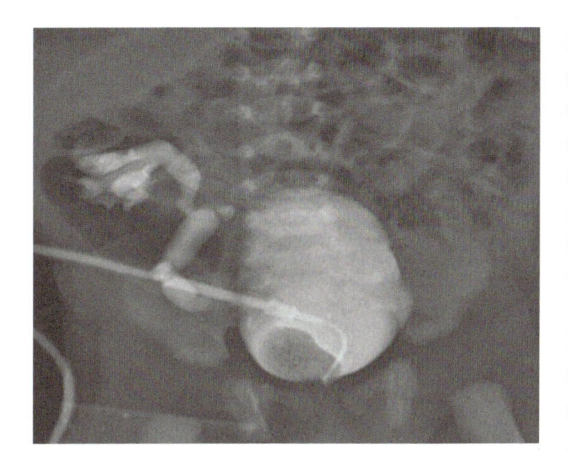

Congenital Anomalies of the Renal Pelvis and Ureter

Fig. 35 VCUG of a typical right duplex. The U-cele is visible as a filling defect, there is a right VUR in the right lower pole

(Fig. 37). The degree of VUR varies from mild to severe and can be graded like VUR into single systems. Massive VUR into a markedly dilated system may be misinterpreted as VUR in a single system. The VUR in the lower pole may be an isolated finding or may coexist with other types of pathologies and especially obstruction of the upper pole (Claudon et al. 1999).

The so-called reflux nephropathy (RN) of the lower pole is commonly associated with VUR (Fig. 37). It may be present already at birth with no preexisting urinary tract infection ("fetal RN"). VUR may occur simultaneously in both moieties (Fig. 38); this implies that the ureteral openings within the bladder are very close or

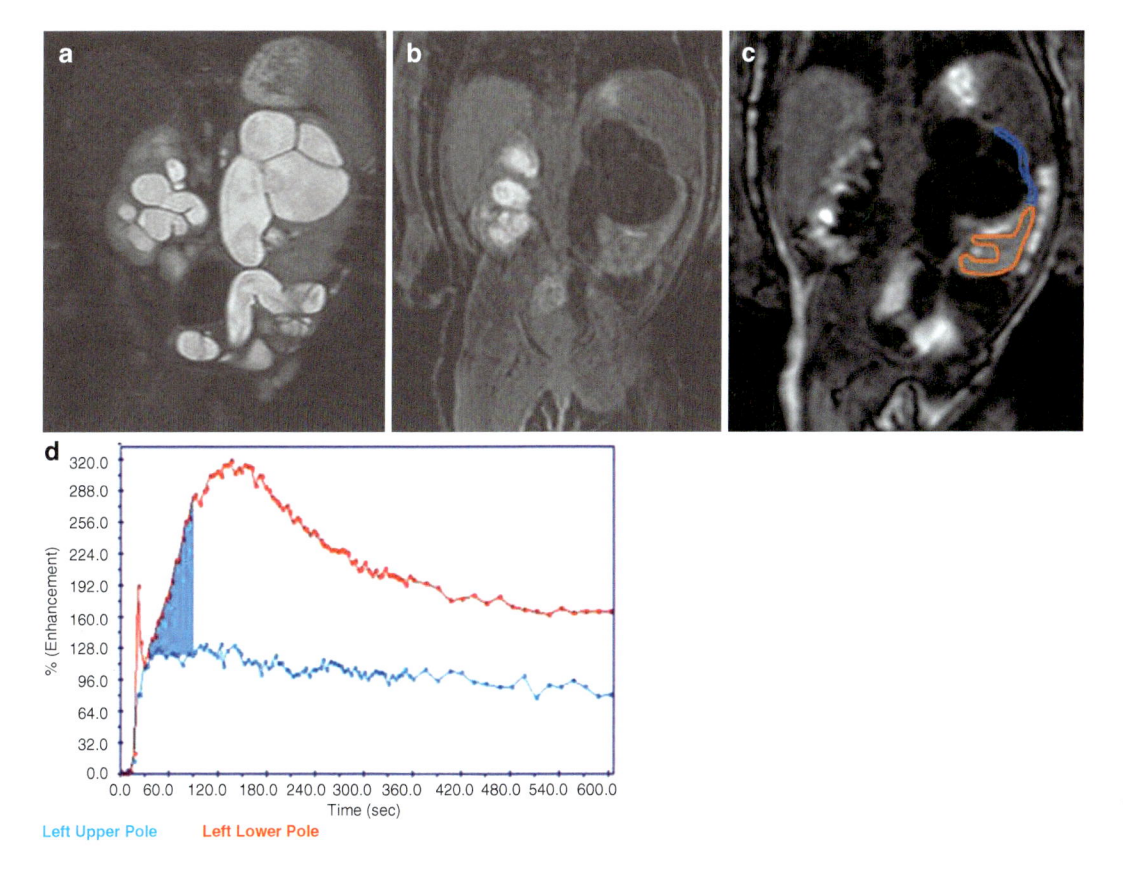

Fig. 36 Complicated duplex and MR urography. (**a**) Coronal T2W sequence: markedly dilated upper pole pyelocalyceal system and ureter. Thinned cortical band. Non-dilated lower pole. Contralateral hydronephrosis. (**b**) Coronal T1+Gd sequence, no enhancement of the upper pole. (**c, d**) Comparative analysis of upper and lower pole enhancement after gadolinium. The curve corresponding to the upper pole demonstrates poor enhancement and probable decreased function

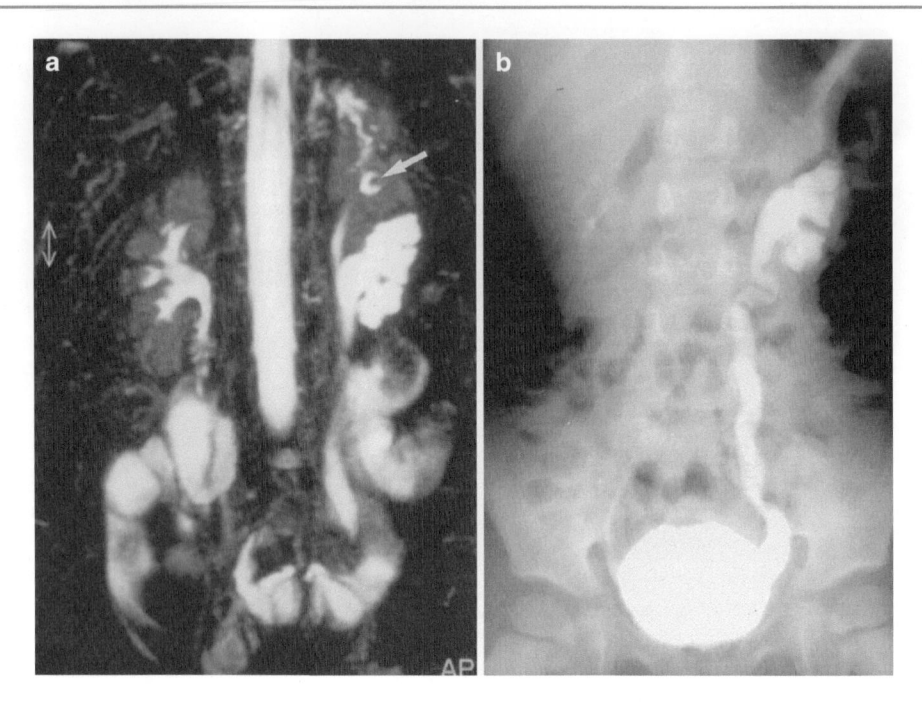

Fig. 37 VUR into the lower pole of a duplex system. (**a**) Left grade III–IV VUR into the lower pole (right grade II VUR). (**b**) MR urography displaying the monocalyceal upper (*arrow*) and dilated lower collecting systems (T2W coronal sequence)

VUR into the upper pole may also occur after inadvertent catheterization of a U-cele or after endoscopic unroofing of a U-cele (Blyth et al. 1993). The natural history of VUR into the lower pole is similar to VUR into a single system; it may resolve spontaneously (Peppas et al. 1991).

4.5 Ureteral Ectopia

Typically, the ureter draining the upper pole develops caudal to the normal location and is often ectopic, somewhere along the pathway of the mesonephric system. In boys, ectopic ureteral orifices open most usually into the posterior urethra but also into the ejaculatory ducts or the epididymis (the condition should therefore be suspected in orchiepididymitis). In girls, the ectopic ureter drains into the bladder neck, the vagina, the uterus, or any Mullerian variant. An ectopic ureter is usually associated with obstruction, with VUR, or both (Fig. 39).

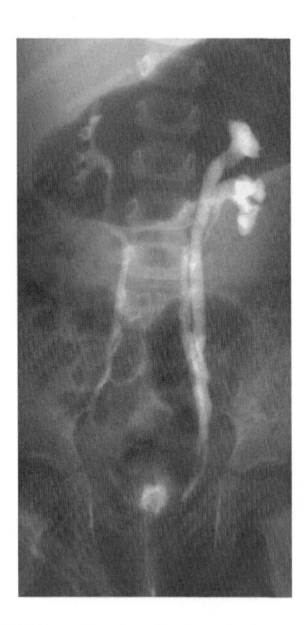

Fig. 38 VCUG – reflux into both moieties of a left duplex system

even common. VUR can occur in the lower pole due to ectopic insertion (at the bladder neck) of the ureter (see below).

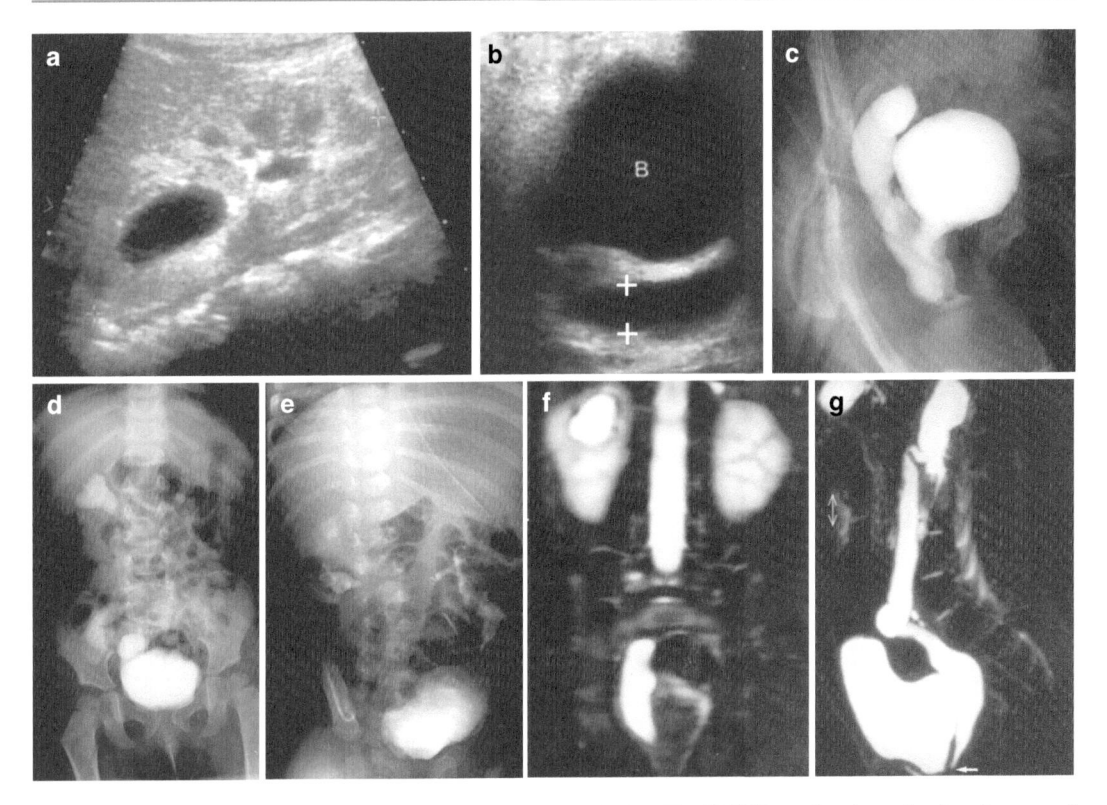

Fig. 39 Right duplex collecting system with ectopic urethral insertion of the upper pole in a 6-month-old baby girl. (**a**) US of the kidney (between crosses): dilatation of the upper pole. (**b**) Right sagittal scan of the bladder (B). The ureter is dilated (between crosses), but its insertion cannot be visualized. (**c**) VCU: during voiding, the ureter opacifies and the insertion seems located in the urethra (there is also a vaginal VUR). (**d**) VUR reaches the pyelocalyceal system of the upper pole. (**e**) IVU: the opacification of the right upper pole is poor. (**f**) MR urography: coronal SPIR T2 sequence showing the right duplication and the inferior insertion. (**g**) MR urography: sagittal inversion-recovery T2 sequence with MIP reconstruction shows the low extravesical insertion of the upper pole ureter (*arrow*)

As mentioned above, more and more cases are diagnosed during obstetrical US and evaluated at birth. In these children, the anomaly will be confirmed by US after birth, and further work-up will include VCUG and MR urography (see Chap. 26). In older children, ectopic ureters may be detected during the work-up of urinary tract infection. Typical clinical presentations include orchiepididymitis in boys and urinary dribbling in girls. Yet, many cases may evolve unrecognized up to late childhood since many ectopic draining upper poles function poorly (Share and Lebowitz 1990). Usually the duplex system is detected on US examination with the dilatation of the lower or the upper pole. The technique can suggest an ectopic insertion but usually cannot demonstrate it, though perineal US sometimes can be helpful for this diagnosis. The ectopic ureter may occasionally opacify during a VCUG (Fig. 39c). MR urography (or – if MR is unavailable and there is sufficient renal function of the respective moiety – contrast-enhanced CT) is able to demonstrate the ectopic extravesical insertion even though the upper pole parenchyma is small or functions poorly (Figs. 41, 42, 43, 44, 45, 46, 47, 48, and 49) (Share and Lebowitz 1990; Braveman and Lebowitz 1991).

Contrast-enhanced CT and better MR urography are both able to demonstrate the ectopic extravesical insertion even though the upper pole parenchyma is small or functions poorly (Figs. 39, 40, 41, 42, and 43) (Share and Lebowitz 1990; Braveman and Lebowitz 1991).

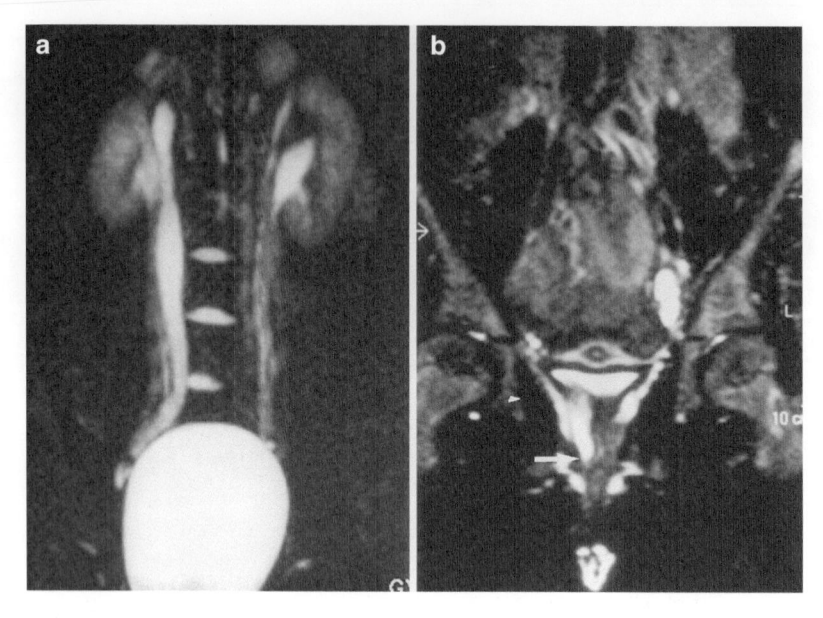

Fig. 40 Ectopic vaginal insertion of an upper pole ureter (7-year-old girl with urinary dribbling). (**a**) MR urography T2W sequence shows bilateral duplication with dilated right upper pole ureter. (**b**) MR urography on the bladder: vaginal ectopia of the ureter corresponding to the upper pole (*arrow*)

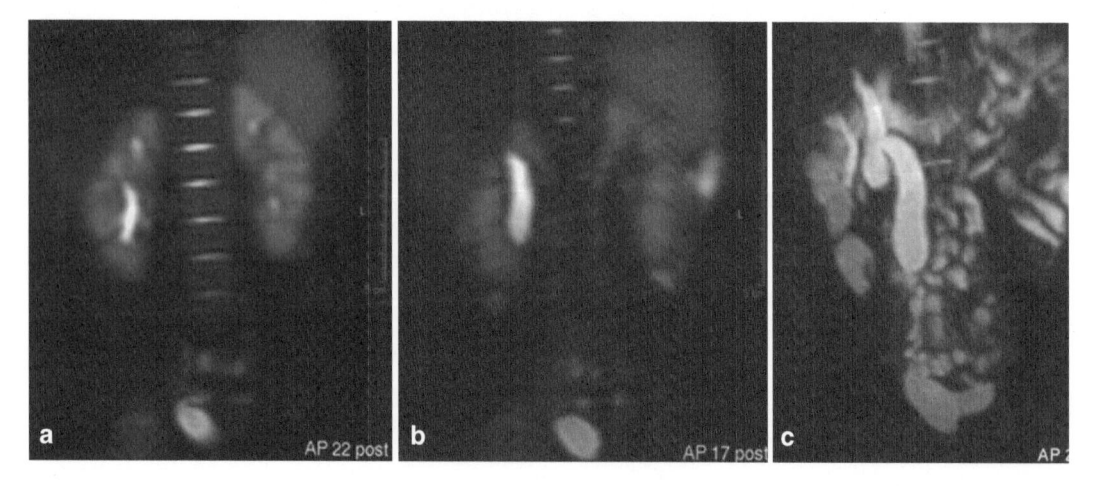

Fig. 41 (**a–c**) Ectopic insertion into a Mullerian remnant – MR urography T2W sequences successively views demonstrating the duplex system, a "dysplastic" upper pole ureter inserting into a retrovesical cystic structure

Upper pole heminephrectomy is required in order to stop the urinary dribbling or recurrent urinary tract infection when the dysplastic upper pole is still functioning. The inferior part of the ureter is usually left in place and may display VUR. MR imaging (with Gd injection) is able to determine the remaining function of the dysplastic parenchyma.

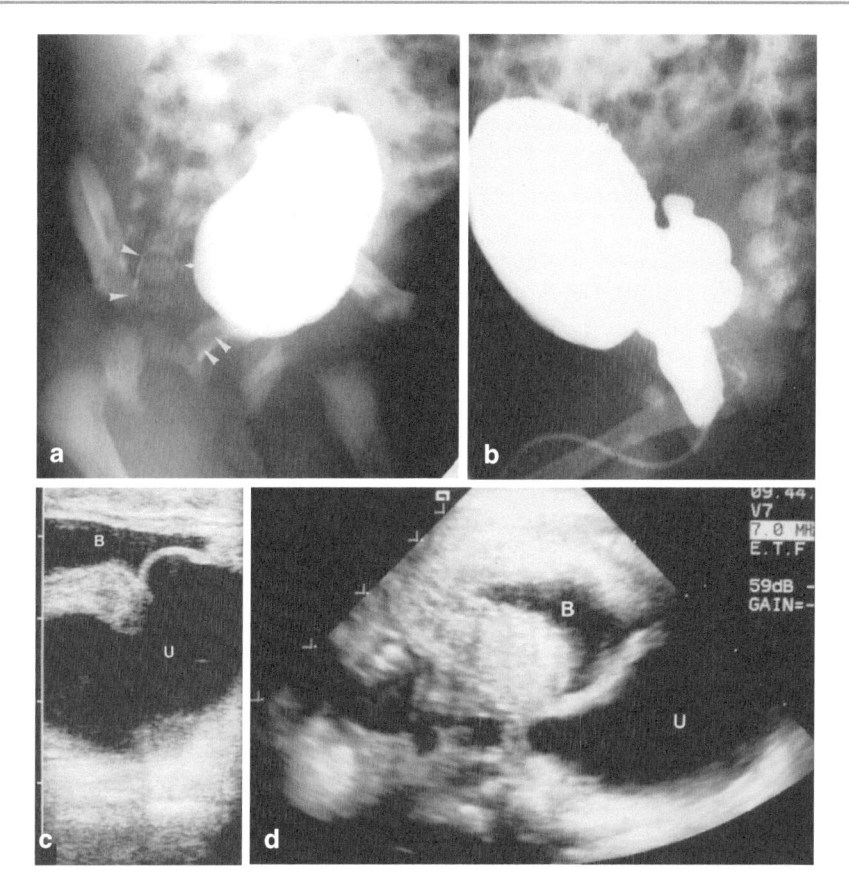

Congenital Anomalies of the Renal Pelvis and Ureter 457

Fig. 42 Cecoureterocele. (**a**) On VCU, the U-cele lies within the posterior urethra (*arrowheads*). (**b**) On a later phase, the ureterocele has everted. (**c**) US of the bladder (B) showing the large ureterocele (U). (**d**) On the postvoiding film, the ureterocele (U) still occupies the posterior urethra. Note the thickened bladder wall

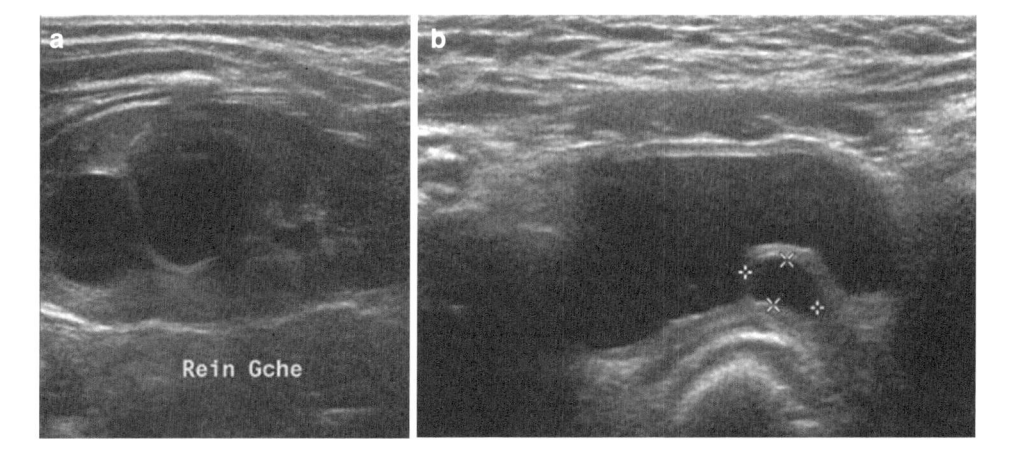

Fig. 43 Small obstructive U-cele. (**a**) Important dilatation (D) of the corresponding upper pole. (**b**) Small intravesical U-cele (*arrow*)

4.6 Ureterocele

U-cele is the other anomaly that can be associated with the upper pole of a duplex kidney. U-celes represent a dilatation of the intravesical portion of the ureter (Figs. 34b and 42c). They may be associated with a wide spectrum of anomalies at the upper pole, in the bladder, and in the urethra. Large U-celes may be in relation with tiny upper poles, whereas small U-celes may be highly obstructive (Fig. 43). U-celes have been classified into stenotic, sphincteric, sphincterostenotic, cecoureterocele, blind U-cele, and non-obstructed U-cele according to their location and degree of obstruction (Lebowitz and Avni 1980; Share and Lebowitz 1989). The cecoureteroceles are located down into the posterior urethra (Fig. 42), and their surgical correction is more difficult. Again, as for ectopic ureter, many U-celes are detected during fetal US allowing rapid evaluation and treatment at birth. They are also detected during the work-up of urinary tract infection and more rarely as an interlabial mass in the baby girl.

U-celes are best visualized on US examination as a cystic structure within the bladder (Figs. 36, 42, and 43). Small low-positioned U-celes may remain unrecognized with this technique. Their differential diagnosis on US includes a Gartner duct cyst and the Wolffian duct cyst, which are extravesical and may be associated with genital or renal anomalies (Trigaux et al. 1991). U-celes are also well visualized on MR urography (Fig. 44) and VCU. On VCU, the differential diagnosis should include air bubble, blood clot, lithiasis, tumor, or balloon catheter (Lebowitz and Avni 1980). US is usually sufficient for this differential. On VCU the U-celes may display varying appearances. During the filling phase, the U-cele may vanish, evert, or prolapse within the urethra and induce bladder outlet obstruction (Figs. 43 and 45) (Lebowitz and Avni 1980; Bellah et al. 1995). The fear of this type of obstruction has led several teams to propose early endoscopic unroofing of the U-cele (Blyth et al. 1993; Shekarriz et al. 1999; Jayanthi and Koff 1999; Husmann et al. 1999). The advantage of the method is that it helps to drain the obstructed urinary tract, providing hope of improving function and rendering heminephrectomy unnecessary. The disadvantage is that secondary VUR into the upper pole may supervene, making reimplantation necessary. After incision, the U-cele collapses and appears as a pseudomass within the bladder (Rypens et al. 1992).

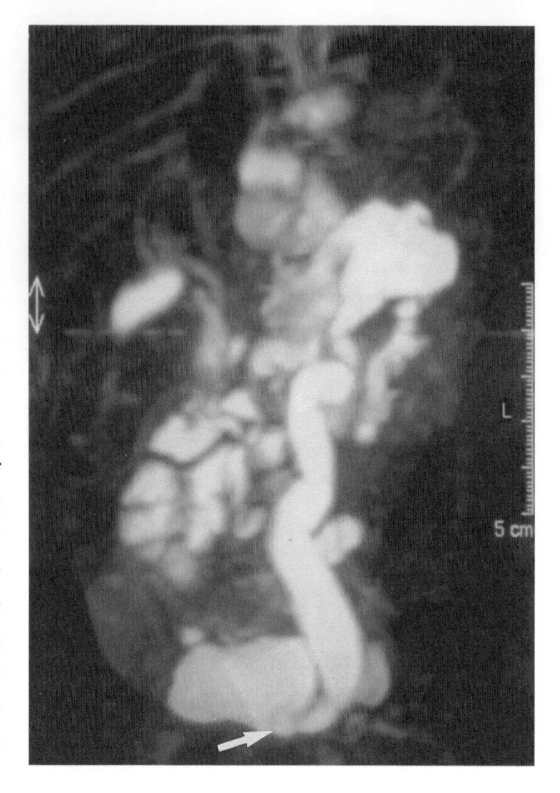

Fig. 44 MR urography of duplex system with ectopic U-cele, T2 inversion-recovery sequence. The small ureterocele (*arrow*) was not visualized by US

4.7 (Cystic) Dysplasia of the Upper Pole

The appearance and function of the parenchyma at the upper pole of a duplex kidney vary widely. It may appear normal with a preserved function; this usually occurs in duplex kidneys with normally or near-normally positioned ureteral openings. On the contrary, the parenchyma may be very thin and poorly functioning in relation with ectopic U-cele or ectopic ureters (Corrales and Elder 1996). The condition is usually detected by US, sometimes in utero. The condition may be recognized later in childhood due to infection or dribbling. CT or MR urography and

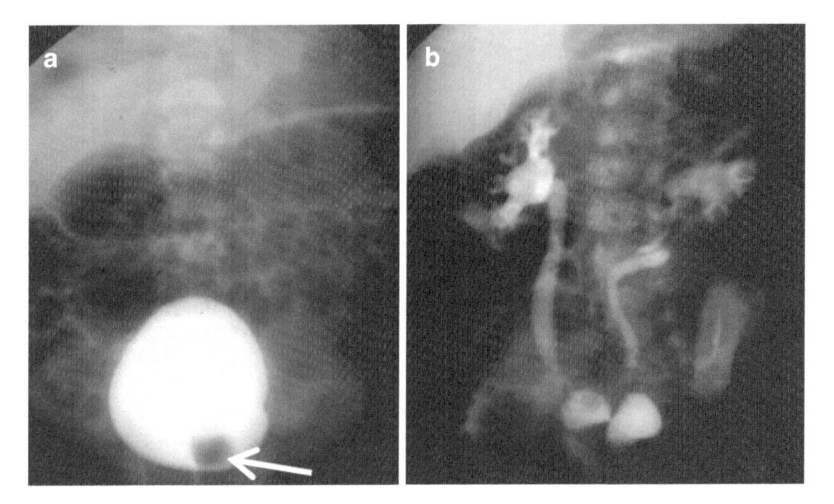

Fig. 45 Eversion of a ureterocele. (**a**) Filling phase of the VCU: the ureterocele is seen within the bladder as a filling defect (*arrow*). (**b**) After voiding, the ureterocele has now everted; bilateral VUR is also present (right grade II; lower left pole grade II)

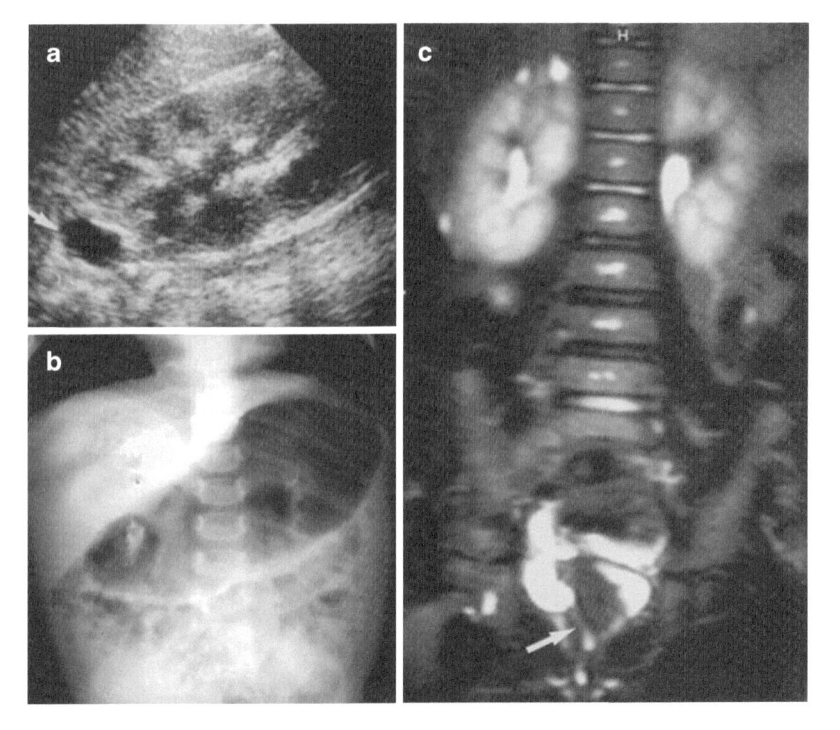

Fig. 46 Cystic dysplasia of the upper pole of a right duplex kidney. (**a**) On US, a single cyst (*arrow*) is visualized on the sagittal scan of the right kidney. (**b**) On IVU, the upper pole does not opacify. (**c**) MR urography displays the cystic upper pole and the extravesical insertion of the corresponding ureter (*arrow*) (SPIR T2 sequence)

isotopes are complementary in demonstrating the morphology and the function of the dysplastic renal moiety (Fig. 46) (Share and Lebowitz 1990; Avni 1997). The dysplastic upper pole may involute progressively, in a way similar to MDKD. Furthermore, MDKD may involve the upper or the lower pole of a duplex system (Fig. 47).

4.8 Other Types of Obstruction in Duplex Kidney

Obstruction may occur at many levels including the PUJ of the upper and lower pole (the latter is the most common) (Fig. 48). Obstruction may also occur at the UVJ of one or both ureters (Fig. 49) (Ulchaker et al. 1996; Ho et al. 1995).

> **Take Away**
> A wide variety of anomalies occur in duplex kidneys. Dedicated and skilful, partially individualized imaging is mandatory in order to characterize the precise anatomy, to decide on treatment, and to orient for surgery.

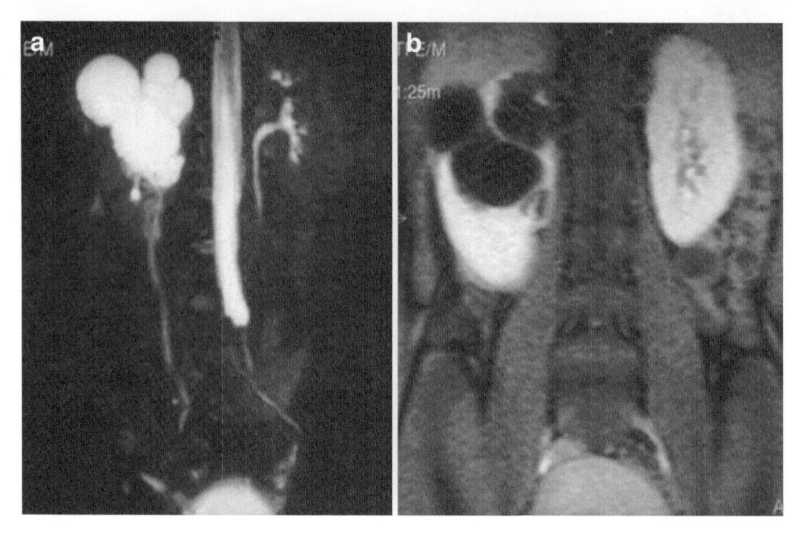

Fig. 47 MCDK of an upper pole – MR urography. (**a**) T2W sequence. (**b**) T1+ Gd sequence

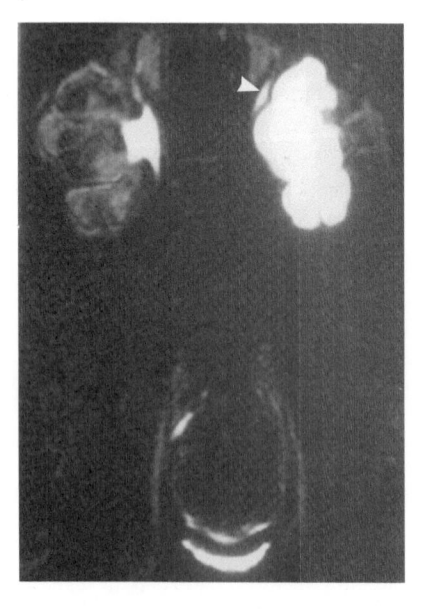

Fig. 48 PUJ obstruction on the lower pole displayed by MR urography (T2W sequence). The arrowhead points to the upper pole system

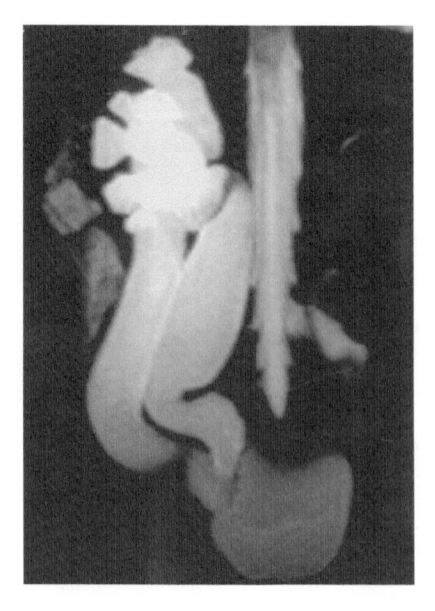

Fig. 49 UVJ obstruction on the upper and lower moieties displayed by MR urography (inversion-recovery sequence with MIP reconstruction)

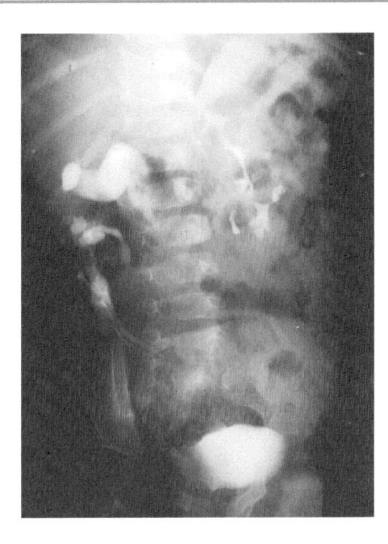

Fig. 50 IVU demonstration of ureteral quadruplication (Courtesy of L. Sourtzis, MD)

5 Triplication and Quadruplication of the Ureter

Triplication and quadruplication of the ureter are very unusual conditions that can be diagnosed on IVU, VCUG, and MRI (Fig. 50) (Hassan 1990; Sourtzis et al. 1994).

Conclusion

Many anomalies occur at any level of the collecting system. The morphology of the anomalies is best evaluated by MR urography, especially if there is no or only poor function. US, however, mostly is a good initial imaging tool and often useful for follow-up, complemented by VCUG (ce-VUS) in the initial diagnostic work-up and isotope studies for functional queries.

References

Avni EF, Matos C, Rypens F, Schulman CC (1997) Ectopic vaginal insertion of an upper pole ureter: demonstration by special sequences of magnetic resonance imaging. J Urol 158(5):1931–1932

Avni EF, Nicaise N, Hall M et al (2001) The role of MR imaging for the assessment of complicated duplex kidneys in children. Pediatr Radiol 31:215–223

Baskin LS, Zderic SA, Snyder HM et al (1994) Primary dilated megaureter: long-term follow-up. J Urol 152:618–621

Bellah RD, Long FR, Canning DA (1995) Ureterocele eversion with VUR in duplex kidneys. AJR 165:409–413

Blyth B, Passerini-Glazel G, Camuffo C et al (1993) Endoscopic incision of ureteroceles: intravesical versus ectopic. J Urol 149:5556–5560

Bomalski MD, Hirsch RB, Bloom DA et al (1997) VUR and UPJ obstruction: association treatment options and outcome. J Urol 157:969–974

Borer JG, Bauer SB, Peters CA et al (1998) A single system ectopic ureter draining an ectopic dysplastic kidney. Br J Urol 81:474–478

Braveman RM, Lebowitz RL (1991) Occult ectopic ureter in girls: diagnosis with CT. AJR 156:365–366

Bude RO, DiPietro MA, Platt JF et al (1992) Age dependency of the renal resistive index in healthy children. Radiology 184:469–473

Calder AD, Hiorns MP, Abhyankar A et al (2007) Contrast-enhanced MR angiography for the detection of crossing renal vessels in children with symptomatic UPJ obstruction. Pediatr Radiol 37:356–361

Cendron M, D'alton ME, Crombleholme TM (1994) Prenatal diagnosis and management of the fetus with hydronephrosis. Semin Perinatol 18:163–181

Claudon M, Ben-Sira L, Lebowitz RL (1999) Lower-pole reflux in children: uroradiologic appearances and pitfalls. AJR 172:795–801

Claudon M, Durand E, Grenier N, Prigent A et al (2014) Chronic urinary obstruction: evaluation of dynamic contrast-enhanced MR urography. Radiology 2014;273: 801–812

Cope RM, Snow BW (1991) Massive cystic ureteral diverticula in infancy. J Urol 146:575–577

Coplen DE, Austin PF, Yan Y, Blanco VM et al (2006) The magnitude of fetal renal pelvic dilatation can identify obstructive postnatal hydronephrosis, and direct post natal evaluation and management. J Urol 176:724–727

Corrales JG, Elder JS (1996) Segmental multicystic kidney and ipsilateral duplication anomalies. J Urol 155:1398–1401

Darge K, Higgins M, Hwang TJ, Delgado J et al (2013) MR and CT in pediatric urology: an imaging overview for daily practice. Radiol Clin N Amer 51:583–598

Duong HP, Piepsz A, Collier F et al (2013) Predicting the clinical outcome of antenatally detected unilateral pelviureteric junction stenosis. Urology 82:691–696

Eskild-Jensen A, Gordon I, Piepsz A et al (2004) Interpretation of the renogram: problems and pitfalls in hydronephrosis in children. BJU Int 94:887–892

Flaschner SC, Mesrobian HJ, Flatt JA et al (1993) Nonobstructive dilatation of upper urinary tract may later convert to obstruction. Urology 42:569–573

Frauscher F, Janetschek G, Helweg G et al (1999) Crossing vessels at the UPJ: detection with contrast enhanced color Doppler imaging. Radiology 210:727–731

Gharagoloo AM, Lebowitz RL (1995) Detection of a poorly functioning malpositioned kidney with single ectopic ureter. AJR 164:957–961

Glassberg KI, Braren V, Duckett JW et al (1984) Suggested terminology for duplex systems, ectopic ureters and ureteroceles. J Urol 132:1153–1154

Gordon I, Colarinha P, Piepsz A et al (2001) Guidelines for standard and diuretic renography in children. Eur J Nucl Med 28:BP21–BP30

Gordon I, Piepsz A, Sixt R (2011) Guidelines for standard and diuretic renogram in children. Eur J Nucl Med Mol Imaging 38:1175–1188

Hassan MA (1990) Ureteral triplication with VUR. Urology 30:78–80

Herbetko J, Hyde I (1990) Urinary tract dilatation in constipated children. Br J Radiol 63:855–857

Ho DS, Jerkins GR, Williams M et al (1995) UPJ obstruction in upper and lower moiety of duplex renal systems. Urology 45:503–506

Husmann D, Strand B, Ewalt D et al (1999) Management of ectopic ureterocele associated with renal duplication. J Urol 162:1406–1409

Ismaili K, Piepsz A (2013) The antenatal detected pelviureteric junction stenosis: advances in renography and strategy of management. Pediatr Radiol 43:428–435

Jayanthi VR, Koff SA (1999) Long-term outcome of transurethral puncture of ectopic ureteroceles. J Urol 162:1077–1080

Jones JA, Perez-Brayfield MR, Kirsch AJ et al (2004) Renal transit time with MR urography in children. Radiology 233:41–50

Keller MS, Weiss RM, Rosenfield NS (1993) US evaluation or ureterectasis in children. J Urol 149:553–555

Koff SA, Campbell KD (1994) The non-operative management of unilateral hydronephrosis. J Urol 152:593–595

Koff SA, Peller PA, Young DC et al (1994) The assessment of obstruction in newborn with unilateral hydronephrosis by measuring the size of the opposite kidney. J Urol 152:596–599

Kraus SJ, Lebowitz RL, Royal SA (1999) Renal calculi in children. Pediatr Radiol 29:624–630

Lautin EM, Haramati N, Frager D et al (1988) CT diagnosis of circumcaval ureter. AJR 150:591–594

Lebowitz RL, Avni EF (1980) Misleading appearances in pediatric uroradiology. Pediatr Radiol 10:15–31

Liu AHY, Dhillon HK, Diamond DA et al (1994) Clinical outcome and management of prenatally diagnosed primary megaureters. J Urol 152:614–617

Maizels M, Reisman ME, Flom LS et al (1992) Grading nephro-ureteral dilatation detected in the first year of life. J Urol 148:609–614

Mandell GA, Snyder HM, Heyman S et al (1986) Association of congenital megacalycosis and ipsilateral segmental megaureter. Pediatr Radiol 17:28–33

Matsumoto JS (1986) Acquired lesions involving the ureter in childhood. Semin Roentgen 21:166–167

McGrath MA, Estroff J, Lebowitz RL (1987) The coexistence of obstruction at the UPJ and UVJ. AJR 149:403–406

Mckie GG, Stephens FD (1975) Duplex kidneys: a correlation of renal dysplasia with position of ureteral orifice. J Urol 114:274–280

Nguyen HT, Herndron CD, Cooper C, Gatti J et al (2010) The society for fetal urology consensus statement on the evaluation and management of antenatal hydronephrosis. J Pediatr Urol 6:212–213

Nogarède C, Tondeur M, Piepsz A (2010) Normalized residual activity and output efficiency in case of early furosemide injection in children. Nucl Med Commun 31:355–358

Nolte-Ernstig C, Bucker A, Adam GB et al (1998) Gadolinium-enhanced excretory MR urography after low dose diuretic injection. Radiology 209:147–157

Nussbaum AR, Lebowitz RL (1983) Interlabial masses in little girls. AJR 141:65–71

Oyen R, Gielen J, Baert L et al (1987) CT demonstration of a ureterosciatic hernia. Urol Radiol 9:174–176

Palmer LS (2006) Pediatric urologic imaging. Urol Clin N Am 33:409–433

Pantuck AJ, Barone JG, Rosenfeld DL, Fleisher MH (1996) Occult bilateral vaginal ureters. Abdom Imag 21:78–80

Patriquin H (1991) Doppler examination of the kidney in infants and children. Urol Radiol 12:220–227

Patti G, Menghini ML, Tordini AR et al (2000) The role of the renal resistive index ratio in diagnosing obstruction and in the follow-up of children with unilateral hydronephrosis. BJU Intern 85:308–312

Peerboccus M, Damry N, Pather S et al (2012) The impact of hydration on renal measurements and on cortical echogenicity in children. Pediatr Radiol 43:1557–1565

Peppas DS, Skoog SJ, Canning DA et al (1991) Nonsurgical management of VUR in complete ureteral duplication. J Urol 146:1594–1595

Peters CA (1995) Urinary tract obstruction in children. J Urol 154:1874–1884

Piepsz A, Ham HR (2006) Pediatric applications of renal nuclear medicine. Semin Nucl Med 36:16–35

Piepsz A, Colarinha P, Gordon I et al (2001) Guidelines for glomerular filtration rate determination in children. Eur J Nucl Med 28:31–36

Piepsz A, Kuyvenhoven J, Tondeur HH (2002) Normalized residual activity: usual values and robustness of the method. J Nucl Med 43:33–38

Piepsz A, Gordon I, Brock J III et al (2009) Round table on the management of renal pelvic dilatation in children. J Pediatr Urol 5:437–444

Piepsz A (2009) The predictive value of the renogram. Eur J Nucl Med Mol Imaging 36:1661–1664

Piepsz A (2011) Antenatal detection of pelviureteric junction stenosis: main controversies. Semin Nucl Med 41:11–19

Piepsz A, Tondeur M, Nogarède C et al (2011) Can severely impaired cortical transit predict which children with pelvi-ureteric junction stenosis detected antenatally might benefit from pyeloplasty? Nucl Med Commun 32:199–205

Pinter AB, Szabo L, Szever ZS et al (1997) Bilateral congenital segmental megaureter. J Urol 158:570–571

Prigent A, Cosgriff P, Gates GF et al (1999) Consensus report on quality control of quantitative measurements of renal function obtained from renogram: International Consensus Committee for the Scientific Committee of Radionuclides in Nephrourology. Semin Nucl Med 29:146–159

Regan F, Bohlman ME, Khazan R et al (1996) MR urography using HASTE imaging in the assessment of ureteric obstruction. AJR 167:1115–1120

Renjen P, Bellah R, Hellinger JC, Darhe K (2012) Advances in uroradiologic imaging in children. Radiol Clin N Amer 50:207–218

Riccabona M, Simbrunner J, Ring E, Ebner F, Fotter R (2002) Feasibility of MR-urography in neonates and infants with anomalies of the upper urinary tract. Eur Radiol 12:1442–1450

Riccabona M, Avni FE, Blickman JG, Dacher JN et al (2009) Imaging recommendations in pediatric uroradiology: Childhood obstructive uropathy, high grades fetal hydronephrosis and childhood haematuria. Pediatr Radiol 39:891–898

Riccabona M, Avni FE, Dacher JN, Damasio B et al (2010) Imaging recommendations in pediatric uroradiology: IVU, uro-CT and MR urography. Pediatr Radiol 40:1315–1320

Rickwood AMK, Godiwalla SY (1997) The natural history of UPJ obstruction in children presenting clinically with the complaint. Br J Urol 80: 793–796

Roarke MC, Sandler CM (1998) Provocative imaging diuretic renography. Urol Clin N Am 25:227–249

Rohrschneider WK, Haufe S, Clorius JH, Troger J (2003) MR to assess renal function in children. Eu Radiol 13:1033–1045

Rypens F, Avni EF, Bank WO et al (1992) The UVJ in children. AJR 158:837–842

Schlotmann A, Clorius J, Clorius SN (2009) Diuretic renography in hydronephrosis: renal tissue tracer predicts functional course and thereby need for surgery. Eur J Nucl Med Mol Imaging 36:1665–1673

Share JC, Lebowitz RL (1989) Ectopic ureterocele without ureteral and calyceal dilatation. AJR 152:567–571

Share JC, Lebowitz RL (1990) The unsuspected duplex collecting system. AJR 155:561–564

Sheih CP, Li Y, Liao Y, Chiang C (1996) Small ureterocele-like Gartner's duct cyst associated with ipsilateral renal dysgenesis. J Clin Ultrasound 24:533–535

Shekarriz B, Upadhyay J, Flemeing P et al (1999) Long-term outcome based on the initial surgical approach to ureterocele. J Urol 162:1072–1076

Sherman C, Winchester P, Brill P et al (1988) Childhood retroperitoneal fibrosis. Pediatr Radiol 18:245–247

Silveri M, Adorisio O, Pane A et al (2002) Fetal monolateral urinoma and neonatal renal function outcome in posterior urethral valves obstruction: the pop-off mechanism. Pediatr Med Chir 24:394–395

Sourtzis S, Damry N, Janssen F et al (1994) Ureteral quadruplication. Pediatr Radiol 24:604–605

Stabin M, Taylor A Jr, Eshima D et al (1992) Radiation Dosimetry for technetium-99m-MAG3, technetium-99m-DTPA, and iodine-131-OIH based on human biodistribution studies. J Nucl Med 33:33–40

Stocks A, Richards D, Frentzen B et al (1996) Correlation of prenatal pelvic antero-posterior diameter with outcome in infancy. J Urol 155:1050–1052

Tondeur M, Nogarede C, Donoso G, Piepsz A (2013) Inter- and intra-observer reproducibility of quantitative renographic parameters of differential function and renal drainage in children. Scand J Clin Lab Invest 73:414–421

Trigaux JP, Van Beers B, Delchambre F (1991) Male genital tract malformations associated with ipsilateral renal agenesis. J Clin Ultrasound 19:3–10

Tsai JD, Huang FY, Lin C et al (2006) Intermittent hydronephrosis secondary to UPJ obstruction: clinical and imaging features. Pediatrics 117:139–146

Uhlenhuth E, Amin M, Harty JL et al (1990) Infundibulopelvic dysgenesis: a spectrum of obstructive renal disease. Urology 35:334–337

Ulchaker J, Ross J, Alexander F et al (1996) The spectrum of UPJ obstruction occurring in duplicated collecting systems. J Ped Surgery 31:1221–1224

Vargas B, Lebowitz RL (1986) The coexistence of congenital megacalyces and primary megaureter. AJR 147:313–316

Vergani P, Ceruti P, Locatelli et al (1999) Accuracy of prenatal US diagnosis of duplex kidney. J Ultrasound Med 18:463–467

Veyrac C, Baud C, Lopez C, Couture A et al (2003) The value of color Doppler US for identification of crossing vessels in children with PUJ obstruction. Pediatr Radiol 33:745–751

Vivier PH, Dolores M, Taylor M, Dacher JN (2010a) MR Urography in children Part 2.: how to use Image MR urography processing software. Pediatr Radiol 40(5):739–746

Vivier PH, Dolores M, Taylor M et al (2010b) MR urography in children. Part 1: how I do the F0 technique. Pediatr Radiol 40:732–738

Vivier PH, Storey P, Rusinek H et al (2011) Kidney function: glomerular filtration rate measurement with MR renography in patients with cirrhosis. Radiology 259(2):462–470

Wilcox D, Mouriquand P (1998) Management of megaureter in children. Eur Urol 34:73–78

Wille S, Von Krobloch R, Klose KJ et al (2002) MR urography in pediatric urology. Scand J Urol Nephrol 37:16–21

Yagci F, Erbagci A, Sarica K et al (1999) The place of diuretic enhanced Doppler US in distinguishing between obstructive and nonobstructive hydronephrosis in children. Scand J Urol Nephrol 33: 382–385

Upper Urinary Tract Dilatation in Newborns and Infants and the Postnatal Work-Up of Congenital Uro-nephropathies

Freddy Avni, Marianne Tondeur, and Rene-Hilaire Priso

Contents

1   Introduction 465
2   **Postnatal Work-Up** 466
2.1 Clinical Situations and Antenatal Diagnoses Necessitating a Rapid Management 468
2.2 Postnatal Work-Up of Uropathies 468
2.3 Further Anatomical Assessment 471
2.4 Functional Assessment: Nuclear Medicine Studies 473
2.5 The Postnatal Work-Up of Nephropathies 474

3   **Long-Term Follow-Up and (Potential Treatment) in the Light of the Natural History of Uro-nephropathies** 475
3.1 Vesicoureteric Reflux 475
3.2 Pelvi-ureteric Junction (PUJ) Obstruction 476
3.3 Ureterovesical Junction (UVJ) Obstruction 477
3.4 Multicystic Dysplastic Kidney (MCDK) 477
3.5 Complicated Duplex Kidneys 477
3.6 Nephropathies 477

Conclusions 478
References 478

F. Avni, MD, PhD (✉) • R.-H. Priso, MD
Department of Pediatric Radiology, Jeanne de Flandre Hospital, Lille University Hospital, 59037 Lille, France
e-mail: favni@skynet.be

M. Tondeur, MD
Department of Radio-Isotopes, CHU Saint-Pierre, Rue Haute 322, 1000 Brussels, Belgium

1 Introduction

In many European countries, obstetric ultrasound (US) is performed routinely during normal pregnancies. This leads to the discovery of many fetal anomalies, and, among them, uro-nephropathies represent one of the largest groups amenable to neonatal management. They are now included in the so-called CAKUT [congenital anomalies of the kidney and urinary tract] group (Renkema et al. 2011; Wiesel et al 2005; Ek et al. 2007).

Changes have occurred in the neonatal management since nowadays these uropathies are detected in mostly asymptomatic patients, and the treatment is mainly preventive. Antenatal detection and postnatal follow-up have yielded new data on the natural history of many uropathies and have shown that a majority of antenatally diagnosed renal dilatations will resolve spontaneously (Barbosa et al. 2012; Ek et al. 2007; Kumar et al. 2012; Quirino et al. 2012; Wollenberg et al. 2005).

The aims of the postnatal work-up will be first to confirm the anomaly, to ascertain the diagnosis (and the prognosis), then to adapt the follow-up to the type of anomaly, and finally to decide on the best treatment (see also chapter "Congenital Urinary Tract Dilatation and Obstructive Uropathy"). The rationale of all the imaging is clearly to prevent further complications on an already damaged kidney (Ismaïli et al. 2004, 2005).

2 Postnatal Work-Up

The ideal postnatal work-up is still debated but it has been markedly standardized. At first the antenatal US findings were standardized (Table 1) differentiating minimal and moderate dilatation from marked dilatation in order to define the proper postnatal management. Secondly the postnatal management has been also standardized depending on the antenatal and postnatal findings (Tables 2a and 2b). All proposed managements are based on the US findings (Riccabona et al. 2008, 2009).

An American consensus panel has recently proposed a further classification and standardization: the UTD (urinary tract dilatation) classification system aimed to describe simultaneously both antenatally and postnatally US findings. It is based on six US findings, anterior-posterior (AP) axial renal pelvic dilatation, calyceal dilatation, renal parenchymal thickness, parenchymal appearance, bladder and ureteral anomalies, as well as the amniotic fluid volume. The system distinguishes whether the findings are antenatal (A) or postnatal (P) followed by a number. UTD A1 represents mild antenatal UTD and UTD P3 marked postnatal dilatation (Nguyen et al. 2014). The examination is intended to confirm the anomaly, differentiate between uro- and nephropathies (knowing that both can be associated), and determine the need for further

Table 1 Sonographic classification of fetal pelvi-calyceal dilatation (Riccabona et al. 2008, updated 2017)

US grading of pelvi-caliceal distention / dilatation / width (PCD) in neonates and infants

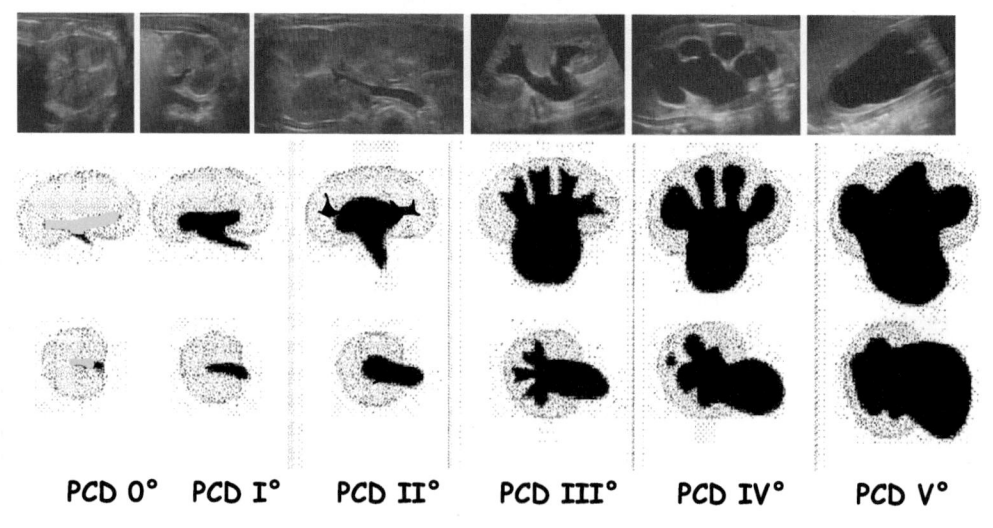

PCD 0°   PCD I°   PCD II°   PCD III°   PCD IV°   PCD V°

PCD 0	=	collecting system not or hardy visible, normal
PCD I	=	just renal pelvis clearly visible, calices not depictable axial plevic diameter less than 7 mm, considered normal
PCD II	=	axial renal pelvis diameter less than 10 mm , (some) calices visible, but with normal forniceal and papillar shape / configuration (often normal variation)
PCD III	=	marked dilatation of calices and pelvis, the pelvic axial width usually >10 mm with flattened papilla and rounded fornices, but without parenchymal narrowing
PCD IV	=	gross dilatation of entire collecting system + narrowing of renal parenchyma
(PCD V	=	additionally used in some places, to describe an extreme PCD IV° with only a thin, membrane-like residual renal parenchymal rim)

Table 2 (a) Mild to moderate) and (b) (severe dilatation). Proposed neonatal work-up of fetal uropathies. (a) Postnatal imaging algorithm in mild or moderate fetal UTD (Riccabona et al. 2008). (b) Postnatal imaging algorithm in severe fetal UTD (Riccabona et al. 2009)

a Postnatal imaging algorithm in mild or moderate foetal urinary tract dilatation (Riccabona et al. 2006)

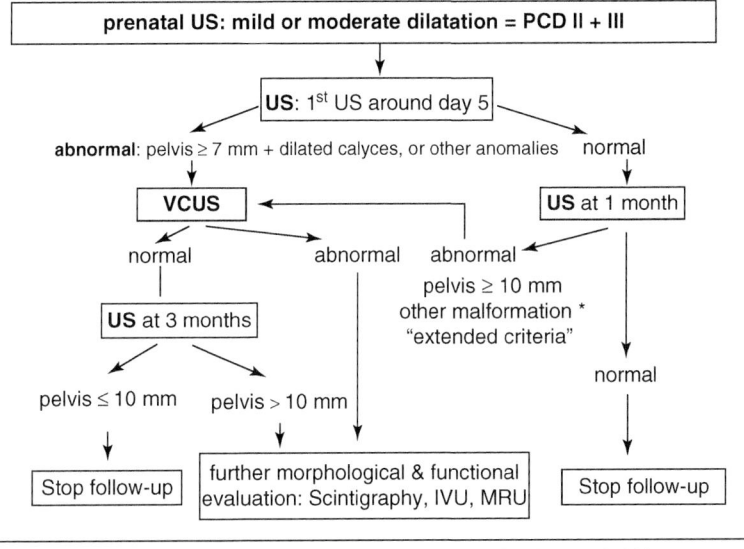

prenatal US: mild or moderate dilatation = PCD II + III

↓

US: 1st US around day 5

- abnormal: pelvis ≥ 7 mm + dilated calyces, or other anomalies → VCUS
- normal → US at 1 month

VCUS:
- normal → US at 3 months
  - pelvis ≤ 10 mm → Stop follow-up
  - pelvis > 10 mm → further morphological & functional evaluation: Scintigraphy, IVU, MRU
- abnormal → further morphological & functional evaluation: Scintigraphy, IVU, MRU

US at 1 month:
- abnormal: pelvis ≥ 10 mm, other malformation *, "extended criteria" → VCUS
- normal → Stop follow-up

* **US genitography**: in all patients with single kidney, MCDK, ectopic kidneys etc ...

b Postnatal imaging algorithm in severe foetal urinary tract dilatation

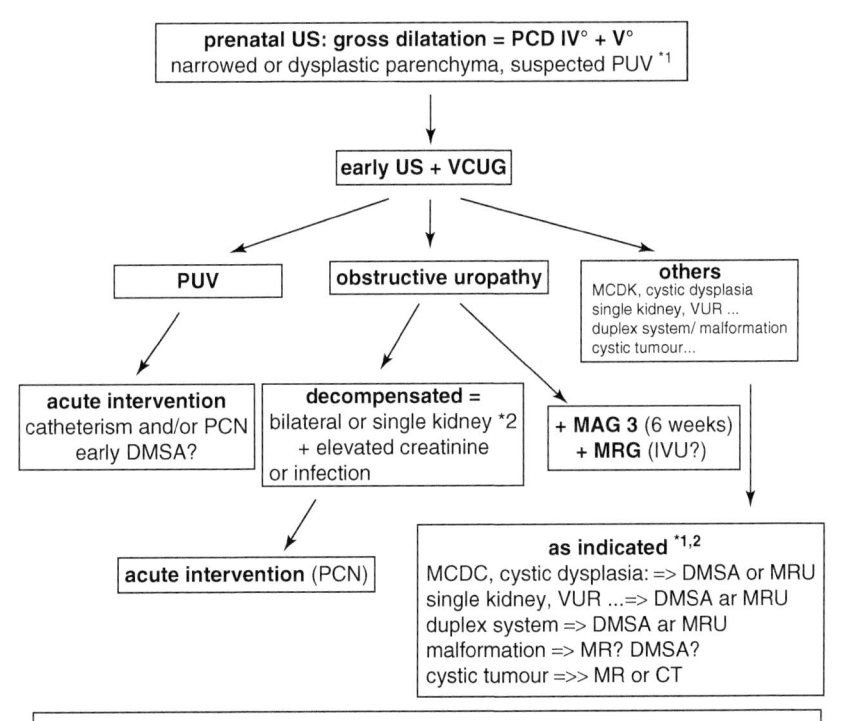

prenatal US: gross dilatation = PCD IV° + V°
narrowed or dysplastic parenchyma, suspected PUV [*1]

↓

early US + VCUG

- **PUV** → acute intervention: catheterism and/or PCN, early DMSA?
- **obstructive uropathy**
  - decompensated = bilateral or single kidney [*2] + elevated creatinine or infection → acute intervention (PCN)
  - + MAG 3 (6 weeks) + MRG (IVU?)
- **others**: MCDK, cystic dysplasia, single kidney, VUR ... duplex system/ malformation, cystic tumour...

as indicated [*1,2]
- MCDC, cystic dysplasia: => DMSA or MRU
- single kidney, VUR ...=> DMSA ar MRU
- duplex system => DMSA ar MRU
- malformation => MR? DMSA?
- cystic tumour =>> MR or CT

[*1] **ce-VUS**: can be considered in all girls with dilated ureters and gross PCD
[*2] **US genitography**: in all patients with single kidney, MCDK, ectopic kidneys etc ...

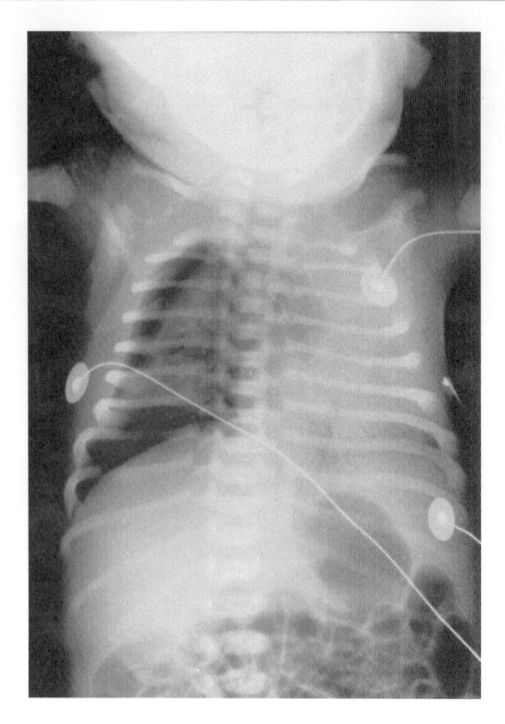

Fig. 1 Right pneumothorax and bilateral lung hypoplasia in a neonate with recessive-type polycystic kidney disease

imaging. Voiding cystourethrography (VCUG) looking for vesicoureteric reflux (VUR) and functional studies (scintigraphy, MRI) will be used afterward as required (Ismaili et al. 2006; Riccabona et al. 2008, 2009; Nguyen et al. 2014).

2.1 Clinical Situations and Antenatal Diagnoses Necessitating a Rapid Management

After birth, severe bilateral renal diseases (renal hypoplasia, posterior urethral valves, polycystic kidney diseases, etc.) can be associated with pneumothorax, lung hypoplasia, and life-threatening respiratory distress (Fig. 1). A respiratory assistance is mandatory even before considering any treatment for the urinary tract anomaly. Conversely, whenever a neonate presents massive – seemingly – spontaneous pneumothorax, an US examination should be performed in order to verify the status of the urinary tract.

Several other conditions could necessitate early management and workup in the immediate neonatal period. In posterior urethral valves (Fig. 2), the rapid placement of a bladder catheter (suprapubic or urethral) will help to decrease the high bladder pressure, before valve resection. An ectopic ureterocele associated with an obstructed upper pole of a duplex kidney is prone to prolapse into the urethra during micturition and to provoke acute bladder outlet obstruction (Fig. 3). Cystoscopic unroofing the ureterocele is therefore advocated as the first step in managing this type of duplex kidneys (Uphadhyay et al. 2002; Van Savage and Mesrobian 1995; Hagg et al. 2000) (Fig. 4). Markedly dilated urinary tract (giant pelvi-ureteric junction obstruction) may cause uncomfortable enlargement of the baby's abdomen and interfere with normal bowel transit, and then early nephrostomy or nephrectomy may become indicated (Fig. 5) (Shimada et al. 2007). Once all necessary therapeutic measures are taken, the work-up can restart more classically.

2.2 Postnatal Work-Up of Uropathies

As mentioned, the aims of postnatal work-up are to ascertain the diagnosis of the uropathy, determine the degree of "obstruction" and/or renal function impairment, as well as the presence of VUR.

For all uropathies, the workup has been markedly standardized. Nowadays, the major workload of an imaging department dealing with neonatal pathology is related to the management of antenatally diagnosed urinary tract dilatation and its significance. Noteworthy, the extensive neonatal workup performed in recent years by many teams has increased mainly the detection of neonatal VUR, with questionable impact on management in quite a few of these infants (Van Eeide et al. 2007; Ismaïli et al. 2006).

Two work-up approaches have been proposed. For some authors, whatever the result of a neonatal US, a VCUG should be performed in case of any antenatal urinary tract dilatation. For them,

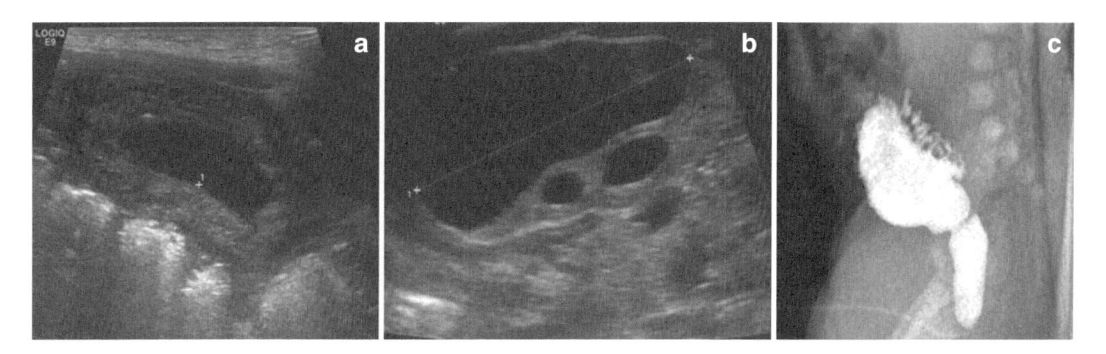

Fig. 2 Posterior urethral valves. (**a**) US of the bladder – sagittal scan of the bladder displaying a marked thickened well. (**b**) Left kidney – sagittal scan – dilated pyelocaly-ceal system and perirenal – urinoma (between the crosses). (**c**) VCU, micturition phase; typical appearance of PUV

Fig. 3 Ureterocele prolapse

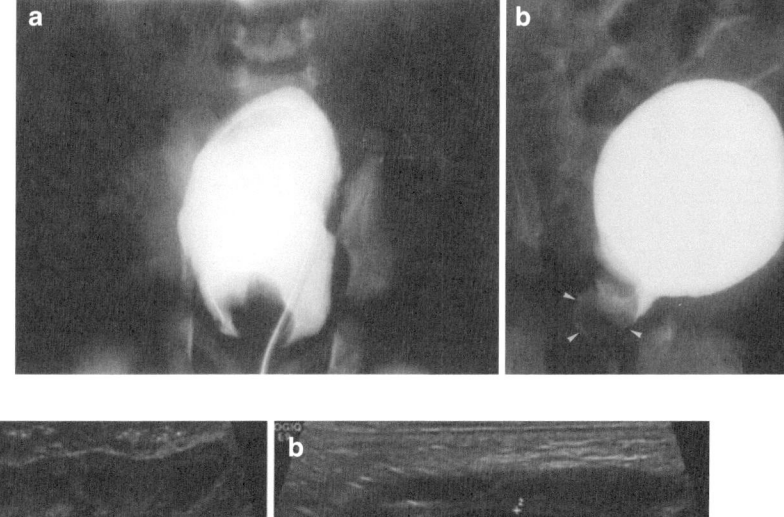

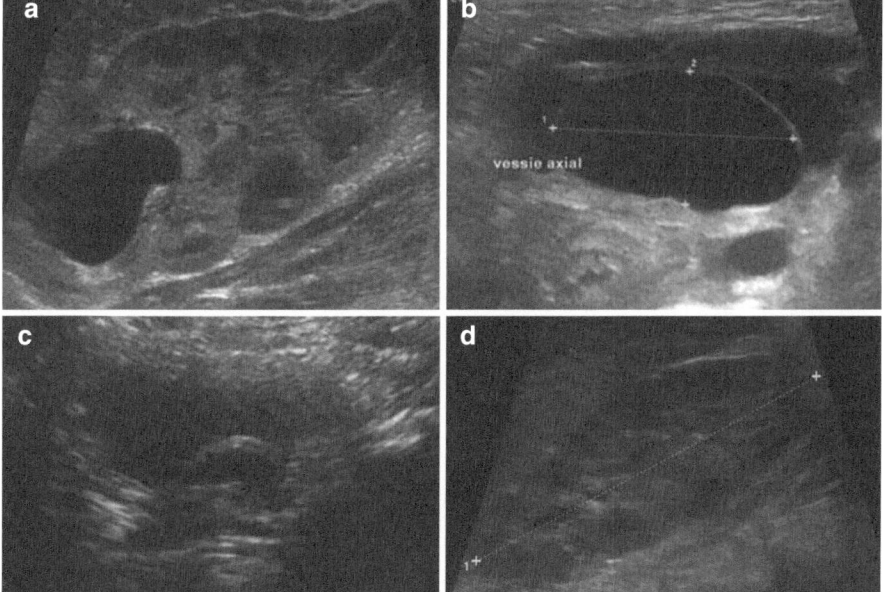

Fig. 4 Neonatal puncture of ureterocele. (**a**) Sagittal scan of the right kidney demonstrating dilatation of the upper pole. (**b**) Transverse scan of the bladder demonstrating a large ureterocele (limited by the crosses). (**c**)Transverse scan of the bladder after unroofing of the ureterocele. (**d**) Sagittal scan of the kidney, the dilatation has resolved

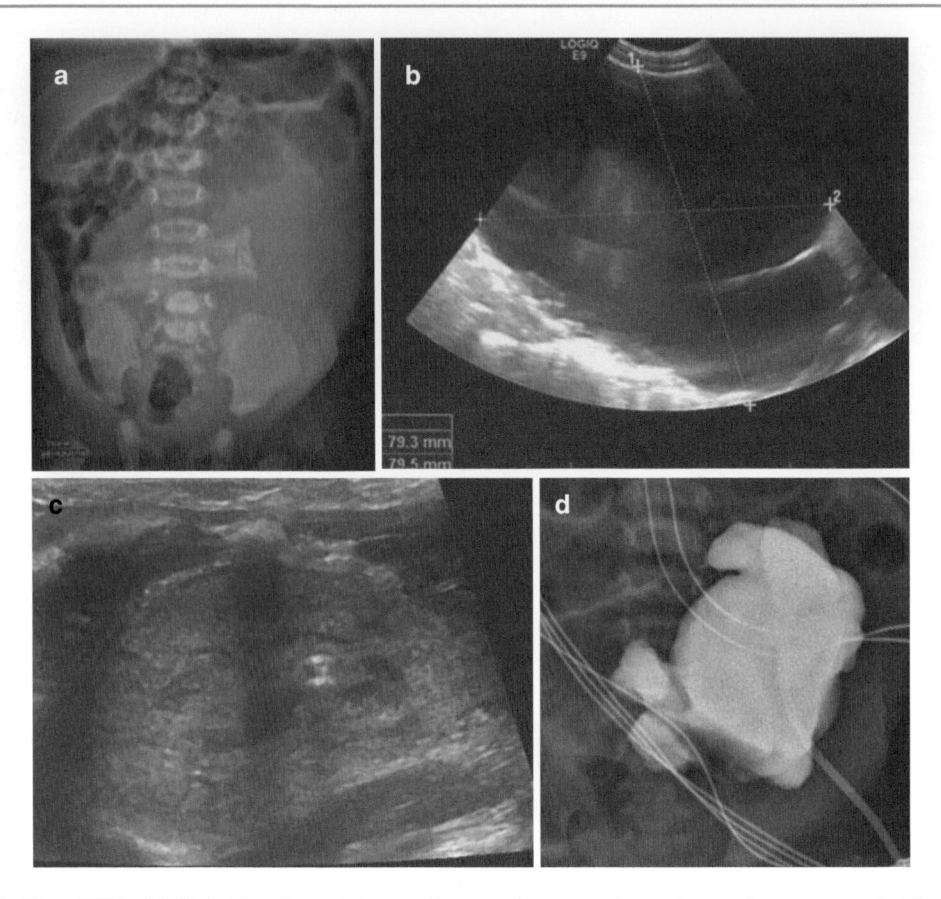

Fig. 5 Giant PUJO. (**a**) Plain film of the abdomen: the bowel is displaced to the right by the distended kidney. (**b**) US: marked dilatation of the left kidney; the limits are hard to define; there is no parenchyma visible. (**c**) US after nephrostomy, the renal parenchyma can now be identified. (**d**) Opacification of the pyelocalyceal system (it corresponded to the left part of a horseshoe kidney) confirming a UPJ obstruction

US is a poor predictor of VUR (Tibballs and De Bruyn 1996; Walsh and Dubbins 1996). For others, a VCUG should not be performed in all neonates; there will be too many unnecessary negative VCUGs. A VCUG should be performed only in those patients in whom the anomaly has been confirmed after birth (Yerkes et al. 1999). We favor the second approach and recommend a decision tree based on the neonatal and follow-up US findings (Riccabona et al. 2008, 2009) (Tables 2a and 2b). Hence, US is performed first in order to confirm the anomaly (Fig. 6) (Marra et al. 1994; Avni et al. 1997; Hulbert et al. 1992). In any urgent situation and in all cases where the dilatation is known to be marked, it can be performed as soon as the clinical condition permits. For all other cases, it should be delayed to the post physiological dehydration period, namely, after the fifth day of life. At that time, the US examination should be as detailed as possible in order to detect every anomaly that would justify continuing the work-up (Table 3). The presence of a urinary tract dilatation is the most important landmark; seven mm is the most widely accepted upper limit of normal (some prefer 5 mm, others 10 mm or even 12 mm) in the second and third trimester, respectively. Higher degrees of dilatation are associated with higher probability of a significant uropathy. Still, dilatation of the renal pelvis is not the only anomaly that should be looked for. Other US features can be associated with VUR or "obstruction" (Table 2b). One should not forget to examine the bladder; a large bladder with a thickened and trabeculated wall

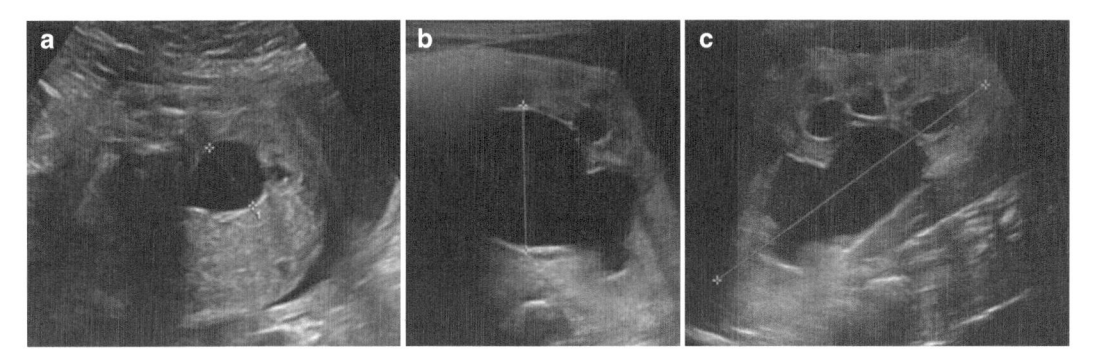

Fig. 6 Ante- and postnatal diagnosis of PUJ obstruction. (**a**) Transverse scan of a fetal abdomen (third trimester). The left pyelocalyceal system is dilated (20 mm between crosses). (**b, c**) Postnatal US ((**b**) transverse scan and (**c**) sagittal scan) confirming the dilatation

Table 3 US findings that may be associated with VUR

• Pelvic dilatation more than 7 mm
• Variable dilatation
• Calyceal dilatation
• Ureteral dilatation more than 3 mm
• Pelvic wall thickening
• Loss of CM differentiation
• Small kidney
• Signs of dysplasia
• Enlarged bladder

could be a sign of VUR (Fig. 7). With a meticulous US examination, one should be able to detect indirect signs for VUR in over 85% of cases. Those VURs that are missed are non-dilating or grade I–II VURs with less clinical significance (Nguyen et al. 2014; Pates and Dashe 2006; Weinberg and Yeung 1998; Ismaïli et al. 2004; Bouzada et al. 2004). Finally, particularly in baby boys, the comprehensive US study should include a perineal scan of the urethra during voiding – particularly if indirect signs suggest a possible posterior urethral valve.

If the initial US examination is entirely normal, it seems reasonable to perform follow-up examinations at 1 or 3 months in order to detect cases that would have escaped the neonatal screening (Riccabona et al. 2008, 2009) (Tables 2a and 2b).

In case of an abnormal US, a VCUG (or ce.-VUS) should be performed, preferably during the first weeks of life. The examination may be performed under prophylactic antibiotic therapy. The aim of the examination is to detect VUR and bladder or urethral anomalies.

If high-grade VUR is demonstrated, the patient is followed up clinically hoping that the VUR will resolve spontaneously. During this period of time, renal growth can be monitored every 3–6 months using US. The persistence of VUR should be verified if infections occur or in the absence of renal growth (Kousidis et al. 2008).

If no VUR is present, marked dilatation can be associated with urinary drainage impairment (possibly obstruction) at the level of the pelvi-ureteric junction, the ureterovesical junction, or below the bladder outlet. US will help to determine the level of obstruction. In some centers, the work-up will be completed by functional studies, including a furosemide nephrogram – especially in cases with severe dilatation (Morris et al. 2009) (see below).

2.3 Further Anatomical Assessment

If drainage impairment seems important and surgery may become indicated, the exact anatomy of the urinary tract must be assessed. Intravenous urography is no longer performed and MR urography is the best technique available to evaluate the anatomy of the urinary tract (Fig. 8). It will assess most precisely the anatomy of the dilated urinary tract (Avni et al. 2000; Darge et al. 2013). Furosemide is usually injected in order to increase diuresis and thus to optimize visualization of the

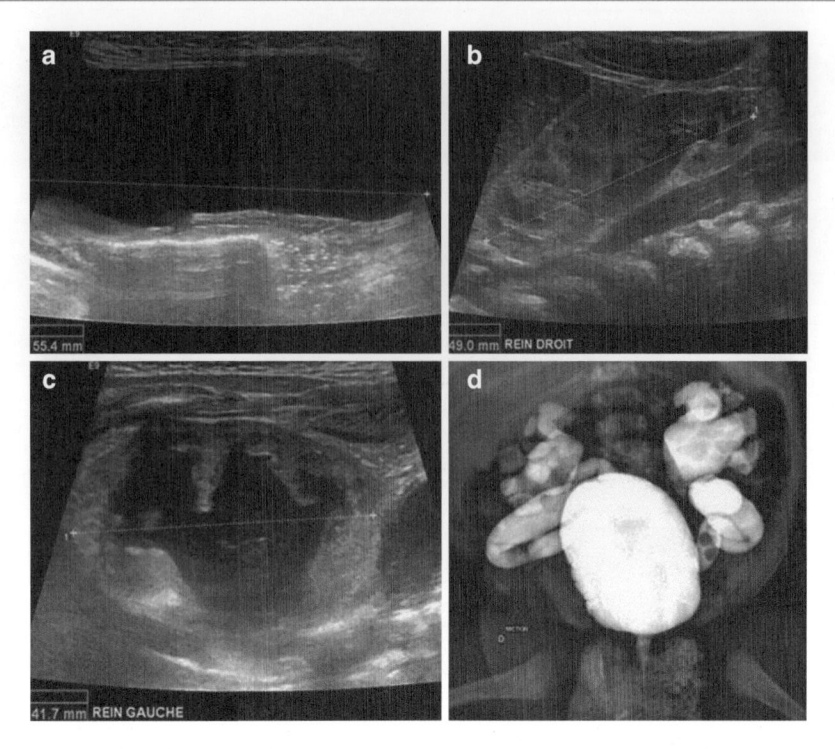

Fig. 7 Neonatal VUR (antenatal diagnosis of a megabladder). (**a**) Sagittal scan of the bladder appearing markedly enlarged. (**b**) Sagittal scan of the right kidney that appears slightly dilated (between crosses). (**c**) Sagittal scan of the left kidney that appears markedly dilated (between crosses). (**d**) VCUG demonstrating bilateral grade IV VUR

Fig. 8 Neonatal MR urography of a left megaureter (T2w sequence)

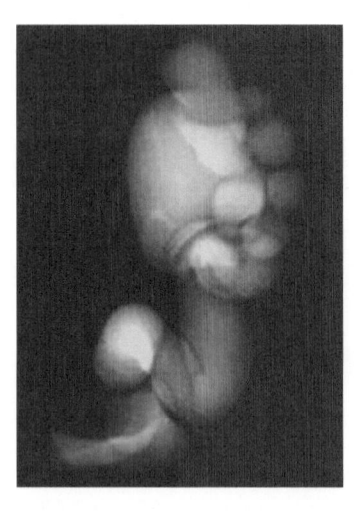

entire collecting and draining system. T2 sequences, inversion recovery sequences, and post-gadolinium enhancement 3D-T1 sequences allow a good evaluation of the entire urinary tract (see chapter "MR of the Urogenital Tract in Children"). The only drawback of the method is that it may require sedation and that it is not widely available.

In case of a duplex collecting system, the work-up is similar to that for obstruction, except that the morphological assessment must be more rapid since an early therapeutic maneuver may become necessary. Again US, VCUG/ce-VUS, and MR urography will optimally evaluate the exact morphology (Fig. 9). MR urography demonstrates accurately the extravesical insertion of an ectopic ureter (Avni et al. 2000; Adeb et al. 2013). An isotope study, using preferably Tc^{99m} MAG 3 or Tc^{99m} ECD, is also mandatory in order to evaluate the remaining function of the two moieties (Piepsz and Ham 2006; Adeb et al. 2013) (see below, and chapter "Nuclear Medicine").

Fig. 9 (**a, b**) MR imaging in complicated duplex kidney. (**a**)Left duplex with obstructed upper pole and ectopic infravesical insertion of the dilated ureter (*arrow*). (**b**) Left duplex with obstructed upper pole and ectopic ureterocele (*arrow*)

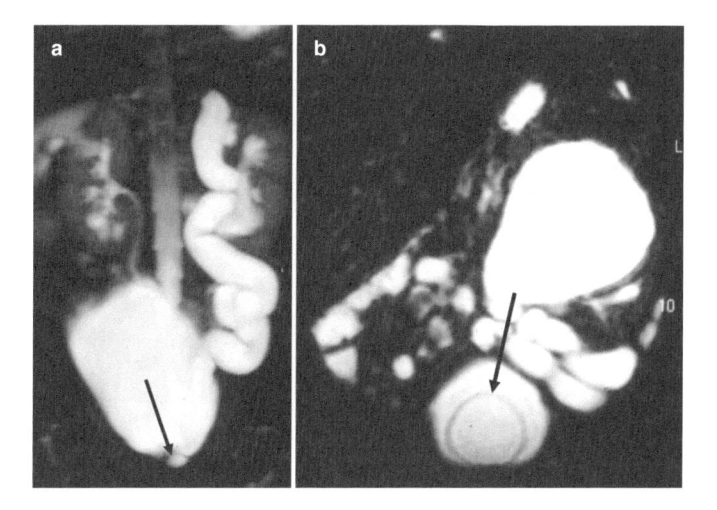

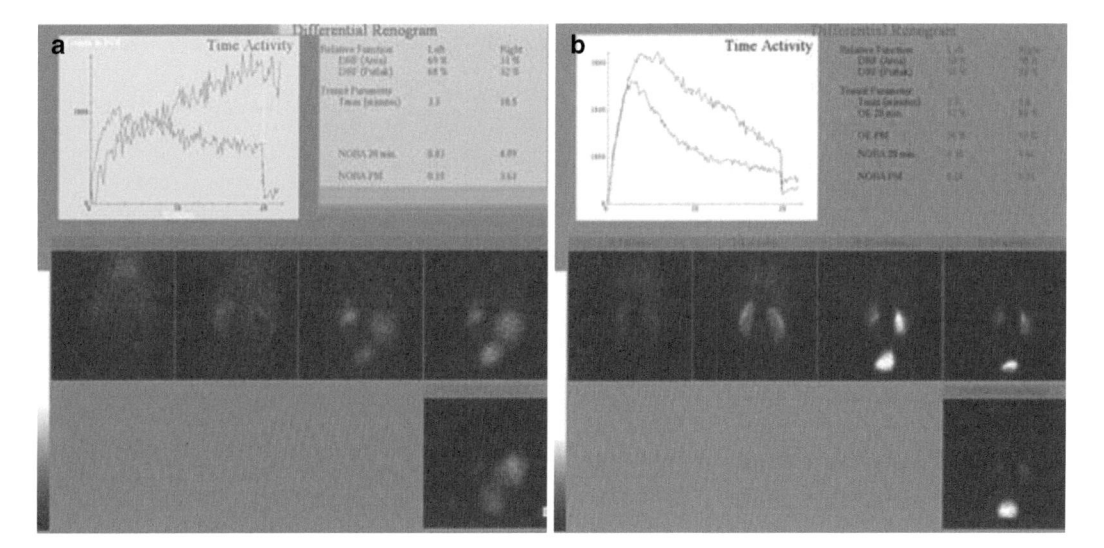

Fig. 10 1 "F0" diuretic renogram (Tc^{99m}-MAG3) of a 1-day-old boy. Antenatal diagnosis of bilateral hydronephrosis. (**a**) Important background activity related to low function (immaturity). Low right kidney DRF; severe impairment of right kidney drainage without emptying after micturition. Delayed cortical transit time. Impaired drainage of the left kidney with partial emptying after micturition. (**b**)Same child after right pyeloplasty at age 2 weeks: Low background activity (functional maturation). Normal DRF values. Normal drainage and complete renal emptying after micturition

2.4 Functional Assessment: Nuclear Medicine Studies

Radionuclide renogram may be performed starting at 4–6 weeks – ideally around 3–6 months – but in cases of severe dilatation, it may be performed as early as 3–4 days of age (Piepsz et al. 2009; Ismaili and Piepsz 2013). In very young infants, in case of impaired overall GFR or in case of important renal pelvic dilatation, the determination of the differential renal function (DRF) has a poor accuracy (Piepsz et al. 2009). In such situations, the aim will essentially be to roughly estimate the function and drainage impairment of the affected kidney (Piepsz et al. 2011) (Fig. 10). Tubular tracers (Tc^{99m} MAG 3 or Tc^{99m} ECD) are currently recommended, especially in young patients, because their high extraction rate allows accurate quantification of the renogram (Ismaili and Piepsz 2013; Piepsz et al. 2009; Gordon et al. 2001, 2011) (Fig. 10). The same radiopharmaceutical should be used for the follow-up studies (Piepsz et al. 2009). The radiation dose delivered is low, between 0.2 and 0.4 mSv (Stabin et al. 1992; Smith and Gordon 1998; Ismaili 2013). Determining DRF in infants is less precise than in older children; DRF are evaluated from the early phase of the renogram. Normal values are between 45 and 55 % (Gordon et al. 2011; Prigent et al. 1999; Eskild-Jensen et al. 2004). Drainage stimulation, using furosemide, is the procedure of choice to obtain information about renal drainage. Furosemide (1 mg/kg body weight, up to 20 mg) is often injected simultaneously with the radiopharmaceutical agent ("F0 protocol"), reducing the duration of the examination and the number of venous punctures (Piepsz et al. 2011); however, it needs sufficient renal maturity and functional capacity to be effective, as well as sufficient/physiological hydration for the study. A full bladder at the end of the renogram may result in a poor drainage; therefore, post-micturition images obtained in an erect position if possible are mandatory (Gordon et al. 2011; Piepsz et al. 2009, 2011; Ismaili and Piepsz 2013). The evaluation of renal drainage is essentially based upon output efficiency (OE) and normalized residual activity (NORA); these quantitative parameters do not depend on the level of the renal function. They are calculated at the end of the dynamic part of the renogram and on the late post-micturition post-erect images. Normal and abnormal values have been determined (Piepsz et al. 2002; Nogarède et al. 2010).

Evaluating the prognosis of these patients on the basis of the analysis of the DRF and drainage remains a challenge and is still controversial (Piepsz et al. 2009; Piepsz 2009; Gordon et al. 2011; Ismaili and Piepsz 2013). Normal drainage strongly suggests the absence of risk for functional deterioration (Piepsz 2009), but impaired drainage does not allow predicting the outcome if a conservative approach is chosen. Several recent studies strongly suggest the importance of the visual analysis of the cortical transit time of the tracer as a prognostic factor (Schlotmann et al. 2009; Piepsz 2011; Duong et al. 2013): severely delayed cortical transit time is associated with a high rate of improvement after surgery (Fig. 10). It also predicts functional deterioration in the absence of surgical treatment. However, a normal cortical transit does not exclude the risk of DRF deterioration.

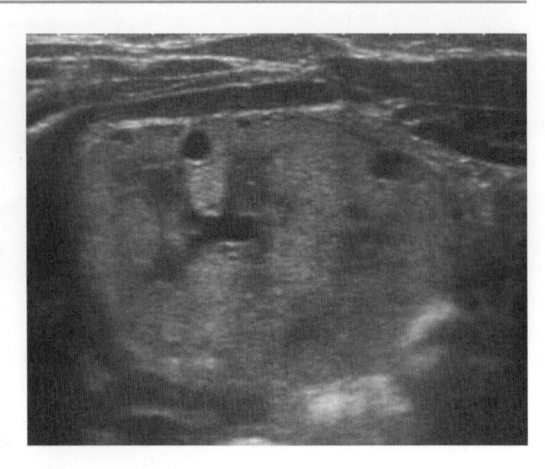

Fig. 11 Case of HNF1β mutation (hyperechoic kidneys in utero) sagittal scan of the right kidney. It appears hyperechoic with small subcortical cysts that were not seen in utero

2.5 The Postnatal Work-Up of Nephropathies

The group of nephropathies with antenatal diagnosis encompasses a large spectrum of diseases with variable degree of renal functional impairment. The largest group includes renal cystic diseases (see chapters "Renal Agenesis, Dysplasia, Hypoplasia and Cystic Diseases of the Kidney" and "Imaging in Renal Agenesis, Dysplasia, Hypoplasia and Cystic Diseases of the Kidney"). The renal involvement will be confirmed by postnatal US. The presence of small cysts is sometimes easier to detect after birth than in utero, and this will help to precise the diagnosis (Fig. 11). US will also be helpful to detect associated malformations especially those occurring in the genital tract, the liver, and the pancreas. The rest of the work-up will mainly be focused on clinical, biological, and genetic data that must be evaluated in order to characterize the diseases or syndromes (Avni et al 2006, 2012). US will be used during childhood in order to follow the renal growth and eventually changing US patterns with time (Fig. 12.).

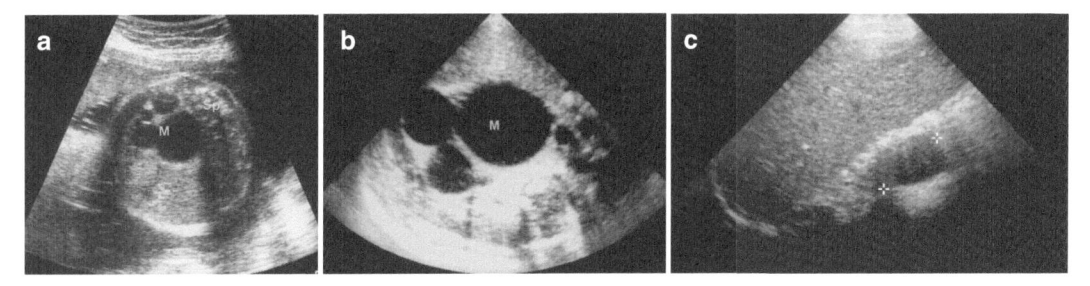

Fig. 12 Spontaneous involution of a multicystic dysplastic kidney. (**a**) In utero at 34 weeks, transverse scan of the fetal abdomen. Typical right multicystic kidney (*M*); *Sp*, spine. (**b**) At birth transverse scan of the right kidney: same appearance of the mass (*M*) as in utero. (**c**) At the age of 2 years, sagittal scan of the right kidney: only one small cyst remains (*between the crosses*)

> **Take away**
> The postnatal work-up of urinary tract anomalies has now been standardized, US being the cornerstone. Depending on the result, VCUG (or ce-VUS), MRI, and/or isotopes will be performed in order to clarify the diagnosis and choose the proper treatment.

For multicystic dysplastic kidney, renal ectopia, or unilateral agenesis, the work-up should also include US and a VCUG, if US is abnormal (see above) in order to detect ipsi- or contralateral VUR. Again, high-grade VURs might require prophylactic antibiotic therapy (Atiyeh et al. 1993; Flack and Bellinger 1993; Selzman and Elder 1995; Ismaïli et al 2005). Also of interest is to search for associated genital anomalies on pelvic US (Tables 2a and 2b).

3 Long-Term Follow-Up and (Potential Treatment) in the Light of the Natural History of Uro-nephropathies

As mentioned above, antenatal diagnosis has led to dramatic changes in the management of uropathies. First, nowadays, most patients are asymptomatic; second, the medical follow-up of many pathologies confirms their potential to resolve spontaneously. Consequently, surgery has been less and less advocated. The main goal of the prophylactic treatment (if applied) is to prevent further renal damage during the period when spontaneous resolution is expected. It should be noted that infection does occur in some cases despite the prophylactic antibiotic therapy; these cases make alternative treatment necessary (Jaswon et al. 1999; Ismaïli et al. 2006; Lee et al. 2006).

3.1 Vesicoureteric Reflux

Many series have shown that two-thirds of neonatal VURs (mainly grades I-III) are likely to resolve or at least to improve during an observation period of 2 years (Fig. 13). Therefore, once the anomaly is detected, the patient is given prophylactic antibiotic therapy (in cases of high-grade VUR) and followed clinically or by imaging as described above. In some circumstances, another therapeutic approach (surgery or endoscopic injection of bulging agents) should be proposed: in the case of breakthrough infection despite therapy, if there is failure to thrive, or if continuing the treatment is problematic for the family (Herndon et al. 1999; Burge et al. 1992; Bouachrine et al. 1996; Assael et al. 1998; Ismaïli et al. 2006; Van Eeide et al. 2007) (see chapters "UTI and VUR" and "Vesicoureteric Reflux").

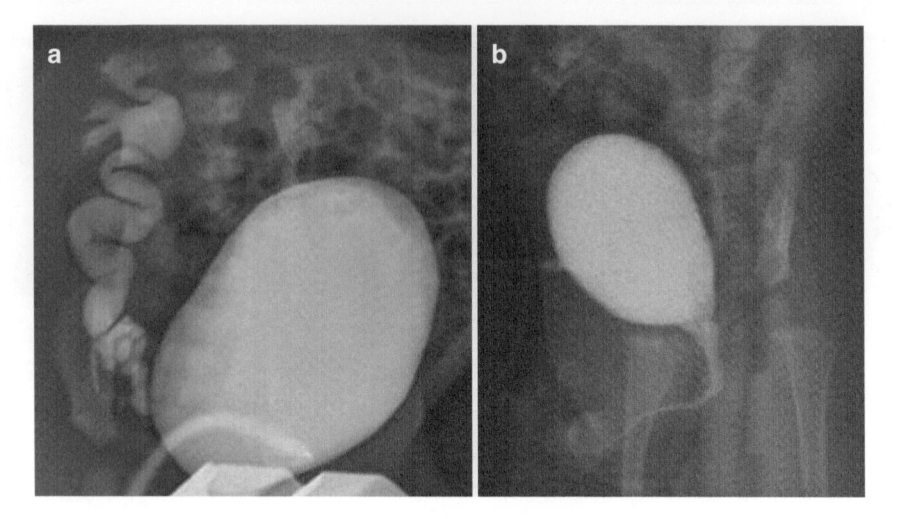

Fig. 13 Spontaneous resolution of VUR. (**a**) At birth, bilateral grade IV VUR. (**b**) At age 10 month, no VUR anymore

Fig. 14 Partial resolution of left UPJ obstruction. Transverse scan of the left kidney. (**a**) At birth, dilated pyelocalyceal system. Renal pelvis measures 27 mm. (**b**) At age 6 months, the renal pelvic dilatation has diminished to 7 mm

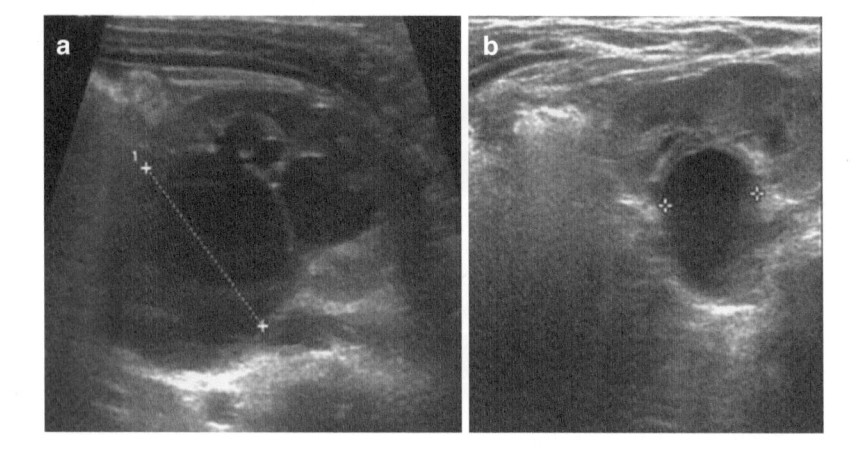

3.2 Pelvi-ureteric Junction (PUJ) Obstruction

The therapeutic management of PUJ obstruction has been even more controversial than for VUR. Advocates and opponents of neonatal surgery have published large amounts of scientific material that shows opposite or contradictory results. For some, early surgery is safe and improves renal function notably. For others, the PUJ obstruction has been present for a long time, and there is only a faint chance of improving the condition by surgery, especially since the dilatation itself may resolve spontaneously (Fig. 14). Others suggest operating only those patients who would show functional deterioration. Finally, some suggest following renal growth on US and operating when the contralateral kidney displays compensatory growth.

On the basis of all the data accumulated, conservative management seems the most adequate in mild or moderate cases. Clinical status, renal anomalies, and renal function must be monitored closely. Regular US examinations should be performed (every 6 months, during the first 2 years; every year later – possibly with standardized and comparable hydration). In most cases, the dilatation will be stable or even resolve. Surgery must be proposed if clinical symptoms appear or if renal function and/or cortical transit deteriorate. In rare and severe cases, spontaneous resolution is less likely to occur and symptoms related to abdominal discomfort are more frequent. For such patients, surgery may be beneficial even

Fig. 15 Resolution of left megaureter, sagittal scan of the bladder. (**a**) At birth, the dilated left ureter measures 14 mm diameter. (**b**) At age 1 year, the ureter measures 7 mm

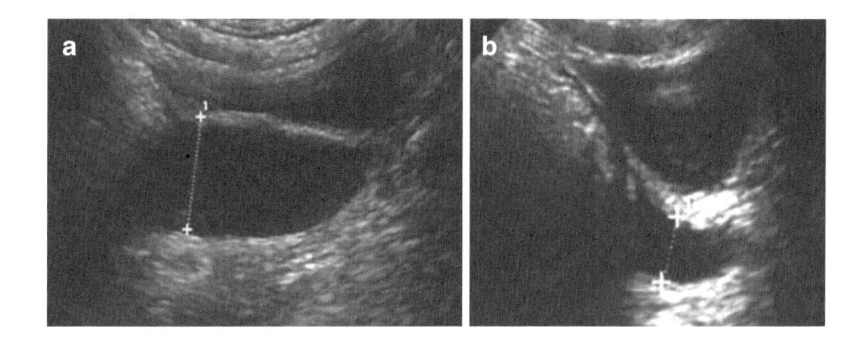

without other signs of deterioration (Docimo and Silver 1997; Duckett 1993; Capolicchio et al. 1999; McAleer and Kaplan 1999; Chertin et al 1999; Salem et al. 1995; Thorup et al. 2003).

3.3 Ureterovesical Junction (UVJ) Obstruction

Like VUR, UVJ obstruction has shown great potential for spontaneous resolution, probably because of the maturation of the UVJ (Fig. 15). Therefore, after completion of the initial work-up, a prophylactic antibiotic therapy should be started and the urinary tract monitored by US (possibly with standardized and comparable hydration and bladder filling) and eventually functional isotope studies (or fMRU). US may underestimate the drainage impairment, especially since the renal pelvis may not be dilated. Therefore, before confirming complete resolution or before surgery particularly in a more complex anatomy, morphological assessment of the urinary tract may be necessary – best achieved by MR urography (Baskin et al. 1994; Liu et al. 1994; Shukla et al. 2005).

3.4 Multicystic Dysplastic Kidney (MCDK)

Once the diagnosis of a MCDK appears highly probable (on the basis of the neonatal US examination and on the lack of function demonstrated by nuclear medicine studies or MRI), a clinical and imaging (US) follow-up is the most widely accepted approach. In two-thirds of cases, a MCDK diagnosed in utero will involute spontaneously within the first 2 years of life; the involution may already start in utero (Fig. 12). Complications are very unusual. Only very large MCDKs causing abdominal discomfort and without resolution on follow-up examinations will require surgical removal (Hrair-Georges et al. 1993; Rabelo et al. 2006; Aslam and Watson 2006).

3.5 Complicated Duplex Kidneys

In case of complicated duplex collecting systems, one of the aims of imaging will be to differentiate between an ectopic ureteral insertion and an ectopic ureterocele. An extravesical ectopic ureter insertion with a functional upper renal pole will lead to the reimplantation of the ureter (with or without modeling) in the bladder or its anastomosis into the lower renal pole ureter. A nonfunctioning upper pole with an extravesical ectopic ureter will bring us to an upper pole heminephrectomy and ureterectomy by lomboscopy in case of significant renal pelvis dilatation or infection. An extravesical or an obstructive ureterocele will be punctured or unroofed by cystoscopy before the child is discharged from the maternity hospital (Fig. 4). In case of a pyelonephritis, depending of the renal moieties function and/or if there is a VUR, an upper or lower heminephrectomy with ureterectomy will be proposed or the removal of the ureterocele and the reimplantation of both ureters (Uphadhyay et al. 2002; Husman et al. 1999; Blyth et al. 1993).

3.6 Nephropathies

Congenital nephropathies will be managed individually; the work-up and follow-up are tailored case-by-case and will depend upon the clinical

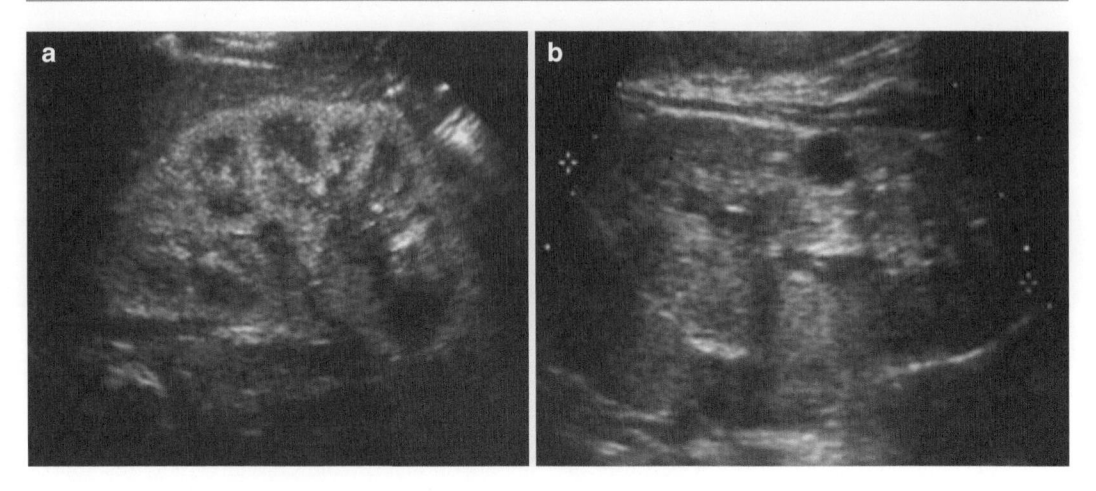

Fig. 16 Evolution of ADPKD. US of the right kidney. (**a**) At birth. (**b**) At age 5 years, first cysts are visible

presentation. Some patients will have signs of renal failure directly at birth, while for others the renal failure will develop progressively later in childhood or even only during adult life. Some patients will display only renal symptoms; for others, other organs and systems may be involved (the brain, pancreas, liver, etc.). For the latter, complementary examinations will be necessary (MRI, CT, etc.).

In most cases, US will be sufficient for the follow-up (Fig. 16). Still, imaging will have to be adapted to the type and degree of the anomaly (Avni et al. 2006, 2012).

> **Take away**
> US is the main imaging technique that will be used for diagnosis and the follow-up of all uro-nephropathies. Depending on clinical and biological data, the management will be adapted. If necessary, MRI and isotopes will be used to provide anatomical and functional information.

Conclusions

US is the cornerstone of the work-up of congenital uropathies at birth and during follow-up. The use of other techniques will depend on the US findings at birth. MR imaging and isotopes will help to determine the anatomy and the function of the urinary tract. Apart from acute conditions requiring immediate treatment, the therapeutic approach to congenital uropathies is less and less surgical. Prophylactic antibiotic therapy may be initiated at birth in severely dilated cases.

References

Adeb M, Daye K, Dihlman JR et al (2013) MR urography in evaluation of duplicated renal collecting systems. MRI Clin N Amer 21:717–730

Aslam M, Watson AR (2006) Unilateral MDK: long-term outcomes. Arch Dis Child 91:820–823

Assael BM, Guez S, Marra E et al (1998) Congenital reflux nephropathy: a follow-up of 108 cases diagnosed perinatally. Br J Urol 82:252–257

Atiyeh B, Husmann D, Baum M (1993) Contralateral renal abnormalities in patients with renal agenesis and non-cystic renal dysplasia. Pediatrics 91:812–815

Avni EF, Ayadi K, Rypens F et al (1997) Can careful ultrasound examination of the urinary tract exclude vesicoureteric reflux in the neonate. Br J Radiol 70:977–982

Avni EF, Bali MA, Regnault M et al (2000) MR urography in children. Eur Radiol 43:154–166

Avni EF, Garel L, Cassart M et al (2006) Perinatal assessment of hereditary cystic renal diseases. Pediatr Radiol 36:405–416

Avni FE, Garel C, Cassart M et al (2012) Imaging and classification of congenital cystic renal diseases. AJR Am J Roentgenol 198:1004–1013

Barbosa JA, Chow J, Benson CB et al (2012) Postnatal longitudinal evaluation of children diagnosed with prenatal hydronephrosis. Prenat Diagn 32:1242–1249

Baskin LS, Zderic SA, Snyder HM et al (1994) Primary dilated megaureter long-term follow-up. J Urol 152:618–621

Blyth B, Passerini Glazel G, Camuffo C et al (1993) Endoscopic incision of ureteroceles intravesical versus ectopic. J Urol 149:556–560

Bouachrine H, Lemelle JL, Didier F et al (1996) A follow-up study of pre-natally detected primary VUR: a review of 61 patients. Br J Urol 78:936–939

Bouzada MCF, Oliveira FA, Pereira AK et al (2004) Diagnostic accuracy of postnatal pelvic diameter as a predictor of uropathy. Pediatr Radiol 34:798–804

Burge DM, Griffiths MD, Malone PG et al (1992) Fetal VUR outcome following conservative management. J Urol 148:1743–1745

Capolicchio G, Leonard MP, Wong C et al (1999) Prenatal diagnosis of hydronephrosis: impact on renal function. J Urol 162:1029–1032

Chertin B, Fridman A, Knizhnik M et al (1999) Does early detection of UPJ obstruction improve surgical outcome? J Urol 162:1037–1040

Darge K, Higgins H, Hway TJ et al (2013) MR and CT in pediatric urology. Radiol Clin N Am 51:583–598

Docimo SG, Silver RI (1997) Renal ultrasonography in newborns with prenatally detected hydronephrosis: why wait? J Urol 157:1387–1389

Duckett JW (1993) When to operate on neonatal hydronephrosis. Urology 42:617–619

Duong HP, Piepsz A, Collier F et al (2013) Predicting the clinical outcome of antenatally detected unilateral pelviureteric junction stenosis. Urology 82:691–696

Ek S, Lindefeldt KJ, Vanicio L et al (2007) Fetal hydronephrosis: prevalence, natural history and postnatal consequences in an unselected population. Acta Obstet Gynecol 86:1463–1466

Eskild-Jensen A, Gordon I, Piepsz A et al (2004) Interpretation of the renogram : problems and pitfalls in hydronephrosis in children. BJU Int 94: 887–892

Flack CE, Bellinger MF (1993) The multicystic dysplastic kidney and contralateral vesicoureteral reflux protection of the solitary kidney. J Urol 150:1873–1874

Gordon I, Colarinha P, Piepz A et al (2001) Guidelines for standard and diuretic renography in children. Eur J Nucl Med 28:BP21–BP30

Gordon I, Piepsz A, Sixt R (2011) Guidelines for standard and diuretic renogram in children. Eur J Nucl Med Mol Imaging 38:1175–1188

Hagg MJ, Mourachov PV, Snyder HM et al (2000) The modern endoscopic approach to ureterocele. J Urol 163:940–943

Herndon CDA, McKenna PH, Kolon TF et al (1999) A multicenter outcomes analysis of patients with neonatal reflux presenting with prenatal hydronephrosis. J Urol 162:1203–1208

Hrair-Georges JM, Rushton HG, Bulas D (1993) Unilateral agenesis may result from in utero regression of MDK. J Urol 150:793–794

Hulbert WC, Rosenberg HK, Cartwright PC et al (1992) The predictive value of ultrasonography in evaluation of infants with posterior urethral valves. J Urol 148:122–124

Husman D, Strand B, Ewalt D et al (1999) Management of ectopic ureterocele associated with renal duplication. J Urol 162:1406–1409

Ismaïli K, Avni FE, Wissing JK et al (2004) Long term outcome of infants with mild and moderate fetal pyelectasis: validation of neonatal US as a screening tool to detect significant nephro-uropathy. J Pediatr 144:759–765

Ismaïli K, Avni FE, Alexander M et al (2005) Routine VCUG is of no value in neonates with unilateral MDK. J Pediatr 146:759–763

Ismaïli K, Hall M, Piefz A et al (2006) Primary VUR detected in neonates with a history of fetal renal pelvis dilatation. J Pediatr 148:222–227

Ismaili K, Piepsz A (2013) The antenatal detected pelviureteric junction stenosis: advances in renography and strategy of management. Pediatr Radiol 43:428–435

Jaswon MS, Dibble L, Puri S et al (1999) Prospective study of outcome in antenatally diagnosed renal pelvis dilatation. Arch Dis Child Fetal Neonatal Ed 80:F135–F138

Kousidis G, Thomas DFM, Morgan H, Haider N et al (2008) The long term follow-up of prenatally detected PUV: a 10 to 23 year follow-up study. BJU Int 102:1020–1024

Kumar S, Walla S, Ikpene O (2012) Post natal outcome of prenatally diagnosed renal pelvic dilatation. Prenat Diagn 32:519–522

Lee RS, Cendron M, Kinnamon DD et al (2006) Antenatal hydronephrosis as a predictor of postnatal outcomes: a meta-analysis. Pediatrics 118:586–593

Liu HYA, Dhillon HK, Yeung CK et al (1994) Clinical outcome of prenatally diagnosed primary megaureters. J Urol 152:614–617

Marra G, Barbieri G, Dell'Agnola CA et al (1994) Congenital renal damage associated with primary vesicoureteral reflux detected prenatally in male infants. J Pediatr 124:726–730

McAleer IM, Kaplan GW (1999) Renal function before and after pyeloplasty: does it improve? J Urol 162:1041–1044

Morris RK, Malin GL, Khan KS, Kitty MD (2009) Antenatal US to predict post natal renal function in congenital lower urinary tract obstruction: systematic review of test accuracy. BJOG 116:1290–1299

Nogarède C, Tondeur M, Piepsz A (2010) Normalized residual activity and output efficiency in case of early furosemide injection in children. Nucl Med Commun 31:355–358

Nguyen HT, Herndon CDA, Cooper C, Gatti J, Kirsch A, Kokorowski P et al (2014) The Society for fetal urology consensus statement on the evaluation and management of antenatal hydronephrosis. J Pediatr Urol 6:212–231

Pates JA, Dashe JS (2006) Prenatal diagnosis and management of hydronephrosis. Early Hum Dev 82:3–8

Piepsz A, Kuyvenhoven J, Tondeur HH (2002) Normalized residual activity: usual values and robustness of the method. J Nucl Med 43:33–38

Piepsz A, Ham HR (2006) Pediatric applications of renal nuclear medicine. Semin Nucl Med 36:16–35

Piepsz A (2011) Antenatal detection of pelviureteric junction stenosis : main controversies. Semin Nucl Med 41:11–19

Piepsz A, Tondeur M, Nogarède C et al (2011) Can severely impaired cortical transit predict which children with pelvi-ureteric junction stenosis detected antenatally might benefit from pyeloplasty ? Nucl Med Commun 32:199–205

Piepsz A, Gordon I, Brock J 3rd et al (2009) Round table on the management of renal pelvic dilatation in children. J Pediatr Urol 5:437–444

Piepsz A (2009). The predictive value of the renogram. Eur J Nucl Med Mol Imaging 36:1661–1664

Prigent A, Cosgriff P, Gates GF et al (1999) Consensus report on quality control of quantitative measurements of renal function obtained from renogram : International Consensus Committee for the Scientific Committee of Radionuclides in Nephrourology. Semin Nucl Med 29:146–159

Quirino IG, Diniz JSS, Bouazada MCF et al (2012) Clinical course of 822 children with prenatally detected nephron-uropathies. Clin J Amer Soc Nephrol 17:444–451

Rabelo EAS, Oliveira EA, Silva JMP et al (2006) US progression of prenatally detected MDK. Urology 68: 1098–1112

Renkema KY, Winyard PJ, Skovorodkin IN et al (2011) Novel perspectives for investigating CAKUT. Nephrol Dial Transplant 26:3843–3851

Riccabona M, Avni FE, Blickman JG, Dacher JN, Darge K, Lobo ML, Willi UV (2008) Imaging recommendations in paediatric uroradiology: minutes of the ESPR workgroup session on urinary tract infection, fetal hydronephrosis, urinary tract US and voiding cystourethrography. Pediatr Radiol 38: 138–145

Riccabona M, Avni EF, Blickman JG et al (2009) Imaging recommendations in paediatric uroradiology. Minutes of the ESPR uroradiology task force session on childhood obstructive uropathy, high-grade fetal hydronephrosis, childhood haematuria, and urolithiasis in childhood. ESPR Annual Congress, Edinburgh, UK, June 2008. Pediatr Radiol 39:891–898

Salem YH, Majd M, Rushton HG (1995) Outcome analysis of pediatric pyeloplasty as a function of patient age presentation and differential renal function. J Urol 154:1889–1893

Schlotmann A, Clorius J, Clorius SN (2009) Diuretic renography in hydronephrosis: renal tissue tracer predicts functional course and thereby need for surgery. Eur J Nucl Med Mol Imaging 36:1665–1673

Selzman AA, Elder JS (1995) Contralateral vesicoureteral reflux in children with a multicystic kidney. J Urol 153:1252–1254

Shimada K, Matsumoto F, Kawagoe M, Matsui F (2007) Urological emergency in neonates with congenital hydronephrosis. Int J Urol 14:388–392

Shukla AR, Cooper J, Paytel RK, Carr MC, Canning DA, Zderic SA, Snyder HM (2005) Prenatally detected primary megaureter: a role for extended follow-up. J Urol 173:1353–1356

Smith T, Gordon I (1998) An update of radiopharmaceutical schedules in children. Nucl Med Commun 19:1023–1036

Stabin M, Taylor A Jr, Eshima D et al (1992) Radiation Dosimetry for technetium-99m-MAG3, technetium-99m-DTPA, and iodine-131-OIH based on human biodistribution studies. J Nucl Med 33:33–40

Thorup J, Jokela R, Cortes D, Nielsen OH (2003) The results of 15-years of consistent strategy in treating antenatally suspected PUJ obstruction. BJU Int 91:850–852

Tibballs JM, De Bruyn R (1996) Primary vesicoureteric reflux: how useful is postnatal ultrasound? Arch Dis Child 75:444–447

Uphadhyay J, Bolduc S, Braga L, Fahrat W et al (2002) Impact of prenatal diagnosis on the morbidity associated with ureterocele management. J Urol 167:2560–2565

Van Savage JG, Mesrobian HG (1995) The impact of prenatal US on the morbidity and outcome of patients with renal duplication abnormalities. J Urol 153:768–770

Van Eeide AM, Hentgent MH, de Jond TPVM et al (2007) VUR in children with prenatally detected hydronephrosis. Ultrasound Obstet Gynecol 29:463–469

Walsh G, Dubbins PA (1996) Antenatal renal pelvis dilatation: a predictor of vesicoureteral reflux? AJR 167:897–900

Weinberg B, Yeung N (1998) US sign of intermittent dilatation of the renal collecting system in ten patients with VUR. J Clin Ultrasound 26:65–68

Wiesel A, Queisser-Luft A, Clementi M, Bianca S, Stoll C (2005) Prenatal detection of congenital renal malformations by fetal ultrasonographic examination: an analysis of 709,030 births in 12 Europeans countries. Eur J Med Genetics 48:131–144

Wollenberg A, Neuhaus T, Willi UV, Wisser J (2005) Outcome of fetal renal dilatation diagnosed during the third trimester. Ultrasound Obstet Gynecol 25: 483–488

Yerkes EB, Adams MC, Pope JC et al (1999) Does every patient with prenatal hydronephrosis need voiding cystourethrography. J Urol 162:1218–1220

Imaging in Prune Belly Syndrome and Other Syndromes Affecting the Urogenital Tract

Gundula Staatz and Wolfgang Rascher

Contents

1 Introduction 481
2 Pathology 482
3 Pathogenesis 483
3.1 A Primary Defect in Mesoderm Formation 483
3.2 A Primary Defect Leading to Urethral Obstruction 484
4 **Clinical Presentation and Diagnosis** 484
4.1 Obstetric Ultrasound and Antenatal Diagnosis 484
4.2 Postnatal Diagnostic Approach 485
5 **Management** 487
6 **Other Syndromes Associated with Urinary Tract Malformations** 488
References 489

G. Staatz, MD (✉)
Department of Radiology, Section of Pediatric Radiology, Medical Center of the Johannes Gutenberg University, Mainz, Germany
e-mail: gundula.staatz@unimedizin-mainz.de

W. Rascher, MD
Kinder- und Jugendklinik, Universitätsklinikum Erlangen, Loschgestrasse 15, 91054 Erlangen, Germany

1 Introduction

The absence of the abdominal musculature, urinary tract dilatation, and bilateral undescended testis is known as prune belly syndrome (PBS) (Eagle and Barrett 1950; Greskovich and Nyberg 1988; Williams 1982). The classical syndrome is also known as triad syndrome, Eagle-Barrett syndrome, or abdominal muscular deficiency syndrome. There is a broad spectrum of malformations with severe dilatation of the urinary tract as a consequence of aplasia of the musculature. The pathogenetic mechanism is different from that of dilatation as a consequence of supra- or infravesical obstruction. Some patients with prune belly syndrome have a real obstruction, such as urethral aplasia with oligohydramnios syndrome. The prognosis of the malformations depends upon the degree of renal dysplasia (Rohrmann and Duckett 2011). There is no consensus as to the pathogenesis of this complex abnormality, although most investigators consider prune belly syndrome a distinct entity.

Unfortunately, the term prune belly syndrome is inconsistently used in the literature. The incomplete form of the syndrome has been occasionally described as pseudo-prune belly syndrome (Bellah et al. 1996). However, the term pseudo-prune belly syndrome in patients with massive, prune belly-like dilatation of the urinary tract but normal abdominal wall examination and incomplete cryptorchidism or normal testes is confusing and should be avoided. Furthermore, diagnosis of severe urinary tract anomalies with oligohydramnios by prenatal ultrasound often results in termination of pregnancies (Hoshino et al. 1998). In these cases the typical pathology of prune belly syndrome has not always been demonstrated sufficiently.

More than 100 years ago, Parker (1895) reported on a male newborn infant with a parchment-thin and flaccid abdominal wall with marked underdevelopment of both the oblique and transverse abdominal muscles and a marked hypertrophy of the bladder with dilatation of the ureters and renal pelves. Obstructing urethral lesions were absent and the testes were undescended. Osler (1901) described a similar pathology in a 6-year-old child and likened the appearance of the abdominal wall to a wrinkled prune. The persistent use of this metaphor led to the unfortunate term prune belly syndrome for patients with this abnormality.

Eagle and Barrett (1950) reported urethral obstruction in five out of nine cases, and surgeons began to try correction of urologic abnormalities. Through the 1970s urologists experimented with detailed reconstruction of the enlarged urinary collecting system, the abdominal wall, and the undescended testes. Poor results and the lack of evidence of intrinsic urinary tract obstruction in many cases favored a more conservative approach. Up to now results have not demonstrated an obvious benefit for either method.

2 Pathology

The incidence of prune belly syndrome is 1 out of 40,000 live births with a male predominance of 97%. By definition affected females cannot have the complete triad, and the urologic manifestations may often be less severe. In females, anomalies of the urethra, uterus, and vagina are usually present (Reinberg et al. 1991). Most cases occur sporadically, although familial occurrence has been described (Ramasamy et al. 2005). In selected cases, an association with trisomies 13, 18, and 21 has been reported.

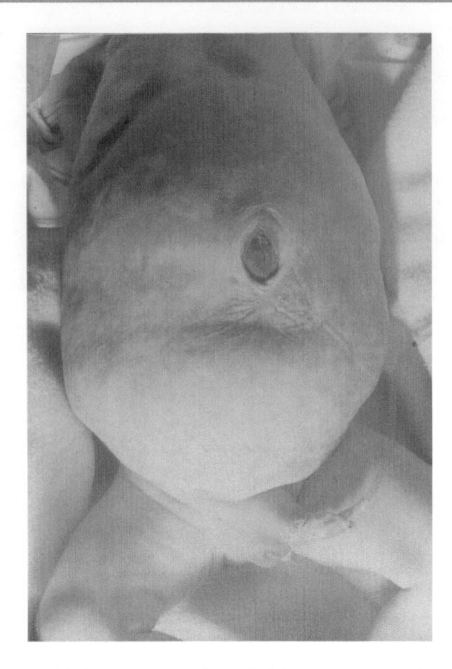

Fig. 1 Clinical presentation of abdominal muscular deficiency syndrome (prune belly syndrome)

The appearance of the abdominal wall is caused by a muscular deficiency (Fig. 1). In severe cases, muscle fibers are absent and replaced by a thick collagenous material. In many, but not all cases, the abdominal wall is simply a cosmetic problem. Urinary tract pathology is highly variable with ureteric dilatation, megacystis, and dilatation of the prostatic urethra. The anterior urethra may be dilated, resulting in a megalourethra, and the prostate is hypoplastic. A urethral stenosis or atresia is seldom present. The ureters are dilated, elongated, and tortuous and may show obstruction at the level of the pelviureteric or the vesicoureteric junction (Wheatley et al. 1996).

Renal involvement ranges from near-normal kidneys to a severe degree of dysplasia with primitive ducts in embryonic mesoderm, cysts, and metaplastic cartilage. Severe renal dysplasia may resemble type II cystic kidneys according to Potter (1972), but also small kidneys with subcortical glomerular and tubular cysts as a consequence of urethral obstruction have been reported, as seen in type IV cystic dysplasia.

3 Pathogenesis

Two main mechanisms have been proposed in the pathophysiology of prune belly syndrome: firstly, a primary defect of abdominal wall mesoderm formation during early embryogenesis and, secondly, overdistension of the abdominal wall and urinary tract as a consequence of severe bladder outlet obstruction. Despite extensive study of clinical and autopsy cases, no single theory can satisfactorily explain the entire spectrum of the prune belly syndrome.

3.1 A Primary Defect in Mesoderm Formation

A primary defect during the embryonic formation of the mesoderm may affect the muscles of the developing abdominal wall and urinary tract as well as the renal and prostatic primordia. Comparison of the bladder, urethra, and genital tract of specimens of patients with prune belly syndrome and of posterior urethral valves revealed differences in the pathologic anatomy (Stephens and Gupta 1994; Workman and Kogan 1990). The seminal ducts and vesicles and the prostatic glands were abnormal in the prune belly syndrome specimens and normally developed in the posterior urethral valve specimens. Figure 2 illustrates the different pathologies. This major difference points to a primary defect of the mesoderm formation in prune belly syndrome.

Bladder histology of fetuses with prune belly syndrome and no evidence of obstruction showed thin bladder walls with increased connective tissue. However, fetuses with posterior urethral valves or with prune belly syndrome and evidence of urinary tract obstruction had increased bladder muscle thickness (Popek et al. 1991). These results suggest that the phenotypic appearance of the prune belly syndrome may result from a mesenchymal defect, but urinary tract obstruction may contribute. Chest wall anomalies, gut malrotation, and orthopedic malformations are secondary to the abdominal wall defect or oligohydramnios.

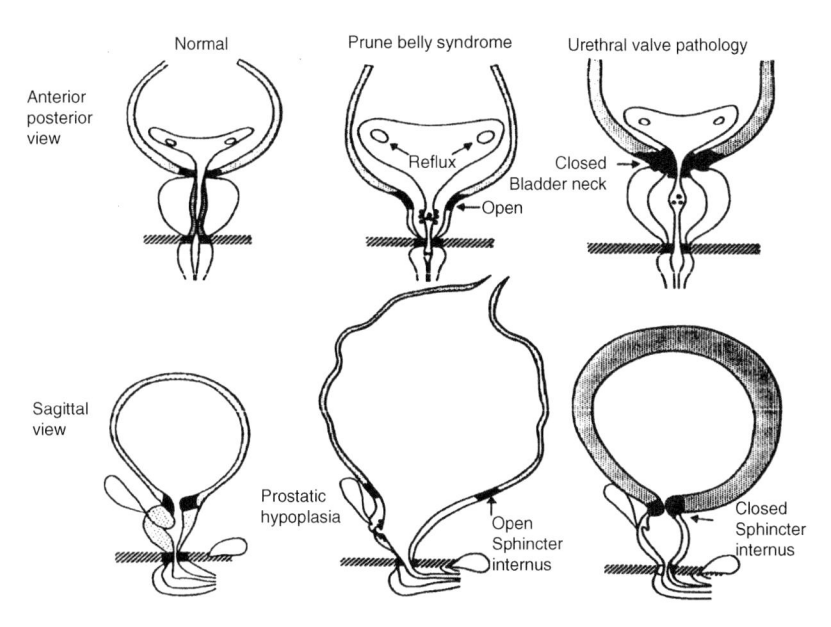

Fig. 2 Comparison between normal anatomy, prune belly pathology, and urethral valve pathology in anterior-posterior and sagittal view. Note the enlarged trigone in both pathologic conditions, whereas the detrusor muscle is thin in prune belly syndrome and hypertrophied in valve pathology (Modified from Sigel and Rösch 1993)

3.2 A Primary Defect Leading to Urethral Obstruction

The basis of the theory of primary obstruction is the existence of a lesion at or distal to the prostatic urethra producing back pressure into the fetal urinary tract. Compression of the prostatic primordia may prevent normal development, and the prostatic urethra dilates. Gross distension of the bladder causes abdominal distension and degeneration of the abdominal wall muscles. The distended bladder prevents access of the testes to the inguinal canal.

Obstructive lesions exist in a considerable number of patients, although the proof of an urodynamically significant obstruction is difficult. As documented in twelve studies comprising 151 patients mainly studied postmortem, 84 had obstructive urethral lesions (Wheatley et al. 1996). If the theory of urethral obstruction as a primary defect in prune belly syndrome is correct, the timing and severity of the obstruction must be distinct from other obstructive uropathies, particularly from posterior urethral valves.

The common observation of an urachal diverticulum or patent urachus points to possible damage from high pressure in the urinary tract before the 15th week of gestation when the urachus closed. At that time urine production in the glomerular tissue has started. The first nephrons form at about 8 weeks after conception, and the human embryo produces urine from the twelfth week of gestation. Distension of the urinary tract at 13–15 weeks gestation may induce degenerative changes of the abdominal wall and urinary tract.

Significant high pressure in patients with posterior urethral valves occurs later when urine is excreted in large amounts. At that time the urachus is closed, and prostatic development and the abdominal wall are normal.

> **Take Away**
> Prune belly syndrome is the combination of the absence of the abdominal musculature, urinary tract dilatation, and bilateral undescended testis as a consequence of aplasia of the musculature.

4 Clinical Presentation and Diagnosis

Diagnostic criteria of the prune belly phenotype are wrinkled skin, thinness, and laxity of the abdominal wall (Fig. 1) in the absence of palpable testes. Urinary tract abnormalities are demonstrable only by diagnostic procedures, e.g., ultrasonography (US), and vary widely in appearance and severity.

4.1 Obstetric Ultrasound and Antenatal Diagnosis

To date, prenatal US screening has resulted in the identification of increasing numbers of patients with suspected prune belly syndrome (Yamamoto et al. 2001). However, it is difficult to define reliably whether urinary tract dilatation during gestation is associated with true prune belly syndrome. It is even more difficult to decide whether severe obstruction is present that will interfere with normal renal development. Obstetric US is unable to give reliable information on functional renal tissue and glomerular and tubular renal function. Whether prenatal vesico-amniotic shunting is beneficial remains to be shown despite positive case reports (Biard et al. 2005).

Reduced urine production with early and persistent oligohydramnios (e.g., before 20 weeks of gestation) is strongly associated with an adverse outcome (Moore et al. 1989). Fetal compression due to a deficiency in amniotic fluid results in a recognizable constellation of clinical findings, including skeletal abnormalities, characteristic facies, pulmonary hypoplasia, and perinatal death due to respiratory insufficiency (Potter's sequence). When this complication (severe persistent oligohydramnios) occurs before 24 weeks of gestation, it is associated with pulmonary hypoplasia. A deficiency in amniotic fluid prevents normal fetal lung expansion. Prognosis is poor if oligohydramnios occurs during early gestation (Mandell et al. 1992).

Although normal fetal kidneys can sometimes be identified by US in the 16th week of gestation, the adrenals are large and may be a source of misinterpretation. After 32 weeks of gestation, both kidneys can usually be visualized during maternal US. The fetal bladder can be seen between 12 and 15 weeks gestation, when active urine production begins. The cyclical increases in size and emptying can often be seen during an examination. Repeat examinations will demonstrate adequate bladder filling.

The key problem in pre- and postnatal US examinations is the limited information about renal function and urodynamics. There is no question that the experienced investigator is able to define anatomical details of urinary tract anomalies reliably. The term prune belly syndrome is frequently used for prenatally diagnosed severe urinary tract malformation that resulted in termination of pregnancy, although the pathologic examination is incomplete, particularly due to lack of histologic examination of the prostate (Cazorla et al. 1997; Hoshino et al. 1998).

Fetal urinary indices, e.g., sodium, creatinine, microproteins, etc., are not precise predictors of subsequent renal function. Therefore, they are not helpful in the prediction of renal function after birth.

4.2 Postnatal Diagnostic Approach

As with other fetal urinary tract anomalies detected prenatally, suspected prune belly syndrome should be monitored by US, and delivery should be carried out at a center where expert neonatal, nephrologic, urologic, and pediatric radiological experience is available. The first postnatal physical examination clearly shows absent abdominal muscle wall (prune belly) syndrome (Fig. 1).

Ultrasound often suggests, in addition to the clinical examination, the diagnosis of prune belly pathology, but complementary radiological and radionuclide imaging is necessary to rule out a significant obstruction that will have to be corrected surgically. Radiological diagnostic procedures are rarely an emergency. Urine output and micturition can be monitored clinically, and serial determination of serum creatinine is important to assess renal function. Serum creatinine at day 1 represents the serum creatinine of the mother and falls to normal values of less than 0.3 mg/dl within 14 days. If serum creatinine remains high or rises, renal insufficiency can be diagnosed. After peaking between 1 and 2 weeks of age, serum creatinine may fall in the case of adequate urine production. If the serum creatinine level remains high under stable conditions, it indicates the degree of renal dysplasia.

4.2.1 Renal and Urinary Tract Ultrasonography

After the physical examination has been completed, US should be performed. A realistic interpretation of an US examination is important since it provides only anatomic information: dilatation of the urinary tract is not necessarily induced by obstruction, particularly in patients with prune belly syndrome.

In typical prune belly syndrome, the kidneys show various degrees of dysplasia, cystic dilatation of the calices, and dilated, enlarged, and tortuous ureters (Fig. 3).

In addition to dilatation of the renal pelvis and the ureters, bladder filling and bladder wall thickness can be determined by US (Fig. 3). Bladder outlet obstruction is usually associated with thickened and hypertrophied bladder wall. Perineal ultrasound may be helpful in case of associated VACTERL for the evaluation of anorectal malformation.

4.2.2 Voiding Cystourethrography

The first additional radiological examination performed in patients with prune belly syndrome should be voiding cystourethrography (VCUG), an investigation that is independent of the degree

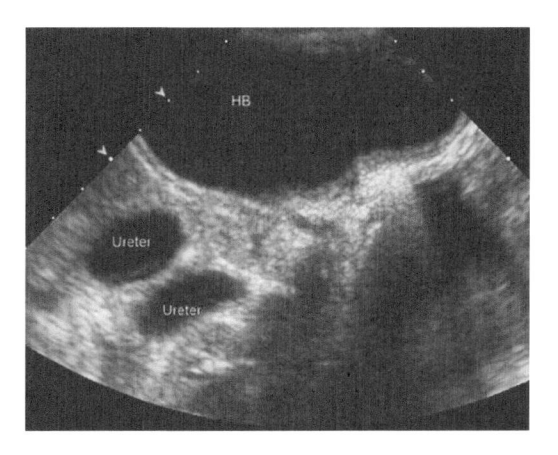

Fig. 3 Ultrasonographic demonstration of a large bladder (HB) with thin bladder wall and a dilated tortuous ureter in a 1-year-old infant with prune belly syndrome

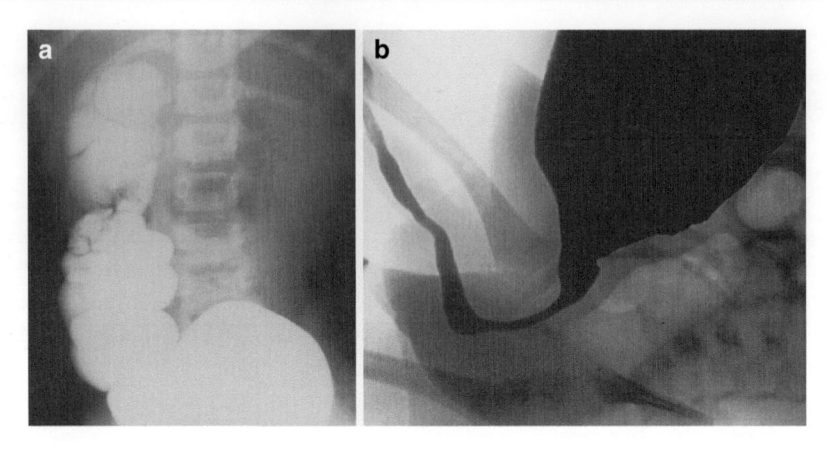

Fig. 4 Voiding cystourethrogram in an infant with prune belly syndrome. (**a**) High-grade VUR into the enlarged ureter; (**b**) a wide bladder neck as a consequence of an open internal urethral sphincter

of renal function and gives valuable information regarding the lower urinary tract (bladder outflow) and whether vesicoureteric reflux (VUR) is present.

Since megacystis can be expected in patients with prune belly syndrome, the investigator should be prepared for a large bladder volume (Fig. 4). A persistent urachus may be seen, and the bladder typically empties slowly and incompletely. Bilateral VUR is commonly observed. The prostatic urethra is often dilated and presents in a V-shaped manner, and the prostatic utricle may be opacified.

With the combination of US and VCUG, adequate morphologic evaluation of the kidneys and collecting systems shortly after birth is possible and permits appropriate management to be instituted immediately (e.g., suprapubic drainage if urethral obstruction is present). Because of the high risk of urinary tract infection, antibiotic prophylaxis should be given at the time of the diagnostic procedure.

4.2.3 Dynamic Renography

Further imaging may be planned when the neonate is stable, and clinical and laboratory findings have been evaluated. Since normal renal function is necessary for further diagnostic procedures, it should be done only after the end of the neonatal period (after 4 weeks of age).

Dynamic renography with 99 m technetium-mercaptoacetyltriglycine (^{99m}Tc-MAG3) is generally characterized by a continuously rising curve reflecting poor drainage of the kidney if a dilatation of the collecting system exists. In this condition furosemide should be administered (diuretic renography), which increases urinary flow and may distinguish between good and impaired drainage (for further details, see chapter "Diagnostic Procedures: Excluding MRI, Nuclear Medicine and Video Urodynamics").

The dynamic renogram is only of diagnostic value if glomerular renal function is normal and both kidneys appear normal on US evaluation. It is important that dynamic renography is performed with an empty bladder to exclude an obstruction at the ureterovesical junction. Therefore, in infants the use of an indwelling bladder catheter that is not clamped is required. Adequate hydration is necessary to yield a reliable examination (Rascher and Rösch 2005).

4.2.4 Static Renal Scan

The ^{99m}Tc-dimercaptosuccinic acid (DMSA) scan, as a static renal scan, binds to functioning proximal tubular cells and indicates functioning renal parenchymal mass. This scan has an important role in identifying small, poorly functioning or nonfunctioning dysplastic kidneys and in obtaining information about split renal function.

In the newborn period, the ^{99m}Tc-DMSA scan is characterized by high background activity and relatively low fixation of the isotope in the renal tubules, but valuable evidence of differential function between the two kidneys can still be obtained during the first months of life, particularly after the first 4 to 6 weeks.

4.2.5 Intravenous Urography

Intravenous urography (IVU) has been previously used for further evaluation of prune belly syndrome, but nowadays it should be replaced by magnetic resonance urography (MRU). Magnetic resonance urography is superior to the conventional IVU in many aspects, particularly in evaluating renal parenchymal disease, for assessment of ureteral anatomy and ureteral orifice, and for evaluation of poorly functioning renal systems (Riccabona et al. 2002). If MRU is not applicable or available, IVU is helpful to assess renal dysmorphy and ureteric pathology, which is typically characterized by bilateral hydroureteronephrosis in children with prune belly syndrome.

Intravenous urography should not be performed in newborns within the first 4 weeks of life, because of the risk of contrast nephropathy, and not in children with impaired renal function.

4.2.6 Computed Tomography and Magnetic Resonance Imaging

Computed tomography is usually not indicated in children with prune belly syndrome. Magnetic resonance urography is the imaging modality of choice for the cross-sectional assessment of upper urinary tract dilatation in children (Nolte-Ernsting et al. 2003; Riccabona 2004; Grattan-Smith and Jones 2006). The combination of heavily T2-weighted (static) MRU and dynamic contrast-enhanced (excretory) T1-weighted MRU after administration of gadolinium and low-dose furosemide provides accurate anatomic information and functional information such as renal transit time or differential renal function (Rohrschneider et al. 2002; Grattan-Smith and Jones 2006; Boss et al. 2014) (for further details, see Sect. 2 in chapter "Diagnostic Procedures: Excluding MRI, Nuclear Medicine and Video Urodynamics").

> **Take Away**
> Postnatal physical examination with wrinkled skin, thinness, and laxity of the abdominal wall in the absence of palpable testes in combination with US and other radiological demonstrations of the massive urinary tract dilatation (VCUG, MRU) establishes the diagnosis of prune belly syndrome.

5 Management

Treatment of prune belly syndrome is primarily conservative, and surgical management is seldom required. When obstruction is absent, the goal of treatment is the prevention of urinary tract infection. When obstruction of the ureters or urethra can be demonstrated or is strongly suspected, temporary drainage procedures, such as pyelostomies or vesicostomies, may help to preserve renal function until the child is old enough for reconstructive surgery.

Chronic renal failure is mostly due to the accompanying renal dysplasia and the deleterious effects of acute pyelonephritis that has been diagnosed and treated too late. Since massive bladder distension and megaureter often promote urinary tract infection, antibiotic prophylaxis is often logical and highly effective. Conservative management is more efficient than an extensive and aggressive surgical approach such as urinary diversion or ureteric remodeling (Burbige et al. 1987; Rohrmann and Duckett 2011). Current practice is to correct the cryptorchidism surgically. Orchidopexy in these children can be quite difficult and is best accomplished at the end of the first year of life. Reconstruction of the abdominal wall may offer cosmetic and functional benefits.

The prognosis depends on the degree of pulmonary hypoplasia and renal dysplasia. Up to one-third of children with prune belly syndrome are stillborn or die in the first few months of life as a consequence of pulmonary hypoplasia.

However, early termination of pregnancies with severe prune belly pathology will reduce the proportion of patients with this syndrome and particularly reduce those cases with a poor outcome.

Of the long-term survivors, one-half will develop chronic renal failure from dysplasia or complications of infection or reflux, and 15 % of all children with PBS will require renal transplantation (Seidel et al. 2014). The results of renal transplantation in these patients are favorable (Fontaine et al. 1997; Fusaro et al. 2004).

> **Take Away**
> Management of prune belly syndrome is primarily conservative (prevention of urinary tract infection, treatment of chronic renal failure when present). Surgical procedures are required only when obstruction is present.

6 Other Syndromes Associated with Urinary Tract Malformations

There are various other syndromes, which are affecting the urinary tract. Often syndromic cystic renal disease is present, but also other urinary tract malformations can be associated with syndromic disease. For many of them, the respective gene defect has been described (Table 1):

In syndromic CAKUT, structural and functional malformations of the urogenital system are associated with other congenital abnormalities, for example, of the central nervous system, whereas in nonsyndromic CAKUT, only the urogenital tract is affected. A typical example for systemic malformations is the well-known VACTERL association. Details of the various changes resemble the individual malformation as detailed in the respective chapters, with the same implications on imaging workup and follow-up.

Table 1 From Rosenblum ND. Overview of congenital anomalies of the kidney and urinary tract [CAKUT] UpToDate®, Wolters Kluwer

Alagille syndrome	*JAGGED1*	Cystic dysplasia
Apert syndrome	*FGFR2*	Urinary tract dilatation
Bardet-Biedl syndrome	*BBS1*	Cystic dysplasia
Beckwith-Wiedemann syndrome	Dysregulation of imprinting in chromosome 11, p15.5	Medullary dysplasia
Branchio-oto-renal syndrome (BOR)	*EYA1*, *SIX1*, *SIX5*	Unilateral/bilateral agenesis/dysplasia, hypoplasia, collecting system anomalies
Campomelic dysplasia	*SOX9*	Dysplasia, hydronephrosis
Fraser syndrome	*FRAS1*	Agenesis, dysplasia
Hypoparathyroidism, sensorineural deafness, and renal anomalies (HDR)	*GATA3*	Dysplasia
Kallmann syndrome	*KAL1*	Agenesis
Ulnar-mammary syndrome	*TBX3*	Dysplasia
Meckel-Gruber syndrome	MKS1, MKS3, NPHP6, NPHP8	Cystic dysplasia
Nephronophthisis	*CEP290, GLIS2, RPGRIP1L, NEK8, SDCCAG8, TMEM 67, TTC21B*	Cystic dysplasia
Okihiro syndrome	*SALL4*	Unilateral agenesis, VUR, malrotation, cross-fused ectopia
Pallister-Hall syndrome	*GLI3*	Agenesis, dysplasia, urinary tract dilatation
Renal coloboma syndrome	*PAX2*	Hypoplasia, VUR

Table 1 (continued)

Renal hypoplasia, isolated	BMP4, RET, DSTYK	Hypoplasia, VUR; DSTYK mutations also associated with UPJO
Renal tubular dysgenesis	Renin, angiotensinogen, ACE, AT1 receptor	Tubular dysgenesis
Rubinstein-Taybi syndrome	CREBBP	Agenesis, hypoplasia
Simpson-Golabi-Behmel syndrome	GPC3	Medullary dysplasia
Townes-Brocks syndrome	SALL1	Hypoplasia, dysplasia, VUR
Zellweger syndrome	PEX1	Cystic dysplasia
Smith-Lemli-Opitz syndrome	DHCR7	Renal hypoplasia, cysts, and aplasia

UPJO = pelviureteric junction obstruction

References

Bellah RD, States LJ, Duckett JW (1996) Pseudoprune-belly syndrome: imaging findings and clinical outcome. Am J Roentgenol 167:1389–1393

Biard JM, Johnson MP, Carr MC et al (2005) Long-term outcomes in children treated by prenatal vesicoamniotic shunting for lower urinary tract obstruction. Obstet Gynecol 106:503–508

Boss A, Martirosian P, Fuchs J, Obermayer F, Tsiflikas I, Schick F, Schäfer JF (2014) Dynamic MR urography in children with uropathic disease with a combined 2D and 3D acquisition protocol-comparison with MAG3 scintigraphy. Br J Radiol 87(1044):20140426. doi:10.1259/bjr.20140426, Epub 2014 Oct 1

Burbige KA, Amodio J, Berdon WE et al (1987) Prune belly syndrome: 35 years of experience. J Urol 137:86–90

Cazorla E, Ruiz F, Abad A, Monleon J (1997) Prune belly syndrome: early antenatal diagnosis. Eur J Obstet Gynecol Reprod Biol 72:31–33

Eagle JF, Barrett GS (1950) Congenital deficiency of abdominal musculature with associated genitourinary abnormalities, a syndrome: reports of nine cases. Pediatrics 6:721–736

Fontaine E, Salomon L, Gagnandoux MF et al (1997) Longterm results of renal transplantation in children with the prune belly syndrome. J Urol 158:892–894

Fusaro F, Zanon GF, Ferreli AM et al (2004) Renal transplantation in prune-belly syndrome. Transpl Int 17:549–752

Grattan-Smith JD, Jones RA (2006) MR urography in children. Pediatr Radiol 36:1119–1132

Greskovich FJ, Nyberg LM (1988) The prune belly syndrome: a review of its etiology, defects, treatment and prognosis. J Urol 140:707–712

Hoshino T, Ihara Y, Shirane H, Ota T (1998) Prenatal diagnosis of prune belly syndrome at 12 weeks of pregnancy: case report and review of the literature. Ultrasound Obstet Gynecol 12:362–366

Mandell J, Peters CA, Estroff JA, Benacerraf BR (1992) Late onset severe oligohydramnios associated with genitourinary abnormalities. J Urol 148:515–518

Moore TR, Longo J, Leopold GR et al (1989) The reliability and predictive value of an amniotic fluid scoring system in severe second-trimester oligohydramnios. Obstet Gynecol 73:739–742

Nolte-Ernsting CC, Staatz G, Tacke J, Gunther RW (2003) MR urography today. Abdom Imaging 28:191–209

Osler W (1901) Congenital absence of the abdominal muscles with distended and hypertrophied urinary bladder. Bull Johns Hopkins Hosp 12:331–333

Parker RW (1895) Absence of abdominal muscle in an infant. Lancet 1:1252–1254

Popek EJ, Tyson RW, Miller GJ, Caldwell SA (1991) Prostate development in prune belly syndrome (PBS) and posterior urethral valves (PUV): etiology of PBS – lower urinary tract obstruction or mesenchymal defect? Pediatr Pathol 11:1–29

Potter EL (1972) Normal and abnormal development of the kidney. Year Book, Chicago

Ramasamy R, Haviland M, Woodard JR, BArone JG (2005) Patterns of inheritance in familial prune belly syndrome. Urology 65:1227–1228

Rascher W, Rösch W (2005) Congenital anomalies of the urinary tract. In: Davison AM, Cameron JS, Grünfeld JP, Ponticelli C, Ritz E, Winearls CG, van Ypersele C (eds) Oxford textbook of clinical nephrology, 3rd edn. Oxford University Press, Oxford, pp 2470–2494

Reinberg Y, Shapiro E, Manivel JC et al (1991) Prune belly syndrome in females: a triad of abdominal musculature deficiency and anomalies of the urinary and genital system. J Pediatr 118:395–398

Riccabona M (2004) Pediatric MRU-its potential and its role in the diagnostic work-up of upper urinary tract dilatation in infants and children. World J Urol 22:79–87

Riccabona M, Simbrunner J, Ring E et al (2002) Feasibility of MR urography in neonates and infants with anomalies of the upper urinary tract. Eur Radiol 12:1442–1450

Rohrmann D, Duckett JW (2011) Prune-belly-Syndrom. In: Stein R, Beetz R, Thüroff JW (eds) Kinderurologie in Klinik und Praxis. Thieme, Stuttgart, pp 395–405

Rohrschneider WK, Haufe S, Wiesel M et al (2002) Functional and morphologic evaluation of congenital urinary tract dilatation by using combined static-dynamic MR urography: findings in kidneys with a single collecting system. Radiology 224:683–694

Seidel NE, Arlen AM, Smith EA, Kirsch AJ (2015) Clinical manifestations and management of prune-belly syndrome in a large contemporary pediatric population. Urology 85:211–215. doi:10.1016/j.urology.2014.09.029

Sigel A, Rösch W (1993) Prune-belly-("Pflaumenbauch") syndrom. In: Sigel A (ed) Kinderurologie. Springer, Berlin Heidelberg, pp 107–114

Stephens FD, Gupta D (1994) Pathogenesis of the prune belly syndrome. J Urol 152:2328–2331

Wheatley JM, Stephens FD, Hutson JM (1996) Prune-belly syndrome: ongoing controversies regarding pathogenesis and management. Semin Pediatr Surg 5:95–106

Williams DI (1982) Prune belly syndrome. In: Williams DI, Johnston JH (eds) Paediatric urology. Butterworths, London, pp 289–297

Workman SJ, Kogan BA (1990) Fetal bladder histology in posterior urethral valves and the prune belly syndrome. J Urol 144:337–339

Yamamoto H, Nishikawa S, Hayashi T et al (2001) Antenatal diagnosis of prune belly syndrome at 11 weeks of gestation. J Obstet Gynaecol Res 27:37–40

Vesicoureteric Reflux

Freddy Avni, Marianne Tondeur,
Frederica Papadopoulou, and Annie Lahoche

Contents

1 Introduction 491
2 **Diagnosing VUR** 492
2.1 Voiding Cystourethrography (VCUG) 492
2.2 Direct Radionuclide Cystography (DRNC) 493
2.3 Indirect Radionuclide Cystography (IRC) 494
2.4 Ultrasound 495
2.5 Contrast-Enhanced Voiding Urosonography (ce-VUS) 498
2.6 MR Urography 499
3 **Detection of VUR: Circumstances** 500
3.1 Postnatal Workup of Antenatally Diagnosed Fetal Uropathies 500
3.2 Urinary Tract Infection 501
3.3 Familial VUR 502
4 **Particular Presentations of VUR** 503
4.1 VUR and Pelvi-Ureteric Junction Obstruction 503
4.2 VUR and UVJ Obstruction 503
4.3 Reflux and Lithiasis 503
4.4 VUR into an Unused Ureter 503
4.5 Yo-yo Reflux 504
4.6 The (So-Called) Megacystis–Megaureter Association 505
4.7 VUR and Duplex Kidneys 506
4.8 VUR into Ectopic Ureter 506
4.9 Iatrogenic VUR 506
4.10 VUR and Bladder Diverticulum 507
4.11 VUR in case of Other Uropathies 507
4.12 Fetal Reflux 508
5 **Natural History, Treatment, and Follow-up of VUR** 508
5.1 Conservative Treatment 508
5.2 Surgical Treatment 508
5.3 Complications of VUR 509
5.4 Fetal Reflux Nephropathy 509
5.5 Imaging RN and the Progression of Renal Disease 510

Conclusion 512

References 512

F. Avni, MD, PhD (✉)
Department of Pediatric Radiology, Jeanne de Flandre Hospital, Lille University Hospital, 59037 Lille, France
e-mail: favni@skynet.be

M. Tondeur, MD
Department of Nuclear Medicine, Saint Pierre Hospital, Brussels, Belgium

F. Papadopoulou, MD
Radiology, Ioannina University, Ioannina, Greece

A. Lahoche, MD
Department of Pediatric Nephrology, Jeanne de Flandre Hospitals, Lille, France

1 Introduction

In case of urinary tract infection (UTI), vesicoureteric reflux (VUR) is considered a significant factor for the recurrence of UTIs and for the development of progressive renal damage. Optimizing its detection is important for the identification of patients at risk. This necessitates a good knowledge of the pathogenesis, the circumstances of occurrence, and the natural history of the disease. In addition, the techniques used for demonstrating VUR must be used at their best and for good purposes (The RIVUR trial investigators 2014; Garin et al. 1998; Hellström and Jacobsson 1999; Jakobsson et al. 1999; Ismaili et al. 2006a, b).

VUR results from the lack of a normal valve-like mechanism of the vesicoureteric orifice (Thomson et al. 1994) (see also chapter "UTI and VUR"). Many factors contribute to the competence of the vesicoureteric orifice, e.g., the location of the orifice, the normal renal function with downhill diuresis, and the hydration of the patient. Refluxing ureters often have a larger diameter, and the ostium is at a more lateral or caudal position. Furthermore, the competence of the vesicoureteric junction is also influenced by the length of the intravesical segment of the ureter: a shorter distance is likely to result in VUR. Primary VUR occurs mainly in neonates and in infants, whereas secondary VUR results from or is associated with various uro-nephropathies. It occurs more often in school-age girls. The exact prevalence of VUR in healthy children is unknown but apparently is between 1 and 2 % (Verrier-Jones 1999).

Table 1 VUR grading

Grade	Findings
Grade I	VUR limited to the ureter
Grade II	VUR up the renal cavities without dilatation
Grade III	VUR into the renal cavities inducing dilatation and eversion of the calyces
Grade IV	Moderate-to-marked dilatation of the ureter and pyelocalyceal system
Grade V	Marked tortuosity and dilatation of the ureter and pyelocalyceal system

2 Diagnosing VUR

2.1 Voiding Cystourethrography (VCUG)

To date, voiding cystourethrography (VCUG) is the central method for the initial diagnosis of VUR in children with UTI (or for workup of an antenatal diagnosis of fetal uropathy) (Fernbach et al. 2000). The method allows the detection of VUR, its precise grading, and the detection of intrarenal reflux. Grading of VUR is based on the work of the International Reflux Study Group and includes VUR from grade I–V (Table 1) (Figs. 1, 2, 3, 4, 5, and 6) (Lebowitz et al. 1985). VURs of higher grades are associated with a greater degree of dysplasia/reflux nephropathy. Also, higher grades of VUR tend to resolve more slowly than milder grades of VUR. A special aspect of VUR, the intrarenal reflux, occurs more often at the upper and lower poles of the kidney and at compound papillae (Fig. 4). It is related to the particular anatomy of the medulla–calyceal complex in these poles that renders intrarenal reflux more prone to occur and scars more likely to develop (Ransley and Risdon 1975; Rolleston et al. 1974).

VCUG is also useful as it provides a simultaneous evaluation of the bladder and urethra. The demonstration of voiding dysfunction, bladder wall thickening, or diverticula may help to characterize and understand certain types of VUR (Fotter et al. 1986; Koff 1992). Urethral obstruction, whatever its origin, may also be associated with secondary VUR (Fig. 7). The drawbacks of the method are that the procedure is invasive, necessitating bladder catheterization or puncture, and that it is an irradiating technique. Fortunately, the newer pulsed fluoroscopy cystographic technique reduces the radiation dose almost as low as radionuclide studies (ovarian dose 0.017–0.052 mGy, mean dose: 0.029 mGy) (Kleinman et al. 1994; Hernandez and Goodsitt 1996).

Another limitation of the technique is that conventional VCUG underestimates the occurrence and degree of VUR. Cyclic filling of the bladder has been shown to improve the detection rate of VUR by 3 % in a second and up to 18 % in a third filling. This is of particular interest in neonates or in other patients with low vesical capacity (Fig. 8) (Gelfand et al. 1999; Papadopoulou et al. 2002; Riccabona 2002).

Pitfalls of VCUG include underestimation of the degree of VUR in case of reflux into an already dilated and obstructed ureter (refluxing megaureter) or when VUR and ureteropelvic obstruction coexist (Bomalaski et al. 1997); due to the obstruction, the refluxing urine may not reach the pyelocalyceal system (see below). Finally, reflux of contrast into the vagina during the micturition phase of the VCUG is commonly observed and

Fig. 1 VUR grading

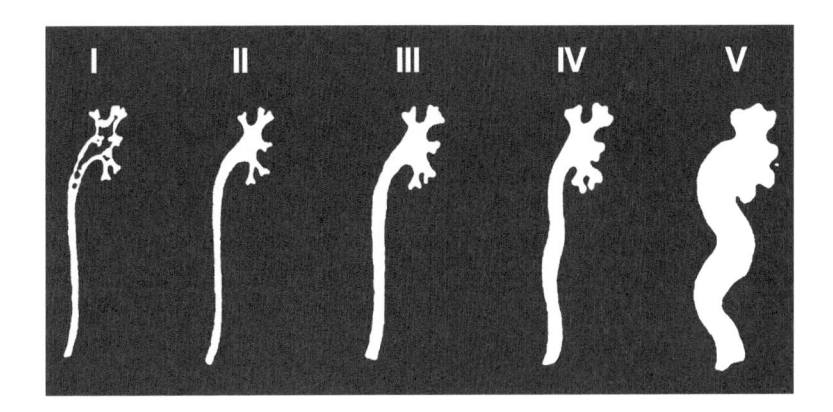

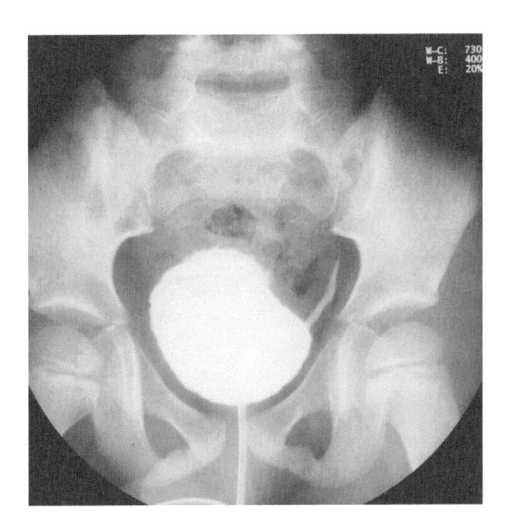

Fig. 2 VCUG: left VUR grade I

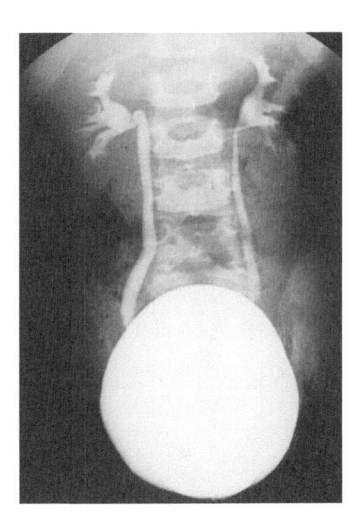

Fig. 3 VCUG: bilateral VUR grade II

should not be regarded as a sign of ectopic insertion or of fistula (Fig. 9) unless the refluxed contrast fills a distended vagina or unless there is no clear separation between the vagina and urethra. In such cases a variant of urogenital sinus must be suspected (Lebowitz and Avni 1980).

2.2 Direct Radionuclide Cystography (DRNC)

Even if DRNC lacks resolution, this approach is attractive since it delivers a lower radiation dose than pulsed fluoroscopy VCUG or continuous fluoroscopy VCUG (Lee et al. 2006a, b; Ward et al. 2008) (see also chapter "Nuclear Medicine").

DRNC requires bladder catheterization as well. Still, numerous studies have demonstrated that DRNC is more sensitive than VCUG in detecting VUR (Dalirani et al. 2014). This is not surprising: VUR is intermittent, and DRNC, by allowing an uninterrupted image registration during a longer duration, detects a higher number of reflux episodes. DRNC is however less sensitive in detecting intrarenal reflux and grade I VUR (Mozley et al. 1994; Unver et al. 2006); it does not provide anatomical information about the bladder or urethra (Fig. 10).

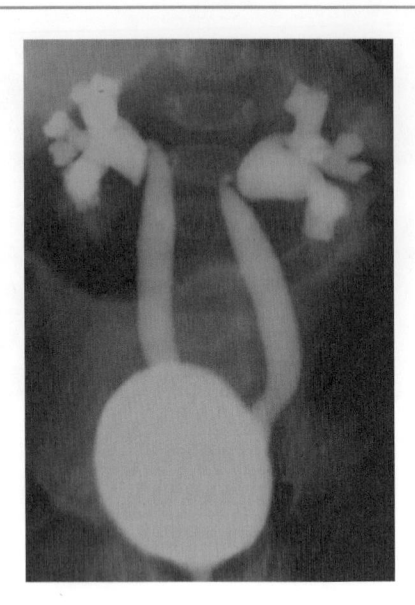

Fig. 4 VCUG: bilateral VUR grade III with left intrarenal reflux

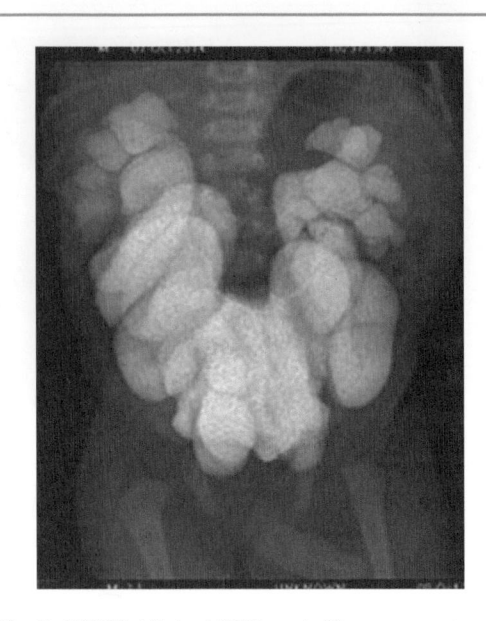

Fig. 6 VCUG: bilateral VUR grade V

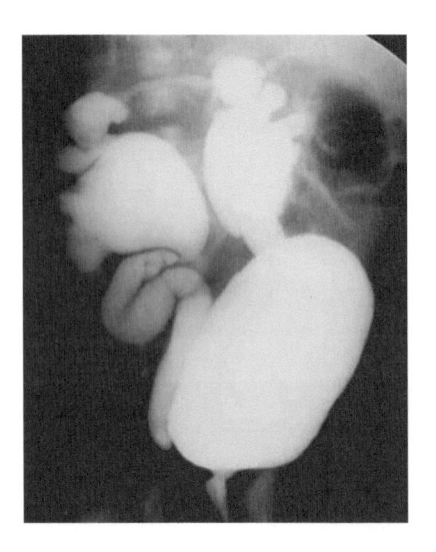

Fig. 5 VCUG: Bilateral VUR grade IV

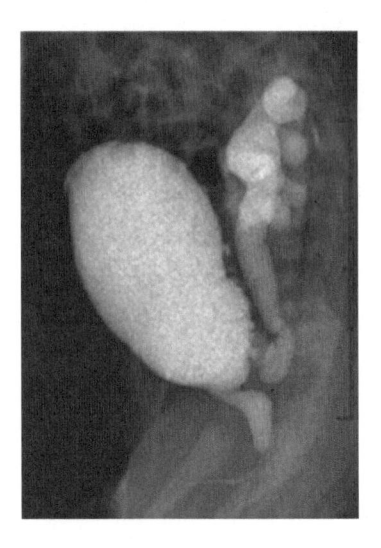

Fig. 7 VUR and PUV. VCUG, micturition phase, showing typical PUV associated with left grade IV VUR

The unquestionable indications of DRNC are the follow-up of patients with previously known VUR and the screening of siblings of patients with VUR as VUR may be present in 25% of these siblings (Wan et al. 1996; Fettich et al. 2003; Piepsz and Ham 2006).

2.3 Indirect Radionuclide Cystography (IRC)

In IRC, the isotopic tracer is injected intravenously in the framework of the measurement of the separate kidney functions; the presence of VUR is

Fig. 8 Cyclic VCUG. (**a**) No VUR is demonstrated at the first filling. (**b**) Left grade III/IV VUR appears during the third filling

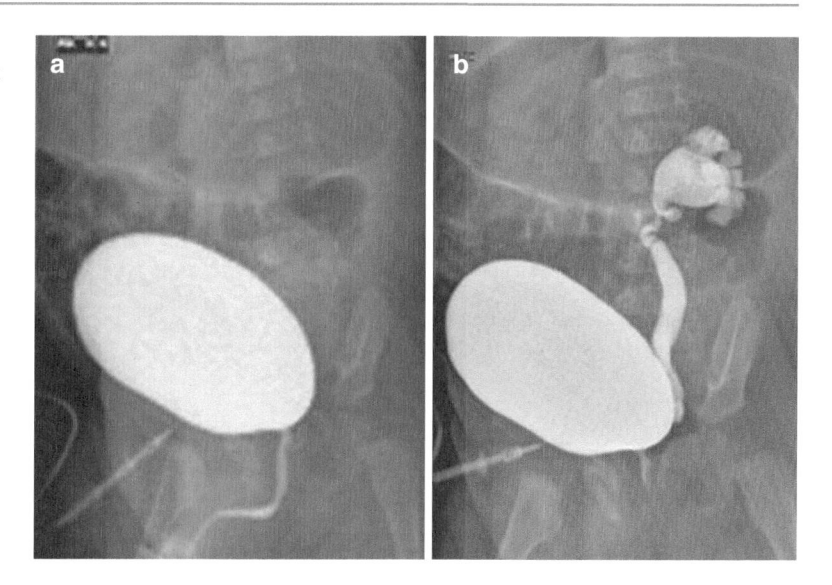

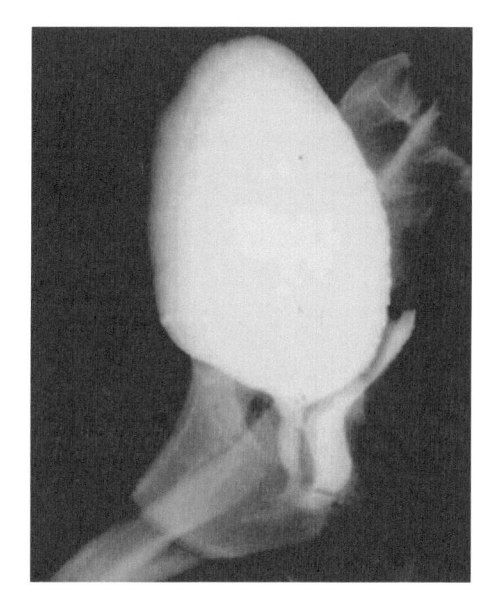

Fig. 9 VCUG (voiding phase): retrograde filling of the vagina

evaluated on the late micturition phase of the procedure (Fig. 11) (see also chapter "Nuclear Medicine"). This technique presents several advantages over the direct procedures: it is noninvasive and more physiological. However, IRC does not study the bladder-filling phase nor it images the micturition phase; the method misses VUR in a significant number of children: a negative examination can therefore not exclude VUR (De Sadeleer et al. 1994); moreover, performing IDRC is possible only in children who are toilet trained, i.e., over 3–4 years of age (Gordon et al. 2001).

2.4 Ultrasound

Ultrasound (US) has gained popularity for the evaluation of the urinary tract in children. It is easily performed, and, since it is a non-irradiating technique, it is well accepted by the parents. Because the patients are small, high-resolution transducers can be used and the urinary tract is nicely displayed (see also chapter "Diagnostic Procedures: Excluding MRI, Nuclear Medicine and Video-Urodynamics").

The role of the technique for screening patients at risk of having VUR has been very controversial. Many authors suggest that conventional US in no way replaces VCUG in patients at risk; for these authors, US detects only 25–45 % of patients with VUR (Di Pietro et al. 1997; Zerin et al. 1993). Unfortunately most of these studies underestimate the value of US because they rely on the presence

Fig. 10 Indirect cystography performed after the end of the renogram; right VUR during the micturition phase

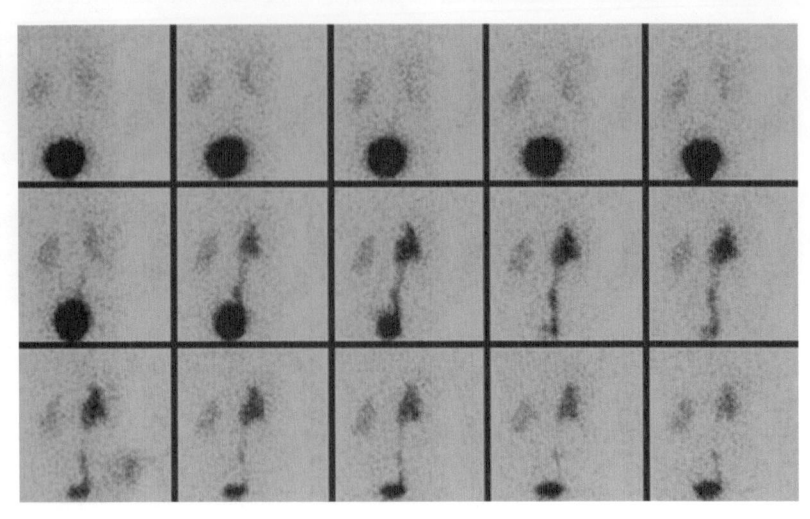

Table 2 US signs that can be associated with VUR

Renal pelvic dilatation
Variable dilatation
Ureteral dilatation
Calyceal dilatation
Loss of corticomedullary differentiation
Signs of dysplasia
Pelvic and ureteral wall thickening
Hyperechoic medulla
Color Doppler turbulence in dilated ureters
Enlarged bladder

of urinary tract dilatation as the only sign of VUR. Many other US signs have been described in association with VUR (Table 2) and should be looked for (Avni et al. 1997; Hiraoka et al. 1994; Hiraoka et al. 1997; Tsai et al. 1998). Renal pelvis dilatation is certainly an important sign of VUR, but the problem is also to determine the degree of dilatation that should be considered abnormal: 7 mm in the newborn and 10 mm in older children seem to be a good cutoff for diagnosing dilatation (Stocks et al. 1996; Marra et al. 1994; Walsh and Dubbins 1996). The detection of calyceal or ureteral dilatation is an important supplementary finding, and both have been shown to be associated with VUR (Newell et al. 1990; Leroy et al. 2010). A varying dilatation of the pelvis is suggestive of VUR (Fig. 11). The lack of corticomedullary differentiation is also commonly associated with VUR (Figs. 12 and 13). These signs, as well as an overall increased cortical hyperechogenicity, could result from high intravesical pressure and ischemic damage, which lead to glomerular ischemic damage and renal dysplasia (Hulbert et al. 1992). Small kidneys or renal cortical thinning, features of renal dysplasia, may also be associated with VUR and with high pressure damage already in utero (Gobet et al. 1999). Another interesting US sign that can be associated with VUR is pelvic and ureteral wall thickening (Fig. 13). The sign is not specific as it can be encountered in cases of UTI, renal transplant rejection, as well as postoperatively. Yet once the other etiologies such as postoperative status are excluded, a VCUG seems justified (Robben et al. 1999). Finally, ureteral dilatation has been shown to be the most accurate sign predicting VUR (Leroy et al. 2010). Using all these US data, one should be able to detect 65–85% of patients with VUR and particularly the high-grade cases (III–V) (Avni et al. 1997; Tsai et al. 1998; Hiraoka et al. 1997).

Color Doppler sonography (CDS) has been proposed as an adjunct to conventional US for the detection of VUR. First, the visualization of the ureteric jet by means of color Doppler US was thought to mean there was no VUR (Salih et al. 1994). Although it might be interesting to localize the ureteric orifices (Strehlau et al. 1997), other studies did not confirm this hypothesis. The

Fig. 11 Direct cystography: left VUR during both the filling and the micturition phases

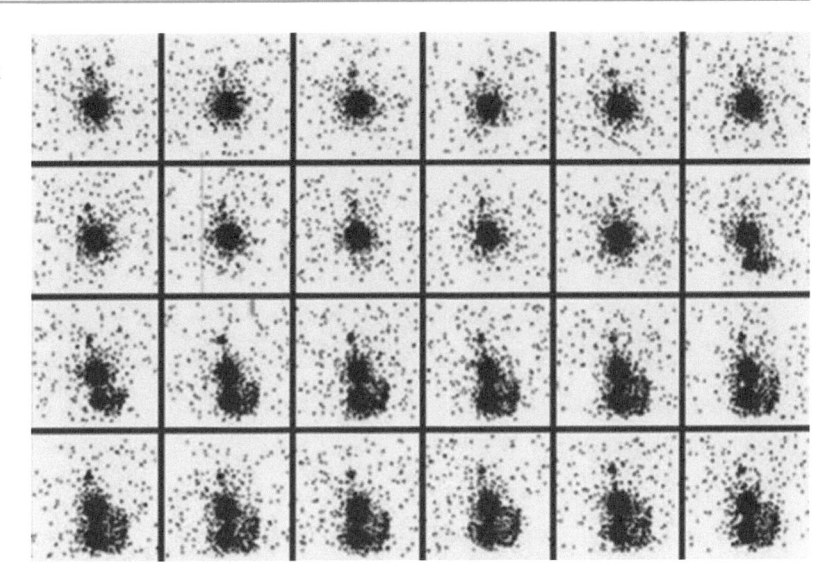

Fig. 12 US anomalies in case of VUR. (**a**) Transverse scan of the right kidney: small kidney and thickening of the renal pelvis wall (*arrow*).
(**b**) VCUG demonstrating a right grade IV VUR

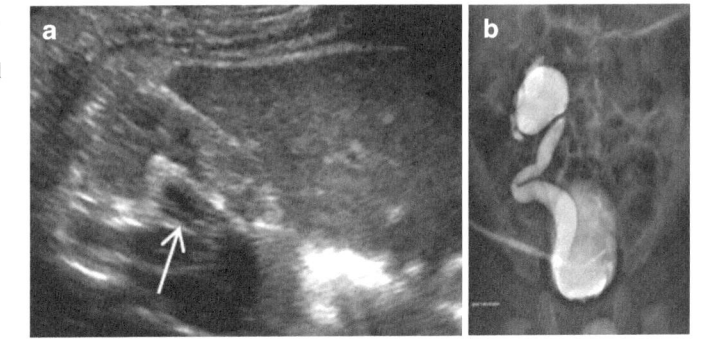

Fig. 13 US anomalies in case and VUR: varying renal pelvic dilatation. Transverse scans of the right renal pelvis. (**a**) With a full bladder, the renal pelvis measures 7 mm.
(**b**) After micturition, the dilatation increased to 13 mm

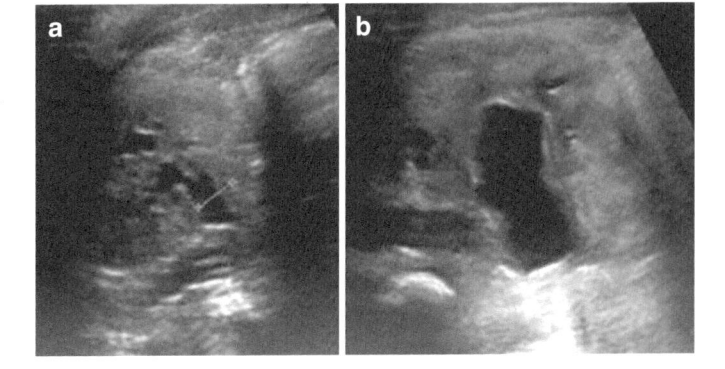

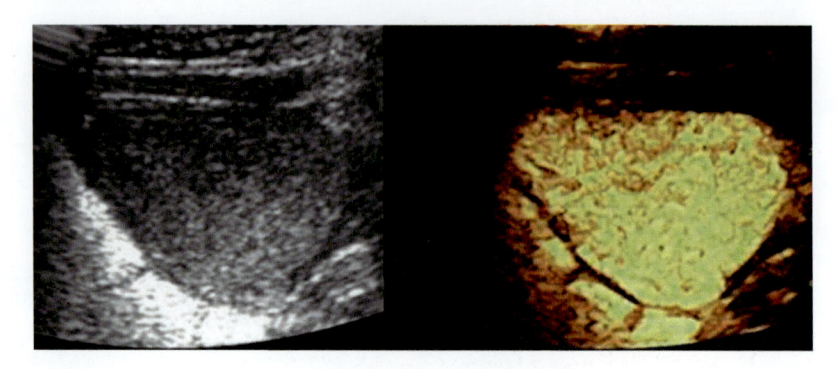

Fig. 14 Simultaneous dual imaging of the bladder during filling, saggital baldder view. Echogenic contrast filling the bladder is better seen on contrast-specific mode (on the *right*) than on conventional gray-scale imaging (on the *left*)

Fig. 15 VUR grades II–III on the left kidney on sagittal view of a 5-year-old girl. Refluxing contrast microbubbles slightly dilate the left ureter (*arrowhead*) and the major calyces (*arrow*), better seen on contrast-specific imaging (on the *right*)

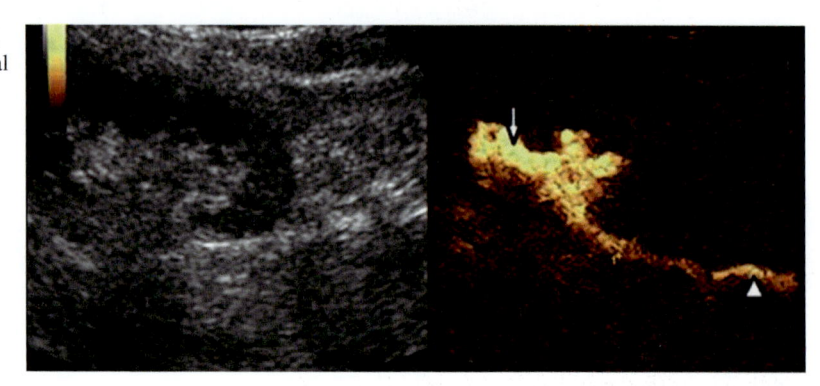

use of CDS for the demonstration of VUR in dilated ureters has also been reported with VUR; the refluxing urine displays different colors related to the variable direction of flow. Unfortunately this can only be obtained when the ureters are dilated (Matsumo et al. 1996).

2.5 Contrast-Enhanced Voiding Urosonography (ce-VUS)

During the last two decades, contrast-enhanced voiding urosonography (ce-VUS) has emerged as a sensitive and radiation-free imaging modality for the detection and follow-up of VUR in children (see also Sect. 4.2). The examination is performed with US and introduction of microbubble-containing US contrast agents in the bladder through a catheter (Fig. 13). During filling and voiding, the bladder, ureters, and kidneys are continuously monitored for possible VUR detection. During voiding the urethra is imaged through a perineal or lower abdominal approach for any structural abnormalities such as posterior urethral valves or stenosis. The diagnosis of VUR is made when echogenic microbubbles are seen entering into the ureters and renal collecting systems (Fig. 14) (Darge et al. 1998). More detailed description of the method can be found in the chapter on "Diagnostic Procedures: Excluding MRI, Nuclear Medicine and Video-Urodynamics". On ce-VUS, VUR can be graded in five grades in a similar manner as on VCUG (Darge and Troeger 2002). Intrarenal reflux can also be clearly seen with contrast-specific imaging mode (Figs. 15 and 16). The diagnostic accuracy of ce-VUS with first- or second-generation ultrasound contrast agents has been assessed in many comparative studies with VCUG or RNC and found high in almost all (Darge et al. 1999; Berrocal et al. 2005; Mentzel et al. 1999; Vassiou et al. 2004; Ascenti et al. 2004; Darge et al. 2005; Kis et al. 2010; Papadopoulou et al. 2012).

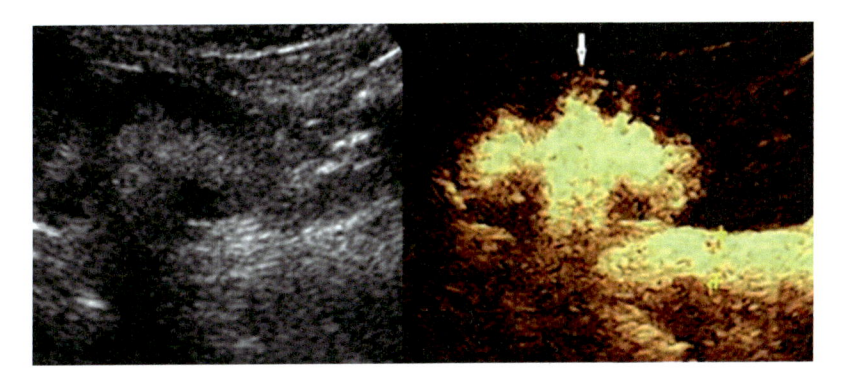

Fig. 16 Grade IV reflux on sagittal view of the left kidney in a 4-month-old girl. The significantly dilated ureter (measured 9 mm between the crosses) and pelvi-calyceal system are better seen on contrast-specific imaging (on the *right*). Intrarenal reflux is also clearly seen in the parenchyma (*arrow*) on the middle part of the left kidney during the second cycle of ce-VUS

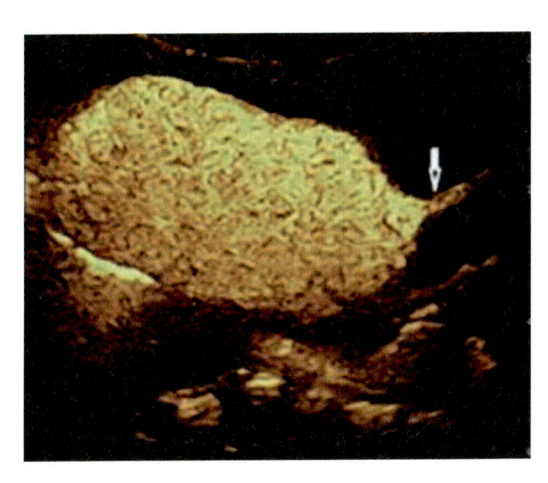

Fig. 17 Urethral imaging during voiding on ce-VUS. Normal female urethra (*arrow*) of a 4-month-old girl is imaged through abdominal approach

and 17) (Papadopoulou et al. 2006; Duran et al. 2009). Due to its complete lack of radiation, the examination can be performed in more than two or three cycles resulting thus in a higher depiction rate of intermittent VUR compared to conventional imaging methods, especially in young infants (Papadopoulou et al. 2006). On top of that, ce-VUS with ultrasound contrast agents has a favorable safety profile reported in several studies (Riccabona et al. 2012; Duran et al. 2012; Papadopoulou et al. 2014). Disadvantages of the method are that catheterization is still required and that US contrast agents are not yet available or approved for pediatric use in all countries.

2.6 MR Urography

Intravenous urography (IVU) should no longer be performed for the anatomical (or functional) assessment of the urinary tract damaged by VUR. Instead, MR urography (MRU) should be performed whenever necessary and available (Koyicigit et al. 2014) (see chapter "MR of the Urogenital Tract in Children" for details).

The increasing awareness of the radiation risks in the pediatric population has resulted in the worldwide acceptance of the ce-VUS as an alternative option in VUR imaging and has been incorporated in imaging recommendations by the Uroradiology Task Force members of the European Pediatric Radiology Society (Riccabona et al. 2008; 2012). Moreover, the availability of more stable second-generation US contrast agents and the advances in US technology with the development of contrast-specific imaging modes resulted in progressive improvement of ce-VUS's diagnostic accuracy both in VUR as well as in urethral morphology imaging (Figs. 16

On MRU, several features may suggest VUR in patients examined for other urological reasons: the discovery of a small irregular kidney, thinned parenchyma, dilated and clubbed pyelocalyceal system, and dilatation of the ureters without obstruction (Fig. 18). Conversely, whenever such findings are encountered, a VCUG should be

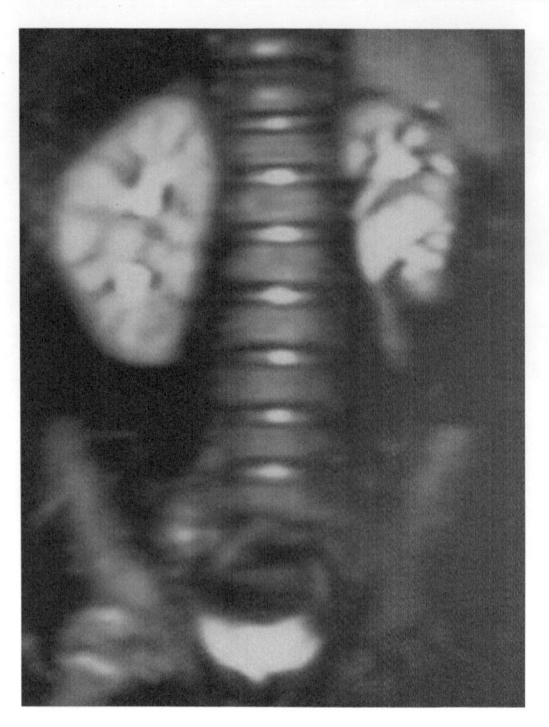

Fig. 18 Fetal reflux nephropathy. MR urography shows a small left kidney in a 2-month-old baby boy with VUR (SPIR T2 sequence)

performed in order to confirm the presence of VUR. It is worth noting that massive VUR occurring during an MR urography may fill the renal cavities. Therefore, a catheter might be introduced into the bladder prior to an MRU performed in a patient with known high-grade VUR (Lebowitz and Avni 1980).

> **Take Away**
> VCUG, using the newest pulsed fluoroscopy technique, is the most suitable technique for characterizing VUR with all important anatomical features additionally allowing for a panoramic overview. US, with all its potential applications, should be utilized as a screening method in patients at risk. Ce-VUS and isotopic cystographies should be used as follow-up techniques but may be considered as a first-line investigation in females potentially complemented by VCUG.

3 Detection of VUR: Circumstances

3.1 Postnatal Workup of Antenatally Diagnosed Fetal Uropathies

Antenatal diagnosis of fetal anomalies by obstetrical US has led to the detection of an increasing number of fetal uro-nephropathies. The attitude toward antenatally diagnosed uropathy has now been standardized (see chapter "Upper Urinary Tract Dilatation in Newborns and Infants and the Postnatal Work Up of Congenital Uro-nephropathies"), leading to increased detection of VUR (Avni et al. 1998; Zerin et al. 1993; Van Eerde et al. 2007; Lee et al. 2006a, b; Ismaili et al. 2006a, b; Riccabona et al. 2008). Furthermore, VCUG is performed selectively in the neonatal period based on obstetric US findings if confirmed on neonatal US.

Primary VUR is demonstrated more and more frequently and has become one of the leading causes of neonatal urinary tract dilatation (Zerin et al. 1993). Noteworthy, making a precise diagnosis of VUR in utero is more difficult, unless variability of the pelvic dilatation is observed during the obstetrical US examination (Hiraoka et al. 1994; Walsh and Dubbins 1996); another circumstance under which VUR is directly diagnosed in utero is the so-called megacystis–megaureter association (see below).

Perinatal VUR differs notably from VUR detected in older children, which occurs mainly in girls. Among patients with perinatal VUR, two groups are encountered: a group with mild VUR and usually normally functioning kidneys and a second group with severe VUR into massively dilated ureters, which is associated with renal damage at birth (the so-called fetal or congenital reflux nephropathy) (Fig. 19). This has led to the CAKUT concept (congenital anomalies of the kidneys and urinary tract) describing the association between renal dysplasia and hypoplasia with urinary tract malformation (Najmaldin et al. 1990; Anderson and Rickwood 1991; Yeung et al. 1997; Ismaili et al. 2006a, b).

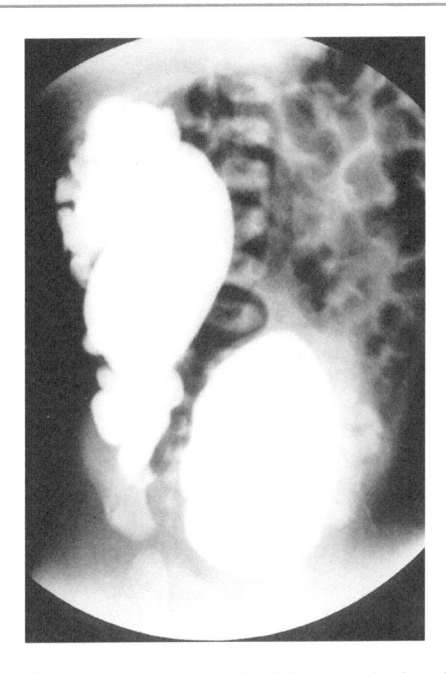

Fig. 19 Massive right grade V VUR in a baby boy. The renal function was impaired

The first type of VUR is often an incidental finding during neonatal VCUG; it is encountered equally in girls and boys. The second most severe type is almost exclusively detected in baby boys already during fetal life, and this particularity has led to a theory associating this frequent occurrence of severe VUR in baby boys with a transient fetal bladder outlet obstruction (Avni and Schulman 1996; Sillen 1999a,1999b). Whatever its grade, VUR in children tends to resolve more often than VUR detected in older patients.

3.1.1 Nonneurogenic Bladder–Sphincter Dysfunction

Voiding dysfunctions are another condition in which VUR is often detected (see also chapters "Non-neurogenic Bladder-Sphincter Dysfunction ("Voiding Dysfunction")" and "Neurogenic Bladder in Infants and Children"). Nonneurogenic voiding dysfunction is a frequent disorder mostly occurring in school-age girls. Most theories hypothesize that in such patients, VUR is not primary but secondary to the bladder–sphincter dysfunction. Treatment of this type of VUR is unsuccessful unless the dysfunction is treated as well (Snodgrass 1998; Sillen 1999a).

Urodynamic studies coupled to a VCUG are mandatory for the proper management of severely affected patients (Fotter et al. 1986; Sillen 1999a; Pfister et al. 1999). On VCUG, the bladder wall appears trabeculated and thickened, diverticula may be present, the urethra is wide (so-called spinning top urethra), and the bladder neck appears tightened (Baunin et al. 1993).

3.2 Urinary Tract Infection

The relation between VUR and UTI has been largely debated (Gordon 1995). It seems that UTI does not cause VUR and that VUR does not cause UTI (Shanon and Feldman 1990), but the prevalence of VUR among children with UTI varies between 18 and 35 % (Finnell et al. 2011); so, if VUR is present, the risk for recurrence of UTI is increased (see also chapter "UTI and VUR") with renal scarring and late renal failure as consequences. As VCUG is an invasive procedure, important work has been performed aiming to define groups of children at risk to develop renal scars in which performing VCUG would be mandatory to choose the appropriate strategy. The respective roles of US and Tc^{99m}-DMSA scan were studied, but there was an important heterogeneity between studies: the age of the children and the timing performing either Tc^{99m}-DMSA or US or both were different. It is therefore not surprising that conflicting results were obtained: while Hansson suggested performing VCUG only in patients with Tc^{99m}-DMSA renal lesions (Hansson et al. 2004), Hoberman et al. concluded that Tc^{99m}-DMSA scan was not useful (Hoberman et al. 2003). Lee observed an important probability of high-grade VUR when both Tc^{99m}-DMSA scan and US were altered (Lee et al. 2009), and Bayram et al. showed that, in the absence of other risk factors for UTI, the association of mild Tc^{99m}-DMSA scarring and normal US excludes high-grade reflux (Fig. 20) (Bayram et al. 2014). Taking into account that patients with low-grade VUR have a very low risk for

Fig. 20 DMSA scan – static mode. Three incidences are usually obtained: left posterior oblique (*LPO*); posterior (*POST*); right posterior oblique (*RPO*). Scars at the left external edge of the left kidney and at the lower part of the right kidney (*arrows*)

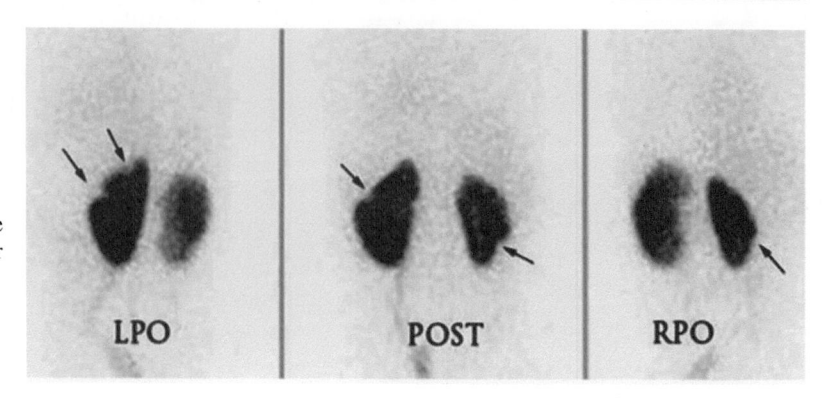

renal scarring, several authors suggested that antimicrobial prophylaxis would be unnecessary in these children (Pennesi et al. 2008; Roussey-Kesler et al. 2008; Montini and Hewitt 2009). Different guidelines were published (Awas et al. 2015; Roberts 2011; Subcommittee on Urinary Tract Infection, Steering Committee on Quality Improvement and Management 2011; Tekgul et al. 2012). Some of these recommendations are discussed by De Palma et al. (De Palma and Manzoni 2013); Springer et al. underline that these guidelines, most of which are based upon nonstandardized diagnostic procedures, do not take into account several parameters such as cost-effectiveness and quality of life (Springer and Subramanian 2014). Recently a large prospective double-blind study including more than 600 children with VUR who received either antimicrobial prophylaxis or placebo showed a significantly lower risk for recurrent UTI in the treatment group (The RIVUR trial investigators 2014; Couthard et al. 2008); the authors concluded that the "watchful waiting" approach without performing VCUG should be questioned. Still, the need for performing VCUG in the workup of febrile or of recurrent urinary tract infection remains controversial.

3.3 Familial VUR

The familial occurrence of VUR may justify the use of a screening procedure in order to detect affected siblings. For this purpose, US and direct radionuclide cystogram or ce-VUS appear to be

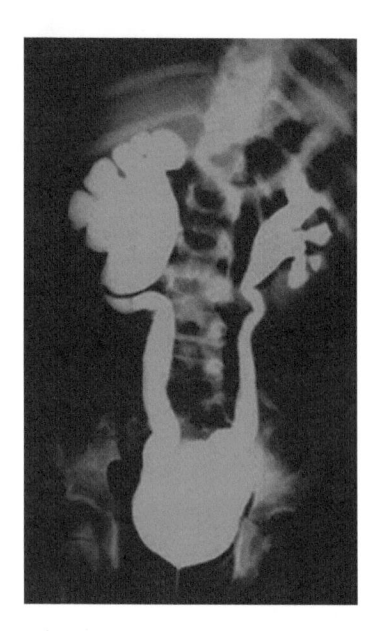

Fig. 21 Bilateral grade III VUR in a 12-year-old boy with neurogenic bladder

the most appropriate techniques (Heale 1997; Fettich et al. 2003).

3.3.1 Secondary VUR

As mentioned above, VUR may be associated with voiding dysfunction; furthermore, VUR is frequently associated with bladder outlet obstruction whatever its origin or with neurogenic bladder disorders (Figs. 21 and 22). Therefore, a VCUG is the best adapted examination for evaluating these patients; furthermore, analysis of the micturition phase and evaluation of the urethra must be part of every VCUG (Van Gool 1995).

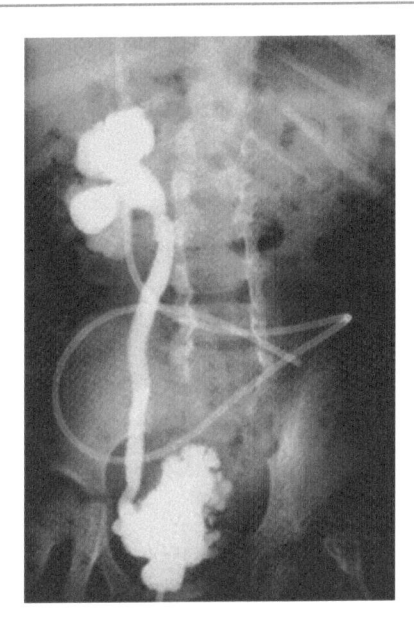

Fig. 22 Right grade III–IV VUR in an 8-year-old patient with neurogenic bladder and ventriculoperitoneal shunt

> **Take Away**
> VUR is mainly detected during the workup of congenital uropathies, UTI, and bladder dysfunction.

4 Particular Presentations of VUR

4.1 VUR and Pelvi-Ureteric Junction Obstruction

The coexistence of VUR and pelvi-ureteric junction (PUJ) obstruction (PUJO) occurs in 10–14% of patients undergoing surgery for PUJO and in 1% of patients in whom VUR is detected (Fig. 23). In these patients, proper medical management will depend upon the accuracy of the evaluation. Imaging has to differentiate between a true PUJO associated with VUR (in which case, pyeloplasty should be performed first) and a pseudo-PUJO secondary to severe VUR, in which case ureteral reimplantation should be performed first (Bomalaski et al. 1997). On the VCUG, the VUR may sometimes hardly reach the dilated pelvi-calyceal system. In case of complete obstruction, no urine will opacify the collecting system, whereas in pseudo-obstruction, some contrast will reach the dilated pelvi-calyceal system (Fig. 24). In such patients, MRU shows at best the obstructed PUJ.

4.2 VUR and UVJ Obstruction

VUR and obstruction at the ureterovesical junction (UVJ) may coexist; therefore, a VCU should be part of the workup of every dilated ureter. Also, the presence of an obstruction at the UVJ may lead to an underestimation of the degree of VUR; the refluxing contrast may show fluid levels and will dilute within the urine already present in the dilated ureter, and it may not be detected at all (Fig. 25). Furthermore, the VUR may not reach the pelvi-calyceal system due to the marked ureteral dilatation. The proper surgical management of this association, if indicated, should include ureteral modeling along with reimplantation using an antireflux procedure.

4.3 Reflux and Lithiasis

The incidence of urolithiasis among patients with VUR is approximately 0.5%, whereas the incidence of VUR among patients with lithiasis is about 8%. Any functional or anatomical abnormality of the urinary tract that favors stasis of the urine facilitates the development of lithiasis (Fig. 26). Removal of the stone alone or removal together with a ureteral reimplantation must be discussed case by case (Kraus et al. 1999).

4.4 VUR into an Unused Ureter

The normal downhill flow of urine from the kidney toward the bladder is one of the mechanisms preventing VUR. In case of diversion, renal transplant, or partial nephron-ureterectomy, urine may reflux from the bladder into the ureteral

Fig. 23 VUR and PUJO on VCUG. (**a**) During the filling phase, the renal pelvi-calyceal system appears markedly dilated compared with the mildly dilated ureter. (**b**) After micturition, the pelvi-calyceal system remains dilated above the PUJ

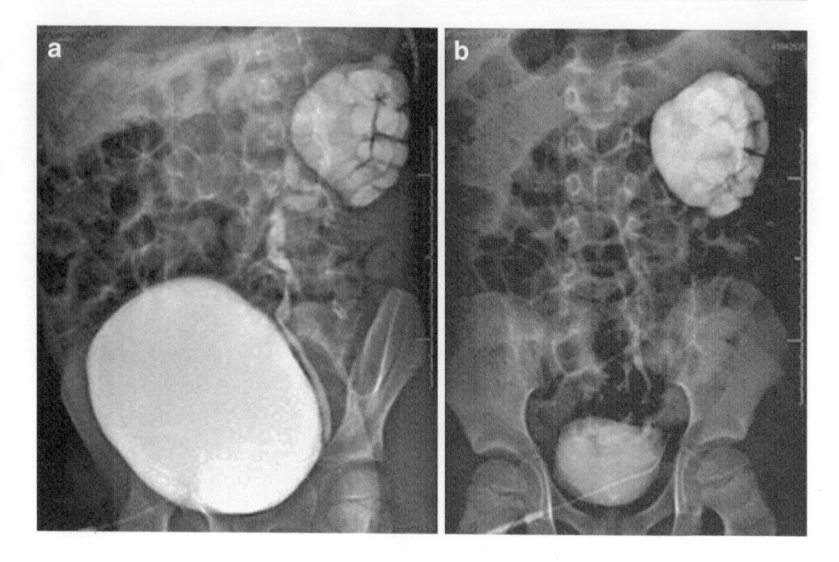

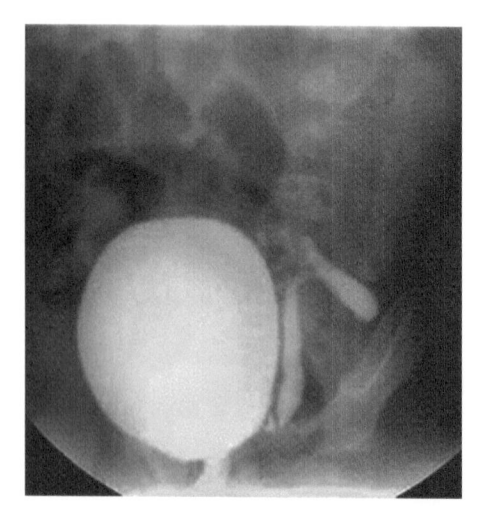

Fig. 24 VUR and PUJO. Neonatal left PUJO and VUR (antenatal diagnosis of UPJ obstruction). The refluxed urine merely reaches the dilated pelvi-calyceal system due to the severe UPJ obstruction. This could be misdiagnosed as grade I

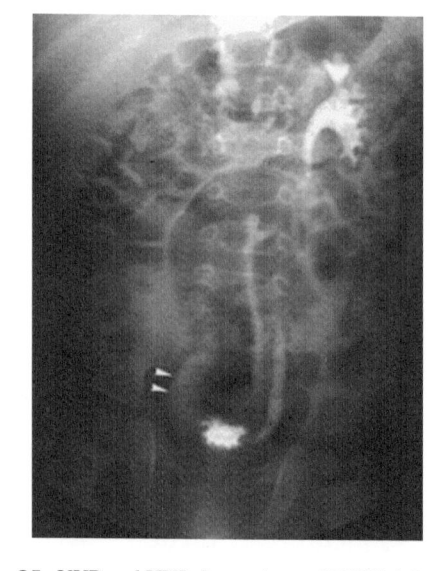

Fig. 25 VUR and UVJ obstruction; at VCUG: left grade II VUR; the right VUR is very subtle (*arrowheads*) because of the dilatation and obstruction of the ureter

stump (Cain et al. 1998). It is best visualized on VCUG, but the condition may sometimes be identified on US (Fig. 27). In most cases, no further complication occurs. Rarely, suprainfection may occur, and in such cases, the stump may have to be removed or occluded by cystoscopic injection of bulcking agents.

4.5 Yo-yo Reflux

Yo-yo VUR refers to uretero-ureteric or pyelo-pelvic reflux occurring into incomplete duplex kidneys. The urine refluxes from one collecting system to the other, and surgery, if necessary, must be aimed at preventing this passage (Gonzales 1992).

Fig. 26 VUR and lithiasis. (**a**) Plain film of the abdomen showing the lithiasis. (**b**) VCUG: left grade II

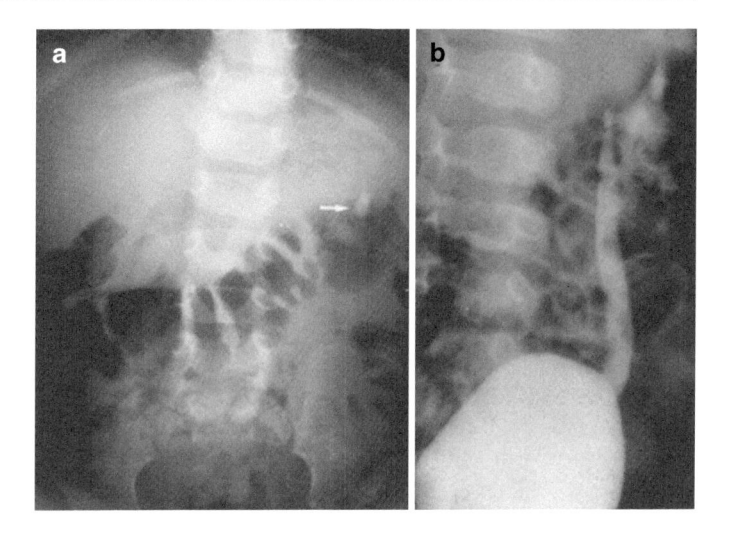

Fig. 27 VUR in unused ureter after upper pole heminephrectomy and partial ureterectomy. (**a**) On US, a dilated blind-ending ureter (*u*) is visualized behind the bladder (*B*); (**b**) On VCUG, reflux into the unused ureter

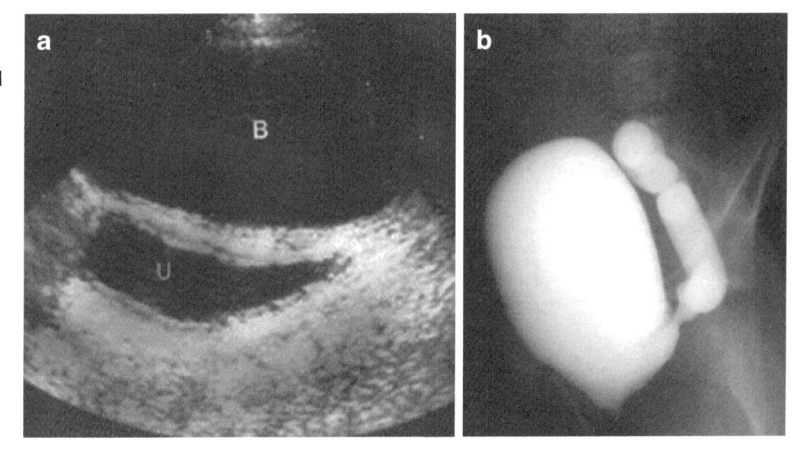

4.6 The (So-Called) Megacystis–Megaureter Association

In the megacystis–megaureter association, massive bilateral grade IV or V VUR is present. During micturition, the bladder empties normally through the urethra but also through reflux into the ureters (Fig. 28a–d). At the end of micturition, the bladder is completely empty, but only for a very short time. It refills immediately with the refluxed urine; as such, the bladder is never really empty, and the volume of urine within the bladder increases continuously. A vicious circle begins, and the bladder wall thickens progressively because of increasing voiding difficulties (Willi and Lebowitz 1979; Lebowitz and Avni 1980). This diagnosis can be made already in the fetus: a large bladder and bilateral fetal ureterohydronephrosis are present. In the megacystis–megaureter association, the amount of amniotic fluid is normal, and this helps to differentiate this entity from urinary dilatation secondary to posterior urethral valves in which oligohydramnios is more often present (Mandell et al. 1992).

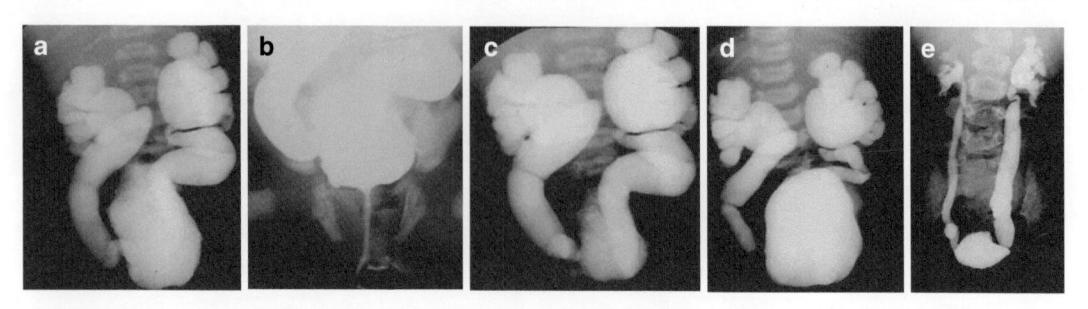

Fig. 28 VCUG, megacystis–megaureter association in a newborn girl. (**a**) Prevoiding: bilateral grade IV–V VUR. (**b**) Voiding: normal urethra. (**c**) Postvoiding: the bladder is almost empty, but the VUR has increased. (**d**) A few seconds later, the bladder has refilled with the refluxed urine. (**e**) At age 2, VUR is still present but has improved

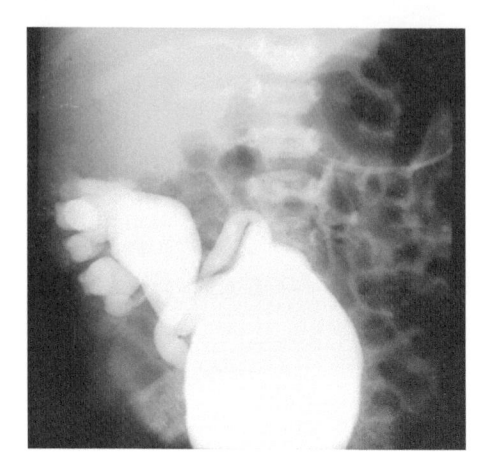

Fig. 29 Grade IV VUR into the lower pole of a right duplex system

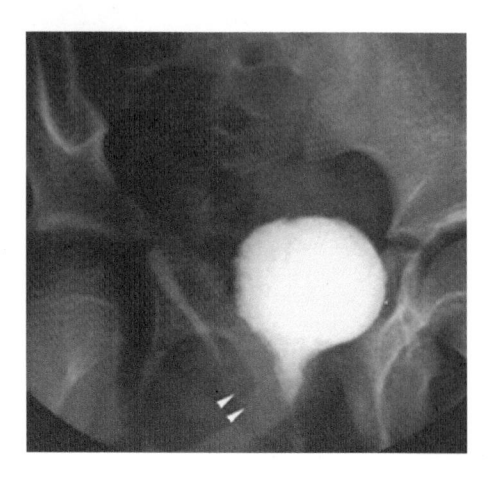

Fig. 30 VUR into a ureter that inserts at the level of the bladder neck

4.7 VUR and Duplex Kidneys

VUR may occur in both moieties of a duplex kidney, but it is much more frequent into the lower pole (Fig. 29). VUR in duplex systems is associated with the more lateral opening of the corresponding ureteral orifice. This type of VUR may be associated with renal damage at the corresponding lower moiety (reflux nephropathy; see below). Severe VUR into the lower pole system may be associated with significant urinary tract dilatation, which may obscure the presence of a duplex system. VUR into a lower moiety has a potential of spontaneous resolution just as VUR can spontaneously resolve into a single collecting system (Claudon et al. 1999).

4.8 VUR into Ectopic Ureter

VUR into an ectopic ureter that opens into the urethra or near the bladder neck may be difficult to visualize during a conventional VCUG (Fig. 30). Cyclic filling of the bladder helps to demonstrate this condition, which is usually, but not always, associated with a duplex collecting system. A single-system ectopic ureter is usually associated with a markedly dysplastic kidney.

4.9 Iatrogenic VUR

Inadvertent catheterization of a ureterocele (Ucele) during a VCU may lead to VUR into an upper pole of a duplex kidney. Reflux into an

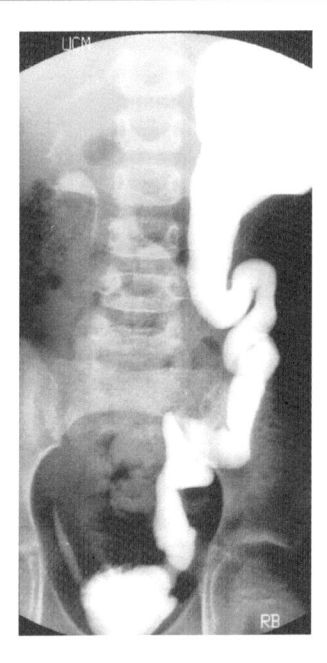

Fig. 31 Iatrogenic VUR. VUR into the left upper pole has occurred after endoscopic incision of an ectopic ureterocele

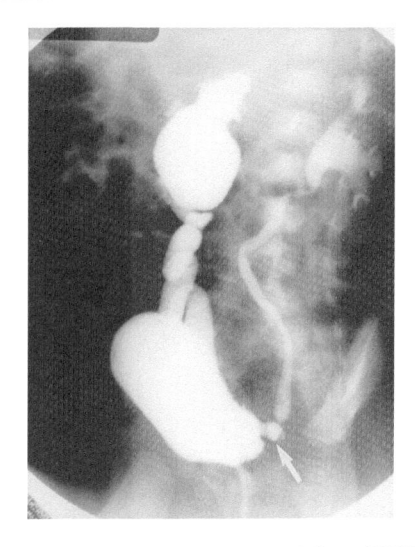

Fig. 32 VUR and bladder diverticulum. Bilateral VUR. Left grade II; a small diverticulum is also present (*arrow*)

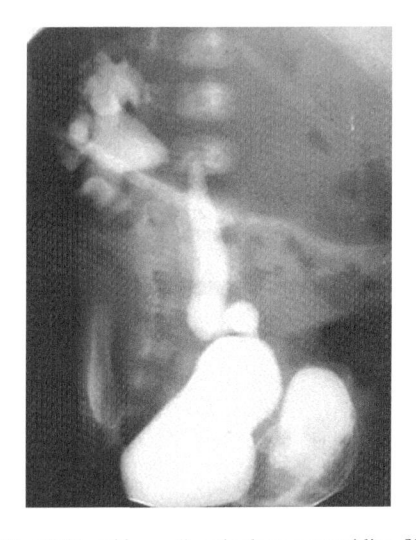

Fig. 33 VUR and large diverticulum; postvoiding film of a VCUG; a large diverticulum is filled along with the right grade III VUR

upper pole also occurs after endoscopic unroofing of an ectopic Ucele (Fig. 31) (Blyth et al. 1993).

4.10 VUR and Bladder Diverticulum

Bladder diverticulum reflects a weakness of the bladder wall. Its presence next to a ureteral orifice may lead to secondary VUR; the ureter is progressively included within the diverticulum (Figs. 32 and 33). In such a case, VUR will not resolve spontaneously and will require surgical correction (Blane et al. 1994).

4.11 VUR in case of Other Uropathies

Contralateral VUR may be present in about 10–20% of patients with multicystic dysplastic kidney (Fig. 34). VUR is also present in a significant number of other uropathies, i.e., horseshoe kidney, crossed fused kidney, PUJ, and UVJ obstruction. Therefore, a VCU should be advised for a complete workup in complicated cases (Atiyeh et al. 1992; Ring et al. 1993; Song et al. 1995; Avni et al. 1997; Cascio et al. 1999).

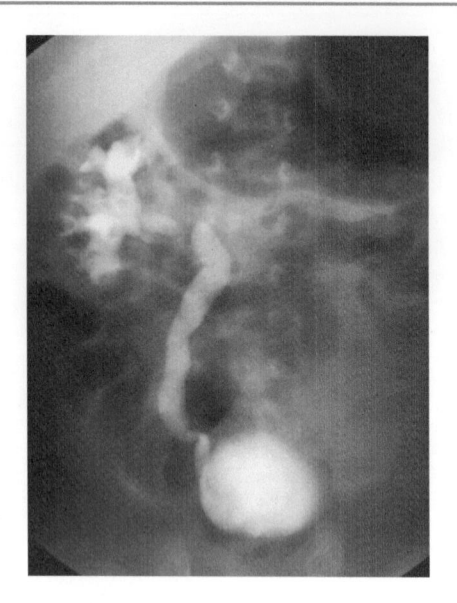

Fig. 34 Right grade II VUR in a case of a left multicystic dysplastic kidney

4.12 Fetal Reflux

Primary fetal reflux is one of the most common causes of fetal renal dilatation. As mentioned above, gross dilatation resulting from high-grade reflux occurs essentially in baby boys. In utero VUR may also be secondary and associated with bladder outlet obstruction and especially with posterior urethral valves (Kaefer et al. 1995; Sillen et al. 1992).

> **Take Away**
> VUR may be an isolated finding, but it may also be encountered in many other circumstances. Its management must be adapted to each individual presentation.

5 Natural History, Treatment, and Follow-up of VUR

5.1 Conservative Treatment

For years, the proper treatment of VUR has been controversial, and attitudes have varied (Weiss et al. 1992; Smellie et al. 1992). Antenatal diagnosis of VUR in asymptomatic patients has brought dramatic modifications in the management of VUR. In infants, several retrospective and prospective studies have shown the potential for spontaneous resolution of a large number of primary VURs (Assael et al. 1998; Yu et al. 1997; Ismaili et al. 2006a, b). Among infants, VUR tends to resolve or at least to improve markedly in 75% of the patients within 2–3 years; higher grades of VUR (grades IV–V) resolve to a lesser extent than VUR of low or moderate grades (I–III) (Fig. 28e) (Herndon et al. 1999).

Following all the data that has been accumulated, the presently accepted attitude tends much more toward medical than surgical management of VUR. Patients with high-grade VUR (III–V in boys, IV–V in girls) are placed under prophylactic antibiotherapy and followed, clinically and with imaging, up to the moment they are toilet trained. Renal growth can be monitored by US every 6–12 months; if needed renal function is controlled by Tc^{99m}-ECD or Tc^{99m}-MAG3 used simultaneously with Cr-EDTA.

The same scheme can be applied to VUR into both moieties of the duplex collecting system or into the lower pole of a duplex system.

After that the patients are toilet trained and if no complication has occurred, no further follow-up is needed (Robinson et al. 2014; Springer and Subramanian 2014; Arlen et al. 2015; Hari et al. 2015).

In older children, the attitude must be adapted to the previous history of the patient and to the clinical data. Medical treatment should be favored as much as possible. However, recurrent UTI, poor renal growth, and poor social environment would be arguments toward proposing an alternative treatment. Whenever a voiding dysfunction is also present, resolution of the VUR will be achieved only if the voiding anomaly is managed at the same time (Sillen 1999a).

5.2 Surgical Treatment

As mentioned above, surgical treatment of VUR should be considered whenever conservative treatment has not been successful or cannot be conducted satisfactorily. This includes patients in whom decreasing renal function is observed, patients presenting recurrent UTI under correct antibiotic therapy, and patients whose family members are unable to follow the conservative treatment. The presence of bladder diverticula would also require surgical treatment of VUR. In all patients with secondary VUR, proper management of the anomaly that has resulted in VUR should be considered before treating the VUR (Jodal et al. 1999; Jodal and Lindberg 1999).

US is usually sufficient for the postsurgical follow-up and demonstrates well the ureteral reimplantation; immediate postoperative dilatation is almost always present but usually transient. In any abnormal clinical course or if the dilatation increases, MRU may be necessary for the proper management of the patients in order to exclude hematoma or urinary leakage (Rypens et al. 1992).

5.2.1 Endoscopic Treatment

The injection under the ureteral orifice bulking agents has been proposed as an alternative to surgery. The results in terms of short-term VUR resolution are similar to the success rate of surgery.

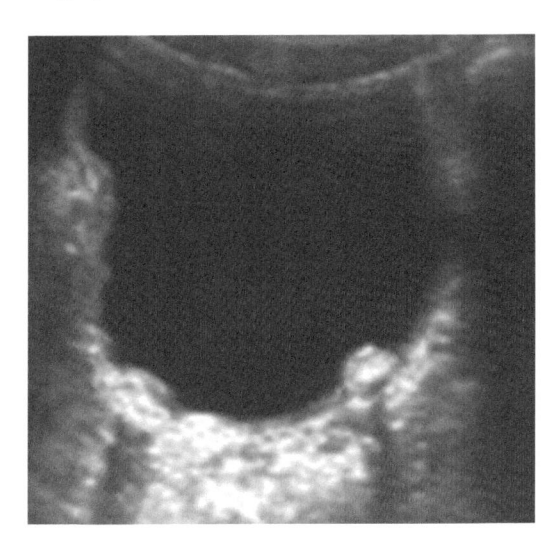

Fig. 35 Injection of antireflux bulcking material on US – transverse scan of the bladder. Echoic nodules are visible at both UVJ with acoustic shadowing

Injections should be proposed to non-resolving low-grade VUR associated with recurrent UTI.

The paste injected under the ureteral orifice is well demonstrated on US studies (Fig. 35). US studies are also helpful in order to demonstrate the rare cases of complications (persisting obstruction). In long-term studies, granuloma-like masses can be found on US studies; they appear as highly dense nodules on CT (Rypens et al. 1992; Läckgren et al. 1999; Schulman et al. 1990).

5.3 Complications of VUR

The aim in detecting VUR and initiating rapidly a prophylactic treatment is to prevent long-term complications (Arant 1991; Olbing et al. 1992; Bailey et al. 1992; Goldraich and Goldraich 1992; Merrick et al. 1995). This topic has been and remains controversial. The main concern remains understanding the factors that lead to the development of renal scars, the so-called reflux nephropathy (RN), and preventing complications such as renal hypertension, complicated pregnancies, renal failure, and finally end-stage renal disease (Jungers et al. 1996). The role of imaging is first to detect all patients at risk (having VUR or congenital dilating uropathies) and then those that have already developed RN (Jakobsson et al. 1999; Gordon 1995; Caione et al. 2004).

> **Take Away**
> VUR tends to resolve spontaneously in a large number of patients; therefore, a conservative treatment of VUR is preferable. Follow-up is achieved by US, isotopes, and optimized VCUG.

5.4 Fetal Reflux Nephropathy

It was long thought that renal scars occur only following a UTI. The antenatal diagnosis of fetal uropathies has revealed that renal damage/ dysplasia already exists at birth with no relation to UTI. In utero, VUR has deleterious effects on renal parenchyma, probably due to backward high pressure. This leads to reduced renal growth (Najmaldin et al. 1990). Many of the kidneys with fetal RN already show reduced function on isotopic studies in the neonatal period (Assael et al. 1998). On imaging, the kidney appears small and irregular with a cortical thinning (Fig. 18). The pyelocalyceal system may be dilated and clubbed. The presence of fetal RN may explain why patients with congenital uropathies that are protected by prophylactic antibiotic therapy nevertheless progress toward renal failure (Mana et al. 2004; Caione et al. 2004; Gobet et al. 1999; Stock et al. 1998).

5.5 Imaging RN and the Progression of Renal Disease

DMSA scanning is considered as the gold standard technique for the demonstration of RN lesions. DMSA has the advantage of being a low-irradiating technique with a high rate of detection of late sequelae (Fig. 20). However, it brings no information on the pelvi-calyceal system. It is less accurate in case of poor renal function. US can demonstrate the typical lesions of RN: cortical thinning and irregularities (Fig. 37). However, compared to DMSA, US is not accurate enough for assessing the number and extent of renal scars (Stokland et al. 1999). Another difficulty for US is to differentiate scars from fetal lobulation and interrenicular fat deposition. The role of US is mainly to monitor renal growth. MR urography can also display the parenchymal lesions (Koyicigit et al. 2014) (Fig. 18).

MRU has been shown to demonstrate RN. The technique appears accurate for demonstrating both the scars and the pelvi-calyceal system (Figs. 35, 36, and 37a). The technique could develop as the gold standard once it becomes more accessible (Chan et al. 1999). Some patients with RN may progress toward renal failure, as progressive glomerulosclerosis and fibrosis develop in the damaged kidney (Matsuoka et al. 1994; Bernstein and Arant 1992). Compensatory hyperfiltration may occur in less damaged areas, detectable on US studies as diffuse or localized cortical hyperechogenicity (Figs. 37b and 38) (Damry et al. 2005). These areas should not be misinterpreted as renal tumors.

Take Away
The role of imaging is to detect not only VUR but also its complications: reflux nephropathy. Presently, DMSA scanning and MRU are the best techniques available for this purpose.

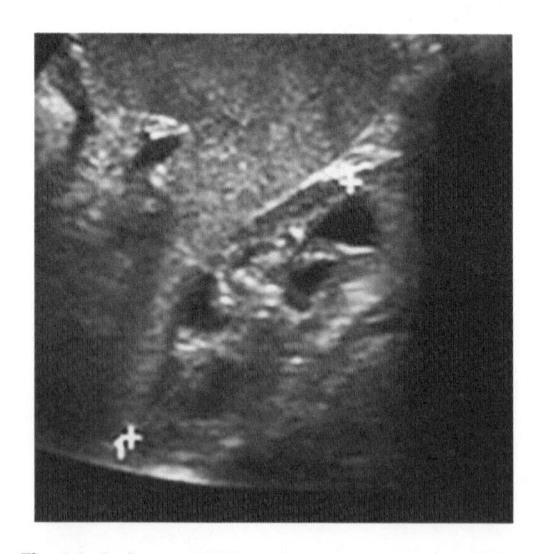

Fig. 36 Reflux and UTI nephropathy. An 8-year-old boy with long history of VUR and recurring UTI. Sagittal scan of the left kidney with irregular thinning of the parenchyma

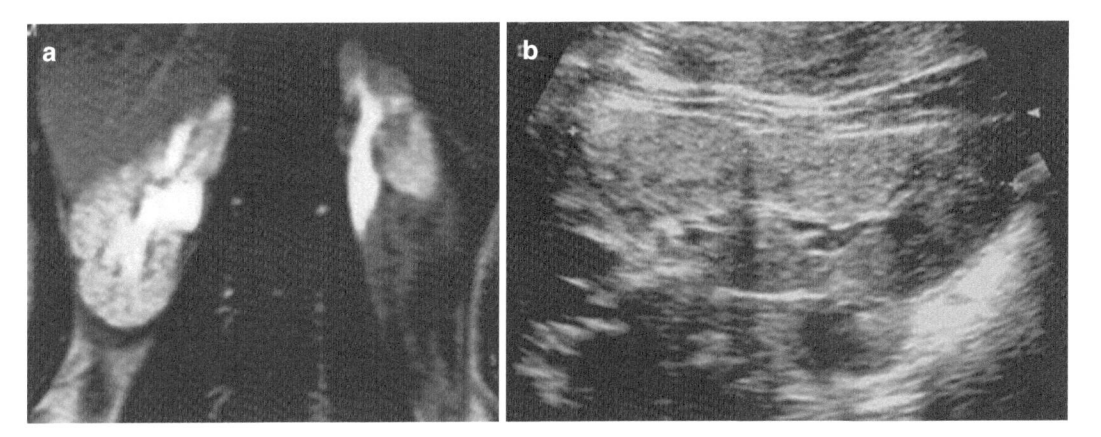

Fig. 37 Reflux nephropathy in a 9-year-old girl with known VUR and hypertension. (**a**) MRU: typical scarred kidney and clubbed pelvi-calyceal system (TFE T1 sequence with gadolinium). (**b**) US: sagittal scan of the right kidney; diffuse hyperechogenicity of the renal cortex in association with glomerular hyperfiltration

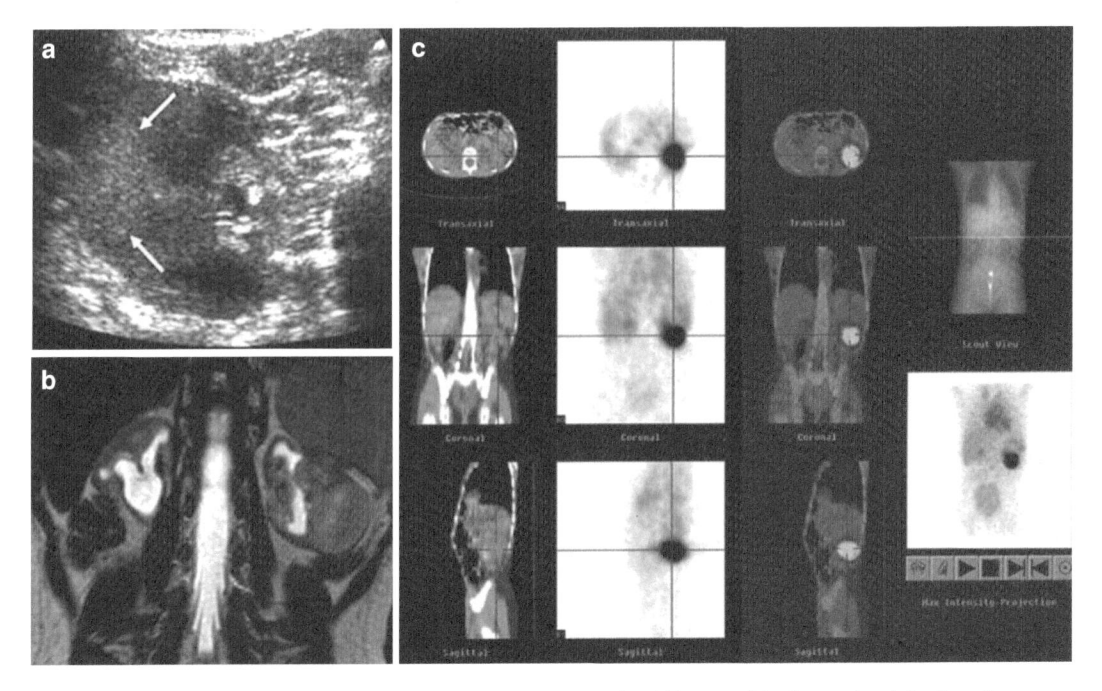

Fig. 38 Localized pseudotumoral pattern of glomerular hyperfiltration in a case of reflux nephropathy. (**a**) US: transverse scan of the left kidney; hyperechoic ill-defined area in the external part of the kidney (marked by *arrows*). (**b**) MRU: T2-weighted sequence displays bilateral small irregular kidneys with distorted pelvi-calyceal systems and a "tumoral" appearance of the left kidney. (**c**) Tc^{99m}-DMSA–SPECT-CT: the outer part of the left kidney highlights suggesting hyperfunction

Conclusion

VCUG is the main investigation that can be used in order to detect VUR. US is used for monitoring renal growth and postoperative settings; however, ce-VUS is an alternative for detecting and documenting as well as grading VUR. DMSA scan, at present, and MRU, probably more in the future, are used as complementary examinations in order to detect the patients at risk for further complications.

References

Anderson PAM, Rickwood AMK (1991) Features of primary VUR detected by prenatal US. Br J Urol 67:267–271

Arant BS (1991) VUR and renal injury. Am J Kidney Dis 17:491–511

Arlen AM, Merriman LS, Kirsch JM et al (2015) Early effects of AAP UTI guidelines on radiographic imaging and diagnosis of VUR in the emergency room setting. J Urol 193:1760–1765

Ascenti G, Zimbaro G, Mazziotti S et al (2004) Harmonic US imaging of vesicoureteric reflux in children: usefulness of a second generation US contrast agent. Pediatr Radiol 34:481–487

Assael BM, Guez S, Marra G et al (1998) Congenital reflux nephropathy: follow-up of 108 cases diagnosed perinatally. Br J Urol 82:252–257

Atiyeh B, Hussman D, Baum M (1992) Contralateral renal abnormalities in MDKD. J Pediatr 121:65–67

Avni FE, Schulman CC (1996) The origin of VUR in male newborns: further evidence in favor of a transient fetal urethral obstruction. Br J Urol 78:454–459

Avni FE, Ayadi K, Rypens F, Hall M, Schulman CC (1997) Can careful US examination of the urinary tract exclude VUR in the neonate? Br J Radiol 70:977–982

Avni FE, Hall M, Schulman CC (1998) Congenital uronephropathies: is routine VCU always warranted? Clin Radiol 53:247–250

Awas M, Rehman A, Zaman MV et al (2015) Recurrent UTI in young children: role of DMSA in detecting VUR. Pediatr Radiol 45:62–68

Bayram MT, Kavucku S, Alaygut D et al (2014) Place of ultrasonography in predicting vesicoureteral reflux in patients with mild renal scarring. Urology 83:904–908

Bailey RR, Lynn KL, Smith AH (1992) Long-term follow-up of infants with gross VUR. J Urol 148:1709–1711

Baunin C, Puget C, Moscvici J, Juskiewenski S et al (1993) Vessie immature de l'enfant: présentation d'un syndrome radiologique à partir de 138 cystographies. Rev Im Med 5:93–97

Bernstein J, Arant BS (1992) Morphological characteristics of segmental scarring in VUR. J Urol 148:1712–1714

Berrocal T, Gayá F, Arjonilla A et al (2001) Vesicoureteral reflux: diagnosis and grading with echo-enhanced cystosonography versus voiding cystourethrography. Radiology 221:359–365

Berrocal T, Gayá F, Arjonilla A (2005) Vesicoureteral reflux: can the urethra be adequately assessed by using contrast-enhanced voiding US of the bladder? Radiology 234:235–241

Blane CE, Zerin MJ, Bloom DA (1994) Bladder diverticula in children. Radiology 190:695–697

Blyth B, Passerini-Glazel G, Camuffo C et al (1993) Endoscopic incision of ureteroceles: intravesical versus ectopic. J Urol 149:556–559

Bomalaski MD, Hirschl RB, Bloom DA (1997) VUR and UPJ obstruction: association, treatment options and outcome. J Urol 157:969–974

Cain MP, Pope JC, Casale AJ et al (1998) Natural history of refluxing distal ureteral stumps. J Urol 160:1026–1027

Caione P, Villa M, Capozza N et al (2004) Predictive risk factors for chronic renal failure in primary high grade VUR. BJU Int 93:1309–1312

Cascio S, Paran S, Puri P (1999) Associated urological anomalies in children with unilateral renal agenesis. J Urol 162:1081–1083

Chan Y, Chan K, Roebuck D et al (1999) Potential utility of MRI in the evaluation of children at risk of renal scarring. Pediatr Radiol 29:856–862

Claudon M, Ben Sira L, Lebowitz RL (1999) Lower pole reflux in children: uroradiologic appearances and pitfalls. AJR Am J Roentgenol 172:795–801

Couthard MG (2008) Is reflux nephropathy preventable and will the NICE childhood UTI guidelines help. Arch Dis Child 93:196–199

Dalirani R, Mahyiar A, Sharifan M et al (2014) The value of direct radionuclide cystography in the detection of vesicoureteral reflux in children with normal voiding cystourethrography. Pediatr Nephrol 29:2341–2345

Damry N, Avni F, Guissard G et al (2005) Compensatory hypertrophy of renal parenchyma presenting as a mass lesion. Pediatr Radiol 35:832–833

Darge K, Duetting T, Zieger B et al (1998) Diagnosis of VUR with echo-enhanced voiding urosonography. Radiology 38:405–409

Darge K, Moeller RT, Trusen A et al (2005) Diagnosis of VUR with low dose contrast enhanced harmonic US imaging. Pediatr Radiol 35:73–78

Darge K, Troeger J (2002) Vesicoureteral reflux grading in contrastenhanced voiding urosonography. Eur J Radiol 43:122–128

Darge K, Troeger J, Duetting T et al (1999) Reflux in young patients: comparison of voiding US of the bladder and retrovesical space with echo enhancement versus voiding cystourethrography for diagnosis. Radiology 210(1):201–207

De Sadeleer C, De Boe V, Keuppens F et al (1994) How good is technetium-99mmercaptoacetyltriglycine indirect cystography? Eur J Nucl Med 21:223–227

De Palma D, Manzoni G (2013) Different imaging strategies in febrile urinary tract infection in childhood. What, when, why? Pediatr Radiol 43:436–443

Di Pietro MA, Blane CE, Zerin JM (1997) VUR in older children: concordance of US and VCU findings. Radiology 205:821–822

Duran C, del Riego J, Riera L et al (2012) Voiding urosonography including urethrosonography: high-quality examinations with an optimised procedure using a second-generation US contrast agent. Pediatr Radiol 42:660–667

Duran C, Valera A, Alguersuari A et al (2009) Voiding urosonography: the study of the urethra is no longer a limitation of the technique. Pediatr Radiol 39:124–131

Fernbach SK, Feinstein KA, Schmidt MB (2000) Pediatric VCU: a pictorial guide. Radiographics 20:155–168

Fettich J, Colarinha P, Fischer S et al (2003) Guidelines for direct radionuclide cystography in children under the auspices of the paediatric committee of the European association of nuclear medicine. Eur J Nucl Med 30(5):B39–B44

Finnell SME, Carroll AE, Downs SM, Subcommittee on Urinary Tract Infection (2011) Diagnosis and management of an initial UTI in febrile infants and young children. Pediatrics 128:e749–e770

Fotter R, Kopp W, Klein E et al (1986) Unstable bladder in children: functional evaluation by modified VCU. Radiology 161:811–813

Garin EH, Campos A, Homsy Y (1998) Primary VUR: review of current concepts. Pediatr Nephrol 12:249–256

Gelfand MJ, Koch BL, Elgazzar AH et al (1999) Cyclic cystography: diagnostic yield in selected pediatric populations. Radiology 213:118–120

Gobet R, Cisek LJ, Chang B et al (1999) Experimental fetal VUR induces renal tubular and glomerular damage and is associated with persistent bladder instability. J Urol 162:1090–1095

Goldraich N, Goldraich IH (1992) Follow-up of conservatively treated children with high- and low-grade VUR: a prospective study. J Urol 148:1688–1692

Gonzales ET (1992) Anomalies of the renal pelvis and ureter. In: Kelalis PP, King L, Belman AB (ed) Clinical pediatric urology, 3rd edn. Saunders, Philadelphia, p 530–579.

Goonasekera CDA, Dillon MJ (1999) Hypertension in reflux nephropathy. Br J Urol 83 [Suppl]:1–12

Gordon I (1995) VUR, UTI and renal damage in children. Lancet 346:489–490

Gordon I, Colarinha P, Fettich J et al (2001) Guidelines for indirect radionuclide cystography. Under the auspices of the paediatric committee of the European association of nuclear medicine. Eur J Nucl Med 28:BP16–BP20

Hari P, Hari S, Sinha A et al (2015) Antibiotic prophylaxis in the management of VUR Pediatr Nephrol 2015;30:479–486

Hansson S, Dhamey M, Sigstrom O et al (2004) Dimercapto-Succinic Acid scintigraphy instead of voiding cystourethrography for infants with urinary tract infection. J Urol 172:1071–1074

Heale WF (1997) Hereditary VUR: phenotypic variation and family screening. Pediatr Nephrol 11:504–507

Hellström M, Jacobsson B (1999) Diagnosis of vesicoureteric reflux. Acta Pediatr 431(Suppl):1–12

Herndon CDA, McKenna PH, Kolon TF et al (1999) A multicenter outcomes analysis of patients with neonatal VUR presenting with prenatal hydronephrosis. J Urol 162:1203–1205

Hernandez RH, Goodsitt M (1996) Reduction of radiation dose in pediatric patients using pulsed fluoroscopy. AJR Am J Roentgenol 167:1247–1253

Hiraoka M, Kasuga K, Hori C et al (1994) US indicators of VUR in the newborn. Lancet 343:519–520

Hiraoka M, Hashimoto G, Hori C et al (1997) Use of US in the detection of VUR in children suspected of having UTI. J Clin Ultrasound 25:195–199

Hoberman A, Charron M, Hickey RW et al (2003) Imaging studies after a febrile urinary tract infection in young children. N Engl J Med 348:195–202

Hulbert WC, Rosenberg HK, Cartwright PC et al (1992) The predictive value of US in evaluation of infants with posterior urethral valves. J Urol 148:122–124

Ismaili K, Avni FE, Piepsz A et al (2006) VUR in children. EAU-EBU update series 4, European Urology Publ p 129–140

Ismaili K, Hall M, Piepsz A et al (2006b) Primary VUR detected in neonates with a history of fetal renal pelvis dilatation. J Pediatr 148:222–227

Jakobsson B, Jacobson SG, Hjälmas K (1999) VUR and other risk factors for renal damage: identification of high- and low-risk children. Acta Paediatr 431 [Suppl]:31–39. Jacobsson SH, Hansson S, Jakobsson B (1999) Vesico-ureteric reflux: occurrence and long-term risks. Acta Paediatr 431 [Suppl]: 22–30

Jodal U, Lindberg U (1999) Guidelines for management of children with UTI and VUR. Recommendations from a Swedish state of the art conference. Acta Paediatr 431(Suppl):87–89

Jodal U, Hansson S, Hjälmas K (1999) Medical or surgical management for children with VUR. Acta Pediatr 431(Suppl):53–61

Jungers P, Houilier P, Chauveau D et al (1996) Pregnancy in women with reflux nephropathy. Kidney Int 50:393–399

Kaefer M, Keating MA, Adams MC et al (1995) Posterior urethral valves, pressure pop-off and bladder function. J Urol 154:708–711

Kis E, Nyitrai A, Várkonyi I et al (2010) Voiding urosonography with 2nd generation contrast agent versus voiding cystourethrography. Pediatr Nephrol 25:2289–2293

Kleinman PK, Diamond DA, Karellas A et al (1994) Tailored low-dose fluoroscopic VCU for the reevaluation of VUR in girls. AJR Am J Roentgenol 162:1151–1154

Koff SA (1992) Relationship between dysfunctional voiding and reflux. J Urol 148:1703–1706

Koyicigit A, Yuksel S, Bayram R et al (2014) Efficacy of MRU in detecting renal scars in children with VUR. Pediatr Nephrol 29:1215–122O

Kraus SJ, Lebowitz RL, Royal SA (1999) Renal calculi in children. Pediatr Radiol 29:624–630

Läckgren G, Wählin N, Sternberg A (1999) Endoscopic treatment of children with VUR. Acta Paediatr 431(Suppl):62–71

Lebowitz RL, Avni EF (1980) Misleading appearances in pediatric uroradiology. Pediatr Radiol 10:15–31

Lebowitz RL, Olbing H, Parkkulainen KV et al (1985) International Reflux Study in children: international system of radiographic grading of vesico-ureteric reflux. Pediatr Radiol 15:105–109

Lee RS, Cendron R, Kinnamon DD et al (2006a) Antenatal hydronephrosis as a prediction of postnatal outcome: a meta-analysis. Pediatrics 118:586–593

Lee H, Hyun Soh B, Hee Hong C et al (2009) The efficacy of ultrasound and dimercaptosuccinic acid scan in predicting vesicoureteral reflux in children below the age of 2 years with their first febrile urinary tract infection. Pediatr Nephrol 24:2009–2013

Lee RS, Diamond DA, Chow JS (2006b) Applying the ALARA concept to the evaluation of vesicoureteric reflux. Pediatr Radiol 36(Suppl 2):185–191

Leroy S, Vantalon S, Larabek A, Ducou Lepointe H, Bensman A (2010) VUR in children with UTI: comparison of diagnostic accuracy of renal US. Radiology 255:890–898

Mana G, Oppezzo C, Ardissino G et al (2004) Severe VUR and chronic renal failure. J Pediatr 144:677–681

Mandell J, Lebowitz RL, Peters CA et al (1992) Prenatal diagnosis of the megacystis-megaureter association. J Urol 148:1487–1489

Marra G, Barbieri G, Moioli C et al (1994) Mild fetal hydronephrosis indicating VUR. Arch Dis Child 70:147–150

Matsumo T, Fukushima Motoyama H, Higushi E et al (1996) Color flow imaging for detection of VUR. Lancet 347:757

Matsuoka H, Oshima K, Sakamoto K et al (1994) Renal pathology in patients with reflux nephropathy. Eur Urol 26:153–159

Mentzel HJ, Vogt S, Patzer L et al (1999) Contrast-enhanced sonography of VUR in children: primary results. AJR Am J Roentgenol 173:737–740

Merrick M, Notghi A, Chalmers N et al (1995) Long-term follow-up to determine the prognostic value of imaging after UTI. 1. Reflux. Arch Dis Child 72:388–392

Montini G, Hewitt I (2009) Urinary tract infection: to prophylaxis or not to prophylaxis. Pediatr Nephrol 24:1605–1609

Mozley PD, Heyman S, Duckett JW et al (1994) Direct vesicoureteral scintigraphy: quantifying early outcome predictors in children with primary reflux. J Nucl Med 35:1602–1608

Najmaldin A, Burge DM, Atwell JD (1990) Fetal VUR. Br J Urol 65:403–406

Newell SJ, Morgan ME, McHugo JM (1990) Clinical significance of antenatal calyceal dilatation detected by US. Lancet 336:372

Olbing H, Claësson I, Ebel K et al (1992) Renal scars and parenchymal thinning in children with VUR. J Urol 148:1653–1656

Papadopoulou F, Efremidis SC, Oiconomou A et al (2002) Cycling VCU: is VUR missed with standart VCU. Eur Radiol 12:666–670

Papadopoulou F, Tsampoulas C, Siomou E et al (2006) Cyclic contrast-enhanced Urosonography for the evaluation of reflux. Can we keep the cost of the examination low? Eur Radiol 16(11):2521–2526

Papadopoulou F, Evangelou E, Riccabona M et al (2012) Contrast enhanced voiding urosonography for diagnosis of vesicoureteric reflux in comparison to conventional methods: a meta-analysis. ECR Book of Abstracts, Insights Imaging 3:SS 1712, B-0860

Papadopoulou F, Ntoulia A, Siomou E, Darge K (2014) ce- VUS with intravesical administration of a second-generation US contrast agent for diagnosis of VUR: propspective evaluation of contrast safety in 1,010 children. Pediatr Radiol 44:719–728

Pennesi M, Travan L, Peratoner L et al (2008) Is antibiotic prophylaxis in children with vesicoureteral reflux effective in preventing pyelonephritis and renal scars? A randomized controlled trial. Pediatrics 121:1489–1494

Pfister C, Dacher JN, Gaucher S et al (1999) The usefulness of a minimal urodynamic evaluation and pelvic floor feedback in children with chronic voiding dysfunction. BJU Int 84:1054–1057

Piepsz A, Ham HR (2006) Pediatric applications of renal nuclear medicine. Semin Nucl Med 36:16–35

Ransley PG, Risdon RA (1975) Renal papillary morphology and intrarenal reflux in young pigs. Urol Res 3:105–109

Riccabona M (2002) Cystography in children and infants. Eur Radiol 12:2910–2918

Riccabona M, Avni FE, Damasio MB et al (2012) ESPR Uroradiology Task Force and ESUR Paediatric Working Group–Imaging recommendations in paediatric uroradiology, part V: childhood cystic kidney disease, childhood renal transplantation and contrast-enhanced ultrasonography in children. Pediatr Radiol 42(10):1275–1283

Riccabona M, Avni FE, Blickman JG et al (2008) Imaging recommendations in paediatric uroradiology: minutes of the ESPR workgroup session on urinary tract infection, fetal hydronephrosis, urinary tract ultrasonography and voiding cystourethrography, Barcelona, Spain, June 2007. Pediatr Radiol 38(2):138–145

Ring E, Peritsch P, Riccabona M et al (1993) Primary VUR in infants with a dilated fetal urinary tract. Eur J Pediatr 152:523–525

Robben SGE, Boesten M, Linmans J et al (1999) Significance of thickening of the wall of the renal collecting system in children an US study. Pediatr Radiol 29:736–740

Roberts KB (2011) Urinary tract infection: clinical practice guideline for the diagnosis and management of the initial UTI in febrile infants and children 2 to 24 months. Pediatrics 128:595–610

Robinson JL, Finlay JC, Lang ME et al (2014) UTI in infants and children: diagnosis and management. Paediatr Child Health 19:315–325

Rolleston GL, Maling TMJ, Hodson CJ (1974) Intrarenal reflux and the scarred kidney. Arch Dis Child 49:531–539

Roussey-Kesler G, Gadjos V, Idres N et al (2008) Antibiotic prophylaxis for the prevention of recurrent urinary tract infection in children with low-grade vesicoureteral reflux: results from a prospective randomized study. J Urol 179:674–679

Rypens F, Avni F, Bank WO et al (1992) The ureterovesical junction in children: US findings after surgical or endoscopic treatment. AJR Am J Roentgenol 158:837–842

Salih M, Baltaci S, Kilic S et al (1994) Color flow Doppler US in the diagnosis of VUR. Eur Urol 26:93–97

Schulman CC, Pamart D, Hall M et al (1990) VUR in children: endoscopic management. Eur Urol 17:314–317

Shanon A, Feldman W (1990) Methodologic limitations in the literature on VUR: a critical review. J Pediatr 117:171–178

Sillen U (1999a) Bladder dysfunction in children with VUR. Acta Paediatr 431(Suppl):40–47

Sillen U (1999b) VUR in infants. Pediatr Nephrol 13:355–361

Sillen U, Hjalmas K, Aili M et al (1992) Pronounced detrusor hypercontractibility in infants with gross bilateral VUR. J Urol 148:598–599

Smellie JM, Tamminen-Mobius T, Olbing H et al (1992) International reflux study in children 5-year study of medical or surgical treatment in children with severe reflux: radiological renal findings. Pediatr Nephrol 6:223–230

Snodgrass W (1998) The impact of treated dysfunctional voiding on the non-surgical management of VUR. J Urol 160:1823–1825

Song JT, Ritchey ML, Zerin JM, Bloom DA (1995) Incidence of VUR in children with unilateral renal agenesis. J Urol 153:1249–1251

Springer A, Subramanian R (2014) Relevance of current guidelines in the management of VUR. Eur J Pediatr 173:835–843

Stock JA, Wilson D, Hanna MN (1998) Congenital reflux nephropathy and severe unilateral reflux. J Urol 160:1017–1018

Stocks A, Richards D, Frentzen B et al (1996) Correlation of prenatal renal pelvic antero-posterior diameter with outcome in infancy. J Urol 155:1050–1052

Stokland E, Hellström M, Jakobsson B et al (1999) Imaging of renal scarring. Acta Paediatr Scand 431(Suppl):13–21

Strehlau J, Winkler P, de la Roche J (1997) The ureterovesical jet as a functional diagnostic tool in childhood hydronephrosis. Pediatr Nephrol 11:460–467

Subcommittee on Urinary Tract Infection, Steering Committee on Quality Improvement and Management (2011) Urinary tract infection: clinical practice guideline for the diagnosis and management of the initial UTI in febrile infants and children 2 to 24 months. Pediatrics 128:595–610

Tekgul S, Riedmiller H, Hoebeke P et al (2012) EAU guidelines on vesicoureteral reflux in children. Eur Urol 62:534–542

The RIVUR trial investigators (2014) Antimicrobial prophylaxis for children with vesicoureteral reflux. N Engl J Med 370:2367–2376

Thomson AS, Dabhoiwala NF, Verbeek FJ et al (1994) The functional anatomy of the ureterovesical junction. Br J Urol 73:284–291

Tsai JD, Huang FY, Tsai TC (1998) Asymptomatic VUR detected by neonatal US screening. Pediatr Nephrol 12:206–209

Unver T, Alpay H, Biyikli NK et al (2006) Comparison of direct radionuclide cystography and voiding cystourethrography in detecting vesicoureteral reflux. Pediatr Int 48:287–291

Van Eerde AM, Mertgent MH, De Jong TPVM et al (2007) VUR in children with prenatally detected hydronephrosis. Ultrasound Obstet Gynecol 29:463–469

Van Gool JD (1995) Dysfunctional voiding: a complex of bladder-sphincter dysfunction, urinary tract infections and VUR. Acta Urol Belg 63:27–33

Vassiou K, Vlychou M, Moisidou R et al (2004) Contrast enhanced US detection of VUR in children. Rofo 176:1453–1457

Verrier-Jones K (1999) Prognosis for vesico-ureteric reflux. Arch Dis Child 81:287–294

Walsh G, Dubbins PA (1996) Antenatal renal pelvis dilatation: a predictor of VUR? AJR Am J Roentgenol 167:897–900

Wan J, Greenfield SP, Ng M et al (1996) Sibling reflux: a dual center retrospective study. J Urol 156677–679

Ward VL, Strauss KJ, Barnewolt CE et al (2008) Pediatric radiation exposure and effective dose reduction during voiding cystourethrography. Radiology 249:1002–1009

Weiss R, Tamminen-Möbius T, Koskimies O et al (1992) Characteristics at entry of children with severe primary reflux recruited for a multicenter international therapeutic trial comparing medical and surgical management. J Urol 148:1644–1649

Willi U, Lebowitz RL (1979) The so-called megauretermegacystis syndrome. AJR Am J Roentgenol 133:409–416

Yeung CK, Godley ML, Dhillon HK et al (1997) The characteristics of primary VUR in male and female infants with prenatal hydronephrosis. Br J Urol 80:319–327

Yu TJ, Chen W, Chen HY (1997) Early versus late surgical management of fetal reflux nephropathy. J Urol 157:1416–1419

Zerin M, Ritchey M, Chang A (1993) Incidental VUR in neonates with antenatally detected hydronephrosis and other renal abnormalities. Radiology 187:157–160

Postoperative Imaging and Findings

Michael Riccabona, Josef Oswald, and Veronica Donoghue

Contents

1	Introduction..	517
2	**Pelvi-ureteric Junction Obstruction (PUJO)**..	518
3	**Congenital Disorders of the Ureter**..............	522
3.1	Non-refluxing Primary Megaureter/ Uretero-vesical Junction Obstruction (UVJO)...	522
3.2	Ureteric Duplication, Ureteric Ectopia, and Associated Anomalies...............................	523
4	**Congenital Anomalies of the Urinary Bladder**...	525
4.1	Congenital Anomalies of the Urethra...............	526
4.2	Vesicoureteric Reflux...	529
5	**Oncological Surgery**.......................................	530
6	**Renal Stone Disease**.......................................	531
	Conclusion..	532
	References..	532

M. Riccabona (✉)
Department of Radiology, Division of Pediatric Radiology, University Hospital LKH Graz, Graz, Austria
e-mail: michael.riccabona@klinikum-graz.at

J. Oswald, FEAPU
Department of Pediatric Urology, Hospital of the Sisters of Charity, Linz, Austria

V. Donoghue, FRCR, FFR.RCSI
Departments of Radiology, Temple Street Children's University Hospital, Dublin, Ireland

National Maternity Hospital, Holles Street, Dublin, Ireland

1 Introduction

The practice of pediatric urology and uroradiology has changed a great deal in recent years. The increase in the clinical use of antenatal ultrasonography (US) and its ability to provide anatomic information about the developing fetus has led to the growth and development of perinatal urology. There has been a significant increase in the number of genitourinary anomalies diagnosed in the prenatal and newborn period, and greater attention is paid to postnatal assessment, diagnosis, and management, including follow-up imaging of these infants. The urological conditions requiring surgery are varied, but the abnormalities that require the most frequent surgical intervention are those that give rise to urinary tract dilatation/distention (UTD). This chapter aims at discussing the short- and long-term postoperative follow-up of common situations including assessment of complications and long-term monitoring; rarer conditions or aspects that are addressed in other chapters of this book (e.g., prune-belly syndrome, renal transplantation, etc.) are omitted and not addressed again.

Following surgery, imaging may be required in three situations: to evaluate the success of the procedure, to assess potential (early) operative complications, and to monitor the subsequent progress of the treated condition. Depending on the underlying condition, all imaging modalities may be required. However, a comprehensive US is the first and often the only imaging tool required.

2 Pelvi-ureteric Junction Obstruction (PUJO)

The pelvi-ureteric junction (PUJ) is by far the most common site of urinary obstruction in children (see also Chaps. 14, 15, and 26) (O'Flynn KJ et al. 1993). When the diagnosis has been made antenatally, improvement or resolution of the "hydronephrosis" (HN) /urinary tract distension/dilatation (UTD) occurs in approximately 30 % of infants (Arnold and Rickwood 1990; Freedman and Rickwood 1994) or more. These and other considerations have led to a more conservative approach to the surgical management of PUJO. Still it is rather challenging to determine which cases of fetal UTD are caused by a significant PUJO stenosis which would benefit from surgery in contrary to a simple dilatation unlikely to cause significant morbidity. The clear indications for active intervention are:

- Impaired renal function. Less than 40 % of the differential function in a unilateral lesion is the general consensus for surgical intervention, or deteriorating function during surveillance; some particularly European centers also see a deteriorating obstructive drainage pattern on MAG3 diuretic scintigraphy or diuretic MR urography as an indication (Gordon et al. 2011).
- Clinical symptoms (pain, infection, hematuria, etc.)
- Complications such as renal calculi or hypertension

Active intervention usually means surgical relief of the obstruction, though there have been some reports of successful balloon dilatation of the PUJ (Wilkinson and Azimy 1996; Doraiswamy 1994; McClinton et al. 1993). The usual outcome (e.g., of such an experimental balloon dilatation) in infants who have unilateral obstruction and where the function of the obstructed kidney is severely compromised at less than 20 % differential function is a kidney that still functions poorly, though perhaps a little less poorly than preoperatively. Sometimes renal function declines further despite technically satisfactory surgery, presumably due to significant vascular changes intrarenally (Grapin et al. 1990). Functional recovery is less likely if the affected kidney is small and the contralateral kidney has undergone compensatory hypertrophy (Koff and Campbell 1992). Percutaneous nephrostomy drainage can be performed in these patients if infected (otherwise the outcome is very poor) and the function reassessed after 4–6 weeks (Fig. 1); nephrectomy is usually the treatment of choice when the function remains poor (Ransley et al. 1990). Percutaneous nephrostomy drainage is also the initial treatment of choice in infants who present with a pyonephrosis before proceeding to surgical correction.

Open pyeloplasty is the usual procedure to correct pelvi-ureteric junction obstruction (see Chaps. 14 and 15). Postoperative drainage may be carried out by extra-anastomotic drainage, nephrostomy with a transanastomotic splint, or a double J pyelovesical stent – the latter being the presently most favored approach in severely dilated kidneys to avoid additional parenchymal damage (Fig. 2). A nephrostography through the extra- or trans-anastomotic stent drain can be performed approximately 7–10 days postoperatively to assess satisfactory drainage down the ureter prior to removal of the drain; an infusion technique can be used with an estimated pressure which will also give information on the leak pressure (Fig. 3). However, today mostly the pyeloplasty catheter is blocked after 6 days and then removed, if the dilatation remains unchanged (documented by US). Nephrostography can also become indicated for assessing urinomas and extravasation/leakage. Early complications are uncommon and usually comprise prolonged urinary drainage where extra-anastomotic drainage has been employed or delayed drainage at the anastomosis site where a nephrostomy plus transanastomotic splint has been used though this latter technique is outdated. Sometimes dislocation of a JJ stent may occur; this can be assessed by US (Fig. 4). Persistence of either complication more than 2 weeks postoperatively can often be treated by retrograde passage of a ureteric catheter. On occasions, part of the renal pelvis may be resected, and in these patients, a reduction in the size of the renal pelvis seen on US does not necessarily imply the success of the procedure. In addition, while a

Postoperative Imaging and Findings

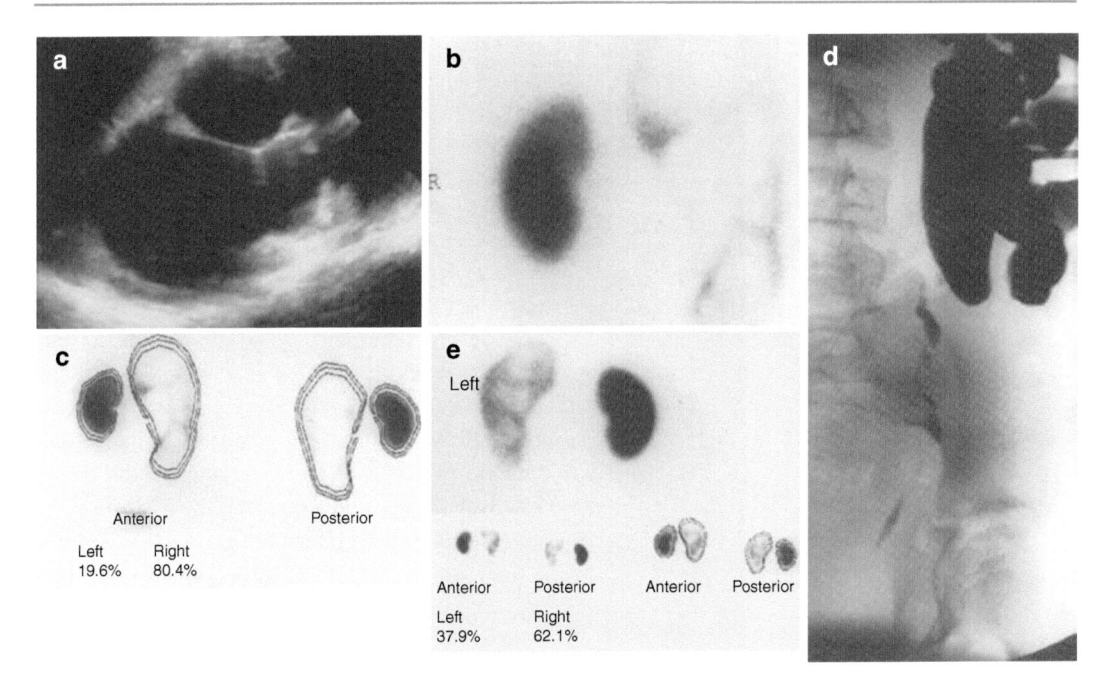

Fig. 1 (**a**) US shows very marked UTD with a thin cortical rim. (**b, c**) DSMA renal scintigraphy shows an enlarged left kidney with very thin rim of functioning renal tissue. The percentage uptake of the radiopharmaceutical on the *left side* is 19.6%. (**d**) Nephrostogram outlining a UTD with drainage down the ureter 4 weeks after nephrostomy drainage. (**e**) DMSA scan 4 weeks after nephrostomy drainage. There is an improvement in left kidney function to 37.91%

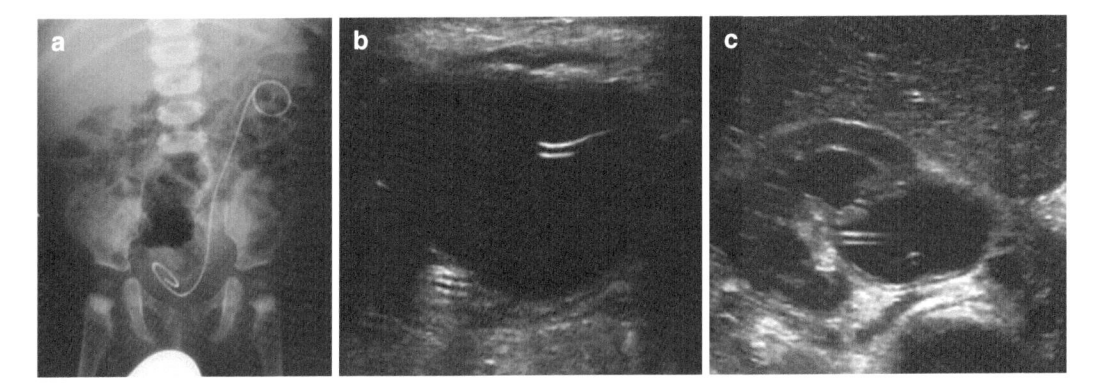

Fig. 2 Double J pyelo-vesical stent in position after open pyeloplasty (**a**) KUB film. (**b**) US of the bladder with the lower end and (**c**) US of the kidney with the upper end of the JJ stent (*arrows*)

postoperative drainage system is in place, obtaining pelvi-caliceal width measurements is not an accurate means of assessing persistent drainage impairment. The renal calices may remain sonographically wide for months and years following surgery, despite excellent drainage, as they have been dilated for a long period of time and may only gradually normalize during future growth.

If significant anastomotic failure is present, retrograde balloon dilatation (McClinton et al. 1993; Wilkinson and Azimy 1996) with insertion of a JJ catheter for a longer period or reoperation in rare cases is carried out. Neither procedure is advisable before 1 month postoperatively, and in the interim, the kidney can – if necessary – be drained by percutaneous nephrostomy or if possible by a JJ catheter. Rarer postoperative complications include urinomas following anastomotic leaks and hemorrhagic collections. These can usually be monitored with US. As the vasculature of the kidney can be variable and anomalous, care must be taken during surgery not to damage the blood supply – particularly in aberrant (e.g., lower pole) vessels causing an extrinsic PUJ stenosis. If this is suspected, it can be monitored with US (amplitude-coded) color and spectral Doppler studies, or even contrast-enhanced US (Fig. 4d–f).

In general, assessment of outcome following pyeloplasty is performed at approximately 6 months following reconstructive surgery.

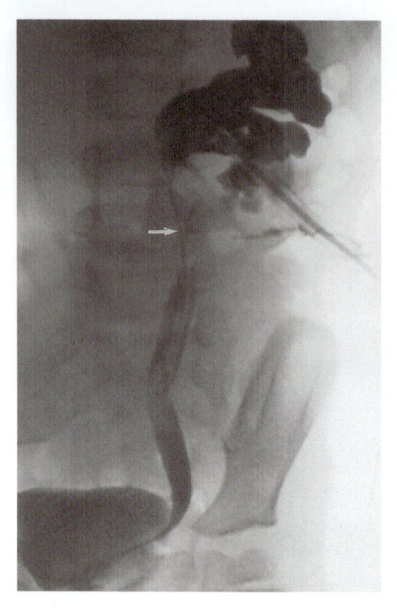

Fig. 3 Nephrostogram through a nephrostomy catheter after pyeloplasty. Contrast flows down the ureter. Trans-anastomotic splint in position (*arrow*)

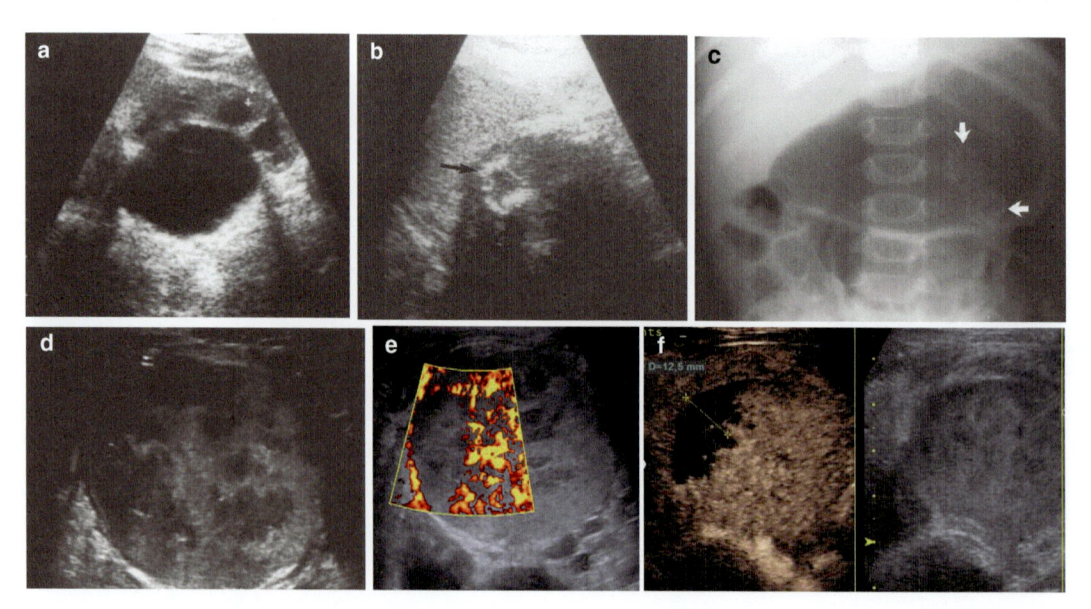

Fig. 4 (**a**) US demonstrating marked dilatation of the renal pelvis with dilatation of the calyces in a child with pelvi-ureteric junction obstruction. (**b**) US 1 month after open pyeloplasty. There was damage to the kidney blood supply at surgery. The kidney is shrunken and is replaced by a rim of increased echogenicity compatible with calcification (*arrow*). (**c**) Plain radiography confirming a shrunken left kidney replaced by calcification (*white arrows*). (**d–f**) postoperative imaging in a child with vascular injury of one of the multiple arteries (*g* gray scale image, *h* power Doppler image that shows the lack of perfusion, and *i* contrast-enhanced US confirms the necrotic, non-perfused area+…+)

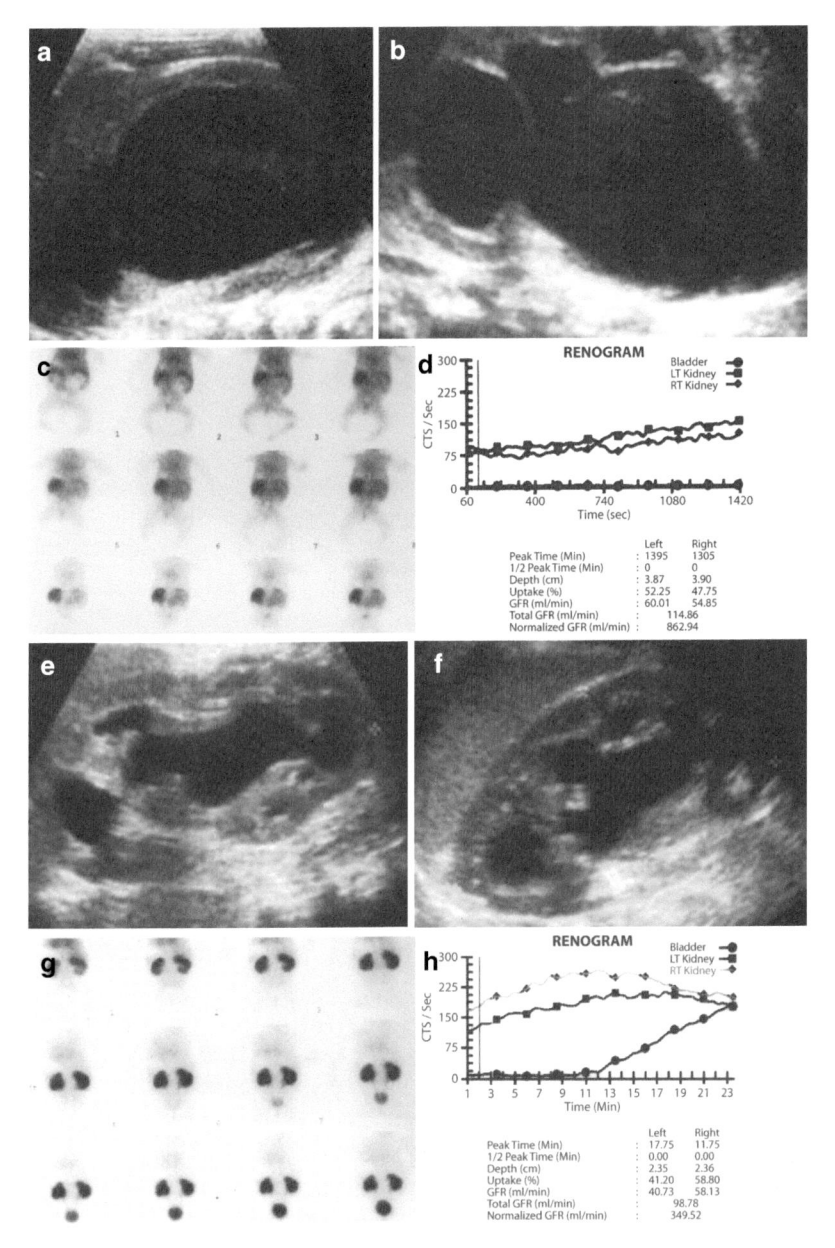

Fig. 5 (a) Right kidney and (b) left kidney outlining bilateral UPJO by US. There is dilatation of the calyces and renal pelvis on both sides. (c, d) Preoperative Tc 99m DTPA scintigraphy showing poor uptake of the radiopharmaceutical bilaterally with no significant detectable excretion. (e) Right kidney and (f) left kidney after pyeloplasty. On US there is a significant reduction in the degree of UTD and an increase in cortical thickness. (g, h) Postoperative Tc 99m MAG 3 renogram 1 year after operation. There is improved function in both kidneys, more on the right than on the left side, with an improvement in excretion

A significant reduction in the degree of UTD and an increase in the parenchymal thickness on US are good indicators of successful surgery (Fig. 5), but the absence of this finding does not necessarily indicate a persistent obstruction (Kis et al. 1998). The use of the IVU to assess postoperative relief of obstruction has largely been replaced by dynamic nuclear scintigraphy using Tc^{99m} MAG 3 or functional diuretic MR urography (fMRU) (Fig. 5). However, in the presence of massive UTD, where there is significantly impaired renal function, or following reconstructive surgery, scintigraphy may not be reliable (Chung et al. 1993). There should therefore be close correlation between the preoperative and postoperative studies. A Whitaker test may be necessary to confirm or exclude residual obstruction (Kass and Majd 1985, Pegolo et al. 2012). In children where renal function is impaired postoperatively and where early postoperative nephrostograms indicate technically satisfactory surgery, reassessment of function can be deferred for up to 2 years because functional recovery before this time is generally slight. As restenosis may occur, these children are usually followed during their growth period by annual US exams. Sufficient hydration prior to these US examinations is mandatory so that re-obstruction is not masked – note that US alone based on dilatation measurements cannot reliably assess or rule out obstruction and functional imaging will be needed for detailed assessment if re-obstruction is suspected.

> **Take Away**
> The outcome in children treated surgically for PUJO is best monitored by means of US and dynamic radionuclide scintigraphy (or increasingly fMRU). The use of IVU to assess postoperative relief of obstruction has largely been abandoned, as have postoperative nephrostograms – as the transrenal percutaneous drains have been mostly replaced by removable transureteric pyeloplasty stents.

3 Congenital Disorders of the Ureter

3.1 Non-refluxing Primary Megaureter/Uretero-vesical Junction Obstruction (UVJO)

In this condition, there is an adynamic segment of the distal ureter just prior to its insertion into the bladder resulting in obstruction to urine flow (Hanna et al. 1977). These patients are prone to collecting system infection, sometimes with atypical bacteria, and even with pyonephrosis. If the patient is ill and not responding well to antibiotic treatment, a percutaneous nephrostomy catheter should be inserted to drain the pus. A functional assessment of the kidney is undertaken in approximately 6 weeks, and a decision is taken as to whether to proceed to nephrectomy or a ureteric reimplantation or maybe even just observation.

If the ureter is very large, a low-end (cutaneous) (loop or Sober) ureterostomy may be performed allowing the ureter to decompress before carrying out a reimplantation; alternatively a temporary JJ stent, an endoscopic balloon dilation, or an endoureterotomy may be an option. Like PUJO, management of UVJO is often nonoperative initially. One study found that 34 % resolved spontaneously, 49 % persisted, and only 17 % required a reimplantation due to infections or deteriorating renal function (Liu et al. 1994). The majority of dilated ureters less than 7 mm in diameter resolved, while 50 % of those greater than 10 mm were treated with surgery. The definite indications for surgery are:

- Deteriorating renal function on scintigraphy
- Recurrent urinary tract infections despite antibiotic prophylaxis
- Pyonephrosis or stones
- Clinical symptoms

The surgical treatment involves resection of the adynamic distal segment of the ureter with reimplantation of the dilated proximal portion possibly following a reduction in the caliber of the ureter by tailoring techniques – the technique of hitching the ureter onto the psoas muscle so that a long tunnel can be obtained which has been abandoned because of the secondary J-hook effect causing significant long-term problems such as recurrent obstruction and bladder function disturbance (see also Chap. 15). Any patient who has had a ureteric tailoring will most likely have the ureter stented and a bladder catheter in position for up to 10 days postoperatively. US or plain radiography can be performed prior to its removal to check the position of the stent (Fig. 6). US is also used to assess the degree of dilatation of the collecting system and ureter. If a tapering technique has been performed, attention should be paid to possible postoperative complications such as urinary leak. There is also a risk to the blood supply of the distal ureter, which results in ischemia and restenosis. After surgery, patients usually remain on antibiotic prophylaxis

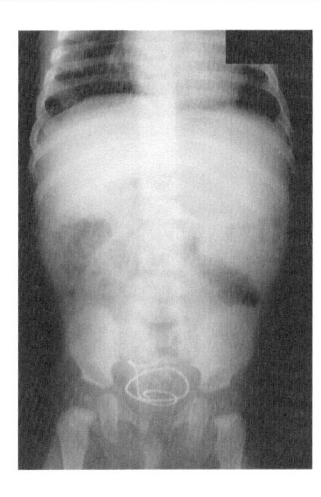

Fig. 6 Plain radiography after ureteric reimplantation. There is malposition of the ureteric stent, which lies completely in the urinary bladder

for some time; in some centers a follow-up voiding cystourethrogram (VCUG) is performed to exclude VUR. In general, follow-up investigations using US and radionuclide imaging are carried out between 3 and 6 months after surgery; some centers perform a dynamic MRU.

> **Take Away**
> Postoperative imaging in children with UVJ obstruction may include a VCUG to rule out VUR. Follow-up US and radionuclide scintigraphy are performed not earlier than 4 months after the procedure.

3.2 Ureteric Duplication, Ureteric Ectopia, and Associated Anomalies

Duplication of the renal collecting system and ureters is a common variant or anomaly. The duplication may range from a bifid pelvis to incomplete or complete duplication. Ureteroceles are cystic dilatations of the distal segment of the ureter. Though they may be associated with single ureter, they most commonly occur at the distal end of the upper ureter draining the upper moiety collecting system in a complete duplication ("Meyer-Weigert rule" – see Chaps. 7, 9, 14, 24).

In most cases, incomplete ureteric duplication is an incidental finding. However, it is occasionally possible that there is "yo-yo" reflux leading to stasis and ureteric dilatation. This can lead to flank pain and infection. In the rare cases which require surgery, the type of operation depends on the level of duplication. If this is very low, it may be possible to carry out a reimplantation of the ureters with separate ureteric orifices into the bladder. If the duplication is higher, a high ureteropyelostomy or ureteroureterostomy with excision of most of the duplicated ureter is the treatment of choice if refluxing; otherwise the distal ureter stump is left in place, sometimes after cystoscopic injection of bulging agents.

Management of a refluxing duplicated ureter depends on the function of the respective (usually lower) moiety. Lower grades of VUR with good function may resolve spontaneously as the child grows. Higher grades of VUR may benefit from reimplantations of the ureter (see Chap. 15). Poor function of the lower (or the upper) moiety (less than 10% of the individual renal function) is usually treated by a hemi-nephroureterectomy. This approach to treatment also applies to ectopic ureters.

The factors taken into account when planning treatment of *ureteroceles* are the renal function, the intravesical or ectopic position of the ureterocele, whether there is a single or duplex system, the degree of ureteric dilatation, the presence of ipsilateral or contralateral VUR, and the degree of detrusor covering of the ureterocele. The treatment of choice for an intravesical ureterocele is a small endoscopic incision just above its base (Fig. 7) (see Chaps. 14 and 15) (Blyth et al. 1993). Using this procedure, the incidence of secondary VUR is about 50%. Other surgical options include a nephrectomy for poor function which is a rare indication nowadays (Prieto et al. 2009). In some centers, this procedure is now performed laparoscopically using either a retroperitoneal or transabdominal approach (Wallis et al. 2006; Sydorak and Shaul 2005). The procedure is safe with a low morbidity, but complications have been reported which include urine leaks next to the bladder, retroperitoneal fluid collections, and functional loss of the remaining ipsilateral moiety in cases with a duplicated kidney; thus, this approach is increasingly under discussion (Fig. 8) (Wallis et al. 2006).

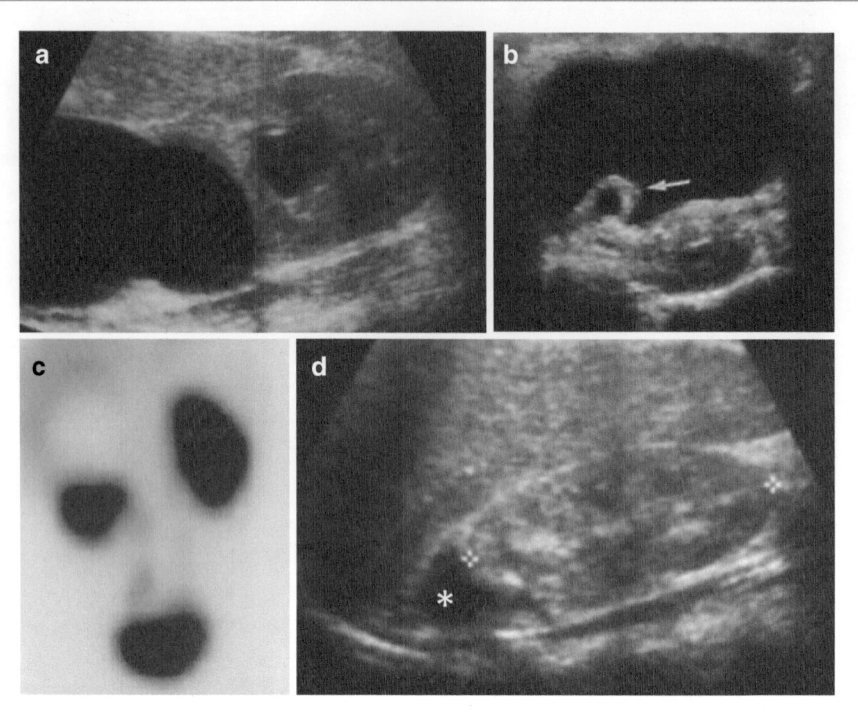

Fig. 7 (**a**) Right renal US outlining a duplex system. On US there is very marked UTD of the upper pole moiety with no significant renal cortex. Mild dilatation of the collecting system of the lower-pole moiety can be seen. (**b**) Post-endoscopic incision of ureterocele US outlines a small residual right ureterocele in the posterior bladder wall (*arrow*). (**c**) MAG 3 renogram shows no function in the upper pole moiety on the right side. (**d**) Follow-up US after incision of the ureterocele showing a significant reduction in the degree of dilatation of the upper pole collecting system (*, lower-pole moiety between cursors)

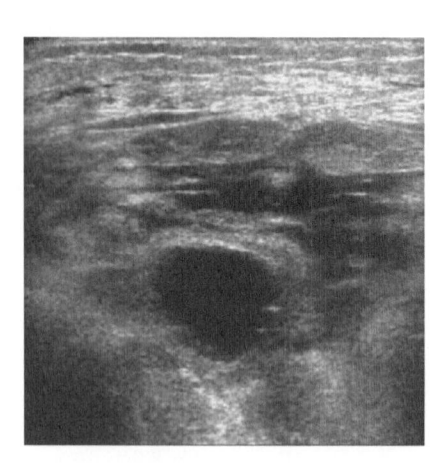

Fig. 8 US shows a postoperative perivesical urinoma after ureterocele unroofing (Courtesy of Riccabona M, Pediatric Ultrasound, Requisites, and Applications, p 362, Fig. 10.33e, Springer 2014)

Documented persistent symptomatic VUR will require reimplantation, and if the ureter caliber is very large, a tapered reimplantation may be required. If there is ureterocele prolapse mimicking a bladder diverticulum due to poor detrusor covering, this should also be repaired (Fig. 9). There are a number of options available to treat ectopic ureteroceles with a trend in recent years toward more conservative management. If the preoperative renal functional imaging shows poor function of the upper moiety of a duplex system with an ectopic ureterocele, its removal with decompression of the ureterocele and a staged approach to surgery at the bladder level is used in some centers. This approach avoids surgery on the ureterocele until it has a chance to reduce in size following decompression. This is best assessed using US. Currently persistent ipsilateral lower-pole VUR is the most common indication for excision of the ureterocele and reimplantation of the lower-pole ureter using a common sheath reimplantation technique. There are other rarer cases where VUR into the ureterocele and upper ureteric stump leads to problems of infection and post-micturition dribbling. In these children, the

Fig. 9 VCUG in a child with bilateral duplex systems. (**a**) There is significant VUR into the lower-pole moiety of a right duplex system and a right ureterocele obstructing the upper pole moiety (*arrow*). (**b**) At the end of micturition, there is relapse of the ureterocele mimicking a bladder diverticulum (*arrowhead*)

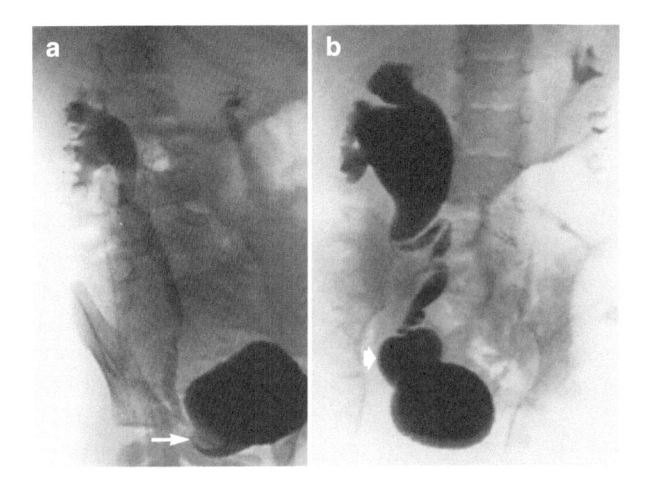

extent of the ureterocele and the ureteric stump may be imaged using US and occasionally MRI, which has replaced CT for this query if available. These patients also require surgery. When the upper moiety associated with an ectopic ureterocele has sufficient function to require a salvage procedure, high ureteroureterostomy or ureteropyelostomy may be undertaken if there is an extrarenal pelvis or a dilated lower-pole ureter. Some surgeons advocate a primary endoscopic incision of the ectopic ureterocele with follow-up investigations to see whether the upper moiety will regain function – though this is a rather old concept – as most upper poles are primarily dysplastic and thus do usually not regain sufficient function and growth potential. However, a secondary surgical procedure for persistent VUR is required in approximately 50 % of these patients (Blyth et al. 1993). As the vasculature to the upper moiety is often variable and anomalous, the blood supply to the lower moiety may be damaged during upper pole partial nephrectomy. It is also important that the entire upper pole calyceal system is excised. This procedure, however, may be associated with significant blood loss.

Bladder dysfunction has been reported in approximately 6 % of children with ureteroceles (Caldamone et al. 1984). The fact that patients treated with upper tract surgery alone have similar rates of incontinence to those who undergo additional lower tract surgery suggests that it is congenital in origin as opposed to surgically acquired (Holmes et al. 2002).

Children who undergo bilateral ureterocele repair have been found to be at increased risk for postoperative voiding dysfunction (Sherman et al. 2003).

Take Away

The treatment of *ureteric duplication* depends on the level of duplication and the presence or absence of clinically symptomatic associated VUR.

The many factors taken into account when planning treatment of *ureteroceles* are the renal function, their intravesical or ectopic position, whether there is a single or duplex system, the degree of ureteric dilatation, the presence of ipsilateral or contralateral VUR, and the degree of detrusor covering of the ureterocele.

4 Congenital Anomalies of the Urinary Bladder

Cloacal exstrophy, bladder exstrophy, and epispadias are developmental abnormalities of ranging severity, as a result of disruption of the formation and opposition of the pelvic bones, the cavitation of the pelvic organs, and the partitioning of the pelvic cavity (see also Chaps. 19, 21, and 22). Urinary tract diversion using an ileal conduit to treat this and other bladder abnormalities is now a practically obsolete procedure. However, children who have had this procedure require follow-up imaging studies. Yearly US and occasionally MRU (or CT) are necessary to detect dilatation due to obstruction and calculus disease (Fig. 10). Treatment now involves closure of the exstrophied bladder, bladder neck reconstruction, and epispadias repair. The upper tracts are usually normal in these infants though there is a high primary VUR incidence due to insertion pathology aggravated by surgery with bladder neck reconstruction; US is used for monitoring the urinary tract supplemented by other imaging as individually indicated – though multiple associated anomalies have been described. The main complication in these children after surgery is fistulation and incontinence – dehiscence of the wound due either to excess tension of the abdominal wall, infection, or bladder prolapse has become a rarity. Repeat closure with possible bladder augmentation is performed, for which a segment of ileum or colon is used. Rarely obstruction at the UVJ occurs (Fig. 11). A technique of percutaneous bladder catheterization is possible by creating a continent urinary stoma either via an appendicovesicostomy (Mitrofanoff stoma) or with a tapered ileum (MONTI technique) which is the method of choice for patients with chronic outlet obstruction or persistent incontinence (Mitrofanoff 1980, Monti et al. 1997). Close and regular monitoring of the upper tracts using US and possibly DMSA scintigraphy is necessary.

4.1 Congenital Anomalies of the Urethra

The commonest congenital abnormality of the urethra is a posterior urethral valve (PUV), which may result in the most severe renal disease in childhood (see also Chap. 18). This condition requires regular follow-up with imaging. Antenatal insertion of a double J stent between the fetal bladder or dilated collecting system of

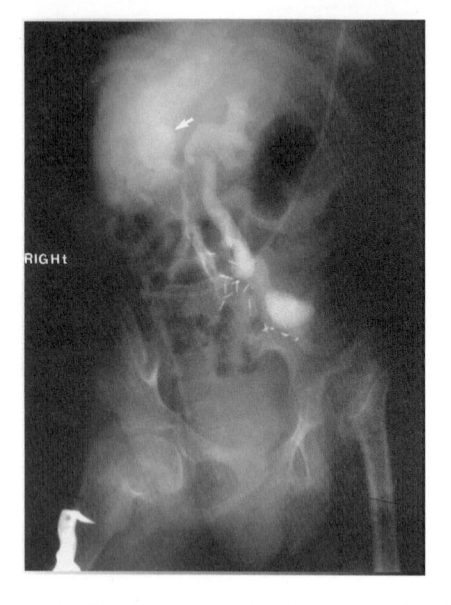

Fig. 10 IVU in a patient with urinary tract diversion using an ileal conduit. There is significant right UTD due to stone development at the PUJ (*arrowhead*)

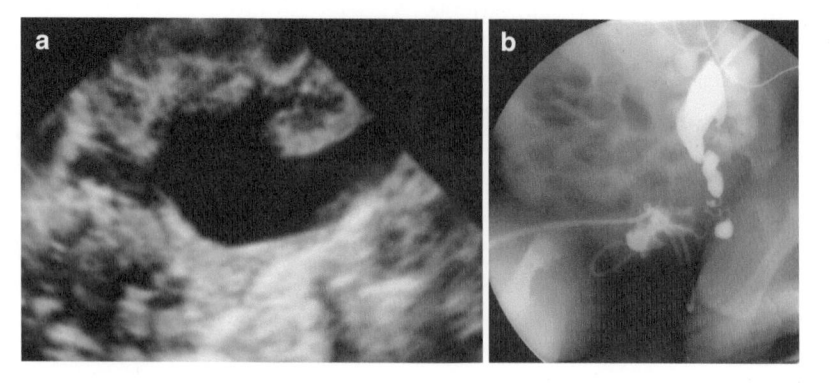

Fig. 11 (**a**) Repair of bladder exstrophy in a patient with a single left kidney. The patient developed subsequent UTD of the single kidney following surgery. (**b**) This required temporary nephrostomy drainage for relief of obstruction. There is narrowing of the distal ureter that resolved spontaneously

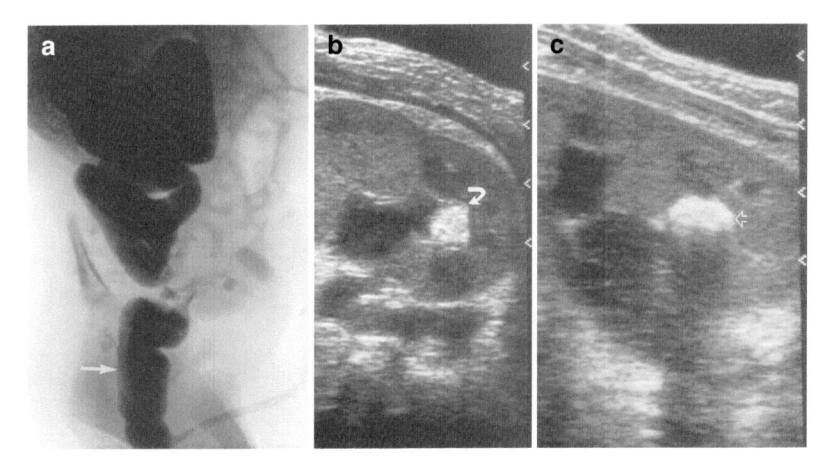

Fig. 12 (**a**) Infant with posterior urethral valves. There is dilatation of the posterior urethra (*arrow*) and marked VUR. (**b**) Patient developed echogenic area in the lower-pole collecting system after valve surgery (*curved arrow*). (**c**) Stone developed at site of a *Candida* ball 1 month after surgery (*open arrowhead*)

the kidneys and the amniotic cavity under US guidance allows decompression of the urinary tract. However, as this procedure is performed rather late in pregnancy, its benefit for the kidney has not yet been demonstrated; it however may enable a better fetal lung maturation. More recently, laser perforation of posterior urethral valves has been performed using fetoscopy. After birth, it is first essential to resuscitate and reassess the infant as necessary and allow free urine drainage, and this is followed by destruction of the valves. Urine drainage can be achieved by inserting a transurethral or a suprapubic catheter. However, a catheter does not always allow complete drainage of the upper tracts because of the increased bladder wall thickness and its poor compliance. Patients who have bilateral VUR, severe ureter dilatation, poor renal function, US evidence of thin renal parenchyma with or without dysplasia/cysts, and poor renal perfusion on (a) CDS are in an unfavorable group and may require vesicostomy. If uremia persists and the child is severely ill, percutaneous nephrostomy may be necessary. Valve destruction is usually achieved via retrograde endoscopy using an electrode or special knives. The use of laser therapy and Fogarty balloon catheter ablation has been practically abandoned. Post-obstructive diuresis or urinary tract infection can occur following relief of obstruction and instrumentation (Fig. 12). In most incidences, there is a progressive improvement in the appearance of the bladder and the upper tracts after complete destruction of the valves, though it can take years for the dilatation to reduce. This progress is best monitored using US and scintigraphy or possibly MRU (McMann et al. 2006) (Fig. 13). VUR, monitored using a VCUG or ce-VUS, may disappear if reasonable renal function is maintained. Dilatation of the posterior urethra also resolves with time (Fig. 14). However, unilateral VUR may act as a pop-off valve and may have a protective effect by reducing intravesical pressure (= VURD syndrome) (Narasimhan et al. 2005). Urodynamic studies are required, therefore, before considering a nephro-ureterectomy or a ureteric reimplantation in such a patient. Reimplantation in a trabeculated bladder is often difficult and unsuccessful and apparently does not affect outcome (Speakman et al. 1987). Endoscopic treatment of VUR in these children is also difficult. Persistent UTD without VUR may be related to a degree of obstruction at the UVJ (Fig. 14). This obstruction may be intermittent or permanent. Bladder augmentation is rarely indicated. It can improve capacity and compliance and may relieve UVJ obstruction. Incontinence is reported in up to 38% of boys after treatment of PUV. Despite adequate relief of urethral obstruction, urodynamic abnormalities such as abnormal detrusor

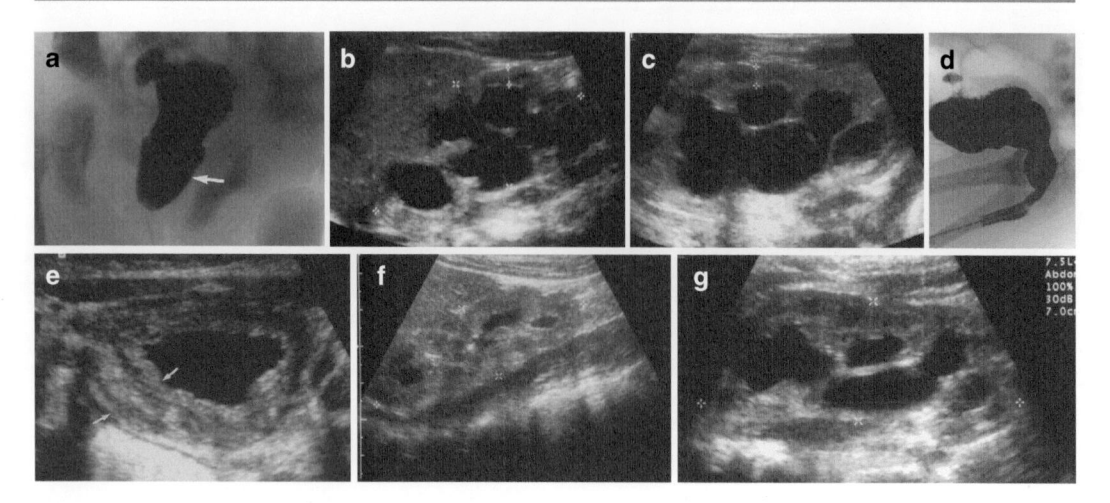

Fig. 13 An infant with posterior urethral valve. (**a**) Marked dilatation of the posterior urethra (*white arrow*) with marked thickening of the bladder wall and a right bladder diverticulum. (**b**) Preoperative sonography of right kidney and (**c**) left kidney demonstrating marked bilateral UTD. (**d**) VCUG at 10 days after valve destruction. The urethra is smaller in caliber, and there is good urine flow on voiding. There is still marked bladder wall thickening with diverticulum formation. (**e**) Bladder US 4 months after operation. There is still significant bladder wall thickening (*arrows*). f, g Postoperative US at 4 months of (**f**) right kidney and (**g**) left kidney shows significant improvement in the UTD

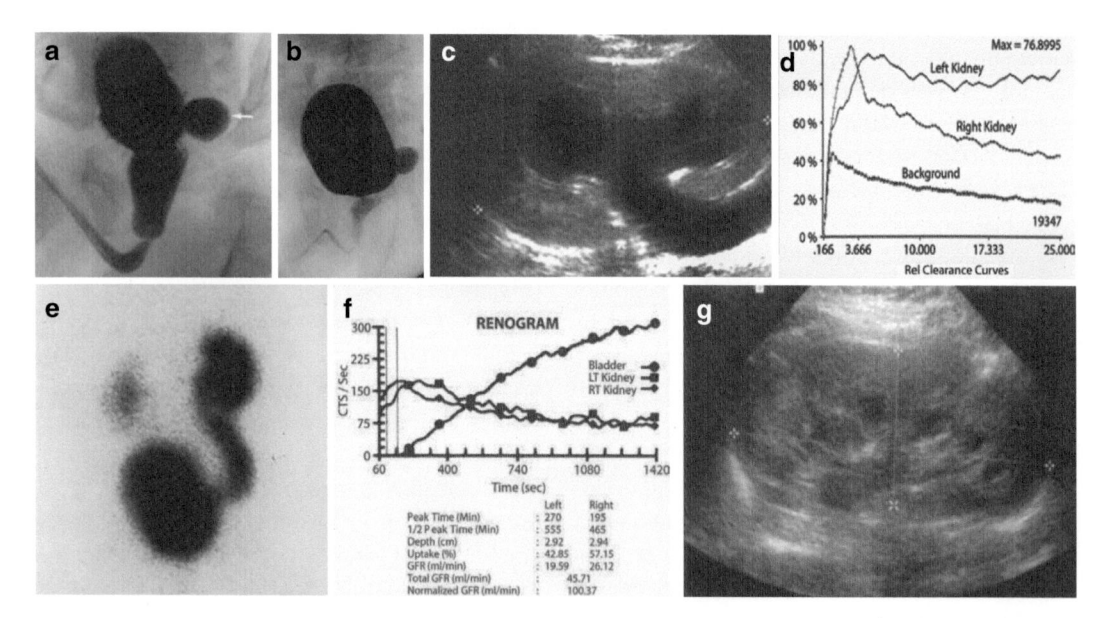

Fig. 14 An infant with PUV. (**a**) There is marked dilatation of the posterior urethra and significant bladder wall thickening and a large left bladder diverticulum (*arrow*). (**b**) Five months after valve destruction. There is almost complete resolution of the dilatation of the posterior urethra, and the bladder wall has a much smoother outline. There is still a large left bladder diverticulum. (**c**) Ten months after surgery. US shows a significant left UTD and a dilated ureter. (**d, e**) Tc 99m DTPA scintigraphy confirms good uptake of the radiopharmaceutical on this left side with poor excretion down a dilated ureter. VCUG was normal. These appearances are compatible with obstruction at the UVJ. (**f, g**) Four years after surgery, US and renography demonstrate complete resolution of the obstruction without surgical intervention

function are thought to be responsible for these symptoms. Growth problems, renal function deterioration, and quite regularly end-stage renal disease can occur at any time during childhood, puberty, or even later (see also Chap. 34). Therefore, all patients should have at least yearly

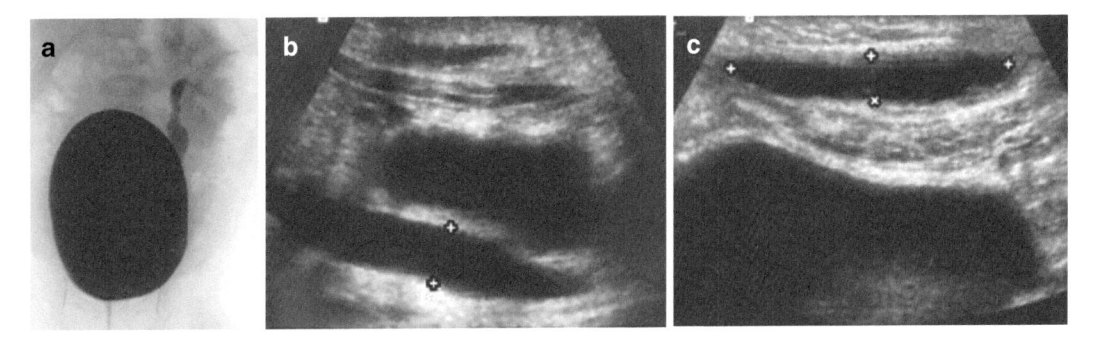

Fig. 15 (**a**) Patient with right multicystic kidney and left intrarenal reflux on VCUG. (**b**) US shows development of ureter dilatation after surgery (*cursors*). (**c**) Patient also developed subcutaneous collection at wound site (*cursors*)

imaging using US for assessment of upper tract dilatation and drainage and residual bladder volume assessment. Renal functional imaging is also necessary using Tc^{99m} DMSA or MAG 3 scintigraphy.

> **Take Away**
>
> In neonates with PUV, it is essential to resuscitate and reassess the child after birth when necessary, ensure unhindered urine drainage, and destroy the valves. Follow-up in all patients should include yearly imaging using US to assess upper tract dilatation, bladder shape and wall, as well as residual bladder volume. Renal functional imaging is also necessary, as most of the severe cases inevitably will progress to end-stage renal failure.

4.2 Vesicoureteric Reflux

Management of VUR should help to prevent renal damage in urinary tract infections. This is usually accomplished by a daily dose of prophylactic antibiotic therapy to maintain sterile urine, although this is increasingly under discussion. VUR may resolve or improve in many incidences (see Chaps. 13 and 28). Surgical correction of VUR may be required with higher grades of reflux (grades IV–V) when a child develops infections while on prophylactic antibiotic therapy, when new or progressive renal scarring develops, where long-term antibiotic use is not practical for medical or social reasons, or where severe VUR persists for years. There are different methods (see Chap. 14 and 15).

Postoperative US demonstrates localized thickening of the bladder wall, and follow-up US is required early in the postoperative period to check the continued correct positioning of the uretero-vesical stent (if inserted, eg., after Hendren procedure) and to monitor the ureter size and exclude the rare complication of stenosis of the distal ureter due to ischemia (Fig. 15). Some degree of ureteral distention is a normal finding postoperatively, in addition to altered ureteral peristalsis as a response to the ureteral splint. However, intrarenal dilatation should be monitored, and an asymmetric increase of the resistive index on Doppler studies may hint at acute drainage impairment then usually associated with other US signs of acute obstruction (but sometimes obscured by the preexisting renal parenchymal alterations in reflux nephropathy).

Submucosal agent injection has become an accepted alternative. It reliably prevents VUR in lower degrees, but the results are variable in higher degrees, and in the severe grades, more than one injection may be required. US shows the echogenic deposit of the bulking agent at the site of the injection adjacent to the transmural part of the ureter with varying amount of acoustic shadowing (depends on the material used) (Figs. 16 and 6 in chapter "Congenital Urinary Tract Dilatation and Obstructive Uropathy"). Nowadays, the success of the procedure is frequently checked intraoperatively by ce-US or by fluoroscopy using a cystoscopic injection.

Fig. 16 (a) Echogenic area with acoustic shadowing at the Teflon injection site (*arrow*); (b) CDS confirms the patency of the ostium/ureter in spite of the impressive deposit protruding into the bladder after bulking agent injection; note that the injection had been performed on both sides in (b)

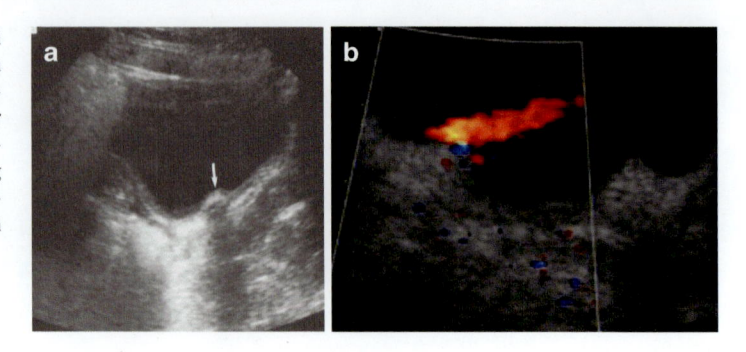

As a result, follow-up VUR tests are less often necessary, particularly in clinically asymptomatic patients. However, late reoccurrence is more common than after open surgery and must be kept in mind.

> **Take Away**
> When surgery is required to treat VUR, the method of choice is ureteric reimplantation with elongation of the submucosal tunnel. Follow-up US is required to check ureteric size and the grade of postoperative upper tract distension. Submucosal injection of bulking agents is increasingly used as an alternative.

5 Oncological Surgery

Surgical excision is still the cornerstone of therapy for Wilms' tumor, the most common malignant neoplasm of the urinary tract, and rhabdomyosarcoma, the most common soft tissue sarcoma in childhood, of which 15–20% arise in the urinary tract. Meticulous surgical technique is necessary because of the risk of tumor spillage, particularly with surgery for Wilms' tumor. In Europe, in patients (particularly with advanced) Wilms' tumor disease and in patients with bilateral disease, the treatment involves percutaneous biopsy for diagnosis (if the diagnosis is not evident) followed by chemotherapy before definitive surgery approximately 14 weeks after successful chemotherapy (Dykes et al. 1991; Weiner et al. 1998). Tumor can be present in adjacent organs in up to 17% of cases. Other authors used a similar regime that reduced tumor size and made it less vascular. In some incidences, subsequent partial nephrectomy was possible. In these series, there was no needle track seeding or tumor rupture (Greenberg et al. 1991; McLorie et al. 1991). However, controversy still exists as to the best approach to the management of these children with regard to neoadjuvant chemotherapy (NWTS, SIOP, and UKCCSG protocols – also see Chap. 36). In patients with a diagnosis of rhabdomyosarcoma, the treatment comprises various combinations of chemotherapy, radiotherapy, and surgical resection depending on the initial staging of the disease. This treatment protocol is determined by the Intergroup Rhabdomyosarcoma Study Group.

Surgical complications encountered in tumor surgery involving the genitourinary tract include small bowel obstruction diagnosed using plain radiography and major hemorrhage for which US and CT are useful. Follow-up imaging using US and CT or MRI should be performed initially at 6 weeks and following this at 3-month intervals to assess response to chemotherapy and to plan the timing of surgery if required (Fig. 17) (see also Chap. 36). Following this, imaging, including chest radiography (or in newer protocols chest CT), is performed every 6 months on two occasions and then yearly as indicated, to check for tumor resolution or recurrence (Fig. 17).

> **Take Away**
> Postoperative imaging in children following tumor surgery of the urogenital tract is performed using US and CT or MRI at time intervals dictated by the treatment protocol used.

Postoperative Imaging and Findings

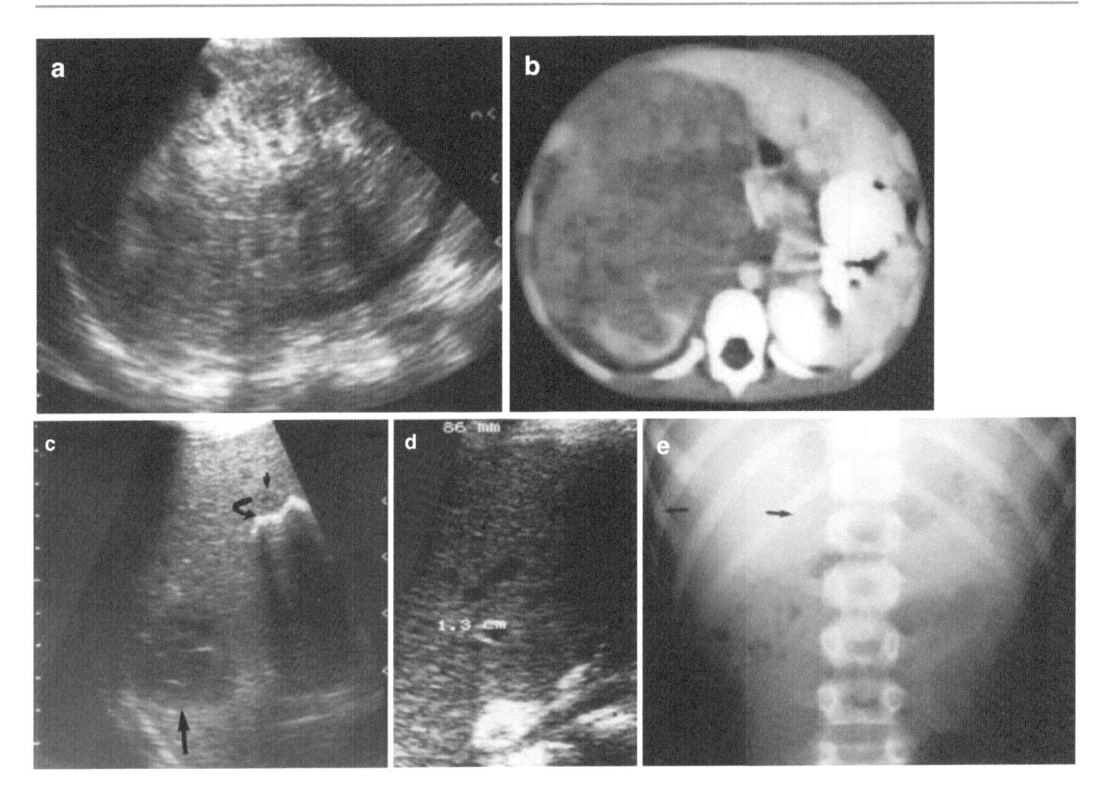

Fig. 17 (**a**) US and (**b**) CT scan show a large mass arising from the right kidney. A Wilms' tumor was confirmed at biopsy. There were also tumor nodules present in the adjacent liver. (**c**) Follow-up US at 6 weeks after chemotherapy shows a residual tumor nodule in the posterior aspect of the right lobe of the liver (*black arrow*). There is an area of increased echogenicity with some shadowing in a more anterior location in keeping with the development of calcification at the site of a second nodule (*curved arrow*) close to the gallbladder (*arrowhead*). (**d**) Follow-up US at 2.5 years. There is an area of increased echogenicity (*between cursors*) in the inferior aspect of the right lobe of the liver, the site of a previous tumor nodule. (**e**) Calcification on plain radiography at two liver tumor nodule sites (*arrows*)

6 Renal Stone Disease

In renal stone disease, surgery is now reserved for cases that cannot be managed using extracorporeal shockwave lithotripsy (ESWL), particularly where stones are in a difficult location or where there is an underlying anatomic abnormality. Percutaneous renal surgery and lithotripsy lithopraxy are also occasionally used (Papanicolaou et al. 1986, Landau 2015). Whatever the treatment, US is used to monitor residual UTD, and US complemented by radiography will monitor the disappearance of stone fragments from the ureter and bladder. Both are also necessary as follow-up investigations to exclude recurrence. CT scanning may be helpful in selected cases. With ESWL renal injury may occur, and this can usually be depicted on US by using additional Doppler techniques or sometimes ce-US (Fig. 18).

> **Take Away**
> Whatever treatment is chosen for renal stone disease, US and plain radiography are used to monitor outcome; only rarely repeated CTs are unavoidable.

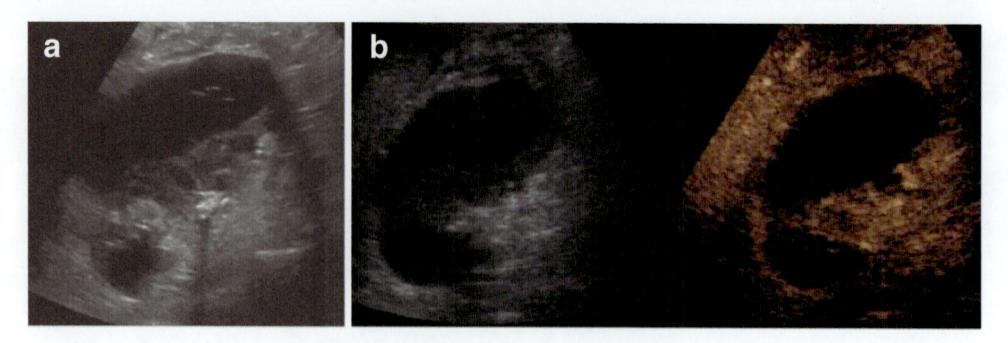

Fig. 18 (a) US depicts a huge urinomatous subcapsular hematoma after ESWL; (a) a residual calculus can be depicted. (b) Contrast-enhanced US demonstrates that the renal parenchyma is at least centrally still perfused, though the periphery is compromised

Conclusion

The surgical procedure undertaken to treat the various renal tract abnormalities may vary from surgeon to surgeon and may also depend on the severity of the conditions with additional regional differences. These influence the complications and the outcome. Therefore, knowledge of the exact surgical procedure is necessary in most instances prior to postsurgical imaging, and close correlation with presurgical studies is mandatory.

References

Arnold AJ, Rickwood AMK (1990) Natural history of pelviureteric obstruction detected by prenatal sonography. Br J Urol 65:91–6

Blyth B, Passerini-Glazel G, Camuffo C et al (1993) Endoscopic incision of ureteroceles: intravesical versus ectopic. J Urol 149:556–60

Caldamone A, Snyder HM, Duckett JW (1984) Ureteroceles in children: follow-up management with upper tract approach. J Urol 131:1130–2

Chung S, Majd M, Rushton HG et al (1993) Diuretic renography in the evaluation of neonatal hydronephrosis: is it reliable? J Urol 150:765–8

Doraiswamy NV (1994) Ureteroplasty using balloon dilatation in children with pelviureteric obstruction. J Pediatr Surg 29:937–40

Dykes EH, Marwaha RK, Dicks-Mireaux C et al (1991) Risks and benefits of percutaneous biopsy and primary chemotherapy in advanced Wilms' tumour. J Pediatr Surg 26:610–2

Freedman ER, Rickwood AMK (1994) Prenatally diagnosed pelviureteric junction obstruction: a benign condition? J Pediatr Surg 29:769–72

Gordon I, Piepsz A, Sixt R (2011) Auspices of Paediatric Committee of European Association of Nuclear Medicine. Eur J Nucl Med Mol Imaging 38:1175–88

Grapin C, Chartier-Kastler E, Audry G et al (1990) Failures observed after repair of the pelviureteric junction in children based on a series of thirteen cases (in French). Ann Pediatr (Paris) 37:26–9

Greenberg M, Burnweit C, Filler R et al (1991) Preoperative chemotherapy for children with Wilms' tumour. J Pediatr Surg 26:949–53

Hanna MK, Jeffs RD, Sturgess JM et al (1977) Ureteral structure and ultrastructure. III. The congenitally dilated ureter (megaureter). J Urol 117:24–7

Holmes NM, Coplen DE, Strand W et al (2002) Are bladder dysfunction and incontinence associated with ureteroceles congenital or acquired? J Urol 168:718–9

Kass EJ, Majd M (1985) Evaluation and management of upper urinary tract obstruction in infancy and childhood. Urol Clin North Am 12:133–41

Kis E, Verebely T, Kovi R et al (1998) The role of ultrasound in the follow-up of postoperative changes after pyeloplasty. Pediatr Radiol 28:247–9

Koff SA, Campbell R (1992) Nonoperative management of unilateral neonatal hydronephrosis. J Urol 148:525–31

Landau EH (2015) Modern stone management in children. Eur Urol Suppl 14(1):12–19 ISSN 1569–9056

Liu A, Dillon HG, Yeung CK et al (1994) Prognosis and management of primary megaureters detected in the newborn period. In: Book of abstracts, American Academy of Pediatrics Annual Meeting, pp 67–68

McMann LP, Kirsch AJ, Scherz HC et al (2006) Uropathy in the evaluation of prenatally diagnosed hydronephrosis and renal dysgenesis. J Urol 176:1786–92

McClinton S, Steyn H, Hussey JR (1993) Retrograde balloon dilatation for pelviureteric junction obstruction. Br J Urol 71:152–5

McLorie GA, McKenna PH, Greenberg M et al (1991) Reduction in tumour burden allowing partial nephrectomy following preoperative chemotherapy in biopsy proved Wilms' tumour. J Urol 146:509–13

Mitrofanoff P (1980) Cystostomie continent transappendeculaire dans le traitement des vessies neurologiques. Chir Pediatr 21:297–305

Monti PR, Lara RC, Dutra MA, de Carvalho JR (1997) New techniques for construction of efferent conduits based on the Mitrofanoff principle. Urology 49:112–5

Narasimhan KL, Mahajan JK, Kaur B, Mittal BR, Bhattacharya A (2005) The vesicoureteral reflux dysplasia syndrome in patients with posterior urethral valves. J Urol 174:1433–5

O'Flynn KJ, Gough DC, Gupta S et al (1993) Prediction of recovery in antenatally diagnosed hydronephrosis. Br J Urol 71:478–80

Papanicolaou N, Pfister RC, Young HH et al (1986) Percutaneous US lithotripsy of symptomatic renal calculi in children. Pediatr Radiol 16:13–6

Pegolo PT, Miranda ML, Kim S, Oliveira Filho AG, Reis LO, Silva JM (2012) Antegrade pressure measurement of urinary tract in children with persistent hydronephrosis. Int Braz J Urol 38:448–55

Prieto J, Ziada A, Baker L, Snodgrass W (2009) Ureteroureterostomy via inguinal incision for ectopic ureters and ureteroceles without ipsilateral lower pole reflux. J Urol 181:1844–8

Ransley PG, Dhillon HG, Gordon I et al (1990) The postnatal management of hydronephrosis diagnosed by prenatal ultrasound. J Urol 144:584–7

Sherman ND, Stock JA, Hanna MK (2003) Bladder dysfunction after bilateral ectopic ureterocele repair. J Urol 170:1975–7

Speakman MJ, Bradling AF, Gilpin CJ (1987) Bladder outflow obstruction: a cause of denervation supersensitivity. J Urol 138:1461–6

Sydorak RM, Shaul DB (2005) Laparoscopic partial nephrectomy in infants and toddlers. J Pediatr Surg 40:1945–7

Wallis MC, Khoury AE, Lorenzo AJ et al (2006) Outcome analysis of retroperitoneal laparoscopic heminephrectomy in children. J Urol 175:2277–80; discussion 2280–2282

Weiner JS, Coppes MJ, Ritchey ML (1998) Current concepts in the biology and management of Wilms' tumour. J Urol 159:1316–25

Wilkinson AG, Azimy A (1996) Balloon dilatation of the pelviureteric junction in children: early experience and pitfalls. Pediatr Radiol 26:882–6

Part VI

Renal Parenchymal and Cystic Disease, Urolithiasis, Renal Failure and Transplantation

Imaging in Urinary Tract Infections

Lil-Sofie Ording Muller, Freddy Avni, and Michael Riccabona

Contents

1 **Introduction** 537
1.1 Background 537
1.2 The Role of Imaging in UTI and Patient Selection 538

2 **Radiological Examinations in UTI and Typical Imaging Findings** 540
2.1 Ultrasonography (US) 540
2.2 DMSA Static Renography 542
2.3 Magnetic Resonance Imaging (MRI) 542
2.4 Computer Tomography (CT) 543
2.5 Voiding Cystourethrography 543
2.6 Intravenous Urography (IVU) 543

3 **Normal Progression of UTI** 544

4 **Complications from Pyelonephritis** 544
4.1 Acute Bacterial Nephritis 544
4.2 Renal Abscess 545
4.3 Renal Scarring 546
4.4 Xanthogranulomatous Pyelonephritis 547

5 **Cystitis** 548

6 **Unusual Infections** 549
6.1 Renal Candidiasis 549
6.2 Tuberculosis 550
6.3 Hydatid Disease 550
6.4 Bilharziasis 550

7 **Summary and Conclusion** 550

References 551

L.-S. Ording Muller, MD, PhD (✉)
Department of Radiology and Nuclear Medicine, Unit for Paediatric Radiology, Oslo University Hospital, Oslo, Norway
e-mail: LIL-SOFIE.ORDING@UNN.NO

F. Avni, MD, PhD
Department of Pediatric Radiology, Jeanne de Flandre Hospital, Lille University Hospital, 59037 Lille, France
e-mail: favni@skynet.be

M. Riccabona, MD
Department of Radiology, Division of Pediatric Radiology, University Hospital Graz, Graz, Austria

1 Introduction

1.1 Background

Urinary tract infection (UTI) is one of the most common bacterial infections in childhood, affecting 8 % of girls and 2 % during the first 8 years of life. Up to 6 months of age, the prevalence is higher in boys than in girls (see also chapter "UTI and VUR"). In school age UTI is two- to fourfold more prevalent in girls and up to 5 % of all girls contract a UTI during their school years (Brandstrom and Hansson 2014).

According to the American Academy of Pediatrics, UTI is defined as growth of >10^5 colony-forming bacteria units per millilitre in a clean urine specimen. The presumptive diagnosis of UTI is often made by microscopic urine analyses. The most frequent uropathogen is *Escherichia coli* (*E. coli*), accounting for 85 % of all UTIs.

Other bacteria accounting for UTI in children are *Klebsiella*, *Proteus*, *Enterobacter*, *Citrobacter* and *Staphylococcus saprophyticus*, and infections with the latter agents are referred to as non-*E. coli* UTI (Chakupurakal et al. 2010). The most common route of infection is ascending pathogens from the perineal flora.

The clinical presentation of UTI varies both with the severity of the infection and with the age of the child. It can either affect the lower urinary tract (cystitis) or ascend to involve the renal pelvis and kidneys (pyelonephritis). The clinical presentation ranges from asymptomatic bacteriuria or symptoms related to cystitis, like pollakiuria and dysuria or fever and malaise or even sepsis. In children under 2 years of age, the clinical presentation of UTI tends to be non-specific and this entity should always be considered in a young child presenting with signs of infection or malaise without other obvious causes (Tullus 2011; Yim et al. 2014).

The risk of renal scarring after the first UTI has been reported to be up to 15 % (Shaikh et al. 2010). In confirmed pyelonephritis renal scarring was confirmed by DMSA in up to 40 % in some studies (Faust et al. 2009). The presence of high-grade vesicourethral reflux (VUR) significantly increases the risk of renal involvement in UTI with subsequent scarring (see also chapters "UTI and VUR" and "Vesicoureteric Reflux"). However, the outcome of high-grade VUR appears to also depend on individual characteristics of the patients and not so much on VUR grade, and renal scarring can even occur in patients without demonstrable VUR (Wennerstrom et al. 2000; Garin et al. 2007; Montini et al. 2008). Important risk factors other than VUR for development of pyelonephritic scars include urinary tract obstruction, low age, recurrent infection with low virulent bacteria and bladder dysfunction.

1.2 The Role of Imaging in UTI and Patient Selection

The imaging and management of children with UTI is one of the most controversial areas in paediatrics. For decades, children with UTI were almost inevitably imaged with intravenous urography and renal technetium-99m dimercaptosuccinic acid (DMSA) scintigraphy to diagnose and localise UTI in the acute phase and, after the infection was treated, with voiding cystourethrography (VCUG) to look for VUR (Tullus 2013). Now clinical tests have emerged to relatively high diagnostic accuracy reducing the role of imaging in diagnosing UTI. With the new identified risk factors and the new knowledge on the impact of VUR for renal scarring, the imaging approach in children after an UTI has also changed. The main focus for imaging tests is no longer detection and monitoring of VUR but rather to focus on the impact of UTI on the kidneys and to detect underlying conditions that would make the patient more susceptible for renal damage caused by the infection like signs of atypical disease, unidentified malformations and voiding dysfunction. There has been a shift from invasive procedures and investigations with a high radiation burden to less invasive and harmless studies where ultrasonography (US) plays the major role.

Numerous studies have tried to define the ideal imaging algorithm in UTI. Several new recommendations for management and treatment of UTI, including directions for patient selection for imaging tests, have been proposed over the last decade in order to reduce unnecessary imaging tests (Fig. 1). All the current guidelines share a more selective approach to imaging based on the patient's age and the clinical presentation of the infection. None of the guidelines recommend VCUG to be routinely performed in all children presenting after the first UTI. The American Academy of Pediatrics revised guidelines from 2011 recommend US of the kidneys and bladder in all patients under 2 years of age (Subcommittee on Urinary Tract Infection SCoQI, Management; Roberts 2011). The UK National Institute of Clinical Excellence (NICE) guidelines from 2007 only recommend routine US of all children under 6 months of age (Mori et al. 2007).

The diagnosis of UTI is most often based on the clinical and laboratory findings and does not

Imaging in Urinary Tract Infections

a

```
                    Suspected UTI
                         ↓
                    US + aCDS
              especially if severe or in an infant
```

Branches:
- Normal + Clinically cystitis → STOP (↑ If normal)
- Normal + Clinically upper UTI → DMSA or MRI with DWI in the acute phase → Normal → Consider repeat US → If normal → STOP
- Pyelitis/Nephritis → Follow-up US; VUR-evaluation (-always in infants, -usually if <4 years, -usually if recurrent UTI); DMSA in 4-6 months (or MRI); Bladder function studies (Urodynamics if over 6 years)
- Pyo/Hydro-nephrosis → Consider nephrostomy → (to VUR-evaluation)

b

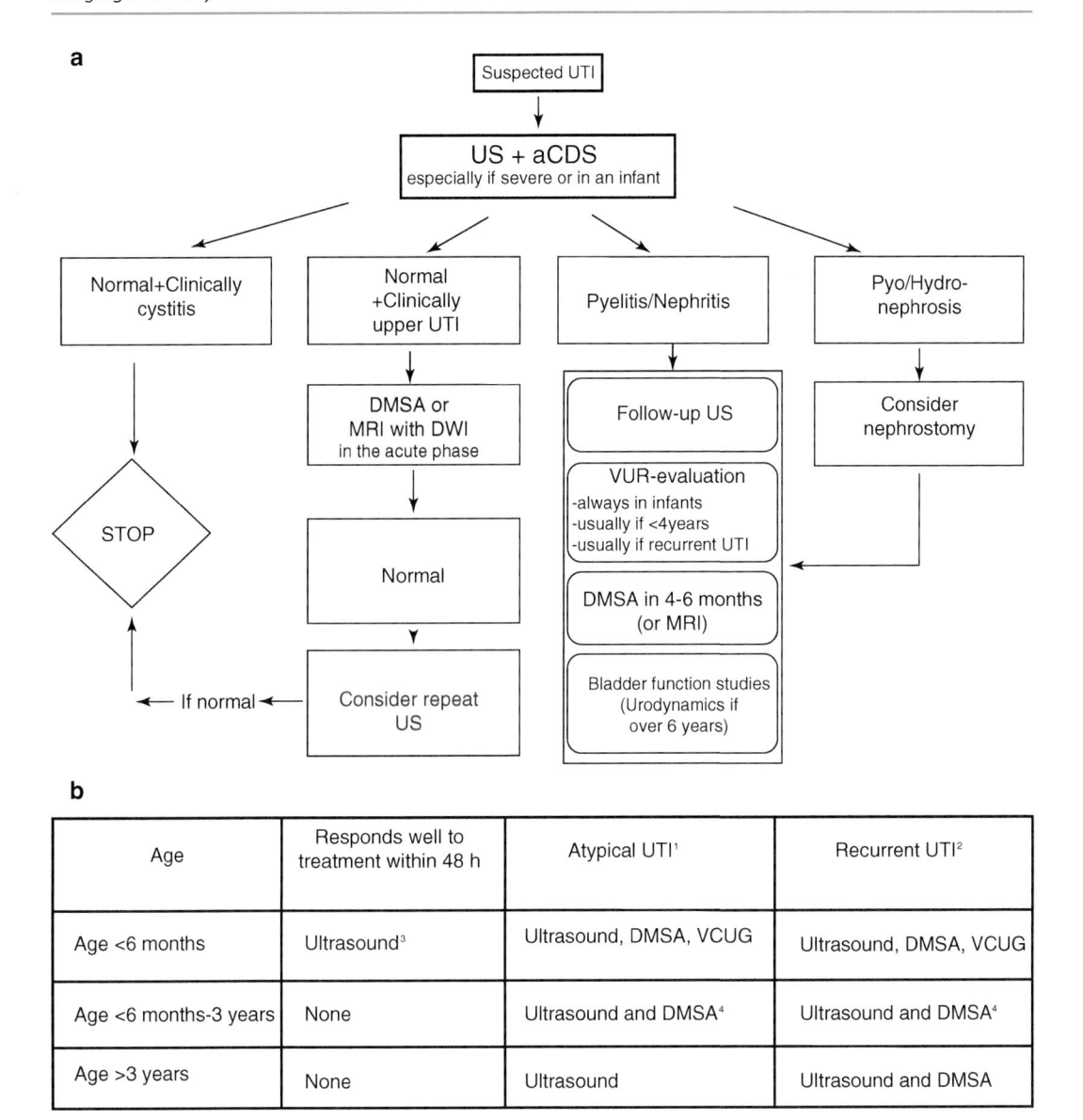

Age	Responds well to treatment within 48 h	Atypical UTI[1]	Recurrent UTI[2]
Age <6 months	Ultrasound[3]	Ultrasound, DMSA, VCUG	Ultrasound, DMSA, VCUG
Age <6 months-3 years	None	Ultrasound and DMSA[4]	Ultrasound and DMSA[4]
Age >3 years	None	Ultrasound	Ultrasound and DMSA

1. Atypical UTI: Non-Escherechia coli UTI: seriously ill, poor urine flow, abdominal or bladder mass, raised creatinine, septicemia, failure to respond to treatment with suitable antibiotics within 48 h

2. Two or more episodes of UTI with acute pyelonephritis/upper urinary tract infection or
One episode of UTI with acute pyelonephritis/upper urinary tract infection plus one or more episode of UTI with cystitis/lower urinary tract infection or Three or more episodes of UTI with cystitis/lower urinary tract infection

3. If ultrasound is abnormal, consider a VCUG

4. Consider VCUG if dilatation on ultrasound, poor urine flow, non-E. coli infection, family history of VUR

Fig. 1 (a) ESPR/ESUR recommendations for imaging in childhood urinary tract infections (Riccabona et al. 2010). (b) Summary of imaging algorithm in childhood UTI according to the NICE guidelines. Subcommittee on Urinary Tract Infection SCoQI, Management, (2011)

routinely include imaging. However collecting urine and interpreting the results can be difficult in young children. It may also be challenging to differentiate lower urinary tract infection from pyelonephritis because the symptoms in this patient group may be non-specific (Garin et al. 2007). Therefore, in selected patients, and preferably in all infants and neonates, imaging is indicated, not just in the follow-up after a UTI but also in the acute phase of suspected pyelonephritis to help diagnose and localise the infection and to detect underlying malformations of the renal tract.

Once the diagnosis is established, selection for further imaging studies is based on the clinical presentation of the UTI, the patient's age and potential findings on US. The timing of the US scan depends on the clinical situation. In patients who are severely ill or when there is no substantial improvement, US is recommended during the first 2 days of treatment to identify serious complications, such as renal or perirenal abscesses or pyonephrosis associated with obstructive uropathy. In children other than neonates and infants, imaging is not needed in the acute phase of infection if the patient responds well to adequate treatment. The imaging findings during an acute infection can even be misleading because *E. coli* endotoxin can cause relaxation of the muscles in the urothelium causing dilatation of the collecting system, which could be confused with hydronephrosis, pyonephrosis or obstruction. DMSA or MRI in the acute phase to diagnose pyelonephritis in equivocal cases is recommended by the European Society for Paediatric Radiology work group on urogenital imaging (Riccabona et al. 2008). This is advocated only as a follow-up examination to look for renal scarring by the other guidelines.

The NICE guidelines have the most restrictive approach to imaging in UTI, and recent studies suggest that a substantive number of children with high-grade VUR or other significant pathologies may be missed if these guidelines are followed strictly (McDonald and Kenney 2014; Ristola and Hurme 2014). Despite all the new knowledge and the recent published guidelines, the optimal approach to imaging in UTI still remains controversial.

2 Radiological Examinations in UTI and Typical Imaging Findings

2.1 Ultrasonography (US)

US is always the first, and sometimes the only, imaging modality required in children selected for further imaging in UTI. US should ideally be performed by an investigator experienced in paediatric US, using an up-to-date protocol for paediatric imaging (Riccabona et al. 2008; Riccabona 2015).

The sonographic signs of acute pyelonephritis include focal or general nephromegaly due to oedema, focal or general increased echogenicity of the renal parenchyma with reduced corticomedullary differentiation. The affected parenchyma will have decreased perfusion due to oedema and ischaemia and therefore the corresponding reduced colour Doppler flow is seen in the affected part of the parenchyma. Other features such as slightly thickened and hyperechoic uroepithelium in the renal pelvis, mild increased AP diameter of the renal pelvis, increased echogenicity of the perirenal fat and sometimes a sliver of subcapsular fluid may also be seen (Muller 2014; Brader et al. 2008) (Figs. 2 and 3; Table 1). Sometimes the urine may be echogenic due to pyuria. In a severely ill child with dilated collecting system containing echogenic urine suggestive of pus (Fig. 4), placement of a nephrostomy tube should be discussed, particularly if the child does not respond to treatment within 24 h. Neither of the sonographic signs of APN are entirely specific, and particularly thickening of the uroepithelium may also be seen in patients with VUR or obstruction; hence the imaging features must of course be correlated with the clinical picture (Sorantin et al 1997; Riccabona 2015/2016).

The most widely accepted role of US in the workup for APN is to determine whether there is an underlying renal malformation that has favoured the UTI. This can normally be done in the subacute phase of the infection or electively. Dilated collecting systems and the level of a potential obstruction are easily seen with US if the child is well hydrated. The most common

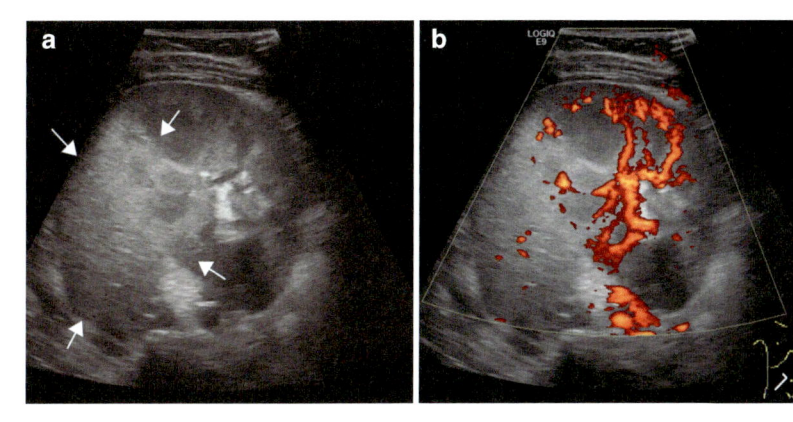

Fig. 2 Ultrasound findings in pyelonephritis include focal nephromegaly with increased echogenicity and loss of corticomedullary differentiation (*arrows*) (**a**). The affected part of the kidney will show reduced perfusion on colour Doppler examination (**b**)

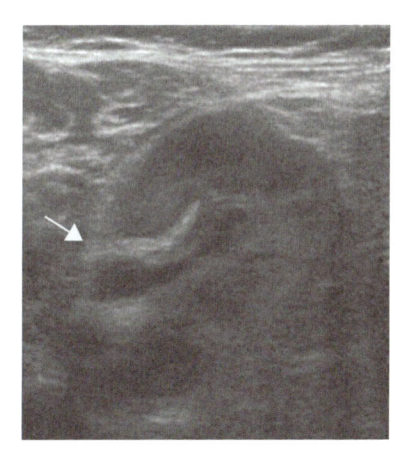

Fig. 3 Thickening and increased echogenicity of the uroepithelium (*arrow*) can be seen in acute pyelitis/pyelonephritis

Table 1 Signs of acute pyelonephritis on US

Focal or general nephromegaly
Focal or general increased or inhomogeneous echogenicity
Loss of corticomedullary differentiation
Increased perirenal echogenicity
Increased hilar echogenicity
Reduced perfusion of the affected area (s) on colour Doppler examination

malformation is a duplex system, which can normally be assessed by US, particularly if dilated. Duplex systems can have associated ureteroceles and/or VUR. Assessment of the bladder pre- and post-micturition to assess the bladder emptying and to look for changes in the collecting system pre-/post-voiding should be included in the workup. The parenchyma should be carefully assessed to reveal signs of renal cystic disease or congenital anomalies of the kidneys and urinary tract (CAKUT). Ultrasound is also useful in the assessment of possible complications from pyelonephritis like the development of a renal abscess.

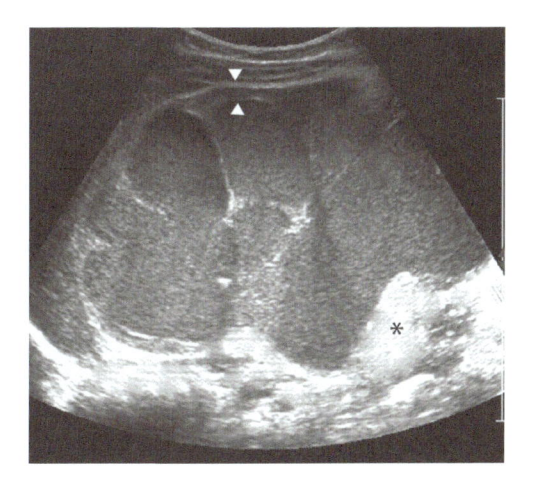

Fig. 4 A severely ill child with dilated collecting system containing echogenic urine suggestive of pus. There is severe pelvicalyceal dilatation and thinning of the renal parenchyma (*arrowheads*). In this setting placement of a nephrostomy tube may be indicated. Note the hyperechogenicity inflamed perirenal fat (*asterisk*)

In the follow-up after a pyelonephritis, US can be used to look for normalisation of the renal parenchyma and the collecting system and for the assessment of renal growth (see also below – Sect. 3). However, US has a limited usefulness for the detection of renal scarring (Sinha et al. 2007).

2.2 DMSA Static Renography

Static renal scintigraphy using DMSA ^{99m}TC as the tracer is considered as the gold standard for the detection of renal involvement in UTI (see also chapter "Nuclear Medicine"). The main feature of renal involvement is lack of uptake of the tracer in diseased areas. This may be localised or more diffuse, but is non-specific and can only be properly interpreted in context with other 'anatomic' imagings and the clinical information. The sensitivity of the technique is over 90%, and it is quite specific. DMSA scanning has the disadvantage of not differentiating old from new lesions; hence the interpretation in the acute phase can be difficult without a previous examination for comparison (MacKenzie 1996). However the diagnosis of acute pyelonephritis is made based on clinical and laboratory data, and DMSA is now normally not advocated, hence rarely used, in the acute phase of suspected pyelonephritis.

The main role of DMSA is to monitor the kidneys after the infection. In selected patients (see guidelines, Sect. 1.2), a DMSA should be performed 4–6 months after the acute infection to look for signs of nephron loss to identify the patients more susceptible to renal scarring from acute pyelonephritis, which is the most important factor to determine further treatment and prophylaxis for UTI.

2.3 Magnetic Resonance Imaging (MRI)

MRI has great potential for detecting areas of infected renal parenchyma. Both experimental and clinical trials have shown a good correlation between MRI and DMSA scanning for the detection of pyleonephritis (Vivier et al. 2014) (see also chapter "MR of the Urogenital Tract in Children"). After contrast injection, the diseased areas appear hypointense on T1 sequences. This corresponds to the areas of decreased Doppler flow on US and represents hypoperfusion of the parenchyma. However, diffusion-weighted imaging is as sensitive to renal involvement in UTI as contrast-enhanced MRI, making contrast injection superfluous in the assessment of acute pyelonephritis (Fig. 5). In equivocal cases a simplified MRI protocol with diffusion-weighted images can confirm or exclude the diagnosis of acute pyelonephritis with high sensitivity and specificity without

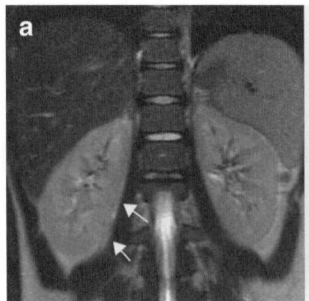

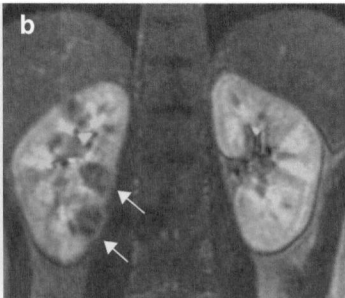

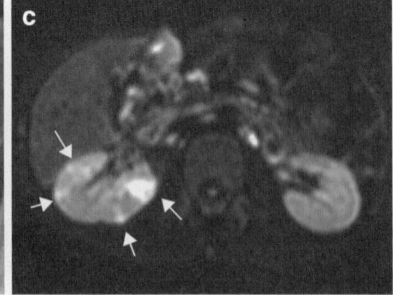

Fig. 5 MRI of a child with pyelonephritis of the right kidney. (**a**) The focal areas of oedema (*arrows*) are not easily depicted on T2-weighted images; only sparse cortical oedema with slightly increased signal is seen. (**b**) T1 fat-saturated images after intravenous contrast administration clearly show the cortical areas of hypoperfusion caused by focal oedema due to the infection. (**c**) Diffusion-weighted images (**b** 1000) show increased signal of the affected areas in the kidney, indicating restricted diffusion due to inflammation and oedema

the use of intravenous contrast (Vivier et al. 2014). MRI has also shown to have equal sensitivity to DMSA in the detection of renal scarring (Kocyigit et al. 2014). To date, the biggest problem with this technique is the relatively low availability and the need for sedation in younger children. Currently MRI has no place in routine workup of UTI in childhood but may gain momentum in the future. The main role of MRI in UTI is the assessment of complex malformations where US cannot give the full overview. Functional MRI is also being increasingly used as a 'one-stop shop' in the workup of both anatomy and function of the urinary tract (see chapter "MR of the Urogenital Tract in Children").

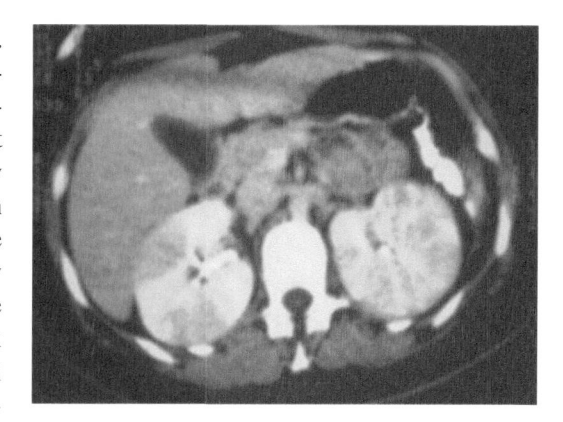

Fig. 6 CT should not be used to diagnose pyelonephritis and should be avoided in general in children with acute abdominal pain due to the large radiation burden. Despite this CT is sometimes still performed; hence the signs of pyelonephritis are important to recognise. Pyelonephritis is most easily depicted on the late postinjection phase and appears as hypodense striated triangular-shaped areas within the renal parenchyma

2.4 Computer Tomography (CT)

CT plays a very limited role in UTIs in children due to ionising hazards and the need of contrast injection and should normally *not* be performed as a diagnostic supplement. CT can be used if there is clinical progression under appropriate therapy or if an abscess is suspected when US does not give a sufficient information and MRI is not available or feasible (Riccabona et al. 2010).

Even if CT is not recommended, it is sometimes still performed in an acutely ill child; hence it is important to recognise the signs of pyelonephritis. Contrast-enhanced CT is sensitive to acute pyelonephritis. The renal changes are best demonstrated on the late postinjection phase and appear as hypodense striated triangular-shaped areas within the renal parenchyma (Fig. 6). There is focal or general nephromegaly and inflammatory changes in the perirenal fat (fatty stranding) may be seen. Due to the corticomedullary differentiation of the early postinjection ('cortical') phase, the extension of the renal disease may be underestimated if the images are obtained too early (Dacher et al. 1996). Sometimes CT is indicated in unusual infections like xanthogranulomatous pyelonephritis or renal tuberculosis.

2.5 Voiding Cystourethrography

VUR assessment by VCUG (or contrast-enhanced voiding urosonography or possibly radionuclide cystography, see chapter "Diagnostic Procedures: Excluding MRI, Nuclear Medicine and Video-Urodynamics") should be performed in selected patients according to the preferred guideline or protocol (see Fig. 1). It is used to diagnose VUR and in follow-up after VUR treatment. The procedure is invasive and includes catheterisation of the patient; hence it should only be performed after successful treatment of the UTI (for details see chapters "UTI and VUR" and "Vesicoureteric Reflux").

2.6 Intravenous Urography (IVU)

This technique has been replaced by more sensitive and less invasive methods and has no longer a place in the acute phase of a UTI. IVU also has a very limited role in the workup after UTI, and only a modified protocol in the excretory phase to look for the level of a suspected obstruction or for the assessment of an (infectious) stone may be used in carefully selected patients (Riccabona et al. 2010).

> **Take Away**
> Ultrasound is always the first – and often the only – modality required for children referred for further imaging workup in UTI. DMSA scintigraphy remains the modality of choice for renal scarring but may be replaced by MRI. VCUG (or ce-VUS/RNC) should only be performed in selectively selected patients based on age and the clinical presentation of the infection. IVU plays a very limited role in UTI. CT and MRI have no role in the routine workup of UTI, but MRI is increasingly used for both anatomical and functional urographies and may even gain momentum in the future to diagnose pyelonephritis, and help with assessment of complications.

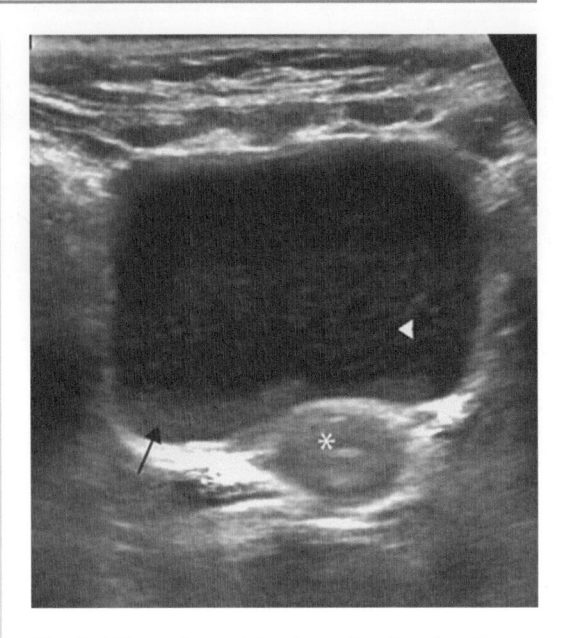

Fig. 7 Echogenic particles (*arrowhead*) and sediments (*arrow*) in the bladder might be seen on ultrasound and are not necessarily a sign of pus. It might be seen after an infection due to concentrated urine and urine sediments but can also be seen as an incidental finding

3 Normal Progression of UTI

In most children, with good response to appropriate treatment of UTI, the clinical symptoms resolve rapidly, even when there is renal involvement. However, the imaging findings, particularly on US, may remain for several weeks and it can take 4–6 weeks before the renal size and corticomedullary differentiation returns to normal. The pelvic wall thickening and hyperechogenicity of the renal sinus and perirenal fat may remain for even longer. This should be taken into account when performing a follow-up US after an acute pyelonephritis, particularly when monitoring renal growth. A significant decrease in renal size some weeks after an episode of acute pyelonephritis does not necessarily mean that there is damage to the renal parenchyma with nephron loss but may rather be due to normalisation of the oedema in a previously inflamed kidney. Note that sometimes echogenic particles are seen sonographically in the urine – this does not necessarily mean persisting puss, but often correlates with concentrated urine and urine sediments (Fig. 7).

> **Take Away**
> Imaging plays no role in evaluating treatment response if the clinical response is adequate. Note that imaging findings of UTI may persist for several weeks even after normal recovery.

4 Complications from Pyelonephritis

4.1 Acute Bacterial Nephritis

Acute bacterial nephritis or acute lobar nephronia is an unusual form of pyelonephritis and refers to a localised haemorrhage or necrosis or pseudo-tumorous swelling and oedema superimposed on the local, segmental bacterial infection. On US the involved area usually appears as a tumorous hyper- or hypoechoic swelling with or without clear limits and loss of corticomedullary differentiation (Cheng et al. 2004). This probably corresponds to a pre-abscess formation stage and can be challenging to differentiate from a renal tumour (Shimizu et al. 2005; Uehling et al. 2000; Cheng et al. 2010).

4.2 Renal Abscess

In delayed or inappropriate treatment of acute pyelonephritis as well as in some aggressive or resistant bacteria, the pyelonephritic lesions may coalesce and form an abscess (Fig. 8). This may remain limited to the kidney or extend first into the renal capsule and successively into the perinephric space (Fig. 9). The progressive extension of the inflammatory process may be demonstrated by US. An increased echogenicity of the retroperitoneal fat or even of the perivesical fat can be seen, sometimes also with focal complex fluid. The abscess itself sonographically appears as a mass with variable central echogenicity depending on the degree of necrosis. Both CT and MR imaging are valuable techniques for the demonstration of the abscess and its extension (Figs. 8 and 9). Large renal abscesses may mimic a renal tumour, but the clinical presentation and the response to treatment will normally lead to the right diagnosis (Wang et al. 2003).

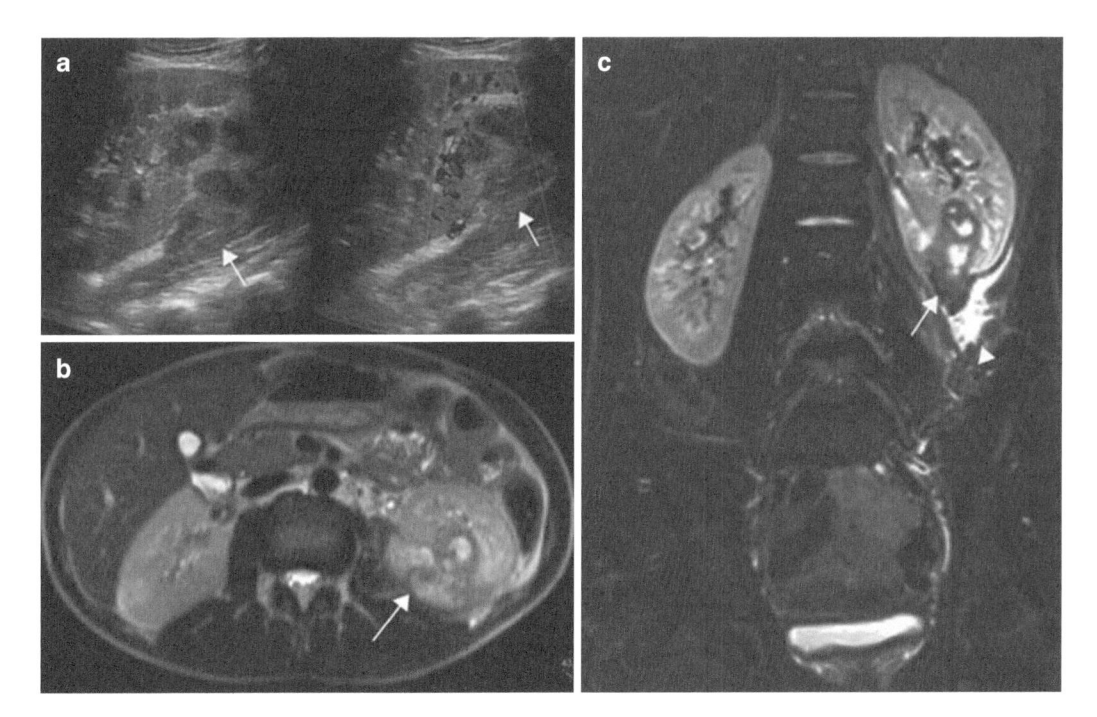

Fig. 8 A 13-year-old boy with type I diabetes presented with flank pain and mild fever. Ultrasound scan revealed a process in the lower pole of the left kidney with extension out of the kidney and hyperemia in the periphery and no flow seen within the lesion suggesting an inflammatory process (**a**). MRI (axial T2 TSE (**b**) and coronal STIR (**c**)) revealed an encapsulated fluid-filled process erupting out of the kidney (*arrows*) and fluid around the lower pole of the kidney (*arrowhead*). A renal abscess was suspected and confirmed by fine needle aspiration

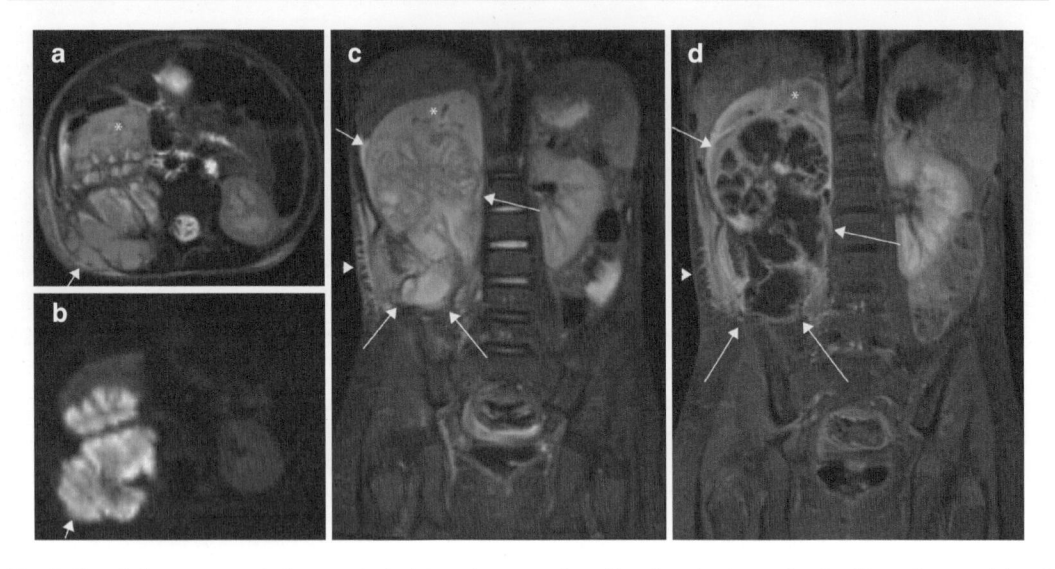

Fig. 9 Renal abscesses may be large and mimic a tumour. However, it is most often possible to make the correct diagnosis based on the clinical picture and the imaging findings. This 18-month-old child presented with a clinical picture of severe infection. There was a palpable mass in the right abdomen and flank. MRI showed a large mass (*arrows*) arising from the right kidney (*asterisk*). An axial (**a**) and coronal (**c**) STIR shows a septated mass with intermediate to high signal invading the posterior abdominal wall and cutis (*arrowhead*). There is a peripheral enhancement on a T1-weighted fat-saturated coronal image (**d**), and the central, non-enhancing areas also show restricted diffusion on a **b** 1000 diffusion-weighted image (**b**) suggestive of pus. A renal tumour would rarely invade adjacent tissue, whereas inflammatory processes typically cross tissue borders. This child responded well to acute drainage of the abscess and adequate treatment with antibiotics (Image courtesy of John Asle Bjørlykke)

4.3 Renal Scarring

Acute pyelonephritis may potentially cause nephron loss and subsequent renal scarring. Patients presenting renal scars are at risk for developing renal hypertension, pregnancy-related complications, renal failure and, rarely, end-stage renal failure (Fidan et al. 2013; Peters and Rushton 2010; see also chapter "UTI and VUR"). Patients with UTI presenting with high temperature (>39 °C), non- *E. coli* infection, pathology on US, cell count of greater than 60 %, CRP > 40 mg/L and the presence of VUR are at higher risk of developing renal scars as are children with recurrent or non-febrile UTI. High-grade VUR (grades IV and V) is thought to be the strongest predictor of renal scarring; however, this degree of VUR is only seen in a small proportion of patients who develop renal scars (Shaikh et al. 2014; Snodgrass et al. 2013). DMSA is the preferred technique for detection of renal scarring (Sinha et al. 2007) (Fig. 5). MRI has equally high sensitivity for renal scarring (Kocyigit et al. 2014) and when feasible this technique can replace DMSA in the assessment of renal scars (Fig. 10). US has a limited potential; even Doppler techniques are limited for this query – although high-resolution detailed scanning can depict scars – and gross scaring can be depicted by US reliably (Fig. 11). In the future, contrast-enhanced US may potentially help to improve the US potential for this application.

Imaging in Urinary Tract Infections

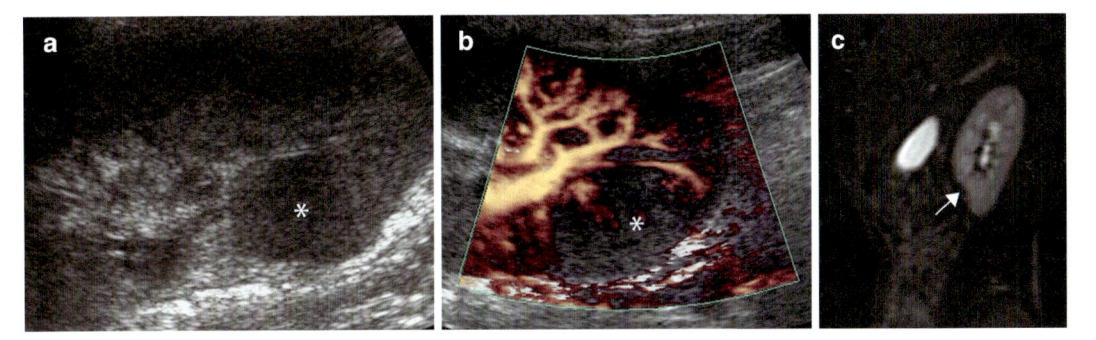

Fig. 10 Ultrasound of an 8-year-old boy with suspected pyelonephritis shows focal nephromegaly in the lower pole of the right kidney (*asterisk*) (**a**), amplitude-coded Doppler examination shows reduced perfusion in the same area in keeping with pyelonephritis (**b**). MRI 7 months after the acute infection shows parenchymal loss in the lower right pole in keeping with renal scar, here shown on a sagittal STIR (**c**) (*arrow*) (Image courtesy of Pierre Hugues Vivier)

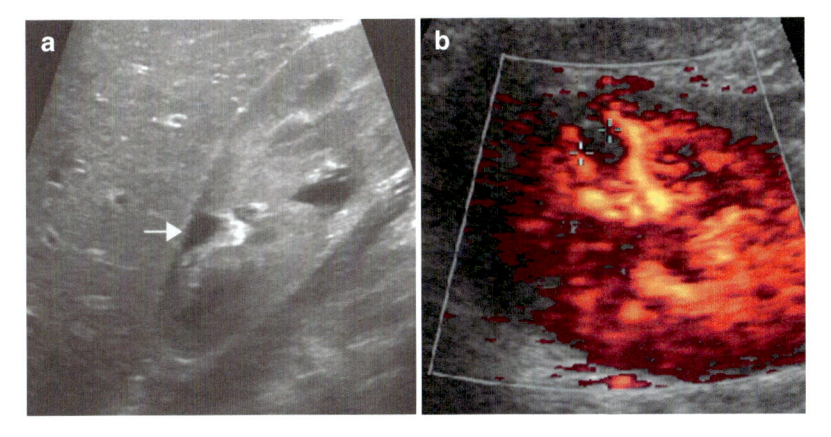

Fig. 11 Ultrasound is not a sensitive method for detection of renal scars, but large scars may however be seen. (**a**) Focal scar with clubbed calix and destroyed cortex acute pyelonephritis of the upper pole. (**b**) Small peripheral scar seen as perfusion defect on aCDS, not easily depicted by greyscale US (Reprinted with permission from: Riccabona (2014))

4.4 Xanthogranulomatous Pyelonephritis

Xanthogranulomatous pyelonephritis (XPN) is a rare form of chronic renal parenchymal infection. Its origin is controversial and probably multifactorial. Pathogenesis includes calculus or non-calculus obstruction, ineffectively treated acute pyelonephritis, ischaemia, a change in renal metabolism and altered immune response to infection. The diagnosis may be suggested in a child with tender flank pain, fever, pyuria, haematuria, weight loss, anaemia and imaging findings suggestive of this condition. The typical finding is a centrally calcified nodule within an otherwise normal-appearing kidney (localised form) or a large space-occupying lesion replacing the entire kidney and containing (often more central) cystic necrotic areas (diffuse form) (Fig. 12). Although typically a central (staghorn) calculus is seen, the mass is, however, not always calcified (Gasmi et al. 2010). The condition is usually mistaken for a neoplasm, and the final diagnosis is sometimes made based on histopathology – particularly as typical findings such as the central calculus and the typical history are often absent. The classic feature is the chronic inflammation and the infiltration of lipid-laden macrophages. This is reflected on MRI where fat often can be seen within the lesion. On diffusion-weighted imaging, the areas of necrosis often show very restricted diffusion (Zugor et al. 2007).

Take Away
Imaging is crucial in the workup of complications from pyelonephritis. Ultrasound is the diagnostic tool to detect focal nephritis and renal abscess. Renal scintigraphy remains the diagnostic tool for renal scarring but may be replaced by MRI. CT or MRI is often used in the rare occasion of suspected xanthogranulomatous pyelonephritis or other rare diseases/complications.

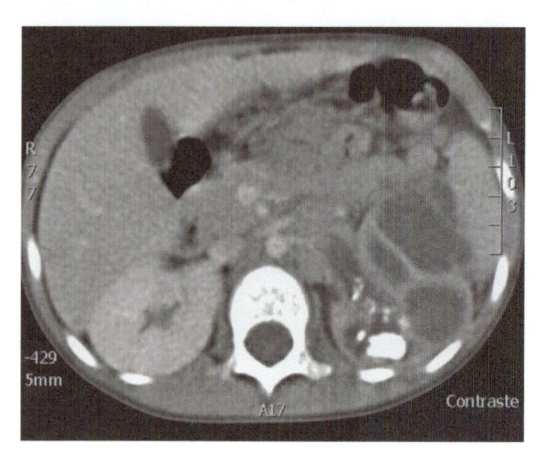

Fig. 12 CT findings of xanthogranulomatous pyelonephritis with loss of normal renal architecture and calcifications in the left kidney. The diagnosis is finally made based on histopathology

5 Cystitis

Cystitis refers to an infection or inflammation confined to the bladder. The classical symptoms are dysuria, pollakisuria and sometimes haematuria, but small children with cystitis may also experience weakness, irritability, reduced appetite and vomiting. Children with cystitis have normal or mildly elevated temperature. Sonographically, the bladder wall is thickened (Fig. 13) and it can be irregular and/or pseudo-tumoral and hence mimic neoplasms (Fig. 14). The urine within the bladder may contain floating echoes. These findings are not specific for a bacterial cystitis, since bladder wall thickening may appear in various conditions (Table 2) and urine echogenicity

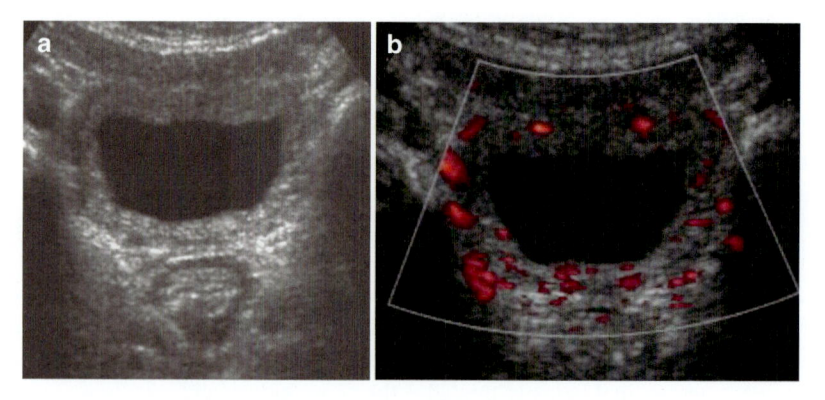

Fig. 13 Ultrasound in cystitis shows irregular thickening of hyperaemic bladder wall

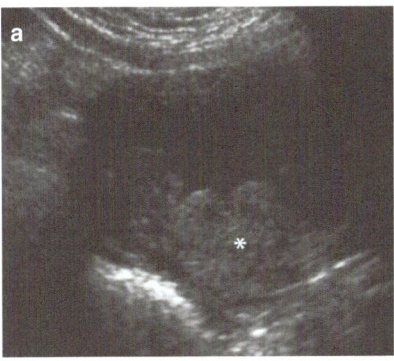

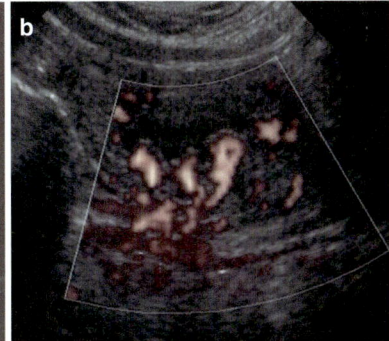

Fig. 14 Cystitis may cause focal thickening of the bladder wall. Greyscale ultrasound (**a**) shows thickening of the posterior bladder wall (*asterisk*), and amplitude-coded Doppler (**b**) shows hyperaemia of the 'lesion'. Imaging alone cannot differentiate focal thickening in cystitis that forms a tumour, but the clinical setting and normalisation of findings on treatment with antibiotic usually give the diagnosis

Table 2 Causes of bladder wall thickening

Infectious cystitis (may be localised pseudo-tumoral)
Eosinophilic cystitis
Drug-induced cystitis
Neurogenic bladder
Nonneurogenic bladder-sphincter dysfunction
Posterior urethral valves
Bladder outlet obstruction
Megacystis-megaureter association

can be present in children without infection due to haemorrhage and urine sediments, sometimes only caused by high concentrated urine. Imaging in bacterial cystitis in children has a limited role, but US can be performed in equivocal cases, in recurrent cystitis and in the assessment of differential diagnosis. If US is performed, indirect signs of bladder dysfunction should be assessed, such as an open bladder neck, a non-physiological bladder tension and shape, pathologic bladder capacity/filling volume or residual urine, as well as bladder wall thickening and trabeculation. However, the signs of bladder dysfunction may be caused by the cystitis itself and the signs could remain false positive weeks after the infection (for bladder dysfunction; please also see chapter "Non-neurogenic Bladder-Sphincter Dysfunction ("Voiding Dysfunction")") (Milosevic et al. 2013; McCarville et al. 2000).

6 Unusual Infections

6.1 Renal Candidiasis

Immunocompromised patients, neonates, patients under massive and long-term antibiotic therapy and patients with complicated uropathies are at particular risk of renal candidiasis (Festekjian and Neely 2011). On US various patterns have been described. The finding of global renal hyperechogenicity, hyperechoic sludge (resembling small lithiasis) and hyperechoic fungal balls without posterior shadowing in the right clinical setting should suggest candidiasis. The fungal balls typically cause obstruction of the collecting system; hence mild hydronephrosis and dilated calyces are a common finding. Lesions may involve the renal vessels with secondary hypertension or even extend into the extrarenal space. Additional imaging usually is not beneficial; the diagnosis is made from urine samples – unless the fungus grows in a heavily obstructed and poorly function system. In such cases diagnostic, image-guided urine sampling from the kidney is necessary.

6.2 Tuberculosis

Tuberculous involvement of the urinary tract is uncommon. The radiological features have mainly been described on IVU and include poor definition of a minor calyx or what is called the 'drooping lily' appearance of pyelocalyceal system. It may evolve towards an acquired infundibular stenosis. It is followed by cavitation into the parenchyma. Finally, the kidney may undergo end-stage autonephrectomy by ulcerocavernous caseation and subsequent calcification (putty kidney) (Das et al. 2014).

6.3 Hydatid Disease

Hydatid disease is a parasitic infection caused by larvae of tapeworms of the genus *Echinococcus*. Renal manifestation is unusual in hydatid disease but should be considered in areas or patients presenting an epidemiological risk. CT or US typically demonstrates a thick-walled multiloculated, cortical, solitary cystic structure. The cyst may sometimes be unilocular and may calcify. The falling snowflakes pattern within the cyst during patient mobilisation is a characteristic of the stages that resemble those reported for the liver and can thus be graded by US (Ghartimagar et al. 2013; Rami et al. 2011; Pedrosa et al. 2000).

6.4 Bilharziasis

Bilharziasis or schistosomiasis determines extensive inflammatory granulomatous reaction in the urinary tract. Renal involvement is usually asymptomatic, whereas ureteral involvement determines obstructive uropathy. Calcified thickening of the bladder wall is typical, and the bladder volume is markedly reduced (Fig. 15).

> **Take Away**
> Unusual infections may occur anywhere in the renal tract in children and the findings, both in the bladder and kidneys, may sometimes mimic neoplasms. Imaging plays an important role in suspecting, and sometimes diagnosing, unusual infections of the renal tract. Image-guided intervention, either biopsy or aspiration of urine, is sometimes required to secure the diagnosis.

7 Summary and Conclusion

The aim of imaging in childhood UTI is to detect underlying conditions that need to be modified to avoid recurrent infections and renal damage. Imaging is also crucial to detect both acute and

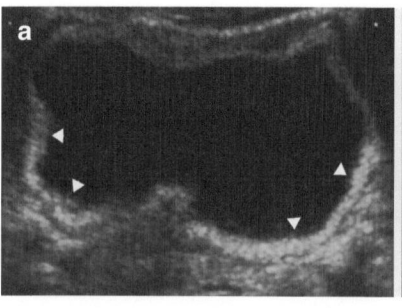

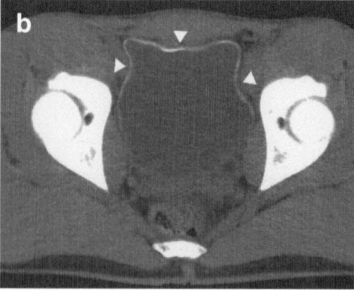

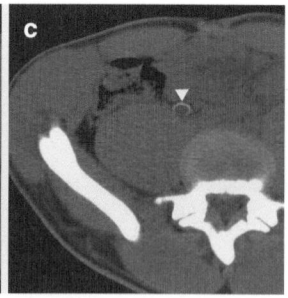

Fig. 15 The granulomatous inflammation caused by schistosomiasis *(bilharzia)* causes calcification of the bladder wall and ureters. (**a**) Ultrasound of a patient with bilharziasis shows hyperechoic calcified bladder wall. CT of another patient with bilharziasis clearly depicts the calcified bladder wall with restricted elasticity (**a**). Calcification of the ureters (**b**) may cause obstructive uropathy

long-term complications from UTI. Ultrasound remains the main modality in both workup of UTI and the detection of complications and of underlying conditions. The diagnosis of UTI is mainly based on clinical and laboratory findings, and patients must be meticulously selected for imaging, particularly for more invasive studies, based on the clinical presentation of the infection and the age of the child. New knowledge, particularly on VUR, is gained in the last decade, but the ideal patient selection and imaging algorithm in childhood UTI remain under discussion.

References

Brader P, Riccabona M, Schwarz T, Seebacher U, Ring E (2008) Value of comprehensive renal ultrasound in children with acute urinary tract infection for assessment of renal involvement: comparison with DMSA scintigraphy and final diagnosis. Eur Radiol 18(12):2981–2989. doi:10.1007/s00330-008-1081-z

Brandstrom P, Hansson S (2014) Long-term, low-dose prophylaxis against urinary tract infections in young children. Pediatr Nephrol. doi:10.1007/s00467-014-2854-z

Chakupurakal R, Ahmed M, Sobithadevi DN, Chinnappan S, Reynolds T (2010) Urinary tract pathogens and resistance pattern. J Clin Pathol 63(7):652–654. doi:10.1136/jcp.2009.074617

Cheng CH, Tsau YK, Hsu SY, Lee TL (2004) Effective ultrasonographic predictor for the diagnosis of acute lobar nephronia. Pediatr Infect Dis J 23(1):11–14. doi:10.1097/01.inf.0000105202.57991.3e

Cheng CH, Tsau YK, Lin TY (2010) Is acute lobar nephronia the midpoint in the spectrum of upper urinary tract infections between acute pyelonephritis and renal abscess? J Pediatr 156(1):82–86. doi:10.1016/j.jpeds.2009.07.010

Dacher JN, Pfister C, Monroc M, Eurin D, LeDosseur P (1996) Power Doppler sonographic pattern of acute pyelonephritis in children: comparison with CT. AJR Am J Roentgenol 166(6):1451–1455. doi:10.2214/ajr.166.6.8633462

Das CJ, Ahmad Z, Sharma S, Gupta AK (2014) Multimodality imaging of renal inflammatory lesions. World J Radiol. 28;6(11):865–873

Faust WC, Diaz M, Pohl HG (2009) Incidence of postpyelonephritic renal scarring: a meta-analysis of the dimercapto-succinic acid literature. J Urol 181(1):290–297. doi:10.1016/j.juro.2008.09.039; discussion 7–8

Festekjian A, Neely M (2011) Incidence and predictors of invasive candidiasis associated with candidaemia in children. Mycoses 54(2):146–153. doi:10.1111/j.1439-0507.2009.01785.x

Fidan K, Kandur Y, Buyukkaragoz B, Akdemir UO, Soylemezoglu O (2013) Hypertension in pediatric patients with renal scarring in association with vesicoureteral reflux. Urology 81(1):173–177. doi:10.1016/j.urology.2012.09.003

Garin EH, Olavarria F, Araya C, Broussain M, Barrera C, Young L (2007) Diagnostic significance of clinical and laboratory findings to localize site of urinary infection. Pediatr Nephrol 22(7):1002–1006. doi:10.1007/s00467-007-0465-7

Gasmi M, Jemai R, Fitouri F, Ben Slama A, Sahli S, Hamzaoui M (2010) Xanthogranulomatous pyelonephritis in childhood: diagnosis difficulties and success of conservative treatment. Tunis Med 88(6):427–429

Ghartimagar D, Ghosh A, Shrestha MK, Talwar OP, Sathian B (2013) 14 years hospital based study on clinical and morphological spectrum of hydatid disease. JNMA J Nepal Med Assoc 52(190):349–353

Kocyigit A, Yuksel S, Bayram R, Yilmaz I, Karabulut N (2014) Efficacy of magnetic resonance urography in detecting renal scars in children with vesicoureteral reflux. Pediatr Nephrol 29(7):1215–1220. doi:10.1007/s00467-014-2766-y

MacKenzie JR (1996) A review of renal scarring in children. Nucl Med Commun 17(3):176–190

McCarville MB, Hoffer FA, Gingrich JR, Jenkins JJ 3rd (2000) Imaging findings of hemorrhagic cystitis in pediatric oncology patients. Pediatr Radiol 30(3):131–138

McDonald K, Kenney I (2014) Paediatric urinary tract infections: a retrospective application of the National Institute of Clinical Excellence guidelines to a large general practitioner referred historical cohort. Pediatr Radiol 44(9):1085–1092. doi:10.1007/s00247-014-2967-3

Milosevic D, Trkulja V, Turudic D, Batinic D, Spajic B, Tesovic G (2013) Ultrasound bladder wall thickness measurement in diagnosis of recurrent urinary tract infections and cystitis cystica in prepubertal girls. J Pediatr Urol 9(6 Pt B):1170–1177. doi:10.1016/j.jpurol.2013.04.019

Montini G, Rigon L, Zucchetta P, Fregonese F, Toffolo A, Gobber D et al (2008) Prophylaxis after first febrile urinary tract infection in children? A multicenter, randomized, controlled, noninferiority trial. Pediatrics 122(5):1064–1071. doi:10.1542/peds.2007-3770

Mori R, Lakhanpaul M, Verrier-Jones K (2007) Diagnosis and management of urinary tract infection in children: summary of NICE guidance. BMJ 335(7616):395–397. doi:10.1136/bmj.39286.700891.AD

Muller LS (2014) Ultrasound of the paediatric urogenital tract. Eur J Radiol 83(9):1538–1548. doi:10.1016/j.ejrad.2014.04.001

Pedrosa I, Saiz A, Arrazola J, Ferreiros J, Pedrosa CS (2000) Hydatid disease: radiologic and pathologic features and complications. Radiographics 20(3):795–817. doi:10.1148/radiographics.20.3.g00ma06795

Peters C, Rushton HG (2010) Vesicoureteral reflux associated renal damage: congenital reflux nephropathy and acquired renal scarring. J Urol 184(1):265–273. doi:10.1016/j.juro.2010.03.076

Rami M, Khattala K, ElMadi A, Afifi MA, Bouabddallah Y (2011) The renal hydatid cyst: report on 4 cases. Pan Afr Med J 8:31

Riccabona M (2014) Ultrasound of the urogenital tract, Fig 10.22. In: Riccabona M (ed) Pediatric ultrasound, requisites and applications. Springer, Berlin/Heidelberg. ISBN 978-3-642-39155-2

Riccabona M (2015/2016). Imaging in childhood urinary tract infection. La Radiologia Medica; e-pblished Nov 2015. doi: 10.1007/s11547-015-0594-1

Riccabona M, Avni FE, Blickman JG, Dacher JN, Darge K, Lobo ML et al (2008) Imaging recommendations in paediatric uroradiology: minutes of the ESPR workgroup session on urinary tract infection, fetal hydronephrosis, urinary tract ultrasonography and voiding cystourethrography, Barcelona, Spain, June 2007. Pediatr Radiol 38(2):138–145. doi:10.1007/s00247-007-0695-7

Riccabona M, Avni FE, Dacher JN, Damasio MB, Darge K, Lobo ML et al (2010) ESPR uroradiology task force and ESUR paediatric working group: imaging and procedural recommendations in paediatric uroradiology, part III. Minutes of the ESPR uroradiology task force minisymposium on intravenous urography, uro-CT and MR-urography in childhood. Pediatr Radiol 40(7):1315–1320. doi:10.1007/s00247-010-1686-7

Ristola MT, Hurme T (2014) NICE guidelines cannot be recommended for imaging studies in children younger than 3 years with urinary tract infection. Eur J Pediatr Surg. doi:10.1055/s-0034-1384646

Shaikh N, Ewing AL, Bhatnagar S, Hoberman A (2010) Risk of renal scarring in children with a first urinary tract infection: a systematic review. Pediatrics 126(6):1084–1091. doi:10.1542/peds.2010-0685

Shaikh N, Craig JC, Rovers MM, Da Dalt L, Gardikis S, Hoberman A et al (2014) Identification of children and adolescents at risk for renal scarring after a first urinary tract infection: a meta-analysis with individual patient data. JAMA Pediatr 168(10):893–900. doi:10.1001/jamapediatrics.2014.637

Shimizu M, Katayama K, Kato E, Miyayama S, Sugata T, Ohta K (2005) Evolution of acute focal bacterial nephritis into a renal abscess. Pediatr Nephrol 20(1):93–95. doi:10.1007/s00467-004-1646-2

Sinha MD, Gibson P, Kane T, Lewis MA (2007) Accuracy of ultrasonic detection of renal scarring in different centres using DMSA as the gold standard. Nephrol Dial Transplant 22(8):2213–2216. doi:10.1093/ndt/gfm155, gfm155 [pii]

Snodgrass WT, Shah A, Yang M, Kwon J, Villanueva C, Traylor J et al (2013) Prevalence and risk factors for renal scars in children with febrile UTI and/or VUR: a cross-sectional observational study of 565 consecutive patients. J Pediatr Urol 9(6 Pt A):856–863. doi:10.1016/j.jpurol.2012.11.019

Sorantin E, Fotter R, Aigner R, Ring E, Riccabona M (1997) The sonographically thickened wall of the upper urinary tract: correlation with other imaging methods. Pediatr Radiol 27:667–671

Tullus K (2011) Difficulties in diagnosing urinary tract infections in small children. Pediatr Nephrol 26(11):1923–1926. doi:10.1007/s00467-011-1966-y

Tullus K (2013) A review of guidelines for urinary tract infections in children younger than 2 years. Pediatr Ann 42(3):52–56. doi:10.3928/00904481-20130222-10

Uehling DT, Hahnfeld LE, Scanlan KA (2000) Urinary tract abnormalities in children with acute focal bacterial nephritis. BJU Int 85(7):885–888

Subcommittee on Urinary Tract Infection SCoQI, Management; Roberts KB (2011) Urinary tract infection: clinical practice guideline for the diagnosis and management of the initial UTI in febrile infants and children 2 to 24 months. Pediatrics 128(3):595–610. doi:10.1542/peds.2011-1330

Vivier PH, Sallem A, Beurdeley M, Lim RP, Leroux J, Caudron J et al (2014) MRI and suspected acute pyelonephritis in children: comparison of diffusion-weighted imaging with gadolinium-enhanced T1-weighted imaging. Eur Radiol 24(1):19–25. doi:10.1007/s00330-013-2971-2

Wang YT, Lin KY, Chen MJ, Chiou YY (2003) Renal abscess in children: a clinical retrospective study. Acta Paediatr Taiwan 44(4):197–201

Wennerstrom M, Hansson S, Jodal U, Stokland E (2000) Primary and acquired renal scarring in boys and girls with urinary tract infection. J Pediatr 136(1):30–34

Yim HE, Yim H, Bae ES, Woo SU, Yoo KH (2014) Predictive value of urinary and serum biomarkers in young children with febrile urinary tract infections. Pediatr Nephrol 29(11):2181–2189. doi:10.1007/s00467-014-2845-0

Zugor V, Schott GE, Labanaris AP (2007) Xanthogranulomatous pyelonephritis in childhood: a critical analysis of 10 cases and of the literature. Urology 70(1):157–160. doi:10.1016/j.urology.2007.02.068

Imaging in Renal Agenesis, Dysplasia, Hypoplasia, and Cystic Diseases of the Kidney

Michael Riccabona, Ekkehard Ring, and Freddy Avni

Contents

1	Introduction..	553
2	Renal Agenesis..	554
3	Renal Hypoplasia...	556
4	Renal Dysplasia..	557
5	Cystic Renal Disease.......................................	559
5.1	Polycystic Kidney Disease.................................	561
5.2	Multicystic Dysplastic Kidney (MCDK)............	565
5.3	Medullary Sponge Kidney (MSK)....................	567
5.4	Simple Renal Cyst and Acquired Renal Cyst...	568
5.5	Complicated Renal Cyst, Multiloculated Cyst, and Cystic Renal Tumor........................	570
6	Summary..	572
References..		572

1 Introduction

Renal malformations represent the most common manifestation of congenital diseases in childhood. Renal agenesis, dysplasia, hypoplasia, and cystic renal diseases are such entities. Causes vary; partially they derive from the complex renal organogenesis, and partially they have a genetic background. Today there is evidence that disturbances of the cilium-centrosome complex form the pathogenetic base of most or many phenotypically different cystic renal diseases on a cellular level; thus, they are summarized under the term "ciliopathies" (Guay-Woodford 2006; Hildebrandt 2005; Hildebrandt et al. 2011). Furthermore, uromodulin – a urinary mucoprotein former known as "Tamm-Horsfall protein" – appears to play an important role in the genesis of cystic kidney diseases (Iorember and Vehaskari 2014). The knowledge of the individual etiology and development helps to understand the disease process, affects further diagnostic and therapeutic management, and helps to properly estimate prognosis of these patients and their families, respectively. The clinical and genetic basics including the relevant queries toward imaging are discussed in chapters "Genetics in Nephrourology" and "Renal Agenesis, Dysplasia, Hypoplasia, and Cystic Diseases of the Kidney".

Diagnosis is often easy; gross renal pathology may already be depicted by prenatal ultrasound (US) (Helin and Persson 1986; Cohen and Haller 1987; Patten et al. 1990; Zejil et al. 1999).

M. Riccabona, MD (✉) • E. Ring, MD (Retired)
Department of Pediatrics, Division of General Pediatrics, University Hospital Graz, Auenbruggerplatz 34, A – 8036 Graz, Austria
e-mail: michael.riccabona@meduni-graz.at

F. Avni, MD, PhD
Department of Pediatric Radiology, Jeanne de Flandre Hospital, Lille University Hospital, 59037 Lille, France
e-mail: favni@skynet.be

However, gradually evolving disease may only manifest later, or subtle pathology can pose some difficulties to imaging. Furthermore, renal pathology may be detected by screening programs after birth or examinations for other reasons such as urinary tract infection, hematuria, nephrolithiasis, wetting, hypertension, or symptoms of developing renal insufficiency; even unrelated symptoms may lead to an US investigation that depicts renal pathology by chance.

Differentiation of various similar entities can be challenging, indicating the need for imaging. The known association with other pathology of the urinary tract may also necessitate additional studies, such as voiding cystourethrography (VCUG). Postnatal imaging usually is governed by prenatal findings, family history, known disease likely to be associated with renal abnormalities, or clinical as well as laboratory findings that indicate renal disease in either symptomatic or otherwise healthy patients.

The task of imaging is to reliably define or rule out a disease state in an economic way at minimal burden to the patient. In general, US is used as the first, noninvasive, nonionizing imaging tool for evaluation of the urinary tract and possible associated malformations, for example, in syndromal conditions. If US, including the modern techniques such as color Doppler (CDS), power Doppler (= amplitude-coded color Doppler sonography, aCDS), and harmonic imaging (HI) combined with high-resolution techniques and transducers, sufficiently answers the clinical query, no further imaging is needed; US may sometimes even offer more information than MRI particularly in small children (due to its high resolution) (Fig. 1). Otherwise, scintigraphy for evaluating renal (relative) function, VCUG (or contrast-enhanced voiding urosonography, ceVUS) for evaluation of vesicoureteral reflux (VUR), and MRI (rarely CT) for assessing calyceal cysts/diverticula, duplex systems, evaluation of complications, and cystic renal tumors, renal calcifications, or (US-guided) renal biopsy may become necessary (Fig. 2). Once the diagnosis is established, follow-up depends on the course of the disease and the implications on management; this can usually be accomplished by repeated US.

2 Renal Agenesis

In patients with unilateral renal agenesis, one usually finds no ipsilateral ureter, as well as associated aplasia, hypoplasia, or anomalies of genital structures originating from the ipsilateral Wolffian and Mullerian duct (Woolf and Allen 1953). The renal vessels are missing, and there may be aplasia of the ipsilateral adrenal gland in 10 % (Frohneberg 1986; Hoyer 1996a; Kiechl-Kohlendorfer et al. 2011). Unilateral renal agenesis has no significant impact on the patient only with a risk of accompanying malformations (Cope and Trickey 1982). The contralateral kidney may be ectopic and malrotated and usually presents with compensatory hypertrophy. However, if

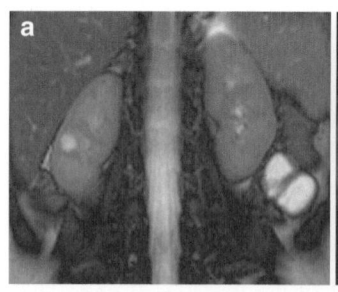

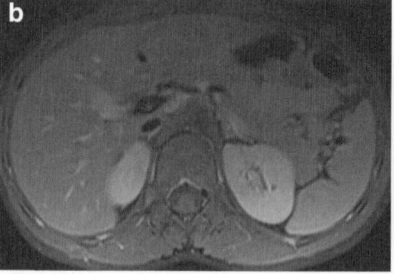

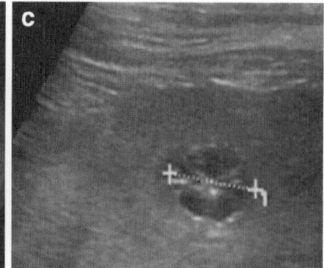

Fig. 1 MRI and US in cystic renal disease - both methods have their advantages: (**a**) MRI (performed for the query "complicated cyst versus cystic nephroma") shows the cyst in the middle section of the right kidney, but additionally depicts a tiny cyst in the contralateral cyst arrow) which was missed on US (**b**, **c**) HR-US of the right kidney of same patients as in Figure 31.1.a nicely demonstrates the multicystic, septated nature of this complicated cyst (+ ....+), with a normal outer cortex – a finding not differentiated by MRI

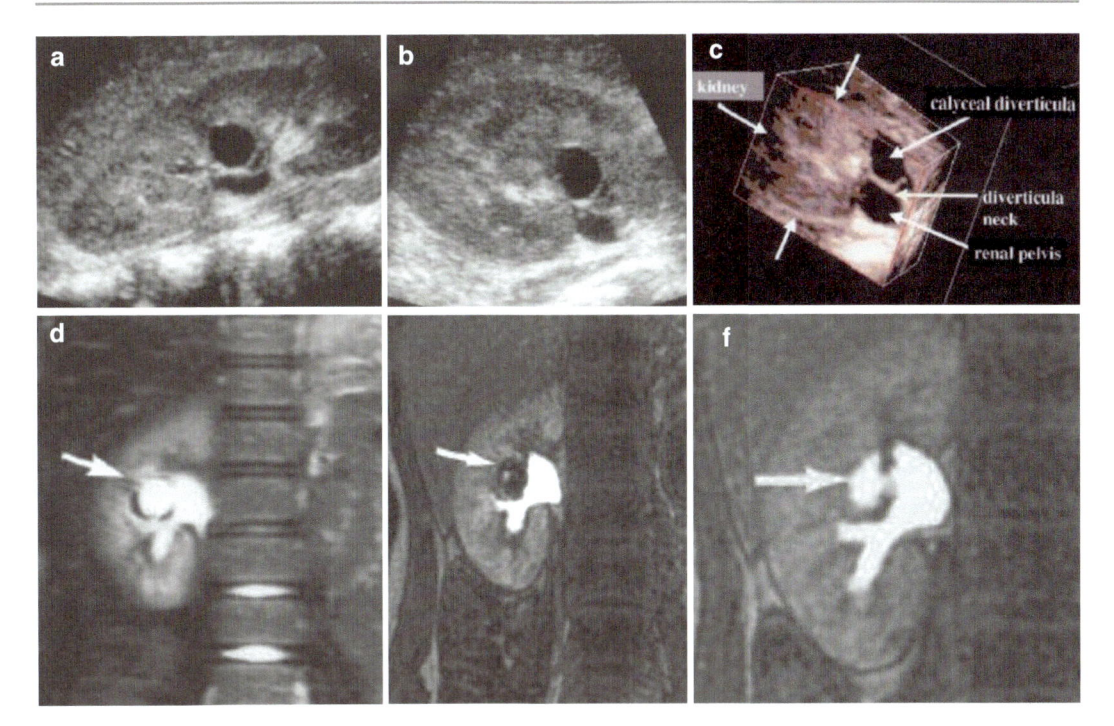

Fig. 2 Multimodal imaging for differential diagnosis, here for diagnosing a calyceal diverticulum: (**a, b**) US of a simple renal cyst close to the renal pelvis in longitudinal and transverse images. (**c**) 3DUS of the same cyst suggesting a connection of the cyst to the urinary collecting system (diverticular neck). (**d–f**) MR-urography images of this calicyeal diverticulum (*arrow*) demonstrating initially the topographic anatomy of the cyst (T2-weighted coronal image, (**d**), then the delayed contrast extravasation into this calyceal diverticulum on dynamic imaging after contrast administration (T1-weighted fast gradient echo 3D sequences/acquisitions; (**e**) = early phase, no contrast in the cyst; (**f**) = delayed scan with gadolinium coming from the collecting system into cyst)

hypertrophy is not present, dysplastic and/or hypoplastic changes of the remaining single kidney must be considered, and these patients need close nephrological follow-up since prognosis is worse. And as close relatives have a slightly increased risk of renal malformations, some propose US screening for them. Bilateral renal agenesis, also called Potter's syndrome, is lethal.

The purpose of postnatal imaging is to search for ectopic kidney parenchyma, to evaluate the contralateral kidney (e.g., to differentiate crossed dystopia), to assure normal renal appearance, and to evaluate associated abnormalities, particularly of the genital structures. In general, US is used as the first step (Fig. 3). Then MRI (or scintigraphy – including an anterior acquisition with a catheterized urinary bladder) and – in risk patients – VCUG or ce-VUS are performed (Riccabona et al. 2012; Riccabona et al. 2004a, b). No additional imaging

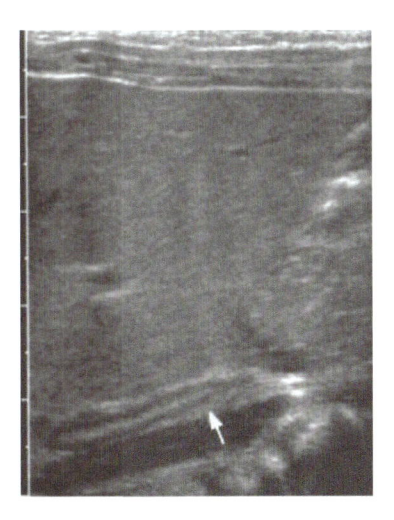

Fig. 3 US of renal agenesis showing the empty renal fossa with a somewhat atypically shaped adrenal gland (*arrow*) in this longitudinal view of the *right upper quadrant*

is used routinely. However, MRI and three-dimensional US (3DUS) can be helpful for evaluating associated genital anomalies, e.g., to find an ectopic testis (by MRI) or to confirm a bicornuate or septate uterus (using 3DUS, with rendering and thick slab coronal reconstructions) (Beomonte-Zobel et al. 1990; Jurkovic et al. 1995; Landry et al. 1999; Nelson et al. 1999; Riccabona 2014). Note that imaging sometimes has restrictions in differentiating real renal agenesis form a shrunken (ectopic) renal bud leaving the patient with a single kidney; cystoscopy confirming only one ureteral orifice will definitely establish the diagnosis – this usually is without consequence on prognosis and management and thus not deemed necessary.

> **Take Away**
>
> In renal agenesis, imaging (primarily US, complemented by MRI, sometimes VCUG or ce-VUS and scintigraphy) is used for confirming the diagnosis and for evaluating and monitoring the contralateral kidney.

3 Renal Hypoplasia

Renal hypoplasia is a mixture of many different conditions, describing a congenital renal anomaly. It is defined as a small kidney (2SD below the normal) with normal morphology and a reduced number of nephrons (Cain et al. 2010). It may be detected by chance in children who are otherwise healthy; in others, it is diagnosed by an examination indicated by symptoms or presentation of a more severe disease state such as urinary tract infection, hypertension, or chronic renal failure. Neonates with oligohydramnios may suffer from bilateral hypoplasia and have neonatal chronic renal failure. The details on etiology and different entities as well as clinical implications and queries for imaging arising for diagnosis and management are discussed in chapters "Genetics in Nephrourology" and "Renal Agenesis, Dysplasia, Hypoplasia, and Cystic Diseases of the Kidney" (Table 1).

Table 1 Renal hypoplasia

Simple renal hypoplasia
Isolated
Syndromal (branchio-oto-renal syndrome, fetal alcohol syndrome, Turner syndrome, Goldenhar syndrome, autosomal syndromes)
Unipapillary kidney and segmental hypoplasia (Ask-Upmark kidney)
Mixed renal hypoplasia (with dysplastic and cystic elements)
Oligomeganephronia
Isolated
Syndromal (branchio-oto-renal syndrome)

Classification and forms of renal hypoplasia, adapted according to Bernstein (1973, 1992) and Watkins et al. (1997)

Imaging usually starts with US. US typically – in pure renal hypoplasia – shows a just small kidney with otherwise often normal sonomorphologic appearance. However, US cannot reliably differentiate hypo- from dysplasia which both can be uni- or bilateral; thus often the term hypodysplastic kidney is used (Fig. 4). Standardized volume calculations are essential as well as calculating relative renal size. Renal growth charts reflect the changes in renal size depending on age and bodyweight, but do not account for regional variations (Avni et al. 1985; Dinkel et al. 1985; Kasiske and Umen 1986; Churg et al. 1987; Hoyer 1996a; Schneider and Fendel 1995) (see chapter

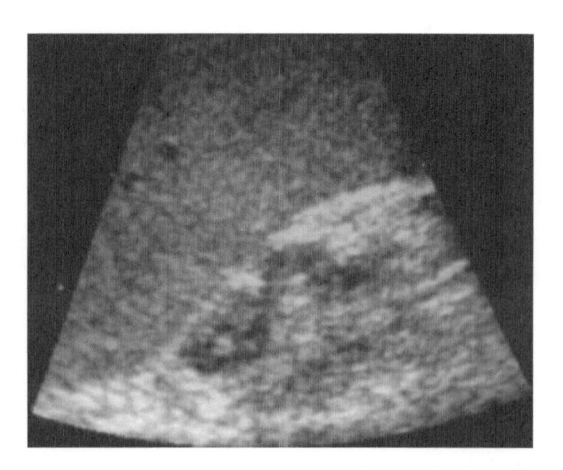

Fig. 4 US of the right upper quadrant showing a small, but otherwise sono-morphologically relatively normal kidney in a longitudinal section, consistent with renal hypo(-dys-)plasia

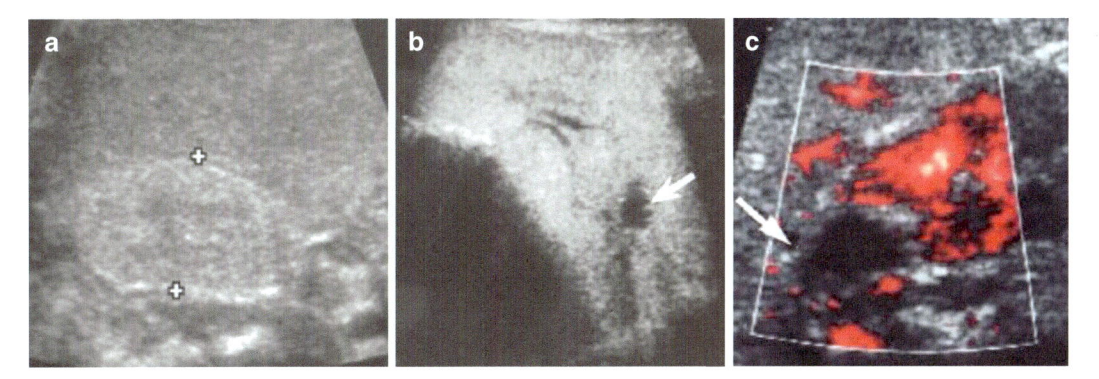

Fig. 5 Renal dysplasia: (**a**) Renal US shows an increased echogenicity of the undifferentiated renal parenchyma in cross-sectional view of a relatively small, dysplastic right kidney (+ +). (**b**) US using HI demonstrates the echogenic, not differentiated parenchyma of a diffusely dysplasic, ectopic kidney of approximately normal size, with a slightly prominent calyx (*arrow*) in the *lower part*. (**c**) ACDS demonstrates reduced vasculature/perfusion in the segmental obstructive dysplasia of the upper moiety in a duplex system (*arrow*), in relation to good perfusion of the normal renal parenchyma of the lower part

"Normal Values"). In segmental – then usually dysplastic – manifestation, aCDS may demonstrate segmental vessel rarefaction in the affected areas (see Fig. 5c). Scintigraphy confirms the lack of focal parenchymal defects in diffuse hypoplasia. IVU is rarely used nowadays and is restricted for situations where no MRI is available and with suspicion of a duplex system, a unipapillary kidney, or a possible segmental manifestation as well as in an additionally dilated urinary tract. It shows a small kidney with reduced concentration of contrast both in the parenchyma and in the otherwise normal urinary tract in diffuse disease or regional parenchymal narrowing with reduced parenchymal contrast in segmental (then usually dysplastic) manifestation.

Sometimes additional workup is performed with VCUG (or ce-VUS) to rule out VUR as a possible cause for a radiologically small kidney and scintigraphy (increasingly replaced by MRI) for determination of relative (split) renal size and function.

Various entities leading to small kidneys have to be considered for the differential diagnosis, especially when disease is discovered later in childhood. These include renal artery stenosis, renal dysplasia, chronic renal parenchymal disease, or postpyelitic "cirrhotic" shrunken kidney/end-stage kidney. CT or MR angiography and (sometimes) captopril scintigraphy are performed in suspected renal artery stenosis after a detailed Doppler US study (Riccabona et al. 2011). In chronic glomerulonephritis, US-guided biopsy may become indicated. Catheter angiography is performed to confirm renal artery stenosis or regional vascular disease and often combined with balloon dilatation/angioplasty in the same session if applicable.

4 Renal Dysplasia

> **Take Away**
> Imaging is used to differentiate pure hypoplasia from other entities that cause a small kidney such as acquired disease, (obstructive) dysplasia, scarring, and "reflux nephropathy." It starts with US (including a Doppler US study) and then generally is complemented by VCUG/ce-VUS and MRI and/or isotope studies.

There is a wide range of manifestations and underlying causes for renal dysplasia (Stockamp 1986). Etiology and classification details are again discussed also in chapter "Genetics in Nephrourology".

The manifestation can vary from focal/segmental dysplasia, such as in duplex kidneys (with or without ectopic ureteroceles), or subtle tissue changes over diffuse severe disease to even nonfunctioning renal units such as in MCDK (see also Sect. 5.2). In general, a disturbed renal ontogenesis results in the presence of histological structures not present during normal nephrogenesis – naturally these cannot be diagnosed by imaging in detail. These changes can be associated with hypoplasia; US may however not always allow differentiation of those, and thus, in these cases the term hypodysplasia is used (see Fig. 4). Dysplasia can be diagnosed if typical signs are observed such as echogenic cortex without normal differentiation or cystic changes and with various syndromes (syndromal dysplasia, e.g., in trisomies 13–15 and 18 or in Meckel-Gruber syndrome) (Table 2; see also Sect. 5.1.5).

Clinical symptoms vary depending on the individual manifestation, the underlying disease, and the amount of renal functional impairment. And diagnostically, imaging plays the most important role in the initial workup.

US can detect tissue changes: it usually shows an echogenic renal parenchyma with reduced corticomedullary differentiation; sometimes small "microscopic" changes cannot be depicted by US. Cysts of varying sizes, mostly small, may be present (Fig. 5a, b). Duplex Doppler may show elevated renal resistance in poorly functioning units; aCDS helps to evaluate reduced peripheral renal vasculature and perfusion, most convincingly displayed in segmental manifestation – but may be poor in differencing the etiology of a cystic structure (Fig. 5c). Additionally, VCUG or ce-VUS – to detect the often-associated VUR – and scintigraphy are performed in part, the latter being increasingly replaced by MRI, not only for patients with complex urinary tract abnormalities (Terrier et al. 1986; Krestin 1990; Sigmund et al. 1991; Hattery and King 1995; Avni et al. 1997; Borthne et al. 1999). Only in some equivocal situations, when disease is found during later childhood and imaging as well as genetics remains inconclusive, diagnosis is made by (US-guided) renal biopsy. Focal dysplasia as found in tuberous sclerosis (renal angiomyolipoma) and von Recklinghausen's neurofibromatosis are discussed in chapter "Neoplasms of the Genitourinary System" (renal neoplasm) and "MR of the Urogenital Tract in Children" usually are listed as benign renal masses (Dodat et al. 1988; Bernstein 1993a, b), as they rather present as a renal mass or tumor than as a focal dysplasia or a renal cyst.

Table 2 Renal dysplasia

Multicystic renal dysplasia
Obstructive renal dysplasia:
With lower urinary tract obstruction
With upper urinary tract obstruction
Segmental renal dysplasia
Diffuse renal dysplasia
Syndromal:
Autosomal dominant: tuberous sclerosis, von Hippel-Lindau syndrome
Autosomal recessive: Meckel-Gruber syndrome, orofacial-digital syndrome, Zellweger syndrome, short limb-polydactyly syndrome, Jeune syndrome
Aneuploidies: trisomies 13–15, 18, 21, Turner syndrome
Non-inherited syndrome: nail patella syndrome, prune belly syndrome, Ehlers-Danlos syndrome, branchio-oto-renal syndrome
Non-syndromal and miscellaneous
Focal renal dysplasia
Miscellaneous
Hereditary:
Angiomyolipoma (tuberous sclerosis)
Neurofibroma (von Recklinghausen's neurofibromatosis)

Various manifestations of renal dysplasia, including cystic and syndromal forms, adapted according to Bernstein (1992), Kissane (1990), Hoyer (1996a), and Watkins (1997)

Take Away

US can be suggestive of (hypo-)dysplasia. Histology establishes the definite diagnosis, particularly in patients with disease detected later in life and not in early infancy. VCUG (or ce-VUS) is obligatory. Other imaging methods are used for additional workup, to confirm an otherwise normal urinary tract and to evaluate (split) renal function (isotope studies, fMRU).

5 Cystic Renal Disease

This includes a variety of entities; numerous classifications exist that have changed over time. The old Potter classification has been abandoned which was rather descriptive and less oriented toward pathogenesis. New proposals either focus on the genesis, or the time of manifestation (Glassberg et al. 1987; Avni and Hall 2010; Vester et al. 2010) (Tables 3 and 4). And for imaging – particularly US – a schematic guide to help differentiation has been developed based on the schema for adults developed by Morcos and adapted toward children and new insights (Morcos 2009; Riccabona et al. 2012) (Fig. 6a).

The causes vary. Inherited diseases as well as a disturbed renal embryogenesis and renal development create a wide spectrum of manifestations that spans from diffuse, severe, bilateral congenital disease to simple, single renal cysts occurring in the adult (Tanago 1975; Stockamp 1986) (Table 3). The main mechanism is a disturbance at the junction between the metanephrogenic tissue and the ureteral bud (Osathanondh and Potter 1964, 1966; Devine 1983). Further details on etiology, development, and genetics as well as clinical implications are addressed in chapters "Urinary Tract Embryology, Anatomy, and Anatomical Variants", "Genetics in Nephrourology", and "Renal Agenesis, Dysplasia, Hypoplasia, and Cystic Diseases of the Kidney".

The various forms and clinical presentations may have different prognoses and may imply different diagnostic and therapeutic strategies. The following pages discuss the most important entities separately.

The role of imaging is to detect or confirm a cystic renal disease, sometimes also to rule out renal involvement in a suspected systemic condition, and to help defining the underlying condition (deBruyn and Gordon 2000; Bisaglia et al. 2006). It can be difficult to differentiate small cysts from other parenchymal diseases or a complicated (e.g., hemorrhagic) renal cyst as well as a segmental polycystic abnormality from cystic renal tumors, thus supporting and enabling differential diagnosis in unclear or other suspected cystic renal findings (Fig. 6a, b).

In general, imaging starts with US, including Doppler facilities, HR imaging, and HI, which significantly improves tissue differentiation and detection as well as delineation of cysts, particularly in difficult scanning conditions (Thomas

Table 3 Cystic renal diseases

Hereditary disease
Polycystic kidney disease
Autosomal recessive polycystic kidney disease (ARPKD)
Autosomal dominant polycystic kidney disease (ADPKD)
Juvenile nephronophthisis and medullary cystic disease complex (MCDC) today also summarised as ADTKD
Glomerulocystic kidney disease (GCKD) HNF1B/TCF2-associated disease
for DD [congenital nephrotic syndrome (Finnish type, autosomal recessive)]: not a real cystic disease
Syndromal cysts: for example, in Meckel syndrome, Laurence-Moon-Biedl-Bardet syndrome, Ivemark syndrome, Zellweger syndrome, tuberous sclerosis, von Hippel-Lindau disease, HNF1B disease, Diabetes and renal cysts, etc.
Nonhereditary cystic renal disease
Multicystic dysplastic kidney (MCDK) (Obstructive) cystic dysplasia
Multiloculated cyst and similar entities
Simple renal cyst
Medullary sponge kidney
Secondary or acquired renal cyst (post-traumatic, chronic renal failure, and dialysis)
Cystic renal tumor

Adapted according to the classification proposal of the American Academy of Pediatrics, Urologic Section (Glassberg et al. 1987)

Table 4 Cystic renal diseases

Before nephrogenesis
Multicystic dysplasia
Early during nephrogenesis
Isolated
As part of syndromes
With obstruction
After nephrogenesis
Systemic renal cystic disease ARPKD, ADPKD, juvenile nephronophthisis/medullary cystic disease complex, glomerulocystic kidney disease
Miscellaneous others
Isolated cyst, acquired renal cysts, cysts in tumors, metabolic diseases (renal cysts and diabetes syndrome)

Classification by time of development in relation to the stage of nephrogenesis (Vester et al. 2010)

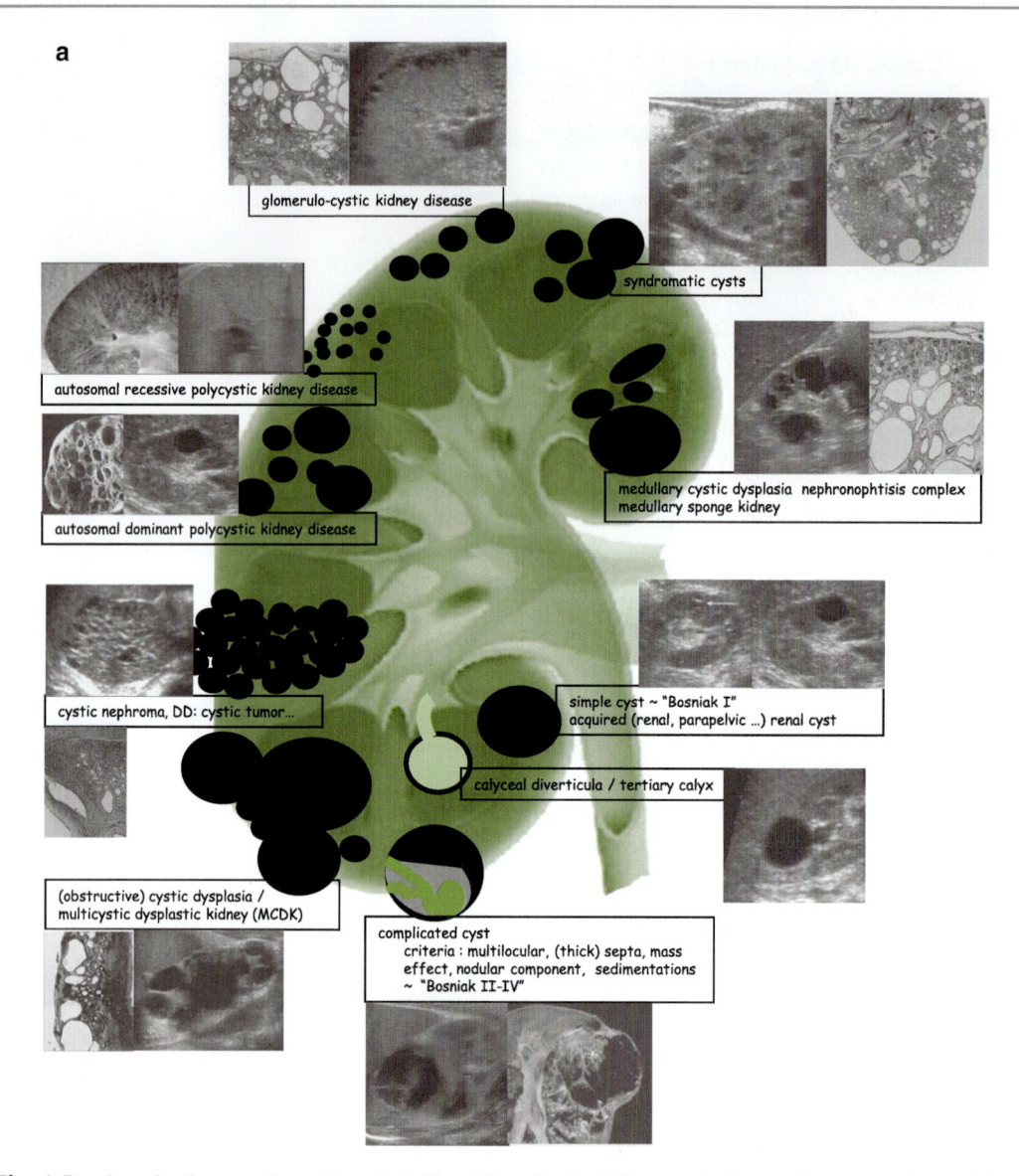

Fig. 6 Renal cystic disease – how things look like: (**a**) Schematic drawing of typical cyst forms and locations in various cystic kidney diseases (adapted from Riccabona et al., Pediatr Radiol 2012) with respective US images and histology: *ARPKD* = autosomal recessive polycystic kidney disease (multiple small cysts, early manifestation, situated mostly cortical or at the cortico-medullary border). *ADPKD* = autosomal dominant polycystic kidney disease (some big cysts, usually during late childhood/adulthood, in all parenchymal areas); *GCKD* = gomerulo-cystic kidney disease (predominantly small cortical or subcapsular cysts); *MCDC* = medullary cystic disease complex (medullary microcysts, centered close to the cortico-medullary junction); *MCDK* = multi-cystic dysplastic kidney; *MSK* = medullary sponge kidney - is included in the medullary cystic dysplasia complex (medullary cystic changes, in a more or less radial pattern, centered towards the papilla) (**b**) US images of various typical other cystic masses important for differential diagnosis: 1 = multicystic dysplastic kidney, with the typical peripheral cysts of different size and some residual central echogenic, non-differentiated dysplastic parenchyma, 2 = a perirenal pop-off urinoma after caliceal rupture in a neonate with a posterior urethral valve, 3 = disproportionally dilated collecting system of the lower moiety of a duplex kidney due to dilating VUR, 4 = hugely dilated cystiform obstructed collecting system of the upper moiety of a duplex kidney with practically no visible parenchyma drained by a megaureter, with only mild distention of the lower moiety's pelvo-caliceal system, 5 = large suprarenal cyst, originating from the adrenal gland (+ .... + indicate the kidney length)

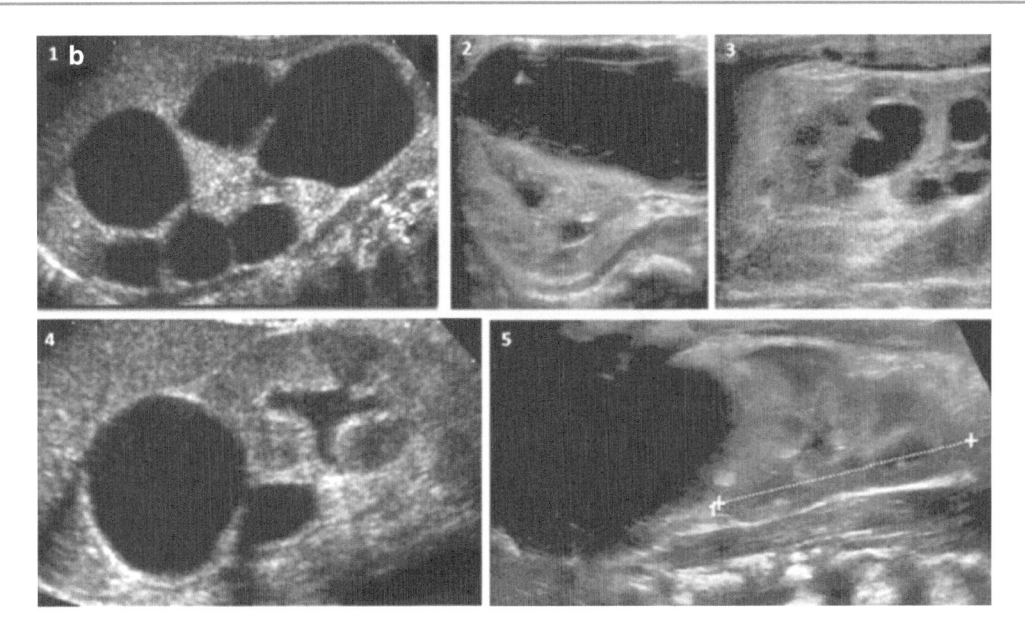

Fig. 6 (continued)

and Rubin 1998; Shapiro et al. 1998; Wittingham 1999). Taking typical imaging features, clinical information, and family history into account, US (supplemented by MRI) can often define the underlying entity (Avni et al. 2006; Avni et al. 2012). VCUG (or ce-VUS) is sometimes used to evaluate potentially associated VUR. MRI is performed in a suspected calyceal diverticula (potentially an adapted IVU if MRI is not available), medullary sponge kidney or duplex systems, and obstructive uropathy. Scintigraphy or fMRU allows for quantification of split renal function which may be essential for follow-up. Contrast-enhanced (multiphasic) spiral CT is helpful for evaluating complicated cysts, complex cystic masses, or cystic renal tumors – but for radiation protection, issues in childhood are only used if ce-MRI is not accessible (Bosniak 1986; Urban 1997; Szolar et al. 1997). In general, MRI is excellent for cyst detection using T2-weighted sequences. In some situations, MRI therefore is applied simply to detect or rule out small lesions and to confirm existing disease or to compare complex changes during follow-up giving a better overall 3D impression of the entire cyst load, number, and size. The latter is becoming increasingly important when monitoring patients under new therapeutic approaches for evaluating response (Hattery and King 1995; Borthne et al. 1999).

5.1 Polycystic Kidney Disease

5.1.1 Autosomal Recessive Polycystic Kidney Disease (ARPKD)

ARPKD, or infantile polycystic kidney disease, is a heredito-familial ciliopathy in the spectrum of hepatorenal fibrocystic diseases. The manifestation and the course of the disease may vary; sometimes, it may first present with extrarenal manifestation such as (congenital) hepatic fibrosis or Caroli disease. In general, ARPKD manifests in early infancy or during childhood, although clinical onset may be delayed into adulthood in some patients with less severe manifestation (Shaikewitz and Chapman 1993; Lieberman et al. 1971; Kaplan et al. 1988, 1989a). However, it leads to renal insufficiency during childhood in 90% of affected patients. Potter's syndrome-like changes secondary to oligohydramnios may be present at birth in severe cases with fetal renal insufficiency, and modern fetal imaging by US (and increasingly also MRI) may detect these early manifestations already in utero (Avni and

Hall 2010). Many of these severely affected neonates die from respiratory failure due to pulmonary hypoplasia. Children surviving the neonatal period may have a prolonged course and may become adolescents before renal replacement therapy is needed (Roy et al. 1997).

Histologically, there are growing numbers of initially very small cysts deriving from dilated collecting tubules with a flattened epithelium. Areas of normal renal structures diminish during the course of the disease, whereas the cysts grow less in size than in number (Cole et al. 1987; Hoyer 1996a; McDonald et al. 1997). ARPKD is associated with hepatic involvement, and histologically dysgenetic periportal biliary ductules with signs of liver fibrosis and duct proliferation are considered obligatory (= congenital hepatic fibrosis); furthermore, cysts can be found in other parenchymal organs (Lieberman et al. 1971; Alvares et al. 1981; Cole et al. 1987; Kaplan et al. 1989a, b).

The first step in imaging usually is US. It (rarely) may show initially sonomorphologically normal-sized kidneys usually with an altered corticomedullary differentiation that quickly become bilaterally enlarged, with normal presentation of the collecting system, but some very small subcapsular cysts of up to 3-mm diameter (Boal and Teele 1980; Zerres et al. 1988; Worthington et al. 1988; Manish et al. 1997). The cysts can be seen unilaterally or bilaterally; often they initially are too small to be detected, creating a bilaterally speckled increased echogenicity of the renal tissue of then usually enlarged kidneys with inhomogenously reduced tissue differentiation, also called the "pepper-salt kidney" (Fig. 7a–e). During the course of the disease, the cysts constantly increase mainly in number, but also in size. After a period of regression with reduction of renal size, a constant enlargement is noted with progressive disease, invariably leading to terminal renal failure.

US is unable to definitely distinguish between ARPKD and ADPKD; but suggestive contributions to diagnosis (and differential diagnosis) can be made based on US features when taking clinical information and family history into account. However, enlarged echogenic kidneys can also be seen in a variety of other conditions such as congenital nephrotic syndrome, fetal malformative syndromes, renal vein thrombosis, or acute renal failure.

With established diagnosis, no further imaging is needed. In equivocal cases, MRI can be used, offering new perspectives in assessing the progress of the disease and associated liver disease (Kern et al. 1999; Riccabona and Avni 2011). IVU is not used any longer – if applied it shows markedly enlarged kidneys with prolonged, persisting, radial streaks and tubular striation as well as delayed cortical brush pattern (Kääriäinen et al. 1988b; Schneider and Fendel 1995). In all patients with ARPKD, imaging of the liver and evaluation of possible portal hypertension are mandatory, particularly also during follow-up.

5.1.2 Autosomal Dominant Polycystic Kidney Disease (ADPKD)

With an incidence of 1:400 to 1:1,000 life births, ADPKD represents one of the most common inherited diseases. Although manifestation usually takes place during adulthood – therefore also called adult polycystic kidney disease – ADPKD may be detected even prenatally or during infancy and childhood by selective family screening or by chance (Porch et al. 1986; Kääriäinen et al. 1988a; Estroff et al. 1991; Fick et al. 1993). Some families as well as siblings of affected patients are predisposed to early manifestation (Kaplan et al. 1977; Sedman et al. 1987; Fick et al. 1994).

Initially, only a few macrocysts may be present with an irregular distribution. Later on, both kidneys are enlarged, with a growing number of large cysts both in the cortex and the medulla. Accompanying cysts of the liver, the pancreas and other organs are common, but congenital hepatic fibrosis is rare. A high incidence of cerebral vessel malformations – particularly of aneurysms of the big cerebral arteries – is reported (in up to 70% of adult patients!) and has been described in pediatric patients as well (Proesmans et al. 1982). Furthermore, some relationship to tuberous sclerosis and the gene localization for tuberous sclerosis is described (Brook-Carter et al. 1994). Chronic renal insufficiency usually develops gradually after the age of 30 years; earlier severe disease is rare (Worthington et al. 1988).

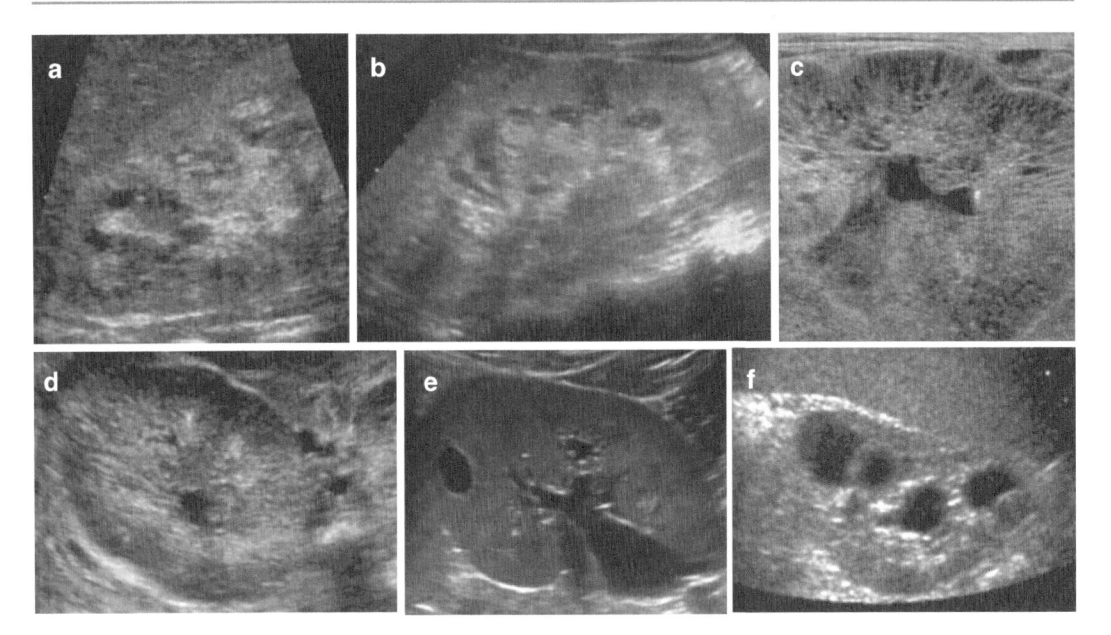

Fig. 7 Ultrasonography in ARPKD (**a–d**) and ADPKD (**f, g**): **a–c** Longitudinal (**a**) and augmented US view (**b**) of an enlarged kidney demonstrating multiple small parenchymal cysts with inhomogenously reduced cortico-medullary differentiation of the very echogenic renal parenchyma in a young girl with ARPKD. (**c**) Massive tubular-cystic changes in a neonate with ARPKD nicely shown by high resolution US, whereas this micro-architecture is less obvious on the normal standard US axial view (**d**), which on the other hand shows that the contralateral kidney also reaches the midline and nearly reaches the right kidney, only separated by the major central abdominal vessels. (**e**) US demonstrates one of a few unspectacular renal cysts – others are scattered throughout the kidney, but not imaged in this axial section – in a child with early onset of ADPKD. Note some reduction in cortico-medullary differentiation and regional inhomogenicity of the renal parenchyma, as well as a slightly prominent collecting system. (**f**) Typical appearance of ADPKD – multiple simple cysts scattered throughout the parenchyma in a school age child (axial section of left kidney)

Clinically, ADPKD usually manifests with loin pain, hematuria, urinary tract infection, nephrolithiasis, hypertension, and chronic renal insufficiency. For evaluation of these symptoms, various imaging modalities are used – depending on the individual, sometimes unspecific symptoms, and the various institutions, though in childhood usually US is the first method and will allow for a diagnosis in the majority of patients then rating other investigations unnecessary.

On US, the kidneys in general look normal during (early) childhood; sometimes one or two parenchymal (even unilateral) renal cysts may be found (Fig. 7f, g). Some rare cases of early manifestation (enlarged fetal kidneys or neonatal renal cysts) have been described (Cole et al. 1987; Boal and Teele 1980; Kääriäinen et al. 1988b). In early stages, two or more cysts in a child with positive family history are considered diagnostic (Zerres 1987). Later on, multiple cysts of varying size, mostly large, in irregular distribution, with varying amounts of normal renal tissue in otherwise hyperechoic renal parenchyma of both enlarged kidneys, represent the typical US finding. These cysts may become complicated by secondary hemorrhage, sedimentation, and infection, sometimes necessitating further imaging or US/CT-guided puncture/drainage. IVU is no longer considered indicated for these queries; if performed it may show indirect signs of calyceal splaying around macrocysts and lucent areas due to cysts replacing normal renal tissue. MRI (and CT, if MRI is not available) is very sensitive in depicting the varying number of cysts. They may be used during follow-up for quantification and comparison, for evaluation of complications, and for differentiation of complicated cysts in cases where US, including (a) CDS and contrast-enhanced studies, is inconclusive (Kääriäinen et al. 1988b; Bosniak 1986; Riccabona et al. 1999a, b; Kim et al. 1999).

5.1.3 Medullary Cystic Disease Complex (MCDC) and Juvenile Nephronophthisis (NPHP)

Medullary cystic disease is an autosomal-dominant inherited disease with a late onset of chronic renal failure. Familial juvenile nephronophthisis (NPHP) is usually transmitted recessively; the sporadic form most probably represents a new mutation (Gadner 1967; Donaldson et al. 1985; Hildebrandt et al. 1992; Avner 1994). The adult form of MCDC is reported to be rare and difficult to diagnose even on renal biopsy specimens, whereas juvenile nephronophthisis is one of the most common genetic causes for ESRD necessitating dialysis and renal transplantation in children and adolescents (see also chapters "Renal Failure and Renal Transplantation" and "Imaging in Renal Failure, Neonatal Oligoanuria, and Renal Transplantation").

Clinically, MCDC is characterized by the insidious onset of chronic renal failure and a relentless progression to ESRD. In 10% of patients with juvenile nephronophthisis, additional liver fibrosis or dysplasia of the bile ducts can be observed similar to the changes seen in ARPKD (Boichis et al. 1973).

On US, no specific changes are seen in early MCDC, except for the more medullary origin of the often relatively large cysts. In NPHP, some reduction in corticomedullary differentiation may be observed initially (Hildebrandt 1997). Then the kidneys become slightly hyperechoic, and renal size decreases, eventually leading to a cirrhotic kidney, with detectable cysts in the corticomedullary junction zone, or subcapsular, predominantly in advanced chronic renal failure (Garel et al. 1984; Blowey et al. 1996). MRI (and CT, if MRI is not available) may be helpful in detecting small medullary cysts earlier than US and for standardized documentation (Elzouki et al. 1996). In general, however, no additional imaging is needed, as it does not contribute significantly to the diagnosis, which is made by family history and molecular genetics (Hildebrandt 1997; Hildebrandt and Otto 2005). Note that today other tubulo-cystic diseases (ADTKD) are also summarised in this group, e.g. medullary sponge kidney.

5.1.4 Glomerulocystic Kidney Disease (GCKD)

GCKD is a rare congenital condition. It can be categorized into a group with hereditary syndromal changes (such as Zellweger syndrome, tuberous sclerosis, or trisomy 13), a group of hereditary nonsyndromal diseases transmitted autosomal dominantly, and sporadic forms (Sellers and Richie 1978; Joshi and Kasznica 1984; Kaplan et al. 1989c; Bernstein 1993a). Some authors also include dysplastic cystic renal disease (see Sect. 4 and 5.2) (Kissane 1990). Today these are also summarised in the group of "HNF1B/TCF2-associated disease".

On US, these often tiny cysts are visualized predominantly in the renal cortex and subcapsular, with a normal-appearing medulla. Possibly signs of interstitial nephropathy can be seen (i.e., accentuated corticomedullary differentiation) in the bilaterally grossly enlarged kidneys with generally increased cortical echogenicity (Hoyer 1996a; Manish et al. 1997) (Fig. 6a). Secondary changes may be observed: inflammation, punctuate calcification, secondary medullary fibrosis, or relative loss of renal size may then confuse the image (Fitch and Stapleton 1986; Fredericks et al. 1989). Differentiation against other entities with bilateral widespread (cortical) small cysts may be difficult, and imaging may present very similar to polycystic kidney disease, particularly ARPKD (Fitch and Stapleton 1986). As diagnosis is made by histology and family history, no additional imaging is performed except for follow-up investigations.

The Finnish type of congenital nephrotic syndrome may be a differential diagnosis in the neonate as dilated proximal renal tubules may be found. Though not a real cystic renal disease, it is often listed in this context. It is a rare autosomal recessive inherited disease caused by a mutation in the podocyte protein nephrin (see chapter "Renal Parenchymal Disease") that manifests at birth and predominantly exists in Finland – there the incidence is 1:8,200 live births (Kestilä et al. 1998; Hallmann et al. 1956; Huttunen 1976). Aside from genetic analysis, diagnosis is made clinically and is very often suspected prenatally based on high alpha-fetoprotein concentration of the amniotic fluid, an enlarged placenta, altered renal echogenicity on fetal US, and severe neonatal proteinuria (Kjessler et al. 1975). On US, initially and prenatally, the kidneys are enlarged with increased cortical echogenicity, and the corticomedullary differentiation disappears during the course of the disease. Other changes such as disturbance of flow pattern with increase of resistive index or variations of corticomedullary differentiation are additionally influenced by renal function, cardiac situation, and medication. US-guided renal biopsy is not necessary, and additional imaging is indicated just for queries related to chronic or end-stage renal failure or for transplantation workup.

5.1.5 Syndromal Cystic Renal Disease

There are a number of hereditary and nonhereditary syndromal cysts as well as cysts in aneuploidies (Table 1, 2, and 3). They can present as multiple renal cysts, as GCKD and MCDC, or as ARPKD and ADPKD (Bernstein 1973, 1976, 1979, 1993b; Donaldson et al. 1985; Kissane 1990; McDonald and Avner 1991; McDonald et al. 1997; Watkins et al. 1997). The pediatric radiologist needs to consider these entities for differential diagnosis and further diagnostic imaging of associated malformations or abnormalities (Fig. 8); otherwise, the presentation and imaging of syndromal renal cysts does not differ from the imaging of the other cystic renal entities and is usually addressed by US only – complemented by MR (or CT) in complications.

Take Away

Cysts within enlarged kidneys and cystic abnormalities of other abdominal parenchymal organs are suggestive of a hereditary polycystic kidney disease. Many of these converge on a common pathogenic pathway centered at the cilium-centrosome complex. However, a broad variation in onset, clinical manifestation and radiological features can make early differential diagnosis difficult. Imaging in pediatric patients usually is accomplished by US; for evaluation of complications, differential diagnosis and evaluation of extrarenal disease as well as follow-up MRI has become the method of choice.

5.2 Multicystic Dysplastic Kidney (MCDK)

This entity represents a subgroup of renal dysplasia (Bernstein 1971). MCDK is the most common cystic renal lesion in pediatric patients and the most common cause for an abdominal mass in neonates. The ipsilateral ureter commonly is abnormal, atretic, and sometimes even absent, supporting the theory that MCDK

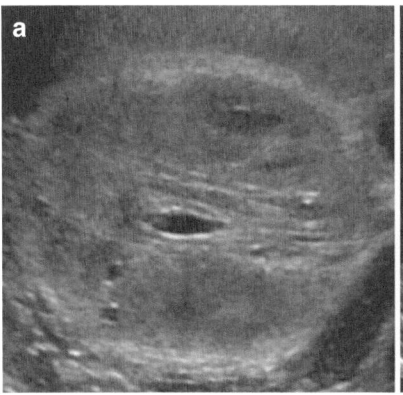

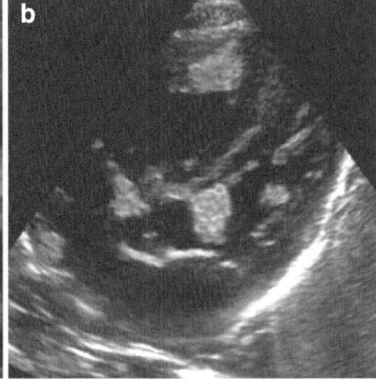

Fig. 8 US in syndromal cystic renal disease: (**a**) A conglomerate of tiny cysts detected by HR-US using HI and image compounding in an otherwise sonographically normal neonatal kidney. (**b**) Echocardiography in the same patient reveals multiple cardiac echogenic tumors consistent with cardiac rhabdomyoma in tuberous sclerosis

results from early ureteral pathology during nephrogenesis and may have a genetic aspect (Huland 1986; Woolf 1997; Srivastava et al. 1999). Floating borders exist to high-grade UPJO and (obstructive) cystic dysplasia. It usually affects the entire kidney, but rarely can also involve only a portion, e.g., in a duplex system, with atresia of the ureter of the upper moiety (Diard et al. 1984; Jeon et al. 1999)

The contralateral kidney is normal in 66 % except for compensatory hypertrophy (if absent, hypo-/dysplasia must be suspected). However, contralateral kidneys are slightly more disposed to positional or rotational anomalies. Associated urinary tract anomalies are present in one third (low degree UPJO in 12 %, VUR in 20 %). Furthermore, associated ipsilateral genital anomalies are found in up to 50 %, such as cystic dysplasia of the rete testis or the seminal vesicle or uterine fusion defects (Greene et al. 1971; Ring et al. 1990; 1993; Kiechl-Kohlendorfer et al. 2011) (Fig. 9c, d). Rare bilateral manifestations (in some series up to 20 %) are incompatible with extrauterine life and may have some underlying genetic preposition (Griscom et al. 1975). Associated additional anomalies of other organs may be present such as atresia of the gastrointestinal tract, impaired cardiac septation, or myelomeningocele. These extrarenal malformations relate to the time of an insult during ontogenesis rather than to the nature of that hypothetical event.

Clinically, MCDK is commonly detected by prenatal US screening or presents neonatally as a palpable abdominal/flank mass. The natural history of MCDK may vary. The mass often shrinks and disappears, making surgery unnecessary (Gordon et al. 1988; Orejas et al. 1992; Ring et al. 1993) (Fig. 9e). Management focuses on monitoring spontaneous regression and/or on detection of complications such as continuing growth with compression of adjacent structures, inflammation, hemorrhage, or even tumors arising within the mass then necessitating surgery (Hoyer 1996b; Krull et al. 1990; Kullendorff 1990).

Imaging is initially focused on establishing the diagnosis, to confirm a normal contralateral renal unit and to rule out associated anomalies. This usually is achieved by US, scintigraphy, and VCUG/ce-VUS. In case of duplex systems or a dilated contralateral collecting renal system or segmental MCDK, as well as in patients with complex malformations or small renal buds as a remnant of such an shrunken MCDK, MR urography (MRU) has become the accepted imaging tool, replacing IVU whenever available (Borthne et al. 1999; Riccabona et al. 2002; Riccabona et al. 2004a, b) (Fig. 9c). Conventional gray-scale US shows a multicystic structure with some big and some smaller cysts that do not communicate and possibly some central echogenic, nondifferentiated tissue components (Avni et al. 1986; Hoyer 1996) (Fig. 9a). Duplex Doppler and (a)CDS may be helpful to depict areas with persisting perfusion, which may be prone to create complications, or may help to establish the differential diagnosis (Riccabona et al. 1993a, b; Hendry and Hendry 1991) (Fig. 9b). Follow-up is usually performed by US. And the initial US study should always include a comprehensive assessment of all other regions with a potentially associated malformation such as the neonatal spinal canal or the genital system – particularly in baby girls, the latter is best assessed already in the neonatal age with physiologic stimulation of the inner female genital structures and using a sophisticated technique in case of suspicion such as US genitography (Riccabona et al. 2014). Additional complications or arising suspicion of malignancy may necessitate further imaging (CT, MRI).

> **Take Away**
> The task of imaging is to establish diagnosis (US, MRI, or scintigraphy), to evaluate the contralateral system and associated disease or (particularly genital) malformation (VCUG/ce-VUS, US genitography, MRI), and to follow-up MCDK (monitoring involution = US, evaluating complications = US, MRI).

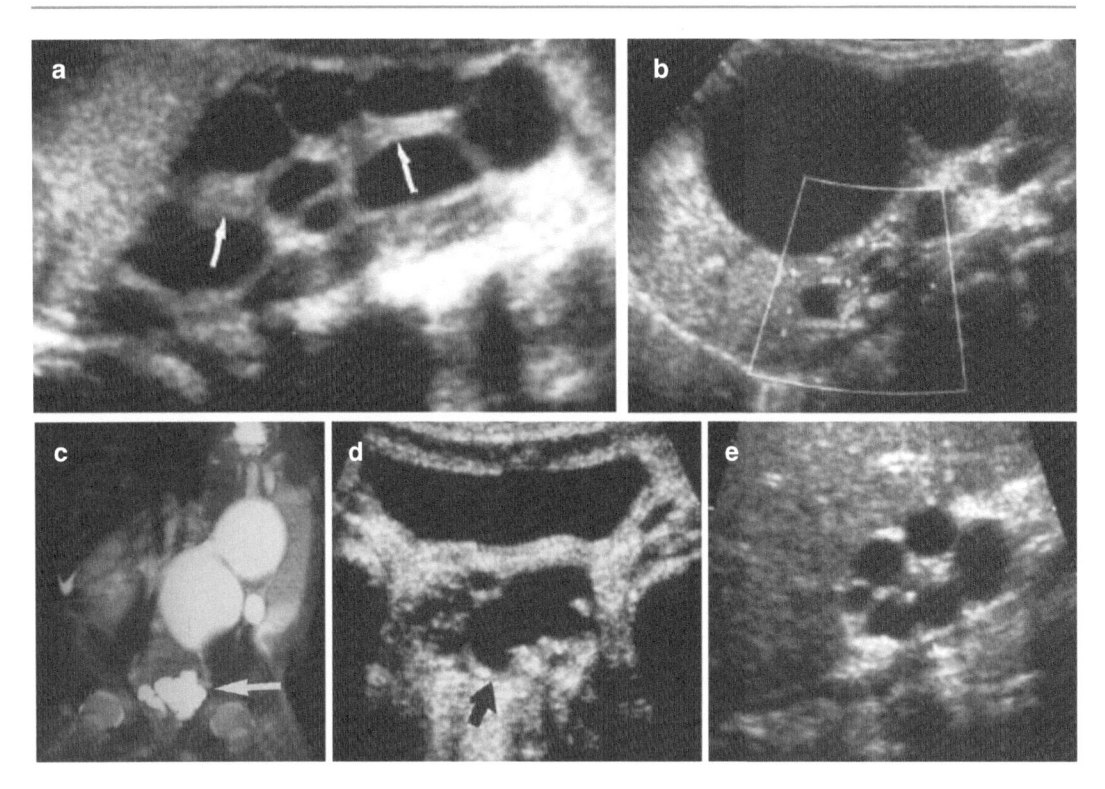

Fig. 9 US (and MRI) in MCDK: (**a**) US images showing longitudinal section of multiple, non-corresponding cystic masses and some echogenic-dysplastic, non-differentiated parenchyma (*arrow*). (**b**) CDS demonstrates vasculature in the echogenic dysplastic parenchymal part of this MCDK. (**c**) 3D reconstructed MRI image of a MCDK with associated cystic dysplastic malformation of the ipsilateral seminal vesicle and rete testis, also demonstrated by US on a transversal section behind the bladder (*arrow*) (**d**). (**e**) US of spontaneous regression/involution of an already relatively small MCDK (*arrow*) in a longitudinal section

5.3 Medullary Sponge Kidney (MSK)

MSK is rare in pediatrics; some cases are familial with an autosomal dominant inheritance; however, it is considered a congenital disorder characterized by cystic dilatation of the collecting tubules (Fabris et al. 2013). It can be segmental or may affect the entire kidney (Yendt 1990; Kissane 1990; Avner 1994; Watkins et al. 1997). Today it is listed within the group of medullary cystic diseases. Usually MSK manifests in adults showing multiple medullary, peripapillary centered cysts with secondary calcifications, hypercalciuria with nephrolithiasis and hematuria, and infection.

US may lack sensitivity in the very early stages: the kidney may look sonomorphologically normal, or – at a slightly delayed stage – the kidney may look similar to early stages of medullary nephrocalcinosis, with normal sonomorphology of the cortex and hyperechoic patches throughout the medulla focusing on the papilla and some ectatic tubuli ("Christmas-tree" phenomenon, Patriquin and O'Regan 1985). Later on, multiple calcifications as well as nephrolithiasis with or without obstruction may be observed on plain films and on US (Fig. 10c). As IVU is an excellent diagnostic tool in the diagnosis particularly of early stages of MSK ("paintbrush-like" appearance) and also of its complications such as an obstructing calculus, US and (as one of the few exceptions) IVU with plain film still form the mainstay of imaging in this query – other imaging is not used routinely (Palubinskas 1963) (Fig. 10a, c). CT shows a typical pattern, with radial patchy contrast in the pyramids on the excretory (late) phase of a multiphasic contrast-enhanced scan, and is increasingly used particularly in adults (Fig. 9b). MRI is very sensitive

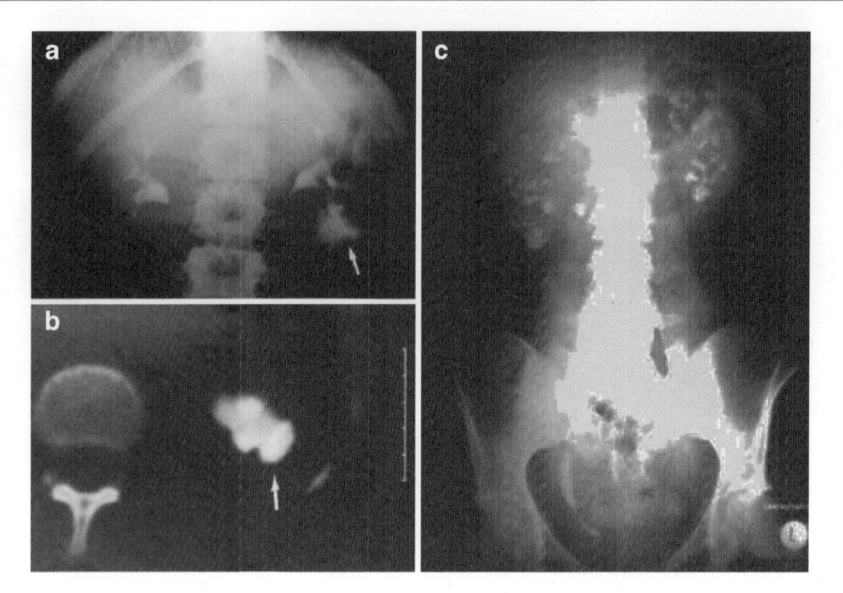

Fig. 10 Medullary sponge kidney: (**a**) IVU of a segmental MSK (*arrow*) in a child, with corresponding late phase CT image (**b**). (**c**) Plain film of severe diffuse disease with bilateral clotty medullary calcifications and distal ureteral calculi in an adolescent patient

toward detecting even small cysts that might be missed on US, but has restrictions in visualizing small calcifications. CT and MRI may become necessary during follow-up, as MSK may be associated with hemihypertrophy syndromes and as such bears a slightly higher risk of Wilms' tumor (Hoyer 1996b).

> **Take Away**
> MSK is diagnosed by US and IVU/plain film, but US may miss subtle changes in very early disease. If complications and malignancy occur, CT and MRI become useful.

5.4 Simple Renal Cyst and Acquired Renal Cyst

Simple renal cyst can occur spontaneously or may be familial. They are rare in childhood with a reported incidence of 0.22% (Baert and Steg 1977; McHugh et al. 1991). Simple cysts do not bare any consequences or associated risks except for a few occasions, when growing cysts lead to hypertension, compression of adjacent structures, and possibly obstruction of the collecting system (Churchill et al. 1975). In these rare cases, US-guided puncture/drainage with instillation of sclerosing agents (alcohol, tetracycline, Gelet et al. 1990; Reiner et al. 1992) may be an alternative to operative treatment or endoscopic surgery (Fig. 11c). In adults, cysts are much more common (up to 50%); therefore, the development of simple renal cysts may be seen as a normal aging phenomenon (Baert and Steg 1977; Tada et al. 1983).

Acquired cysts can occur in post-traumatic and post-inflammatory (tuberculous, etc.) settings or spontaneously develop in kidney parenchyma during chronic renal failure and dialysis (Dunill et al. 1977; Leichter et al. 1988; Hogg 1992; see also chapters "Renal Agenesis, Dysplasia, Hypoplasia, and Cystic Diseases of the Kidney" and "Renal Failure and Renal Transplantation"). As malignancy may develop in kidneys with acquired cysts such as in ESRD, even in the wall of such cysts, they need to be monitored (Bretan et al. 1986; Levine 1992).

On US, simple cysts show clear, sharp margins and central anechoic fluid, with dorsal gain amplification. Some compression of the adjacent tissue may occur in big cysts (Fig. 11a, see also Figs. 7a, and 8a). Usually they are detected incidentally; only rarely they present with clinical

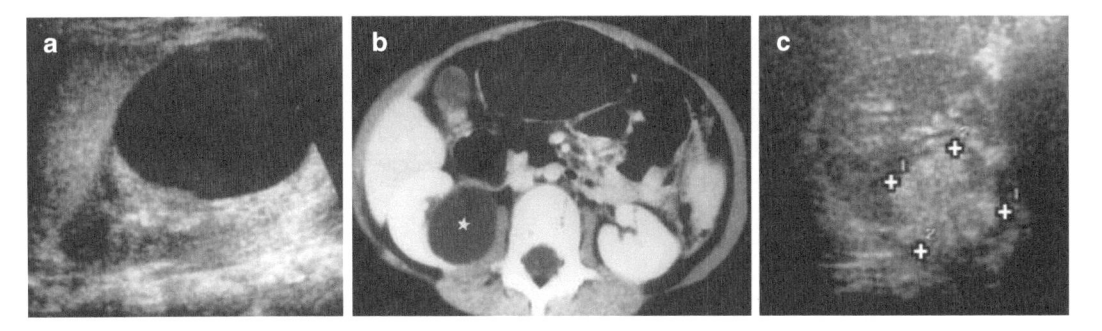

Fig. 11 Simple renal cyst: (**a**) A radiologically simple, but big renal cyst of the lower pole of the left kidney on US with compression of parenchyma, in a longitudinal section, in a 4-year-old boy. (**b**) CT demonstrates a simple cyst (*asterisk*) with compression of the renal hilus/hilar structures in an 8-year-old girl who was consecutively operated on. (**c**) US of the postoperative situation of patient in Fig b with echogenic (= fatty) tissue in the former cyst (+ +) on a transverse section

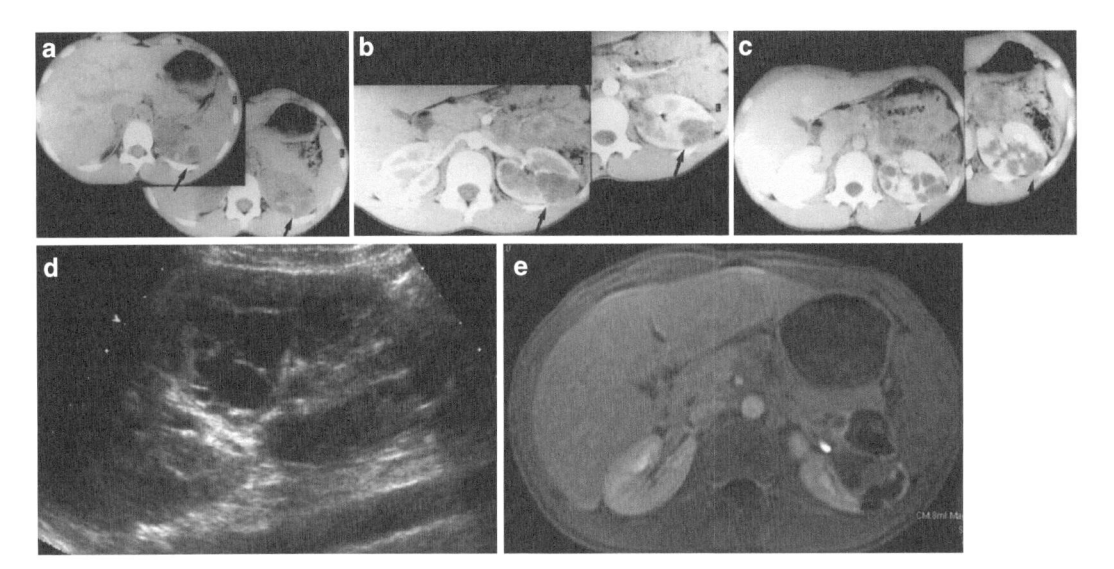

Fig. 12 Cystic nephroma Segmental cystic nephroma (*arrows*) on multiphasic contrast-enhanced CT (**a-c**), longitudinal US section (**d**), and axial MRI (T1-weighted contrast-enhanced image) (**e**); this was discovered incidentally after blunt abdominal trauma when US and then CT was performed, the MRI was during follow-up before surgery

signs of a renal mass (Siegel and McAlister 1980). However, if cysts are multilocal, multiloculated, or bilateral, differentiation against ADPKD may be difficult (Davidson and Hartman 1994; Hoyer 1996b). If a CT is performed (as may become necessary in complicated cases if MRI is not available, or for other reasons), the localized spherical fluid accumulation has between 0 to 20 Hounsfield units (HU) and sharp borders without any contrast enhancement when using 120 kV (Bosniak 1986) (Fig. 11b). On MRI, the typical fluid signal without gadolinium enhancement is observed (Bosniak 1991).

Differentiation against a calyceal cyst may be difficult on US. MRI may be helpful for this differential diagnosis demonstrating a delayed filling (of the cyst) with contrast material relative to the renal excretion into the collecting system; thus, delayed scans are necessary to avoid missing the contrast filling of such a calyceal cyst (Fig. 2a–f). If MRI is not available, this phenomenon with the same procedural implications will be diagnostic also on IVU or CT.

Acquired cysts look similar to normal cysts on US, except for post-traumatic and inflammatory cysts – the latter two may be multiloculated or septated, may show sedimentation, and may demonstrate somewhat irregularly shaped margins (Hoyer 1996 a, b) (Fig. 12, see also Figs. 6 and 11). These cysts must be treated like complicated renal cysts necessitating follow-up or – in cases without adequate history – MRI (or CT). Definite differentiation against cystic renal tumors may sometimes only be achieved by (CT- or US-guided) biopsy, particularly in case of (secondary) hemorrhage into the cyst with consequently higher HU values on CT or enhancing septae on MRI (Fig. 12) (see also chapter "Neoplasms of the Genitourinary System").

Take Away
Simple and acquired renal cysts are rare in infancy and childhood. US usually detects them as an incidental finding. Possible manifestation of a polycystic or dysplastic renal disease must be considered necessitating at least a follow-up and nephrourologic checkup.

5.5 Complicated Renal Cyst, Multiloculated Cyst, and Cystic Renal Tumor

Complicated cyst is a term deriving from descriptive radiology. The exact definition varies depending on the imaging modality applied and the age of the patient. A complicated cyst is defined as a cystic lesion with some abnormalities, therefore not matching all criteria necessary for a simple cyst, which are small size, clear and sharp margins, no echoes or contents in the clear fluid, no parenchymal part or inclusion, and no contrast enhancement (if ce-CT/ce-MRI is used for assessment; see also Bosniak's CT-based classification of renal cysts) (Figs. 1c, 6a, and 11). The radiological changes of such a complicated cyst may originate from secondary hemorrhage or sedimentation of proteins and of membrane cells; calcifications may also occur, or infection may be present (Fig. 12b, d). Differentiation of these cysts, usually discovered by US, is essential and achieved in part by ce-MRI (ce-CT), in part in conjunction with clinical and laboratory findings (Table 5).

Table 5 Differential diagnosis of a complicated renal cyst

"Simple cyst" aggravated by:
Secondary hemorrhage
Sedimentation
Inflammation
Acquired cysts
Posttraumatic
Inflammatory cyst (abscess, tuberculoma)
Infected calyceal cyst with sedimentation and calculi
Partially thrombosed vascular aneurysm
Necrotic area after infarct, abscess
Cystic malformation:
Segmental MCDK
Dysplastic cysts (obstructive dysplasia)
Multilocular cyst and multilocular cystic nephroma
Manifestation of congenital (poly-)cystic kidney disease (particularly ADPKD)
Cystic renal tumor
Necrotic hamartoma, capillary hemangioma, vascular malformation, bleeding in an angiomyolipoma, and other cystic benign renal tumors
Cystic Wilms' tumor, cystic mesoblastic nephroma
Cystic carcinoma and other, partially necrotic or cystic, malignant renal tumors

This table lists the most important entities that have to be considered for differential diagnosis of complicated renal cysts

On CT, a renal cyst is usually categorized into three classes of suspicion using the Bosniak classification (Bosniak 1986): a single, sharp bordered cyst with clear fluid (= I°, = simple cyst); a slightly complicated cyst with either septations or complicated fluid (HU > 20), but without parenchymal structures and without contrast enhancement (= II°); and an already very suspicious cyst with additional nodular wall irregularities (= III°). A cystiform structure with contrast enhancement should be handled as a renal mass (= IV°) (Bosniak 1991). As even CT can sometimes not rule out malignancy, only histology can precisely categorize the lesion in these situations and then is compulsory to find or rule out malignancy. The same general appearances also apply to MRI, which is more eagerly used in children due to its lack of radiation burden and its higher soft tissue differentiation potential.

The *multicystic nephroma and multiloculated cysts* often pose a diagnostic problem; various classifications of these closely related entities have been suggested (Takeuchi et al. 1984; Theissig et al. 1986; Upadhyay and Neely 1989; Strand et al. 1989; Domizio and Risdon 1991; Wood 1992). Histology is not definite and is only used to rule out malignancy; often it demonstrates some amount of dysplasia, thus suggesting a form of cystic dysplasia with secondary changes similar to segmental MCDK or Ask-Upmark kidney (i.e., segmental renal dysplasia) (Arant et al. 1979). There are no clinical symptoms, although microscopic hematuria may occur, or an abdominal mass may be palpable.

In multiloculated cysts, US shows multiple, non-confluent, cystic areas, with relatively sharp margins, and compression of the adjacent tissue creating an increased echogenicity of the less differentiated adjacent tissue that may be difficult to evaluate and differentiate even on multiphasic contrast-enhanced CT or ce-MRI (Fig. 13). The remaining rest of the kidney has a normal parenchyma, yet may show disturbed perfusion due to compression; sometimes these changes are detected prenatally (Riccabona et al. 1999a,b).

Various *renal tumors* may present as a cystic renal mass (Takeuchi et al. 1984; Fitch et al. 1985; Dodat et al. 1988; Babut et al. 1993). Unclear or nodular margins, increased echogenicity of the content or areas of (atypically) perfused tissue and septations within the cystic mass, as well as (local) contrast enhancement on MRI or CT may indicate a cystic renal tumor and necessitate further diagnostic workup. Sonographic methods such as CDS and aCDS as well as HI or the use of ultrasound contrast-enhancing agents can be helpful already in the initial sonographic workup (Riccabona et al. 1993a, b; 1999b; Kim et al. 1999) (see also Fig. 11c, d). The important task of imaging is to help to differentiate other similar entities such as unilateral presentation of polycystic kidney disease, inflammation, cystic aneurysm of the renal artery, arteriovenous fistula or arteriovenous malformation, abscess formation, or hemorrhage into a renal infarction. It is used to rule out progressive disease or malignancy. Differentiation of sonographically questionable findings usually is addressed by performing additional dynamic contrast-enhanced MRI. In modern pediatric imaging, multiphasic contrast-enhanced helical CT is used more reluctantly due to the relatively high radiation exposure and the increasing availability of MRI. US is then again used for monitoring these patients. In cases with equivocal findings, US- or CT-guided biopsy and puncture/drainage may be of diagnostic value; sometimes primary surgical intervention, open biopsy, and removal become necessary (see chapters "Surgical Procedures and Indications for Surgery" and "Neoplasms of the Genitourinary System").

Tumors have to be recognized and imaged appropriately. Many tumor entities can present as a cystic renal tumor; the histology ranges from benign renal neoplasm to cystic Wilms' tumor,

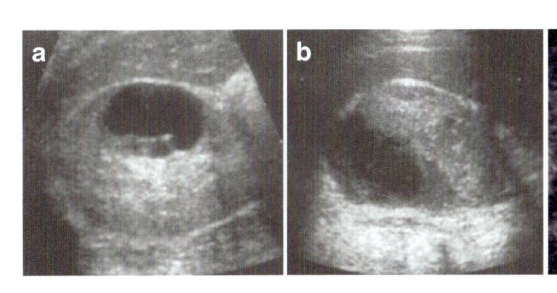

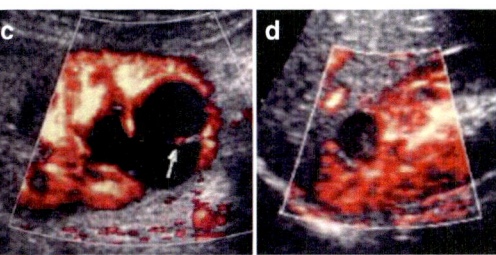

Fig. 13 Complicated renal cyst: (**a**) US demonstration of a complicated cysts with septations and internal daughter cysts; (**b**) US demonstrates sedimentation and inhomogeneity within a complicated renal cyst after hemorrhage into a septic embolic renal infarction; (**c**) vascularization within a septum in a septated renal cyst, demonstrated by aCDS (*arrow*); (**d**) contrast-enhanced aCDS (Levovist®, Schering, Berlin, Germany) demonstrates lack of perfusion and – much better than initial grey scale US – delineates the small renal abscess (= complicated cyst with sedimented echogenic material, without perfusion) in the upper pole of a right kidney on this longitudinal section

cystic mesoblastic nephroma, and cystic renal adenocarcinoma (Theissig et al. 1986; Babut et al. 1993; Upadhyay and Neely 1989). The detailed and definite diagnosis is often only made histologically as imaging features may not be characteristic in the individual case (see chapter "Neoplasms of the Genitourinary System").

> **Take Away**
> In pediatric patients, renal cysts are generally detected by US. If they look like complicated cysts and do not match any entity of congenital polycystic renal disease, they should be studied by additional imaging such as ce-MRI (for complicated cysts and suspected malignancy or for differentiation of calyceal diverticula). If there are still equivocal findings, they should be monitored or – particularly when showing growth or atypically vascularized areas – should undergo biopsy/operation.

6 Summary

Renal hypoplasia, dysplasia, and cystic renal diseases comprise many entities that sometimes are diagnostically challenging. However, many of them have a common pathogenetic pathway on a cellular and genetic level centered at the cilium-centrosome complex ("ciliopathies"); additionally the composition of the uromucoprotein "uromodelin" appears to play a major role. With the help of the clinical information, the onset and patient age, the family history, and the genetic results, diagnosis can be made in the majority of cases without invasive procedures. The location and size, distribution and onset of cysts, and parenchymal abnormalities (as usually described on US) can help to narrow the list of differential diagnoses (Fig. 6a); still suspicion of chronic glomerulonephritis with end-stage renal disease or of a renal cystic tumor/malignancy may necessitate US- or CT-guided biopsy.

Usually US (and sometimes VCUG/ce-VUS) are sufficient as a first imaging step; only sometimes MRI or even CT or angiography may become necessary. IVU has been replaced by MRI; only rarely it is still used for differential diagnosis and some specific conditions – particularly if MRU is not available. New findings in molecular genetics will further improve non-imaging diagnostic capabilities, but variations in expression of the same genetic condition will still necessitate individual imaging in assessing the state and/or manifestation of a disease. Furthermore, rapid improvement in MRI techniques will probably more and more entitle these entities to MR diagnosis in the pre- and postnatal setting. At diagnosis, US may also help in assessing associated malformations.

Once the diagnosis is established, the task of imaging is to help monitor these patients – either the progression or resolution of disease, or the state of the contralateral kidney as well as of potentially associated disorders. Although no curative treatment exists for many cystic renal disorders to date, modern treatment and supportive means help to avoid complications in most children, thus enabling adequate growth and delayed onset of renal insufficiency and in end-stage renal disease improving the chances for dialysis and renal transplantation.

> **Take Away**
> As the "simple renal cyst" is – unlike in the adult population – rather uncommon in childhood, a thorough workup and follow-up of even incidental findings are compulsory.

References

Alvares F, Bernhard O, Brunelle F (1981) Congenital hepatic fibrosis in children. J Pediatr 99:370–375

Arant BS Jr, Soteol-Avila C, Bernstein J (1979) Segmental "hypoplasia" of the kidney (Ask-Upmark). J Pediatr 95:931–939

Avner ED (1994) Medullary cystic disease and medullary sponge kidney. In: Greenberg A (ed) NFK nephrology primer. Saunders, Philadelphia, pp 174–181

Avni EF, Thova Y, Van Gansbeke G et al (1985) The development of hypodysplastic kidney: contribution of antenatal ultrasound. Radiology 154:123–126

Avni EF, Thoua Y, Laimand B et al (1986) Multicystic dysplastic kidney: evolving concepts. In utero diagnosis and post-natal follow-up by ultrasound. Ann Radiol 29:663–668

Avni F, Matos C, Rypens F, Schulman CC (1997) Ectopic vaginal insertion of an upper pole ureter: demonstration by special sequences of magnetic resonance imaging. J Urol 158:1931–1932

Avni EF, Garel L, Cassart M et al (2006) Perinatal assessment of hereditary cystic renal diseases: the role of sonography. Pediatr Radiol 36:405–415

Avni EF, Hall M (2010) Renal cystic diseases: new concepts. Pediatr Radiol 40:939–946

Avni FE, Garel C, Cassart M, D'Haene N, Hall M, Riccabona M (2012) Imaging and classification of congenital cystic renal diseases. AJR Am J Roentgenol 198:1004–1013

Babut JM, Bawab F, Jouan H et al (1993) Cystic renal tumours in children–a diagnostic challenge. Eur J Pediatr Surg 3:157–160

Baert L, Steg A (1977) On the pathogenesis of simple renal cysts in the adult. Urol Res 5:103–108

Beomonte-Zobel B, Vicentini C, Masciocchi C et al (1990) Magnetic resonance imaging in the localization of undescended abdominal testes. Eur Urol 17:145–148

Bernstein J (1971) The morphogenesis of renal parenchymal maldevelopment (renal dysplasia). Pediatr Clin North Am 18:395–407

Bernstein J (1973) The classification of renal cysts. Nephron 11:91–100

Bernstein J (1976) A classification of renal cysts. In: Gardner KD Jr (ed) Cystic diseases of the kidney. Wiley, New York, pp 7–30

Bernstein J (1992) Renal hypoplasia and dysplasia. In: Edelman CM (ed) Pediatric kidney disease. Little & Brown, Boston, pp 1121–1137

Bernstein J (1993a) Renal cystic disease in the tuberous sclerosis complex. Pediatr Nephrol 7:490–495

Bernstein J (1993b) Glomerulocystic kidney disease-nosological considerations. Pediatr Nephrol 7: 464–470

Bisaglia M, Ca G, Senger C, Stallone C, Sessa A (2006) Renal cystic diseases: a review. Adv Anat Pathol 13:26–56

Blowey DL, Querfeld U, Geary D et al (1996) Ultrasound findings in juvenile nephronophthisis. Pediatr Nephrol 10:22–24

Boal DK, Teele R (1980) Sonography of infantile polycystic kidney disease. AJR Am J Roentgenol 135:575–580

Boichis H, Passwell J, David R et al (1973) Congenital hepatic fibrosis and nephronophthisis. Q J Med 42:221–233

Borthne A, Nordshus T, Reiseter T et al (1999) MR urography: the future gold standard in pediatric urogenital imaging. Pediatr Radiol 29:694–701

Bosniak MA (1986) The current radiological approach to renal cysts. Radiology 158:1–10

Bosniak MA (1991) Difficulties in classifying cystic lesions of the kidney. Urol Radiol 13:91–93

Bretan PN Jr, Bush MP, Hricak H et al (1986) Chronic renal failure: A significant risk factor in the development of acquired renal cysts and renal cell carcinoma. Case report and review of the literature. Cancer 57:1871–1879

Brook-Carter PT, Peral B, Ward CJ et al (1994) Deletion of TSC2 and PDK1 genes associated with severe infantile polycystic kidney disease – A contiguous gene syndrome. Nat Genet 8:328–332

Cain JE, Di Giovanni V, Smeeton J et al (2010) Genetics of renal hypoplasia: insights into the mechanisms controlling nephron endowment. Pediatr Res 68:91–98

Churchill E, Kimoff R, Pinshy M et al (1975) Solitary intrarenal cyst: correctable cause of hypertension. Urology 6:485–488

Churg J, Bernstein J, Risdon RA et al (1987) Renal disease. Classification and atlas. Part II: developmental and hereditary disease. Igaku-Shoin, New York

Cohen HL, Haller JO (1987) Diagnostic sonography of the fetal genitourinary tract. Urol Radiol 9:88–98

Cole BR, Wonley SB, Stapelton FB (1987) Infantile polycystic disease in the first year of life. J Pediatr 11:693–699

Cope JR, Trickey FD (1982) Congenital absence of the kidney: problems in diagnosis and management. J Urol 127:10–12

Davidson AJ, Hartman DS (1994) Radiologic anatomy of the kidney and the ureter. In: Davidson AJ, Hartman DS (eds) Radiology of the urinary tract. Saunders, Philadelphia, pp 53–96

deBruyn R, Gordon I (2000) Imaging in cystic renal disease. Arch Dis Child 83:401–407

Devine C (1983) Embryologie des Urogenitaltraktes. In: Hohenfellner R, Zing EJ (eds) Urologie in Klinik und Praxis. Thieme, Stuttgart, pp 833–849

Diard F, LeDosseur P, Cadier L et al (1984) Multicystic dysplasia of the upper component of the complete duplex kidney. Pediatr Radiol 14:310–313

Dinkel E, Ertel M, Dittrich M et al (1985) Kidney size in childhood: sonographical growth charts for kidney length and volume. Pediatr Radiol 15:38–43

Dodat H, Galifer RB, Montupet P et al (1988) Renal tumors in children, excluding Wilm's tumor. J D Urol 94:67–82

Domizio P, Risdon RA (1991) Cystic renal neoplasms of infancy and childhood: a light microscopical lectin histochemical and immunohistochemical study. Histopathology 19:199–209

Donaldson MDC, Warner AA, Trompeter RS et al (1985) Familial juvenile nephronophthisis, Jeune's syndrome, and associated disorders. Arch Dis Child 60:426–443

Dunill MS, Millard PR, Oliver D (1977) Acquired cystic disease of the kidneys: a hazard of long term intermittent maintenance haemodialysis. J Clin Pathol 30:868–877

Elzouki AY, al-Suhaibani H, Mirza K et al (1996) Thin-section computed tomography scans detect medullary

cysts in patients believed to have juvenile nephronophthisis. Am J Kidney Dis 27:216–219
Estroff JA, Mandell J, Benacerraf BR (1991) Increased renal parenchymal echogenicity in the fetus: Importance and clinical outcome. Radiology 181:135–139
Fabris A, Antonio Lupo A, Ferraro PM et al (2013) Familial clustering of medullary sponge kidney is autosomal dominant with reduced penetrance and variable expressivity. Kidney Int 83:272–277
Fick GM, Johnson AM, Strain JD et al (1993) Characteristics of very early onset autosomal dominant polycystic kidney disease. J Am Soc Nephrol 3:1863–1870
Fick GM, Duley IT, Johnson AM et al (1994) The spectrum of autosomal dominant polycystic kidney disease in children. J Am Soc Nephrol 4:1654–1660
Fitch S, Parvey LS, Wiliams J et al (1985) Developmental cystic renal neoplasms in children: Diagnostic imaging characteristics. Comput Radiol 9:149–158
Fitch SJ, Stapleton FB (1986) Ultrasonographic features of glomerulocystic disease in infancy: similarity to infantile polycystic kidney disease. Pediatr Radiol 16:400–402
Fredericks BJ, de-Campo M, Chow CW et al (1989) Glomerulocystic renal disease: ultrasound appearances. Pediatr Radiol 19:184–186
Frohneberg D (1986) Agensie, Hypoplasie und Dysplasie. In: Hohenfellner R, Thüroff JW, Schulte-Wissermann H (eds) Kinderurologie in Klinik und Praxis. Thieme, Stuttgard/New York, pp 236–240
Gadner KD Jr (1967) Juvenile nephronophthisis and renal medullary cystic disease. In: Gadner KD Jr (ed) Cystic diseases of the kidney. Wiley, New York
Garel LA, Habib R, Pariente D et al (1984) Juvenile nephronophthisis: sonographic appearance in children with severe uremia. Radiology 151:93–95
Guay-Woodford LM (2006) Renal cystic diseases: diverse phenotypes converge on the cilium/centrosome complex. Pediatr Neprol 21:1369–1376
Gelet A, Sanseverino R, Martin X et al (1990) Percutaneous treatment of benign renal cysts. Eur Urol 18:248–252
Glassberg KL, Stephens FD, Lebowitz RL et al (1987) Renal dysgenesis and cystic disease of the kidney: a report on terminology, nomenclature, and classification. Section of urology, American Academy Of Pediatrics. J Urol 138:1085–1092
Gordon AC, Thomas DFM, Arthur RJ et al (1988) Multicystic kidney–is nephrectomy still appropriate? J Urol 140:1231–1234
Greene LF, Feinzwig W, Dahlin D (1971) Multicystic dysplasia with special reference to the contralateral kidney. J Urol 105:482–487
Griscom NT, Vawter GF, Fellers FX (1975) Pelvoinfundibular atresia: the usual form of multicystic kidney: 44 unilateral and 2 bilateral cases. Semin Roentgenol 10:125–131
Hallmann N, Hjelt L, Ahvenainen EK (1956) Nephrotic syndrome in newborn and young infants. Ann Pediatr Fenn 2:227–241

Hattery R, King BF (1995) Technique and application of MR urography. Radiology 194:25–27
Helin I, Persson PH (1986) Prenatal diagnosis of urinary tract abnormalities by ultrasound. Pediatrics 78:879–883
Hendry PJ, Hendry GMA (1991) Observations on the use of Doppler ultrasound in multicystic dysplastic kidneys. Pediatr Radiol 21:203–204
Hildebrandt F, Waldherr R, Kutt R et al (1992) The nephronophthisis complex: clinical and genetic aspects. Clin Invest 70:802–808
Hildebrandt F (1997) Nephronophthisis. In: Barrat MT, Avner ED, Harmon WE (eds) Pediatric nephrology. Lippincott Williams & Wilkins, Baltimore, pp 453–458
Hildebrandt F, Otto F (2005) Cilia and centrosomes: a unifying pathogentic concept for cystic kidney disease? Nat Rev Genet 6:928–940
Hildebrandt F, Benzing T, Katsanis N (2011) Ciliopathies. N Engl J Med 364:1533–1543
Hogg RJ (1992) Acquired cystic kidney disease in children prior to the start of dialysis. Pediatr Nephrol 6:176–178
Hoyer PF (1996a) Niere. In: Hoffman V, Deeg KH, Hoyer PF (eds) Ultraschalldiagnostik in der Pädiatrie und Kinderchirurgie. Thieme, Stuttgart/New York, pp 345–361
Hoyer PF (1996b) Nierentumoren. In: Hoffman V, Deeg KH, Hoyer PF (eds) Ultraschalldiagnostik in der Pädiatrie und Kinderchirurgie. Thieme, Stuttgart/New York, pp 406–412
Huland H (1986) Hydronephrotische Atrophie. In: Hohenfellner R, Thüroff JW, Schulte-Wissermann H (eds) Kinderurologie in Klinik und Praxis. Thieme, Stuttgart/New York, pp 18–29
Huttunen NP (1976) Congenital nephrotic syndrome of Finnish type. Study of 75 cases. Arch Dis Child 51:344–348
Iorember FM, Vehaskari MV (2014) Uromodelin: a old friend with new roles in health and disease. Pediatr Nephrol 29:1151–1158
Jeon A, Cramer BC, Walsh E et al (1999) A spectrum of segmental multicystic renal dysplasia. Pediatr Radiol 29:309–315
Joshi VV, Kasznica J (1984) Clinicopathologic spectrum of glomerulocystic kidneys: report of two cases and a brief review of literature. Pediatr Pathol 2:171–186
Jurkovic D, Geipel A, Gruboeck K et al (1995) Three-dimensional ultrasound for the assessment of uterine anatomy and detection of congenital anomalies: a comparison with hysterosalpingography and two-dimensional sonography. Ultrasound Obstet Gynecol 5:233–237
Kaplan BS, Rabin I, Nogrady MB et al (1977) Autosomal dominant polycystic renal disease in children. J Pediatr 90:782–783
Kaplan BS, Kaplan P, Dechadarievan JP et al (1988) Variable expression of autosomal recessive polycystic kidney disease and congenital hepatic fibrosis within one family. Am J Med Genet 29:639–647
Kaplan BS, Fay J, Shah V et al (1989a) Autosomal recessive polycystic kidney disease. Pediar Nephrol 3:43–49

Kaplan BS, Kaplan P, Rosenberg HK et al (1989b) Polycystic kidney diseases in childhood. J Pediatr 115:867–880

Kaplan BS, Gordon I, Pincott J et al (1989c) Familial hypoplastic glomerulocystic kidney disease: a definite entity with dominant inheritance. Am J Med Genet 34:569–573

Kasiske BL, Umen AJ (1986) The influence of age, sex, race and body habitus on kidney weight in humans. Arch Pathol Lab Med 110:55–60

Kääriäinen H, Koskinies O, Norio R (1988a) Dominant and recessive polycystic kidney disease in children: evaluation of clinical features and laboratory data. Pediatr Nephrol 2:296–302

Kääriäinen H, Jääskelainen J, Kivisaari L et al (1988b) Dominant and recessive polycystic kidney disease in children: classification by intravenous pyelography, ultrasound, and computed tomography. Pediatr Radiol 18:45–50

Kern S, Zimmerhackl LB, Hildebrandt F et al (1999) Rare MR urography: a new diagnostic method in autosomal recessive polycystic kidney disease. Acta Radiol 40:543–544

Kestilä M, Lenkkeri U, Lamerdin J et al (1998) Positionally cloned gene for a novel glomerular protein – nephrin – is mutated in congenital nephrotic syndrome. Mol Cell 1:575–582

Kiechl-Kohlendorfer U, Geley T, Maurer K, Gassner I (2011) Uterus didelphys with unilateral vaginal atresia: multicystic dysplastic kidney is the precursor of "renal agenesis" and the key to early diagnosis of this genital anomaly. Pediatr Radiol 41:1112–1116

Kim AY, Kim SH, Kim YJ et al (1999) Contrast-enhanced power Doppler sonography for the differentiation of cystic renal lesions: preliminary study. J Ultrasound Med 18:581–588

Kissane JM (1990) Renal cysts in pediatric patients: a classification and overview. Pediatr Nephrol 4:69–70

Kjessler B, Johansson SOG, Sherman MS et al (1975) Alphafetoprotein in antenatal diagnosis of congenital nephrosis. Lancet 1:123–124

Krestin GP (1990) Morphologic and functional MR of the kidneys and adrenal glands. Field & Wood, Philadelphia

Krull E, Hoyer PF, Habenicht R et al (1990) Multicystic kidney dysplasia. Mschr Kinderheilkd 138:202–205

Kullendorff CM (1990) Surgery in unilateral multicystic kidney. Z Kinderchir 45:235–237

Landry JL, Dodat H, Pelizzo G et al (1999) Dysplasie kystique du rete testis et agenesie renale ipsilaterale chez l'enfant. Arch Pediatr 6:416–420

Leichter HE, Dietrich R, Salusky IB et al (1988) Acquired cystic kidney disease in children undergoing long-term dialysis. Pediatr Nephrol 2:8–11

Levine E (1992) Renal cell carcinoma in uremic acquired renal cystic disease: incidence, detection and management. Urol Radiol 13:203–210

Lieberman E, Salinas-Madeigal L, Gwinn JL et al (1971) Infantile polycystic disease of the kidney and the liver: clinical, pathological and radiological correlation and comparison with congenital hepatic fibrosis. Medicine 50:277–318

Manish J, LeQuesne GW, Bourne AJ et al (1997) High resolution ultrasonography in the differential diagnosis of cystic diseases of the kidney in infancy and childhood: preliminary experiences. J Ultrasound Med 16:235–240

McDonald RA, Avner ED (1991) Inherited polycystic kidney disease in children. Semin Nephrol 11:632–642

McDonald RA, Watkins SL, Avner ED (1997) Polycystic kidney disease. In: Barrat MT, Avner ED, Harmon WE (eds) Pediatric nephrology. Lippincott Williams & Wilkins, Baltimore, pp 459–474

McHugh K, Stringer D, Hebert D (1991) Simple renal cyst in children: diagnosis and follow-up with US. Radiology 178:383–385

Morcos SK (2009) Non-neoplatsic cystic renal lesions. In: Morcos SK, Thomson H (eds) Urogenital imaging: a problem-oriented approach. Wiley-Blackwell, Oxford, pp 75–97

Nelson TR, Downey DB, Pretorius DH et al (1999) Three-dimensional ultrasound. Lippincrott Williams & Wilkins, Philadelphia, pp 111–127

Orejas G, Malaga S, Santos S et al (1992) Multicystic dysplastic kidney: absence of complications in patients treated conservatively. Child Nephrol Urol 12:35–39

Osathanondh V, Potter EL (1964) Pathogenesis of polycystic kidneys: survey of results of microdissection. Arch Pathol 77:510–519

Osathanondh V, Potter EL (1966) Development of human kidney as shown by microdissection. Arch Pathol 82:391–411

Palubinskas AJ (1963) Renal pyramidal structure opacification in excretory urography and its relation to medullary sponge kidney. Radiology 81:963–970

Patriquin HB, O'Regan S (1985) Medullary sponge kidney in childhood. AJR Am J Roentgenol 145: 315–319

Patten RM, Mack LA, Wang KY et al (1990) The fetal genitourinary tract. Radiol Clin North Am 28:115–130

Porch P, Noe HN, Stapleton FB (1986) Unilateral presentation of adult-type polycystic kidney disease in children. J Urol 135:744–746

Proesmans W, Van Damme B, Casaer P et al (1982) Autosomal dominant polycystic kidney disease in the neonatal period: association with a cerebral arteriovenous malformation. Pediatrics 70:971–975

Reiner I, Donell S, Jones M et al (1992) Percutaneous sclerotherapy for simple renal cysts in children. Br J Radiol 65:281–282

Ring E, Petritsch P, Riccabona M et al (1990) Therapie und Prognose von Kindern mit pränatal diagnostizierten Harnwegsfehlbildungen. Wien Klin Wochenschr 102:463–466

Ring E, Petritsch P, Riccabona M et al (1993) Welche Therapie erfordert die pränatal diagnostizierte multizystische Nierendysplasie? Klin Padiatr 205: 150–152

Riccabona M, Ring E, Petritsch G et al (1993a) Colour Doppler sonography in the differential diagnosis of congenital unilateral cystic renal malformations. Z Geburtsh Perinatol 197:283–287

Riccabona M, Ring E, Fueger G et al (1993b) Doppler sonography in congenital ureteropelvic junction obstruction and congenital muticystic kidney disease. Pediatr Radiol 23:502–505

Riccabona M, Ring E, Häusler M et al (1999a) Prenatally recognised multicystic segmental nephroma. Z Geburtsh Neonatol 203:255–257

Riccabona M, Szolar DH, Preidler KW et al (1999b) Renal masses–evaluation by amplitude coded colour Doppler sonography and multiphasic enhanced contrast CT. Acta Radiol 40:457–461

Riccabona M, Simbrunner J, Ring E, Ebner F, Fotter R (2002) Feasibility of MR-urography in neo-nates and infants with anomalies of the upper urinary tract. Eur Radiol 12:1442–1450

Riccabona M, Ruppert-Kohlmeier A, Ring E, Maier C, Lusuardi L, Riccabona M (2004a) Potential impact of pediatric MR-urography on the imaging algorithm in patients with a functional single kidney? AJR Am J Roentgenol 183:795–800

Riccabona M, Michael R, Koen M et al (2004b) Magnetic resonance urography – a new gold standard for evaluation of solitary kidneys and renal buds. J Urol 171:1642–1646

Riccabona M, Avni F, Dacher JN et al (2011) ESPR uroradiology task force and ESUR paediatric working group: imaging recommendations in paediatric uroradiology, part IV Minutes of the ESPR uroradiology task force mini-symposium on imaging in childhood renal hypertension and imaging of renal trauma in children. Pediatr Radiol 41(7):939–944

Riccabona M, Avni FE (2011) MR imaging of the paediatric abdomen. In: Gourtsonyiannis N (ed) Clinical MRI of the abdomen. Why, how, when. Springer, Heidelberg/Dordrecht/London/New York, pp 639–676, ISBN 978-3-540-85689-4

Riccabona M, Avni F, Damasio B et al (2012) ESPR Uroradiology Task Force and ESUR Paediatric Working Group – Imaging recommendations in Paediatric Uroradiology, Part V: childhood cystic kidney disease, childhood renal transplantation, and contrast-enhanced ultrasound in children. Pediatr Radiol 42:1275–1283

Riccabona M (2014) Paediatric 3D-Ultrasound (3DUS). J Ultrasound 14:5–20

Riccabona M, Lobo ML, Willi U et al (2014) ESPR Uroradiology Task Force and ESUR Paediatric Working Group – imaging recommendations in Paediatric Uroradiology, Part VI: childhood renal biopsy and imaging of neonatal and infant genital tract. Minutes from the Task Force session at the annual ESPR Meeting 2012 in Athens on childhood renal biopsy and imaging neonatal genitalia. Pediatr Radiol 44:496–502

Roy S, Dillon MJ, Trompeter RS et al (1997) Autosomal recessive kidney disease: long term outcome of neonatal survivors. Pediatr Nephrol 11:302–306

Schneider K, Fendel H (1995) Urogenitaltrakt. In: Ebel KD, Willich E, Richter E (eds) Differentialdiagnostik in der pädiatrischen Radiologie, Band II. Thieme, Stuttgart/New York, pp 343–392

Sedman A, Bell P, Manco-Johnson M et al (1987) Autosomal dominant polycystic kidney disease in childhood: a longitudinal study. Kidney Int 31:1000–1005

Sellers B, Richie JP (1978) Glomerulocystic kidney: proposed etiology and pathogenesis. J Urol 119:678–680

Shaikewitz ST, Chapman A (1993) Autosomal recessive polycystic kidney disease: issues regarding the variability of clinical presentation. J Am Soc Nephrol 3:1858–1862

Shapiro SS, Wagreich J, Parsons RB et al (1998) Tissue harmonic imaging sonography: evaluation of image quality compared with conventional sonography. AJR Am J Roentgenol 171:701–707

Siegel MJ, McAlister WH (1980) Simple cysts of the kidney in children. J Urol 123:75–78

Sigmund G, Stöver B, Zimmerhackl LB et al (1991) RARE MR urography in the diagnosis of upper urinary tract abnormalities in children. Pediatr Radiol 21:416–420

Strand WR, Rushton HG, Markle BM et al (1989) Autosomal dominant polycystic kidney disease in infants: asymmetric disease mimicking a unilateral renal mass. J Urol 141:1151–1153

Stockamp K (1986) Zystische Nierenerkrankungen. In: Hohenfellner R, Thüroff JW, Schulte-Wissermann H (eds) Kinderurologie in Klinik und Praxis. Thieme, Stuttgart/New York, pp 262–266

Srivastava T, Garola RE, Hellerstein S (1999) Autosomal dominant inheritance of multicystic dysplastic kidney. Pediatr Nephrol 13:481–483

Szolar DH, Kammerhuber F, Altziebler S et al (1997) Multiphasic helical CT of the kidney: Increased conspicuity for detection and characterisation of small (<3 cm) renal masses. Radiology 202:211–217

Takeuchi T, Tanaka T, Tokuyama H et al (1984) Multilocular cystic adenocarcinoma: a case report and review of the literature. J Surg Oncol 25:136–140

Tada S, Yamagishi J, Kobayashi H et al (1983) The incidence of simple renal cysts by computed tomography. Clin Radiol 34:437–439

Tanago EA (1975) Embryology of the genitourinary system. In: Smith R (ed) General urology. Lange, Los Altos

Terrier F, Hricak H, Justich E et al (1986) The diagnostic value of renal cortex-to-medulla contrast on magnetic resonance imaging. Eur J Radiol 6:121–126

Theissig F, Hempel J, Schubert J (1986) Multilocular cystic nephroma simulating kidney carcinoma. Ztschr Urol Nephrol 79:263–267

Thomas JD, Rubin DN (1998) Tissue harmonic imaging: why does it work? J Am Soc Echocardiogr 11:803–808

Upadhyay AK, Neely JA (1989) Cystic nephroma: an emerging entity. Anal Royal Col Surg England 71:381–383

Urban BA (1997) The small renal mass: what is the role of multiphasic helical sacnning. Radiology 202:22–23

Vester U, Kranz B, Hoyer PF (2010) The diagnostic value of ultrasound in cystic kidney disease. Pediatr Nephrol 25:231–240

Watkins SL, McDonald RA, Avner ED (1997) Renal dysplasia, hypoplasia and miscellaneous cystic disorders. In: Barrat MT, Avner ED, Harmon WE (eds) Pediatric nephrology. Lippincott Williams & Wilkins, Baltimore, pp 415–426

Wittingham TA (1999) Tissue harmonic imaging. Eur Radiol 9:323–326

Wood BP (1992) Renal cystic disease in infants and children. Urol Radiol 14:284–295

Woolf AS (1997) The kidney: embryology. In: Barrat MT, Avner ED, Harmon WE (eds) Pediatric nephrology. Lippincott Williams & Wilkins, Baltimore, pp 1–17

Woolf R, Allen W (1953) Concomitant malformations: the frequent simultaneous occurrence of congenital malformations of the reproductive and the urinary tract. Obstet Gynecol 2:236–265

Worthington JL, Shackelford GD, Cole BR et al (1988) Sonographically detectable cysts in polycystic kidney disease in newborn and young infants. Pediatr Radiol 18:287–293

Yendt ER (1990) Medullary sponge kidney. In: Gadner KD, Bernstein J (eds) The cystic kidney. Kluwer, Dordrecht, pp 379–392

Zejil C, Roefs B, Boer K et al (1999) Clinical outcome and follow-up of sonographically suspected in utero urinary tract anomalies. J Clin Ultrasound 27: 21–28

Zerres K (1987) Genetics of cystic kidney diseases: criteria for classification and genetic counseling. Pediatr Nephrol 1:397–404

Zerres K, Hansmann M, Mallman R et al (1988) Autosomal recessive polycystic kidney disease: problems of prenatal diagnosis. Prenat Diagn 8:215–229

Imaging in Renal Parenchymal Disease

Michael Riccabona and Ekkehard Ring

Contents

1	Introduction	579
2	**Renal Parenchymal Disease and Renal Failure**	580
3	**Primary Imaging Management**	583
4	**Specific Imaging Findings**	587
4.1	Glomerular Disease	587
4.2	Vascular and Tubulointerstitial Disease	588
5	**Advanced Imaging**	593
5.1	Advanced Ultrasonography and Doppler Sonography	593
5.2	Renal Biopsy	595
	Conclusions	598
	References	598

M. Riccabona, MD (✉)
Department of Radiology, Division of Pediatric Radiology, University of Graz, 8036 Graz, Austria
e-mail: michael.riccabona@meduni-graz.at

E. Ring, MD (Retired)
Department of Paediatrics, Division of General Paediatrics, University of Graz, 8036 Graz, Austria

1 Introduction

The renal parenchyma is divided into three main compartments:

- The cortex with glomeruli which create the primary ultrafiltrate, the juxtaglomerular apparatus and the cortical proximal and distal tubules, which are responsible for processing the primary urine, thereby maintaining body homeostasis
- The medulla including the Henle loop performing salt and water reabsorption, involved in concentrating and diluting mechanisms, and medullary collecting ducts for final reabsorption draining the urine through the papilla into the renal collecting system
- The interstitium, i.e. connective tissue and vasculature, of both compartments (cortex and medulla), including lymphatic tissue

Renal parenchymal disease (RPD) is defined as a disease that involves one or more compartments of the renal parenchyma (see also chapter "Renal Parenchymal Disease"). Although different segments of the nephron, the interstitium and the vasculature may be affected simultaneously or may become secondarily involved, RPD is generally classified into glomerular, tubular, interstitial and vascular disease and will be discussed in this order. The causes for similar histological changes and similar imaging appearances of affected kidneys may vary; the same disease can manifest in different ways with a wide range of histology. Furthermore, renal parenchyma may be affected by inherited diseases or may become secondarily involved in systemic disease such as metabolic disease, storage disease, infection (e.g. HIV) or sepsis, perfusional disturbances, autoimmune disease and malignant disease (metastasis, leukaemic infiltration, etc.).

Some of the many causes for RPD are discussed and described in other chapters of this book, e.g. infection and abscess (see chapters "UTI and VUR and Imaging in Urinary Tract Infections"), renal failure (see chapters "Renal Failure and Renal Transplantation and Imaging in Renal Failure, Neonatal Oligoanuria, and Renal Transplantation"), cystic and dysplastic renal disease (see chapter "Imaging in Renal Agenesis, Dysplasia, Hypoplasia and Cystic Diseases of the Kidney"), nephrocalcinosis (see chapters "Urolithiasis and Nephrocalcinosis and Imaging of Urolithiasis and Nephrocalcinosis"), changes in congenital urogenital malformations (including obstructive dysplasia, see chapters "Anomalies of Kidney Rotation, Position and Fusion, Congenital Urinary Tract and Obstructive Uropathy, Congenital Anomalies of the Renal Pelvis and Ureter, and Upper Urinary Tract Dilatation in Newborns and Infants and the Postnatal Work up of Congenital Uronephropathies"), traumatic changes (see chapter "Urinary Tract Trauma") or malignant lesions (see chapter "Neoplasms of the Genitourinary System"). This chapter concentrates on imaging in the "classic entities" of RPD and only briefly addresses miscellaneous entities such as involvement in metabolic and autoimmune disease. The clinical background including presentation and symptomatology is discussed in chapter "Renal Parenchymal Disease".

This chapter aims to follow the clinical practice in a paediatric radiology department. The main findings on initial/primary imaging are listed – generally performed by ultrasonography (US) – as established in paediatric radiology literature and paediatric US textbooks (Babcock 1989; Deeg et al. 2014; Gordon and Riccabona 2003; Hoyer 1996; Kettriz et al. 1996; Mettler and Guiberteau 1998; Riccabona et al. 2000, 2001, 2002, 2008; Riccabona 2000, 2006a, b, Riccabona 2013, 2014a; Riccabona and Fotter 2006; Siegel 1991, 1999; Slovis et al. 1989; Teele and Chare 1991; Toma 1991). Furthermore, these US findings are correlated with the presenting clinical symptom(s) and the clinical query, also with respect to the potential to offer important differential diagnostic clues. The possibilities and indications for useful additional and advanced imaging are discussed, and eventually the role of renal and extra-renal imaging during treatment or follow-up of patients with (chronic) RPD is described.

2 Renal Parenchymal Disease and Renal Failure

The clinical aspects of renal failure or pathologic urine sample findings are discussed in chapter "Renal Failure and Renal Transplantation". The role of imaging in impaired renal function is to help define the origin (prerenal, intrinsic, postrenal – see Fig. 2 in chapter "Renal Failure and Renal Transplantation"), help with differential diagnosis (Fig. 1a), monitor the disease, detect complications (Fig. 1b) and follow up thereafter/during treatment. Imaging heavily relies on US, and in many conditions, the imaging findings are unspecific but somewhat typical (Fig. 2). However, there are conditions where typical, nearly pathognomonic changes can be detected quite early by high-resolution (HR) US and may help to narrow the list of differential diagnoses (Fig. 3).

In acute presentation many RPD patients present with some degree of acute renal failure (ARF – nowadays named "acute kidney

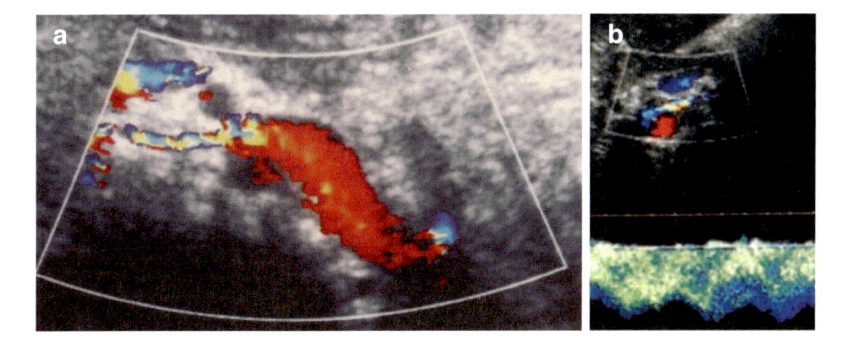

Fig. 1 Ultrasound in pseudo-nutcracker syndrome (= narrow crossing of left renal vein between the aorta and the superior mesenteric artery). (**a**) Colour Doppler sonography shows turbulent flow at the crossing of the left renal vein between the aorta and upper mesenteric artery. Note the marked change in diameter of the left renal vein. (**b**) Colour Doppler sonography-guided duplex Doppler evaluation at the side of the venous compression shows elevated flow velocity with arterialised pulsation in the left renal vein caused by propagation of aortal pulsations (Courtesy Riccabona M, Pediatric Ultrasound. Fig 10.6b, Springer 2014)

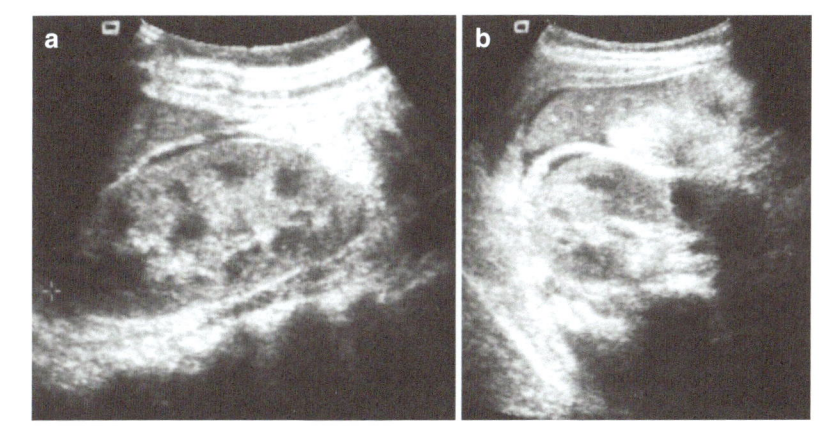

Fig. 2 Ultrasound findings in glomerulonephritis. Longitudinal (**a**) and axial (**b**) section of the right kidney showing renal enlargement and increased cortical echogenicity (compared to the adjacent liver) with broadened cortex, relatively small medulla and consequently accentuated cortico-medullary differentiation in glomerulonephritis. Note the perirenal and perihepatic fluid accumulation

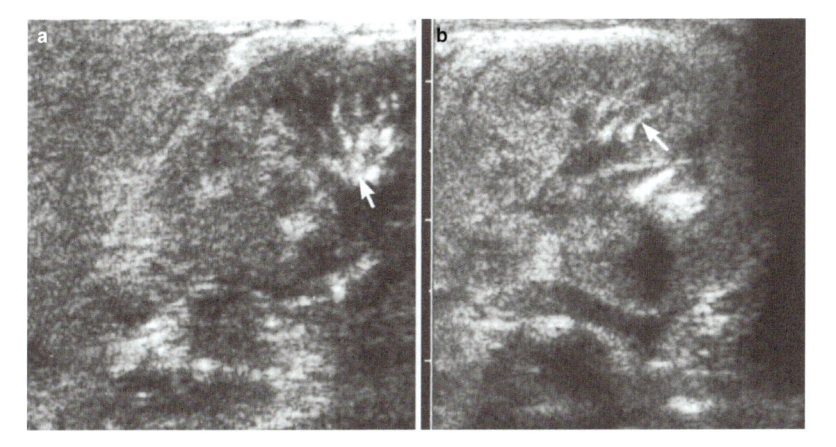

Fig. 3 High-resolution US of a neonatal left kidney. US demonstrates stringlike areas of increased echogenicity (*arrow*) in the renal medulla demonstrating early changes of tubular calcification using a 15-MHz high-resolution linear transducer and image compounding. The baby turned out to suffer from tyrosinosis. (**a**) Longitudinal section. (**b**) Axial section

injury" = AKI, see chapter "Renal Failure and Renal Transplantation"). AKI is defined as the sudden loss of renal function with or without oliguria, commonly due to acute tubular damage resulting from an ischemic/hypoxic or toxic insult. The decrease in glomerular filtration rate is an adaptive response to prevent massive losses of salt and water. Prerenal ARF results from renal hypoperfusion, often secondary to volume contraction. It implies that the kidneys are intrinsically normal and that renal function will normalise with restoration of renal perfusion. Intrinsic ARF due to acute tubular necrosis (ATN) may evolve from prolonged prerenal ARF or after a severe primary renal insult. Except for very severe injuries with the vasculature involved in microthrombi formation leading to cortical necrosis, the prognosis of ATN is good. Postrenal ARF (acute obstructive uropathy) may develop into acute bilateral obstructive uropathy due to acute pressure elevation and subsequent reduction of renal blood flow (see also chapters "Renal Failure and Renal Transplantation and Imaging in Renal Failure, Neonatal Oligoanuria, and Renal Transplantation"). As a rule, the mechanisms of renal injury are complex. For example, in myoglobinuria ARF (crush kidney) may occur as a consequence of renal vasoconstriction, endogenous toxin-induced stress to tubular cells and precipitation of the pigment in the tubular lumen resulting in obstruction. ARF results in azotaemia, acidosis, perturbation of electrolyte balance and often fluid retention with hypertension. ARF in neonates, infants, children and adolescents has many different and diverse causes (Table 1).

Some causes of ARF such as cortical necrosis and renal vein thrombosis occur more commonly in neonates, whereas haemolytic-uraemic syndrome (HUS) is more common in young children, and rapidly progressive glomerulonephritis (GN) generally occurs in older children and adolescence. Besides differentiating between these typical causes of ARF, imaging (i.e. mostly US) should try to answer whether this is likely to be even first single acute ("acute onset"), a manifestation of a chronic disease or an acute deterioration on the base of a chronic condition ("acute or chronic kidney injury"). Usually imaging starts with US and is complemented by modern US techniques and Doppler sonography [such as spectral Doppler analysis, colour Doppler sonography (CDS), amplitude-coded CDS (aCDS)]. Rarely, additional imaging such as MR or MR angiography and isotope studies (with the typical pattern of delayed and flattened tracer uptake into the renal parenchyma by more or less impaired perfusion – depending on the underlying disease – and usually delayed and prolonged tracer transit into the collecting system and flattened/delayed tracer washout curves from the renal pelvis) are used, particularly for follow-up and for confirmation or evaluation of equivocal US findings. The initial imaging in RF should address the following basic questions (Table 2):

(a) Renal size (enlarged = acute, small = chronic, but may be normal in early disease stage).
(b) Renal parenchymal alterations (may hint to a certain disease entity; Table 2).
(c) Dilatation of the urinary tract (obstruction, calculi $\geq$ postrenal RF) (see also Sect. 3).
(d) Renal perfusion (aCDS and spectral Doppler for additional information on DDx, normal vasculature or compromised perfusion, homogeneous/diffuse disease or focal impairment, resistive index [RI]) (see also Sect. 5).
(e) Intravascular volume (size of inferior cava vein, hepatic veins, right atrium, etc.), extravascular fluid collections (ascites, pleural and pericardial effusion, etc.).
(f) Do the information from items a–e allow a narrowing of the DDx or a differentiation of acute versus chronic RF and/or RPD (Table 2)?

A congenital or acquired renal disease leading to a substantial reduction of functioning nephrons results in chronic renal failure (CRF). A progressive decline of renal function ensues and CRF ultimately leads to end-stage renal failure. As renal function deteriorates, various clinical symptoms emerge. As detailed in chapter "Renal Failure and Renal Transplantation", acidosis, growth failure, renal osteodystrophy,

Table 1 The most common causes of ARF with regard to the major pathogenetic mechanisms: prerenal causes, intrinsic RF and postrenal aetiology

Prerenal failure
Dehydration
Gastrointestinal losses
Salt-wasting disease
Third space losses (sepsis, trauma and nephrotic syndrome)
Congestive heart failure
Intrinsic renal failure
Acute tubular necrosis
Prolonged (irreversible) prerenal failure
Ischemic/hypoxic
Drugs and contrast media
Toxins
Urate nephropathy and tumour lysis syndrome
Tubulointerstitial nephritis
Glomerulonephritis
Vascular lesions
Haemolytic-uraemic syndrome (HUS)
Cortical necrosis
Renal artery thrombosis, renal vein thrombosis
Infectious causes
Obstructive uropathy (=postrenal failure)
Obstruction in a solitary kidney
Bilateral ureteral obstruction
Urethral obstruction

Modified from Andreoli (1999) – see also Table 2 in chapter "Renal Failure and Renal Transplantation"

hypertension and anaemia are common manifestations and indicate more extensive and also extra-renal imaging – particularly during follow-up and when preparing for transplantation (see chapter "Imaging in Renal Failure, Neonatal Oligoanuria, and Renal Transplantation").

> **Take Away**
> Clinical presentation and symptomatology of renal parenchymal disease vary widely; in-depth knowledge about the various clinical pictures and the implications on imaging is essential to understand the task of imaging and to properly serve our clinical colleagues as well as our small patients.

3 Primary Imaging Management

In general patients with clinical symptoms and laboratory findings suspicious of renal disease are initially sent to US as the primary imaging modality, mostly before the final diagnosis is established. The role of this initial study is to rule out other diseases like obstructive or refluxive uropathy, acute obstruction, nutcracker syndrome and renal tumours (that all might cause, e.g. haematuria), cystic renal disease and renal dysplasia (that might present with hypertension, proteinuria, tubular symptoms or even haematuria, e.g. in case of a medullary sponge kidney or nephrocalcinosis) or other pre-existing urinary tract malformations. The typical pattern of transient renal medullary hyperechogenicity in neonates represents a well-known neonatal physiological and transient condition that may aggravate under certain circumstances such as long-term frusemide application or antibiotic treatment, indometacin administration, hyperviscosity or dehydration (Avni et al. 1983; Howlett et al. 1977; Riebel et al. 1993; Nakamura et al. 1999; Schulz et al. 1991; Slovis et al. 1993; Starinsky et al. 1994). We shall not discuss this entity here, as this is described in the respective chapters.

Furthermore, the clinician may expect additional information for differential diagnosis and disease status as provided by renal size (e.g. acute versus chronic disease, acute or chronic RF) and renal parenchymal echogenicity/sonomorphology (Table 2) or by renal perfusion (see Sect. 5). One of the key findings for most RPD is bilateral renal involvement; sometimes one may observe secondary extra-renal findings such as ascites and pleural effusion (Fig. 2). The combined information on renal size, bilateral or unilateral involvement, structural pattern and clinical data may point out the differential diagnosis (Toma 1991; Piaggo et al. 1999). Information on intravascular volume and potential effusions will help judge the severity of the condition and is valuable for selecting respective treatment measures. Generally, cortical hyperechogenicity (compared to the adjacent liver or spleen) with consecutively increased cortico-medullary differentiation in an enlarged

Table 2 Differential diagnosis of sonographic renal changes (Adapted from Perale 1992; Hoyer 1996). The typical sonomorphical appearances of various renal diseases with some hints for differential diagnosis are listed in three tables (Table 2a, normal parenchymal pattern but different renal size; Table 2b, diffuse parenchymal abnormalities; Table 2c, focal renal parenchymal alterations). Some entities are listed in more than one column; the other locations are then indicated by letters (A–C in Table 2a) and numbers (1–6 in Table 2b; 7–11 in Table 2c). Note that these tables try to create a systematic approach using usual ("general") US appearance as a guide for differential diagnosis. However, cases with atypical presentation mimicking other entities may well be encountered

Table 2a Differential diagnosis of sonographic renal changes: varying renal size with normal sonographic renal parenchymal pattern

A. *Normal renal size*
- Normal kidney (5, 10)
- VUR (C)
- Non-cystic neonatal nephropathy
- Renal arterial thrombosis
- Trauma (7, 8, 10)
  - Contusion
  - Vascular interruption
- HUS★ (5)
- CDG-Sy★ (5, 6)
- Acute PN (B, 4, 7, 8)
- NS★ (B)
- Acute GN★ (B, 5)
- Nephroblastomatosis (B, 4, 7, 8, 9)
- Acute tubular necrosis★ (5, 10)

B. *Increased renal size*
- Compensatory hypertrophy
- In contralateral disease, e.g. hypo-/dysplasia, RNP, cystic disease, nephrectomy
- Obstructive uropathy, neoplasm, agenesis
- Uncomplicated duplication
- Organomegaly (9)
- Meckel syndrome
- Zellweger syndrome
- Beckwith-Wiedemann sy
- Crossed fused ectopia
- Horseshoe kidney (C)
- Acute PN (A, 4, 7, 8)
- NS★ (A)
- Acute GN★ (A, 5)
- Leukaemia (2, 5, 8)
- Nephroblastomatosis (A, 4, 7, 8, 9)

C. *Reduced renal size*
- Simple hypoplasia
- RNP/VUR (A)
- Partial nephrectomy
- Ectopic kidney
- Supernumerary kidney
- Other hypodysplasia
  - Non-cystic dysplasia (3)
  - Oligomeganephronia
- In utero drug exposure and infections
- Horseshoe kidney (B)
- Chronic glomerular disease★ (3, 10)

Table 2b Differential diagnosis of sonographic renal changes: diffuse abnormality of sonographic renal parenchymal pattern

1. *Large kidney with subcapsular hypoechoic rim*
- ARPKD★ (2, 9)
- (Finnish) congenital NS★ (2)
- Acute cortical necrosis★
- Renal vein thrombosis (3, 5, 7, 10, 11)

2. *Diffusely increased echogenicity: large*
- ARPKD★ (1, 9)
- ADPKD★ (9)
- GCKD★ (9)
- Congenital NS★ (1)
- Bardet-Biedl syndrome★ (9)
- Lesch-Nyhan syndrome
- Foetal hamartomatosis
- Urate NP★ (6)
- Acute medullary necrosis★
- Candida infection (6, 7)
- Renal dysplasia (dilated urinary tract)
- Lymphangioma (intrarenal, mostly★)
- Acute lymphoblastic leukaemia

3. *Diffusely increased echogenicity: small*
- MCDKD (9)
- Non-cystic
- Hypodysplasia (C)
- Tamm-Horsfall sy (and TMHN, 6)★
- Renal atrophy
  - Obstructive NP (5)
  - Renal vein thrombosis (late, 1, 5, 7, 10, 11)
  - Chronic glomerular KD (C, 10) ★
  - Chronic PN (7, 10)
  - RASt
  - Any chronic RPD
- Diffuse NC★
  - Hyperparathyroidism (chronic) (6)
  - Fanconi KD (9)
  - Hypophosphataemic X-1 rickets (chronic)
  - Cystinuria
  - Oxalosis
  - Acute lymphoblastic leukaemia

Table 2 (continued)

4. *Diffuse hypoechogenicity*	**Table 2c Differential diagnosis of sonographic renal changes: focal abnormality and submersion of sonographic renal parenchymal pattern**
Acute PN (A, B, 7, 8)	
Lymphoma (5, 7, 8, 10)	
Nephroblastomatosis (A, B, 7, 8, 9)	7. *Focal hyperechoic or complex abnormality*
5. *Increased cortical echogenicity*	All entities of (6)
Normal newborn (A, 10)	Intrarenal reflux in VUR
Obstructive NP (B)	Juvenile xanthogranuloma
Renal amyloidosis★ (10)	Elastic pseudoxanthoma★
Diabetic NP★	Renal vein thrombosis (1, 3, 5, 10, 11)
Myoglobinuria★	Segmental infarct (8)
Haemoglobinuria★	Acute segmental PN (lobar nephronia; A, B, 4, 8)
HUS★ (A)	Chronic PN (including pseudotumoural glomerular sclerosis; 3, 7, 10)
Acute:	(Micro)cystic KDs
Renal vein thrombosis (1, 3, 7, 10, 11)	Abscess (8)
Tubular necrosis★ (A, 10)	Candida infection (2, 6)
GN★ (A, B)	Trauma (A, 8, 10)
Interstitial nephritis★	Neoplasm
CDG syndrome★ (A, 6)	Benign (6, 9, 11) including angiomyolipoma
Glomerulosclerosis★ (7)	Malignant (4, 5, 7, 8, 10, 11) including Wilms' tumour
Hepatorenal syndrome★	
Burkitt lymphoma (4, 7, 8, 10)	Nephroblastomatosis (A, B, 4, 8, 9)
Acute leukaemia (B, 2, 8)	8. *Focal hypoechoic abnormality*
6. *Increased medullary echogenicity*	Segmental infarct (7)
Medullary NC★	Acute focal PN (A, B, 4, 7)
Hypercalciuria	Abscess (7)
Hypercalcaemia	Trauma (A, 7, 10)
Williams syndrome	Hamartomas
Distal tubular acidosis	Lymphomas (4, 5, 7, 10)
Hyperparathyroidism (3)	Myolipoma (rare)
Bartter syndrome	Nephroblastomatosis (A, B, 4, 7, 9)
Cystinuria	9. *Anechoic/cystic lesion*
Xanthinuria	Cystic hypodysplasia
Malignancies	MCDKD (3)
Drugs (Ca, ACTH, vit. D, frusemide, etc.)	ARPKD★ (1, 2)
Others★	ADPKD★ (2)
Sickle cell disease	GCKD★ (2)
Tyrosinaemia	MSKD★ (6)
Glycogenosis	Cystic KDs
Multiple myeloma	Juvenile nephronophthisis★ (6, 10)
Urate NP (2)	Multiple malformations syndrome★
Shock, asphyxia	Tuberous sclerosis (7)
Blood transfusion	Meckel sy (B)
Candida infection (2, 5)	Jeune syndrome
TMHN★ (3)	Zellweger syndrome (2)
CDG syndrome★ (A, 5)	Von Hippel-Lindau syndrome
Juvenile nephronophthisis★ (9, 10)	Bardet-Biedl syndrome (2)
MSKD★ (9)	
Multiple angiomas (7)	

(continued)

Table 2 (continued)

	Fanconi syndrome
	And many other syndromes
Cysts	
	Simple cyst
	Complicated cysts
	Cystic end-stage KD ("acquired cystic KD")★
	Hydatid cyst
	Multilocular cyst
Mesoblastic nephroma (7, 11)	
Nephroblastomatosis (A, B, 4, 7, 8)	
Cystic renal lymphangioma	
Wilms' tumour (7, 11)	
10. *Focal reduction of parenchymal thickness*	
	Normal kidney (A, 5)
	Lobar segmentation
	Lobulation
	Parenchymal junction line/defect
Non-cystic congenital NP (A)	
Juvenile nephronophthisis★ (6, 9)	
Renal amyloidosis★ (5)	
Chronic glomerular KD (★C, 3)	
Chronic PN (3, 7)	
Tuberculosis	
Renal vein thrombosis (late; 1, 3, 5, 7, 11)	
Late stage of acute neonatal tubular necrosis★ (A, 5)	
Trauma (A, 7, 8)	
Treated lymphoma (4, 5, 7, 8)	
11. *Submersion of parenchymal pattern*	
Renal vein thrombosis (1, 3, 5, 7, 10)	
Xanthogranulomatous pyelonephritis	
Neoplasm	
	Malignant (7, 9)
	Mesoblastic nephroma (7, 8, 9)

★ bilateral, *NS* nephrotic syndrome, *Sy* syndrome, *KD* kidney disease, *chron* chronic, *PN* pyelonephritis, *GN* glomerulonephritis, *PN* pyelonephritis, *HUS* haemolytic-uraemic syndrome, *RNP* reflux nephropathy, *VUR* vesicoureteral reflux, *CDG-Sy* carbohydrate-deficient glycoprotein syndrome *NP* nephropathy, *GCKD* glomerulocystic kidney disease, *TMHN* transient medullar hyperechogenicity of the newborn, *MSKD* medullary sponge kidney disease, *NC* nephrocalcinosis, *RASt* renal artery stenosis, *MCDKD* multicystic dysplastic kidney disease

kidney corresponds with acute glomerular disease. Reduction in size as well as a more or less inhomogeneously increased echogenicity with reduced cortico-medullary differentiation hint towards chronic RPD, particularly with both glomerular and tubulointerstitial involvement (Fredericks et al. 1989; Perale et al. 1988; Perale 1992). Loss of cortico-medullary differentiation with normal cortical echogenicity may hint towards medullary disease, particularly in cases with medullary or papillary hyperechogenicity and consecutively reversed echogenicity pattern as seen in hypercalciuria, nephrocalcinosis, nephrotoxicity of some drugs (e.g. chemotherapy), cystinosis and oxalosis. Dilatation and differentiation of the collecting urinary system depends on renal function – in polyuric RF the renal pelvis can be prominent; in poor functioning units, the renal pelvis may collapse and thus be invisible for US. Knowledge of hydration and diuresis is essential for adequate interpretation of particularly slight calyceal and pelvic dilatation, as even in severe acute obstruction, only little distension may be seen. Furthermore – in some diseases – US changes may precede clinical recurrence (e.g. HUS, IgA nephropathy), and the severity of changes (e.g. degree of hyperechogenicity of the renal cortex) may correlate with the severity of the disease (Hricak et al. 1982; Rosenfield and Siegel 1981). Advanced US such as high-resolution imaging or Doppler evaluation may still offer more potential for differential diagnosis and may provide valuable information during the course of the disease (see Sect. 5). Some centres use standardised diagnostic flow charts and imaging algorithms to evaluate typical clinical presentations; however, they are more commonly applied to other entities such as congenital urinary tract malformations than to RPD.

Other modalities such as intravenous urography (IVU), CT or MRI are rarely used in the initial assessment, as they partially are expensive, invasive and not generally available, bare the risk of contrast-induced nephropathy or nephrogenic systemic fibrosis and yet are not specific to date (Diettrich 1990; Kettriz et al. 1996; Riccabona and Fotter 2006; Riccabona et al. 2010; Riccabona 2015; Siegel 1999). Depending on the patient's history and the initial US finding (e.g. dilated collecting system with enlarged ureter, increased echogenicity of renal parenchyma, decreased renal size), voiding cysto-urethrography (VCUG) may be indicated to find or to rule out VUR associated with RPD. In suspected obstructive RPD/uropathy, dynamic isotope studies may be performed and may show a flattened dynamic curve with delayed tracer uptake as well as prolonged tracer washout and diffusely speckled tracer rarefaction over the renal parenchyma (Mettler and Guiberteau 1998).

Seldom renal parenchymal abnormalities consistent with RPD are picked up as an incidental finding on a study performed because of a different query, such as interstitial (septic) renal involvement and parainfectious GN in a septic patient, or RPD in a dystrophic child. Contrast-enhanced CT studies may demonstrate delayed and prolonged parenchymal enhancement with reduced cortico-medullary differentiation of enlarged kidneys in acute GN – but in general radiopaque intravenous contrast agents as administered for IVU or CT should be avoided in RPD with renal functional impairment; if these studies are performed, good hydration as well as diuretic measures are compulsory to prevent possible contrast-induced nephropathy with renal damage such as papillary necrosis or even ARF (Erley and Bader 2000; Morcos 1998; Murphy et al. 2000; Riccabona 2014b).

> **Take Away**
> Clinical manifestation of RPD is unspecific, and symptoms vary. Primary imaging in RPD is generally accomplished by US and helps in the initial differential diagnosis but mainly rules out other disease entities. IVU and contrast-enhanced CT should be avoided to prevent contrast-induced nephropathy in cases with compromised renal function.

4 Specific Imaging Findings

4.1 Glomerular Disease

In most *congenital* and *inherited glomerular disease* entities, imaging studies are normal or uncharacteristic. US is used in the primary assessment and for renal biopsy; during follow-up radiology may additionally serve in imaging of potential complications such as leiomyomatosis. These sequelae point out the role of imaging in dealing with some of these patients; furthermore, one has to consider these entities in patients with unilateral Wilms' tumour and contralateral renal abnormalities and/or gonadal alterations/dysgenesis and male pseudohermaphroditism, Wilms' tumour, isolated diffuse mesangial sclerosis and focal and segmental glomerulosclerosis (Barbaux et al. 1997; Denamur et al. 1999; Jeanpierre et al. 1998; Little and Wells 1997).

In *post-/parainfectious GN* (renal), imaging plays a rather unimportant role, is restricted to US (including CDS) and shows findings just as in any type of GN with more or less enlarged kidneys with a varying degree of altered parenchymal echotexture (Fig. 2) but never is diagnostic.

Rapidly progressive GN defines a variety of severe glomerular diseases histologically defined by proliferation within Bowman's space and formation of crescents ("crescentic nephritis"). Clinical presentation is an acute nephritic/nephrotic syndrome with pronounced oliguric renal failure, hypertension and signs of volume overload. Underlying diseases include nearly all primary renal or systemic diseases with possible renal manifestation including IgA nephropathy, Henoch-Schönlein purpura, membranoproliferative nephritis, systemic lupus erythematodes (SLE), Wegener's granulomatosis and polyarteritis nodosa. The classical disease with crescentic nephritis and pulmonary haemorrhage is Goodpasture syndrome (Kluth and Rees 1999) caused by autoantibodies against the alveolar and glomerular basement membranes (GBM), but haemoptysis is not restricted to this specific disease. Any patient presenting with nephritis and pulmonary haemorrhage may be in a nephrological emergency situation acutely requiring renal biopsy for correct diagnosis, as US and all other imaging are non-diagnostic. Additionally, (HR) CT of the lung may be performed for differential diagnosis of the pulmonary manifestation; renal granulomas ("pseudotumours," e.g. in Wegener's granulomatosis) must not be mistaken for renal neoplasm. Otherwise, US may not show much but bilaterally increased renal size and some increase of the cortical echogenicity; Doppler indices usually are normal – only a halo sign (= reduced peripheral/cortical perfusion demonstrated as a lack of colour on aCDS in the periphery of the renal parenchyma, creating a halo-like impression) may be seen in patients with severe GN (Hoyer et al. 1999; Riccabona 2000, 2002, 2006a, b, c; Riccabona et al. 1997, 2001) (Fig. 4). Even during therapy imaging plays a marginal role, except for monitoring biopsy and renal size and eventually in the pretransplantation workup.

In *IgA nephropathy* imaging again is nondiagnostic and only used to rule out other diseases or to monitor renal changes during the course of the disease, where relapses may be predicted by US changes.

Henoch-Schönlein purpura (HSP) is a systemic vasculitis affecting the skin, joints, gut and kidneys. Nephritis in HSP and IgA nephropathy seems to be related diseases. US may show unspecific changes, may even be normal and probably reflects more the severity of the disease than the individual entity. Renal biopsy is indicated in cases presenting with acute nephritic/nephrotic syndrome suggesting a rapid progressive nephritis, and if significant proteinuria persists for more than 3 months. No other imaging is used for diagnosis but may well be indicated for monitoring the patients during treatment.

Some patients with *idiopathic nephrotic syndrome* are prone to disease-related complications, such as acute renal failure due to hypovolemia, infections, thrombosis, hypertension and growth failure. Imaging is generally restricted to US that demonstrates bilaterally increased renal volume and unspecific diffuse changes of the parenchyma with usually increased echogenicity specifically of the cortex, as well as ascites and pleural effusion. The US changes correspond with the clinical course and sonographic normalisation may even precede clinical improvement. In persisting disease renal biopsy is performed.

Membranoproliferative GN and *membranous glomerulopathy* are chronic glomerular diseases with typical findings on renal biopsy specimen and a questionable prognosis in many cases. As diagnosis is made by renal biopsy, there is no specific role for further imaging – however, US and CDS studies are usually performed initially and during follow-up.

4.2 Vascular and Tubulointerstitial Disease

Vasculitis (such as polyarteritis nodosa, microscopic polyarteritis or Takayasu's disease) occurs in different diseases and syndromes in childhood. It is the predominant manifestation in certain rare disorders, and the pathogenetic mechanisms involved may be immune complexes, autoantibodies, cell adhesion molecules or miscellaneous factors. US including (a)CDS serves as the initial imaging tool and includes other abdominal organs and vessels; renal (and hepatic as well as cerebral) (MR) angiography is recommended in some of them (e.g. *polyarteritis nodosa*) and then frequently shows arterial aneurysms, segmental narrowing, variation in vascular calibre and infarctions (McLain et al. 1972). Ischaemia and infarctions may as well be visible as patchy areas of decreased isotope uptake on DMSA scanning. In *microscopic polyarteritis*, renal involvement as a rapidly progressive GN soon predominates the clinical picture, and there is also an association with lung disease, including pulmonary haemorrhage. In *Wegener's granulomatosis* (a necrotising granulomatous vasculitis of the upper and lower respiratory tract, and GN, at times with a rapidly progressive course, nowadays renamed "granulomatosis with polyangiitis"), radiology, including CT and MRI, of paranasal sinus and

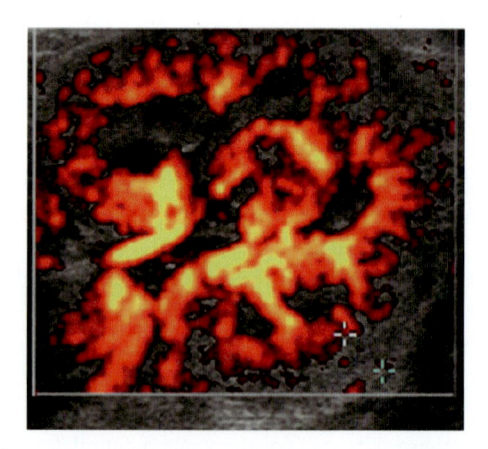

Fig. 4 Amplitude-coded colour Doppler sonography in glomerulonephritis ("halo sign"). Amplitude-coded colour Doppler sonography demonstrates a small cortical peripheral rim- or halo-like layer (+ ... +) with no colour signals, indicating peripherally reduced flow (in spite of normal RI values) in a patient with glomerulonephritis

chest contributes to the diagnosis, whereas renal US only shows non-specific tissue alterations. However, histological evaluation of affected tissue from the respiratory tract or kidneys is often needed. Furthermore, the disease may present as a renal pseudotumour on initial scans ("renal granuloma") or may develop secondary bladder and/or prostatic disease (cystitis, cancer, etc.) due to treatment with cyclophosphamide (Verwijvel et al. 2000; Talar-Williams et al. 2000) and therefore indicate regular imaging follow-up. *Giant cell arteritis* is an inflammatory vasculitis of the large arteries especially affecting the aorta and its major branches (D'Souza et al. 1998). Doppler US of the kidney, but also of other organs and vessels (sometimes additional transcranial CDS), echocardiography and (MR) angiography are essential for diagnosis, therapeutic decisions and prognostic.

The *haemolytic-uraemic syndromes* (HUS) are a heterogeneous group of similar entities with variable expression and severity. Renovascular endothelial cell injury is central to the pathogenesis, leading to platelet activation and intravascular coagulation, haemolytic anaemia with fragmented erythrocytes, thrombocytopenia and renal failure.

Imaging usually starts with abdominal and renal US (including Doppler investigations). Depending on the underlying entity and the severity of the disease, it may show more or less enlarged kidneys with increased parenchymal echogenicity as well as extra-renal changes of the bowel wall and ascites (Fig. 5b); alterations in renal perfusion are depicted as reduced vasculature on (a)CDS and increased RI (Garel et al. 1983; Hoyer et al. 1999; Patriquin et al. 1989; Platt et al. 1991; Riccabona 2000). These Doppler findings may be valuable for predicting relapses or improvement and may even serve for prognostic considerations (Scholbach 1999a). CT, MRI and isotope studies are rarely used, although new reports on MRI evaluation of renal blood flow and perfusion may emphasise the future possible role of other imaging modalities in the initial differential diagnosis and prognosis, as well as for following up these patients (Vallee et al. 2000). However, depending on extra-renal manifestations such as stroke or pancreatitis, additional imaging for the respective symptoms may become necessary and then may involve US, MR and even sometimes CT or angiography.

Acute *tubulointerstitial nephritis* is a multifactorial inflammatory disorder affecting the renal tubules and the interstitial space. Glomeruli and vessels may be affected secondarily. The contribution of radiology is restricted to US showing marked enlargement of the kidneys and

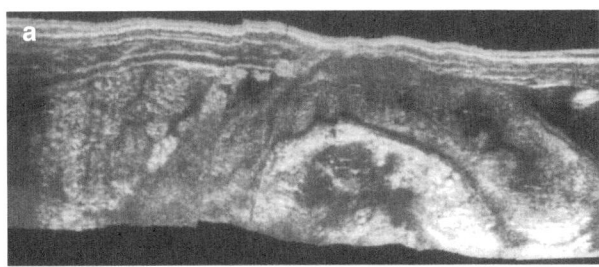

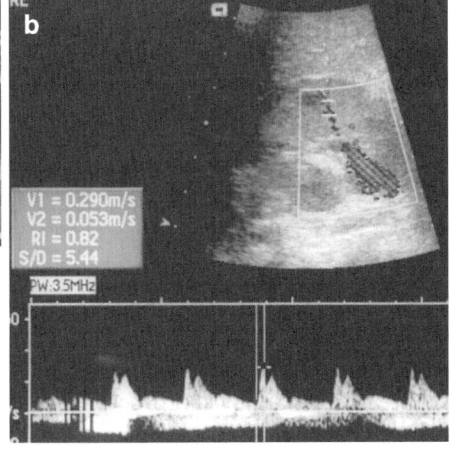

Fig. 5 Sonography in haemolytic-uraemic syndrome (HUS). (**a**) Severe thickening of the bowel wall caused by severe *E. coli* enteritis (extended view sonography with tissue harmonic imaging). (**b**) Alteration of renal parenchymal echogenicity in HUS, with duplex Doppler sonography showing elevated RI (RI=0.82) due to reduced diastolic flow velocity and increased renal vascular resistance

a more or less diffuse cortical hyperechogenicity (Hiraoka et al. 1996). Normalisation of kidney size seems to parallel improvement of renal function; Doppler findings are unspecific and reflect primarily systemic changes and functional improvement. However, renal interstitial disease may be associated with elevated RI value.

Numerous *tubular disorders* mostly are inherited diseases. Diagnosis is made by clinical, laboratory and genetic evaluation. There is little contribution of diagnostic imaging for primary diagnosis, but during the course of the disease, US is of value to show secondary parenchymal lesions or to detect side effects of therapy, as most tubulopathies important for imaging lead to nephrocalcinosis and/or urolithiasis. *Cystinuria* may serve as an example of a hereditary aminoaciduria leading to urolithiasis. *Bartter syndrome* and distal renal tubular acidosis (*d-RTA*) are disorders mostly characterised by nephrocalcinosis. The severe polyuria of *nephrogenic diabetes insipidus* may cause impressive dilatation of the upper urinary tract similar to urinary obstruction ("pseudo-obstructive" pattern). *X-linked hypophosphatemic rickets* are treated with calcitriol and phosphate supplementation – this again may lead to nephrocalcinosis; therefore, repeated skeletal radiographs are necessary to show adequacy of therapy concerning rickets, and renal US is recommended at regular intervals for early detection of nephrocalcinosis.

4.2.1 Renal Parenchymal Involvement in Systemic Disease

In *SLE* a generalised autoimmunity is present with autoantibodies directed against a variety of cell components. Renal manifestation is present in nearly two-thirds of children. Renal biopsy is crucial in all children with SLE who have abnormal urine findings and/or reduced renal function, because of its impact on initial treatment and prognosis. Since SLE is a systemic disease, a wide range of extra-renal manifestations may be present. The central nervous system, lungs, musculoskeletal system, skin, heart or gastrointestinal tract may be affected. Some patients with lupus nephritis have antiphospholipid antibodies which have been associated particularly with renal arterial, venous and glomerular capillary thrombosis, valvular heart disease and cerebral thrombosis (Asherson et al. 1996). All these might indicate respective imaging in severe extra-renal manifestation, such as MR and CT in cerebral involvement or echocardiography and cardiac MR in valvular heart disease. Renal imaging usually is performed by US. Depending on the state and severity of the disease, the kidneys may look normal or appear as in GN; in severe renal involvement, one may observe rarefaction of vasculature on aCDS with elevated RI values in duplex Doppler (Fig. 6). Improvement and normalisation of Doppler findings correlate with clinical improvement.

Sickle cell disease is an inherited haemoglobinopathy with various renal manifestations. The increased blood viscosity, functional venous engorgement and interstitial oedema predispose the kidneys to ischaemia and infarction. Segmental scarring, interstitial fibrosis, dilatation of veins and capillaries and renal papillary necrosis are the result. Rupture of vessels may be the reason for severe haematuria, with the left kidney four times more frequently involved; furthermore, renal papillary necrosis may often be discovered in patients with macrohaematuria. Renal medullary carcinoma is associated with sickle cell disease and may also present with haematuria and flank pain, with the right kidney involved more often (Davis et al. 1995). When looking at these renal and extra-renal complications, the role of imaging becomes evident. The task of paediatric radiology is not the initial diagnosis, but rather the reliable monitoring, yet as noninvasively as possible, to detect any of these sequelae. Radiological investigations include US and (a)CDS as basic investigations to show alterations of the renal perfusion (including screening for renal infarctions, Fig. 7; or transcranial CDS for cerebral complications, etc.) and to exclude other causes of haematuria such as urolithiasis. Increased echogenicity of renal pyramids in the absence of hypercalciuria is suggestive of sickle cell nephropathy. US may help to detect papillary necrosis or show renal medullary carcinoma that usually exhibits a lobulated pattern of the tumour, located within the

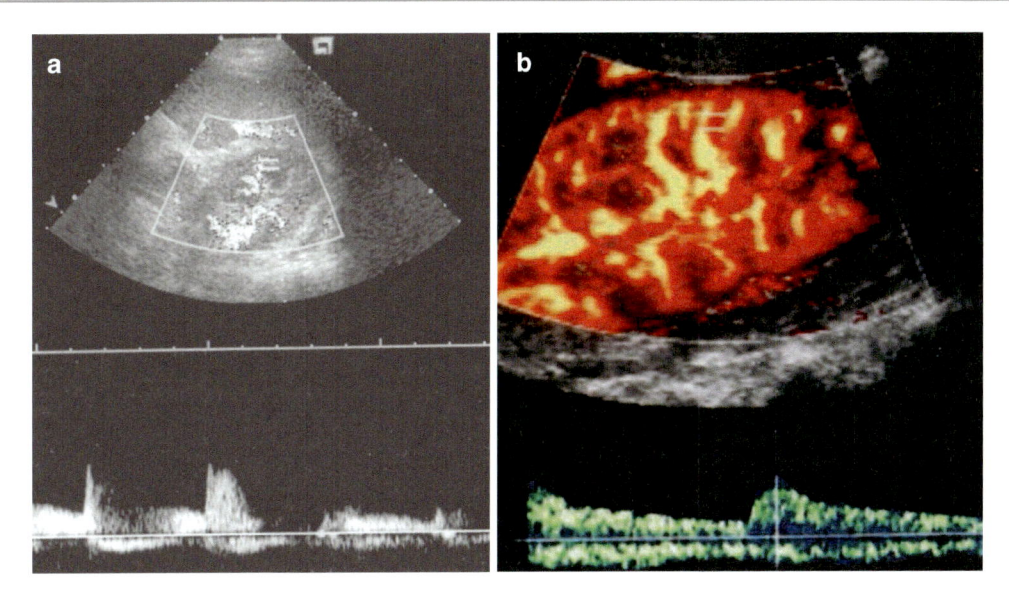

Fig. 6 Sonographic findings in lupus nephritis. (**a**) Unspecific changes of the renal parenchyma with reduced vasculature on colour Doppler sonography and increased RI (peripheral RI = 0.75) on duplex Doppler in acute severe lupus nephritis. (**b**) Normalisation of renal vasculature on amplitude-coded colour Doppler sonography with improvement of peripheral RI during treatment (prior to clinical normalisation)

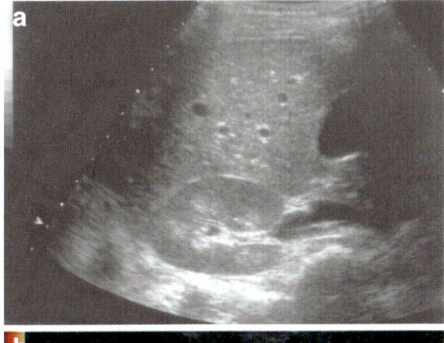

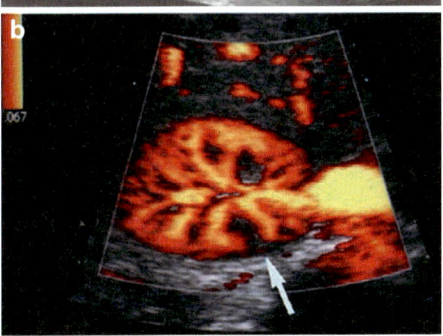

Fig. 7 Renal US in sickle cell disease. (**a**) Increased echogenicity of the medulla with consecutively inverted cortico-medullary differentiation. In the absence of hypercalciuria, this pattern is typical for sickle cell nephropathy. (**b**) Amplitude-coded colour Doppler sonography of the right kidney (cross section) shows a segmental parenchymal area without colour signals (*arrow*), consistent with a renal infarction in sickle cell disease

renal medulla, with areas of necrosis and haemorrhage and satellite nodules in the renal cortex (Davidson et al. 1994). These entities definitely must be confirmed and evaluated by CT or MRI. DMSA scans, CT or MRI can be of value in special situations such as renal infarction or scarring as well as extra-renal sequelae of the disease (e.g. auto-splenectomy, cerebral infarction, vascular aneurysm and bleeding, etc.). Uncontrollable severe renal bleeding may require angiography and selective embolisation.

There are miscellaneous other systemic diseases with renal involvement. *Renal sarcoidosis* is a granulomatous disease of unknown aetiology, with multiorgan involvement. Renal involvement is mainly attributed to granulomatous interstitial infiltration and hypercalcaemia/hypercalciuria (Casella and Allon 1993). US appearances are unspecific; other imaging (CT/MRI) is used to assess not only renal granulomas and pseudotumours but also manifestations in other body compartments (Herman et al. 1997).

Hereditary amyloidosis encompasses a group of rare autosomal dominant disorders associated with deposition of protein fibrils in beta-pleated sheet configuration. Particularly in *familial*

Mediterranean fever, renal amyloidosis may present. Since amyloidosis is a systemic disease, other organs such as the thyroid gland may be involved as well (Mache et al. 1993). US shows a varying degree of diffusely increased echogenicity in bilaterally enlarged kidneys; the other findings (CDS, spectral Doppler, isotope studies) depend on the disease status and actual renal function.

A variety of metabolic disorders may affect the kidneys and cause *renal manifestations of metabolic disorders*. The basic metabolic abnormality – eventually with a toxic metabolic product – can cause tubular dysfunction and tissue changes. Other disorders primarily lead to glomerular damage with hyperfiltration, glomerular hypertrophy and progressive glomerulosclerosis. Metabolic disorders frequently do not present as primary renal diseases but show involvement of the central nervous system, the liver and the haematopoietic system. Most renal lesions are not specific for any metabolic disease. Nevertheless, the changes may be pronounced like the enlarged, hyperechoic kidneys sometimes with additional nephrocalcinosis or tubular crystal deposits in the medulla found in *hereditary tyrosinaemia* (Forget et al. 1999) (see Fig. 3). Another example are the *CDG syndromes* (= carbohydrate-deficient glycoprotein Sy), often showing kidney involvement with hyperechoic cortex or medulla and poor cortico-medullary differentiation at normal renal size (Hertz-Pannier et al. 2000). One disorder with deleterious effects for the kidneys is primary *hyperoxaluria type I* which manifests as nephrocalcinosis and/or urolithiasis. *Diabetic nephropathy* is the most important single disorder leading to CRF during adulthood. As functional markers seem to correlate well with an increase of kidney volume on US (Cummings et al. 1998; Lawson et al. 1996), US could give valuable information for long-term monitoring of diabetic nephropathy that is mainly used in adults, but there is no indication for further renal radiological investigation particularly in children except for the initial diagnostic workup when the disease is diagnosed. *Glycogen storage diseases* (GSD) represent several enzymatic defects of glucose metabolism with GSD type I as a main type for renal involvement. The metabolic derangement leads to hepatic storage of glycogen, hypoglycaemia, lactic acidaemia, hyperlipidaemia and growth failure. US can demonstrate hepatic and renal enlargement with unspecific diffuse alteration of the parenchymal echogenicity and texture. Furthermore, imaging with US, CT and/or MRI is used during follow-up, as focal hepatic lesions usually representing hepatic adenomas may undergo carcinomatous transformation as a serious long-term complication (Wolfsdorf and Crigler 1999). In *nephropathic cystinosis* radiological investigations contribute little to the primary diagnosis. Renal echogenicity may not be specifically increased on renal US; skeletal radiography can show rickets. Repeated US can contribute to monitoring therapy and – by detection of early changes of renal parenchymal/medullar echogenicity and cortico-medullary differentiation – help to prevent severe nephrocalcinosis (Saalem et al. 1995; Theodoropoulos et al. 1995). Further, renal and extra-renal imaging is needed in CRF and after transplantation. Cystinosis encephalopathy is a long-term problem in patients reaching adulthood after renal transplantation. Cerebral atrophy and cystine deposition – especially in the basal ganglia – are the predominant findings; there, CT and MRI can contribute significantly to diagnosis and follow-up (Broyer et al. 1996).

Take Away
RPD represents a vast variety of entities differentiated only by clinical, laboratory, histologic and genetic findings. US including (a)CDS as initial imaging usually is unspecific but contributes to the differential diagnosis and to monitoring. Imaging furthermore helps in renal biopsy, in evaluation of associated extra-renal disease and in detection of complications during the course of the disease – it then also involves all other imaging modalities.

5 Advanced Imaging

5.1 Advanced Ultrasonography and Doppler Sonography

Modern US techniques have widened the sonographic diagnostic potential in paediatric nephrourology (Riccabona 2000a, b, 2002; Riccabona et al. 2001, 2002, 2004, 2006a, b, c). High-resolution transducers allow for better tissue differentiation and depiction of tiny structures, helpful to early visualisation of subtle renal parenchymal changes (e.g. tiny cysts, dilated tubules, small or tubular calcifications, etc.) (Fig. 3). (Tissue) harmonic imaging improves delineation of cysts and of the collecting urinary system; it furthermore enhances tissue differentiation and particularly improves visualisation of corticomedullary differentiation (Choudhry et al. 2000; Desser et al. 1999; Girard et al. 2000). Contrast-enhanced US with new contrast-specific imaging techniques may further improve tissue evaluation by enabling dynamic studies of contrast inflow, uptake and washout; however, these techniques have not yet been evaluated extensively for application in paediatric RPD (Burke et al. 2000; Claudon et al. 1999; Girard et al. 2000; Riccabona et al. 2014a). Duplex Doppler and (a)CDS are applied to visualise vasculature and evaluate flow as well as flow pattern. In general, diseases limited to the glomeruli do – relatively regardless of the severity of the disease – not affect the RI significantly or may even decrease RI (particularly inflammatory disease), whereas tubulointerstitial and vascular diseases may increase RI (Piaggo et al. 1999; Platt et al. 1990, 1991, 1997; Riccabona et al. 1993; Siegel 1995; Taylor 1994; Vade et al. 1993). However, all these findings still are affected by many other (systemic) factors and by renal function; therefore, they are just another part in the puzzle of the differential diagnosis; furthermore, there are age-related variations (Gill et al. 1994; Mostbeck et al. 1991; Vade et al. 1993). aCDS (and other modern flow imaging techniques such as "B-flow" or "SMI-flow") improves visualisation of peripheral/cortical renal vasculature/perfusion that may help to evaluate focal disease or diffuse alteration with reduced renal perfusion (Babcock et al. 1996; Bude et al. 1994; Gainza et al. 1995; Preidler et al. 1996; Riccabona et al. 1997, 2000, 2001; Rubin et al. 1994; Scholbach 1999a) (Figs. 4 and 7). US elastography is being the most novel of these approaches – at present it is being studied for applications in paediatric RPD and particularly for monitoring renal transplants, but no definite information is yet available on its reliability and clinically useful applications. It seems as if renal US elastography is much more difficult and cumbersome than its well-established liver applications and influenced by a number of systemic factors such as hydration, body activity, size of the respective measured compartment (medulla or cortex) and US access (= US beam direction in relation to the main ultrastructural fibres and vessels). However, the combination of all these new and advanced modalities enables a noninvasive diagnosis of various parenchymal and perfusional disturbances, as some examples may demonstrate:

- Renal vein thrombosis may be an essential differential diagnosis in neonatal RPD. In renal vein thrombosis, arterial RI of the enlarged kidney with increased echogenicity is increased due to congestive changes and the backflow from the obstructed outflow tract, with better identification of this entity using high-frequency transducers (Wright et al. 1996). The central renal vein may still be patent in early stages of peripheral renal vein thrombosis or may show flow disturbances such as increased flow velocity and spectral broadening in partially thrombosed veins. In central renal vein thrombosis, no venous flow can be visualised. CDS can demonstrate regression of thrombosis and improvement of arterial perfusional waveforms during thrombolytic treatment much earlier than clinical improvement or regression of greyscale findings. Remnants after renal vein thrombosis may be difficult to diagnose sonographically and may require additional imaging such as MR and (MR) angiography.

- In (pseudo-)nutcracker syndrome the left renal vein is compressed. This leads to venous congestion of the left kidney creating intermittent haematuria and pain. The left kidney consecutively is asymmetrically enlarged; the left renal vein shows a marked change in diameter at the pre- or retro-aortal crossing, with elevated flow velocity, turbulent flow and arterialised pulsatility of the flow pattern due to propagation of the pulsation of the abdominal aorta [and superior mesenteric artery in pseudo-nutcracker syndrome (Scholbach 1999b, c)] (Fig. 1).
- In inflammatory RPD (e.g. GN) the parenchyma of the more or less enlarged kidney usually shows an altered cortico-medullary differentiation with varying changes of parenchymal echogenicity. In early stages or in mild disease, perfusion patterns can be normal, or RI may be decreased due to increased diastolic flow velocity. In severe disease with compromised renal function, RI increases and eventually even systolic flow velocities may decrease (Figs. 5 and 6). These findings reflect a complex system: various renal compartments may be affected in different diseases such as vasculitis, inflammation, oedema or interstitial fibrosis. Doppler findings are furthermore influenced by extra-renal factors such as heart rate and function, medication or blood concentration and therefore may vary and are not specific (Gill et al. 1994; Knapp et al. 1995; Kuzmic et al. 2000; Mostbeck et al. 1991).
- In HUS, severe GN and acute obstruction, RI is increased due to high renal parenchymal or vascular resistance (Garel et al. 1983; Patriquin et al. 1989; Platt et al. 1990, 1991; Riccabona et al. 1993). RI changes correlate well with the course of the disease and may be used as a prognostic factor. Differentiation of single event or recurrent disease in HUS with poorly differentiated, hyperechogenic kidneys may be supported by flow volume measurements that demonstrate reduced renal perfusion in patients with bad prognosis and poor outcome (Scholbach 1999b). However, note that in a chronic state, the RI may return to (pseudo-)normal values again.
- Evaluation of the amount of renal perfusion and assessment of flow profiles may be helpful for studying A/CRF. Phenomena such as the cortical halo, diffuse/focal vessel rarefaction on aCDS, increased RI values, reduced flow velocities or atypical venous flow profiles in cardiac/congestive renal failure are as unspecific as those changes observed in renal transplants (Figs. 4, 5 and 6). However, they may help in the differential diagnosis and hint towards a certain disease entity (Hoyer et al. 1999; Platt et al. 1991; Riccabona et al. 1997). They may furthermore serve as an additional valuable parameter for follow-up, as normalisation of these sonographic findings may precede clinical improvement.
- Focal renal infarction, e.g. in sickle cell disease or in vascular disorders that sometimes also cause hypertension, as well as other focal renal disease, can be detected using (a)CDS, in some cases even supported by administration of intravenous echo-enhancing agents (Riccabona et al. 2000, 2014a) (Fig. 7). Other focal renal parenchymal changes such as papillary calcinosis or renal calcifications may be picked up by CDS using the "twinkling artefact" as a diagnostic tool (Cehfouh et al. 1998; Rahmouni et al. 1996). Thus, equivocal echogenic spots on greyscale US without definite shadowing may be differentiated, reducing the need for ionising imaging in some patients and helping to narrow down the list of differential diagnoses (e.g. papillary necrosis, dysplastic calcifications and nephrocalcinosis). Another example is the multifocal regional perfusion defect observed as a nearly pathognomonic but short and transient phenomenon using aCDS in exercise-induced ARF.

All these modern US modalities may also be incorporated in the initial imaging. This depends on local circumstances, diagnostic algorithms and individual facilities, equipment and staff. The more complex this modality becomes, the more these specific investigations need high-end equipment and sonographers who are skilled and experienced in properly handling this task in the paediatric population – therefore, often these modern options are only used at specialised referral centres.

5.2 Renal Biopsy

As discussed above, histological classification of RPD remains essential for therapeutic and prognostic assessment as well as for monitoring complications during treatment of RPD (e.g. cyclosporine A toxicity). Therefore, renal biopsy still is an essential tool in paediatric nephrology (see also chapter "Pediatric Genitourinary Intervention"). After the introduction of (usually sonographically) guided renal biopsy, the incidence of complications during and after the procedure has been reduced. Nevertheless, there still exists a considerable risk for possible complications such as intrarenal, perirenal, abdominal (in transplanted kidneys) and urinary tract bleeding (especially dangerous if a clot threatens to congest the urinary collecting system) as well as post-biopsy arteriovenous fistula (AVF) with its implicated potential sequelae (Diaz and Donadio 1975; Dodge et al. 1962; Karafin et al. 1970; Merkus et al. 1993; Pälvänsalo et al. 1984; Proesmans et al. 1982; Riccabona and Ring 1995, 1998; Zeis et al. 1976). Various contraindications for percutaneous needle biopsy have to be considered: coagulopathies, uncontrolled hypertension and severe hydronephrosis as absolute contraindications. Relative contraindications are abscesses, large cysts, severe pyelonephritis, tumours, some variants of abnormal vascular supply and single, ectopic or horseshoe kidneys. In these situations "open," surgical renal biopsy allows a safe procedure and viewing of the kidney with specific selection of certain areas of interest. It furthermore avoids the spread of malignant cells or infection.

US-guided renal biopsy should be performed in a standardised fashion; respective recommendations are available (Riccabona et al. 2014b, see also chapter "Imaging in Renal Failure, Neonatal Oligoanuria, and Renal Transplantation"). It is performed in prone position, with a percutaneous dorsal access to the lower pole of the left kidney, often using a needle guide and potentially a coaxial technique; for renal transplants an anterior access in supine position is used (Fig. 8). One to three specimens are obtained under systemic analgosedation and ECG and pulsoxymetric monitoring using a 16–20 gauge core biopsy needle with real-time visualisation of the needle and the major vessels during the procedure. The adequacy of the sample should be evaluated immediately by visual inspection and – if available – by microscopy. Small red dots (representing the glomeruli) should be present in the sample. The sample size is particularly important in focal sclerosing GN, SLE and crescentic nephritis.

Post-biopsy evaluation of possible complications is recommended. US is usually performed immediately after the procedure, after 4 to 8 h, and 24 h after the intervention, as well as on demand (e.g. clinical deterioration of the patient or clinical symptoms of bleeding, etc.). Some degree of subcapsular or perirenal haematoma is considered "physiological"; more extensive haemorrhage needs proper immobilisation and monitoring of the patient, as well as treatment if symptomatic (Fig. 9). CDS with adequate scale settings should be applied to detect post-biopsy AVF, as these need an altered post-biopsy regime (antihypertensive

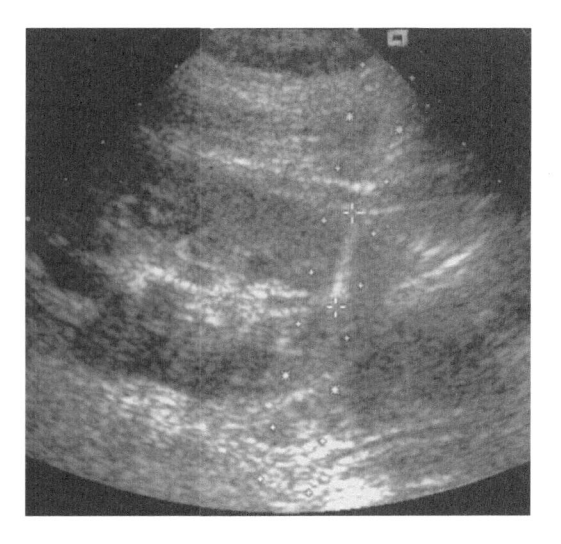

Fig. 8 Sonographically guided renal biopsy using the needle guide attached to the transducer: the dotted lines show the path of the needle and help to guide the biopsy needle (18 gauge core cut needle, performed with a biopsy gun) for safe puncture as well as retrieval of sufficient specimen material. The image is retrospectively taken from the cine-loop analysis of the needle movement during biopsy (useful for documentation and analysis of the procedure): The callipers mark the length of the intraparenchymal needle track (1.7 cm)

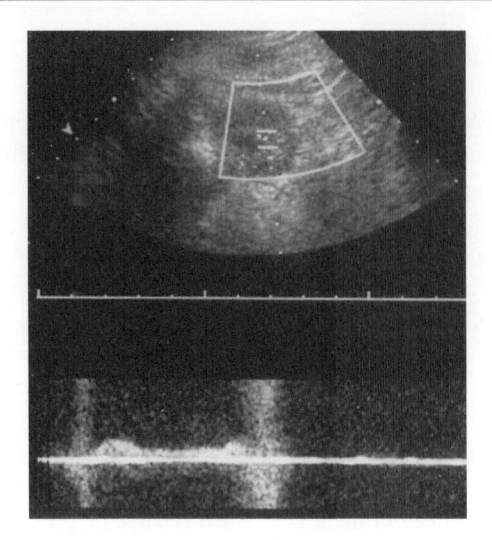

Fig. 9 Imaging of complications after renal biopsy. Colour Doppler sonography depicted an area with atypical colour signals and colour aliasing suspicious for an arteriovenous fistula. Duplex Doppler sonography trace confirms the shunt flow of a post-biopsy arteriovenous fistula

medication, drugs that do not affect competence of renal vascular regulation, prolonged immobilisation and careful mobilisation, clinical monitoring). CDS findings should always be confirmed by spectral Doppler evaluation that demonstrates shunt flow at the AVF as well as various flow changes of the feeding and draining vessel, such as decreased arterial RI and arterialised flow pattern in the draining vein with higher flow velocities (Middleton et al. 1989; Riccabona et al. 1998) (Fig. 9). Usually these AVFs are asymptomatic and diminish spontaneously. However, some persist and may become symptomatic with macrohaematuria and hypertension. Uncontrolled bleeding and symptomatic AVF usually then indicate catheter angiography with embolisation; acute clotting with urinary tract obstruction may require percutaneous drainage. In patients with equivocal sonographic findings, CT or MR angiography should be performed to establish the definite diagnosis. Note that in childhood, CT-guided renal biopsy should be for radiation issues – except for selected cases with insufficient sonographic visualisation of the kidney or with specific (multi)focal pathology not adequately picked up on US.

5.2.1 Role of Other Imaging Modalities

Plain film (for renal calculi and nephrocalcinosis), IVU (e.g. for diagnosis of medullary sponge kidney, otherwise today replaced by MRI – if available), contrast-enhanced CT and isotope studies are rarely used for the diagnosis or differential diagnosis of RPD, except for nephropathy secondary to urinary tract malformations or infections. However, imaging findings such as enlarged kidneys, flattened take-up and washout curves on isotope studies, delayed contrast enhancement with vague cortico-medullary differentiation on CT or calcifications may be noticed in some patients as an incidental finding. These must be properly recognised to initiate further diagnostic workup. MRI is not used in RPD to date; however, there might be a future role for advanced MR techniques (e.g. perfusion or diffusion imaging, BOLD techniques, new and/or intracellular contrast agents such as USPIO and spectroscopy) in differentiating various entities or quantifying vital renal tissue, thus perhaps reducing the need for renal biopsies in some diseases.

5.2.2 Imaging of Renal and Extra-Renal Complications, for Motoring Chronic Disease and in Treatment-Induced Changes

Renal complications are rare except for deterioration during the course of the disease. However, de novo disease may evolve such as tumour in end-stage kidneys or complications such as increasing calcifications in tubular disorders with obstructive calculi and renal colic may occur. Infection may occur, renal artery stenosis may develop in vasculitis or a post-biopsy AVF may be present. Depending on the individual query, these entities have to be evaluated and considered. This necessitates at least a minimal imaging follow-up strategy that should be adapted to the individual situation. In general, regular US is sufficient; some queries necessitate scintigraphy (relative renal function, scars, etc.), MRI (tumour, infarction, etc.), MR angiography (major renal vessel anomaly) or catheter angiography (diagnosis of particularly peripheral and percutaneous treatment of renal artery stenosis, AVF embolisation, etc.). Furthermore, as RPD may lead to end-stage renal failure and to renal transplantation, imaging (US and particularly VCUG) is important to assess the urinary bladder situation, as this will be a prerequisite for successful future treatment.

Depending on the underlying disease, various extra-renal complications may occur; involvement of other organs, primarily or secondary to therapy, may be present. These changes may influence patient management, prognosis, outcome and quality of life. Therefore, they have to be considered when treating these patients and following them during the course of their disease. The most important aspects are skeletal changes during corticosteroid therapy or as a manifestation of the ongoing disease (e.g. osteoporosis, avascular necrosis, extra-renal calcifications and hyperostosis, etc.) evaluated by plain film and MRI (Fig. 10). Rarely CT is used for differential diagnosis in a suspicious lesion to define the entity (Table 3). Furthermore, associated changes in systemic or syndromal disease must be evaluated appropriately necessitating a wide range of imaging in the individual case. The detailed description and discussion of all these findings and the various modalities used for imaging cannot be included in this chapter due to space restrictions.

For imaging of various complications and during follow-up under treatment, US may need to be complemented by CT, MRI and plain film – in particular for extra-renal changes related to RPD or medical treatment.

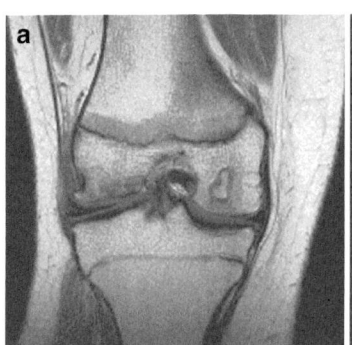

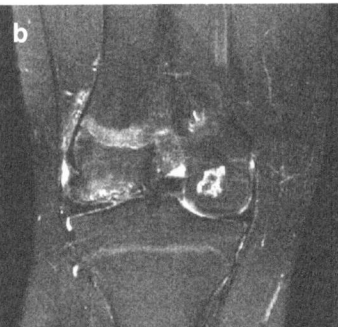

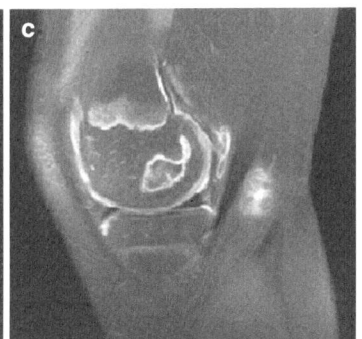

Fig. 10 Imaging of extra-renal complications. Series of MRI images (**a**) T1-weighted coronal image, (**b**) T2-weighted coronal image with fat suppression, (**c**) T2-weighted sagittal image with fat suppression of the knee, demonstrating an avascular necrosis secondary to corticosteroid treatment for chronic renal parenchymal disease

Table 3 Imaging of extra-renal complications and manifestation in renal parenchymal disease

Skeletal anomaly (including hyperostosis, calcifications, etc.)	Plain film
Renal osteodystrophy (osteoporosis, etc.)	Plain film DEXA, CT (osteodensitometry)
Avascular necrosis (bone)	Plain film, MRI, scintigraphy
Cardiac disease (valvular disease, effusion, myocardial hypertrophy, associated malformation, etc.)	Echocardiography, chest film, cardiac MR
Vascular anomalies (AVM, aneurysm, vasculitis, etc.)	US, MR/catheter angiography
Malignant transformation (e.g. liver adenomas) and other extra-renal manifestation of a systemic disease (e.g. Goodpasture syndrome, etc.)	US, CT/MRI
CNS involvement (e.g. infarction in sickle cell disease, cranial haemorrhage, central venous thrombosis)	MR, CT, transtemporal CDS

This table gives a short overview of the various imaging methods used for imaging of extra-renal changes and complications arising during treatment or as a complication during the course of the disease with regard to the affected compartment or organ and the clinical query

> **Take Away**
> Advanced imaging consists mainly of US focusing on modern US techniques. However, diagnosis is often established only by histology necessitating US-guided renal biopsy.

Conclusions

A variety of histologically different RPDs and pathogenetically different entities with varying prognosis and therapy may clinically present in a similar way. Here imaging is needed, may help in the differential diagnosis or – as often is the primary task – can rule out other diseases such as malignancy, obstructive uropathy or congenital conditions. Other diseases such as vascular disorders may be depicted; this ability to help to define the diagnosis gives particularly US with (a)CDS an essential role in the early diagnostic workup of patients with clinically suspected RPD. However, even modern imaging modalities to date cannot properly define the individual underlying entity; thus, renal biopsy remains necessary. Here again imaging helps to monitor the procedure and to reduce or to detect complications. Finally, imaging is helpful for monitoring the disease process, not only with regard to renal changes but also to extra-renal-associated pathology. Thus, imaging can play a significant role for the clinician dealing with RPD, although these renal diseases do not represent a major imaging domain and in general cannot precisely be diagnosed or reliably be ruled out by imaging.

References

Andreoli SP (1999) Management of acute renal failure. In: Barratt TM, Avni ED, Harmon DE (eds) Pediatric nephrology, 4th edn. Lippincott Williams & Wilkins, Baltimore, pp 119–1134

Asherson RA, Cervera R, Piette J-C, Schoenfeld Y (1996) The antiphospholipid syndrome. CRC Press, Boca Raton

Avni EF, Robberecht MS, Lebrun D et al (1983) Transient acute tubular disease in the newborn: characteristic ultrasound pattern. Ann Radiol 26:175–182

Babcock DS (1989) Neonatal and pediatric ultrasonography. Churchill-Livingstone, New York

Babcock DS, Patriquin H, LaFortune M, Duazat M (1996) Power Doppler sonography: basic principles and clinical applications in children. Pediatr Radiol 26:109–115

Barbaux S, Niaudet P, Gubler MC et al (1997) Donor splice site mutations in the WT1 gene are responsible for Frasier syndrome. Nat Genet 17:467–469

Broyer M, Tête MJ, Guest G et al (1996) Clinical polymorphism of cystinosis encephalopathy. Results of treatment with cysteamine. J Inher Metab Dis 19:65–75

Bude RO, Rubin JM, Adler RS (1994) Power versus conventional color Doppler sonography: comparison in the depiction of normal intrarenal vasculature. Radiology 192:777–780

Burke BJ, Pellerito JS, Miller DH, Armand RG (2000) Comparative value of pulse inversion Harmonic Imaging in renal sonography. J Ultrasound Med 19:S80

Casella FJ, Allon M (1993) The kidney in sarcoidosis. J Am Soc Nephrol 3:1555–1562

Cehfouh N, Grenier N, Higueret D et al (1998) Characterization of urinary calculi: in vitro study of twinkling artefact revealed by color-flow sonography. Am J Radiol 171:1055–1060

Choudhry S, Gorman B, Charboneau JW et al (2000) Comparison of tissue harmonic imaging with conventional US in abdominal disease. Radiographics 20:1127–1135

Claudon M, Barnewolt CE, Taylor GA et al (1999) Renal blood flow in pigs: changes depicted with contrast-enhanced harmonic US imaging during acute urinary obstruction. Radiology 212:725–731

Cummings EA, Sochett EB, Dekker MG et al (1998) Contribution of growth hormone and IGF-I to early diabetic nephropathy in type 1 diabetes. Diabetes 47:1341–1346

Davidson AJ, Choyke PL, Hartman DS et al (1994) Renal medullary carcinoma associated with sickle cell trait: Radiological findings. Radiology 195:83–85

Davis CJ Jr, Mostofi FK, Sesterhenn IA (1995) Renal medullary carcinoma: the seventh sickle cell nephropathy. Am J Surg Pathol 19:1–11

Deeg KH, Hofmann V, Hoyer PF (2014) Ultarschalldiagnostik min Pädiatrie und Kinderchirurgie. Thieme, Stuttgart. ISBN 978-3-13-100954-8

Denamur E, Bocquet N, Mougenot B et al (1999) Mother-to-child transmitted splice-site mutation is responsible for distinct glomerular diseases. J Am Soc Nephrol 10:2219–2223

Desser TS, Jeffrey RB, Lane MJ, Ralls PW (1999) Tissue harmonic imaging: utility in abdominal and pelvic sonography. J Clin Ultrasound 27:135–142

Diaz Buxa JA, Donadio JV (1975) Complications and percutaneous renal biopsy: an analysis of 1000 consecutive biopsies. Clin Nephrol 4:223–227

Diettrich RB (1990) Genitourinary system. In: Cohen MD, Edwards MK (eds) Magnetic resonance imaging in children. B.C. Decker, Philadelphia, pp 679–723

Dodge WF, Daeschner CW, Brennan JC et al (1962) Percutaneous renal biopsy in children – general considerations. Pediatrics 30:287–296

D'Souza SJA, Tsai W, Silver MM et al (1998) Diagnosis and management of stenotic aorto-arteriopathy in childhood. J Pediatr 132:1016–1022

Erley CM, Bader BD (2000) Auswirkungen einer intravasalen Röntgenkontrastmittelgabe auf die Nierenfunktion – Risiken und Prävention. Fortschr Röntgenstr 172:791–797

Forget S, Patriquin HB, Dubois J et al (1999) The kidney in children with tyrosinemia: sonographic, CT and biochemical findings. Pediatr Radiol 29:104–108

Fredericks BJ, de Campo M, Chow CW et al (1989) Glomerulocystic renal disease: ultrasound appearances. Pediatr Radiol 19:184–186

Gainza FJ, Minguela I, Lopez-Vidaur I et al (1995) Evaluation of complications due to percutaneous renal biopsy in allograft and native kidneys with color – coded Doppler sonography. Clin Nephrol 43:303–308

Garel L, Habib R, Babin C et al (1983) Hemolytic uremic syndrome. Diagnosis and prognostic value of ultrasound. Ann Radiol 26:169–174

Gill B, Palmer LS, Koenigsberg M, Laor E (1994) Distribution and variability of resistive index values in undilated kidneys in children. Urology 44:897–901

Girard MS, Mattrey RF, Baker KG et al (2000) Comparison of standard and second harmonic B-mode sonography in the detection of segmental renal infarction with sonographic contrast in a rabbit model. J Ultrasound Med 19:185–192

Gordon I, Riccabona M (2003) Investigating the newborn kidney – update on imaging techniques. Semin Neonatol 8:269–278

Herman ET, Shackelford DG, McAlister WH (1997) Pseudotumoral sarcoid granulomatous nephritis in a child: case presentation with sonographic and CT findings. Pediatr Radiol 27:752–754

Hertz-Pannier L, DeLonlay P, Nassogne Mc et al (2000) The kidneys of CDG syndromes. ESPR 2000, Pediatr Radiol 30:S

Hiraoka M, Hori C, Tsuchida S et al (1996) Ultrasonographic findings of acute tubulointerstitial nephritis. Am J Nephrol 16:154–158

Hoyer PF (1996) Niere. In: Hoffmann V, Deeg KH, Weitzel D (eds) Ultraschall in Pädiatrie und Kinderchirurgie. Thieme, Stuttgart/New York, pp 340–381

Hoyer PF, Schmid R, Wünsch L, Vester U (1999) Colour Doppler Energy – a new technique to study tissue perfusion in renal transplants. Pediatr Nephrol 13:559–563

Howlett DC, Greenwood KL, Jarosz JM et al (1977) The incident of transient renal medullary hyperechogenicity in neonatal ultrasound examination. Br J Radiol 70:140–143

Hricak H, Cruz C, Romansky R et al (1982) Renal parenchymal disease: sonographic-pathologic correlation. Radiology 144:141–147

Jeanpierre C, Denamur E, Cabanis MO et al (1998) Identification of constitutional WT1 mutations in patients with isolated diffuse mesangial sclerosis (IDMS) and analysis of genotype-phenotype correlations using a computerized mutation database. Am J Hum Genet 62:824–833

Karafin L, Lendall AR, Felisher DA (1970) Urologic complications in percutaneous renal biopsy in children. J Urol 103:332–335

Kettriz U, Semelka RC, Brown ED et al (1996) MR findings in diffuse renal parenchymal disease. J Magn Reson Imaging 6:136–144

Kluth DC, Rees AJ (1999) Anti-glomerular basement membrane disease. J Am Soc Nephrol 10:2446–2453

Knapp R, Plötzender A, Frauscher F et al (1995) Variability of Doppler parameters in the healthy kidney. J Ultrasound Med 14:427–429

Kuzmic AC, Brkljacic B, Ivankovic D, Galesic K (2000) Doppler sonographic renal resistive index in healthy children. Eur Radiol 10:1644–1648

Lawson ML, Sochett EB, Chait PG et al (1996) Effect of puberty on markers of glomerular hypertrophy and hypertension in IDDM. Diabetes 45:51–55

Little M, Wells C (1997) A clinical overview of WT1 gene mutations. Hum Mutat 9:209–225

Mache CJ, Schwingshandl J, Riccabona M et al (1993) Ultrasound and MRI findings in a case of childhood amyloid goiter. Pediatr Radiol 23:565–566

McLain LG, Kelsch RC, Bookstein JJ (1972) Polyarteritis nodosa diagnosed by renal arteriography. J Pediatr 80:1032–1035

Merkus JW, Zebregts CJ, Hoitsma AJ et al (1993) High incidence of arteriovenous fistula after biopsy of kidney allografts. Br J Surg 80:310–312

Middleton WD, Kellman GM, Nelson GL, Madrazo BL (1989) Postbiopsy renal transplant arteriovenous fistulas: color Doppler characteristics. Radiology 171:253–257

Mettler FA, Guiberteau MJ (1998) Essentials of nuclear medicine imaging: genitourinary system. WB Saunders, Philadelphia, pp 335–368

Mostbeck GH, Kain R, Mallek R et al (1991) Duplex Doppler sonography in renal parenchymal disease. Histopathologic correlation. J Ultrasound Med 10:189–194

Morcos SK (1998) Contrast media induced nephrotoxicity – questions and answers. Br J Radiol 71: 357–365

Murphy SW, Barrett BJ, Parfrey PS (2000) Contrast nephropathy. J Am Soc Nephrol 11:177–182

Nakamura M, Yokota K, Chen C et al (1999) Hyperechoic renal papillae as a physiological finding in neonates. Clin Radiol 54:233–236

Pälvänsalo M, Järvy J, Sumaru I (1984) Occurrence of hematoma after renal biopsy – systemic follow up study by sonography. Clin Nephrol 21:302–303

Patriquin HB, O'Regan S, Robitaille P et al (1989) Hemolytic-uremic syndrome: intrarenal arterial Doppler patterns – a useful guide to therapy. Radiology 172:625–628

Perale R, Talenti E, Lubrano G (1988) Ultrasound for the diagnosis of the uric acid nephropathy in children. Pediatr Radiol 18:265–268

Perale R (1992) Ultrasonographic gamuts of renal parenchyml disease. In: Thomsen HS (ed) European uroradiology '92. FADL Publishers, Copenhagen, pp 148–1551

Piaggo G, Degl'Innocenti ML, Perfumo F (1999) Il ruolo dell'echografia nell'insufficienza renale acuta e cronica in eta' pediatrica. Gaslini 31:165–172

Platt JF, Ellis JH, Rubin JM et al (1990) Intrarenal arterial Doppler sonography in patients with nonobstructive renal diseases: correlation of resistive index with biopsy findings. Am J Radiol 154:1223–1227

Platt JF, Rubin JM, Ellis JH (1991) Acute renal failure: possible role of duplex Doppler US in distinction between acute prerenal failure and acute tubular necrosis. Radiology 179:419–423

Platt JF, Rubin JN, James HE (1997) Lupus nephritis: predictive value of conventional and Doppler US and comparison with serologic and biopsy parameters. Radiology 203:82–86

Preidler KW, Riccabona M, Szolar DM et al (1996) Nachweis der Perfusion in Nierentransplantaten. Ultraschall Med 17:243–246

Proesmans W, Marchal G, Snoeck L, Snoes R (1982) Ultrasonography for assessment of bleeding after percutaneous renal biopsy in children. Clin Nephrol 18:257–262

Rahmouni A, Bargoin R, Herment A, Bargoin N, Vasile N (1996) Color Doppler twinkling artifact in hyperechoic regions. Radiology 199:267–271

Riccabona M, Ring E, Fueger G et al (1993) Doppler sonography in congenital ureteropelvic junction obstruction and congenital multicystic kidney disease. Pediatr Radiol 23:502–505

Riccabona M, Ring E (1995) Sonographisch gezielte Nierenbiopsie im Kindesalter – Rolle der Farbdopplersonographie. Wien Klin Wochenschr 107:252–255

Riccabona M, Preidler K, Szolar D et al (1997) Beurteilung der renalen Vaskularisation mittels amplitudenkodierter Farbdopplersonographie. Ultraschall Med 18:244–248

Riccabona M, Schwinger W, Ring E (1998) Arteriovenous fistula after renal biopsy in children. J Ultrasound Med 17:505–508

Riccabona M (2000) Amplitudenkodierte Farbdopplersonographie im Kindesalter. Ultraschall Med 21:273–283

Riccabona M, Uggowitzer M, Klein E et al (2000) Contrast enhanced color Doppler sonography in children and adolescents. J Ultrasound Med 19:783–788

Riccabona M (2000a) "Checkliste Sonografie in der Pädiatarie und Kinderchirurgie", Stuttgart – NewYork: August Thieme Verlag. ISBN 3-13118471-X

Riccabona M, Rossipal E (2000b) Perikarderguß bei der Coeliakie – ein Zufallsbefund? WiKliWo 112: 27–31

Riccabona M, Schwinger W, Ring E, Aigner R (2001) Amplitude coded color Doppler sonography in pediatric renal disease. Eur Radiol 11:861–866

Riccabona M (2002) Potential of modern sonographic techniques in paediatric uroradiology. Eur J Radiol 43:110–121

Riccabona M, Lindbichler F, Sinzig M (2002) Conventional imaging in paediatric uroradiology. Eur J Radiol 43:100–109

Riccabona M (2004) Ultrasound's potential expands in abdomen – Modern ultrasound techniques in the paediatric abdomen. Diagnostic Imaging Europe, 20(3):16–20

Riccabona M (2006a) Imaging if the neonatal genitourinary tract. Eur J Radiol 60:187–198

Riccabona M (2006b) (Acute) renal Failure in neonates, infants, and children – the role of ultrasound, with respect to other imaging options. Ultrasound Clin 1:457–469

Riccabona M, Fotter R (2006) Radiographic studies in children with kidney disorders: what to do and when. In: Hogg R (ed) Kidney disorders in children and adolescents. Taylor and Francis, Birmingham, pp 15–34

Riccabona M (2006c) Modern pediatric ultrasound: potential applications and clinical significance. A review. Clin Imaging 30(2):77–86

Riccabona M, Avni FE, Blickman JG, Darge K, Dacher JN, Lobo LM, Willi U (2008) Imaging recommendations in paediatric uroradiology: minutes of the ESPR workgroup session on urinary tract infection, fetal hydronephrosis, urinary tract ultrasonography and voiding cysto-urethrography. ESPR-Meeting, Barcelona/Spain, June 2007. ESUR Paediatric guideline subcommittee and ESPR paediatric uroradiology work group. Pediatr Radiol, in press. doi:10.1007/s00247-007-0695-7

Riccabona M, Avni FE, Dacher JN, Damasio B, Darge K, Lobo ML, Ording-Müller LS, Papado-polos F, Willi U (2010) ESPR uroradiology task force and ESUR paediatric working group: Im-aging and procedural recommendations in paediatric uroradiology, Part III. Minutes of the ESPR uroradiology task force mini-symposium on intravenous urography, uro-CT and MR-urography in childhood. Pediatr Radiol 40:1315–1320

Riccabona M (2013) "Pediatric Imaging Trainer" (ed.), Thieme, Stuttgart – New York. ISBN 978-3-13-166191-3

Riccabona M (2014a) Pediatric Ultrasound – requisites and applications (editor and main author). Springer, Berlin/Heidelberg. ISBN 978-3-642-39155-2

Riccabona M (2014b) Chapter 17: Contrast media use in pediatrics: safety issues. In: Thomson HS, Webb AW (eds) Contrast media: safety issues and ESUR guidelines, 3rd edn. Springer, Berlin/New York, pp 245–251

Riccabona M, Vivier HP, Ntoulj A, Darge K, Avni F, Papadopoulou F, Damasio B, Ording-Mueller LS, Blickman J, Lobo ML, Willi U, ESPR Uroradiology Task Force – Imaging Recommendations in Paediatric Uroradiology (2014a) Part VII: standardized terminology, impact of existing recommendations, and update on contrast-enhanced ultrasound of the paediatric urogenital tract. Report on the mini-symposium at the ESPR meeting in Budapest, June 2013. Pediatr Radiol 44:1478–1484

Riccabona M, Lobo ML, Willi U, Avni F, Blickmann J, Damasio B, Ordning-Mueller LS, Darge K, Papadopoulou F, Vivier PH, ESPR Uroradiology Task Force and ESUR Paediatric Working Group (2014b) Imaging recommendations in Paediatric Uroradiology, Part VI: childhood renal biopsy and imaging of neonatal and infant genital tract. Pediatr Radiol 44:496–502

Riccabona M (2015) The pediatric kidney. In: Quaia E (ed) Radiological imaging of the kidneys, 2nd edn. Springer, Heidelberg/New York. ISBN 978-3-540-87596-3

Riebel TW, Abraham K, Wartner R et al (1993) Transient renal medullary hyperechogenicity in ultrasound studies of neonates: is it normal phenomenon or what are the causes? J Clin Ultrasound 21:31–35

Rosenfield AT, Siegel MJ (1981) Renal parenchymal disease: histo-pathologic-sonographic correlation. Am J Radiol 137:793–798

Rubin JM, Bude R, Carson PL, Bree LR, Adler RS (1994) Power Doppler ultrasound: a potential useful alternative to mean frequency based Doppler US. Radiology 190:853–856

Saalem MA, Milford DV, Alton H et al (1995) Hypercalciuria and ultrasound abnormalities in children with cystinosis. Pediatr Nephrol 9:45–47

Scholbach T (1999a) Color Doppler sonographic determination of renal blood flow in healthy children. J Ultrasound Med 18:559–564

Scholbach T (1999b) Prognostische Bedeutung der farbduplex-sonographischen Nierenperfusionsmessung beim hämolytisch-urämischen Syndrom. Ultraschall Med 20:S33

Scholbach T (1999c) Farbduplexsonographie des Nußknacker Syndroms bei Kindern. Ultraschall Med 20:S33

Schultz PK, Stife JL, Strife CF et al (1991) Hyperechoic renal medullary pyramids in infants and children. Radiology 181:163–167

Siegel MJ (1991) Pediatric sonography. Raven Press, New York

Siegel MJ (1995) Urinary tract. In: Siegel MJ (ed) Pediatric sonography. Raven Press, New York, pp 357–435

Siegel MJ (1999) Kidney. In: Siegel MJ (ed) Pediatric body CT. Lippincott, Williams & Wilkins, Philadelphia, pp 226–254

Slovis TL, Sty JR, Haller O (1989) Imaging of the pediatric urinary tract. Saunders, Philadelphia

Slovis T, Bernstein J, Gruskin A (1993) Hyperechoic kidneys in the newborn and young infant. Pediatr Nephrol 7:294–302

Starinsky R, Vardi O, Batasch D, Goldberg M (1994) Increased renal medullary echogenicity in neonates. Pediatr Radiol 25:S43–S45

Talar-Williams C, Hijaz YM, Walther MM et al (2000) Cyclophosphamide induced cystitis and bladder cancer in patients with Wegener's granulomatosis. Ann Intern Med 124:477–484

Taylor GA (1994) Comparison of color Doppler amplitude and frequency shift: Imaging of children and experimental correlation. Radiology 193:372

Teele RL, Chare JC (1991) Ultrasonography in infants and children. Saunders, Philadelphia

Theodoropoulos DS, Shawker TH, Heinrichs C et al (1995) Medullary nephrocalcinosis in nephropathic cystinosis. Pediatr Nephrol 9:412–418

Toma P (1991) Diagnostici per immagini. In: Gusmano R, Perfumo F (eds) Malattie renali nel bambino. Editore, Milano, pp 15–34

Vade A, Subbaiah P, Kalbhen CL, Ryva JC (1993) Renal resistive indices in children. J Ultrasound Med 12:655–658

Vallee JP, Lazeyras F, Khan HG, Terrier F (2000) Absolute renal blood flow quantification by dynamic MRI and Gd-DTPA. Eur Radiol 10:1245–1252

Verwijvel G, Eerens I, Messiaen T, Oyen R (2000) Granulomatous renal pseudotumor in Wegener's granulomatosis. Eur Radiol 10:1265–1267

Wolfsdorf JI, Crigler JF Jr (1999) Effect of continuous glucose therapy on metabolic control, occurrence of severe hypoglycemia, physical growth and development, and complications of glycogen storage disease type I (GSD I). J Pediatr Gastroenterol Nutr 29:136–143

Wright NB, Blanch G, Walkinshaw S et al (1996) Antenatal and neonatal renal vein thrombosis: new ultrasonographic features with high frequency transducers. Pediatr Radiol 26:686–689

Zeis PM, Spigos DS, Samayoa C (1976) Ultrasound localization for percutaneous renal biopsy in children. J Pediatr 89:263–265

Imaging of Urolithiasis and Nephrocalcinosis

Michael Francavilla, Kassa Darge, and Gabriele Benz-Bohm

Contents

1   Background.. 603

2   **Imaging of Urolithiasis**.. 604
2.1   Ultrasound... 604
2.2   Computed Tomography.. 608
2.3   Magnetic Resonance Urography.............................. 610
2.4   Radiography and Intravenous Urography................ 610

3   **Imaging of Nephrocalcinosis**................................. 611
3.1   Ultrasound... 611
3.2   Computed Tomography.. 611
3.3   Magnetic Resonance Urography, Radiography, and Intravenous Urography............ 612

Conclusion.. 612

References... 612

M. Francavilla • K. Darge (✉)
Department of Radiology, The Children's Hospital of Philadelphia, Philadelphia, PA, USA
e-mail: francavilm@email.chop.edu; darge@email.chop.edu

G. Benz-Bohm, MD, (Retired)
Department of Radiology, The Children's Hospital of Philadelphia, Philadelphia, PA, USA
e-mail: g.benz-bohm@t-online.de

1 Background

Urolithiasis is macroscopic calcification in the urinary collecting system, whereas nephrocalcinosis is microscopic calcification in the tubules, tubular epithelium, or interstitial tissue of the kidney. Urolithiasis and nephrocalcinosis are common indications for imaging in children. The clinical and laboratory findings in urolithiasis and nephrocalcinosis are described in chapter "Urolithiasis and Nephrocalcinosis".

The demand for imaging of urolithiasis is rising with the increase in urolithiasis. A recent comprehensive review of the literature revealed that the incidence of urolithiasis has increased in children by about 6–10% in the last 25 years (Tasian and Copelovitch 2014). In the United States alone, the pediatric patient population with urolithiasis rose from 18.4/100,000 in 1999 to 57.0/100,000 in 2008, corresponding to an adjusted annual increase of 10.6% (Routh et al. 2010). It is reported that 1 in 685 hospitalizations of children is for urolithiasis (Bush et al. 2010). Nephrectomy was performed in 1% of pediatric patients hospitalized for urolithiasis (Bush et al. 2010). It is important to note that 100% of children with urolithiasis are regarded as high risk for recurrent disease (Straub et al. 2010).

Imaging is necessary in the initial diagnosis and follow-up evaluations after both conservative and surgical managements. The primary imaging modality for urolithiasis is ultrasound (US). Computed tomography (CT) plays a secondary role. Other imaging modalities currently have only subordinate roles. The need of repeated follow-up imaging studies and the radiation risk, particularly with CT, put US in the forefront of the imaging choices for urolithiasis and nephrocalcinosis. US is the primary diagnostic imaging choice in children. CT should only be considered when the US examination turns out to be equivocal in the presence of high clinical suspicion for urolithiasis or the US is nondiagnostic as in cases of morbid obesity or severe scoliosis. CT is significantly more sensitive for the detection of urolithiasis than US. In a prospective study on children, Passerotti et al. (2009) showed that US was only 76 % sensitive compared to CT in children. The average size of missed stones was 2.3 mm. However, the findings did not affect management (Passerotti et al. 2009). This is of significant practical importance in children. A similar but larger, multi-institutional study in adults showed higher sensitivity for CT, but no difference in primary or secondary outcomes (Smith-Bindman et al. 2014).

The incidence of *nephrocalcinosis* in children is unknown. Certain conditions predispose children to develop nephrocalcinosis, such as prematurity and very low birth weight. About 20 % of very low birth weight infants develop nephrocalcinosis during the first three months of life. In half of the affected infants, the changes are transient, but extensive forms may persist for several years (Saarela et al. 1999). Nephrocalcinosis should not be confused with fleeting medullary hyperechogenicity noted in the first week of life in newborns and known as transient stasis nephropathy. The etiology of nephrocalcinosis can be elucidated by its classification. Classification of nephrocalcinosis depends on the anatomic area involved: medulla, cortex, or diffuse (both cortex and medulla). The imaging of nephrocalcinosis is almost exclusively conducted with US.

2 Imaging of Urolithiasis

2.1 Ultrasound

Diagnostic imaging evaluation in children with suspected urolithiasis should begin with US (Riccabona et al. 2009). US is widespread, easily accessible, and free of ionizing radiation. US is a practical screening tool in both acute and outpatient presentations. Ideally, for the US study, the patient should be hydrated and have a well-distended bladder. This may not be possible in the acute state in a symptomatic patient. Hydration can lead directly not only to better delineation of the renal pelves and calyces but also to bladder distention (Morin and Baker 1979). Thus, possible urinary tract dilation due to stone is not obscured. The assessment of the location, number, contour, and size of renal stones is improved with hydration (Chau and Chan 1997). A distended urinary bladder not only allows for better delineation of intravesical stones but also permits better access for evaluation of the ureters, in particular the distal ureters. The US examination for urolithiasis starts with the evaluation of the urinary bladder, ureterovesical junctions, and the distal ureters. Subsequently, the kidneys and proximal ureters are imaged in both the supine and prone positions. A negative scan in one position may turn out to be positive in the opposite position. Grayscale and color Doppler sonography (CDS) are performed with age- and size-appropriate high- and low-frequency transducers.

2.1.1 Grayscale Ultrasound

Urinary tract stones are universally echogenic on US regardless of their composition. They may also have posterior acoustic shadowing (Fig. 1). However, the absence of a posterior acoustic shadow does not rule out the presence of a stone. The formation of the posterior acoustic shadow is dependent on a number of technical and patient-related factors. In vitro experiments have demonstrated the smallest size of a stone with acoustic shadow to be 3.5–4 mm (King et al. 1985). However, using modern high-frequency US scanners with high resolution, it may be possible to depict acoustic shadowing in stones with even smaller sizes. Other influential factors are focal zone placement and distance from the transducer. The latter is affected by both the scan position and body habitus of the patient. The US modality used for the scan also affects the formation or visualization of the posterior acoustic shadow. Spatial compound imaging is increasingly applied for optimizing the images and has the

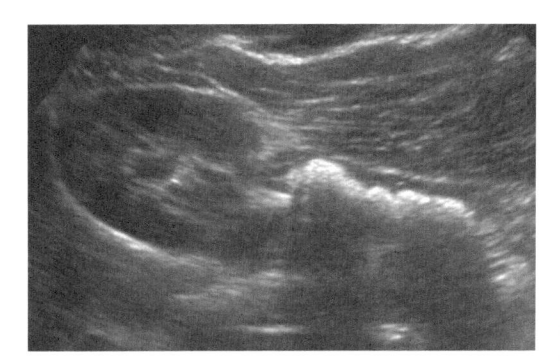

Fig. 1 Greyscale US image of the kidney and proximal ureter showing multiple stones with posterior shadowing and uroepithelial thickening in the proximal ureter

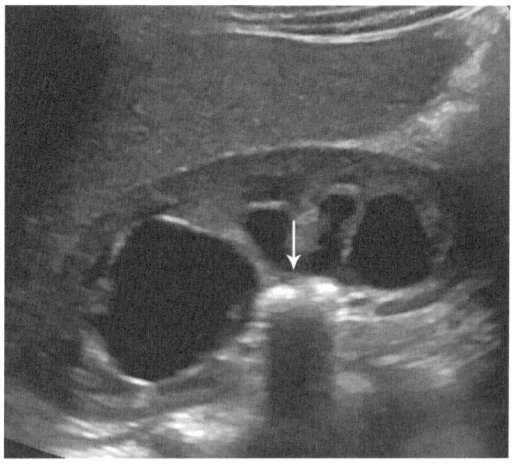

Fig. 2 Greyscale US of the kidney in sagittal plane showing obstructive renal calculi (*arrow*) with posterior acoustic shadowing at the ureteropelvic junction causing pelvicalyceal dilation

advantage of reducing angle-dependent US artifacts, i.e., speckle artifacts. It does so by combining US beams steered at different angles into a single composite image in real time. However, posterior acoustic shadowing was present in only 43% of US examinations with spatial compound imaging compared to 86% with conventional imaging (Heng et al. 2012). Harmonic imaging, another commonly used modern US technique, is based on the nonlinear propagation of US waves and the generation of harmonics, i.e., multiples of the transmitted frequency. It reduces reverberation and side-lobe artifacts and increases the resolution, resulting in clearer better-quality US images (Bartram and Darge 2005). With harmonic imaging, the posterior acoustic shadow appears more conspicuous (Darge and Heidemeier 2005). Note that image compounding may decrease the shadowing artifact; furthermore frequency and transducer affect shadowing. A combination of all the above factors may determine the presence or absence of the posterior acoustic shadow of a urinary tract stone.

It is necessary to measure the diameter of the stone for the purpose of prediction of potential passage of the stone or selection of the type of surgical management (Fig. 2) (Straub et al. 2010). The echogenic focus is measured on the plane with its longest diameter. In children, spontaneous passage of stones is rare for those with a diameter greater than five mm (Pietrow et al. 2002). In up to 41% of renal stones and 63% of ureteral stones, spontaneous passage can occur (Pietrow et al. 2002). Secondary findings in the presence of urolithiasis include dilation of the calices, pelvis, or ureter, uroepithelial thickening of the renal pelvis or ureter, and enlargement of the kidney (Fig. 2). However, in acute obstruction without preexisting dilatation, only very little distention may be present.

There are a number of mimics on US of renal stones (Durr-E-Sabih et al. 2004). The vascular structures, particularly when presenting orthogonally to the US beam, may appear as bright echogenicities. If they have "rail-road track" appearance, it may be possible to differentiate them from stones. At times, it may be difficult to separate the echogenic stone from the echogenic renal sinus fat or an echogenic papilla (Fig. 3). Milk of calcium is a semiliquid suspension of calcium salts in a calyceal cyst or diverticulum (Fig. 4). It amasses in the dependent portion of the cystic structure and can cause reverberations. The posterior acoustic shadow from gas collections tends not to be clear, having internal echoes and indistinct margins rather than posterior acoustic shadowing (Sommer and Taylor 1980). Calcifications in the renal parenchyma or pelvic wall and echogenic medullary pyramids may at times be difficult to differentiate from stones. This may also be the case in the presence of echogenic fungal ball. In these cases, high-resolution US of the kidneys in both the supine and prone positions may be helpful in the differentiation. Without adequate distention of the

Fig. 3 Grayscale (**a**) and color Doppler (**b**) images of the kidney. The small renal calculi difficult to delineate on the grayscale image due to the echogenic sinus fat are easily depicted on color Doppler, at high setting of the pulse repetition frequency, due to the presence of twinkling sign

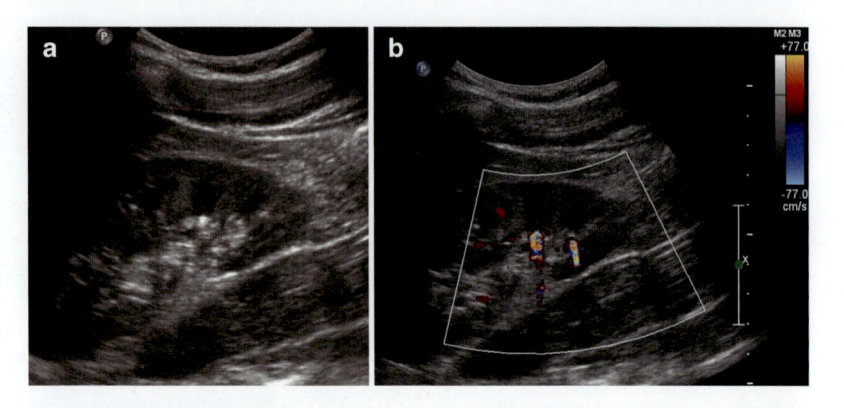

Fig. 4 Greyscale US images of a calyceal diverticulum with milk of calcium without acoustic shadowing with the patient in supine (**a**) and prone (**b**) positions

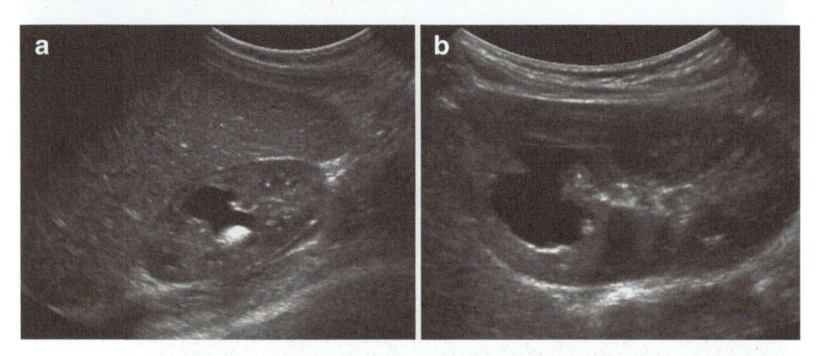

Fig. 5 Transverse US images of the bladder without and with color Doppler. Two stones are present (*calipers*) and demonstrate posterior acoustic shadowing and positive twinkling sign

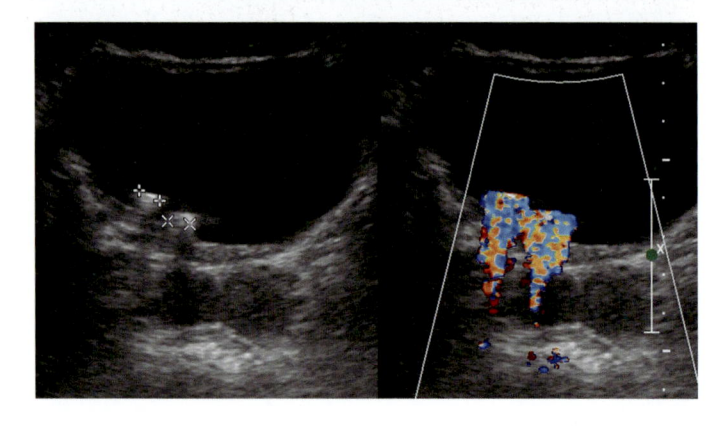

bladder, it may not only be difficult to visualize an intravesical stone, but one may overlook a stone in the distal ureter. Phleboliths or even coprolites may be mistaken for ureteral stones if the bladder is not well distended.

2.1.2 Color Doppler US

The twinkling sign is a CDS or power Doppler artifact, visible as a rapidly changing mixture of different colored pixels behind a reflecting structure at the site where an acoustic shadow is expected (Fig. 5) (Rahmouni et al. 1996). The twinkling sign is particularly useful for detection of small stones and follow-up after lithotripsy (Fig. 6). The twinkling sign may also help differentiate calculi from sonographic mimics of calculi (Fig. 7). The etiology of the twinkling sign is uncertain. Two theories are commonly accepted. The first holds that rough surfaces have multiple reflectors that increase the pulse duration,

Imaging of Urolithiasis and Nephrocalcinosis

Fig. 6 Sagittal US images of the bladder with minimally dilated right distal ureter in which a small stone (*arrow*) is present. On the grayscale image (**a**) it is less conspicuous than on the color Doppler (**b**) with positive twinkling sign

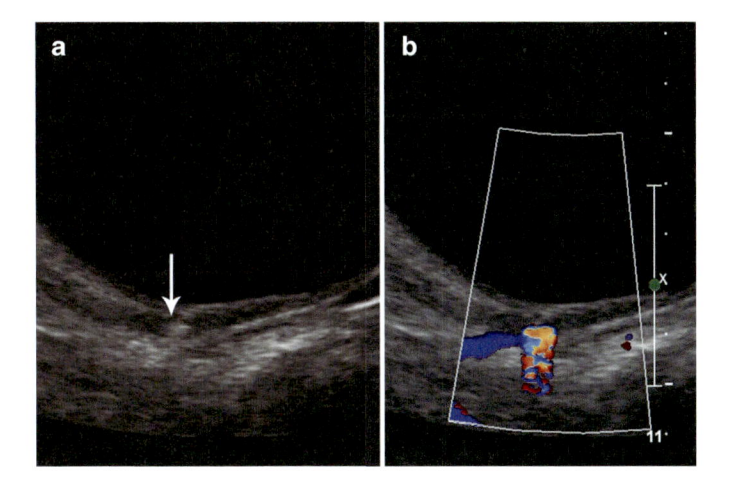

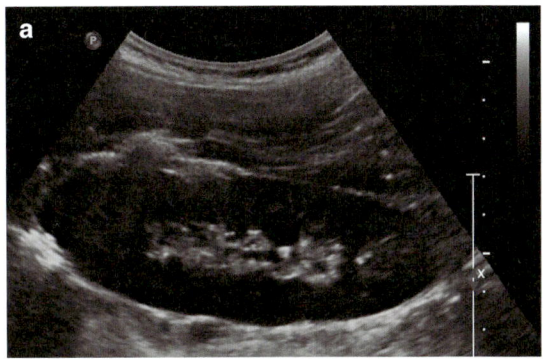

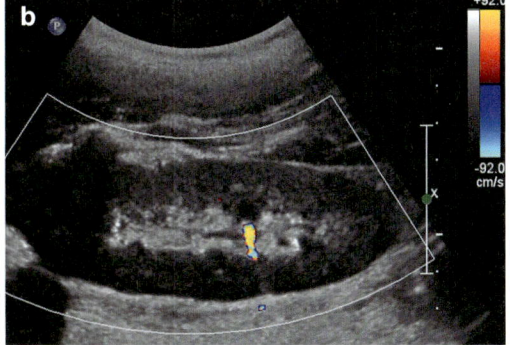

Fig. 7 Grayscale (**a**) and color Doppler (**b**) images of the kidney. The small renal calculi difficult to delineate on the grayscale image due to the echogenic sinus fat are easily depicted on color Doppler, at high setting of the pulse repetition frequency, due to the presence of twinkling sign

which is interpreted as Doppler shift (Rahmouni et al. 1996). The second theory is that intrinsic machine noise is caused by intrinsic "jitter" of the electronic clock (Kamaya et al. 2003).

Many, but not all, calculi will demonstrate a twinkling sign when CDS is applied, and the reasons for this are multifactorial. The choice of US equipment affects the sensitivity of the sign. Aytaç and Ozcan (1999) showed that new digital machines were much more sensitive than older and analog ones, detecting 96% of stones in 65 patients versus only 39%, respectively. The strength of the twinkling sign signal is strongly influenced by the color write priority; lower priority diminishes the artifact (Kamaya et al. 2003).

The depth of the stone, transducer frequency, position of focal zone, and power settings also make a difference in the detection. The most influential factor, and one of great practical significance, is the level of the pulse repetition frequency (PRF). For each transducer used in CDS mode, it is necessary to select the highest PRF with the focus placed at the level of the suspected stone (Fig. 7). It is important not just to rely on choosing a "high flow" setting but to actually set the PRF at its maximum. In most instances, such a PRF setting eliminates the depiction of vascular structures in the CDS mode. However, the twinkling sign becomes conspicuously visible. Spectral Doppler analysis behind the echogenic stone, in the region of twinkling sign, shows no typical flow signal (Kamaya et al. 2003). It is important to note that not all structures demonstrating the twinkling sign are stones, e.g., air or echogenic deposits in the distal medulla as seen in neonates.

US has limitations for imaging calculi. The patient's body habitus, e.g., obese or scoliotic, can limit visualization of the kidneys and ureters. The sonographic detection rate of calculi relative to unenhanced helical CT is only 90 % for intrarenal stones, 75 % for stones in both the kidney and ureter, and only 38 % for stones in the ureter alone (Palmer et al. 2005). One study found that ureteral stones were found in the proximal ureter in 26 %, mid-ureter in 22 %, and distal ureter in 43 % (Akay et al. 2006). The mid-ureter is particularly difficult to visualize by US; a dedicated search for this ureteral portion, particularly at the level of the iliac vessel crossing, is advisable. Urinary tract dilation can be a helpful secondary sign for identifying a calculus, but is present in only 45–73 % of cases (Smergel et al. 2001; Strouse et al. 2002).

2.2 Computed Tomography

Unenhanced CT should be the second line of investigation in children when US evaluation is uncertain or abnormal or when CT may add further information which will contribute to the diagnosis (Riccabona et al. 2009). CT should be employed as an adjunct to US, in cases where there are only secondary signs of an obstructing calculus with no visible stone, when there is high clinical suspicion and no stone on US or when US is nondiagnostic. CT is of particular importance when there is a suspected stone in the mid-ureter, a relative blind spot for US. However, when considering CT to detect urolithiasis in children, certain differences compared to adults need to be understood. Unlike adults, children tend to have small and potentially less calcified stones. The ureter is frequently difficult to identify as it is small and has relatively little surrounding fat. Additionally, children often have nonspecific, poorly localizing symptoms. These factors can decrease the yield of diagnostic CT.

The advantages of CT with its short examination time and relatively high diagnostic yield are counterbalanced by its high dose of ionizing radiation. Care should be taken to follow the "As Low (i.e., little radiation) As Reasonably Achievable (ALARA)" principle when considering CT for evaluation of urolithiasis. Body weight-adapted ("ultra") low-dose CT protocols need to be employed to optimize the radiation dose to the patient (Kluner et al. 2006). Automatic exposure control and iterative reconstruction methods can further reduce dose. However, a dose too low for proper anatomic definition is also not useful.

Consider scanning with the patient in the prone position. This may help differentiate a calculus impacted at the ureterovesicular junction from a stone freely floating in the bladder. Multiplanar reformatted images, especially the coronal reformation, are helpful for accurate localization of a suspected stone within or external to the ureter (Eisner et al. 2011). The window and level should be manipulated to near that of bone for better visualization of the calculi. The size of the stone is reported in the largest diameter, as larger stones are less likely to pass spontaneously (Pietrow et al. 2002). Axial images need to be obtained with 2–3 mm slice reconstructions. Thinner (<5 mm) slices improve detection and density characterization of stones (Eisner et al. 2011). This may entail the use of higher dose to reduce the image noise to a diagnostic range. Sagittal and coronal reconstructions improve reader confidence (Eisner et al. 2011). Maximum intensity projection (MIP) reconstructions in the coronal plane with 3–5 mm slice thickness can be helpful for improved detection of urolithiasis (Fig. 8) (Corwin et al. 2013). Contrast-enhanced CT is rarely performed and only in cases when delineation of ureteral obstruction and additional detailed anatomy of the urinary tract prior to surgical intervention is necessary and magnetic resonance urography (MRU) cannot be performed.

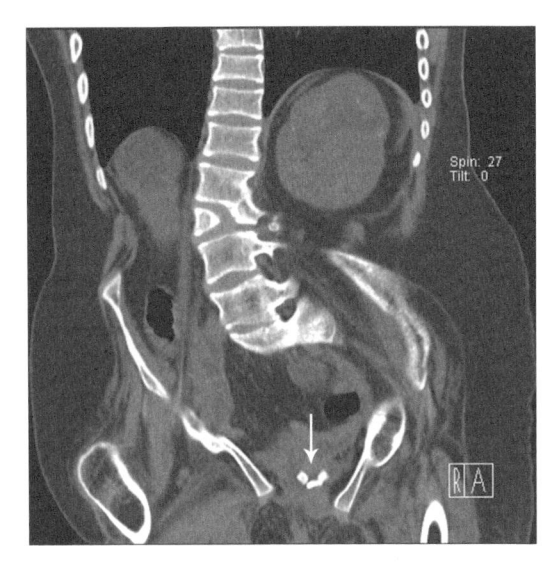

Fig. 8 Coronal reformatted unenhanced CT image of a non-distended, augmented bladder containing 3 bladder calculi (*arrow*) in a patient with spina bifida

An emerging CT modality for urolithiasis diagnostic is dual-energy or dual-voltage CT. This method exploits the differences in attenuation by the same material imaged at two different photon energies, usually 80 kVp and 140 kVp (Chiro et al. 1979). Although it is possible to perform dual-energy CT using a single-source scanner utilizing fast kVp switching, dual-source CT (using two different radiation sources) is more common. Data from acquisition of the two energies is used to create a composite image, which is then used for interpretation (Kaza et al. 2013). The individual datasets can further be analyzed for differences in attenuation. Materials with large atomic numbers, such as calculi, have higher attenuation at 80 kVp than at 140 kVp. The ratio between the attenuation values is referred to as the dual-energy index. The index is then plotted against the attenuation profile of known calculi to determine the stone's composition. Studies have shown that the chemical composition of calculi can be accurately determined, based on the stone's characteristic dual-energy index (Motley et al. 2001; Manglaviti et al. 2011). However, the dual-energy technique has limited accuracy for small (<3 mm) stones and stones of mixed composition. Furthermore, dual-energy CT allows the subtraction of the contrast from contrast-enhanced CT, so-called virtual contrast technique, allowing the possibility of performing contrast CT in cases of suspected obstruction due to urolithiasis and subsequently subtracting the contrast to depict the stone. These applications still require further pediatric adaptations and comparative evaluations, particularly about their management impact and dose implications, prior to becoming integrated in the diagnostic work-up in children.

The primary and most specific sign of urolithiasis is direct visualization of the urinary calculus within the kidney, ureter, or bladder (Fig. 8). Nearly all stones are hyperdense on CT (Federle et al. 1981). Secondary signs in urolithiasis arise from obstruction of the urinary tract, with the prominent signs being pelvicalyceal and ureteral dilation, unilateral renal enlargement, decreased renal density, unilateral absence of dense pyramids, perinephric edema, the "tissue rim sign," periureteral edema, and prominence of the perirenal fascia (Fig. 9) (Preminger et al. 1998; Strouse et al. 2002; Akay et al. 2006). The perirenal and periureteral findings may not be conspicuously visible in young children and those with little body fat. Unilateral renal enlargement can be seen in recent acute obstruction and, if no stone is visible on CT, may indicate a recently passed stone, a stone with low density, or a clot (Preminger et al. 1998). Renal size is best measured in sections traversing the mid-zone planes. Perinephric edema manifests as strands of soft tissue attenuation in the perirenal fat (i.e., fat stranding) (Strouse et al. 2002). The tissue rim sign is a sign specific to CT in which a ureteral calculus is surrounded by a rim of soft tissue density (Fig. 9). The tissue rim sign has been reported to aid in distinguishing calculus from extra-urinary calculus such as phlebolith, a mimic of urolithiasis. However the sign is found substantially less frequently in children than in adults (Strouse et al. 2002; Akay et al. 2006). Fortunately, phleboliths are less common in children than in adults. Decreased renal density

Fig. 9 Axial (**a**, **b**) and sagittal (**c**, **d**) CT images showing right proximal ureteral calculi causing obstruction and pelvicalyceal dilation (*arrows*). There is uroepithelial thickening at the level of the ureteric calculi (soft tissue rim sign). The right kidney is also enlarged and hypodense

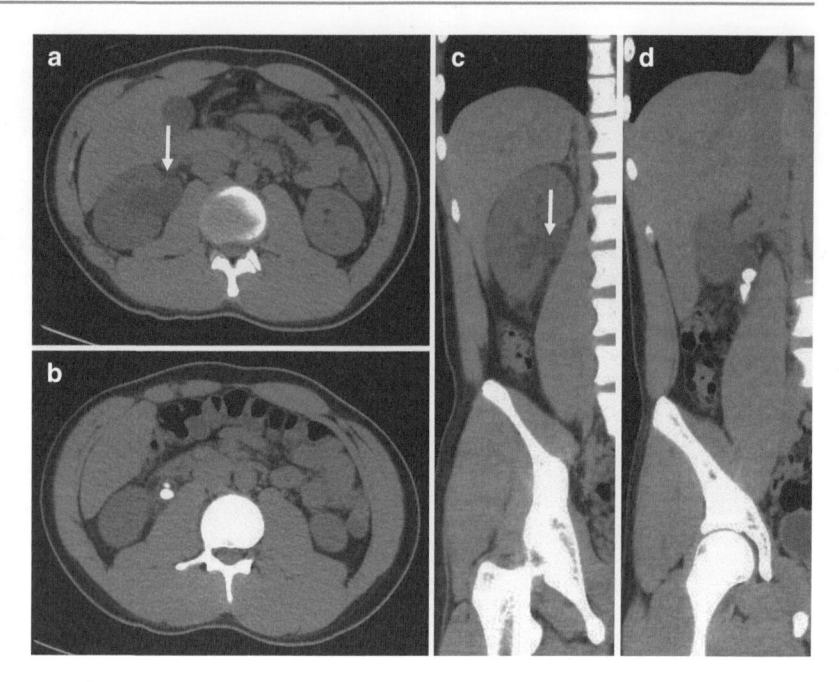

suggests edema and, while nonspecific, can be present in urolithiasis (Strouse et al. 2002; Akay et al. 2006). Periureteral edema is seen as fat stranding, surrounding the ureter due to inflammation. In many cases, these secondary findings are unilateral, and it is helpful to compare to the opposite side.

2.3 Magnetic Resonance Urography

MRU currently has a very limited role in the evaluation of urolithiasis. The foremost limiting factor is that small calculi are generally not well seen on routine sequences. Additional limitations are the lack of widespread availability of MRU, it is expensive to perform, young children usually require sedation, patients must be hydrated, and gadolinium contrast may be required. Advantages MRU has over other modalities are lack of ionizing radiation, excellent anatomic detail, and possibility for evaluation of renal function. MRU may have a role in non-emergent evaluation of obstructive uropathy, particularly when improved preoperative anatomic delineation or functional analysis are important or in patients with underlying or additional malformations/conditions (Grattan-Smith et al. 2008).

2.4 Radiography and Intravenous Urography

Radiography in the form of kidney-ureter-bladder (KUB) film nowadays plays only a minimal role in the diagnosis of urolithiasis in children. It may be a prerequisite for some forms of lithotripsy (Riccabona et al. 2009). Intravenous urography (IVU) is rather obsolete in the era of CT and CT urography (Shine 2008). It may be used in resource-limited setting, but even in such settings, it is recommended to perform a targeted IVU – e.g., focusing only on the pathological side, without an additional scout film, and timing the films in such a way that only the least number of studies is required to make a diagnosis (Riccabona et al. 2009).

> **Take Away**
> 1. Urolithiasis is increasing in children.
> 2. US is the primary imaging modality for urolithiasis in children.
> 3. CT is performed in pediatric urolithiasis only when the US is equivocal in the presence of high clinical suspicion or detailed preoperative anatomic depiction or delineation of the obstruction is necessary.

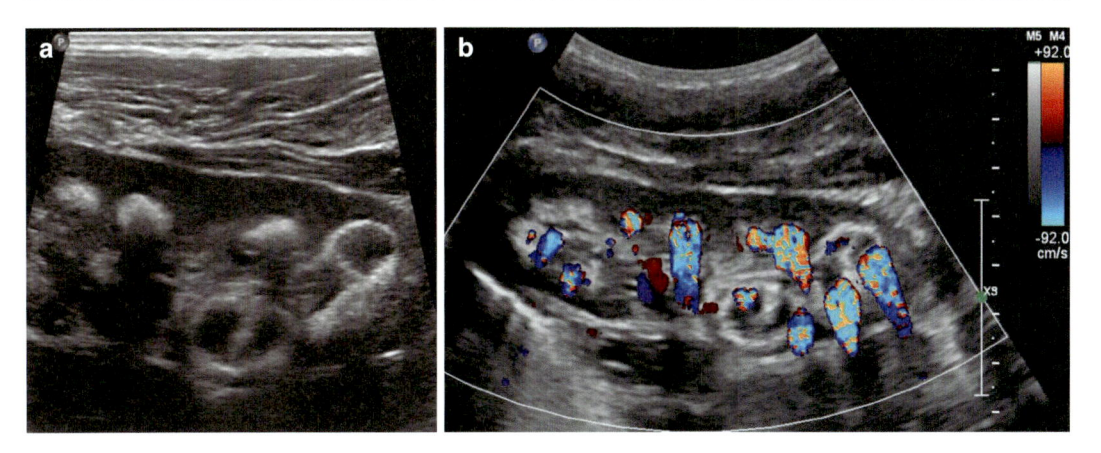

Fig. 10 Greyscale (**a**) and color Doppler (**b**) images of the kidney demonstrating echogenic medullary pyramids with twinkling signs compatible with nephrocalcinosis in a child with hypercalcemia

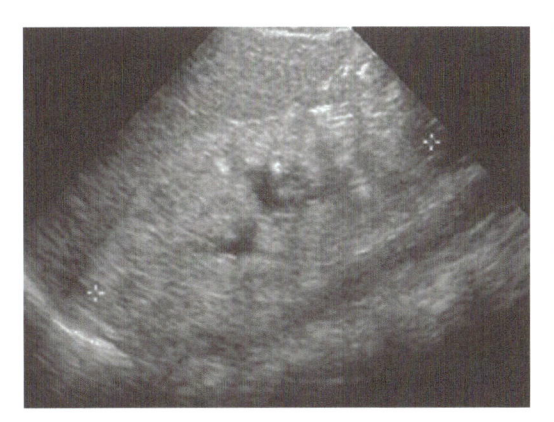

Fig. 11 Diffuse nephrocalcinosis in an infant with primary hyperoxaluria I

Fig. 12 Diffuse cortical nephrocalcinosis and nephrolithiasis in a 7-year-old boy with oxalosis

3 Imaging of Nephrocalcinosis

3.1 Ultrasound

High-resolution US is the best method for identification and classification of nephrocalcinosis in children (Fig. 10). Imaging is performed with a high-frequency transducer to optimize spatial resolution (Fig. 11). Harmonic mode will further increase the spatial resolution of the images. The kidneys are also interrogated with CDS to search for the twinkling sign, which increases sensitivity of the evaluation (Fig. 10). The twinkling sign will appear identical to that seen with nephrolithiasis. Medullary (and not cortical) nephrocalcinosis is graded according to the degree of hyperechogenicity with high interobserver reliability (Dick et al. 1999). Grade 1 corresponds to mild peripheral medullary hyperechogenicity. Grade 2 is mild hyperechogenicity of the entire medulla. Grade 3 nephrocalcinosis is marked hyperechogenicity of the entire medulla. Some studies have found a correlation between the grade of nephrocalcinosis and its treatment outcome (Dick et al. 1999). Renal stones are found in the setting of nephrocalcinosis; the differentiation and depiction however may be challenging (Fig. 12).

3.2 Computed Tomography

Nephrocalcinosis can be depicted on CT (Manz et al. 1980). However, in the era of high-resolution US, CT is no longer the diagnostic modality of choice (Boyce et al. 2013). CT has excellent specificity (96%) and only modest sensitivity (64%) for nephrocalcinosis when compared to US (specificity 85% and sensitivity 86%) (Cramer et al. 1998; Strouse et al. 2002; Palmer et al. 2005). CT may be required for further evaluation when US examination is limited, such as by poor or non-visualization of the kidneys or markedly diffuse nephrocalcinosis. Additionally, nephrocalcinosis may be seen as an incidental finding during CT evaluation for other indications. Nephrocalcinosis appears as high-density, often irregularly shaped, areas in the renal cortex, medulla, or both. It should not be confused with papillary deposits or calcifications or residual contrast after an intravenous contrast-enhanced study.

3.3 Magnetic Resonance Urography, Radiography, and Intravenous Urography

MRU is not employed as a first-line diagnostic modality for nephrocalcinosis as the resolution is not as high as that of US. However, nephrocalcinosis may be an incidental finding on MRU. Depending on the severity, nephrocalcinosis distorts the normal signal intensity of the affected parts. In the presence of a preceding US finding, the resulting change in MRU is easily explained.

Radiographs and intravenous urography (IVU) are frequently unrevealing in nephrocalcinosis. Severe forms may be visible as opacity that conforms to the expected contour of the renal cortex, medulla, or the entire kidney. Although historically the initial study of choice, radiographs currently have no role in the diagnostic evaluation (Manz et al. 1980). Again, nephrocalcinosis may be incidentally seen and its appearance should not be confusing. On both radiography and IVU, nephrocalcinosis presents as calcification of the cortex, medulla, or both.

Take Away
1. Nephrocalcinosis can be medullary, cortical, or both.
2. High-resolution US is the main imaging modality. Others only have minimal or no role in the imaging.

Conclusion

Urolithiasis and nephrocalcinosis are common indications for imaging in children. Pediatric urolithiasis is on the rise. For both conditions, US is the primary imaging modality. US, by virtue of the high resolution coupled with the smaller body size in the majority of children, easily allows the diagnosis or exclusion of urolithiasis or nephrocalcinosis. Large or distorted body habitus may necessitate the use of CT. Stones limited to the ureter are best depicted on CT, too. Other imaging modalities like MR urography, radiography, and intravenous urography are seldom indicated in the diagnosis of urolithiasis and nephrocalcinosis.

References

Akay H, Akpinar E, Ergun O et al (2006) Unenhanced multidetector CT evaluation of urinary stones and secondary signs in pediatric patients. Diagn Interv Radiol 12:147–150

Aytaç SK, Ozcan H (1999) Effect of color Doppler system on the twinkling sign associated with urinary tract calculi. J Clin Ultrasound JCU 27:433–439

Bartram U, Darge K (2005) Harmonic versus conventional US imaging of the urinary tract in children. Pediatr Radiol 35:655–660

Boyce AM, Shawker TH, Hill SC et al (2013) US is superior to computed tomography for assessment of medullary nephrocalcinosis in hypoparathyroidism. J Clin Endocrinol Metab 98:989–994

Bush NC, Xu L, Brown BJ et al (2010) Hospitalizations for pediatric stone disease in United States, 2002–2007. J Urol 183:1151–1156

Chau W-K, Chan S-C (1997) Improved sonographic visualization by fluid challenge method of renal lithiasis in the nondilated collecting system experience in seven cases. Clin Imaging 21:276–283

Chiro GD, Brooks RA, Kessler RM et al (1979) Tissue signatures with dual-energy computed tomography. Radiology 131:521–523

Corwin MT, Hsu M, McGahan JP et al (2013) Unenhanced MDCT in suspected urolithiasis: improved stone detection and density measurements using coronal maximum-intensity-projection images. Am J Roentgenol 201:1036–1040

Cramer B, Husa L, Pushpanathan C (1998) Nephrocalcinosis in rabbits–correlation of US, computed tomography, pathology and renal function. Pediatr Radiol 28:9–13

Darge K, Heidemeier A (2005) Modern US technologies and their application in pediatric urinary tract imaging. Radiologe 45:1101–1111

Dick PT, Shuckett BM, Tang B et al (1999) Observer reliability in grading nephrocalcinosis on US examinations in children. Pediatr Radiol 29:68–72

Durr-E-Sabih KAN, Craig M, Worrall JA (2004) Sonographic mimics of renal calculi. J Ultrasound Med Off J Am Inst Ultrasound Med 23:1361–1367

Eisner BH, McQuaid JW, Hyams E, Matlaga BR (2011) Nephrolithiasis: what surgeons need to know. Am J Roentgenol 196:1274–1278

Federle M, McAninch J, Kaiser J et al (1981) Computed tomography of urinary calculi. Am J Roentgenol 136:255–258

Grattan-Smith JD, Little SB, Jones RA (2008) MR urography evaluation of obstructive uropathy. Pediatr Radiol 38:49–69

Heng HG, Rohleder JJ, Pressler BM (2012) Comparative sonographic appearance of nephroliths and associated acoustic shadowing artifacts in conventional vs. spatial compound imaging: spatial compound appearance of nephroliths. Vet Radiol Ultrasound 53:217–220

Kamaya A, Tuthill T, Rubin JM (2003) Twinkling artifact on color Doppler sonography: dependence on machine parameters and underlying cause. Am J Roentgenol 180:215–222

Kaza RK, Platt JF, Megibow AJ (2013) Dual-energy CT of the urinary tract. Abdom Imaging 38:167–179

King W, Kimme-Smith C, Winter J (1985) Renal stone shadowing: an investigation of contributing factors. Radiology 154:191–196

Kluner C, Hein PA, Gralla O et al (2006) Does ultra-low-dose CT with a radiation dose equivalent to that of KUB suffice to detect renal and ureteral calculi? J Comput Assist Tomogr 30:44–50

Manglaviti G, Tresoldi S, Guerrer CS et al (2011) In vivo evaluation of the chemical composition of urinary stones using dual-energy CT. Am J Roentgenol 197:W76–W83

Manz F, Jaschke W, van Kaick G et al (1980) Nephrocalcinosis in radiographs, computed tomography, sonography and histology. Pediatr Radiol 9:19–26

Morin ME, Baker DA (1979) The influence of hydration and bladder distension on the sonographic diagnosis of hydronephrosis. J Clin Ultrasound 7:192–194

Motley G, Dalrymple N, Keesling C et al (2001) Hounsfield unit density in the determination of urinary stone composition. Urology 58:170–173

Palmer JS, Donaher ER, O'Riordan MA, Dell KM (2005) Diagnosis of pediatric urolithiasis: role of US and computerized tomography. J Urol 174:1413–1416

Passerotti C, Chow JS, Silva A et al (2009) US versus computerized tomography for evaluating urolithiasis. J Urol 182:1829–1834

Pietrow PK, Pope JC, Adams MC et al (2002) Clinical outcome of pediatric stone disease. J Urol 167:670–673

Preminger GM, Vieweg J, Leder RA, Nelson RC (1998) Urolithiasis: detection and management with unenhanced spiral CT–a urologic perspective. Radiology 207:308–309

Rahmouni A, Bargoin R, Herment A et al (1996) Color Doppler twinkling artifact in hyperechoic regions. Radiology 199:269–271

Riccabona M, Avni FE, Blickman JG et al (2009) Imaging recommendations in paediatric uroradiology: Minutes of the ESPR uroradiology task force session on childhood obstructive uropathy, high-grade fetal hydronephrosis, childhood haematuria, and urolithiasis in childhood. ESPR Annual Congress, Edinburgh, UK, June 2008. Pediatr Radiol 39:891–898

Routh JC, Graham DA, Nelson CP (2010) Epidemiological trends in pediatric urolithiasis at United States free-standing pediatric hospitals. J Urol 184:1100–1105. doi:10.1016/j.juro.2010.05.018

Saarela T, Vaarala A, Lanning P, Koivisto M (1999) Incidence, ultrasonic patterns and resolution of nephrocalcinosis in very low birthweight infants. Acta Paediatr 88:655–660

Shine S (2008) Urinary calculus: IVU vs. CT renal stone? A critically appraised topic. Abdom Imaging 33:41–43

Smergel E, Greenberg SB, Crisci KL, Salwen JK (2001) CT urograms in pediatric patients with ureteral calculi: do adult criteria work? Pediatr Radiol 31:720–723

Smith-Bindman R, Aubin C, Bailitz J et al (2014) Ultrasonography versus computed tomography for suspected nephrolithiasis. N Engl J Med 371:1100–1110

Sommer FG, Taylor KJ (1980) Differentiation of acoustic shadowing due to calculi and gas collections. Radiology 135:399–403

Straub M, Gschwend J, Zorn C (2010) Pediatric urolithiasis: the current surgical management. Pediatr Nephrol 25:1239–1244

Strouse PJ, Bates GD, Bloom DA, Goodsitt MM (2002) Non-contrast thin-section helical CT of urinary tract calculi in children. Pediatr Radiol 32:326–332

Tasian GE, Copelovitch L (2014) Evaluation and medical management of kidney stones in children. J Urol 192:1329–1336

# Imaging in Renal Failure, Neonatal Oligoanuria, and Renal Transplantation

Maria Beatrice Damasio, Christoph Mache, and Michael Riccabona

Contents

1 Introduction 615

2 Definitions 616
2.1 Childhood Renal Failure 616
2.2 Urine Production After Birth and Neonatal Oligoanuria 616

3 Basic Considerations on Imaging in Renal Failure and Neonatal Oligoanuria 616
3.1 Renal Imaging in Renal Failure 616
3.2 Diagnostic Workup and Imaging in Neonatal Oligoanuria 618
3.3 Role of Imaging in Planning and During Dialysis 618
3.4 Imaging for Planning Transplantation 621
3.5 Extrarenal Imaging in Chronic Renal Failure 621

4 Imaging Methods and Findings 622
4.1 Basic Situation 622
4.2 Ultrasound 623
4.3 Doppler Sonography and Other Modern Sonographic Imaging Methods 623
4.4 Plain Films/Radiography, Isotope Investigations, Computerized Tomography, and Intravenous Pyelography 624
4.5 Use of Contrast Agents in Renal Failure 624
4.6 Voiding Cystourethrography 625
4.7 Magnetic Resonance Imaging 626

5 Renal Transplantation 626
5.1 Basic Considerations 626
5.2 Surgical Technique 627
5.3 Postoperative and Surveillance Imaging 627
5.4 The Normal Renal Allograft 628
5.5 Posttransplant Complications 629
5.6 Mass Lesions: *Posttransplant Lymphoproliferative Disorder* 635

Conclusion 636

References 636

M.B. Damasio (✉)
Department of Radiology, Division of Radiology, Giannina Gaslini Institute, Genoa, Italy
e-mail: beatricedamasio@gmail.com

C. Mache
Department of Padiatrics, University Hospital LKH Graz, Graz, Austria

M. Riccabona
Department of Radiology, Division of Pediatric Radiology, University Hospital LKH Graz, Graz, Austria
e-mail: michael.riccabona@meduni-graz.at

1 Introduction

Many children who suffer from congenital, hereditary, or severe acquired renal disease have a substantially diminished number of functioning nephrons. Loss of nephrons cannot be replaced by new units, and recovery is impossible. Consequently, according to the patient's age, different diseases enter a common pathway of progressive renal dysfunction called chronic renal failure (CRF). Further deterioration is associated with clinical symptoms and loss of metabolic control. End-stage renal disease (ESRD) is reached when survival is possible with only renal replacement therapy. Aside from all medical and psychosocial care during CRF and ESRD, renal transplantation is the ultimate goal to optimize rehabilitation and lifestyle. This chapter is devoted to these children who need lifelong multidisciplinary care and treatment, including pediatric radiology.

2 Definitions

2.1 Childhood Renal Failure

Loss of one kidney during life or being born with a single kidney may cause slight renal dysfunction but, in general, does not lead to CRF even in late adulthood (Wikstad et al. 1988). Renal failure can occur acute or chronic; CRF can be defined as a disease state with the loss of more than 50% of nephrons, persistently increased serum creatinine above +2 SD of the age-adjusted mean, and a decreased glomerular filtration rate (GFR). It is important to note that serum creatinine must be adjusted for age as, for example, a value of 1.0 mg/dl (88 μmol/l) is normal for an adolescent, but means CRF for an infant. CRF implicates a relentless progression to ESRD without the possibility of cure; incidence and causes vary with age group (Ardissino et al. 2003). In the early stages, it is a silent disease mostly defined by biochemical values. When GFR is reduced to 25% of normal and correspondingly the number of functioning nephrons is reduced to 12% of normal, clinical symptoms of uremia appear and dominate in ESRD. To improve the detection and the treatment of children with renal disorders, the term chronic kidney disease (CKD) was established (Hogg et al. 2003). Patients suffer from CKD if kidney damage – with or without a reduced GFR – is present for at least 3 months, characterized by abnormalities in the composition of the blood or urine, abnormalities on imaging tests, or lesions on renal biopsy. CKD is classified into five stages with stage G1 having a normal GFR and stage G5 meaning the need for renal replacement therapy (KDIGO CKD Work Group 2013). Additionally, albuminuria (stages A1–A3) significantly impacts prognosis.

Acute renal failure (ARF) is an acute event with an increase of creatinine; it can be oligoanuric, normuric, or polyuric. There are a number of reasons that have to be differentiated and then govern treatment; these may be prerenal and systemic (e.g., severe hypoperfusion), intrarenal (e.g., acute glomerulonephritis, hemolytic uremic syndrome=HUS), or postrenal (i.e., obstruction to urine outflow). For further details on the incidence, laboratory findings, entities, pathophysiology, and clinical information, see chapters Renal Parenchymal Disease and Renal Failure and Renal Transplantation.

2.2 Urine Production After Birth and Neonatal Oligoanuria

First voiding often takes place in the delivery room. Healthy newborns pass urine during the first 24 h of life in 92–97% of cases and nearly all void within 48 h (Clark 1977; Wang and Huang 1994). Normal urine volume is 1–3 ml/kg and hour. Thus, polyuria is defined as urine output of more than 4 ml/kg and hour and oliguria as less than 0.5–1.0 ml/kg and hour. ARF is rare in apparently healthy neonates with a normal fetal ultrasound (US). The incidence of ARF in a neonatal intensive care unit (NICU) ranges from 1.5 to 23%. Oligoanuria is the leading symptom in about 40% of cases, and 60% suffer from non-oliguric ARF (Andreoli 2004; Hentschel et al. 1996; Karlowicz and Adelman 1995; Kupferman 1994).

3 Basic Considerations on Imaging in Renal Failure and Neonatal Oligoanuria

3.1 Renal Imaging in Renal Failure

In *CRF*, diagnostic imaging is extremely helpful in unraveling the underlying renal disease, and often an essential part already of the initial diagnosis of a chronic progressive disease, as well as for following up during the evolving process that leads to CRF. US is the basic investigation focusing on renal size and structure as well as potential collecting system pathology; further imaging depends on these US findings. In some situations complementing imaging by voiding cystourethrography (VCUG) or MR becomes necessary – usually in the initial work-up (e.g., high-grade vesicoureteric reflux with renal dysplasia or "reflux nephropathy" as cause of the CRF) or for assessing complications during treatment, monitoring treatment response (e.g., observe development of renal perfusion in HUS) as well as for preparing a potential renal transplantation (rTX).

On US – in chronic disease – the kidneys are generally more or less echodense, but may be small, normal sized, enlarged, or cystic; small echodense kidneys, possibly with a size difference, indicate hypodysplasia or renal scarring (Fig. 1). Focal compensatory hypertrophy may have a nodular tumor-like aspect. Concomitant dilatation of the ureter and/or renal pelvis can reflect vesicoureteric reflux (VUR) or urinary tract obstruction, but may also be caused by long-standing polyuria. In general, (bilateral) renal dysplasia with or without congenital uropathy is the most probable diagnosis in CRF. VCUG and isotope studies are recommended to complete the work-up.

In *ARF*, also US is usually the initial and often the only imaging modality (Gordon and Riccabona 2003). It will help to detect postrenal problems such as a bladder outlet obstruction or an upper tract obstruction in a single kidney – though one must consider that after renal function has ceased and no urine production is present as well as in peracute upper obstruction, no urinary tract dilatation must be present.

In the rare other typical findings in children with RF, nearly normal-sized or enlarged kidneys are found with intrarenal causes of ARF or on early follow-up of many acquired diseases such as glomerulonephritis and HUS. Loss of renal volume mostly indicates progressive CRF.

Fig. 1 Sonography (**a–c**) and VCUG (**d**) congenital reflux nephropathy/dysplasia in a newborn presenting with CRF and bilateral high-grade VUR. The initial US shows bilateral small kidneys with undifferentiated echogenic parenchyma and a dilated collecting system with thickened pelvic wall (**a** = axial view, **b** = sagittal section) and dysplastic cysts (**c**); VCUG depicts bilateral gross VUR without valve (**d**). Note that the left-sided VUR was only seen in the second filling on the cyclic VCUG

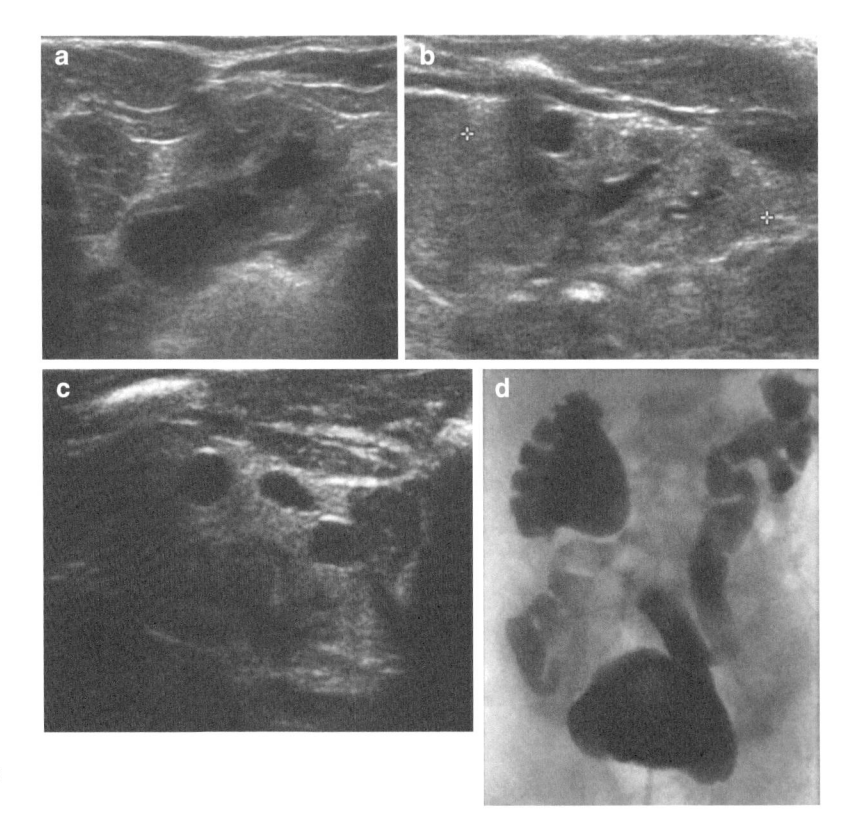

The most probable diagnoses in patients presenting with an as yet unrecognized CRF are Alport syndrome, juvenile nephronophthisis, oligomeganephronia, autosomal recessive polycystic kidney disease (ARPKD), and various syndromes with renal dysplasia. The nephronophthisis-medullary cystic disease complex is a distinct entity of inherited diseases with insidious onset of CRF. Again US contributes most to the diagnosis. On US these kidneys are normal or slightly reduced in size, echodense, and without corticomedullary differentiation. Corticomedullary cysts are characterized and are found predominantly in advanced CRF (Garel et al. 1984; Blowey et al. 1996; Chuang and Tsai 1998). Sometimes medullary cysts can be demonstrated also by CT or MRI (Elzouki et al. 1996); however, the latter investigations probably contribute little to the diagnosis of juvenile nephronophthisis as molecular genetic diagnosis is available (Hildebrandt et al. 1997; Hildebrandt and Otto 2005; Saunier et al. 2005).

If renal cysts are found, cystic disease must be defined as unilateral or bilateral and localized or diffuse (see chapters Renal Agenesis, Dysplasia, Hypoplasia and Cystic Diseases of the Kidney, Renal Parenchymal Disease and Imaging in Renal Agenesis, Dysplasia, Hypoplasia and Cystic Diseases of the Kidney). Extrarenal manifestations such as hepatic or pancreatic cysts should be sought as well as evidence of portal hypertension. CRF in unilateral cystic disease means renal hypodysplasia of the contralateral kidney even if the parenchyma appears relatively normal. Large bilateral cysts favor autosomal dominant polycystic disease, while enlarged and echodense kidneys are found in ARPKD (see chapter Imaging in Renal Agenesis, Dysplasia, Hypoplasia and Cystic Diseases of the Kidney). Glomerulocystic disease may have a similar appearance on US (Fitch and Stapleton 1986). Further differentiation is based on familial history, clinical, and genetic findings (El-Merhi and Bae 2004; Guay-Woodford 2006; Avni et al. 2012; Riccabona et al. 2012). Please note that renal cysts do not necessarily reflect the underlying disorder. Acquired renal cystic disease is a known complication of ESRD (Leichter et al. 1988) and may occur in CRF already before the start of dialysis (Hogg 1992).

3.2 Diagnostic Workup and Imaging in Neonatal Oligoanuria

If oligoanuria is recognized, many urgent questions arise, and the potentially underlying conditions should be recognized (Table 1). Before starting extensive investigations, pitfalls should be excluded. Previous voiding may have been missed; urine collection may be inappropriate with loss around the collection bag. Urine can be mixed with stool, and a previously inserted bladder catheter may be displaced or blocked. If true oligoanuria is combined with an increased serum creatinine, RF is proven. It is traditionally classified as prerenal, intrinsic, or postrenal failure. The term "prerenal" or "functional" implies a systemic disease with normalization of urine flow and of renal function after appropriate therapy. Intrinsic RF occurs in congenital or acquired renal diseases or by transition from prolonged prerenal failure; CRF may be the long-term consequence. Postrenal failure is mostly found in obstructive uropathy. Besides assessing anatomy, morphology, and potential malformations, US is commonly used as the most easily available and only bedside imaging method which is usually diagnostically sufficient; in applying Doppler techniques, US also allows for functional information on renal perfusion very helpful for differentiating prerenal from intrinsic RF and for judging the severity of the condition (Gordon and Riccabona 2003; Riccabona 2006).

3.3 Role of Imaging in Planning and During Dialysis

Once ESRD is reached, survival is possible with only blood purification, performed as peritoneal dialysis (PD) or hemodialysis (HD). According to a joint decision also including the family and

Table 1 Differential diagnosis of neonatal oligoanuria

1. Primary non-renal diseases (prerenal failure)
   (a) Hypovolemia
       Dehydration, reduced intake, increased losses (VLBW infant, phototherapy, stool, polyuria, third space as in peritonitis or NEC)
   (b) Blood loss (placental, umbilical)
   (c) Hemodynamic compromise
       Cardiac failure, surgery, hypotension, shock, PDA, AIST
   (d) Respiratory failure (IRDS, high mean airway pressure)
   (e) Septicemia
   (f) Asphyxia, hyperviscosity, anemia
2. Primary renal diseases (intrinsic failure)
   (a) Congenital (dysplasia, hypoplasia, agenesis, ARPKD)
   (b) Acquired
       Acute cortical, medullary, tubular necrosis, prolonged prerenal failure
       Renovascular accident (arterial, venous, DIC, HUS)
       UTI-pyelonephritis
       Toxic effects, drugs (indomethacin, ACE inhibitors, aminoglycosides), contrast agents, myoglobin, uric acid
3. Urinary tract obstruction (postrenal failure)
   (a) Congenital
       PUJO, UVJO, ureterocele, prune-belly syndrome, pelvic tumor, hydrometrocolpos, neurogenic bladder
   (b) Acquired: fungus balls, urolithiasis, urinary ascites
4. Miscellaneous causes
   (a) Maternal drugs (such as NSAID, ACE inhibitors, immunosuppressants)
   (b) Twin-to-twin transfusion syndrome
   (c) Neonatal (syndrome of inappropriate ADH release)
5. Pitfalls
       Inappropriate collection, blocked bladder catheter, inability to void (sedation, relaxation)

Adapted from Brion et al. (1997)
Abbreviations: *ACE* angiotensin-converting enzyme, *AIST* aortic coarctation, *ADH* antidiuretic hormone, *ARPKD* autosomal recessive polycystic kidney disease, *IRDS* ideopathic respiratory distress syndrome, *DIC* disseminated intravascular coagulopathy, *NSAID* nonsteroidal antiinflammatory drug, *HUS* hemolytic-uremic syndrome, *NEC* necrotising enterocolitis, *PDA* persistent ductus arteriosus, *PUJO* pelvi-ureteric junction obstruction, *UVJO* ureterovesical junction obstruction, *VLBW* very low birth weight

the patient, vascular access for HD or placement of a catheter must be planned. It is the steady state from which early and even preemptive rTX are planned and performed in children in most situations and to which patients return in the case of graft failure. Diagnostic imaging is mostly requested if complications such as a blocked peritoneal catheter or insufficient blood supply of Brescia-Cimino fistula are present. Interpretation of imaging in a disease state is problematic if no comparison with the normal situation is possible. Consequently, diagnostic imaging should be performed at regular intervals even if no problems are present and the diagnostic value of imaging is questionable at first sight.

3.3.1 Peritoneal Dialysis (PD)

PD is the preferred treatment in children with ESRD, and approximately 67% of patients are maintained on continuous PD (Lerner et al. 1999). It is the treatment of choice for infants (Fig. 2). A permanent PD catheter is placed surgically into the peritoneal cavity with the tip in the lower abdomen and a long subcutaneous tunnel. A plain abdominal radiograph can show the position that can be compared in case of catheter dysfunction. US (for subcutaneous) and T2-weighted MR (for retroperitoneal defects) can be used to assess peritoneal leaks in PD failure (Prischl et al. 2002) (Fig. 2).

PD complications can be divided into acute or chronic and infectious or noninfectious. Imaging with US, CT, and eventually MRI can contribute significantly to appropriate treatment of many situations (Taylor 2002). Acute catheter dysfunction may be caused by malposition and can be seen on a plain abdominal radiograph. Development of inguinal hernias is caused by the permanently increased intra-abdominal pressure, and herniotomy is frequently needed. Acute respiratory distress should raise suspicion of hydrothorax caused by thoracic leakage of peritoneal fluid (Rose and Conley 1989); US can easily depict it, and the conventionally performed chest X-ray can show this complication too (Fig. 3). Infections of the exit site, the subcutaneous tunnel, and peritonitis are the most common infectious complications. Tunnel infections typically show pericatheter fluid collection, and US is important for early detection and follow-up (Plum et al. 1994; Vychtytil et al.

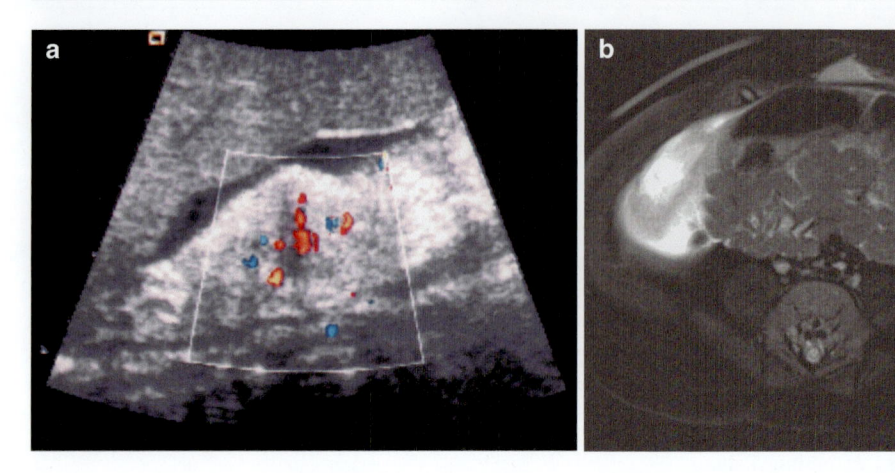

Fig. 2 Imaging in peritoneal dialysis: CDS of a shrunken, nearly non-perfused end-stage kidney in an infant with peritoneal dialysis. Peritoneal fluid within Morrison's pouch (**a**) and T2-weighted MRI image with fat saturation for depiction of leakage of peritoneal dialysis fluid in a child with dialysis failure (**b**)

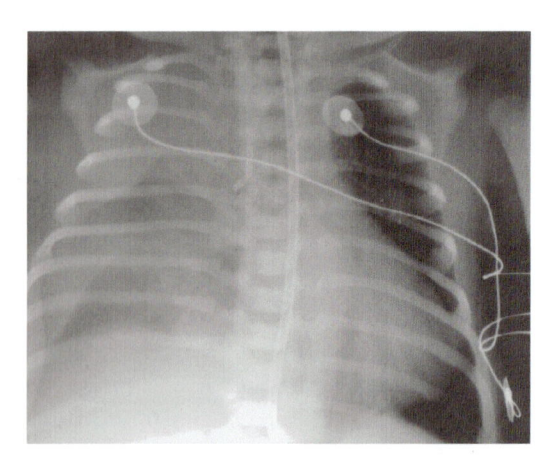

Fig. 3 Chest film: thoracic leak of peritoneal dialysate during peritoneal dialysis

1999). Peritoneal thickening and calcifications, loculated fluid collections, and tethering of the small bowel are diagnostic for peritonitis complicating PD and shown by US, CT, or MRI (Stafford-Johnson et al. 1998; Krestin et al. 1995). Normal values for parietal peritoneal thickness have been reported, enabling early detection of structural changes in the peritoneum by US (Faller et al. 1998).

3.3.2 Hemodialysis

Hemodialysis is a safe and effective treatment for children with ESRD and is performed in 46 % of such children aged more than 12 years (Lerner et al. 1999). Technical refinements enable HD even in small children and infants (Bunchman 1995; Al-Hermi et al. 1999). In this age group, HD is mostly indicated if PD fails or is contraindicated (Rödl et al. 2012a and b).

Vascular access is of utmost importance in pediatric HD. Central venous catheters, internal arteriovenous fistulas (Brescia-Cimino fistula), and synthetic grafts are used. Placement of central venous catheters is the preferred vascular access in many centers (Lerner et al. 1999; Neu et al. 2002). Arteriovenous fistulas are an alternative with a lower rate of complications compared to central venous catheters and sometimes with an improved metabolic control of the patient (Brittinger et al. 1997; Chand et al. 2005; Ramage et al. 2005). On the other hand, a rapid access to rTX may favor central venous catheters. US may be of value in guidance for placing the catheter and detecting thrombosis around the catheter. Doppler sonography or angiography can show stenosis of internal fistula and influence surgical therapy. Development of malignancy in acquired renal cystic disease on long-term dialysis is well recognized in adult patients and has also been reported in children (Levine 1992; Mattoo et al. 1997; Querfeld et al. 1992). Thus, a regular survey of the native kidneys with US and selective use of CT or MRI must be advised for children on dialysis and even after successful rTX.

3.4 Imaging for Planning Transplantation

There are different needs for imaging when planning a renal transplantation (rTX): basically these can be summarized by assessment of the recipient as well as of the donor.

The recipient needs a thorough work-up to grant success of the rTX and to minimize risks. Urological disorders frequently need nephrectomy or nephrecto-ureterectomy before considering transplantation. Assessment of bladder function with VCUG and eventually with cystomanometry is mandatory to prevent bladder problems after transplantation. An augmented bladder is no contraindication for transplantation (Koo et al. 1999; Fontaine et al. 1998; Rigamonti et al. 2005). Renal and abdominal US, VCUG, and eventually MR angiography to show the vascular situation in the region of transplantation are performed; sometimes, however, the higher resolution of CT angiography (CTA) without the risk of nephrogenic systemic fibrosis in children, ESRF will indicate a CTA for vascular pre-transplant assessment.

The donor also needs imaging, and respective recommendations are available (Riccabona et al. 2012; Damasio et al. 2017). A living-related donor must undergo extensive clinical, laboratory, and imaging investigations to ensure that no undue risks are incurred by removal of one kidney; furthermore, it must be granted that the kidney which will be transplanted is healthy and suitable. This imaging is achieved by US, scintigraphy, and sometimes MR; rarely a CT is necessary. A deceased donors' kidney also usually is checked for unrecognized disease and suitability – at least an US study (preferably including CDS to assess vascular supply thus reducing the risk of vascular injury during explantation) is recommended; in childhood rTX this study should include renal size assessment to allow for finding a suitable size match. If (as suggested in some countries for establishing brain death) a CTA/perfusion CT of the brain is performed, the abdominal organs (including the kidneys) can also easily be assessed by extending this contrast-enhanced CT study to the abdomen, e.g., in the late post-bolus phase.

3.5 Extrarenal Imaging in Chronic Renal Failure

The cardiovascular system and the bones are prone to lesions in CRF and ESRD. Cardiac dysfunction is present in most patients and is a major cause of death in ESRD and after renal transplantation (Ehrich et al. 1992; Parekh and Gidding 2005). Chest X-ray may show pulmonary edema, an enlarged vascular pedicle, and cardiac dilatation in volume overload, but can be normal despite severe cardiac dysfunction. Dilative uremic cardiomyopathy is characterized by an increased cardiac volume, a decreased number of cardiomyocytes, and an expanded interstitium. Left ventricular hypertrophy is an early prognostic sign for cardiac compromise (Schärer et al. 1999). Hypervolemia, hypertension, and anemia worsen cardiac function. Cardiac US including Doppler sonography, cardiac CT to look for coronary calcium in young adults (Oh et al. 2002), and functional evaluation can unravel these changes, and a dilated vena cava inferior indicates volume overload. Recently, cardiac MRI has gained an important role in assessing cardiac function, too.

The kidneys have a major contribution in mineral and bone homeostasis. Renal osteodystrophy (ROD) is a serious consequence of CRF and ESRD. Untreated ROD is critical especially in the years of skeletal growth with growth retardation and osseous deformities as a disabling consequence. Bone pain, fractures, slipped epiphyses, muscle weakness, and extraskeletal calcifications (vascular, cardiac, pulmonary, renal, periarticular) are signs of severe ROD. Impaired renal calcitriol synthesis (1,25-dihydroxyvitamin D), phosphate retention, Vitamin D deficiency, hypocalcemia, secondary hyperparathyroidism, alterations of parathyroid hormone action and catabolism, and alterations in the calcium-sensing receptor are the main pathogenetic factors. A broad spectrum from high-turnover to low-turnover bone lesions can be distinguished by laboratory and radiographic findings. High-turnover disease (osteitis fibrosa) is characterized by secondary hyperparathyroidism and by increased bone resorption located in the subperiosteal and endosteal surface of cortical bone. Radiographically, the clavicles, pelvic bones, meta-diaphyseal junction of long bones, and phalanges preferably show these lesions. Focal radiolucencies and sclerotic areas are additional findings. Low-turnover disease (adynamic bone) is characterized by widening of the epiphyseal growth plate and wide radiolucent bands within the cortex indicating pseudofractures and Looser zones. In the past, adynamic lesions were mostly related to aluminum toxicity caused by administration of aluminum-containing phosphate binding agents. Up to 50 % of patients with ESRD have low-turnover disease, and aggressive therapy of ROD contributes in part (Salusky and Goodman 1996; Rigden 1996). Guidelines for prevention and treatment of ROD were published (Klaus et al. 2006; KDIGO CKD-MBD Work Group 2009). Usually, plain films/digital radiographs are sufficient for these purposes, rarely a CT or a MRI may become necessary – mostly for differential diagnosis in some rare situations. Bone densitometry (mostly using CT or a DEXA system or US-based devices) may be helpful in directing treatment of these sequelae of CRF.

> **Take Away**
> Imaging is an essential part of handling children with RF and neonates with oligoanuria. It heavily relies on US; other methods are less frequently necessary and useful. Imaging also is essential for following up these patients, monitoring treatment, and assessing complications also in other regions than the urinary tract. Furthermore, it is important for planning and preparing for rTX.
>
> Knowledge of the various entities, the pathophysiology as well as the clinical implications is essential to properly indicate, plan, perform and read these studies – thus a close collaboration with the pediatric nephrourologist is essential.

4 Imaging Methods and Findings

4.1 Basic Situation

Renal US has dramatically changed and improved the diagnostic and therapeutic possibilities in renal disease. Fetal renal US is available in most pregnancies. Thus, we are aware in advance that many newborns have significant renal and urinary tract pathology. Yet a normal fetal and a normal neonatal US do not exclude renal disease, and the severity of prenatal and postpartal findings may be different. The basic approach to *neonates with oligoanuria* is (1) stabilize the baby; (2) get basic imaging with US, including Doppler sonography (DS) and amplitude-coded color Doppler sonography (aCDS) as noninvasive bedside investigations; and (3) adjust therapy according to the findings (e.g., suprapubic catheter in suspected posterior urethral valve). If the definite diagnosis is not yet established, one has time to consider further imaging. As a rule, the impact of imaging on therapy at a given time must be weighed against the risk of compromising the baby by transport or delay of medical therapy.

For *CRF later in childhood* imaging has usually played an important role in establishing the diagnosis and follow-up. The task of imaging in these children is to monitor the disease process, to assess potential complications, and to evaluate extrarenal implications (see above).

In *ARF*, imaging often is essential to define the cause (and the severity) with all its prognostic implications and thus help to direct treatment. This is usually achieved by US, complemented by other imaging if necessary. In some situations, only histology will clarify and define the disease – then imaging again is essential for providing a safe and effective renal biopsy (Riccabona et al. 2014) (see also chapters Imaging in Renal Parenchymal Disease and Pediatric Genitourinary Intervention).

And finally imaging may be important to *support therapeutic measures* such as image guidance for central line placement (e.g., for fluid balance and hemofiltration/dialysis), for assessing complications, or for guiding a percutaneous drainage of an obstructed system.

4.2 Ultrasound

Normal values for renal size are available (see chapter Normal Values). The normal US appearance depends on age – in neonates it shows a high cortical echogenicity, probably related to the high proportion of glomeruli compared to tubular structures and almost anechoic pyramids (Scott et al. 1990; Slovis et al. 1993). Transient medullary hyperechogenicity are found in 13–58 % of neonates (Riebel et al. 1993; Starinsky et al. 1995; Howlett et al. 1997; Nakamura et al. 1999). It seems to be a transient phenomenon depending on urine flow, protein excretion, or protein cast deposition and is not a sign of renal failure. The term "hyperechoic papillae of the newborn" has been introduced and will eventually replace other nomenclature (Nakamura et al. 1999). Five US appearances are associated with neonatal oligoanuria: (1) no kidney present, (2) uni- or bilateral hydronephrosis, (3) cystic lesions, (4) focal or generalized hyperechogenicity, and (5) focal accumulation of echodense material. These appearances, more than one of which can be present in a single patient, combined with determination of renal size (small or enlarged), and evaluation of clinical data will point to or establish the correct diagnosis in most cases (Figs. 1 and 4). For example, bilateral hydroureteronephrosis with echodense kidneys and cortical cysts in a boy with a trabeculated bladder wall is almost diagnostic for oliguric RF in posterior urethral valves. The differential diagnosis of oligoanuria in enlarged hyperechoic kidneys without corticomedullary differentiation is shown in Table 2. In older patients with RF, there are a variety of US findings that depend on the underlying disease and duration (see respective chapters and Sect. 3.1).

4.3 Doppler Sonography and Other Modern Sonographic Imaging Methods

Both (color) Doppler sonography (CDS) and amplitude-coded color Doppler sonography (aCDS) investigations add functional imaging to the anatomic-morphologic description of US and are mandatory in neonatal oligoanuria and RF (Gordon and Riccabona 2003). Reduced renal systolic flow velocity in asphyxiated neonates on the first day of life has been reported to have 100 % sensitivity for subsequent development of RF (Luciano et al. 1998). These and further findings can influence therapy significantly. Normal renal architecture with a normal perfusion may indicate a favorable outcome in prerenal failure, while focal non-perfused areas are found in renal cortical or medullary necrosis or renovascular accidents. Decreased systolic flow velocity and an increased resistive index (RI) are found in cystic dysplastic kidneys (Riccabona et al. 1993).

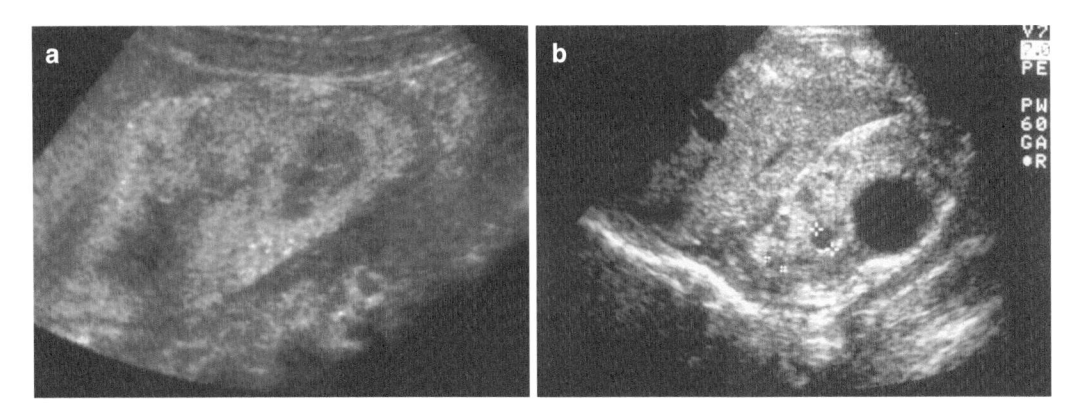

Fig. 4 Sonography: (**a**) echodense kidneys in acute renal failure, (**b**) renal dysplasia with cortical cysts and a dilated renal pelvis in prune-belly syndrome

Table 2 The differential diagnosis of oligoanuria in enlarged hyperechoic kidneys without corticomedullary differentiation

Acute tubular necrosis
Renal venous thrombosis
Autosomal recessive polycystic kidney disease
Diffuse cystic dysplasia
Septicemia including renal candidiasis
Contrast nephropathy

Note that the (C)DS findings including the flow spectrum are mostly influenced by the impairment of renal function and not so much specific of an underlying disease (Riccabona 2006); the same applies, e.g., for aCDS and the cortical non-perfused "halo" that can often be observed in kidneys with ARF (Riccabona 2014a, b).

A specific though rare phenomenon is neonatal renal vein thrombosis; the US appearance of renal venous thrombosis – being unilateral in the majority of neonates – may vary with the stage of disease (Wright et al. 1996; Hibbert et al. 1997). Initially, the interlobular or interlobar thrombus (or regional hemorrhagic infraction) may be visible as an echogenic streak (sometimes this is only the remnant of the neonatally echogenic distal medulla). Calcification of the thrombus at diagnosis supports an antenatal onset of thrombosis being present in at least some cases. Swelling of the kidney leads to increased echogenicity – potentially with prominent hypoechoic pyramids. An increased renal size/length (e.g., above 60 mm or more in the neonate) at presentation strongly predicts permanent kidney damage as outcome (Winyard et al. 2006). Later, the kidney becomes heterogeneous with loss of corticomedullary differentiation. Focal scarring or an atrophic kidney, documented by US follow-up investigations or a DMSA scan, may be the result. If renovascular supply is compromised, CDS with spectral analysis of the renal and the great vessels must be performed and may show thrombosis of the vena cava inferior in renal venous thrombosis or of the abdominal aorta in renal artery thrombosis (Ellis et al. 1997). Typically there is a missing venous flow intrarenally and a high resistance flow profile in the artery – with often inverted diastolic flow – as the blood is returned from the obstructed renal venous outflow; these flow alterations have to be distinguished from systemic flow alteration (e.g., in cardiac conditions and malformations) by comparison with other parenchymal perfusion areas (e.g., contralateral kidney, the brain, the liver). aCDS may add valuable information concerning the general blood supply of the kidney or the presence of focal non-perfused areas. This sensitive investigation is to a great extent dependent on the skill of the investigator and the quality of the equipment.

4.4 Plain Films/Radiography, Isotope Investigations, Computerized Tomography, and Intravenous Pyelography

Isotope investigations are widely performed in various renal diseases and give valuable results even in infants (Wong et al. 1995; Gordon and Riccabona 2003). There seems to be no indication in acute oliguric renal failure, but results are important during follow-up for split renal function, renal scarring, and urinary obstruction.

CT and intravenous pyelography require the use of contrast medium and are contraindicated in renal failure.

Plain films can be of use in cases associated with calcification or urolithiasis (Fig. 5).

4.5 Use of Contrast Agents in Renal Failure

Use of most contrast agents (CA) is contraindicated in RF, as they need a functioning kidney for clearance. In general, particularly iodinated CAs may decrease renal blood flow and cause contrast-induced nephropathy (CIN) with ARF (Murphy et al. 2000; Thomsen et al. 2014). CA should be avoided whenever possible in neonates even with normal renal function. If indicated (e.g., for cardiac catheterization), adequate hydration is mandatory. Administration of the adenosine antagonist theophylline seems to be a promising means of preventing contrast-induced nephropathy (Kolonko et al. 1998; Huber et al. 2006); this also applies for

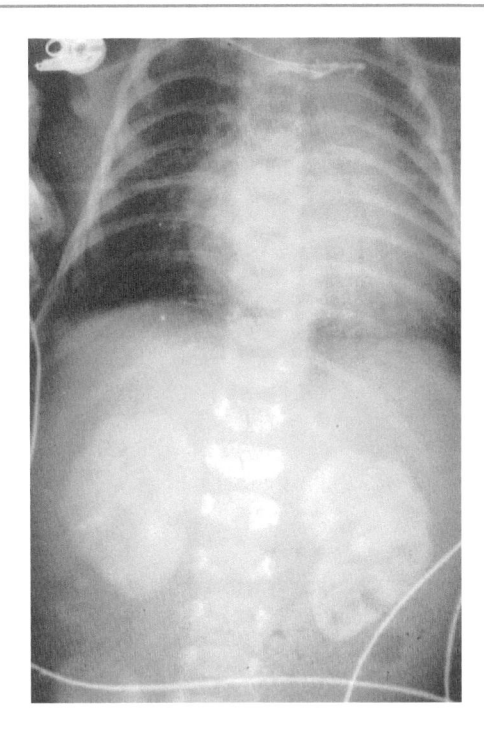

Fig. 5 Plain radiograph. Bilateral nephrocalcinosis in an infant with primary hyperoxaluria type 1 presenting with oliguria during the first weeks of life

acetylcysteine – however, there are no dedicated data or studies in larger pediatric cohorts. However, this may be also of value in neonates and preterm neonates, where theophylline was reported to improve renal function in neonates with respiratory distress syndrome (Huet et al. 1995; Cattarelli et al. 2006). Recommendations and guidelines on the use of all kinds of CAs in neonates, infants, and children and in RF are available (see also chapters Diagnostic Procedures: Excluding MRI, Nuclear Medicine and Video-Urodynamics and Contrast Agents in Childhood: Application and Safety Considerations) (Riccabona 2014a, b); GRF calculation for assessment of renal function is suggested in all patients particularly those with risks for renal impairment prior to intravenous CA application; adapted pediatric equations must be used (Schwartz et al. 1976, 1984). Recently some discussion arose on the real impact of iodinated CA on renal function, and CIN is under discussion – at least in adults with a GFR above 40 (Newhouse et al. 2008; Davenport et al. 2013; McDonald et al. 2013a, b; Thomsen et al. 2014). Nevertheless, although radiopaque CA by themselves obviously do not cause acute renal injury in healthy kidneys, they remain a cofactor for inducing renal damage particularly in patients with coexisting risks such as diabetes mellitus or other medication with nephrotoxic drugs. Thus – even considering these new insights – the use of iodinated CA should be avoided in neonates and children with RF.

Particular caution should be used with gadolinium (Gd)-based CAs in neonates and in all children with reduced renal clearance; in fact our knowledge – but our knowledge on the depositions in the body is yet limited, and no information is available on potential long-term effects of those deposits (e.g., as recently been found in the brain, the bone marrow, in the skin – and not only in patients with renal impairment) as known for nephrogenic systemic fibrosis already for some time (McDonald et al. 2015; Sanyal et al. 2011).

US-CA are not approved for pediatric use – however, these pose a promising option if a contrast-enhanced study is necessary, as they are not excreted by the kidney and thus are applicable in RF; reports on their successful pediatric use (even in RF) for both, the intravesical administration and the intravenous route, describe their potential benefit (Stenzel and Mentzel 2014; Rosado and Riccabona 2016).

4.6 Voiding Cystourethrography

VCUG is an integrative part of investigating neonates with urinary tract malformations. It may be indicated in oliguric neonates with postrenal failure due to posterior urethral valves or bilateral megaureters to differentiate obstructive and reflexive units and to determine the site of intervention (vesical or supravesical). It furthermore is used for pretransplant assessment or for completing work-up of end-stage uropathies of unknown origin. Contrast-enhanced voiding urosonography (ce-VUS) has been established as an alternative reliable modality (see chapter Diagnostic Procedures: Excluding MRI, Nuclear Medicine and Video-Urodynamics); this enables bedside investigations and is of value especially in severely compromised NICU patients. Another rare indication for VCUG is postrenal failure in neonates with suspected posterior urethral valves or infants and children with pelvic tumors, potentially with a congenital bladder or caliceal rupture, where VCUG can exquisitely show urine extravasation (Zaninovic et al. 1992). In most situations, however, VCUG can be delayed and is performed after stabilization.

4.7 Magnetic Resonance Imaging

MRI can be performed even in neonates and provides excellent anatomic imaging in this special group of patients (Avni et al. 2002; Riccabona et al. 2002). Additionally, diffusion-weighted MRI and other modern techniques such BOLD imaging offer new functional information without the need for contrast administration (see chapter MR of the Urogenital Tract in Children). Although eventually applied, we are not aware of valuable data concerning MRI in neonates with renal failure. There is no restriction to perform renal MRI without Gd-containing CA even in oligoanuric neonates and RF patients. However, application of Gd-containing CA for MRI to patients with RF is of major concern nowadays and also in neonates. Development of nephrogenic systemic fibrosis (NSF) is a serious and life-threatening adverse event (see chapter Contrast Agents in Childhood: Application and Safety Considerations, and Sect. 4.5). NSF is directly correlated to Gd (mostly to linear compounds such as gadodiamide), which was found to be deposited in various and affected tissues (Thomsen 2006; Broome et al. 2007). Thus, aside from emergency situations, we currently do not recommend MRI with routine application of intravenous CA in neonates and infants during the first 2 months of life, even with a normal renal function (also see above – Sect. 4.5). An informed consent of the parents for intravenous application of CA for MRI has to be obtained like in CT with CA, particularly if there is renal functional impairment. In addition, serum creatinine representing actual renal function has to be known before the investigation, and age-adapted GFR estimations should be performed (see chapters Contrast Agents in Childhood: Application and Safety Considerations, Renal Parenchymal Disease, and Normal Values). Future research will show whether the CA-associated side effects are proven to be cumbersome and whether MRI can offer valuable information on neonatal renal disease (potentially applying non-enhanced MR techniques) with oligoanuria or in pediatric RF patients in addition to (ce-)US, (C)DS, and aCDS. The latter investigations are performed much more easily, at the bedside, and at a lower cost.

> **Take Away**
> US, (C)DS, and aCSDS are essential for differential diagnosis of neonates with oligoanuria and pediatric patients with RF; furthermore they are useful to monitor therapy. If indicated, further investigations such as VCUG, ce_VUS, MRI, or isotope studies can be delayed and are performed after stabilization in most cases. Long-term follow-up is mandatory, even in cases with apparent complete recovery of (neonatal) renal failure.

5 Renal Transplantation

5.1 Basic Considerations

Renal transplantation (rTX) is universally accepted as the therapy of choice in children with ESKD. Transplantation results in better survival than dialysis for pediatric patients of all ages; furthermore, successful rTX ameliorates metabolic and hormonal control, skeletal growth, sexual maturation, and cognitive and psychosocial performance better than both hemodialysis and peritoneal dialysis (Tsai 2010).

Allograft transplants can be harvested from living or diseased donors, while living donor grafts are associated with substantially improved outcomes in the pediatric population. Children with irreversible CDK stage G4 should be preemptively transplanted if a donor is available (Hardy et al. 2009).

Many aspects of clinical handling in rTX are comparable in children and adults (see also chapter Renal Failure and Renal Transplantation). Similar immunosuppressive medications and regimens are used, creatinine is the major serum biomarker, acute rejection is determined primarily by means of biopsy with the use of Banff criteria for the classification of rejection and allograft pathology (Solez et al. 2008), and the rejection mechanisms of the kidney graft are generally similar. However, many other aspects differ between children and adults, for example, the primary kidney diseases leading to RF differ and are often associated with urologic issues. In addition, immunologic factors and the immunizations that are required before transplantation differ considerably in the pediatric age.

Allocation policies regarding kidneys from deceased donors, surgical techniques in small children, and drug metabolism have distinctive aspects in children. The frequency of primary viral infection after transplantation is higher for children than for adults. Furthermore, children are actively developing so their linear-height growth needs to be optimized and their neurocognitive development fostered (Nankivell and Alexander 2010; Harmon 2010; Dharnidharka et al. 2014).

Current success in pediatric rTX is attributed to improvements in transplantation technology and surgical techniques, immunosuppressive therapy, and age-appropriate clinical care; however, these patients are also prone to complications from surgery and immunosuppression, and therefore accurate imaging assessment is critical for implementing effective treatment.

> **Take Away**
> Renal transplantation is the therapy of choice in children with ESKD.

5.2 Surgical Technique

Renal transplants in children are almost always heterotopic allografts. Grafts can be placed in either an intra- or extraperitoneal location, even though the second is preferred since surgical complications associated with the peritoneal cavity are minimized with the extraperitoneal location. In older children, the allograft is placed in the right or left iliac fossa, as it is in adults. Vascular supply is typically established with end-to-side anastomosis of the transplant renal artery and vein to the ipsilateral external iliac artery and vein, respectively, or – if these vessels are too small – the distal abdominal aorta and inferior cava vein.

If there is considerable difference in sizes between the donor and infant or small pediatric recipient, an intra-abdominal location can be used, with an end-to-side anastomosis of the transplant renal artery to the aorta, to maximize graft perfusion. The transplant ureter is typically directly implanted into the native bladder with a ureteroneocystostomy, only sometimes a reflux-protective implantation technique is used. Nephroureteral stent placement is often performed at the time of surgery to mitigate the risk of early ureteral obstruction (Nixon et al. 2013).

> **Take Away**
> Renal transplants are heterotopic. Extraperitoneal location is preferred, usually in the right or left iliac fossa.

5.3 Postoperative and Surveillance Imaging

US, including gray-scale US with CDS and spectral DS (CDUS), is the gold standard for anatomic imaging of renal transplants in children (Kolofousi et al 2012). An immediate postoperative CDUS examination (performed within 24–48 h) after transplantation is recommended to investigate early complications and to serve as a baseline for future imaging. Additional early postoperative CDUS imaging examinations are performed, depending on the results of the initial postoperative CDUS and the patient's clinical course. Abnormalities in renal function or specific complaints referable to the graft may trigger additional diagnostic imaging or renal biopsy. And for some specific indications, ce-US may serve as a valuable bedside imaging tool (Fig. 6). And in some centers, early (protocol) biopsies

Fig. 6 Contrast-enhanced ultrasound (ce-US): a child after en bloc rTX of two neonatal grafts and acute early posttransplant graft failure – intravenous ce-US confirms the lack of perfusion in both grafts (due to occlusion at the common vascular anastomoses because vessel size mismatch). Split/dual image display with the contrast image on the left side, the basic gray-scale image on the right side showing the en bloc graft as a pair of neonatal kidneys

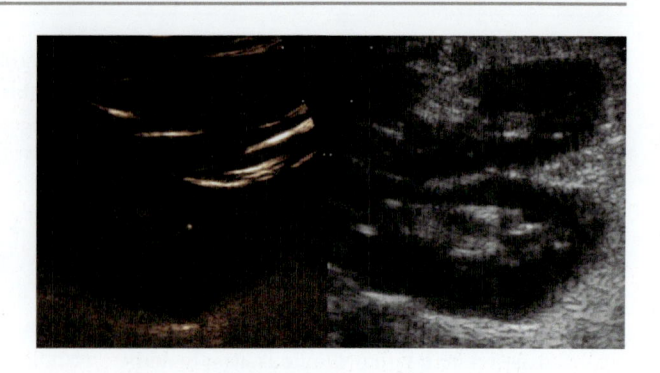

are used or may become necessary for adaptation of immunosuppression (Bruel et al. 2014).

Cross-sectional imaging and renal perfusion scintigraphy are used for further evaluation only in selected cases. MRI without or with concomitant CA application, enhanced or non-enhanced MR angiography, and static and excretory MR urography are increasingly used in the evaluation of posttransplant complications.

CT is rarely the examination of choice in the evaluation of rTX complications in children because of concerns regarding radiation dose and exposure of the allograft to iodinated CA and most of all today because of existing alternative examinations.

Renal scintigraphy with 99mTc-mertiatide is used adjunctively for functional allograft assessment on a case-by-case basis.

Conventional angiography remains the reference standard for confirmation and treatment of vascular complications and can be indicated provided there is sufficient time without risking the graft and particularly if there is an inherent (interventional) treatment option which then can be performed in the same session (Barba et al. 2011; Bou Matar et al. 2012).

> **Take Away**
> CDUS is the main imaging modality in rTX follow-up. Abnormalities in renal function or specific complaints may trigger additional diagnostic imaging (MR, MRA, CT) or renal biopsy.

5.4 The Normal Renal Allograft

A detailed examination protocol includes measurement of renal size and echogenicity, collecting system and ureter condition, and evaluation of any postoperative collections. CDU should assess presence of flow and flow velocity in the renal and iliac vessels as well as evaluate intrarenal vessels.

The collecting system of a well-functioning transplant is often slightly dilated (Fig. 7), presumably because of a combination of an increased volume of urine production and loss of the ureter's tonicity from denervation. However, in the unobstructed transplant, filling should be minor and confined to the renal pelvis, while filling of the infundibula or the calyces is suspicious of significant outflow obstruction.

DS evaluation of the kidney involves global assessment of renal flow by using CDS or aCDS, as well as investigation of the intra- and extrarenal vasculature supplemented by a spectral Doppler analysis (Fig. 7). Although the evaluation is purely qualitative, parenchymal perfusion assessed with CDS or aCDS should be uniform throughout the graft. RI values of 0.8 or lower are expected, although the clinical context should be considered in case of abnormal values, too.

The main renal artery is usually readily visualized, but is often much more tortuous than that of the native kidneys (Fig. 7d). Spectral Doppler analysis of the renal vein will demonstrate continuous antegrade flow with variable phasicity depending on the functional distance from the right atrium (Nixon et al. 2013).

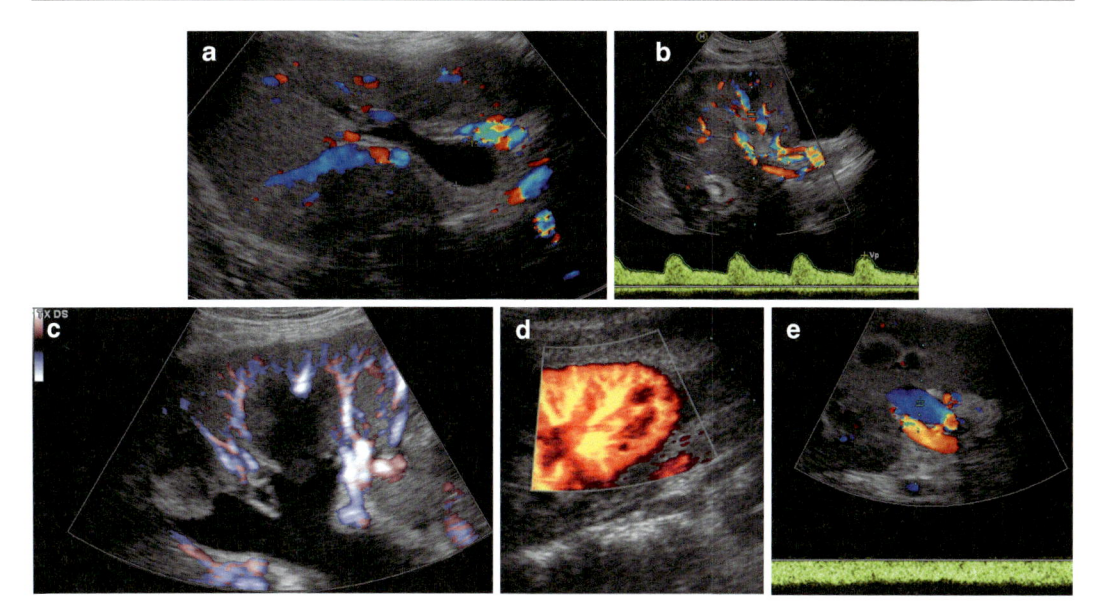

Fig. 7 The US evaluation of a renal allograft demonstrates an intrapelvic kidney with US features identical to those of a native one. The collecting system is often slightly dilated because of loss of tonicity from denervation – however, in the non-obstructed transplant, the filling should be confined to the renal pelvis (+ +) without dilatation of the collecting system unless already preexisting (**a**); spectral Doppler analysis from the interlobar vessels shows the normal fast systolic upstroke with a subsequent slow decay in diastole and a sufficient end-diastolic antegrade flow, thus RI values <0.8 in central vessels are to be expected (**b**); color flow fills out to the peripheral renal parenchyma right till to the renal capsule when using power Doppler (**c**); power Doppler may be useful to assess peripheral cortical perfusion (**d**); the main renal vein is easily accessible for (*color*) Doppler studies (**e**)

> **Take Away**
> The CDUS protocol in rTx includes measurement of renal size and echogenicity, evaluation of the collecting system and ureter, and evaluation of any postoperative collections. Color/power and spectral Doppler imaging should assess flow in the renal and iliac vessels, the respective flow velocities, as well as evaluate the intrarenal vessels.

5.5 Posttransplant Complications

Based on a compartmental morphologic and functional assessment, posttransplant complications can be categorized by entity and cause as (a) nephrologic complications causing graft dysfunction, (b) surgical problems, (c) drug toxicity, (d) infections, and (e) mass lesions (Table 3).

5.5.1 Nephrologic Complications Causing Graft Dysfunction

Several clinical syndromes of graft dysfunction have been defined relative to the time elapsed following transplantation.

Primary graft nonfunction describes a graft that never recovers function. Primary graft nonfunction is typically the result of (a) hyperacute or acute humoral rejection or (b) early vascular thrombosis, rarely of ischemic damage of the graft prior to implantation. Delayed graft dysfunction is defined by the requirement for dialysis within the first week after renal transplantation (Siedlecki et al. 2011). The central pathologic condition underlying delayed graft dysfunction is acute tubular necrosis (ATN). Acute graft dysfunction can occur at any time after recovery

Table 3 Pediatric renal transplant complications

Nephrologic complications causing early graft dysfunction
ATN
Rejection
Toxic effects of calcineurin inhibitors
Recurrence
Chronic allograft injury
Surgical complications
Perinephric fluid collections
Hematoma and seroma
Lymphocele
Urinoma
Abscess
Vascular complications
Renal vascular (artery, vein) thrombosis
Renal artery stenosis
Arteriovenous fistula
Pseudoaneurysm
Urologic complications
Urinoma
Urinary tract obstruction
Vesicoureteral reflux
Extrarenal drug toxicity
Infections
Mass lesion
Posttransplant lymphoproliferative disease

Abbreviations: *ATN* acute tubular necrosis

of graft function and most commonly results from acute rejection. A common alternative cause of parenchymal acute graft dysfunction is the acute toxic effect of calcineurin inhibitor therapy.

Chronic allograft injury refers to the progressive irreversible loss of graft function that results from chronic rejection, toxic effects of drug therapy, hypertensive nephropathy, or chronic graft infection.

The CDUS features of ATN, acute rejection, and nephrotoxicity are nonspecific and include renal enlargement with heterogeneous echogenicity of the thickened renal cortex, less evident corticomedullary differentiation, relative hypo-echogenicity of the renal pyramids in relation to a rather hyperechoic cortex and particularly in acute rejection uroepithelial thickening. Reduced diastolic flow with a resistive index (RI) higher than 0.9 is sensitive for pathology, but this is often not specific and must be interpreted in the context of clinical and laboratory findings. Differentiation between ATN, acute rejection, or drug nephrotoxicity cannot be based on imaging findings alone, and renal biopsy is often necessary.

Graft dysfunction may also be the consequence of recurrence of the primary disease such as in FGS and atypical HUS (Valoti et al. 2012; Cravedi et al. 2013).

Similar imaging findings are observed in chronic allograft injury regardless of cause. Anatomic imaging demonstrates progressive volume loss with diffuse cortical atrophy, often with superimposed focal cortical scarring. Mild to moderate collection system dilatation may be revealed, even in the absence of obstruction; CDS may reveal reduced peripheral perfusion, sometimes with patchy appearance. Renal scintigraphy demonstrates a small graft with poor perfusion and globally decreased function, findings that are similar to those of chronic obstruction or long-standing renal artery stenosis. As, however, differentiation of the most common entities for late and chronic allograft injury, i.e., drug toxicity and rejection, is only possible by histology, and renal biopsies are often necessary – some centers perform "protocol" biopsies in regular intervals, whereas others only perform a biopsy on clinical demand.

5.5.2 Surgical Complications

Perinephric fluid collections are a frequent complication of renal transplantation, occurring in as many as one-half of posttransplant patients at any time after graft placement. Perinephric collections include hematoma, lymphocele, seroma, abscess, and urinoma. The timing of occurrence is predictive of the cause. Most of these collections are small and asymptomatic, requiring no treatment. Cases should be followed over time to ensure resolution because enlarging fluid collections can reflect evolving infection or continuing vascular or urinary extravasation. Perinephric fluid collections are readily imaged by using CDS, with cross-sectional and functional imaging reserved for selected cases. *Perinephric hematoma* can also commonly occur as a complication after renal biopsy (Fig. 8). Subcapsular hematoma can cause parenchymal compression with resulting hypoperfusion, the so-called Page kidney.

Lymphoceles are encapsulated collections of lymphatic fluid that accumulate in the surgical bed, most commonly between 4 and 8 weeks after transplantation. They are believed to result from disruption of normal lymphatic channels during perivascular dissection or from disruption of hilar lymphatic vessels at the time of transplantation. As with perinephric hematomas, small lymphoceles tend to be asymptomatic. Larger collections can cause mass effect, with the possibility of vascular or ureteral obstruction, parenchymal compression, and graft dysfunction. The imaging appearance of a posttransplant lymphocele at CDS is that of a perinephric fluid collection that is largely anechoic. It may contain multiple thin septa and can appear multilocular (Fig. 9). MRI shows a perinephric collection that is hyperintense on T2-weighted images and hypointense on T1-weighted images, sometimes with internal loculation. The septa depicted by CDS and MRI are typically not apparent with CT, and there is no septal enhancement. *Urinoma*s are usually caused by urine leaks at the uretero-vesical anastomosis or as a consequence of a focal renal infarction with collecting system involvement and subsequent leak of urine. Antegrade pyelography or ce-MRU can be used to demonstrate the urine leak; if a percutaneous renal drain is in place, diluted US-CA (as for ce-VUS) can also be instilled to visualize the connection of the collecting system to the perinephric fluid collection (Riccabona 2014b).

Even if quite rare, *abscesses* remain an important complication of renal transplantation, usually in the first postoperative month. Perinephric abscesses can result from infection of the surgical site, spontaneous or iatrogenic infection of a previously sterile fluid collection, or complicated pyelonephritis. In a febrile patient, any perineph-

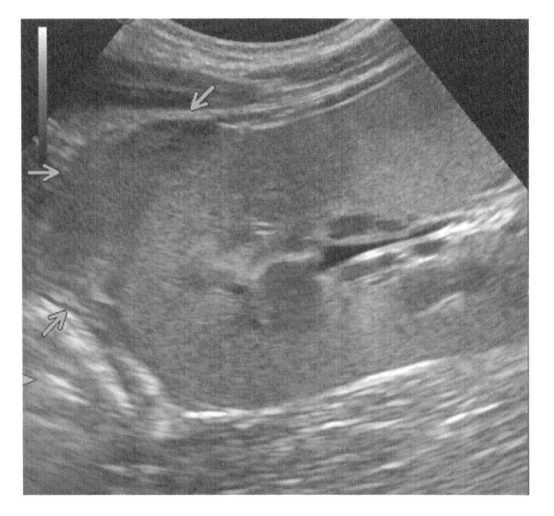

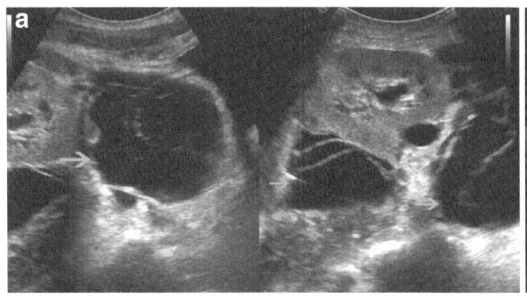

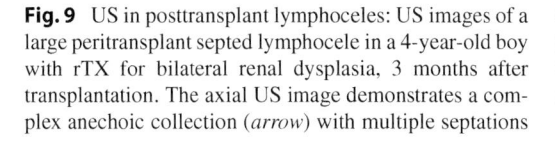

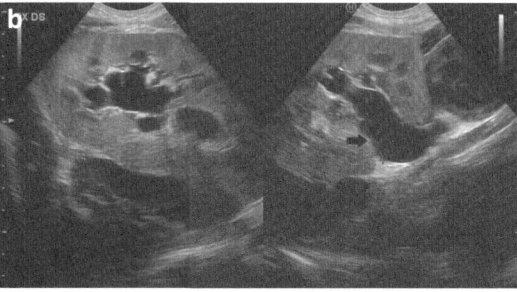

Fig. 8 US in posttransplant perinephric hematoma: A post-biopsy perinephric hematoma (*arrows*) in a 7-year-old boy with renal transplant for reflux nephropathy. Longitudinal gray-scale US shows a crescent echogenic middle complex and perirenal fluid collections around the upper pole of the renal graft

Fig. 9 US in posttransplant lymphoceles: US images of a large peritransplant septed lymphocele in a 4-year-old boy with rTX for bilateral renal dysplasia, 3 months after transplantation. The axial US image demonstrates a complex anechoic collection (*arrow*) with multiple septations at the medial aspect of the renal transplant (**a**); the lymphocele exerts a mass effect on the collecting system of the graft resulting in dilatation of the collecting system (*arrow*, + += renal pelvis) (**b**)

ric fluid collection should be considered infected until proved otherwise; rarely also intrarenal abscesses can develop. On US abscesses appear as a hypoechoic mass with thick irregular walls or capsule. Ce-MRI (or ce-CT) will show a peripheral membrane-like enhancement (as does in ce-US) with a central necrotic complex fluid collection (nicely demonstrated by DWI on MRI); treatment can be image (US)-guided puncture and drainage in addition to the proper antibiotic regime (see also below – Sect. 5.5.4) (Nixon et al. 2013).

Vascular complications include renal artery thrombosis with parenchymal infarction, renal vein thrombosis, and renal artery stenosis. Vascular complications represent an important cause of morbidity after pediatric renal transplantation, affecting between 5 and 10 % of patients. An increased risk of early vascular thrombosis has been observed in children because of their small body habitus and the discrepant donor-recipienst vessel sizes, with the greatest risk occurring in the youngest patients (Fig. 10). Arteriovenous fistula and pseudoaneurysms are additional vascular complications that can result from graft biopsy. CDUS imaging and renal perfusion scintigraphy are the primary modalities used to assess vascular complications after transplantation. Although MR angiography can be helpful in equivocal cases, conventional angiography remains the reference standard for confirmation and often also for management of vascular complications (El Atat et al. 2010).

The most *common urological complication* is a dilated collecting system caused by urinary tract obstruction that may be the consequence of ureteral kinking, stenosis at the ureteral implantation, ureteral necrosis, or large lymphocele. Ureteral necrosis may be secondary to damage the vascular supply. It is important to note that children with ARF caused by severe urinary obstruction may present with just minimal or moderate renal pelvic dilatation due to a diminished urine production (Fig. 11a–c). In addition, these situations are painless as the transplant and the ureter are not innervated. Close follow-up is mandatory, especially in patients with bladder dysfunction or an augmented bladder (Dharnidharka et al. 2014). Most urological problems can be visualized by US in most situations. If requested, isotope studies, fluoroscopy, and CT or preferably MRI may add valuable information – indicated only if relevant for treatment decisions.

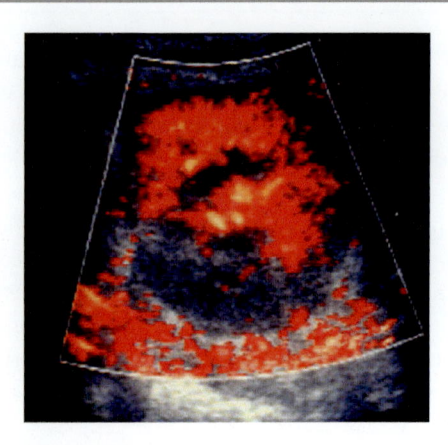

Fig. 10 Amplitude-coded Doppler sonography: renal transplant with perfusion defect due to occlusion renal arterial infarction

> **Take Away**
> Differentiation of nephrologic graft complications cannot be based on imaging findings alone, and renal biopsy is often necessary. Perinephric fluid collections (hematoma, lymphocele, seroma, abscess, and urinoma) and vascular complications are readily imaged with CDS; cross-sectional and functional imaging are reserved for selected cases.

5.5.3 Drug Toxicity

The dosage of calcineurin inhibitors (CNI = cyclosporine and tacrolimus) must be adjusted frequently to obtain sufficient immunosuppression and to avoid nephrotoxicity. Unfortunately, they are potentially nephrotoxic, causing vasoconstriction of the afferent glomerular arterioles, and with long-term use they may cause interstitial fibrosis. US can be either normal or nonspecific; increased RI values may be found on Doppler

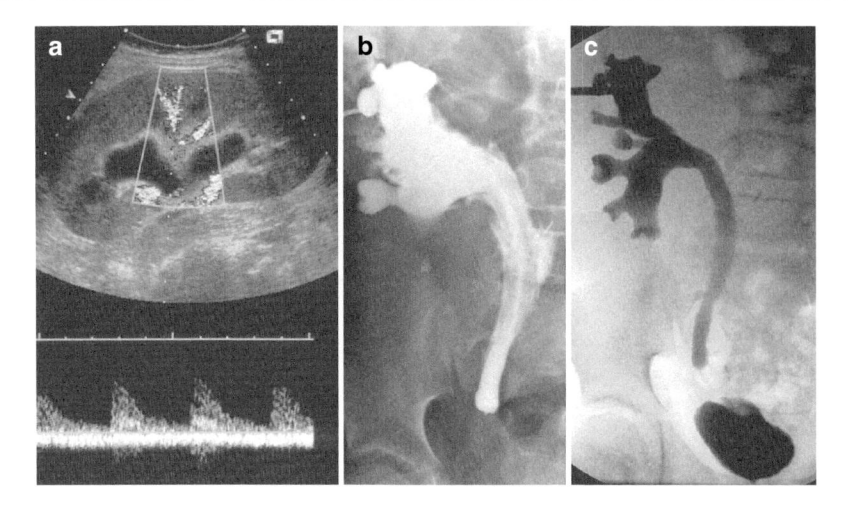

Fig. 11 Acute rise in serum creatinine and oliguria 8 weeks after successful rTX. CDUS (**a**) shows a moderate distension of the renal pelvis without severe impairment of end-diastolic renal perfusion. Immediate percutaneous nephrostomy with antegrade filling (**b**) confirms distal ureteral stenosis caused by ureteral necrosis. Antegrade filling before surgical reconstruction and after stabilization of the renal function confirms this finding (**c**)

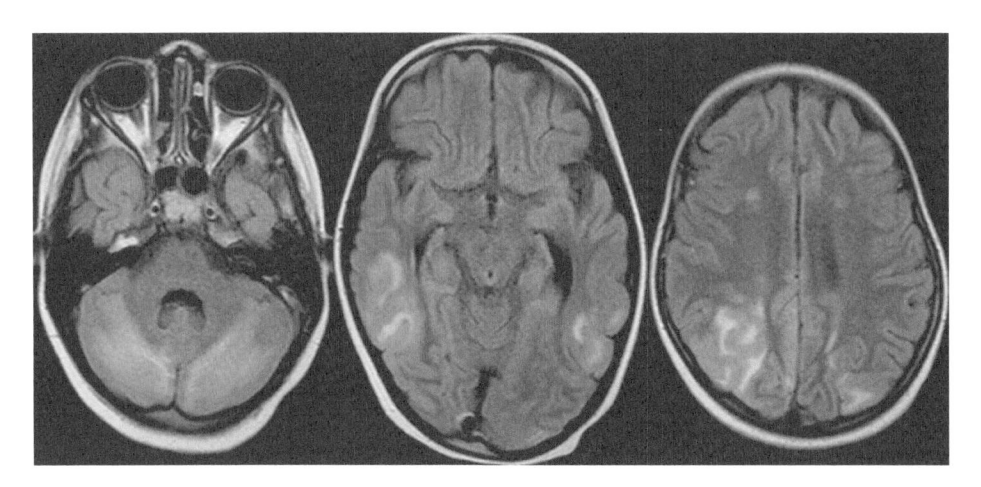

Fig. 12 Axial FLAIR images in an 8-year-old girl with PRES show hyperintense patchy areas involving the cortico-subcortical regions of the temporal and parietal lobes bilaterally as well as the cerebellum

examination (Drake et al. 1990). Findings should be related to the serum drug levels, and eventually only renal biopsy may establish the diagnosis, particularly in chronic changes with intermittently normal blood levels.

Seizures and altered mental status may be signs of CNI-induced neurotoxicity (Potluri et al. 2014). Cerebral MRI can show reversible patchy hyperintense lesions on T2-weighted-FLAIR images in a predominantly occipital pattern, thereby establishing the diagnosis of posterior reversible encephalopathy syndrome (PRES) (Fig. 12). Aside from arterial hypertension, immunosuppressive drugs are another main cause of PRES; note that not even toxic blood levels are required (Lamy et al. 2004).

CDS of the transplant and the native kidneys (if left in situ) as well as echocardiography are recommended at regular intervals, together with the clinical and laboratory surveillance; again some do perform protocol biopsies at regular intervals – although there is a not neglectable risk to the graft because of the potential biopsy complications.

> **Take Away**
> CNI are potentially nephrotoxic. PRES may be secondary to immunosuppressant's toxicity and hypertension. Diagnosis can be suspected clinically and based on laboratory findings, but it is eventually made by histology.

5.5.4 Infections

As a result of immunosuppression, patients are prone to viral and bacterial infections. As with the native kidney, the US appearance of transplant infections is quite variable and nonspecific. Urothelial thickening and focal or diffuse areas of altered echogenicity with impaired corticomedullary differentiation, sometimes even with a pseudotumorous aspect are recognized findings (Fig. 13). Note that some of these features can also be present in the early stages of rejection; thus laboratory and clinical information have to be considered. Any echogenicity within a dilated pyelocaliceal system is usually clinically significant and may be suggestive of pyonephrosis, while rounded weakly shadowed foci and echogenic structures within the collecting system are suggestive of fungus balls. CDS and particularly aCDS are very sensitive for focal perfusion impairment and may support the US diagnosis of a focal transplant infection.

Opportunistic viruses have emerged as great challenges to clinical management after rTX and are probably related to the immunosuppressive regimens currently used, which are more potent than those used in the past. Since the mid-1990s, the incidence of the Epstein-Barr virus (EBV)-driven cancer known as posttransplantation lymphoproliferative disorder (PTLD) has dramatically increased, and polyomavirus BK (BKV) has emerged as a new cause of infection; BKV may cause an interstitial nephropathy or be responsible for ureteral stenosis. These two viruses typically infect people early in life, when they are immunocompetent and cause mild disease, but leave behind a pool of latent virus in the graft. Since kidneys transplanted in children are usually from adult donors, there is an increased chance that a kidney from a seropositive donor (with latent virus) will be transplanted into a seronegative recipient. Thus, as compared with adults, children are at higher relative risk for severe disease from *Cytomegalovirus*, EBV, or BKV, with higher rates of complications, graft loss, and death (Comoli and Ginevri 2012; Dharnidharka et al. 2011a and b). Pneumocystis carinii pneumonitis may occur during the first 6 months after transplantation; however with appropriate prophylaxis this infection has been effectively eliminated in transplant recipients.

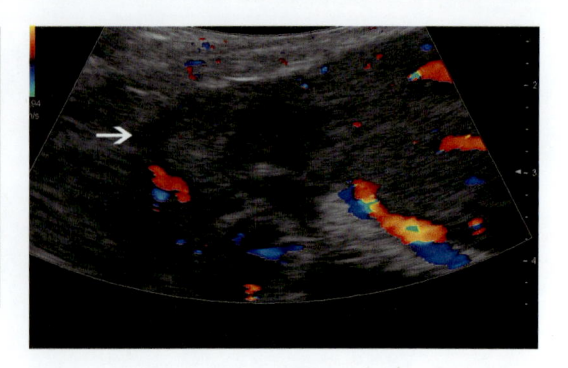

Fig. 13 Acute focal pyelonephritis in a 9-year-old girl with a renal transplant for bilateral reflux nephropathy who presented with fever and dysuria. The longitudinal US image shows a focal, ill-defined area of altered echogenicity in the renal parenchyma with decreased flow on CDS examination

Approximately 50 % of transplanted patients have urinary tract infections. Symptomatic infections are found predominantly during the first 3 months after transplantation. Patients with preexisting urological disorders may have recurrent infections, and kidney transplants seem to be prone to scarring in the case of VUR (Coulthard and Keir 2006). Aside from US, isotope investigations (increasingly replaced by MRI) and VCUG (or ce-VUS) to detect VUR then are recommended.

> **Take Away**
> Transplanted children are at higher risk of viral opportunistic infections (CMV, EBV, BKV) with higher rates of complications, graft loss, and death compared to adults. US appearance of transplant infection is nonspecific. In case of recurrent infections particularly with scarring, VCUG (or ce-VUS) is recommended.

5.6 Mass Lesions: *Posttransplant Lymphoproliferative Disorder*

Long-term immunosuppressive therapy predisposes to the development of neoplastic mass lesions, both within the allograft parenchyma and in other organ systems. Inhibition of native cytotoxic T-cell activity has been implicated as the underlying cause. Both PTLD and (inflammatory) pseudotumors have been described.

Development of *PTLD* is a well-known and serious complication after transplantation. PTLD develops within the context of immunosuppression. It mostly occurs early after rTX and is strongly associated with EBV. The reported incidence of lymphoproliferative disorders after pediatric rTX is approximately 1–4 %, which is more than 20-fold the incidence in the general population, and approximately 94 % of PTLD are non-Hodgkin lymphomas. Early PTLD (within the first year after rTX) is associated with younger recipient age, frequent graft involvement and extranodal disease, and severe immunosuppression and are mostly EBV-driven B-cell lymphomas (Schober et al. 2013). Late PTLD often resembles isolated tumors with nodal appearance (e.g., Burkitt's lymphoma, Hodgkin's disease).

The imaging appearance of PTLD depends on the site of involvement. In case of allograft involvement, the disease typically manifests as multiple ill-defined parenchymal nodular masses that are hypoechoic on gray-scale US images, hypoattenuating relative to the surrounding renal parenchyma on contrast-enhanced CT (ce-CT) and hypointense on contrast-enhanced MR (Fig. 14) (Shroff and Rees 2004; Comoli et al. 2005). Alternatively, diffuse graft enlargement may be the only clue to the disease. Diagnosis is eventually based on histology unless proven elsewise; differential diagnostic considerations include focal or diffuse infection and other soft-tissue or mesenchymal tumors.

In recent years, application of hybrid positron emission tomography (PET)-CT (or even PET-MRI) resulted to be more sensitive and specific than imaging with ce-CT (or MRI) for Hodgkin and non-Hodgkin lymphoma staging

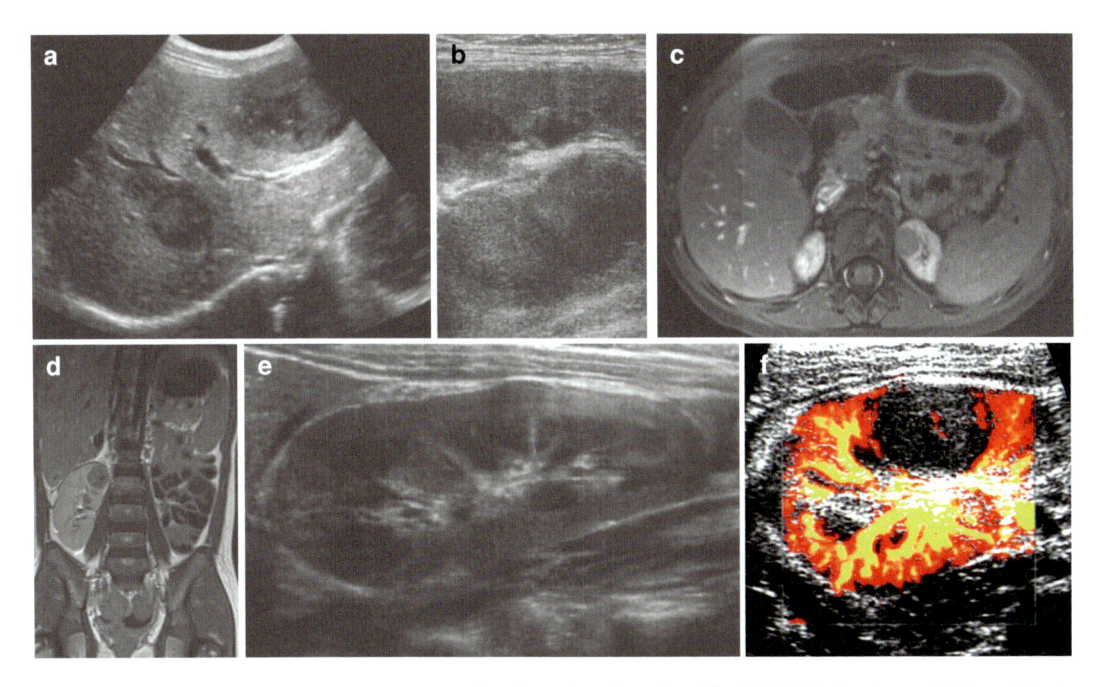

Fig. 14 PTLD in a 13-year-old girl 14 months after she had undergone rTX for nephronophthisis. The longitudinal US scan of the liver shows multiple hypoechoic, well-defined parenchymal nodules (**a**). Coexisting multiple hypoechoic nodules within the renal parenchyma (**b**), MR imaging of a girl with PTLD showing multiple nodules in the graft and the original kidney (**c**, **d**); corresponding gray-scale US (**e**) and aCDS (**f**) image demonstrating that these nodules may show up much more evident on power Doppler than on the basic gray-scale image

and in evaluating treatment response after therapy, especially in patients with persistent lesions in whom FDG uptake can help to differentiate between residual tumor and fibrosis (Shroff and Rees 2004; Hirsch et al. 2013; Purz et al. 2014).

Take Away

In case of PTLD, US will usually reveal multiple hypoechoic well-defined parenchymal masses in the affected organ(s), sometimes only diffuse graft enlargement, sometimes just adenopathy. Diagnosis is based on histology. PET-CT/PET-MRI is increasingly used for staging and the evaluation of treatment response.

Conclusion

Imaging with US, including (C)DS and aCDS, is essential for diagnosis of CRF and to monitor therapy. Further imaging is needed to detect cardiac compromise or renal bone disease and to plan rTX. During dialysis, imaging is mostly requested when complications arise. US with CDS and aCDS is helpful to monitor graft function after transplant. Further imaging with VCUG, isotope studies, or MRI (sometimes CT or even fluoroscopy and catheter angiography) can become necessary or complementary in selected cases before and after rTX.

References

Al-Hermi BE, Al-Saran K, Secker D et al (1999) Hemodialysis for end-stage renal disease in children weighing less than 10 kg. Pediatr Nephrol 13:401–403

Andreoli SP (2004) Acute renal failure in the newborn. Sem Perinatol 28:112–123

Ardissino G, Dacco V, Testa S et al (2003) Epidemiology of chronic renal failure in children: data from the ItalKid project. Pediatrics 111:382–387

Avni FE, Bali MA, Regnault M et al (2002) MR urography in children. Eur J Radiol 43:154–166

Avni FE, Garel C, Cassart M, D'Haene N, Hall M, Riccabona M (2012) Imaging and classification of congenital cystic renal diseases. AJR Am J Roentgenol 198:1004–1013

Barba J, Rioja J, Robles JE, Rinco'n A, Rosell D, Zudaire JJ, Berian JM, Pascual I, Benito A, Errasti P (2011) Immediate renal Doppler ultrasonography findings (<24 h) and its association with graft survival. World J Urol 29:547–553

Blowey DL, Querfeld U, Geary D et al (1996) Ultrasound findings in juvenile nephronophthisis. Pediatr Nephrol 10:22–24

Bou Matar R, Warshaw B, Hymes L et al (2012) Routine transplant Doppler ultrasonography following pediatric kidney transplant. Pediatr Transplant 16:607–612

Brion LP, Bernstein J, Spitzer A (1997) Diseases of the fetus and infant–kidney and urinary tract. In: Fanaroff AA, Martin RJ (eds) Neonatal-perinatal medicine. Mosby Year Book, St Louis, pp 1564–1636

Brittinger WD, Walker G, Twittenhoff WD et al (1997) Vascular access for hemodialysis. Pediatr Nephrol 11:87–95

Broome DR, Girguis MS, Baron PW et al (2007) Gadodiamide-associated nephrogenic systemic fibrosis: why radiologists should be concerned. Am J Roentgenol 188:586–592

Bruel A, Allain-Launay E, Humbert J, Ryckewaert A, Champion G, Moreau A, Renaudin K, Karam G, Roussey-Kesler G (2014) Early protocol biopsies in pediatric renal transplantation: interest for the adaptation of immunosuppression. Pediatr Transplant 18:142–149

Bunchman TE (1995) Chronic dialysis in the infant less than 1 year of age. Pediatr Nephrol 9:S18–S22

Cattarelli D, Spandrio M, Gasparoni A et al (2006) A randomized, double blind, placebo controlled trial of the effect of theophylline in prevention of vasomotor nephropathy in very preterm neonates with respiratory distress syndrome. Arch Dis Child Fetal Neonatal Ed 91:F80–F84

Chand DH, Brier M, Strife CF (2005) Comparison of vascular access type in pediatric hemodialysis patients with respect to urea clearance, anemia management, and serum albumin concentration. Am J Kidney Dis 45:303–308

Chuang YF, Tsai TC (1998) Sonographic findings in familial juvenile nephronophthisis-medullary cystic disease complex. J Clin Ultrasound 26:203–206

Clark DA (1977) Time of first void and first stool in 500 newborns. Pediatrics 60:457–459

Comoli P, Ginevri F (2012) Monitoring and managing viral infections in pediatric renal transplant recipients. Pediatr Nephrol 27:705–717

Comoli P, Maccario R, Locatelli F, Valente U, Basso S, Garaventa A, Tomà P, Botti G, Melioli G, Baldanti F, Nocera A, Perfumo F, Ginevri F (2005) Treatment of EBV-related post-renal transplant lymphoproliferative disease with a tailored regimen including EBV-specific T cells. Am J Transplant 5:1415–1422

Coulthard MG, Keir MJ (2006) Reflux nephropathy in kidney transplants, demonstrated by dimercaptosuccinic acid scanning. Transplantation 82(2):205–210

Cravedi P, Kopp JB, Remuzzi G (2013) Recent progress in the pathophysiology and treatment of FSGS recurrence. Am J Transplant 13:266–274

Damasio B, Ording LS, Marks St, Riccabona M (2017) Imaging in paediatric renal transplantation. Pediatr Transplantation 21 (3):e12885. DOI:10.1111/petr.12885

Davenport MS, Khalatbari S, Dillamn JR et al (2013) Contrast-material induced nephrotoxicity and intravenous low-osmolality iodinated contrast material. Radiology 267:94–105

Dharnidharka VR, Martz KL, Stablein DM, Benfield MR (2011a) Improved survival with recent post-transplant lymphoproliferative disorder (PTLD) in children with kidney transplants. Am J Transplant 11:751–758

Dharnidharka VR, Abdulnour HA, Araya CE (2011b) The BK virus in renal transplant recipients — review of pathogenesis, diagnosis, and treatment. Pediatr Nephrol 26:1763–1774

Dharnidharka VR, Fiorina P, Harmon WE (2014) Kidney transplantation in children. N Engl J Med 371:549–558

Drake DG, Day DL, Letourneau JG, Alford BA, Sibley RK, Mauer SM, Bunchman TE (1990) Doppler evaluation of renal transplants in children: a prospective analysis with histopathologic correlation. AJR Am J Roentgenol 154:785–787

Ehrich JHH, Loirat C, Brunner FP et al (1992) Report on management of renal failure in children in Europe XXII, 1991. Nephrol Dial Transplant 7(Suppl 2):36–42

El Atat R, Derouiche A, Guellouz S, Gargah T, Lakhoua R, Chebil M (2010) Surgical complications in pediatric and adolescent renal transplantation. Saudi J Kidney Dis Transpl 21:251–257

Ellis D, Kaye RD, Bontempo FA (1997) Aortic and renal artery thrombosis in a neonate: recovery with thrombolytic therapy. Pediatr Nephrol 11:641–644

El-Merhi FM, Bae KT (2004) Cystic renal disease. Magn Reson Imaging Clin N Am 12:449–467

Elzouki AY, al Suhaibani H, Mirza K et al (1996) Thin-section computed tomography scans detect medullary cysts in patients believed to have juvenile nephronophthisis. Am J Kidney Dis 27:216–219

Faller U, Stegen P, Klaus G et al (1998) Sonographic determination of the thickness of the peritoneum in healthy children and paediatric patients on CAPD. Nephrol Dial Transplant 13:3172–3177

Fitch SJ, Stapleton FB (1986) Ultrasonographic features of glomerulocystic disease in infancy: similarity to infantile polycystic kidney disease. Pediatr Radiol 16:400–402

Fontaine E, Gagnadoux MF, Niaudet P et al (1998) Renal transplantation in children with augmentation cystoplasty: long-term results. J Urol 159:2110–2113

Garel LA, Habib R, Pariente D et al (1984) Juvenile nephronophthisis: sonographic appearance in children with severe uremia. Radiology 151:93–95

Gordon I, Riccabona M (2003) Investigating the newborn kidney: update on imaging techniques. Sem Neonatol 8:269–278

Guay-Woodford LM (2006) Renal cystic diseases: diverse phenotypes converge on the cilium/centrosome complex. Pediatr Nephrol 21:1369–1376

Hardy BE, Shah T, Cicciarelli J, Lemley KV, Hutchinson IV, Cho YW (2009) Kidney transplantation in children and adolescents: an analysis of United Network for Organ Sharing Database. Transplant Proc 41:1533–1535

Harmon WE (2010) Pediatric renal transplantation. In: Himmelfarb J, Sayegh MH (eds) Chronic kidney disease, dialysis and transplantation. Elsevier, Philadelphia, pp 591–608

Hentschel R, Lödige B, Bulla M (1996) Renal insufficiency in the neonatal period. Clin Nephrol 46:54–58

Hibbert J, Howlett DC, Greenwood KL et al (1997) The ultrasound appearances of neonatal renal vein thrombosis. Br J Radiol 70:1191–1194

Hildebrandt F, Otto E (2005) Cilia and centrosomes: a unifying pathogenic concept for cystic kidney disease? Nat Rev Genet 6:928–940

Hildebrandt F, Strahm B, Nothwang HG et al (1997) Molecular genetic identification of families with juvenile nephronophthisis type 1: rate of progression to renal failure. Kidney Int 51:261–269

Hirsch FW, Sattler B, Sorge I, Kurch L, Viehweger A, Ritter L, Werner P, Jochimsen T, Henryk Barthel H, Bierbach U, Till H, Sabri O, Kluge R (2013) PET/MR in children. Initial clinical experience in paediatric oncology using an integrated PET/MR scanner. Pediatr Radiol 43:860–875

Hogg RJ (1992) Acquired renal cystic disease in children prior to the start of dialysis. Pediatr Nephrol 6:176–178

Hogg RJ, Furth S, Lemley KV et al (2003) National Kidney Foundation's kidney outcomes quality initiative clinical practice guidelines for chronic kidney disease in children and adolescents: evaluation, classification, and stratification. Pediatrics 111:1416–1421

Howlett DC, Greenwood KL, Jarosz JM et al (1997) The incidence of transient medullary hyperechogenicity in neonatal ultrasound examination. Br J Radiol 70:140–143

Huber W, Eckel F, Henning M et al (2006) Prophylaxis of contrast material-induced nephropathy in patients in intensive care: acetylcysteine, theophylline, or both? A randomized study. Radiology 239:793–804

Huet F, Semama D, Grimaldi M et al (1995) Effects of theophylline on renal insufficiency in neonates with respiratory distress syndrome. Intensive Care Med 21:511–514

Karlowicz MG, Adelman RD (1995) Nonoliguric and oliguric acute renal failure in asphyxiated term neonates. Pediatr Nephrol 9:718–722

Kidney Disease: Improving global outcomes (KDIGO) CKD Work Group. (2013) KDIGO (2013) Clinical practise guidelines for the evaluation and management of chronic kidney disease. Kidney Int 3(Suppl): 1–150

Kidney Disease: Improving global outcomes (KDIGO) CKD-MBD Work Group (2009) KDIGO clinical practice guideline for the diagnosis, evaluation, prevention, and treatment of chronic kidney disease – mineral and bone disorder (CKD-MBD). Kidney Int 76(Suppl 113):S1–S130

Klaus G, Watson A, Edefonti A et al (2006) Prevention and treatment of renal osteodystrophy in children on chronic renal failure: European guidelines. Pediatr Nephrol 21:151–159

Kolofousi C, Stefanidis K, Cokkinos DD, Karakitsos D, Antypa E, Piperopoulos P (2012) Ultrasonographic features of kidney transplants and their complications: an imaging review. ISRN Radiol 2013:480862

Kolonko A, Wiecek A, Kokot F (1998) The nonselective adenosine antagonist theophylline does prevent renal dysfunction induced by radiographic contrast agents. J Nephrol 11:151–156

Koo HP, Bunchman TE, Flynn JT et al (1999) Renal transplantation in children with severe lower urinary tract dysfunction. J Urol 161:240–245

Krestin GP, Kacl G, Hauser M et al (1995) Imaging diagnosis of sclerosing peritonitis and relation of radiologic signs to the extent of disease. Abdom Imaging 20:414–420

Kupferman JC (1994) Acute renal failure in newborn infants: incidence, management and outcome. Clin Res 42:449A

Lamy C, Oppenheim C, Méder JF, Mas JL (2004) Neuroimaging in posterior reversible encephalopathy syndrome. J Neuroimaging 14:89–96

Leichter HE, Dietrich R, Salusky I et al (1988) Acquired cystic kidney disease in children undergoing long-term dialysis. Pediatr Nephrol 2:8–11

Lerner GR, Warady BA, Sullivan EK et al (1999) Chronic dialysis in children and adolescents. The 1996 Annual Report of the North American Pediatric Renal Transplant Cooperative Study. Pediatr Nephrol 13:404–417

Levine E (1992) Renal cell carcinoma in uremic acquired renal cystic disease: incidence, detection, and management. Urol Radiol 13:203–210

Luciano R, Gallini F, Romagnoli C et al (1998) Doppler evaluation of renal blood flow velocity as a predictive index of acute renal failure in perinatal asphyxia. Eur J Pediatr 157:656–660

Mattoo TK, Greifer I, Geva P et al (1997) Acquired renal cystic disease in children and young adults on maintenance dialysis. Pediatr Nephrol 11:447–450

McDonald JS, McDonald RJ, Comin J et al (2013a) Frequency of acute kidney injury following intravenous contrast administration: a systemic review and meta-analysis. Radiology 267:119–128

McDonald RJ, McDonald JS, Bida JP et al (2013b) Intravenous contrast-induced nephropathy: causal or coincident phenomenon? Radiology 267:106–118

McDonald RJ, McDonald JS, Kallmes DF, Jentoft ME, Murray DL, Thielen KR, Williamson EE, Eckel LJ (2015) Intracranial gadolinium deposition after contrast-enhanced MR imaging. Radiology 275:772–782

Murphy SW, Barrett BJ, Parfrey PS (2000) Contrast nephropathy. J Am Soc Nephrol 11:177–182

Nakamura M, Yokota K, Chen C et al (1999) Hyperechoic renal papillae as a physiological finding in neonates. Clin Radiol 54:233–236

Nankivell BJ, Alexander SI (2010) Rejection of the kidney allograft. N Engl J Med 363:1451–1462

Neu AM, Ho PL, McDonald RA et al (2002) Chronic dialysis in children and adolescents. The 2001 NAPRTCS annual report. Pediatr Nephrol 17:656–663

Newhouse JH, Kho D, Rao QA, Starren J (2008) Frequency of serum creatinine changes in the absence of iodinated contrast material: implications for studies of contrast nephropathy. Am J Radiol 191:376–382

Nixon JN, Biyyam DR, Stanescu L, Phillips GS, Finn LS, Parisi MT (2013) Imaging of pediatric renal transplants and their complications: a pictorial review. Radiographics 33:1227–1251

Oh J, Wunsch R, Turzer M et al (2002) Advanced coronary and carotid arteriopathy in young adults with childhood onset chronic renal failure. Circulation 106:100–105

Parekh RS, Gidding SS (2005) Cardiovascular complications in pediatric end-stage renal disease. Pediatr Nephrol 20:125–131

Plum J, Sudkamp S, Grabensee B (1994) Results of ultrasound-assisted diagnosis of tunnel infections in continuous ambulatory peritoneal dialysis. Am J Kidney Dis 23:99–104

Potluri K, Holt D, Hou S (2014) Neurologic complications in renal transplantation. Handb Clin Neurol 121:1245–1255

Prischl FC, Muhr T, Seiringer EM, Funk S, Kronabethleitner G, Wallner M, Artmann W, Kramar R (2002) Magnetic resonance imaging of the peritoneal cavity among peritoneal dialysis patients, using the dialysate as "contrast medium". J Am Soc Nephrol 13:197

Purz S, Sabri O, Viehweger A, Barthel H, Kluge R, Sorge I, Hirsch FW (2014) Potential pediatric applications of PET/MR. J Nucl Med 55:1–8

Querfeld U, Schneble F, Wradzilo W et al (1992) Acquired cystic kidney disease before and after renal transplantation. J Pediatr 121:61–64

Ramage IJ, Bailie A, Tyerman KS et al (2005) Vascular access survival in children and young adults receiving long-term hemodialysis. Am J Kidney Dis 45:708–714

Riccabona M (2006) Renal failure in neonates, infants, and children: the role of ultrasound. Ultrasound Clin 1:457–469

Riccabona M (2014a) Chapter 17. Contrast media use in pediatrics: safety issues. In: Thomson HS, Webb AW (eds) Contrast media: safety issues and ESUR guidelines, 3rd edn. Springer, Berlin, pp 245–251

Riccabona M (2014b) Ultrasound guided interventions – other intracavitary contrast applications. In: Riccabona M (ed) Pediatric ultrasound – requisites and applications. Springer, Heiderlber/Dordrecht, pp 67–68. ISBN 978-3-642-39155-2

Riccabona M, Ring E, Petritsch P (1993) Farbdopplersonographie in der Differentialdiagnose unilateraler kongenitaler zystischer Nierenmissbildungen. Z Geburtshilfe Perinatol 197:283–286

Riccabona M, Simbrunner J, Ring E et al (2002) Feasibility of MR urography in neonates and infants with anomalies of the upper urinary tract. Eur Radiol 12:1442–1450

Riccabona M, Avni F, Damasio B, Ordning-Mueller LS, Lobo ML, Darge K, Papadopoulou F, Willi U, Blickmann J, Vivier PH (2012) ESPR Uroradiology Task Force and ESUR Paediatric Working Group – imaging recommendations in paediatric uroradiology, part V: childhood cystic kidney disease, childhood renal transplantation, and contrast-enhanced ultrasound in children. Pediatr Radiol 42:1275–1283

Riccabona M, Lobo ML, Willi U, Avni F, Blickmann J, Damasio B, Ordning-Mueller LS, Darge K, Papadopoulou F, Vivier PH (2014) ESPR Uroradiology Task Force and ESUR Paediatric Working Group – imaging recommendations in paediatric uroradiology, part VI: childhood renal biopsy and imaging of neonatal and infant genital tract. Minutes from the Task Force session at the annual ESPR Meeting 2012 in Athens on childhood renal biopsy and imaging neonatal genitalia. Pediatr Radiol 44:496–502

Riebel TW, Abraham K, Wartner R et al (1993) Transient medullary hyperechogenicity in ultrasound studies of neonates: is it a normal phenomenon and what are the causes? J Clin Ultrasound 21:25–31

Rigamonti W, Capizzi A, Zacchello G et al (2005) Kidney transplantation into bladder augmentation or urinary diversion: long-term results. Transplantation 80: 1435–1440

Rigden SPA (1996) The treatment of renal osteodystrophy. Pediatr Nephrol 10:653–655

Rödl S, Marschitz I, Mache CJ, Nagel B, Koestenberger M, Zobel G (2012a) Hemodiafiltration in infants with complications during peritoneal dialysis. Artif Organ 36:590–593

Rödl S, Marschaitz I, Mache CJ, Nagel B, Koesetnberger M, Zobel G (2012b) Hemodiafiltration in infants with complications during peritoneal dialysis. Artif Organs 36:590–593

Rosado E, Riccabona M (2016) Off-label use of ultrasound contrast agents for intravenous applications in children – a meta-analysis. J Ultrasound Med 35(3):487–496

Rose GM, Conley SB (1989) Unilateral hydrothorax in small children on chronic continuous peritoneal dialysis. Pediatr Nephrol 3:89–91

Salusky IB, Goodman WG (1996) The management of renal osteodystrophy. Pediatr Nephrol 10:651–653

Sanyal S, Marckmann P, Scherer S, Abraham JL (2011) Multiorgan gadolinium (Gd) deposition and fibrosis in a patient with nephrogenic systemic fibrosis— an autopsy-based review. Nephrol Dial Transplant 26:3616–3626

Saunier S, Salomon R, Antignac C (2005) Nephronophthisis. Curr Opin Genet Dev 15:324–331

Schärer K, Schmidt KG, Soergel M (1999) Cardiac function and structure in patients with chronic renal failure. Pediatr Nephrol 13:951–996

Schober T, Framke T, Kreipe H, Schulz TF, Großhennig A, Hussein K, Baumann U, Pape L, Schubert S, Wingen AM, Jack T, Koch A, Klein C, Maeker-Kolhoff B (2013) Characteristics of early and late PTLD development in pediatric solid organ transplant recipients. Transplantation 95:240–246

Schwartz GJ, Haycock GB, Edelman CM Jr et al (1976) A simple estimate of glomerular filtration rate in children derived from body length and plasma creatinine. Pediatrics 58:259–263

Schwartz GJ, Feld LG, Langford DJ (1984) A simple estimate of glomerular filtration rate in full-term infants during the first year of life. J Pediatr 104: 849–854

Scott JES, Hunter EW, Lee REJ et al (1990) Ultrasound measurement of renal size in newborn infants. Arch Dis Child 65:361–364

Shroff R, Rees L (2004) The post-transplant lymphoproliferative disorder-a literature review. Pediatr Nephrol 19:369–377

Siedlecki A, Irish W, Brennan DC (2011) Delayed graft function in the kidney transplant. Am J Transplant 11:2279–2796

Slovis TL, Bernstein J, Gruskin A (1993) Hyperechoic kidneys in the newborn and young infant. Pediatr Nephrol 7:294–302

Solez K, Colvin RB, Racusen LC et al (2008) Banff 07 classification of renal allograft pathology: updates and future directions. Am J Transplant 8:753–760

Stafford-Johnson DB, Wilson TE, Francis IR et al (1998) CT appearance of sclerosing peritonitis in patients on chronic ambulatory peritoneal dialysis. J Comput Assist Tomogr 22:295–299

Starinsky R, Vardi O, Batasch D et al (1995) Increased renal medullary echogenicity in neonates. Pediatr Radiol 25(Suppl 1):S43–S45

Stenzel M, Mentzel HJ (2014) Ultrasound elastography and contrast-enhanced ultrasound in infants, children and adolescents. Eur J Radiol 83:1560–1569

Taylor PM (2002) Image-guided peritoneal access and management of complications in peritoneal dialysis. Semin Dial 15:250–258

Thomsen HS (2006) Nephrogenic systemic fibrosis: a serious late adverse reaction to gadodiamide. Eur Radiol 16:2619–2621

Thomsen HS, Stacul F, Webb JAW (2014) Contrast induced nephropathy. In: Thomson HS, Webb AW (eds) Contrast media: safety issues and ESUR guidelines, 3rd edn. Springer, Berlin, pp 81–104. ISBN 978-3-642-36723-6

Tsai EW and Ettenger RB (2010) Kidney transplantation in children in Handbook of kidney transplantation. 5th edn. Edited by Danovitch GM by Lipincott Williams&Wilkins

Valoti E, Alberti M, Noris M (2012) Posttransplant recurrence of atypical hemolytic uremic syndrome. J Nephrol 25:911–917

Vychtytil A, Lilay T, Lorenz M et al (1999) Ultrasonography of the catheter tunnel in peritoneal dialysis patients: what are the indications? Am J Kidney Dis 33:722–727

Wang PA, Huang FY (1994) Time of first defecation and urination in very low birth weight infants. Eur J Pediatr 153:279–283

Wikstad I, Celsi G, Larsson L et al (1988) Kidney function in adults born with unilateral renal agenesis or nephrectomized in childhood. Pediatr Nephrol 2:177–182

Winyard PJD, Bharucha T, De Bruyn R et al (2006) Perinatal renal venous thrombosis: presenting renal length predicts outcome. Arch Dis Child Fetal Neonatal Ed 91:F273–F278

Wong JC, Rossleigh MA, Farnsworth RH (1995) Utility of technetium-99m-MAG3 diuretic renography in the neonatal period. J Nucl Med 36:2214–2219

Wright NB, Blanch G, Walkinshaw S et al (1996) Antenatal and neonatal renal vein thrombosis: new ultrasonic features with high frequency transducers. Pediatr Radiol 26:686–689

Zaninovic AC, Westra SJ, Hall TR et al (1992) Congenital bladder rupture and urine ascites secondary to a sacrococcygeal teratoma. Pediatr Radiol 22:509–511

Renovascular Hypertension

Frederica Papadopoulou and Melanie P. Hiorns

Contents

1	Introduction	641
2	Definition	641
3	Clinical Presentation	642
4	Causes	642
5	Imaging	643
5.1	Ultrasonography with Doppler	643
5.2	Post-captopril Renal Scintigraphy	645
5.3	Computed Tomographic Angiography (CTA)	645
5.4	Magnetic Resonance Angiography (MRA)	647
5.5	Digital Subtraction Angiography (DSA)	647
6	Endovascular Treatment	648
Conclusion		648
References		648

F. Papadopoulou, MD (✉)
Radiology, Ioannina University, Ioannina, Greece
e-mail: fpapadopoulou@hotmail.com

M.P. Hiorns, MBBS, MRCP, FRCR
Great Ormond Street Hospital for Children,
London WC1N 3JH, UK

1 Introduction

Hypertension in children is usually secondary, although primary (essential) hypertension is progressively increasing along with increasing childhood obesity (Gomes et al. 2011). The more severe the hypertension and the younger the child, then the more likely it is to be secondary hypertension. Secondary hypertension is most commonly due to renal parenchymal diseases and congenital abnormalities (Wyszynska et al. 1992). Renovascular disease (RVD) is an unusual cause of secondary hypertension in children accounting for less than 10% of hypertension cases (Gill et al. 1976; Wyszynska et al. 1992). However, it is important to be diagnosed as it is potentially curable with transcatheter angioplasty and/or surgery (Tullus et al. 2008). RVD is now well recognized in pediatrics, but the etiology and management are very different to adult practice (Sadowski and Falkner 1996).

2 Definition

Hypertension is defined as average systolic and/or diastolic blood pressure (BP) that is ≥95th percentile for gender, age, and height on at least three occasions. Stage 1 hypertension is the designation for BP levels that range from the 95th percentile to 5 mmHg above the 99th percentile. Stage 2 hypertension is the designation for BP levels that are >5 mmHg above the 99th percentile (National High Blood Pressure 4th Report 2004). Renovascular hypertension (RVH) is caused by arterial lesions impeding blood flow to one or both kidneys or to one or more intrarenal segments (Watson et al. 1985; Dillon 1997). Hypoperfusion results in increased renin release from the juxtaglomerular apparatus of the kidney and activation of the renin-angiotensin cascade pathway. Renin-mediated hypertension is often refractory to conventional medical therapy and, if untreated, can lead to serious complications, including hypertensive encephalopathy and stroke, left ventricular hypertrophy with diastolic dysfunction and congestive heart failure, and diminished renal function (Castelli et al. 2013). In RVH, the BP is usually markedly high usually exceeding the 97th percentile. BP measurements should always be compared with published standards for age, sex, and height (National High Blood Pressure 4th Report 2004; Goonasekera and Dillon 2000; Rosner et al. 1993) (see also chapter "Normal Values").

> **Take Away**
> There are three different stages of hypertension in childhood, and age-matched normal values have to be used.

3 Clinical Presentation

The presentation of RVD in childhood is variable. Occasionally a child is incidentally found to have high blood pressure (BP) on routine examination. The diagnosis is often delayed due to technical problems in measuring the BP and a low index of suspicion in children (Tullus et al. 2008). Other presentations may relate to secondary effects of hypertension, such as cardiac failure, an isolated lower motor neuron facial palsy, severe headaches, or failure to thrive.

4 Causes

Renovascular disease (RVD) must first be distinguished from other, more common, causes of secondary childhood hypertension such as renal scarring and glomerular disease in children older than 1 year of age and coarctation of the aorta in infants (Table 1). Occasionally obstructive uropathy such as bilateral ureteropelvic junction obstruction or posterior urethral valves may also present with hypertension. Endocrine diseases and tumors (neuroblastoma, pheochromocytoma,

Table 1 Causes of secondary hypertension

Renal
Glomerulonephritis or any nephritis (acute and chronic)
Pyelonephritis
Obstructive uropathy
Polycystic kidney disease
Renal dysplasia
Renal injury
Vascular
Renal artery stenosis
Coarctation of aorta (commonest cause in children aged <1 year)
Middle aortic syndrome
Renal vein or artery thrombosis
Neonatal aortic thrombosis
Umbilical artery catheterization
Vasculitis (Takayasu's disease, polyarteritis nodosa, Kawasaki disease)
Transplant renal artery stenosis
Genetic syndromes
Neurofibromatosis
Williams syndrome
Tuberous sclerosis
Endocrine/tumors
Primary hyperaldosteronism
Cushing syndrome
Neuroblastoma
Wilms' tumor
Mesoblastic nephroma
Pheochromocytoma
Other causes
Radiation
Medications
Idiopathic hypercalcemia of infancy

or Wilms' tumor) are other potential causes of hypertension in children. Fibromuscular dysplasia (FMD) is the commonest cause of RVD in children, although Takayasu's disease is more common than FMD in some eastern countries (Slovut and Olin 2004; McCulloch et al. 2003). Fibromuscular dysplasia differs from that in adults and is now considered as a part of the developmental arterial dysplasia (Srinivasan et al. 2011). Histopathologically it is a combination of intimal fibroplasia, medial thinning, and excessive external elastic lamina (Srinivasan et al. 2011). Neurofibromatosis type 1 is another common cause of RVH, but other less common entities are also encountered such as William's syndrome and idiopathic hypercalcemia of infancy. Middle aortic syndrome is a morphological pattern in which the abdominal aorta and one or more of its major branches are stenosed. In children, especially those with an identifiable underlying cause such as neurofibromatosis type 1, arterial involvement tends to be more extensive than in adults with multiple vascular lesions including mid-aortic narrowing as well (Srinivasan et al. 2011). Bilateral disease and involvement of the intrarenal vasculature occur in more than 30–50 % of children with RVD (Deal et al. 1992; Shroff et al. 2006; Tullus et al. 2010; Srinivasan et al. 2011).

Take Away
There are many causes for RVD that may induce hypertension in childhood; they do differ partially from adults. Particularly childhood RAS often involves more distal vessels than the typical arteriosclerotic adult-type RAS – with its implication on the imaging approach.

5 Imaging

There are several imaging modalities for the diagnosis of RVD. Noninvasive methods include ultrasonography (US) with Doppler techniques,

Table 2 High clinical suspicion of renovascular disease

Extremely high blood pressure at presentation
Antihypertensive treatment
Hypertension not controlled on one or two drugs
Unacceptable adverse effects of antihypertensive drugs
Secondary symptoms (e.g., neurological symptoms, cardiac failure)
Syndrome associated with renovascular disease
Neurofibromatosis type 1
Williams syndrome
Tuberous sclerosis
Evidence of large vessel vasculitis
History of renal trauma or radiation
Umbilical artery catheterization
Renovascular thrombosis
High renin levels
Abdominal bruit
Renal transplant

scintigraphy, CT angiography (CTA), and MR angiography (MRA). None of these methods can rule out RVD (Vo et al. 2006; Tullus et al. 2008). However, these techniques are useful in cases of low probability for RVD, for follow-up cases, and for depicting or excluding other causes of hypertension. So in children with severe or symptomatic hypertension and in children with the presence of positive findings on imaging techniques or with high clinical suspicion of RVD (Table 2), catheter-based digital subtraction angiography (DSA) is still considered as the gold standard for both the diagnosis and therapeutic intervention (Tullus et al. 2010; Riccabona et al. 2011).

5.1 Ultrasonography with Doppler

Ultrasonography (US) is a first-line imaging modality widely available, easy and safe. It can depict most renal causes of hypertension such as a small scarred or dysplastic kidney, polycystic kidney disease, hydronephrosis, or tumor. Renal Doppler techniques are most useful in diagnosing RVD; it is however operator dependent and requires operator's experience (Castelli et al. 2013). Moreover, it is difficult to visualize directly the stenosis of small vessels in children such as the renal branches and accessory renal arteries or even the main renal artery in small infants (Brun et al. 1997; Tullus et al. 2010). For this reason, the diagnosis is usually based on indirect findings such as the very low intrarenal resistive index, and the tardus-parvus spectral Doppler waveform usually depicted in more distal vessels (Patriquin et al. 1992; Brun et al. 1997; Li et al. 2006; Castelli et al. 2014). Several Doppler findings and flow parameters have been widely used for RVD diagnosis in adults. A recent analysis of 88 published studies involving 8,147 adult patients and evaluating four parameters (peak systolic velocity, acceleration time, acceleration index, and renal-aortic ratio) showed that sonography is a moderately accurate screening test for renal artery stenosis (RAS) (Williams et al. 2007). The single measurement, peak systolic velocity, has the highest performance characteristics, an expected sensitivity of 85% and specificity of 92% (Williams et al. 2007). However, it is not clear whether the accepted criteria in adults, i.e., a peak systolic velocity >180–200 cm/s, acceleration time >80 ms (both parameters show age-dependent variations in early childhood), side difference of resistive index >0.05, and renal artery to aortic flow velocity ratio >3–3.5, are applicable to children (Bud et al. 1999; Riccabona et al. 2011). Only the typical distal tardus-parvus waveform, which is seen unilaterally, distal to a severe RAS, or bilaterally in aortic coarctation or middle aortic syndrome (Fig. 1), and the direct visualization of the stenosis on color Doppler sonography such as the turbulent flow at increased velocity causing aliasing (Figs. 2 and 3) are reliable predictors for childhood RAS (Tullus et al. 2010; Riccabona et al. 2011; Castelli et al. 2013). Despite many recent advances in US, however, false-positive and false-negative studies for branch artery or even main renal artery stenosis may still occur (Brun et al. 1997; Castelli et al. 2014). A normal US study does not exclude a single renal scar, renovascular pathology, or a small pheochromocytoma (especially if it is extra-adrenal), and so further imaging is needed. The current recommendation is that children with a diagnosis of RVD on US and Doppler sonography and children with a negative US study but with a high probability of RVD or severe hypertension (stage 2 in all ages and stage 1 in less than 1-year-old) should be referred for catheter angiography with renal vein sampling, potentially with simultaneous endovascular treatment (Tullus et al 2010; Riccabona et al 2011). Further noninvasive imaging by CTA or MRA has no significant benefit in these children, only creating additional costs and delays (Riccabona et al 2011). In children, however, with negative Doppler US and a low clinical suspicion of RVD (see Table 2), further imaging with other noninvasive techniques is indicated. If US shows other pathologies to be the cause of hypertension, further appropriate imaging will be needed such as a diuretic renogram with 99mTc-

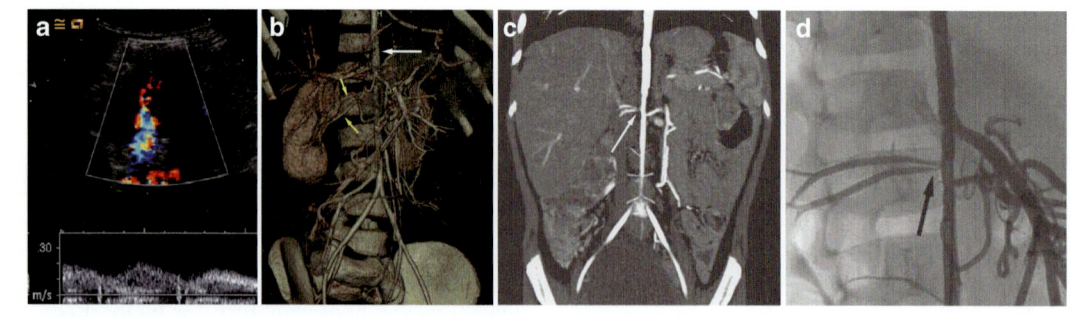

Fig. 1 A 7-year-old male with neurofibromatosis type 1 and middle aortic syndrome. (**a**) Doppler ultrasound shows a "tardus-parvus" pattern with prolonged acceleration time and low velocity systolic peak in an artery at the right renal hilum. This was also present on the left side, suggesting aortic and/or bilateral renal artery stenosis. (**b**) Volume-rendered CT image shows an aortic stent (*large arrow*). There are two arteries to the right kidney (*small arrows*). (**c**) Coronal reformatted CT image shows that these two arteries have a common origin, which may be narrow (*arrow*). (**d**) Aortography confirms that the right renal arteries have a common origin (*arrow*) and shows that both have mild focal stenoses

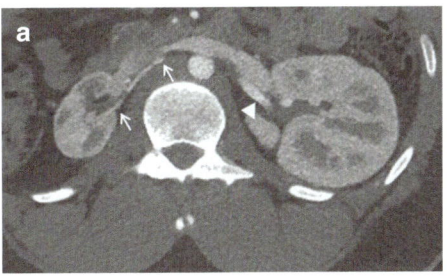

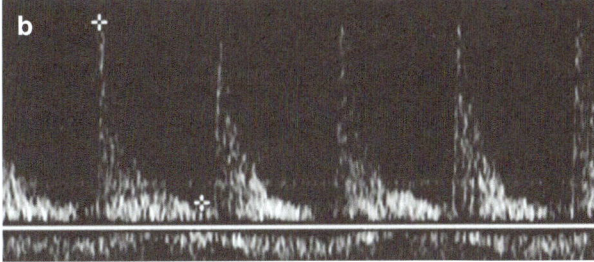

Fig. 2 CT of the abdomen of a 17-year-old male with hypertension. (**a**) Long segment of narrowing in the right renal artery (between *arrows*). The caliber of the left renal artery is normal (*arrowhead*). The right kidney is diffusely atrophied with cortical thinning. There is compensatory hypertrophy of the left kidney. (**b**) Spectral Doppler ultrasound. Corresponding spectral Doppler ultrasound shows decreased diastolic flow and increased peak systolic velocities in the main renal artery with resulting aliasing in the long stenotic segment and elevated resistive index (0.88) indicative of the stenosis. Note that the peak systolic velocity is not very high probably because of the reduced flow volume due to the increased renal vascular resistance (Bud et al. 1999) (Courtesy of A. Ntoulia, MD, PhD; Children's Hospital of Philadelphia, Pennsylvania, USA)

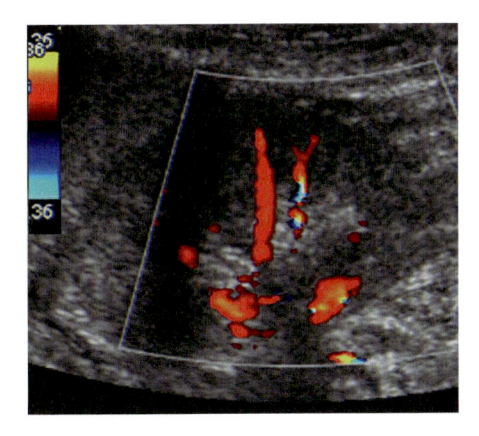

Fig. 3 Color Doppler ultrasound of a young child with intrarenal artery stenosis. The site of stenosis can be seen as aliasing due to turbulent blood flow via the reduced lumen of the vessel (Courtesy of M. Riccabona, MD, Prof. University Hospital of Graz, Austria)

labeled mercaptoacetyltriglycine (MAG3) in hydronephrosis (to assess function and drainage) or a dimercaptosuccinic acid (DMSA) study and a cystogram in a small and/or scarred kidney (to assess function and possible VUR).

5.2 Post-captopril Renal Scintigraphy

Renal scintigraphy using 99mTc-labeled DMSA or MAG3, before and after administration of an angiotensin-converting enzyme inhibitor such as captopril, is potentially a very elegant method of revealing RVD in children (Fig. 4). However captopril scintigraphy has poor accuracy in diagnosing RVD in children especially in bilateral or segmental disease (Ng et al. 1997; Abdulsamea et al. 2010; Reusz et al. 2010; Tullus et al. 2010). So its role as a part of a rational algorithm for the evaluation of hypertension in children remains controversial. In practice, the results of this technique have not been good enough to identify with sufficient accuracy which children with severe hypertension do not need angiography. The sensitivity and specificity for RVD are reported to be 48–73 % and 68–88 %, respectively (Ng et al. 1997; Minty et al. 1993; Abdulsamea et al. 2010). Although detection of segmental abnormalities is sometimes possible with this technique (Cheung et al. 2004), the high prevalence of bilateral and/or branch artery RVD may well limit its utility in children.

5.3 Computed Tomographic Angiography (CTA)

Computed tomographic angiography (CTA) provides excellent resolution, allowing high-quality multiplanar 2D/3D reconstructions; it is rapid resulting in fewer motion-related artifacts and less need for sedation and it is ssreproducible (Castelli et al. 2013; Kurian et al. 2013). Disadvantages of CTA include the need for IV iodinated contrast material and ionizing radiation exposure, although pediatric appropriate

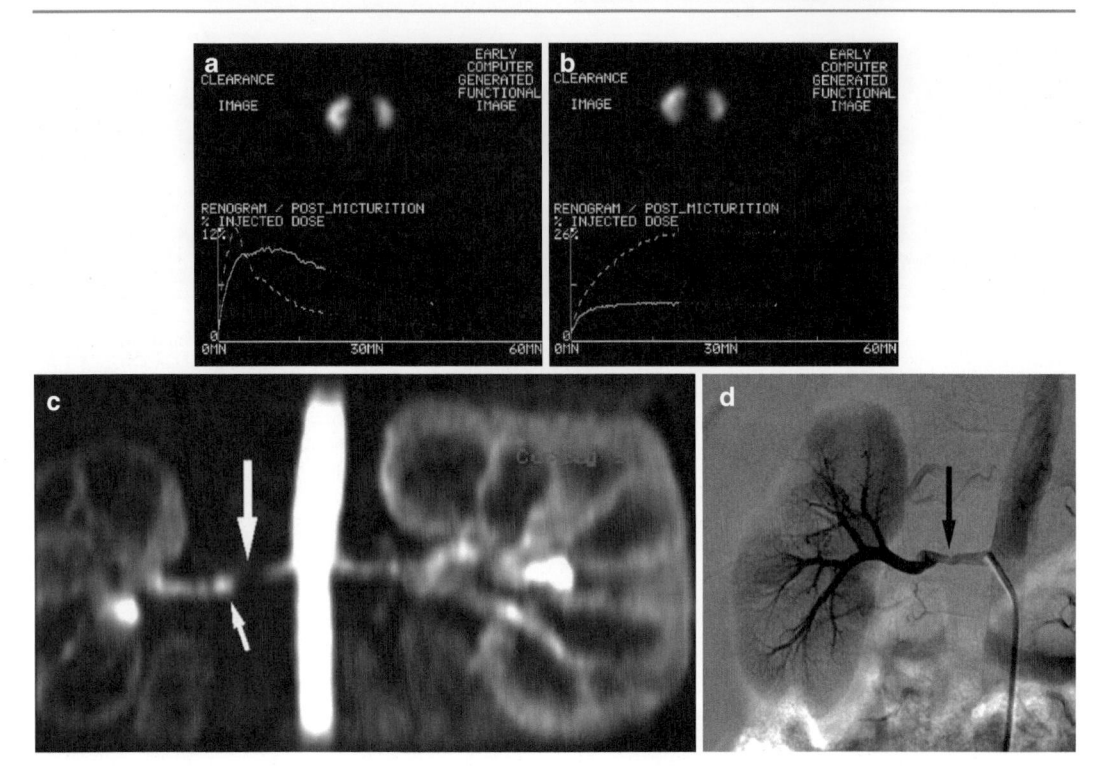

Fig. 4 A 5-year-old male with right renal artery stenosis. (**a**) Pre-captopril scintigraphy with ^{99m}Tc-labeled mercaptoacetyltriglycine (*MAG3*). The left kidney (*dashed line*) shows normal handling of the tracer. The right kidney shows slow transit and only 40% of total renal function. (**b**) Post-captopril MAG3 scintigraphy. There was a significant hypotensive response to captopril (systolic blood pressure fell from 170 to 100 mmHg). This accounts for the delayed transit on the left side. The right kidney shows more prolonged transit than before and a small fall in divided function to 37%. These findings suggest right renal artery stenosis. (**c**) Contrast-enhanced magnetic resonance angiography (*MRA*) shows stenosis of the right main renal artery (*large arrow*) and suggests that there may be a poststenotic dilatation (*small arrow*). (**d**) Digital subtraction angiography confirms the stenosis (*arrow*) and poststenotic dilatation. Note that the MRA underestimates the extent of intrarenal disease (*old numbering 22.2a–d*)

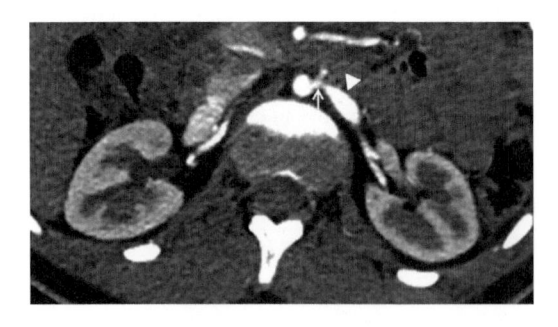

Fig. 5 CT angiography of 16-year-old male with Williams syndrome. High-grade stenosis is noted at the origin of the left renal artery (*arrow*) with poststenotic dilatation (*arrowhead*). Mild diffuse cortical thinning of the left kidney compared to the right kidney (Courtesy of A. Ntoulia MD, PhD; Children's Hospital of Philadelphia, Pensylvania, USA)

low-dose radiation exposures can be used with high-quality renal CTA examinations (Castelli et al. 2013; Kurian et al. 2013). CTA has been used with high efficacy in the diagnosis of renovascular disease in adults; however, in children, its diagnostic accuracy is unknown (Visrutaratna et al. 2009). CT angiography clearly is adequate for most patients with disease of the aorta and main renal arteries (Fig. 5), (Vade et al 2002). At present CTA should not be used to screen for RAS because the site of stenosis in children is frequently in second-order vessels and CTA might not be able to evaluate these small caliber vessels. Due to these technical challenges, and the high radiation dose of CTA, catheter-based digital subtraction angiography is still the preferred option in children with a high probability for RVD (Visrutaratna et al. 2009). Furthermore, conventional angiography offers the opportunity for angioplasty, if appropriate, at the same time as the diagnostic study.

5.4 Magnetic Resonance Angiography (MRA)

Magnetic resonance angiography (MRA) is currently adequate for assessment of the aorta and main renal arteries. Some studies in adults report very high accuracy (up to 90%) in significant RVD; however, in children, there are no published studies comparing MRA with DSA in meaningful numbers (Tullus et al. 2008, 2010). Advantages of MRA include excellent contrast resolution, the ability to obtain three-dimensional images either without or with IV contrast material, and the lack of ionizing radiation exposure (Castelli et al. 2013). Disadvantages of MRA compared with CTA include lower spatial resolution limiting successful evaluation of intrarenal branches and small accessory renal arteries, the potential to exaggerate areas of arterial narrowing, and the presence of movement and flow artifacts (Castelli et al. 2013; Tullus et al. 2010). Despite these limitations, new techniques, including quantification of renal blood flow and perfusion imaging, may increase the ability of MRA to identify RVD in the future (Tullus et al. 2010).

5.5 Digital Subtraction Angiography (DSA)

Digital subtraction angiography (DSA) is considered as the gold standard for diagnosing renovascular causes of hypertension, primarily because of its excellent spatial, contrast, and temporal resolution (Castelli et al. 2013; Tullus et al. 2010). DSA has the additional advantages of potential renal vein renin sampling for lateralizing an ischemic focus (or even localizing it within a kidney), and for the endovascular treatment of some lesions, both of which can be performed at the same time as diagnostic DSA (Deal et al. 1992; Teigen et al. 1992; Tullus et al. 2010). Disadvantages of DSA are that it generally entails a higher radiation dose than a CTA, it carries a small risk of arterial damage, it almost always requires general anesthesia, and it does not give direct information about arterial wall (Tullus et al. 2010). In younger children, less than about 10 years of age, DSA is exclusively performed under general anesthesia, especially if angiography is being performed with a view to immediate intervention. Muscle relaxants are used to allow the suspension of ventilation during acquisition, to minimize subtraction artifacts. Diagnostic angiography is usually performed following US-guided puncture of the common femoral artery. Biplane aortography provides views of the origins of the renal and visceral arteries (Fig. 1). Selective renal angiography with oblique projections is performed to provide detailed images of the renal arteries and their branches without opacification of overlying superior mesenteric artery branches (Fig. 4). Views of the pelvis and celiac branches are included for surgical planning when required. Modern centers are increasingly using rotational angiography to acquire CT-like 3D volumes which allow multiplanar reconstructions and three-dimensional reconstructions of the vascular tree and specifically of affected vessels (see also chapter "Pediatric Genitourinary Intervention").

> **Take Away**
> For imaging in childhood hypertension, US is the first imaging test, but may be equivocal and insufficient; particularly US has limitations in ruling out RAS. Scintigraphy and CTA or MRA may offer an alternative in children with low probability for RVD; however, only DSA is able to reliable find or rule out vascular pathology. Thus all children with a high probability of RAS should undergo DSA directly after US – potentially with simultaneous intravascular treatment.

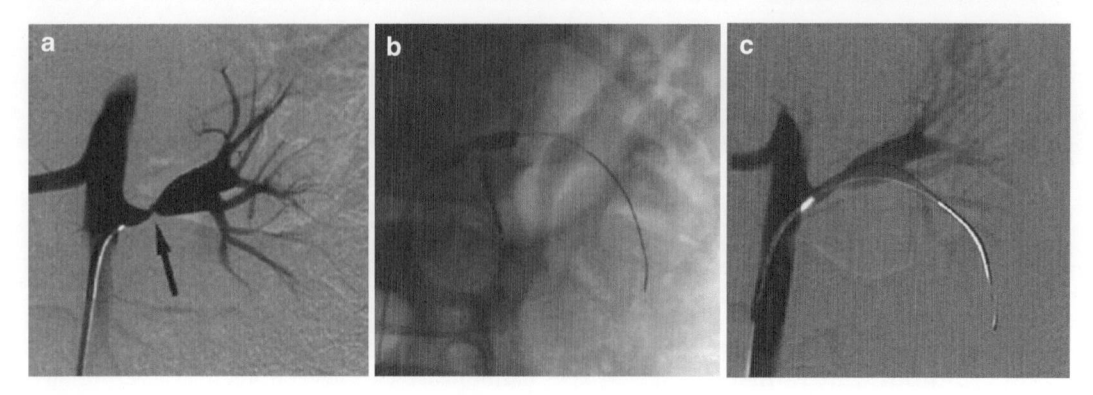

Fig. 6 A 9-year-old girl with left renal artery stenosis. (**a**) Digital subtraction angiography shows a tight stenosis of the left renal artery (*arrow*). (**b**) The waist on the 4-mm angioplasty balloon (*arrow*) corresponds to the stenosis. (**c**) Following further inflation and abolition of the waist on the balloon, there is a good angiographic result. Note that the balloon was selected according to the size of the normal renal artery and not the poststenotic dilatation

6   Endovascular Treatment

The decision to proceed to angioplasty or stenting is best made by a multidisciplinary renovascular team (Tullus et al. 2008), and further reading is suggested in chapter "Pediatric Genitourinary Intervention" of this book by Towbin et al., regarding genitourinary interventions. The common femoral artery is the usual access point, with an appropriately sized sheath size according to the size of the child and the planned procedure. Adult coronary angioplasty systems are particularly useful for small children and segmental renal artery stenoses. These can be introduced through a 4-F sheath or a 6-F guiding catheter. Angioplasty is often successful, particularly in simple main renal artery stenoses (Fig. 6) (Shroff et al. 2006). In children, stenting is still controversial and is therefore usually reserved for treatment of complications or for stenoses that recur rapidly following initial clinical success (Shroff et al. 2006). Embolization may be appropriate if DSA and renal vein renin sampling localize a segmental ischemic focus. Ethanol is injected into a segmental artery in order to destroy the appropriate area of renal parenchyma by causing irreversible endothelial damage (Teigen et al. 1992). There are many surgical options for RVD in childhood, but these are usually reserved for children in whom endovascular therapy is not feasible or has failed (Tullus et al. 2008).

Conclusion

RVD is an important cause of childhood hypertension. US may be a first imaging test, but has significant limitations. CTA and MRA also have restrictions in children; thus DSA is the gold standard test and should be performed in children with a high probability of RAS/RVD without other previous imaging studies even if US is negative. When certain clinical and/or imaging findings suggest RVD, children with hypertension should be referred to a multidisciplinary pediatric renovascular team for consideration of endovascular therapy.

References

Abdulsamea S, Anderson P, Biassoni L et al (2010) Pre- and postcaptopril renal scintigraphy as a screening test for renovascular hypertension in children. Pediatr Nephrol 25:317–322

Brun P, Kchouk H, Mouchet B et al (1997) Value of Doppler ultrasound for the diagnosis of renal artery stenosis in children. Pediatr Nephrol 11:27–30

Bud RO, Larson RG, Nichols WW et al (1999) Stenosis of the main artery supplying an organ: effect of end-organ vascular resistance on the poststenotic peak systolic velocity in an in vitro hydraulic model at Doppler US. Radiology 212:79–87

Castelli PK, Dillman JR, Smith EA et al (2013) Imaging of renin-mediated hypertension in children. AJR 200(6):W661–W672

Castelli PK, Dillman JR, Kershaw DB, Khalatbari S, Stanley JC, Smith EA (2014) Renal sonography with

Doppler for detecting suspected pediatric renin-mediated hypertension – is it adequate? Pediatr Radiol 44(1):42–49

Cheung WS, Wong KN, Wong YC, Ma KM (2004) Segmental renal artery stenosis diagnosed with captopril renography in a child. Pediatr Radiol 34:636–639

Deal JE, Snell MF, Barratt TM, Dillon MJ (1992) Renovascular disease in childhood. J Pediatr 121:378–384

Dillon MJ (1997) The diagnosis of renovascular disease. Pediatr Nephrol 11:366–372 (PR)

Gill DG, de Mendes CB, Cameron JS et al (1976) Analysis of 100 children with severe and persistent hypertension. Arch Dis Child 51:951–956

Gomes RS, Quirino IG, Pereira RM et al (2011) Primary versus secondary hypertension in children followed up at an outpatient tertiary unit. Pediatr Nephrol 26:441–447

Goonasekera CD, Dillon MJ (2000) Measurement and interpretation of blood pressure. Arch Dis Child 82:261–265

Kurian J, Epelman M, Darge K et al (2013) The role of CT angiography in the evaluation of pediatric renovascular hypertension. Pediatr Radiol 43(4):490–501

Li JC, Wang L, Jiang YX et al (2006) Evaluation of renal artery stenosis with velocity parameters of Doppler sonography. J Ultrasound Med 25(6):735–742

McCulloch M, Andronikou S, Goddard E et al (2003) Angiographic features of 26 children with Takayasu's arteritis. Pediatr Radiol 33(4):230–235

Minty I, Lythgoe MF, Gordon I (1993) Hypertension in paediatrics: can pre- and post-captopril technetium-99m dimercaptosuccinic acid renal scans exclude renovascular disease? Eur J Nucl Med 20:699–702

National High Blood Pressure Education Program Working Group on High Blood Pressure in Children and Adolescents (2004) The fourth report on the diagnosis, evaluation, and treatment of high blood pressure in children and adolescents. Pediatrics 114:555–576

Ng CS, de Bruyn R, Gordon I (1997) The investigation of renovascular hypertension in children: the accuracy of radio-isotopes in detecting renovascular disease. Nucl Med Commun 18:1017–1028

Patriquin HB, Lafortune M, Jequier JC et al (1992) Stenosis of the renal artery: assessment of slowed systole in the downstream circulation with Doppler sonography. Radiology 184:479–485

Reusz GS, Kis E, Cseprekal O, Szabo AJ (2010) Captopril-enhanced renal scintigraphy in the diagnosis of pediatric hypertension. Pediatr Nephrol 25:185–189

Riccabona M, Lobo NL, Papadopoulou F et al (2011) ESPR uroradiology task force and ESUR paediatric working group: imaging recommendations in paediatric uroradiology, Part IV: minutes of the ESPR uroradiology task force mini-symposium on imaging in childhood hypertension and imaging of renal trauma in children. Pediatr Radiol 41(7):939–944

Rosner B, Prineas RJ, Loggie JM, Daniels SR (1993) Blood pressure nomograms for children and adolescents, by height, sex, and age, in the United States. J Pediatr 123:871–886

Sadowski RH, Falkner B (1996) Hypertension in pediatric patients. Am J Kidney Dis 27:305–315

Shroff R, Roebuck DJ, Gordon I et al (2006) Angioplasty for renovascular hypertension in children: 20-year experience. Pediatrics 118:268–275

Slovut DP, Olin JW (2004) Fibromuscular dysplasia. N Engl J Med 350(18):1862–1871

Srinivasan A, Krishnamurthy G, Fontalvo-Herazo L et al (2011) Spectrum of renal findings in pediatric fibromuscular dysplasia and neurofibromatosis type 1. Pediatr Radiol 41:308–316

Teigen CL, Mitchell SE, Venbrux AC, Christenson MJ, McLean RH (1992) Segmental renal artery embolization for treatment of pediatric renovascular hypertension. J Vasc Interv Radiol 3:111–117

Tullus K, Brennan E, Hamilton G et al (2008) Renovascular hypertension in children. Lancet 371:1453–1463

Tullus K, Roebuck DJ, McLaren CA, Marks SD (2010) Imaging in the evaluation of renovascular disease. Pediatr Nephrol 25:1049–1056

Vade A, Agrawal R, Lim-Dunham J, Hartoin D (2002) Utility of computed tomographic renal angiogram in the management of childhood hypertension. Pediatr Nephrol 17:741–747

Visrutaratna P, Srisuwan T, Sirivanichai C (2009) Pediatric renovascular hypertension in Thailand: CT angiographic findings. Pediatr Radiol 39:1321–1326

Vo NJ, Hammelman BD, Racadio JM et al (2006) Anatomic distribution of renal artery stenosis in children: implications for imaging. Pediatr Radiol 36:1032–1036

Watson AR, Balfe JW, Hardy BE (1985) Renovascular hypertension in childhood: a changing perspective in management. J Pediatr 106:366–372

Williams G, Macaskill P, Chan S et al (2007) Comparative accuracy of renal duplex sonographic parameters in the diagnosis of renal artery stenosis: paired and unpaired analysis. AJR 188:798–811

Wyszynska T, Cichocka E, Wieteska-Klimczak A, Jobs K, Januszewicz P (1992) A single pediatric center experience with 1,025 children with hypertension. Acta Paediatr 81:244–246

Part VII

Urinary Tract Tumors, Trauma and Intervention

Neoplasms of the Genitourinary System

Eline Deurloo, Hervé Brisse, and Anne Smets

Contents

1	**Renal Tumors**	654
1.1	Introduction	654
1.2	Wilms' Tumor or Nephroblastoma	654
1.3	Non-wilms' Malignant Tumors	666
1.4	Benign Tumors	674
1.5	Pseudotumoral Conditions	679
1.6	Diagnostic Strategy of Renal Neoplasms in Children	679
2	**Neoplasms of the Lower Genitourinary Tract**	682
2.1	Rhabdomyosarcoma	682
2.2	Differential Diagnosis	687
	References	689

List of Abbreviations

ADC	Apparent diffusion coefficient
ALK	Anaplastic lymphoma kinase
A-RMS	Alveolar-type rhabdomyosarcoma
BP RMS	Bladder-prostate rhabdomyosarcoma
CCSK	Clear cell sarcoma of the kidney
CDS	Color Doppler sonography
CMN	Congenital mesoblastic nephroma
CPDN	Cystic partially differentiated nephroblastoma
CXR	Chest X-ray
DWI	Diffusion weighted imaging
EFS	Event-free survival
EpSSG	European paediatric Soft tissue Sarcoma Study Group
E-RMS	Embryonal-type rhabdomyosarcoma
FDG-PET	Fludeoxyglucose positron emission tomography
GU	Genitourinary
ILNRs	Intralobar nephrogenic rests
IVC	Inferior vena cava
MA	Metanephric adenoma
MRTK	Malignant rhabdoid tumor of the kidney
NRs	Nephrogenic rests
NSS	Nephron-sparing surgery
NWTSG	North American National Wilms' Tumor Study Group
PLNRs	Perilobar nephrogenic rests
pPNET	Peripheral primitive neuroectodermal tumor

E. Deurloo, MD, PhD (✉) • A. Smets, MD
Department of Radiology, Academic Medical Center,
Meibergdreef 9, 1105 AZ Amsterdam,
The Netherlands
e-mail: e.e.deurloo@amc.uva.nl

H. Brisse, MD, PhD
Department of Radiology, Institut Curie,
26 rue d'Ulm, Paris 75005, France

PT RMS	Paratesticular rhabdomyosarcoma
RCC	Renal cell carcinoma
RMS	Rhabdomyosarcoma
RTSG	Renal Tumour Study Group
SIOP	International Society of Pediatric Oncology
US	Ultrasound
VOD	Veno-occlusive disease
WT	Wilms' Tumor

1 Renal Tumors

1.1 Introduction

Nephroblastoma or Wilms' tumor (WT) is the most common renal neoplasm in children accounting for 90 % of pediatric renal tumors (Pastore et al. 2006). It is a tumor with a good prognosis and with well-established treatment strategies. Other rare malignant renal tumors, such as clear cell sarcoma and rhabdoid tumor of the kidney, have a poor prognosis despite aggressive treatment. Renal cell carcinoma occurs in older children, while mesoblastic nephroma is the most frequent renal tumor in the neonate. Hematological malignancies, the most frequent neoplasms in children, may also involve the kidney, most often as part of a multi-organ involvement. Renal infections and malformations are much more common in children than renal tumors and may show a pseudotumoral pattern mimicking a renal tumor. In all cases, close collaboration among radiologists, pediatricians, and pathologists is essential so as to avoid diagnostic pitfalls due to atypical presentations.

1.2 Wilms' Tumor or Nephroblastoma

1.2.1 Epidemiology

Wilms' tumor accounts for 6 % of childhood cancers but for 90 % of renal tumors in childhood (Grundy et al. 2002). It is the fourth most common pediatric cancer after acute leukemia, brain tumors, and neuroblastoma. The incidence of WT is 8.1/106 in Caucasian children under the age of 15 (Breslow et al. 1994). Most WTs are solitary lesions, but about 12 % of children develop multifocal tumors within a single kidney and almost 7 % have bilateral involvement at diagnosis or later on (Pastore et al. 2006).

The most common unilateral form occurs at a mean age of 3.5 years (mostly between 1 and 5 years, 98 % before 7 years) with a male to female ratio of 0.92:1 (Grundy et al. 2002). Neonatal or prenatal WTs are extremely rare (Isaacs 2008). Familial cases are rare (1–2 %) (Breslow et al. 1996). In 9–17 % of WT patients, there is a predisposing syndrome, specifically WT1-associated syndromes and overgrowth syndromes such as WAGR syndrome (Wilms' tumor, aniridia, genitourinary malformations, and mental retardation) and Denys-Drash syndrome (DDS; mesangiosclerosis, Wilms' tumor, and pseudohermaphroditism/genitourinary malformations). The most common overgrowth syndrome is Beckwith-Wiedemann syndrome (hemihypertrophy, macroglossia, macrosomia, neonatal hypoglycemia, abdominal wall defects, and increased risk for Wilms' tumor and other embryonal tumors).

Bilateral synchronous WT is more frequent in girls (sex ratio: 0.6:1), at a younger age (mean: 2.5 years), and the association with nephrogenic rests, congenital malformations, and/or predisposing genetic syndromes is higher than in unilateral WT (Scott et al. 2006a; Segers et al. 2012) (Table 1).

1.2.2 Pathology

1.2.2.1 Wilms' Tumor

The typical form is a large lesion, surrounded by a pseudocapsule and sharply delineated from the adjacent renal parenchyma. The internal structure is usually heterogeneous, with hemorrhagic and/or necrotic cystic areas (Fig. 1). The typical "triphasic" tumor is composed of blastemal, epithelial, and stromal cells, but variable patterns may be observed (Schmidt and Beckwith 1995). Regarding correlation between the histological features and survival, three histological risk groups were defined by the International Society of Pediatric Oncology (SIOP), based on

Table 1 Major genetic syndromes associated with Wilms' tumor

	WT1 gene (11p13)		WT2 gene (11p15.5)		Other				
Syndromes	WAGR	Denys-Drash	Frasier	Beckwith-Wiedemann	Perlman	Simpson-Golabi-Behmel (type 1)	Sotos	Fanconi anemia D1	Mosaic variegated aneuploidy
Genetics	Constitutional microdeletion WT1 and PAX6	Constitutional mutation exons 8 and 9	Constitutional mutation intron 9	H19 hypermethylation, uniparental disomy	?	Xq26 GPC3 gene mutation	5q35 (NSD1) deletion mutation	13q12.3 biallelic mutation BRCA2	BUB1B gene mutation
Nephrogenic rests	Intralobar	Intralobar	Intralobar	Perilobar	Perilobar				
Estimated tumor risk	50%	>50%	8%	5–10%	?	10%	4%	?	>20%
Other renal abnormalities	Genitourinary malformation	Glomerular disease: mesangial sclerosis		Nephromegaly, medullary cysts, calyceal diverticula, hydronephrosis, nephrolithiasis	Nephromegaly, renal dysplasia, cortical hamartomas, hydronephrosis				
Associated features	Aniridia, mental retardation	Male pseudohermaphroditism, gonadal dysgenesis, gonadoblastoma		Macrosomia, macroglossia, hemihypertrophy, abdominal wall defects, pancreatic islet cell hyperplasia, hepatoblastoma, rhabdomyosarcoma, adrenocortical tumor		Macrosomia, heart and skeletal abnormalities	Macrosomia, CNS abnormalities	Hematologic malignancies	Growth retardation, microcephalia
					Facial dysmorphism, diffuse muscular hypotonicity, cryptorchidism, pancreatic islet cell hyperplasia, mental retardation				

DeBaun and Tucker (1998), Bliek et al. (2004), Cooper et al. (2005), Rump et al. (2005), Scott et al. (2006a), Scott et al. (2006b)

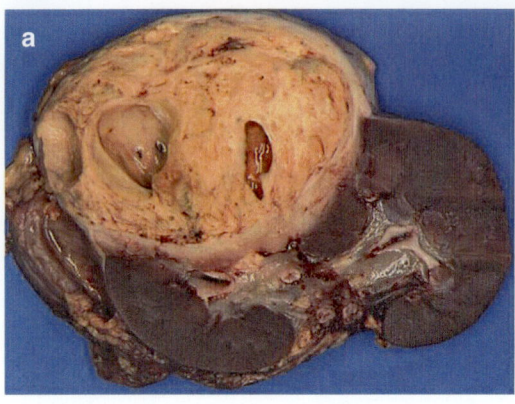

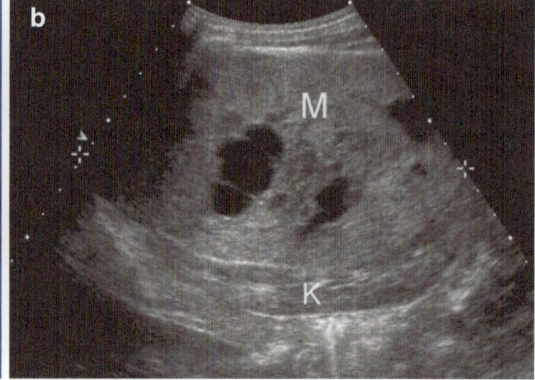

Fig. 1 Wilms' tumor in a 5-year-old girl. (**a**) Gross specimen: large, well-demarcated mass containing cystic areas (courtesy Prof. M. Peuchmaur, Hopital R Debré, Paris, France). (**b**) Corresponding abdominal ultrasound showing a heterogeneous mass (*M*) containing fluid-filled areas and surrounded by the residual normal parenchyma of the kidney (*K*)

Table 2 SIOP working classification of pretreated renal tumors

Low risk	Intermediate risk	High risk

Cystic partially differentiated nephroblastoma (CPDN)
Completely necrotic nephroblastoma
Mesoblastic nephroma
	Nephroblastoma
	  Epithelial type
	  Stromal type
	  Mixed type
	  Regressive type (>2/3 nonviable tumor)
	  Focal anaplasia
		Nephroblastoma
		  Blastemal type
		  Diffuse anaplasia
		Clear cell sarcoma of the kidney (CCSK)
		Rhabdoid tumor of the kidney (MRTK)

Vujanic et al. (2002)

histological findings after pretreatment with chemotherapy (SIOP 2001) (Table 2). "Low-risk" tumors are tumors that have become completely necrotic after neoadjuvant chemotherapy and cystic partially differentiated nephroblastoma (CPDN), a variant that usually occurs in children less than 2 years of age. It is defined by tumors composed entirely of cysts with thin septa (<5 mm) containing blastemal cells in any amount, with or without other embryonal stromal or epithelial cell types. The prognosis of CPDN is excellent (Luithle et al. 2007).

The difference between the various types of "intermediate-risk" tumors is based on the amount of remaining viable tumor and on the predominance (66 %) of histological elements in the remaining viable tumor: epithelial, stromal, mixed, regressive, or focal anaplasia. A peculiar and rare histological variant is teratoid Wilms' tumor. This tumor contains heterologous tissues (fat, glial tissue, muscle, cartilage, or bone) (Inoue et al. 2006). This variant may be bilateral and may present with pyeloureteral obstruction, uremia, and hypertension (Fernandes et al. 1988).

"High-risk" tumors include blastemal and diffuse anaplasia types. Blastemal WT is defined by a residual viable component consisting of at least 2/3 of blastema. This type is associated with a worse prognosis and resistance to chemotherapy. WT with diffuse anaplasia is the other high-risk type. Three histological criteria are necessary to meet the diagnosis of anaplasia: the presence of atypical mitotic figures, marked nuclear enlargement, and the presence of hyperchromatic tumor cell nuclei. WT with diffuse anaplasia is a high-grade malignancy subtype, uncommon in infants, observed at a mean age of 5 years (Vujanic et al. 1999) and is more frequent in black children.

Focal anaplasia consists of only a few discrete sharply demarcated foci (a single focus not larger than 15 mm, two or more foci not larger than 5 mm) within a primary intrarenal tumor. As mentioned above, tumors with only focal anaplasia are classified as "intermediate risk."

1.2.2.2 Nephrogenic Rests and Nephroblastomatosis

Nephrogenic rests (NRs) are persistent microscopic or macroscopic clusters of embryonal metanephric blastema within the kidney. The two main types are perilobar nephrogenic rests (PLNRs), sharply demarcated at the periphery of the renal cortex, occurring frequently in hemihypertrophy and Beckwith-Wiedemann syndromes and intralobar nephrogenic rests (ILNRs) situated within the renal lobe and associated with WT1 gene, sporadic aniridia, WAGR, and Denys-Drash syndromes (Beckwith et al. 1990; Lonergan et al. 1998). NRs are histologically classified as: dormant, sclerosing, hyperplastic, or neoplastic. Hyperplastic nodules are considered precursor lesions to WT (Beckwith 1993) and are difficult to distinguish from WT, both on imaging and pathology (Beckwith 1998; Subhas et al. 2004; Cox et al. 2014; Charlton et al. 2015).

NRs are discovered incidentally in about 1% of normal infant's kidneys (Beckwith 1998) but in 41% of unilateral WT specimens, in 99% of synchronous bilateral WT, and in 94% of metachronous bilateral WT (Beckwith 1993).

Nephroblastomatosis is defined by diffuse or multifocal involvement of the kidneys with NRs. Diffuse perilobar nephroblastomatosis results in bilateral enlarged kidneys with loss of corticomedullary differentiation. NRs are an important clue in the differential diagnosis of a renal tumor in a child since they have only rarely been described in association with a renal tumor of childhood other than WT (Vujanic et al. 1995).

1.2.3 Clinical Features

1.2.3.1 Sporadic Wilms' Tumor

WT is a very rapidly growing tumor with a doubling rate estimated at 11 days (Zoubek et al. 1999). Sporadic tumors usually present with nonspecific clinical symptoms: abdominal mass, pain, or swelling. Hematuria, fever (20%), and hypertension (25%) are other frequent findings. Varicocele may be associated with renal vein or IVC thrombosis. WT-associated abnormalities are cryptorchidism (prevalence: 4.7%), hypospadias (2%), and sporadic hemihypertrophy (2.5%) (Grundy et al. 2002; Breslow et al. 1993).

1.2.3.2 Wilms' Tumor Screening in Patients with Predisposing Syndromes

Screening for WT in children with predisposing syndromes (Table 1) is based on the hypothesis that the detection of a tumor at an early stage may decrease morbidity and permits curative nephron-sparing surgery. This more conservative type of surgery is considered in these patients with predisposing genetic syndromes who are at risk of developing metachronous renal tumors, in bilateral WT, in unilateral WT with contralateral urological or nephrological disorders, and in carefully selected patients with non-syndromic unilateral WT (Wilde et al. 2014; Cozzi and Zani 2006; Kieran et al. 2014). Surveillance should be offered after evaluation by a clinical geneticist to assess the tumor risk according to the individual genetic abnormalities. Ultrasound (US) is the primary screening examination recommended for children at more than 5% risk of developing a WT. US screening is recommended every 3 or 4 months until the age of 5 or 7 years, depending on the genetic profile. As false-positive examinations may result in unnecessary surgery, therefore screening-detected lesions should be managed in reference centers (Owens et al. 2008; Scott et al. 2006a).

1.2.4 Imaging of Wilms' Tumor

1.2.4.1 Common WT Radiological Pattern

Since WT is a rapidly growing tumor, the mass is usually large at diagnosis (>5–10 cm) (Fig. 2). US typically shows a solid noncalcified heterogeneous lesion containing various amounts of anechoic areas representing hemorrhage, necrosis, and/or epithelial cysts (Fig. 1). CT scan

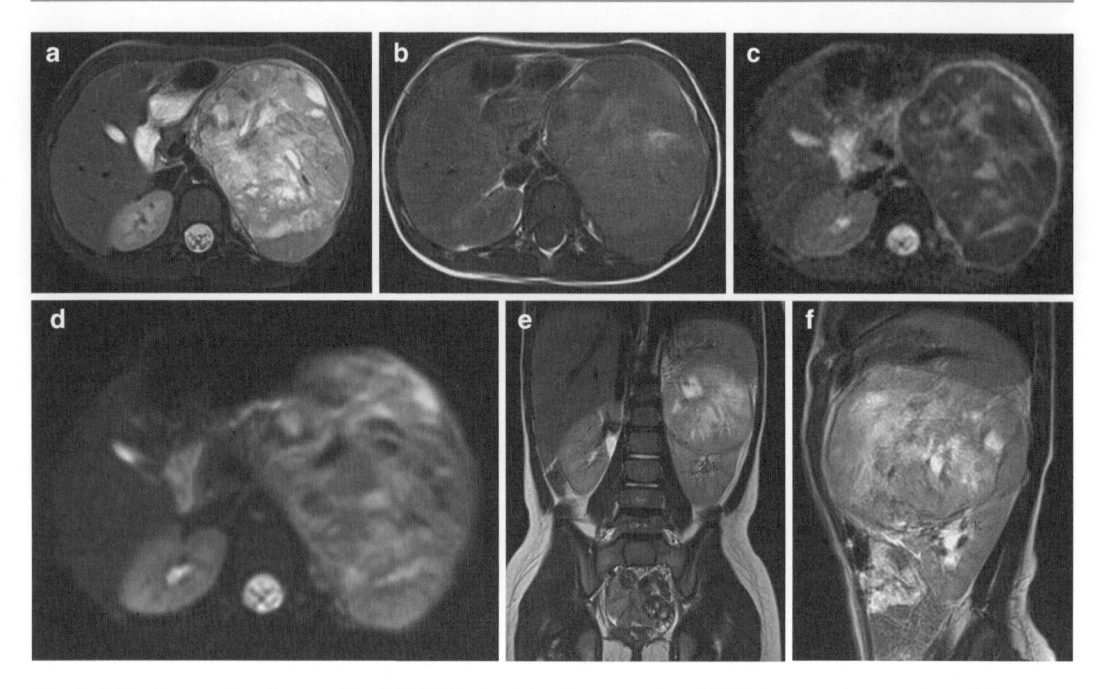

Fig. 2 Wilms' tumor in a 5-year-old girl. MRI (**a**) axial T1-weighted image, (**b**) axial T2-weighted image with fat saturation, (**c**) axial DWI with b value of 800 (**d**) axial ADC, (**e**) sagittal and (**f**) coronal T2-weighted images: these MRi images show a large inhomogeneous mass in the left kidney. ADC shows restricted diffusion, indicating a high cell density

shows a heterogeneous and low attenuating lesion. With intravenous injection of contrast agent, the lesion enhances heterogeneously and to a lesser degree than the normal renal cortex (Brisse et al. 2008b; Smets and de Kraker 2010; Goske et al. 1999). MRI demonstrates a heterogeneous lesion with relatively low signal intensity on T1-weighted sequences and low or intermediate signal intensity compared to the renal cortex with hyperintense necrotic or cystic areas on T2-weighted images (Fig. 2). WTs have a high cellularity and show diffusion restriction on diffusion weighted imaging (DWI) with high b-values. Because of the heterogeneity of WT and the fact that ADC values vary with the different cellular subtypes, the overall mean ADC value does not reflect the tumor composition nor the predominant histology (Hales et al. 2015).

1.2.4.2 Atypical Patterns
Curvilinear intratumoral calcifications may be observed in 5–10% of WT (Navoy et al. 1995). Macroscopic fatty components are rarely observed (Parvey et al. 1981) but may occur in teratoid forms (Park et al. 2003). CPDN presents as a well-limited, purely cystic mass with multiple septations (Fig. 3) (Agrons et al. 1995). This form has to be recognized because it is treated with primary surgery and has an excellent prognosis. "Botryoid" forms have been reported as WT with primary intrapelvic development and exceptional extension down the ureter into the bladder (Fig. 4) (Xu et al. 2013; Nagahara et al. 2006).

1.2.4.3 Bilateral Disease
Bilateral and/or multifocal nodules may correspond to either bilateral WT and/or nephrogenic rests. Macroscopic NRs are occasionally observed, either in the remaining parenchyma or within the contralateral kidney. On sonography, the conspicuousness of these lesions is low because their echogenicity is close to that of renal cortex. The sensitivity of the technique can be enhanced with high-frequency transducers and tools such as harmonic imaging, Power Doppler, or contrast-enhanced

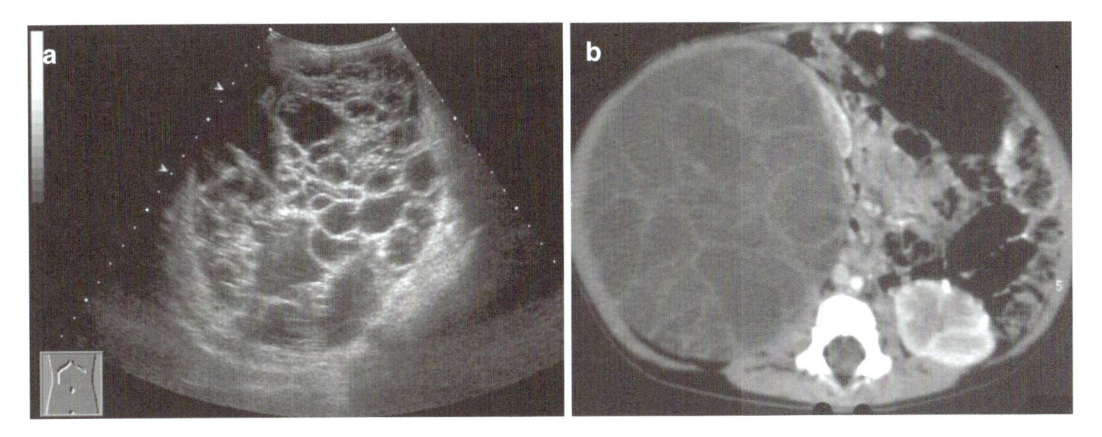

Fig. 3 Cystic partially differentiated nephroblastoma (CPDN) in an 8-month-old boy. Both ultrasound (**a**) and enhanced CT scan (**b**) show a well-demarcated, purely cystic mass with multiple septations

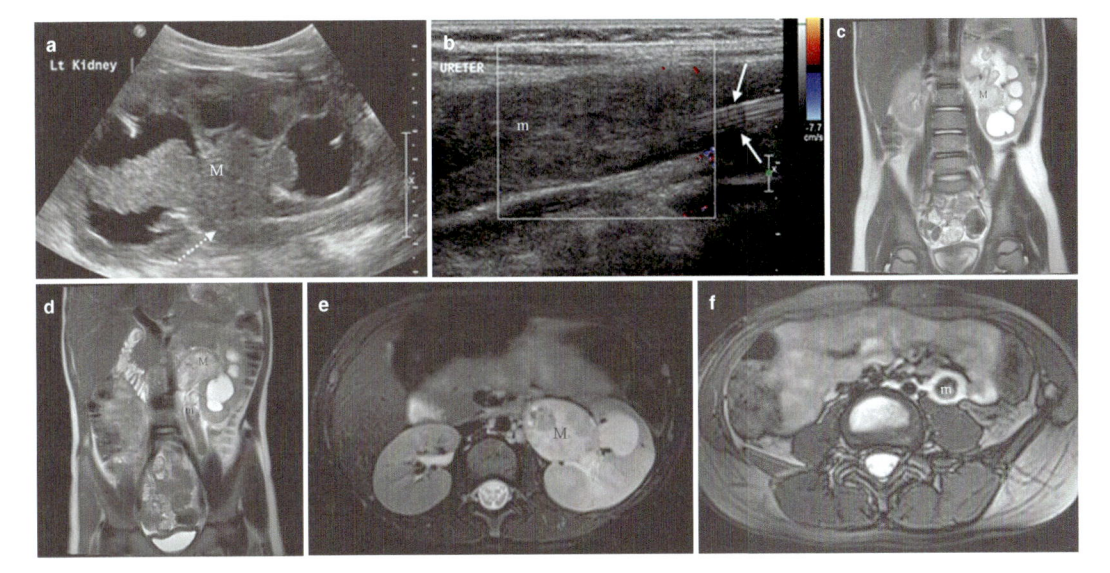

Fig. 4 Botryoid type of Wilms' tumor in a 6-year-old girl, presenting with dysuria and urine containing fragments of tissue. (**a**) Ultrasound of the kidney. (**b**) Ultrasound of the mid-ureter. MRI (**c, d**) coronal T2-weighted images, ((**e, f**) axial T2-weighted fat-saturated images). There is dilatation of the renal collecting system with a central mass (*M*) extending into the dilated ureter (*m*). A JJ stent was positioned in the ureter (*short arrows*)

US. Corticomedullary differentiation may be lost with diffuse nephroblastomatosis (Lonergan et al. 1998). On CT, NRs appear as homogeneous peripheral plaque-like foci or nodules with a slightly higher attenuation value than the normal renal parenchyma on unenhanced images. Nodules enhance homogeneously after intravenous injection of contrast, but to a lesser degree than the normal renal cortex (Fig. 5). On MRI, nephroblastomatosis cannot be differentiated from the normal renal parenchyma on T1-weighted images, but after gadolinium injection, hyperplastic NRs are hypointense to normal renal tissue. On T2-weighted images, hyperplastic NRs are isointense or slightly hyperintense to renal cortex, while sclerotic nephrogenic rests are hypointense. On all images, the signal intensity of nephrogenic rests is homogeneous (Fig. 6) (Gylys-Morin et al. 1993).

In patients with a WT, the additional macroscopic NRs in the ipsilateral kidney are more accu-

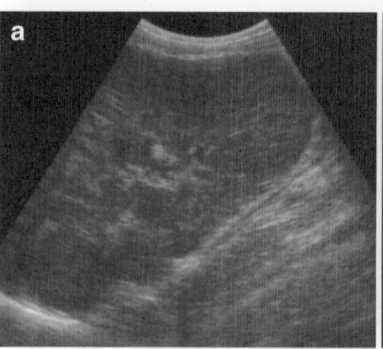

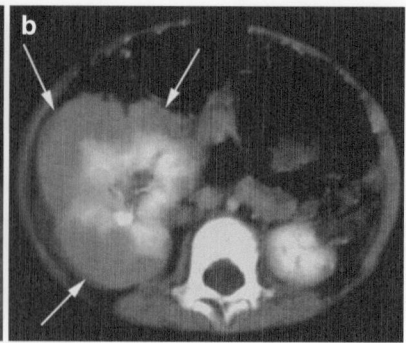

Fig. 5 Diffuse nephroblastomatosis in a 2-year-old girl with a predisposing syndrome (hemihypertrophy). Ultrasound (**a**) shows diffuse enlargement of the right kidney with loss of corticomedullary differentiation. Enhanced CT scan (**b**) shows low attenuating homogeneous peripheral plaque-like masses. Pathological analysis revealed diffuse nephroblastomatosis and three focal stage I WT

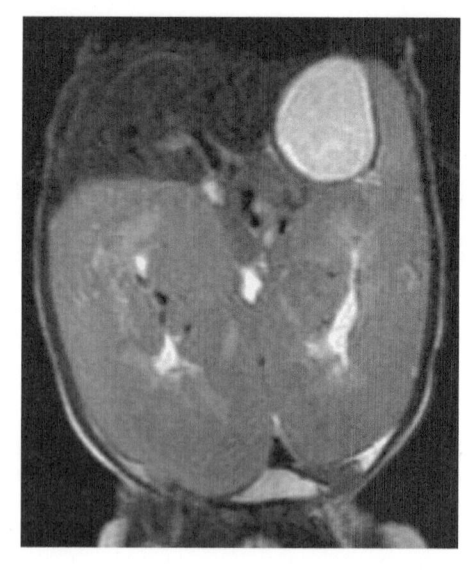

Fig. 6 Diffuse nephroblastomatosis. Coronal T2-weighted MRI showing diffuse enlargement of both kidneys and diffuse thickening of renal cortex

rately depicted with CT or MRI (sensitivity: 57% and 67%, respectively) than with ultrasound (sensitivity: 6%). The most reliable criterion to differentiate NRs from WT is their overall homogeneity (Rohrschneider et al. 1998). However, the differentiation between small WT and NRs cannot rely on imaging only (Fig. 7) (Subhas et al. 2004; Cox et al. 2014). DWI might play a role in the differentiation of WT from NRs; however, its value is still unknown. In imaging reports the term "bilateral disease" should hence be used instead of "bilateral tumors."

1.2.4.4 Locoregional Tumor Extent

The most relevant information is the vascular extension of tumor through the renal vein (Fig. 8) and IVC (Fig. 9), occurring in 5–10% of cases. Patency of the renal vein is assessed preferably with color Doppler sonography (CDS), whereas IVC thrombosis is usually identifiable on grayscale ultrasound. The superior extent of the thrombus should be identified, and the hepatic veins and right atrium must be checked for possible intravascular or intracardiac extension.

Hilar or para-aortic lymph nodes are to be mentioned in reports but carefully interpreted, since small lymph nodes may be invaded by tumoral cells, whereas large lymph nodes may only be inflammatory at pathology (Gow et al. 2000). The final local staging is obtained after surgery, on the basis of histopathological findings (Table 3).

Although rare, intraperitoneal tumor rupture is a major risk factor of abdominal recurrence (Shamberger et al. 1999). Tumor rupture may occur spontaneously, after minor abdominal trauma, during a surgical biopsy procedure or during surgery. Preoperative occurrence of tumor rupture is a rare event, and the incidence of emergency surgery related to preoperative tumor

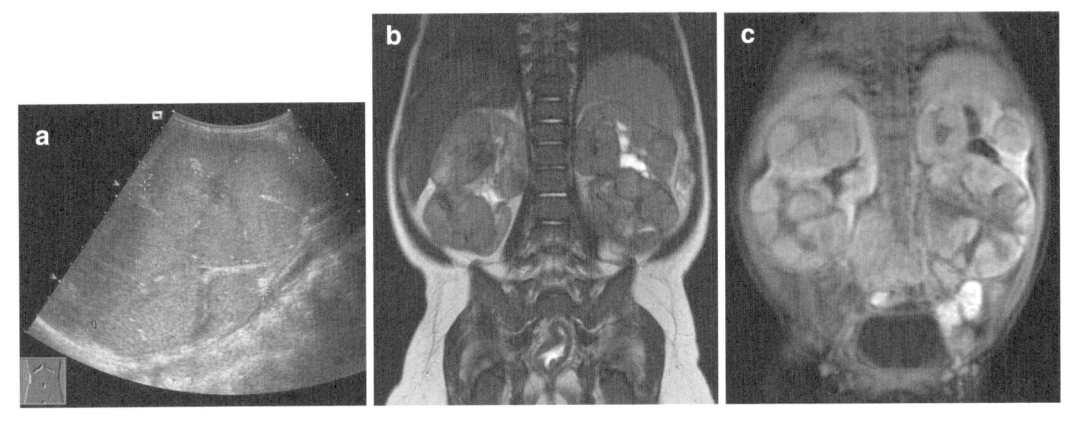

Fig. 7 Macroscopic nephrogenic rests and Wilms' tumors in a 7-month-old girl. Ultrasound (**a**) and MRI (**b**) coronal T2-weighted, and (**c**) coronal contrast-enhanced T1-weighted images show multiple bilateral heterogeneous nodules. After bilateral nephrectomy, pathological analysis showed two stage I WT and three macroscopic nephrogenic rests on the right side and eight stage I WT and two nephrogenic rests on the left side

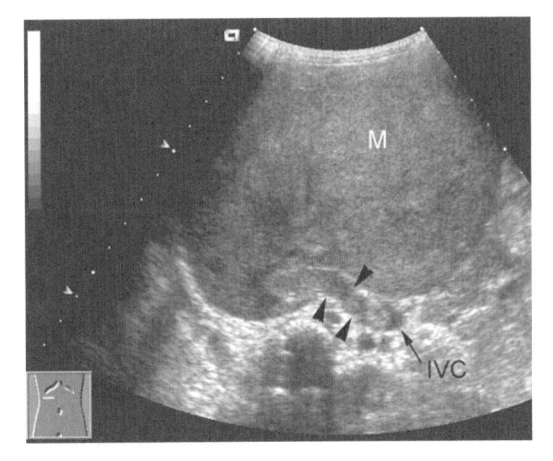

Fig. 8 Right renal vein tumor thrombosis associated with Wilms' tumor (*M*). Ultrasound shows an enlargement of the renal vein (*arrowheads*) filled with echogenic material

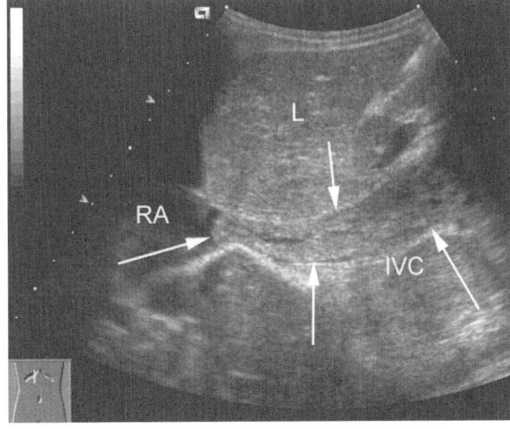

Fig. 9 Inferior vena cava thrombosis related to Wilms' tumor. Ultrasound (sagittal image) shows enlargement of the IVC (*arrows*). The thrombosis reaches the right atrium (*RA*). *L* liver

rupture was estimated at 1.8 % (Godzinski et al. 2001). Isolated peritoneal effusion is not a reliable sign of rupture. An isolated small amount of peritoneal fluid, usually located in the Douglas recess, is frequently observed at diagnosis in patients with WT. It is thought to correspond to a nonspecific inflammatory reaction of the peritoneum due to the rapid tumor growth or to IVC compression or thrombosis. The presence of ascites beyond the cul-de-sac, irrespective of attenuation, was reported to be the most useful indicator on enhanced CT of preoperative Wilms tumor rupture in a recent study (Khanna et al. 2013). Patients with retroperitoneal tumor rupture demonstrate intratumoral, subcapsular, or perirenal hemorrhage (Fig. 10) (Byerly et al. 2006). Hemoperitoneum and/or intraperitoneal, mesenteric, and/or omental masses are related to

Table 3 Histological staging criteria for renal tumors of childhood with exception of RCC according to UMBRELLA SIOP-RTSG 2015 protocol

Stage I	(a) The tumor is limited to the kidney or surrounded with a fibrous (pseudo) capsule if outside of the normal contours of the kidney. The renal capsule or pseudocapsule may be infiltrated by the tumor, but it does not reach the outer surface
	(b) The tumor may be protruding ("bulging") into the pelvic system and "dipping" into the ureter but is not infiltrating their walls
	(c) The vessels or the soft tissues of the renal sinus are not involved
	(d) Intrarenal vessel involvement may be present
	Necrotic tumor in the renal sinus or perirenal fat does not upstage if completely excised
	Fine needle aspiration or percutaneous core needle (tru-cut) biopsy does not upstage but size of needle should be reported to the pathologist
Stage II	(a) Viable tumor penetrates through the renal capsule and/or fibrous pseudocapsule into the perirenal fat but is completely resected
	(b) Viable tumor infiltrates the soft tissues of the renal sinus
	(c) Viable tumor infiltrates blood and lymphatic vessels of the renal sinus or in the perirenal tissue but is completely resected
	(d) Viable tumor infiltrates the renal pelvic or ureter's wall
	(e) Viable tumor infiltrates adjacent organs or IVC but is completely resected
Stage III	(a) Viable tumor extends to the resection margins. If there is only nonviable tumor at inked resection line, it is regarded as stage III if viable tumor is closer than 5 mm to the inked margin. If viable tumor is more than 5 mm distant from the resection line and only regressive changes are found at inked margin, it does not upstage the tumor
	(b) Any abdominal lymph nodes are involved
	(c) Intraoperative tumor rupture
	(d) Tumor penetration through the peritoneal surface
	(e) Tumor implants are found on the peritoneal surface
	(f) Tumor thrombi present at resection margin of vessels or ureter, transected or removed piecemeal by surgeon
	(g) The tumor has been surgically biopsied (wedge biopsy) prior to preoperative chemotherapy or surgery
Stage IV	Hematogenous metastases (lung, liver, bone, brain, etc.) or lymph node metastases outside the abdominopelvic region
Stage V	Bilateral renal tumors at diagnosis (each side should be substaged according to the above criteria)

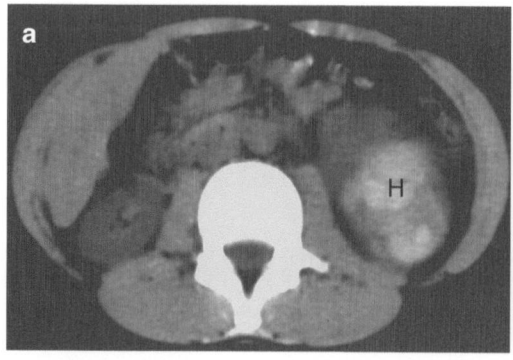

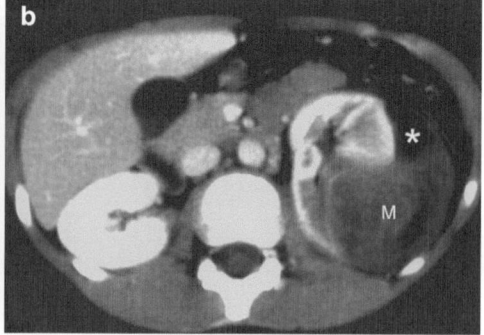

Fig. 10 Retroperitoneal Wilms' tumor rupture in a 9-year-old girl presenting with acute abdominal pain. Unenhanced CT scan (**a**) shows a perirenal hematoma (*H*). Enhanced CT (**b**) shows subcapsular effusion related to tumor rupture (*). Wilms' tumor (*M*)

intraperitoneal dissemination (Fig. 11) (Slasky et al. 1997). Tumor rupture is reported to be clinically silent in 33% of patients (Brisse et al. 2008a). Since treatment of intraperitoneal rupture includes whole abdomen radiotherapy, the diagnosis should rely on relevant findings such as

Fig. 11 Intraperitoneal Wilms' tumor rupture in a 4-year-old girl presenting with a painless right abdominal mass. Enhanced CT scan (**a, c**) with sagittal reconstruction (**b**) shows direct peritoneal extension (*arrows* in **a** and **b**) and pouch of Douglas peritoneal location (*arrows* in **c**)

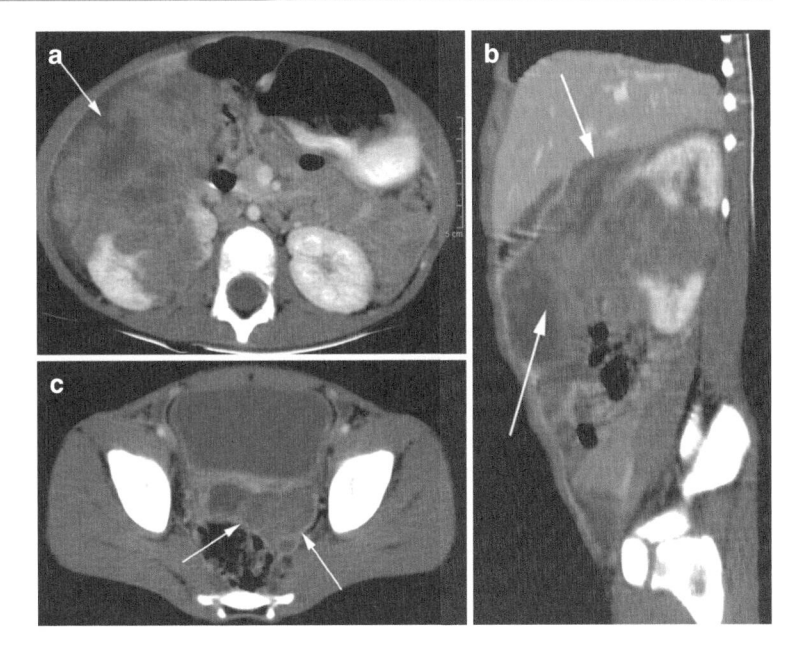

peritoneal lesions observed during surgery or obvious macroscopic intraperitoneal nodules on initial imaging.

1.2.4.5 Distant Metastases

Distant metastases at diagnosis are observed in about 10% of cases. The lungs are usually the only metastatic site. In the last decade, the standard diagnostic tool for the detection of lung metastasis has shifted from chest X-ray (CXR) to chest CT in children with a renal tumor. Chest CT will be the mandatory technique for the evaluation of lung metastasis in the new SIOP protocol (UMBRELLA SIOP-RTSG 2015 protocol). However, the low specificity of CT for lung nodules (McCarville et al. 2006), the variability in interpretation (Wilimas et al. 1997), and the higher radiation exposure of CT compared to CXR must be kept in mind. Although there is no evidence yet that the use of chest CT will improve overall outcome, CT might help identify a subgroup of patients with metastases undetectable on CXR, who may benefit from intensified treatment (Smets et al. 2012; Grundy et al. 2012).

Liver metastases occur in only about 2% of patients (Szavay et al. 2006; Ehrlich et al. 2009). Bone metastases are exceptional and observed in only 0.8% (Gururangan et al. 1994). Bone scintigraphy is therefore not required as a staging tool in typical WT.

1.2.4.6 Preoperative Imaging

US is sufficient in most unilateral WT patients to assess tumor size reduction during neoadjuvant chemotherapy. Lack of tumor response may be related to histological type (high-risk form or stromal type). Progression of localized WT is rarely seen in patients during preoperative chemotherapy. However, these patients are known to have poorer survival (Ora et al. 2007).

In a preoperative stage, cross-sectional imaging, preferably with MRI, provides valuable information for the surgeon to determine the degree of complexity of the operation (Schenk et al. 2008). Of importance are the extent of the tumor, venous involvement, invasion of surrounding organs and structures (liver, diaphragm, spleen, pancreas, and adrenal glands), enlarged lymph nodes, and involvement of the contralateral kidney. Imaging studies are of special interest when nephron-sparing surgery (NSS) is considered (Brisse 2005). Virtual simulation of tumor resection may help surgeons in planning the surgical procedure (Fuchs et al. 2011). Whenever possible, NSS is standard of care for bilateral WT. The benefit of NSS in unilateral WT is currently being evaluated (Wilde et al. 2014; Cost et al. 2014b). In the SIOP protocol, guidelines for NSS for unilateral non-syndromic WT have been formulated: unifocal tumor, tumor restricted to one pole or peripherally situated at mid-kidney, tumor volume smaller than 300 ml at diagnosis, no preoperative or intraoperative rupture, no tumor in calyces or renal pelvis, no invasion of surrounding organs or structures, no thrombus in renal vein or IVC, excision that can be performed with safe oncologic margins, and a kidney remnant of at least 66 % that is expected to be functional. Information on the location and the number of renal arteries is crucial. Intraoperative US can be useful during NSS.

1.2.5 Principles of Treatment

1.2.5.1 Unilateral Wilms' Tumor

According to SIOP protocols, treatment is based on preoperative chemotherapy to reduce the risk of perioperative tumor rupture and to reduce the local stage (de Kraker et al. 1982). Chemotherapy regimens consist of vincristine and actinomycin D for localized disease and with the addition of doxorubicin for metastatic disease. Conversely, the North American National Wilms' Tumor Study Group (NWTSG) approach is based on primary nephrectomy. Total nephroureterectomy remains the surgical reference treatment (de Kraker and Jones 2005).

In the SIOP protocol, partial nephrectomy is considered in unilateral WT when the child has a contralateral nonfunctioning kidney or associated renal disease or an associated predisposing syndrome in order to preserve as much renal function as possible. After surgery and pathological analysis, postoperative treatment is stratified according to stage and histological risk group and consists of adjuvant chemotherapy and abdominal radiation therapy ("flank RT") for stage III patients. Children with pre- or perioperative intraperitoneal tumor rupture, hence peritoneal spillage, are given radiotherapy of the whole abdomen. Children with stage IV tumors with residual pulmonary nodules have lung wedge resections to assess histological response. In case of incomplete response, they will receive adjuvant chemotherapy and lung radiotherapy.

A well-known complication of actinomycin D is hepatic veno-occlusive disease (VOD). The reported incidence ranges between 1.2 and 8 %, and it is more frequent in young children, in children with lower body weight, in right-sided WT, and when radiotherapy was given previously. The diagnosis relies on the combination of clinical signs and symptoms such as hepatomegaly, ascites, weight gain, hyperbilirubinemia, and upper abdominal pain (Cesaro et al. 2011). The role of US and Doppler US in the diagnosis and the evaluation of the severity of VOD has been investigated: only reversal of portal venous flow was reported to be a relatively specific parameter, but it seldom occurs (McCarville et al. 2001).

1.2.5.2 Bilateral Wilms' Tumor

The SIOP and NWTSG experiences have converged on the same strategy for bilateral disease (i.e., bilateral WT, bilateral nephroblastomatosis, unilateral WT with contralateral nephroblastomatosis, and WT in a single kidney or horseshoe kidney): primary chemotherapy in order to decrease tumor volume, followed by NSS in order to preserve the maximum amount of functional renal tissue. Chemotherapy for more than 12 weeks rarely shows ongoing response (Furtwangler et al. 2014; Sudour et al. 2012; Hamilton et al. 2011). The risk of end-stage renal disease is important (Aronson et al. 2011). It is recommended that an experienced team should manage these rare cases. The goal is bilateral partial nephrectomy or wedge resection, performed in one single or two separate operations with an interval of no more than two postoperative chemotherapy courses. The less involved kidney is operated on first. Imaging plays an important role in the detection of bilateral disease, monitoring during chemotherapy and follow-up. Since these patients will need to be imaged very frequently, special attention should be paid to reduction of ionizing radiation, and follow-up imaging should be performed with US and MRI.

1.2.6 Prognosis and Follow-Up

1.2.6.1 Prognostic Factors

The most important prognostic factors are tumor stage and histological risk group. Tumor shrinkage under preoperative chemotherapy is also considered a prognostic factor. A preoperative volume of more than 500 ml is associated with poorer survival (Graf et al. 2012). The prognostic significance of various genetic abnormalities is currently being studied (loss of heterozygosity (LOH) on chromosomes 16q, 1p, and 22q, TP53 mutation or overexpression, telomerase activity, gain of 1q, expression of TRKB) (Maschietto et al. 2014; Gratias et al. 2013). In the group of patients with a WT of NWTSG-favorable histology, tumor-specific LOH for both chromosomes 1p and 16q identifies a subset of patients who have a significantly increased risk of relapse and death (Grundy et al. 2005).

1.2.6.2 Survival

The therapeutic management of WT is a model for successful cancer treatment. Thanks to consecutive clinical trials conducted by the SIOP-RTSG, the NWTSG, and national study groups, overall survival (OS) rates are nowadays exceeding 90%. Despite this, certain patient groups, including those with bilateral disease, unfavorable histologic and molecular features, and recurrent disease, still have an OS well below 90%. Together, these groups represent 25% of patients with WT (Dome et al. 2015).

1.2.6.3 Relapses

Approximately 15% of patients with favorable-histology WT and 50% of patients with anaplastic or post-chemotherapy blastemal-type WT, experience a recurrence (Spreafico et al. 2009). Most first recurrences occur within 2 years of the initial diagnosis. The most common site of recurrence is the lung (58%), sometimes with pleural involvement, whereas abdominal recurrences represent 29% of all relapses. Favorable prognostic factors for children with relapsed WT include favorable histology, interval from nephrectomy to relapse ≥ 12 months, pulmonary relapse only, initial treatment with only vincristine and actinomycin D, and no prior radiation therapy (Grundy et al. 1989). The risk factors for local recurrence are local stage III and high-risk histology (Shamberger et al. 1999). Abdominal recurrences may arise in the lumbar fossa, in the liver, in the regional lymph nodes, and in the peritoneal cavity when peritoneal spillage had occurred before or during surgery (Fig. 12). The 5-year overall survival of children after local recurrence varies between 40 and 80% (Green et al. 2007; Malogolowkin et al. 2008; Dome et al. 2002).

Metachronous contralateral WT is rare. The percentage of patients who develop contralateral disease is 1.5% at 5 years after diagnosis (Coppes et al. 1999). Recognized risk factors are nephrogenic rests detected with either initial imaging or pathological analysis of the non-tumoral part of the kidney and age at initial diagnosis less than 12 months (Coppes et al. 1999; Daw et al. 2002; Bergeron et al. 2001).

1.2.6.4 Imaging During Follow-Up

The overall prognosis of WT is excellent, and follow-up imaging must be done with minimally invasive techniques but carefully and with knowledge of both recurrence patterns and risk factors. Detection of recurrences is important, since relapsed patients have a good chance of being cured with salvage therapies. Ninety percent of relapses occur during the first 4 years after diagnosis (Grundy et al. 2005).

Abdominal US surveillance for 3 years after end of treatment is considered to reveal most abdominal recurrences (Daw et al. 2002). During surveillance, the remaining kidney is screened for metachronous contralateral tumor. Evaluation of normal (compensatory) growth of the remaining kidney is also part of the nephrological surveillance, together with monitoring of blood pressure and serum creatinine.

CXR is the imaging modality used for follow-up of the lungs, supplemented with chest CT when pulmonary recurrence is suspected (Table 4).

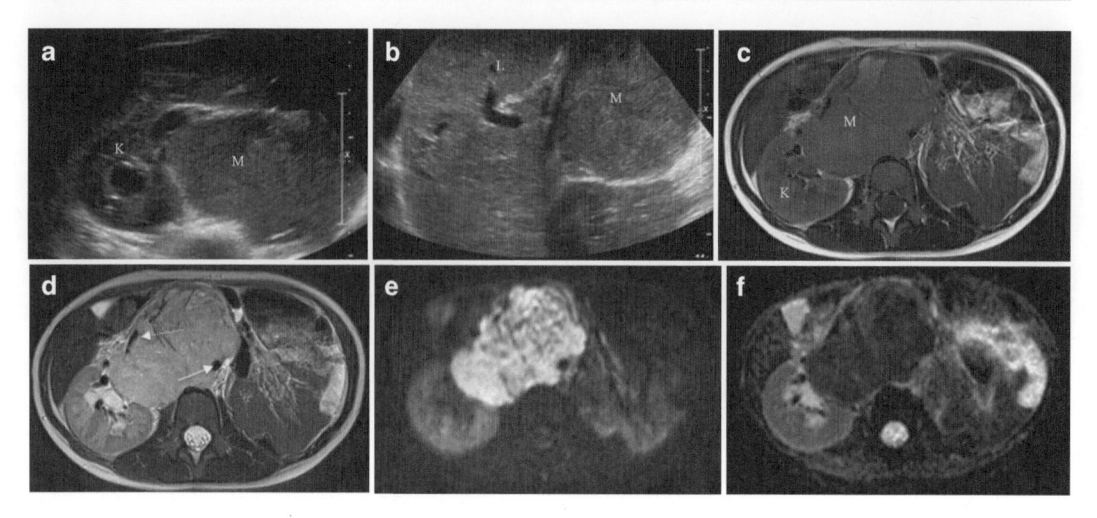

Fig. 12 Four-year-old girl with previous treatment (chemotherapy and nephrectomy) for a Wilms' tumor stage II of the left kidney. Eight months post-nephrectomy, ultrasound ((**a**) axial, (**b**) sagittal) showed a large aorto-caval mass (*M*), extending to the right renal hilum. L liver, K right kidney. MRI ((**c**) axial T1-weighted image, (**d**) axial T2-weighted image, (**e**) DWI with b value 800, (**f**) ADC) shows a large mass with internal hemorrhage (high signal on axial T1-weighted image) and displacement of the aorta (*solid arrow*) and inferior vena cava (*dashed arrow*)

Table 4 Radiological investigations during follow-up of children with Wilms' tumor (UMBRELLA SIOP-RTSG 2015 protocol)

Investigation	Frequency after end of treatment
Abdominal ultrasound	First and second years: every 3 months Third to fifth years: every 6 months After 5 years: once a year
Chest X-ray	First and second years: every 3–4 months Third to fifth year: every 6 months After 5 years: once a year

Take Away

Wilms' tumor (WT) is by far the most frequent renal neoplasm in children between 1 and 5 years.

Wilms' tumor (WT) has an overall good prognosis.

Children with syndromes predisposing for Wilms' tumor (WT) should be screened by US every 3–4 months.

Distant metastases occur mainly in the lungs.

Nephrogenic rests cannot be differentiated from small Wilms' tumor (WT) with imaging with certainty.

1.3 Non-wilms' Malignant Tumors

1.3.1 Clear Cell Sarcoma of the Kidney

Clear cell sarcoma of the kidney (CCSK) accounts for approximately 3–5% of renal neoplasms in childhood and is the second most common renal malignancy in children. Mean age at diagnosis is 36 months (range of 2 months to 14 years), with more than 85% of patients diagnosed before the age of 5 (Zhuge et al. 2010). The male to female ratio is 2:1. Unlike WT, CCSK is always unilateral and unicentric. At histology, typical gross features included large size (mean diameter 11.3 cm), a mucoid texture, foci of necrosis, and prominent cyst formation. Nine major histological patterns are identified (classic, myxoid, sclerosing, cellular, epithelioid, palisading, spindle, storiform, and anaplastic); virtually all tumors contain multiple patterns that blend with one another (Argani et al. 2000). CCSK is a high-risk tumor (SIOP). Overall 10-year survival is 70% (Zhuge et al. 2010). Patients present with abdominal distention or a mass, abdominal pain, hematuria, vomiting, decreased oral intake, fever, constipation, and hypertension (Gooskens et al. 2012).

Fig. 13 Clear cell sarcoma of the kidney in an 18-month-old girl. Ultrasound (**a**) and MRI ((**b**) axial T2-weighted image with fat saturation, (**c**) coronal T1-weighted image, and (**d**) coronal T2-weighted image) show a large heterogeneous tumor arising in the left kidney

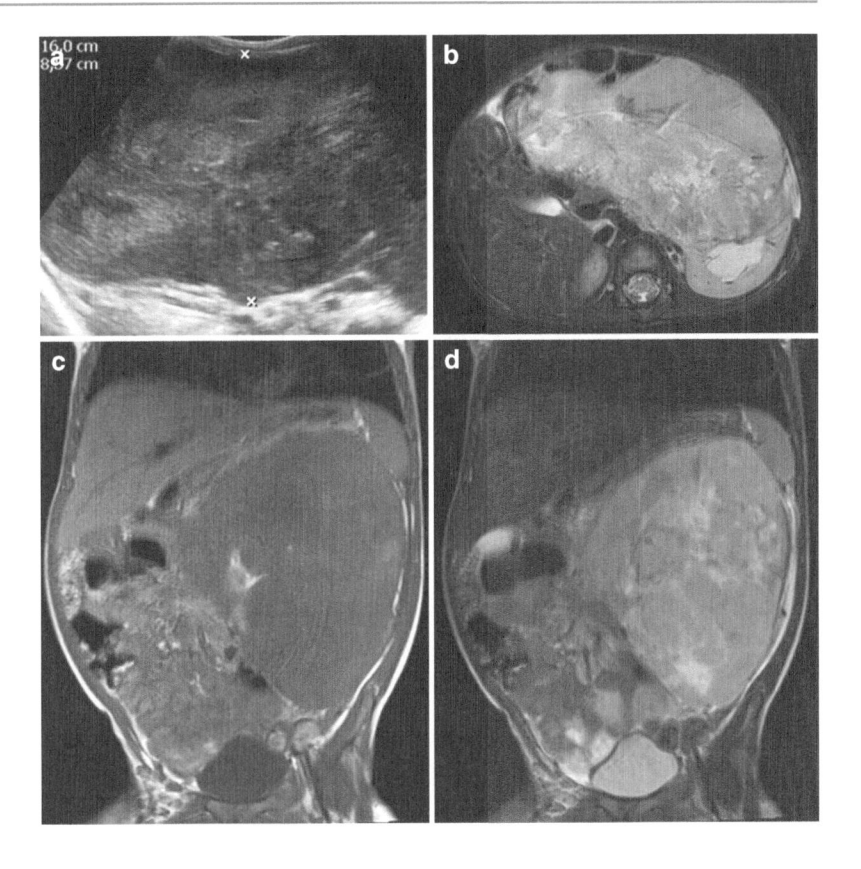

CCSK does not show imaging patterns that can differentiate it from WT (Fig. 13) (Lowe et al. 2000). Like WT, CCSK may have features that simulate those of benign conditions, such as renal abscess. Rarely CCSK shows invasion of the inferior vena cava (5 %) with extension into the right atrium (Gooskens et al. 2012). Extracapsular spread is common (70 %). Less than 10 % of patients present with distant metastases at diagnosis (Zhuge et al. 2010), but metastases of CCSK may also occur several years after treatment. Metastases at diagnosis mainly involve the skeleton, lungs, lymph nodes, and liver (Marsden et al. 1978; Morgan and Kidd 1978; Gooskens et al. 2012). Bone metastases are highly suggestive of CCSK (Fig. 14). Reports from both SIOP and NWTSG indicate that the pattern of relapse is changing since the introduction of intensified chemotherapy: brain metastases are now more common than bone metastases.

Bone scintigraphy, MRI of the brain, and chest CT are recommended for staging (Smets and de Kraker 2010).

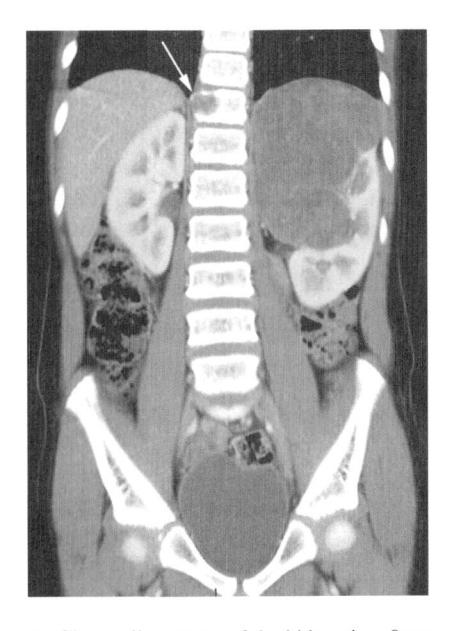

Fig. 14 Clear cell sarcoma of the kidney in a 9-year-old boy presenting with hematuria. Contrast-enhanced CT (coronal reconstruction) shows a left upper pole renal mass and a bone metastasis in a vertebral body (*arrow*) (courtesy Dr. J.-L. Ferrand, Clinique Saint-Jean, Montpellier, France)

1.3.2 Rhabdoid Tumor of the Kidney

Malignant rhabdoid tumors of the kidney (MRTK) are rare, highly aggressive cancers of early childhood. Malignant rhabdoid tumors can occur in various locations, mainly the liver, genitourinary tract, gastrointestinal tract, and central nervous system (atypical teratoid/rhabdoid tumors). In some cases, abnormalities of chromosome 22 and 11p13 have been described. MRTK accounts for about 1 % of all renal neoplasms in childhood (Vujanic et al. 1996; Tomlinson et al. 2005). They can develop sporadically or occur as part of the hereditary rhabdoid tumor predisposition syndrome (RTPS) (Sredni and Tomita 2015). Median age at diagnosis is 11 months (range from 0 up to 9 years) with more than 85 % of cases diagnosed before the age of five (Zhuge et al. 2010; Tomlinson et al. 2005). The male to female ratio is 1.5:1. Several findings suggest that rhabdoid tumors might arise from primitive cells involved in formation of the renal medulla (Weeks et al. 1989). Gross features include a characteristic involvement of perihilar renal parenchyma. There is a wide histological spectrum that may cause confusion with other renal neoplasms. MRTK is not associated with conditions predisposing to WT or with nephrogenic rests. Although clinical features are nonspecific, a combination of clinical presentation with fever, hematuria, and high-tumor stage at presentation in very young children suggests the diagnosis (Amar et al. 2001). About 20 % may have associated hypercalcemia (Vujanic et al. 1996). On imaging, these tumors may resemble WT, but subcapsular fluid collections, tumor lobules separated by areas of necrosis or hemorrhage and linear calcifications outlining tumor lobules, are suspicious for MRTK, especially if the patient is an infant (Fig. 15) (Chung et al. 1995; Han et al. 2001; Lowe et al. 2000; Prasad et al. 2005; Smets and de Kraker 2010).

Metastases are observed in up to 50 % of children at diagnosis (lung, abdomen, lymph nodes, liver, bone, and brain) (Vujanic et al. 1996; van den Heuvel-Eibrink et al. 2011; Zhuge et al. 2010; Tomlinson et al. 2005; Warmann et al. 2012). Up to 20 % of patients – mostly infants – have synchronous or metachronous brain tumors (Fig. 15) (Tomlinson et al. 2005). The prognosis of rhabdoid tumor of the kidney is poor, and up to

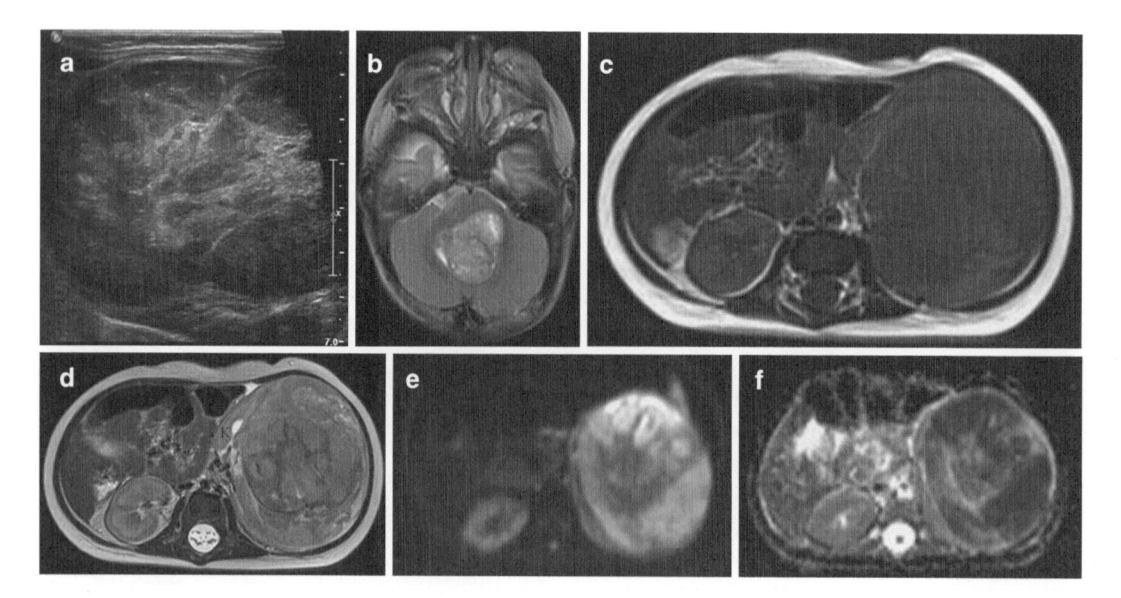

Fig. 15 Malignant rhabdoid tumor of the kidney in a 7-month-old girl with a synchronous intracranial mass. Abdominal ultrasound (**a**) shows a large heterogeneous mass in the left kidney. MRI of the brain (**b** axial T2-weighted image) shows a large mass in the fourth ventricle. Abdominal MRI ((**c**) axial T1-weighted image, (**d**) axial T2-weighted image, (**e**) axial DWI b value 800, (**f**) axial ADC) shows a large heterogeneous mass arising from the left kidney (*K*) with restricted diffusion

80 % of patients die within a year of diagnosis, despite aggressive treatment (Weeks et al. 1989; van den Heuvel-Eibrink et al. 2008; Zhuge et al. 2010; Tomlinson et al. 2005).

1.3.3 Renal Cell Carcinoma

Renal cell carcinoma (RCC) accounts for 2–6 % of all malignant renal tumors in childhood. Although rare in children, it is the most common renal tumor in adolescents with a median age at diagnosis of 11–13 years (Selle et al. 2006; Rialon et al. 2015). Recent studies have shown that RCC in children is different from the adult type with regard to tumor biology as well as clinical behavior. The most common type of RCC in children is tRCC (translocation type), involving the transcription factor E3 (TFE3) gene at Xp11.2. The adult clear cell type also occurs in children, but less frequently (Geller et al. 2015).

Clinical findings are gross painless hematuria, flank pain, and abdominal mass; less often fever and weight loss are reported (Sausville et al. 2009).

Von Hippel-Lindau syndrome predisposes to the development of various endocrine and non-endocrine tumors (hemangioblastomas of the neuraxis and retina, tumors of the membranous labyrinth, renal cell carcinomas (clear cell type) or cysts, pheochromocytomas, pancreatic cysts or tumors, epididymal cystadenomas). It is the commonest cause of hereditary renal cancer, with a prevalence of up to 75 % (Monsalve et al. 2011). Patients with von Hippel-Lindau syndrome are screened with abdominal US from the age of 5 years for early detection of renal tumors, although renal tumors are rarely detected in children (Maher et al. 2011; Priesemann et al. 2006).

RCC has been reported as a late-occurring complication in pediatric patients treated for a malignancy, presumably related to the chemotherapeutic treatment they received (Schafernak et al. 2007; Dhall et al. 2007; Argani et al. 2006). A subtype of RCC has also been reported in patients who had neuroblastoma at a young age (between 10 weeks and 2 years) and even in neuroblastoma patients who were not exposed to chemotherapy (Fleitz et al. 2003; Medeiros et al. 1999). The RCC developed at an average of 14.7 years after the diagnosis of neuroblastoma. A genetic predisposition seems likely but has not been proven (Wallace et al. 2015).

In pediatric patients who have had a renal transplantation, the reported incidence of renal cell carcinoma is more than 15-fold increased, compared to the general pediatric population. The majority of these tumors occur in a native kidney and not in the transplanted kidney. Most likely the increased risk is due to chronic renal disease because the risk is comparable between transplanted patients and patients on dialysis (Mynarek et al. 2014).

RCC tends to be smaller than WT at diagnosis (Fig. 16). Enlarged lumbar-aortic lymph nodes are frequently observed. Most tumors are large, heterogeneous solid masses enhancing after contrast injection but to a lesser degree than the normal renal parenchyma (Lee 2007). There can be hemorrhage in or around the tumor, and up to 40 % show calcifications (Downey et al. 2012). Compared to WT, RCC more often presents bilaterally and is more likely to metastasize to bone (Smets and de Kraker 2010). With respect to the primary tumor, imaging techniques cannot confidently distinguish renal cell carcinoma from WT.

More than half of the pediatric patients with RCC present with stage I or II with an excellent survival following surgical resection of the tumor (Rialon et al. 2015). However, about 40 % of patients present with lymphatic or hematogenous spread of the tumor, leading to worse overall survival (Sausville et al. 2009; Geller et al. 2015; Rialon et al. 2015). The lung, liver, brain, and bone are the most common sites of distant metastases. The 4-year overall survival lies between 14 and 92 %, depending on the stage of the tumor (Dome et al. 2013).

1.3.4 Renal Medullary Carcinoma

Renal medullary carcinoma is a rare and aggressive tumor occurring in black adolescents and in young adults. The majority of patients with renal medullary carcinoma have sickle cell trait or less frequently hemoglobin sickle cell disease (Swartz

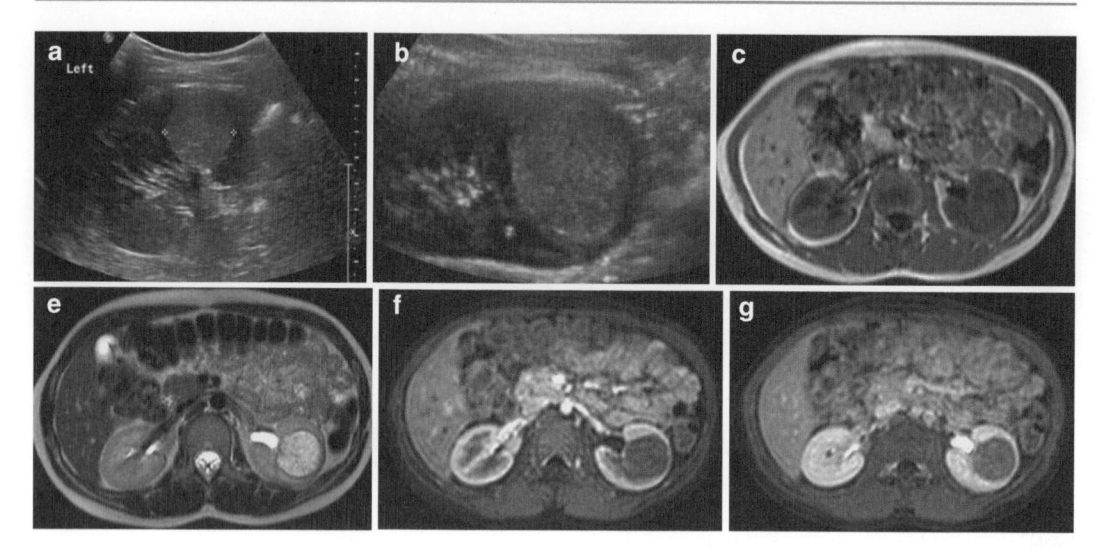

Fig. 16 Renal cell carcinoma in an 8-year-old girl presenting with hematuria. Ultrasound (**a**, **b**) shows a round hyperechoic mass within the renal parenchyma. On MRI, the lesion is well demarcated and shows less enhancement than the surrounding parenchyma ((**c**) axial T1-weighted image, (**d**) axial T2-weighted image, (**e**) early and (**f**) late enhancement on T1-weigthed image with fat saturation after gadolinium)

et al. 2002). Fifty percent of patients are 21 years or younger. Male to female ratio is 2.4:1 (Alvarez et al. 2015). Immunohistologic findings (strong vascular endothelial growth factor and hypoxia-inducible factor expression and positivity for TP53) suggest that medullary hypoxia, chronic ischemic changes, and vaso-occlusion may be involved in the pathogenesis (Alvarez et al. 2015; Swartz et al. 2002).

The most common presenting signs and symptoms include hematuria, abdominal or flank pain, and weight loss. On imaging, an ill-defined, infiltrative heterogeneous lesion within the renal medulla is seen invading the renal sinus, with caliectasis as a result (Prasad et al. 2005; Lee 2007). Regional lymphadenopathy and invasion of the renal vein are often seen (Smets and de Kraker 2010; Lee 2007). Contrast enhancement is heterogeneous (Davidson et al. 1995). Calcifications have not been described in this type of tumor. At diagnosis, many patients have metastatic disease in the lymph nodes, lungs, liver, adrenal glands, and/or bone (Alvarez et al. 2015).

Survival is poor, with an overall mortality of 95 % (mean: 4 months) (Swartz et al. 2002; Alvarez et al. 2015).

1.3.5 Ewing's Sarcoma Family of Tumors (Extraosseous Ewing Sarcoma/Peripheral Primitive Neuroectodermal Tumor (pPNET))

Ewing's sarcoma family of tumors of the kidney is a very rare entity with high malignant potential. Median age at diagnosis is around 27 years, with a wide range (months to late adulthood) (Parham et al. 2001; Zollner et al. 2013). pPNETs are small round blue cell tumors derived from the neural crest. The diagnosis is based on histopathology with subsequent demonstration of typical chromosomal translocations of pPNET/Ewing tumor family (Doerfler et al. 2001; Vicha et al. 2002; Lam et al. 2003). pPNET has a greater level of neural differentiation compared to Ewing's sarcoma. At histology, markers for pPNET/Ewing's sarcoma are t(11;22) (q24;q12) or the associated EWS/FLI1 fusion (Parham et al. 2001).

Patients present with nonspecific signs and symptoms such as pain, a palpable mass, and/or hematuria (Zollner et al. 2013). CT shows a

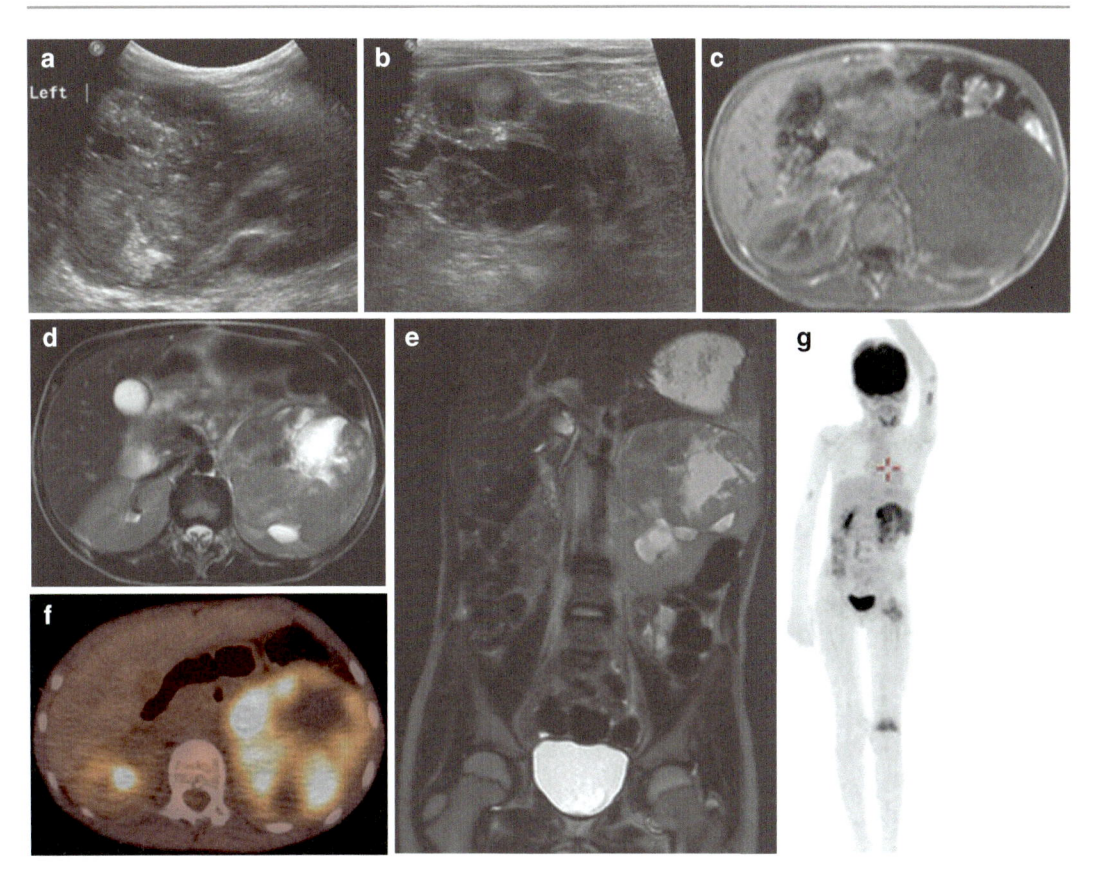

Fig. 17 Ewing's sarcoma of the kidney in an 8-year-old girl, presenting with a painful hip and knee and with a urinary tract infection. Ultrasound of the left kidney (**a**, **b**) shows a heterogeneous mass with calcifications and necrotic areas. MRI ((**c**) axial T1-weighted image, (**d**) axial T2-weighted image, (**e**) coronal T2-weighted image with fat saturation) shows a heterogeneous mass with necrotic areas. FDG-PET-CT scan was performed, showing increased FDG uptake in the renal mass, as well as in skeletal metastases ((**f**) axial fused image, (**g**) whole-body reconstruction)

large and heterogeneous tumor, commonly containing calcifications, internal hemorrhage or necrosis, and peripheral hypervascularity (Lalwani et al. 2011; Smets and de Kraker 2010). On MRI, the tumors are heterogeneous and of intermediate to high signal intensity on T2-weighted sequences (Fig. 17) (Lalwani et al. 2011). The tumor can extend into the renal vein, inferior vena cava, and right atrium (Parham et al. 2001; Zollner et al. 2013). Patients often present with metastases at diagnosis (34 %) mainly in the bones, lungs, and liver. Therapy consists of a combination of chemotherapy, surgery, and radiation therapy. Overall 3-year survival is 92 % in patients with localized disease and 58 % in patients with metastatic disease (Zollner et al. 2013).

1.3.6 Anaplastic Sarcoma

Recently, anaplastic sarcoma of the kidney has been described as a distinct entity. It is a very rare tumor, with only 20 cases occurring among about 13,000 pediatric renal tumors. There is a slight female predominance (1.5: 1). Most patients presenting with anaplastic sarcoma are under 15 years of age (median age of 5 years). About 50 % of the tumors contain a cystic component. At histology, a spindle cell component is found with widespread anaplastic changes. Chondroid differentiation is often seen. Histologically, this tumor shows similarity to the pleuropulmonary blastoma and undifferentiated sarcoma of the liver. Lung, liver and bone metastases can be found (Vujanic et al. 2007).

1.3.7 Malignant Hematologic Diseases

Primary unilateral renal lymphoma is exceptional: it presents as a solid renal tumor without distinctive characteristics (Hugosson et al. 1997). Lymphoma of the kidneys is usually bilateral and associated with other sites of disease. It affects children at an older age (usually between 7 and 10 years) than patients with bilateral WT. It is observed in less than 20 % of abdominal non-Hodgkin lymphomas (Ng et al. 1994) and occurs most frequently in Burkitt's lymphoma, lymphoblastic lymphoma, or large cell lymphoma, while renal involvement in Hodgkin's disease is exceptional (Chepuri et al. 2003). Several patterns may be encountered: bilateral multiple nodules of varying size, diffuse renal infiltration with nephromegaly or retroperitoneal infiltration with encasement of the kidneys (Strauss et al. 1986; Weinberger et al. 1990; Prasad et al. 2005). Lymphoma locations usually appear homogeneously hypoechoic on US (Fig. 18). On CT, bilateral diffuse symmetric enlargement of the kidneys is most often seen with a decreased corticomedullary differentiation (Lee 2007). Sometimes multiple low-density lesions can be seen. At MRI the lesions are hyperintense on T2-weighted imaging and show restricted diffusion (Figs. 18 and 19).

Patients with leukemia may also show diffuse infiltration of the kidneys (Fig. 20). The same imaging features as with lymphoma involvement may be seen.

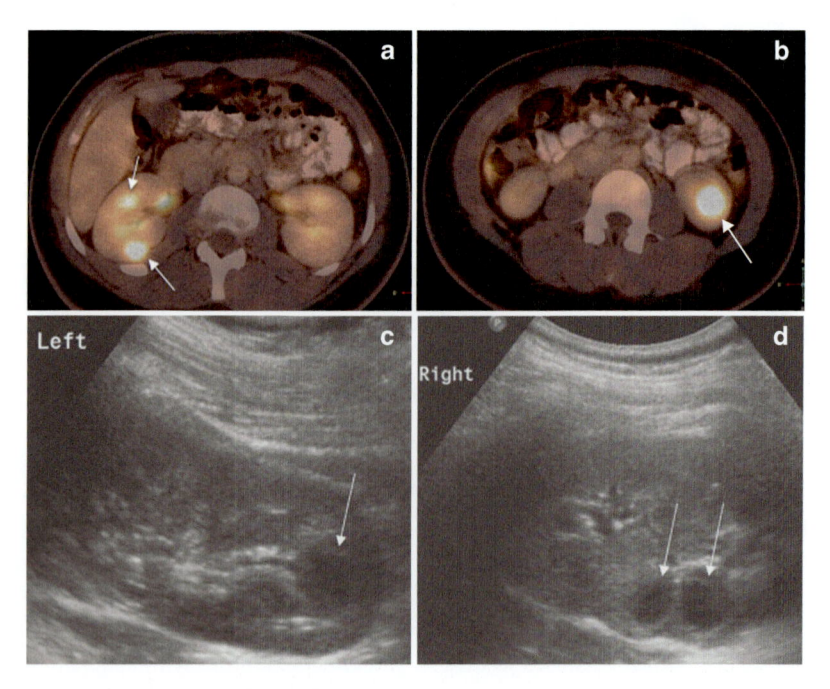

Fig. 18 16-year-old girl with non-Hodgkin lymphoma of the proximal tibia. A staging FDG-PET-CT scan (**a**, **b**) revealed bilateral renal lesions (*arrows*). Ultrasound (**c**, **d**) shows bilateral hypoechoic lesions (*arrows*). MRI (**e** coronal T2-weighted image) shows enlarged kidneys with hypointense lesions on both T1- and T2-weighted images (**f**, **g**), quite difficult to discern. DWI and ADC clearly show restricted diffusion (**h–k**)

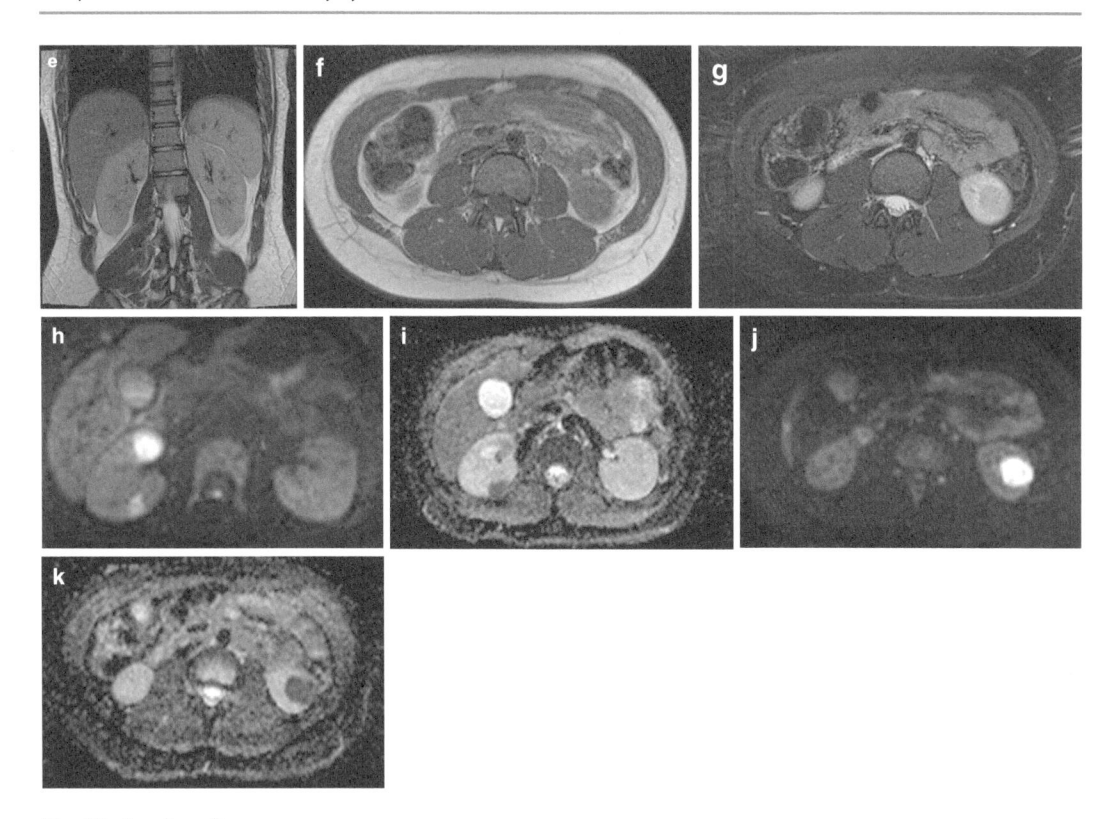

Fig. 18 (continued)

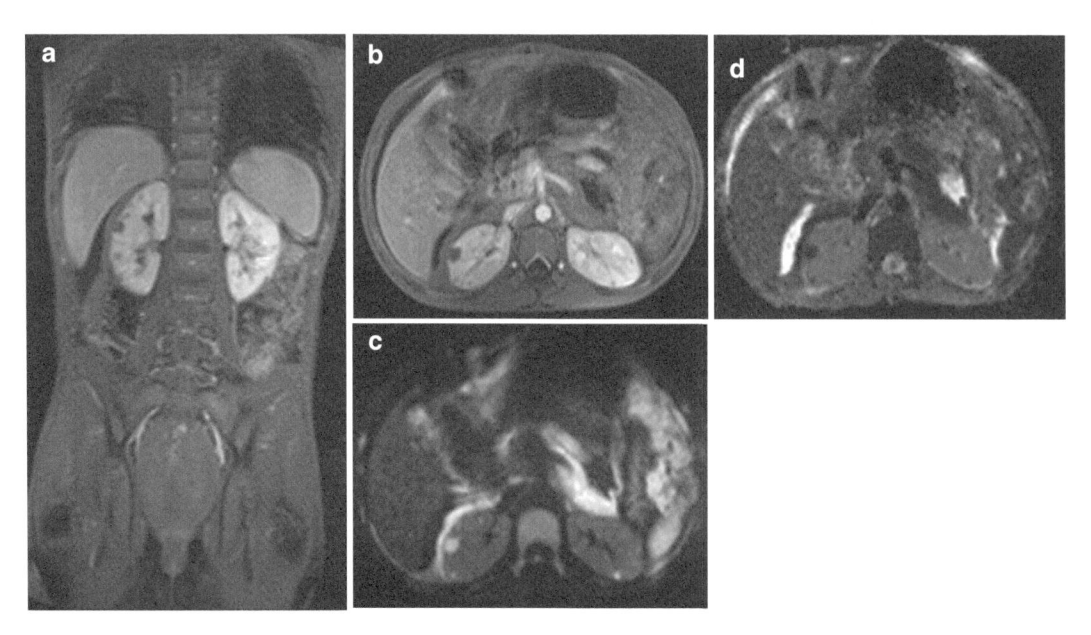

Fig. 19 Burkitt's lymphoma in a 9-year-old boy presenting with increasing abdominal volume. MRI of the abdomen shows multiple nodules in the kidneys. (**a**) Coronal and (**b**) axial T1-weighted images after gadolinium with fat suppression. (**c**) DWI with b value 800. (**d**) ADC

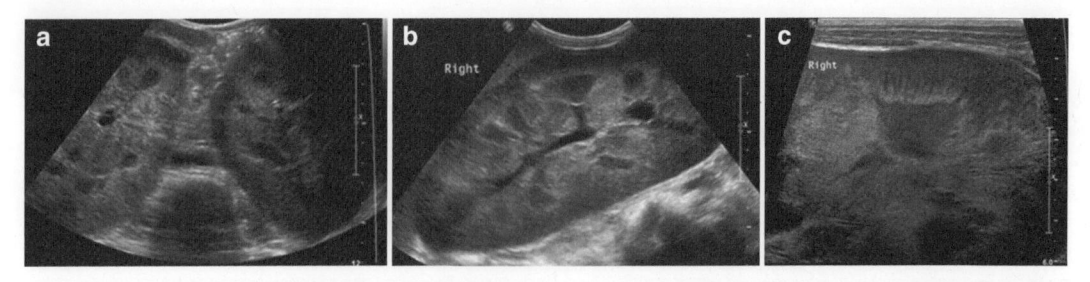

Fig. 20 Six-year-old boy with T-ALL. Ultrasound shows massively enlarged kidneys with diffuse infiltration. (**a**) Axial image showing both kidneys, (**b**) longitudinal image of the right kidney, (**c**) high-resolution image of the right kidney

1.3.8 Renal Metastases

Renal metastases are exceptional in children. Few cases have been described in metastatic neuroblastoma (Filiatrault et al. 1987; Panuel et al. 1992).

> **Take Away**
>
> Bone metastases in young pediatric patients with a renal neoplasm are suggestive of clear cell sarcoma.
>
> Rhabdoid tumor affects young children. Hypercalcemia and metastases at diagnosis are frequent in this highly aggressive tumor.
>
> Pediatric renal cell carcinoma occurs in the second decade and is frequently calcified and smaller than Wilms' tumor (WT).
>
> Renal medullary carcinoma occurs in adolescents with sickle cell trait.
>
> Renal lymphoma is usually bilateral and associated with other sites of involvement.

1.4 Benign Tumors

1.4.1 Congenital Mesoblastic Nephroma or Bolande's Tumor

Congenital mesoblastic nephroma (CMN) is the most frequent solid renal tumor in the neonate (Isaacs 2008). The median age is 1 month (England et al. 2011), and about 75 % of patients are diagnosed during the first 4 months of life (Furtwaengler et al. 2006). The male to female ratio is 1.5:1 (England et al. 2011). At gross analysis, congenital mesoblastic nephroma is an infiltrative mass with ill-defined margins and no capsule. This tumor predominantly contains bundles of spindle cells resembling fibroblasts and myofibroblasts which present many histological features evocative of infantile fibromatosis (Bolande et al. 1967). The tumor border is irregular, and long radial finger-like extensions of tumor tissue into the adjacent renal tissue are a characteristic finding (Hartman et al. 1981).

CMN usually presents as an abdominal mass in a neonate, sometimes with hematuria. Some cases have been discovered on prenatal US examination (Furtwaengler et al. 2006; England et al. 2011; Irsutti et al. 2000; Kelner et al. 2003; Murthi et al. 2003). Sometimes polyhydramnios or neonatal hypercalcemia can be an associated complication (Daskas et al. 2002; Ferraro et al. 1986). US shows a large solid renal mass, often heterogeneous with cystic areas and sometimes containing calcifications. The tumor typically involves the renal sinus (Wang et al. 2014; Bayindir et al. 2009; Smets and de Kraker 2010). A distinctive "ring sign" (concentric hyperechoic and hypoechoic rings) is a suggestive pattern (Fig. 21) (Chan et al. 1987). With CDS it can be shown that the anechoic ring surrounding the tumor contains abnormal vessels (Kelner et al. 2003). On MRI, the lesion is hypointense both on T1- and T2-weighted sequences (Prasad et al. 2005). CT scan demonstrates a homogeneous solid renal mass with low attenuation (Christmann et al. 1990; Prasad et al. 2005). The solid parts of the tumor tend to enhance less than normal renal parenchyma (Lee 2007). During the arterial phase and the excretory phase, a suggestive pattern can be that of residual renal cortex trapped into the tumor resulting from the infiltrative

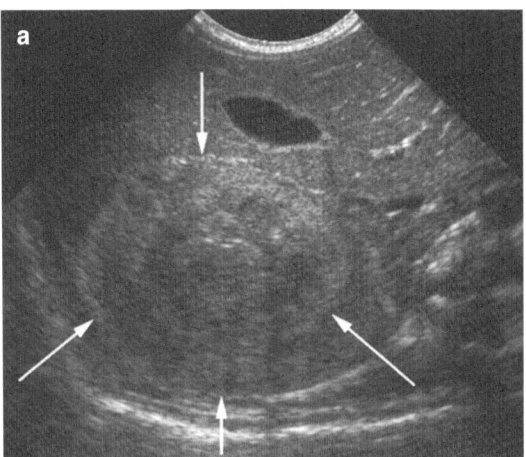

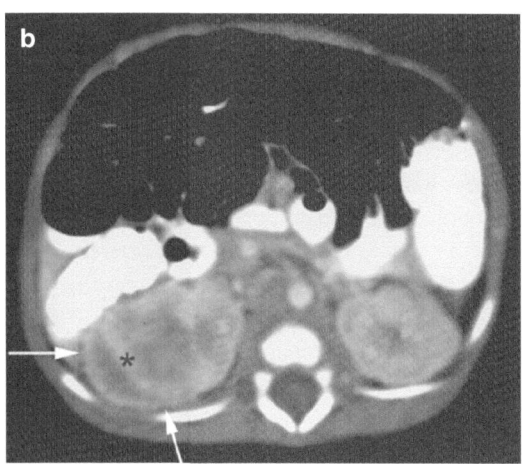

Neoplasms of the Genitourinary System

Fig. 21 Congenital mesoblastic nephroma in a neonate. Ultrasound (axial image, **a**) shows a large solid renal mass (*arrows*) with concentric hyperechoic and hypoechoic rings. Enhanced CT scan (**b**) shows residual renal cortex (*) trapped within the tumor (*arrows*) resulting from the infiltrative growth pattern

growing pattern of the tumor (Kelner et al. 2003; Hartman et al. 1981). The prognosis is excellent, with no tumor recurrence (England et al. 2011).

A more aggressive form, called "cellular" or "atypical" congenital mesoblastic nephroma (Fig. 22), is characterized by a dense fibroblastic proliferation with increased cellularity and numerous mitoses. A close link between cellular congenital mesoblastic nephroma and congenital fibrosarcoma has been identified: they show an identical chromosomal translocation t(12;15)(p13;q25) resulting in the ETV6/NTRK3 gene fusion. Therefore, they are likely to represent the same neoplasm but occurring at different locations (Knezevich et al. 1998; Henno et al. 2003). These tumors occur at a significant later age than those with a classical or mixed subtype (median 149 days versus 43 and 17 days, respectively (England et al. 2011)). It has been suggested that the cellular type of congenital mesoblastic nephroma is more prone to cross the midline than WT and also to displace and encase vessels (Bayindir et al. 2009). Patients with a cellular mesoblastic nephroma may develop local recurrence or metastases (Schlesinger et al. 1995). Paraneoplastic syndromes, especially hypertension, have been reported (Bayindir et al. 2009). Nephrectomy is the radical and only treatment prescribed for these benign tumors. In children with a renal tumor under 6 months of age, primary surgery is recommended since the incidence of non-Wilms' tumor in this age group is relatively high (van den Heuvel-Eibrink et al. 2008) (UMBRELLA SIOP-RTSG 2015 protocol).

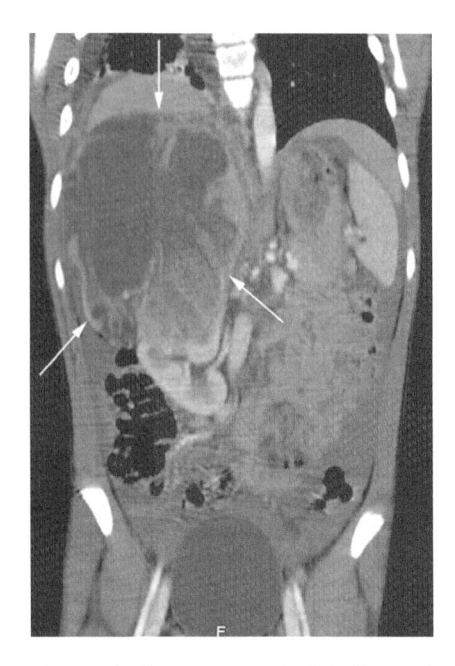

Fig. 22 Renal fibrosarcoma ("cellular" mesoblastic nephroma) in a 14-year-old boy. Enhanced CT scan (coronal reconstruction) shows a large necrotic tumor of the upper pole of the right kidney (*arrows*) with ascites related to tumor rupture

1.4.2 Multilocular Cystic Nephroma

Multilocular cystic nephroma is a segmental, purely cystic tumor characterized by multiple septations composed entirely of differentiated tissues, without blastemal elements. The majority of these tumors occur in children under the age of two with a male predominance. Patients usually present with a painless mass. Hypertension, hematuria, and flank pain may be part of the symptoms (Wootton-Gorges et al. 2005). Multilocular cystic nephroma may be observed in patients with constitutional DICER 1 mutation, a genetical predisposing condition also associated with pleuropulmonary blastoma and other tumors (Bahubeshi et al. 2010).

On imaging, a well-defined, multi-septated mass with cysts and septa, but without solid components, is seen. The septations show moderate contrast enhancement. Calcification is uncommon. Hydronephrosis can occur due to herniation of the mass into the renal pelvis (Wootton-Gorges et al. 2005; Prasad et al. 2005; Riccabona et al. 1999).

Multilocular cystic nephroma and cystic partially differentiated nephroblastoma (CPDN) cannot be distinguished on imaging, and biopsy is not recommended because it is usually noninformative. The only difference between these two entities is the presence of embryonal cells within the septa in CPDN. Therefore, it is recommended that purely cystic renal tumors should be treated primarily with surgery (SIOP 2001 and UMBRELLA SIOP-RTSG 2015); the final diagnosis will be obtained after pathological analysis.

The differential diagnosis of multicystic renal masses also includes WT with cyst formation, cystic clear cell sarcoma, cystic mesoblastic nephroma, cystic renal cell carcinoma, and multicystic dysplasia. Imaging is usually not able to discriminate between these entities (Wootton-Gorges et al. 2005; van den Hoek et al. 2009).

1.4.3 Benign Stromal Tumors

1.4.3.1 Metanephric Adenoma

Metanephric adenoma (MA) is a very rare benign tumor that predominates in females and is very uncommon in children (Davis et al. 1995; Navarro et al. 1999). The mean age at diagnosis is 41 years, (range 15 months to 83 years). The mean size at diagnosis is 5.5 cm (range 0.3–15 cm) (Davis et al. 1995). Microscopically, MA consists of very small epithelial cells that form very small acini in an acellular stroma. Less often, it forms tubular, glomeruloid, or polypoid and papillary formations. These lesions seem histogenetically related to epithelial WT, and, in fact, the two may occur together. They are histologically very similar to the metanephric hamartomatous element of nephroblastomatosis. In a series of 29 cases of metanephric adenoma in adults, 90 % showed a BRAF V600E mutation (Choueiri et al. 2012). Interestingly, the patients without BRAF mutation in this study were significantly younger than the patients with the mutation. In a series of three cases of metanephric adenoma in children, two out of three showed a BRAF V600E mutation, whereas pediatric cases of renal cell carcinoma and WT did not show the mutation (Chami et al. 2015).

Most cases are asymptomatic and detected incidentally. Presenting signs and symptoms are flank pain, hematuria, and palpable mass. Polycythemia is a suggestive sign but observed in only 12 % of cases. This tumor is more commonly calcified than other renal neoplasms. On US, the mass is well circumscribed and hypo- or hyperechoic, the latter suggesting hemorrhage. The lesion may or may not be vascularized. Unenhanced CT scan shows a hyperdense mass, in some cases containing punctuate calcifications. On MRI, the lesion appears isointense on both T1- and T2-weighted sequences (Fig. 23).

1.4.3.2 Metanephric Stromal Tumor

Metanephric stromal tumor was first described in 2000, in a series of 31 cases (Argani and Beckwith 2000). Mean patient age at diagnosis is 2 years. Gross examination typically shows a fibrous lesion centered in the renal medulla containing smooth-walled cysts. Metanephric stromal tumor is histologically identical to the stromal component of metanephric adenofibroma. The most common presentation is an

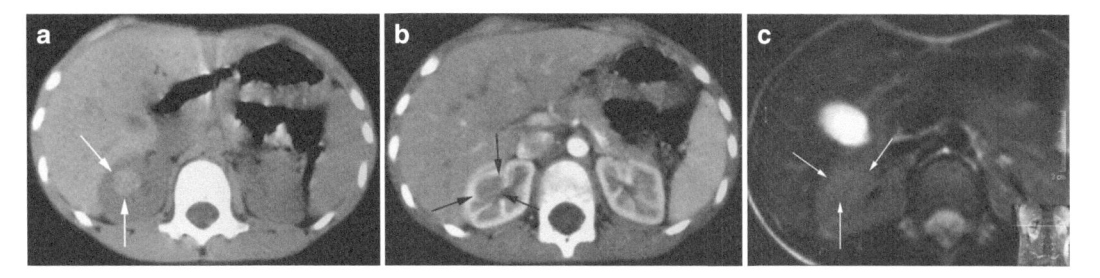

Fig. 23 Metanephric adenoma in a 7-year-old boy. Unenhanced CT scan (**a**) shows a hyperdense small mass. (**b**) On enhanced CT scan, the lesion is difficult to delineate. On MRI T2-weigthed images (**c**), the lesion is almost isointense to the normal parenchyma (courtesy Dr. C. Treguier, Hôpital de Pontchaillou, Rennes, France)

abdominal mass detected on imaging. On imaging this tumor usually appears solid but can sometimes be partly or completely cystic (Fig. 24). Patients may be treated with surgical excision alone.

1.4.3.3 Metanephric Adenofibroma

Metanephric adenofibroma (previously termed nephrogenic adenofibroma) is a very rare benign tumor, containing a variable amount of a bland spindle cell stroma (Arroyo et al. 2001). It is a biphasic tumor that spans the morphologic spectrum between benign pure stromal and pure epithelial lesions, and can merge with the morphology of WT, supporting the concept that these are all related lesions. A relationship to papillary renal cell carcinoma is also suspected. One study reported a BRAF V600E mutation in a case of pediatric metanephric adenofibroma (Chami et al. 2015); further studies are needed to confirm this relationship.

1.4.4 Ossifying Renal Tumor of Infancy

Ossifying renal tumor of infancy is a very rare, benign tumor of infancy. Age range is 6 days to 2½ years (Lee et al. 2014). The male to female ratio is 3:1. The mass arises in the renal medulla, involving the collecting system (Lowe et al. 2000). It contains varying proportions of osteoid, osteoblastic cells, and spindle cells. The proportion of osteoid and the degree of osseous maturation increases with increasing age of the patient. Patients typically present with gross hematuria

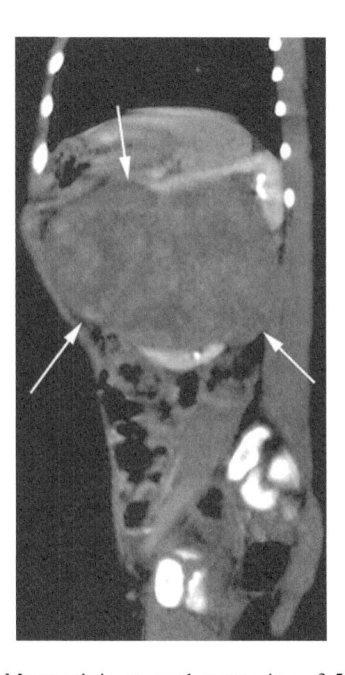

Fig. 24 Metanephric stromal tumor in a 3.5-year-old girl. Contrast-enhanced CT (sagittal reconstruction). Renal mass incidentally discovered during ultrasound performed for enuresis. Pathological diagnosis obtained after neoadjuvant chemotherapy (30% volume response only) and nephrectomy for presumed Wilms' tumor

and show on US a (frequently calcified) renal pelvis mass. Due to the obstructing tumor, widening of the collecting system occurs. Imaging usually shows a small-sized mass located within the kidney with the outline of the kidney maintained, sometimes associated with dilatation of the collecting system (Fig. 25). On US the tumor is hyperechoic with shadowing due to the osteoid formation. The tumor shows poor enhancement

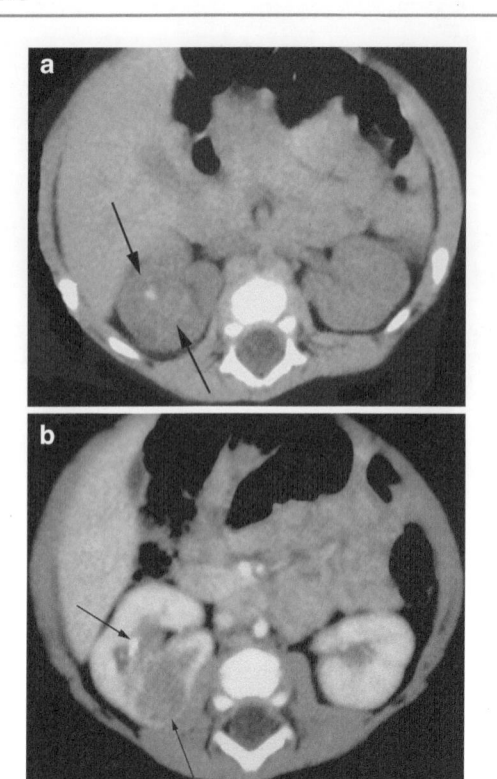

Fig. 25 Ossifying renal tumor of infancy in a neonate with seizures, hypercalciuria, and microscopic hematuria. CT scan ((**a**) enhanced, (**b**) unenhanced) shows a calcified intrarenal mass (*arrow*) (Courtesy Dr. C. Baunin, Hôpital des Enfants, Toulouse, France)

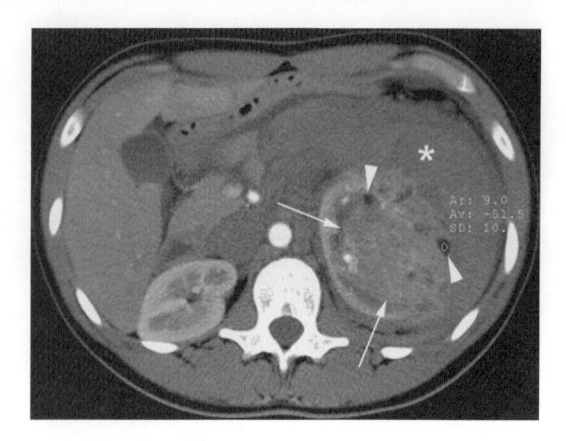

Fig. 26 Angiomyolipoma in a 15-year-old girl with tuberous sclerosis and acute abdominal pain related to tumor rupture. CT scan shows a vascularized intrarenal mass (*arrows*) containing fatty areas (*arrowheads*) and perirenal hematoma (*) (courtesy Prof. H. Ducou-Lepointe, Hôpital A Trousseau, Paris, France)

after contrast administration. Calcifications are frequent (Sotelo-Avila et al. 1995; Ito et al. 1998; Vazquez et al. 1998). The tumor may mimic a staghorn calculus (Schelling et al. 2007; Lowe et al. 2000).

1.4.5 Angiomyolipoma

Angiomyolipoma in childhood is almost always associated with tuberous sclerosis complex (Bourneville's disease). The male to female ratio for angiomyolipomas in tuberous sclerosis complex is 1:1.7, probably related to the sensitivity for progesterone of these lesions. Both cysts, and more frequently angiomyolipoma, occur commonly in pediatric patients and tend to increase in size and number with increasing age (Avni et al. 1984; Casper et al. 2002). Most often, multiple bilateral lesions are present. They show rapid growth during childhood and adolescence. Angiomyolipomas are benign tumors composed of abnormal blood vessels, immature smooth muscle cells, and mature adipose tissue (De Waele et al. 2015). The abnormal vasculature is associated with the development of aneurysms, increasing the risk of spontaneous hemorrhage. Renal angiomyolipomas larger than four cm in diameter have a substantial risk for severe hemorrhage. Other risk factors for bleeding are growth and aneurysm size >0.5 cm (De Waele et al. 2015). Angiomyolipomas larger than four cm will be treated by arterial embolization. Active bleeding is also managed by arterial embolization. As in adults, the fatty component appears hyperechoic on US and shows as low attenuation on CT scan (Fig. 26). Other fat-containing renal masses in children are teratoid WT and xanthogranulomatous pyelonephritis.

1.4.6 Juxtaglomerular Cell Tumor or Reninoma

Juxtaglomerular cell tumor is typically discovered in the second decade of life, when hypertension and hyperaldosteronism suggest the diagnosis. It is a very rare diagnosis in young children; only a few case reports have been published (e.g., Garel et al. 1993; Trnka et al. 2014). The tumor produces excessive amounts of renin, leading to secondary hyperaldosteronism and resulting in severe hypertension, potassium wasting, and hypokalemia (Trnka et al. 2014). US shows a hypoechoic mass. On contrast-enhanced CT, the tumor can be seen as a well circumscribed mildly hyperattenuating lesion (Karaosmanoglu et al. 2015). MRI combined with MR angiography is recommended in this context to detect the tumor and to evaluate the status of the renal artery (Agrawal et al. 1995).

> **Take Away**
>
> Mesoblastic nephroma is the most common renal tumor in the neonate.
>
> Other benign tumors of the kidney are very rare in childhood.
>
> Multilocular cystic nephroma is indistinguishable from cystic partially differentiated nephroblastoma on all imaging modalities.
>
> Metanephric adenoma is strongly associated with polycythemia.
>
> Ossifying tumor of infancy is typically calcified, deeply located within the kidney.
>
> Multiple angiomyolipomas are seen in tuberous sclerosis.
>
> Juxtaglomerular tumor is revealed by hypertension and hyperaldosteronism.

1.5 Pseudotumoral Conditions

1.5.1 Infectious Diseases

Pseudotumoral acute pyelonephritis also called "lobar nephronia" (Fig. 27), renal abscess (Fig. 28), and a necrotic renal tumor may have similar imaging features. Inflammatory clinical and biological signs may also be observed in WT or another renal malignancy. Abdominal wall infiltration, when visible, is more suggestive of infectious disease. Fine needle aspiration and response to antibiotic treatment as well as laboratory signs may help in such circumstances (see also Chapter "Imaging in Urinary Tract Infections").

Xanthogranulomatous pyelonephritis is a specific form of chronic inflammatory kidney disease that occurs at any age. It usually occurs in association with urinary tract obstruction, infection, and/or renal stones. The most common organisms are *E. coli* and *Proteus mirabilis* (Marteinsson et al. 1996). On CT, involvement is typically unilateral and more focal than diffuse (Lee 2007). Focal pseudotumoral xanthogranulomatous pyelonephritis may be confused with a renal tumor. Mass effect, multiple microcysts within the mass, the presence of a pelvic lithiasis, associated triangular areas in the renal parenchyma, and obliteration of fatty tissue in the perirenal space are suggestive signs for xanthogranulomatous pyelonephritis instead of a tumor (see also Section "Ossifying Renal Tumor of Infancy").

1.5.2 Malformations

Renal malformations should always be part of the differential diagnosis when there are cystic lesions. A history of urinary tract infection and an associated ureterocele suggests a segmental multicystic dysplasia (Agrons et al. 1995; Jeon et al. 1999). Neonatal urinoma related to urinary tract obstruction (posterior urethral valve) may be misleading. Vascular malformations such as lymphangioma are a rare cause of a multiloculated renal mass (Farb and Lee 2006).

1.5.3 Miscellaneous

Granulomatous nephritis with renal masses is a very uncommon complication of sarcoidosis. One pediatric case was reported with echogenic masses on US and low-density lesions with mottled contrast enhancement on CT (Herman et al. 1997).

> **Take Away**
>
> Infectious diseases of the kidney and renal cystic malformations can mimic a necrotic tumor.

1.6 Diagnostic Strategy of Renal Neoplasms in Children

Step 1: Always start with noninvasive techniques
 US is the first-line imaging technique. It is available in all centers and does not require

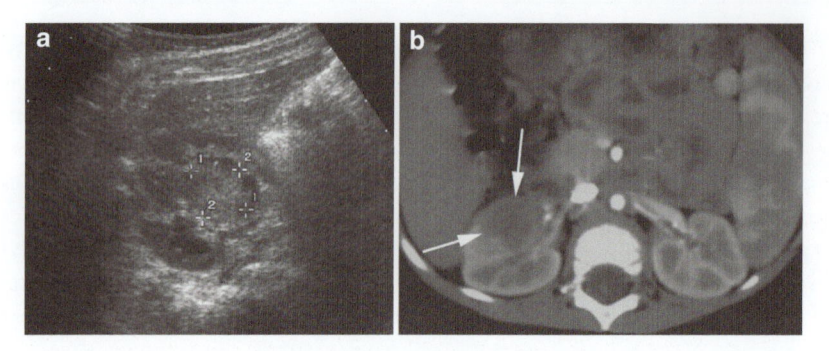

Fig. 27 Focal pseudotumoral pyelonephritis in a 15-month-old girl presenting with fever. Homogeneous small hyperechoic area on ultrasound (**a**) and hypoattenuating area on enhanced CT scan (**b**) without mass effect. Biopsy was not performed. Urinary tract infection diagnosis was based on bacteriuria (*E. coli*) and disappearance of the lesion on ultrasound during antibiotic therapy

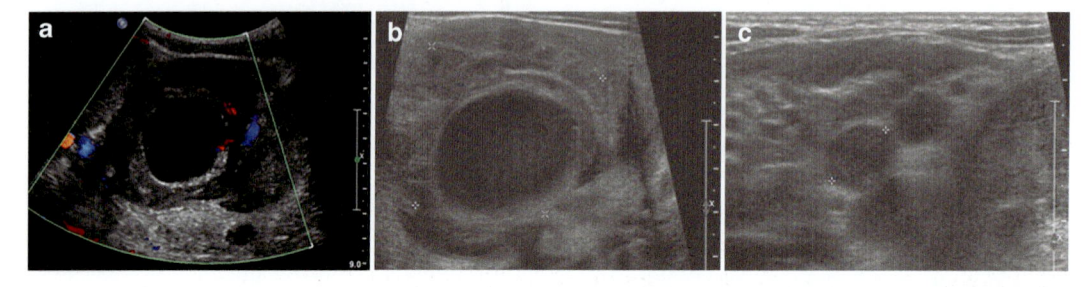

Fig. 28 Renal abscess in a 2-year-old girl. Ultrasound shows a thick-walled cystic intrarenal lesion (**a, b**) and enlarged neighboring lymph nodes (**c**)

sedation or injection of contrast agents. US rapidly confirms the location of the mass, assesses its volume, and depicts critical situations such as vascular invasion or obvious peritoneal rupture.

Step 2: *Confirm the renal origin of the mass*

The mass is often very large, and radiologists should look for the residual normal renal parenchyma in order to confirm the renal origin of the mass (Fig. 29). CDS may be helpful in equivocal cases: normal parenchyma around the mass will show more vascularization than the mass.

Step 3: *Depict relevant tumor extent*

Vascular extension can occur in the renal vein and IVC.

Peritoneal dissemination is associated with hemoperitoneum and/or intraperitoneal masses.

Step 4: *Assess the contralateral kidney*

Use high-frequency (linear) probes (at least 10 MHz, if applicable) and search for abnormalities in the contralateral kidney, such as bilateral tumor, nephroblastomatosis, dysplasia (mesangial sclerosis), or malformation.

Step 5: *Perform additional cross-sectional imaging with MRI or CT*

- To confirm the renal origin of the tumor in difficult cases (images in sagittal or coronal planes or multiplanar reconstructions may be helpful)
- To precisely measure the three tumor diameters (sometimes not possible with US)
- To confirm a suspected tumor rupture
- To depict contralateral disease

Step 6: *Be aware of pitfalls*

- An adrenal neuroblastoma may invade the upper pole of the kidney (Fig. 30).
- A ruptured WT may present as a renal fracture.
- Renal infection, notably xanthogranulomatous pyelonephritis and lobar nephronia, may mimic WT.

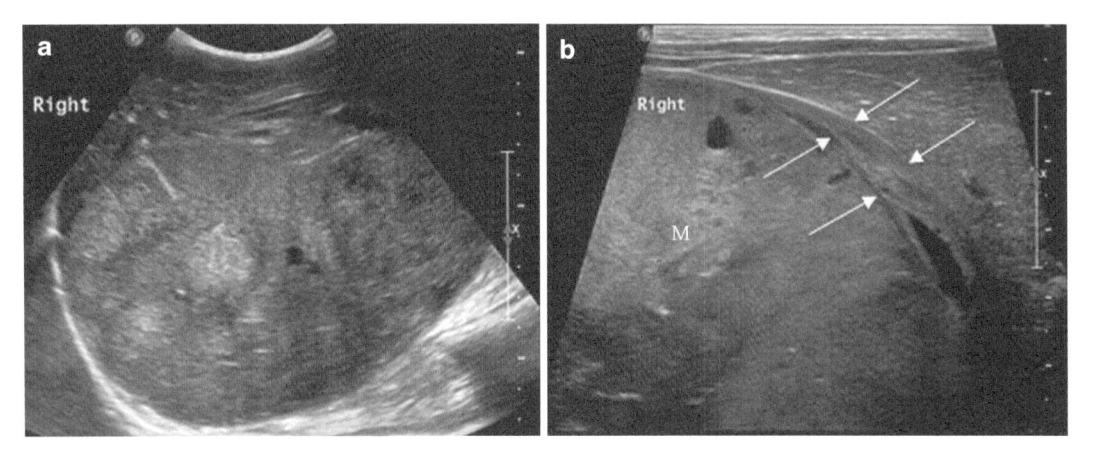

Fig. 29 Wilms' tumor in a 2-year-old girl. Ultrasound (**a**) shows a large tumor arising from the right kidney. With high-frequency linear transducer, normal renal parenchyma (*arrows*) is seen surrounding the mass (*M*) confirming its renal origin

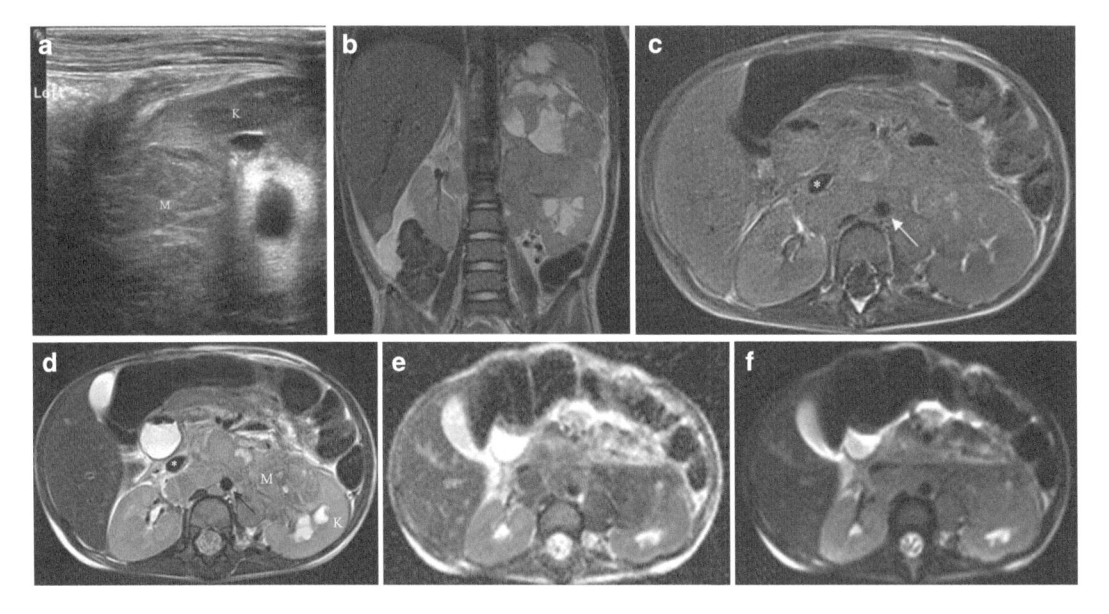

Fig. 30 Adrenal neuroblastoma in a 2-year-old boy invading the upper pole of the left kidney. Ultrasound (**a**) shows a mass (*M*) in direct contact with the central part of the kidney (*K*). MRI ((**b**) coronal T2-weighted image, (**c**) axial T1-weighted image, (**d**) axial T2-weighted image, (**e**) axial DWI with b value 800, (**f**) ADC) shows a large tumor extending into the left kidney. The tumor encases the aorta (*arrow*) and inferior vena cava (*). These features are suggestive of neuroblastoma and rarely observed in WT

Step 7: Check the relevant criteria for the diagnosis of Wilms' tumor
- Age ranges between 1 and 6 years
- No clinical sign of infectious disease
- Classic radiological features
- No extrapulmonary metastasis

Step 8: Check if there is an indication for core needle biopsy

The question of tumor biopsy at diagnosis is relevant for patients treated with primary chemotherapy (SIOP strategy) and not for patients treated by primary surgery (NWTSG strategy). Since WT has a very high prevalence in children, in most countries the diagnosis is usually based on clinical and radiological criteria only. The attitude toward the necessity of biopsy in the new UMBRELLA SIOP-RTSG 2015 protocol is as follows: core needle biopsy at diagnosis is not recommended for all renal masses but must be considered in cases of atypical presentation, i.e.:

- Age >6 years (higher risk of non-Wilms' histology)
- Urinary infection or septicemia (differential diagnosis with pseudotumoral or xanthogranulomatous pyelonephritis)
- Psoas infiltration
- Pulmonary metastasis in children under 2 years (suspicious for MRTK)
- Hypercalcemia (observed in rhabdoid tumor or bone metastases in clear cell sarcoma)
- Increased LDH level (suspicious for neuroblastoma or malignant hematologic disease)
- Uncommon radiological findings: extensive calcification (renal cell carcinoma, neuroblastoma), large lymph nodes (renal carcinoma, clear cell sarcoma, rhabdoid tumor), renal parenchyma not visible or an almost totally extra-renal process (neuroblastoma invading the kidney)
- Extrapulmonary and extrahepatic metastasis

Biopsy must always be performed under general anesthesia, at least in young children, under US guidance (or – in difficult anatomy – by CT), by a trained radiology/pathology team. Blood coagulation tests must be normal (paraneoplastic factor VIII deficiency may occur in nephroblastoma). A posterior/retroperitoneal approach is mandatory to avoid peritoneal dissemination. The coaxial technique should be preferred to allow multiple samples and to reduce the risk of a local complication. The currently recommended maximum diameter of core needle is 1.2 mm (18G). Part of the tissue sample must always be appropriately frozen (or put in culture medium) to allow genetic and biological studies. Currently, several tumors may be identified on the basis of genetic abnormalities, notably juvenile renal cell carcinoma, rhabdoid tumor, and renal fibrosarcoma. The most common complication associated with core needle biopsy is hemorrhage/transient hematuria (20%) (Vujanic et al. 2003). (Fatal) massive tumor bleeding, tumor rupture, and needle track recurrences have been infrequently reported (Dykes et al. 1991; Saarinen et al. 1991; Skoldenberg et al. 1999; Vujanic et al. 2003) and are exceptional in trained hands. Needle biopsy is unnecessary in some situations: bilateral disease (differential diagnosis between NRs and WT is usually not possible on small samples), in patients requiring primary surgery, i.e., in children less than 3 months old (congenital mesoblastic nephroma is highly probable and chemotherapy tolerance is low), or in purely cystic tumors (differential diagnosis with CPDN and benign cystic nephroma is usually impossible on a biopsy specimen, and both tumors do not respond to chemotherapy and are therefore operated upfront).

2 Neoplasms of the Lower Genitourinary Tract

2.1 Rhabdomyosarcoma

2.1.1 Introduction and Epidemiology

The most common primary malignant tumor of the lower genitourinary (GU) tract in the first two decades of life is rhabdomyosarcoma (RMS). It occurs most frequently in children between 2 and 4 years old (2/3 of all RMS arise before the age of 6) with a second peak during adolescence. RMS in newborn babies is extremely rare and there are just a few case reports describing neonatal and prenatally detected genitourinary RMS (Matsunaga et al. 2003; Esfahani et al. 2009; Lobe et al. 1994; Orbach et al. 2013; Marietti et al. 2013). Familial predisposition for RMS has been observed in familial cancer syndromes like Li-Fraumeni, Beckwith-Wiedemann, and Gorlin syndrome. In RMS, neurofibromatosis type 1 has a prevalence of 0.5–1% and is associated with a genitourinary tumor location (Ferrari et al. 2007; Sung et al. 2004). However, most cases are sporadic.

In the genitourinary tract, RMS commonly affects the bladder, prostate, and paratesticular sites but also, less commonly, the vulva, vagina, uterus, pelvic muscles, and perineum. For RMS arising from the bladder or prostate, the term bladder-prostate (BP) RMS is being used because this tumor often infiltrates both structures. In girls, bladder and vagina may also be infiltrated synchronously. The term paratesticular RMS (PT RMS) comprises primary tumors originating in the spermatic cord, penis, and epididymis. PT RMS comprises 7% of all RMS patients (Raney et al. 1987). In adolescents, PT RMS is the most common genitourinary location, representing 15% of all RMS diagnoses, followed by BP RMS (5%) (Cost et al. 2014a).

2.1.2 Histopathology and Genetics

Rhabdomyosarcoma is a solid tumor that grows from immature mesenchymal cells from which the striated musculature originates. However, RMS also grows in sites where no striated musculature is present. Histology and cytology of RMS ranges from undifferentiated "small blue round cell tumor" (like neuroblastoma, Ewing's sarcoma, and lymphoma) to tumors with advanced cytohistology like rhabdomyoma (Kodet et al. 1991). In children, RMS has two main histopathological variants: the embryonal and the alveolar type. A third subtype, pleomorphic RMS, is found in adults and very rarely in children. The embryonal type (E-RMS) is predominant (60–70%) in general and also in the primary GU sites and is subdivided into spindle cell and botryoid sarcoma subtypes. The spindle cell type is most often encountered in the paratesticular location. The growth pattern of the botryoid type is typically exophytic and noninvasive, which has a positive impact on cure and prognosis; it is found most often at vaginal sites. The alveolar type (A-RMS) has a less favorable prognosis. It occurs more often in adolescents and has a higher rate of local recurrence, impairing the chance of cure. Karyotypic studies show chromosomal translocations that distinguish A-RMS from E-RMS and other solid tumors. In A-RMS the most common translocation is t(2;13)(q35;q14) and t(1;13) (p36;q14). These translocations almost never occur in E-RMS, and gains of chromosome 2, 8, 12, and 13 are found more frequently in E-RMS. Genetic testing has shown that the poor outcome of A-RMS is possibly associated with the presence of PAX-FOXO1 fusion genes and not to histologic features. Genetic testing for RMS is currently being researched and will become more and more important in the selection of high-risk patients (Parham and Barr 2013).

2.1.3 Clinical Features

Clinical symptoms of genitourinary RMS depend on the anatomic site of the tumor and are usually related to mass effect and/or obstruction. Paratesticular RMS presents as a sudden appearance of a rapidly growing painless scrotal or inguinal mass distinct from the testis, sometimes fortuitously palpated. Bladder or prostatic RMS usually causes urinary retention due to bladder outlet obstruction or urinary problems such as pollakiuria, dysuria, and hematuria and sometimes also constipation, tenesmus, and a palpable abdominal mass. The purely endovesical variant usually causes hematuria and urinary symptoms mimicking cystitis. Painless hematuria is often considered a benign condition, especially in adolescents, hence may delay the diagnosis. RMS in the vagina or uterine cervix presents with vaginal bleeding or discharge and sometimes a prolapse of a polypoid or grape-like (botryoid) mucosanguineous mass through the vulva. Rarely patients with RMS initially have symptoms related to metastatic disease such as bone pain from skeletal metastases.

2.1.4 Imaging of Rhabdomyosarcoma of the Lower Urinary Tract

2.1.4.1 Locoregional Tumor Extent

Both endoscopic evaluation of bladder and vagina and imaging play a major role in staging at diagnosis, monitoring during treatment, assessment of complications and during follow-up. Persistent hematuria without a history of infection or trauma should prompt an US examination of the urinary tract with a decently filled urinary bladder. If necessary, it should be complemented by a perineal approach. Detection of bladder wall thickening or a mural nodule or mass should initiate further investigations. The features of RMS on US are nonspecific and vary with the tumor presenting as a homogeneous or heterogeneous hypoechoic or hyperechoic mass showing vascularization unless the tumor is necrotic (Fig. 31). CDS and mobilization of the patient can be helpful in differentiating a neoplasm from a blood clot or debris. A tumor may show focal anechoic areas, representing necrosis or cysts. The exact site of origin of the tumor may be difficult to define with US. The excellent soft tissue contrast and the lack of ionizing radiation make MRI the best next step in the imaging workup. For BP RMS, MRI will yield information on infiltration of the bladder wall and invasion of the prostatic bed (Fig. 31). Invasion of the different parts of the bladder must be evaluated: the trigone, the lateral bladder walls, the dome, and the ureters. It may be difficult to distinguish bladder wall thickening due to tumoral invasion from hypertrophy from outlet obstruction.

In the paratesticular form, US with a high-frequency (linear) probe (>7.5 MHz) will confirm an extratesticular location of a solid mass, with increased vascularity (Fig. 32), hence differentiating it from a teratoma or a dysplastic rete testis (Fig. 33). With MRI, the entire abdomen must be screened for enlarged, possibly metastatic, lymph nodes.

MRI is the best imaging modality to depict utero-vaginal forms of RMS: the site of origin will be determined (vagina, uterus, or parametria) as well as the extension into the surrounding tissues and spaces such as the ischiorectal fossa (Fig. 34).

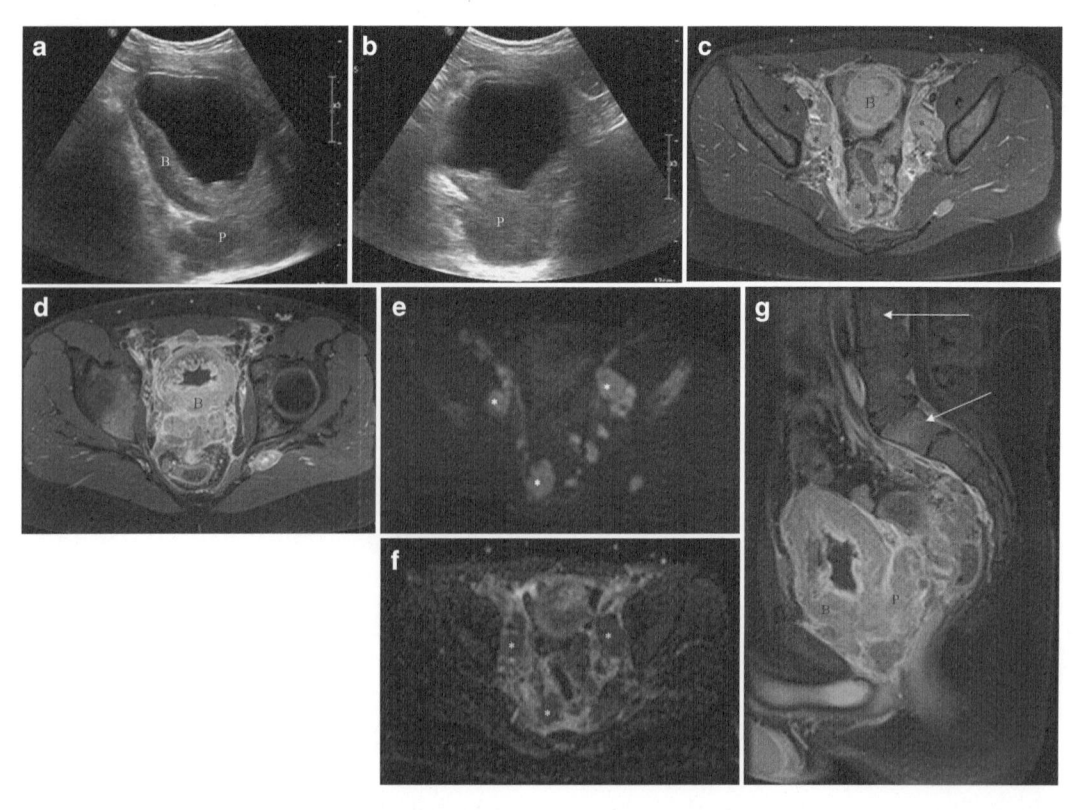

Fig. 31 Rhabdomyosarcoma of the bladder/prostate in a 16-year-old boy. Ultrasound ((**a**) sagittal, (**b**) axial) shows a thickened bladder wall (*B*) and a prostatic mass (*P*). MRI ((**c, d**) axial T1-weighted fat-saturated images with gadolinium, (**e**) axial DWI b value of 800, (**f**) axial ADC, (**g**) sagittal T1-weighted fat-saturated image with gadolinium) shows the thickened bladder wall, as well as multiple lymph node metastases (*) and skeletal metastases (*arrows*)

Tumor volume and locoregional extension are part of the factors that will define the prognosis and treatment: the type of surgery, chemotherapy, and brachytherapy. Imaging will also help in guiding biopsy, i.e., avoiding necrotic parts of the tumor.

2.1.4.2 Distant Metastases

Between 10 and 20 % of patients with RMS have metastases at diagnosis, most commonly in the lungs, cortical bone, and lymph nodes and less commonly in bone marrow and liver (Fig. 31). The pattern of metastatic spread varies with the anatomic site of the primary tumor. Prostate RMS is more likely to spread to the lungs and bone marrow than bladder RMS. Hepatic metastases are rare and must be searched for by US or MRI. Lung metastases occur in less than 10 % of patients at the time of diagnosis, and a chest CT scan is part of the initial workup.

Malignant cells may spread to all neighboring lymphatic chains: inguinal, femoral, obturator, iliac, and lumbo-aortic lymph nodes can be invaded (Fig. 31).

2.1.4.3 Staging

Full initial staging consists of cross-sectional imaging of the primary tumor, the entire abdomen and pelvis, and the chest. US is always performed at diagnosis: if the local disease can be well appreciated, US can be used for monitoring during chemotherapy. According to the EpSSG 2005 protocol, MRI is mandatory for abdominal staging, including contrast-enhanced images. Lymph nodes are suspicious for malignancy if

Fig. 32 (a–d) Paratesticular rhabdomyosarcoma in a 9-year-old boy with a painless scrotal mass since 2 weeks. Ultrasound shows a large heterogeneous, well-vascularized mass (*M*) in the left scrotum, displacing the normal left testicle (*T*)

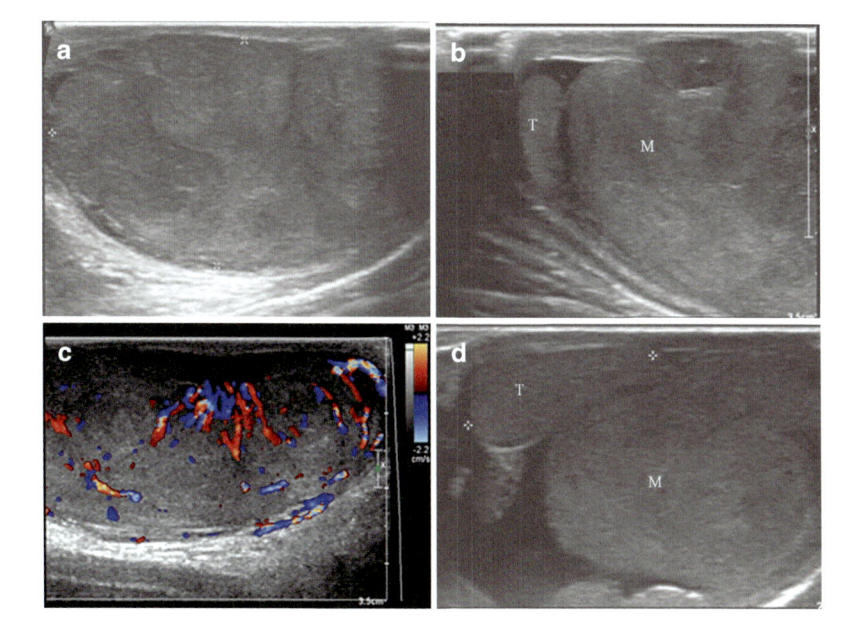

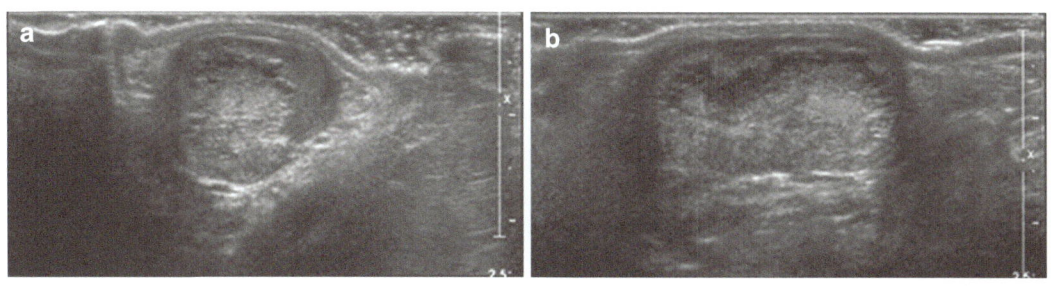

Fig. 33 (a, b) Cystic dilatation of the rete testis in a 7-year-old boy, with an enlarged, painless right testicle since 3 weeks

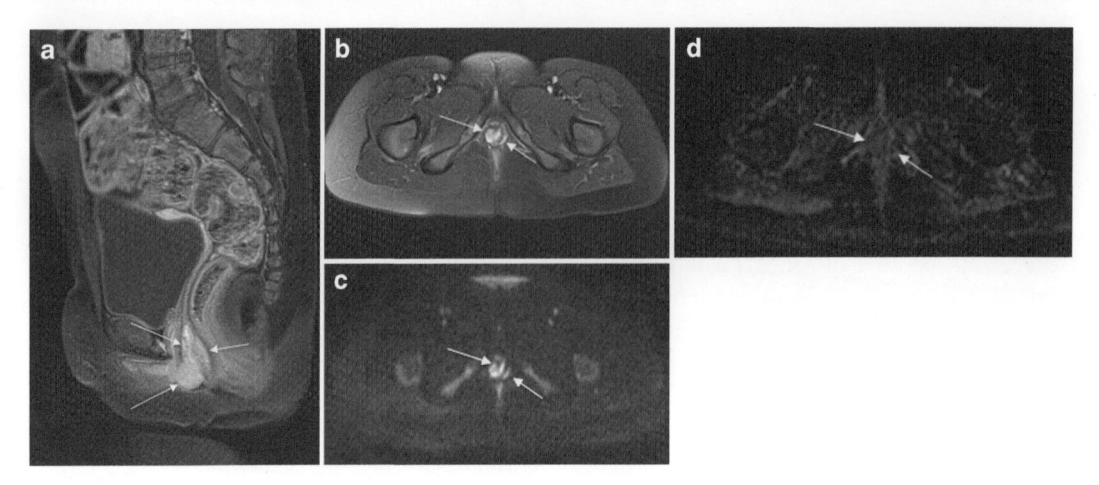

Fig. 34 Vaginal rhabdomyosarcoma in a 4-year-old girl, with intermittently protruding tissue from the vagina since several months. MRI shows a vaginal mass that enhances with gadolinium and shows restricted diffusion (*arrows*) (**a**) sagittal T1-weighted image with fat saturation after gadolinium, (**b**) axial T1-weighted image with fat saturation after gadolinium, (**c**) DWI b value 800, (**d**) ADC

they have a short axis >1.5 cm, if they have a heterogeneous appearance, and if they only show peripheral enhancement. Chest CT is mandatory for evaluation of lung metastasis. It is common practice to search for bone metastasis with bone scintigraphy and perform bone marrow aspiration to exclude bone marrow invasion. A report from the Children's Oncology Group Soft tissue Sarcoma Committee suggests that staging studies can be tailored to the patients' presenting characteristics: chest CT and bone scan might not be necessary in all patients (Weiss et al. 2013). PET-CT is increasingly used as a staging tool in patients with RMS. There seems to be evidence that PET-CT (/MRI) is better than conventional imaging for identifying patients with nodal involvement at diagnosis. However, there is still only limited evidence on the role of PET-CT for treatment response and end of treatment evaluation (Norman et al. 2015).

2.1.5 Principles of Treatment and Prognosis

The presence of metastases at diagnosis is the strongest adverse prognostic factor. Also, alveolar histology, BP RMS, tumor size >5 cm, tumor involving one or more contiguous organs or tissues, clinical or pathological nodal involvement, incomplete surgery, and patient age <1 year and ≥10 years are unfavorable factors (Bisogno and Ferrari 2012; Oberlin et al. 2008). Paratesticular, vaginal, and uterine sites are considered "favorable."

Treatment for RMS is traditionally risk adapted:

Low risk: small (<5 cm) tumor, completely resected at diagnosis, with favorable histology and site. This group consists mainly of paratesticular RMS. The EFS is approximately 90%. In the EpSSG protocol, children with low-risk tumors are treated with a short course of non-intensive chemotherapy.

Intermediate risk: patients with favorable histology and site. EFS is between 70 and 80%.

High risk: patients with large E-RMS in an unfavorable site or with nodal involvement and most A-RMS. EFS is below 60%.

Very high risk: mainly patients with metastatic RMS. EFS is between 20 and 30%. Surgery, radiotherapy, and chemotherapy are and have been combined in different ways by different international groups. There is concordance on the use of intensive chemotherapy and aggressive but non-mutilating surgery. Controversies exist on timing and method of local treatment and on the place of radiotherapy (Bisogno and Ferrari 2012). For BP RMS, retainment of bladder function is one of the goals of treatment. No differences in morbidity or functional outcome for the different treatment philosophies of the different international trials have yet been demonstrated (Raney et al. 2006). In younger children the risks of pelvic radiotherapy are very important, with long-term bladder fibrosis and dysfunction as well as the effect on the growth plates (Krasin et al. 2005; Raney et al. 2006; Alexander et al. 2012). Bladder-sparing surgery in combination with brachytherapy is the treatment of choice for BP RMS (Haie-Meder et al. 2013).

2.1.5.1 Survival
Collaboration between international clinical trials has led to dramatic improvement in survival of patients with low-risk and intermediate-risk disease, but it remains poor for patients with metastatic, relapsed, or refractory disease (Harel et al. 2015).

2.1.5.2 Relapse
Most patients with recurrent RMS have a poor long-term prognosis but survival rates are related to histology. Estimated 5-year survival after relapse is 64% for botryoid RMS, 26% for other E-RMS, and 5% for A-RMS and undifferentiated sarcoma (Pappo et al. 1999).

2.1.6 Follow-Up
According to the EpSSG-RMS-2005 protocol, tumor relapse surveillance is performed during 5 years after end of treatment with (cross-sectional) imaging (US and MRI) of the primary tumor site and with CXR.

> **Take Away**
> Rhabdomyosarcoma (RMS) is the most common primary malignant tumor of the lower GU tract in the first two decades of life.
>
> Distant metastases occur most commonly in the lungs, bone, and lymph nodes.
>
> The prognosis of RMS depends on the location and size of the primary tumor, the presence of metastasis, histology and genetics, age of the patient, and surgical resection.

2.2 Differential Diagnosis

2.2.1 Other Malignant Bladder Tumors
Urothelial neoplasms, also known as transitional cell carcinomas, originate from mesodermal cells in the bladder wall. This tumor type is most frequently found in elderly people and rarely occurs in children and adolescents. In contrast to adults, pediatric urothelial tumors are most often of low-grade malignancy, they tend not to invade the bladder muscle, and they have a low tendency for recurrence (Di Carlo et al. 2014). Inverted papilloma, polypoid bladder wall lesions, common in adults, has also been described in children, although very rarely (Isaac et al. 2000). Several cases of leiomyosarcoma of the bladder have been described in patients previously treated for retinoblastoma (Brucker et al. 2006). These patients have a genetic risk for developing other tumors and also the treatment with cyclophosphamide has been recognized as a cause of hemorrhagic cystitis and bladder cancer.

2.2.2 Benign Bladder Tumors
In general, bladder wall lesions in children are usually benign neoplasms or reactive in nature, but they can present in a similar way to malignancies.

Hemangiomas represent 0.6% of all bladder tumors and are the most frequent benign tumors of the urinary bladder. It is difficult and often impossible to distinguish a bladder hemangioma from bladder RMS, and biopsy is usually required (Ashley and Figueroa 2010; Jahn and Nissen 1991).

Although patients with neurofibromatosis are at higher risk for developing genitourinary RMS, they may also develop neurofibroma in the bladder and prostate or, more rarely, in the internal genital organs in girls (Scheithauer et al. 2008; Mong and Bellah 2006). These tumors are benign but infiltrating, and in the bladder they can cause obstruction leading to renal function impairment.

Bladder lesions such as fibromatous polyps may also mimic a malignant tumor and will often require biopsy. There are a few case reports of leiomyoma of the bladder in children. These benign tumors cannot be differentiated from other tumors with imaging (Chen et al. 2012).

Pheochromocytoma of the bladder is a rare tumor. It occurs most often in young adults but has been described in children as young as 11 years old (Beilan et al. 2013).

2.2.3 Reactive, Inflammatory, and Infectious Lesions of the Bladder (See also Chapter "Imaging in Urinary Tract Infections")

Nephrogenic adenoma and cystitis glandularis are papillary lesions resulting from a metaplastic reaction of the urothelium to chronic inflammation, trauma (catheterization injury, bladder surgery), immunosuppression, or radiation (Waisman et al. 1990; Huppmann and Pawel 2011; Heidenreich et al. 1999). A bladder wall abscess can occur in a context of previous instrumentation or urinary tract infection, an urachal remnant (Fig. 35) or inflammatory bowel disease and has also been described secondary to a bladder wall hematoma (Defoor et al. 2002; Kuo and Cain 2004). During an episode of cystitis, a diffuse bladder wall thickening is not unusual. Focal thickening of the bladder has been described with eosinophilic cystitis: the thickened wall may mimic a bladder wall tumor, hence the term pseudotumoral cystitis (Fig. 36) (Thompson et al. 2005). It has been described in children with food and drug allergies, bacterial or parasitic infections, malignancies such as leukemia, subsequent to surgery and in chronic granulomatous disease, suggesting it is a response of the immune system (Rossi et al. 2011; Barese et al. 2004; Chang et al. 2003). Inflammatory myofibroblastic tumor is characterized by proliferation of spindle cells (myofibroblast) mixed with inflammatory cells (lymphocytes, plasmocytes). It can occur in any organ and has also been described in the bladder. It is a neoplasm with unconstant somatic ALK-gene mutation and malignant potential. It can appear as a polypoid mass or a focal wall thickening (Fuller et al. 2015).

2.2.4 Other Tumors of the Prostate

Prostate adenocarcinoma, a tumor typically occurring in older men, has been described in boys under 17, although this paper dates from 1980, and no other case reports have been described since (Shimada et al. 1980). Non-Hodgkin lymphoma can involve any organ or tissue. Although rare, cases have been reported where the prostate was primarily involved (Sinclair et al. 2014).

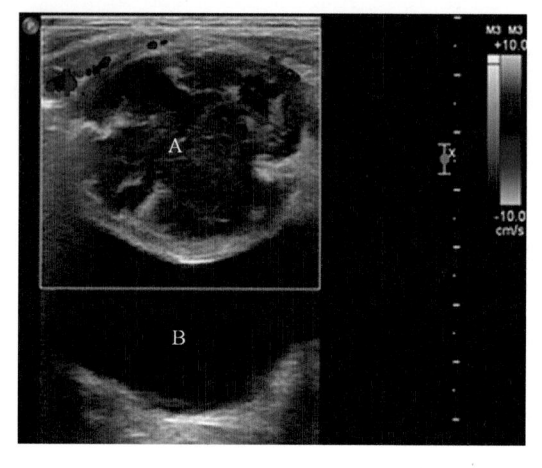

Fig. 35 Two-year-old girl with an abscess in an urachal remnant. Axial ultrasound of the lower abdomen shows a heterogeneous, lobulated fluid-filled mass (*A*) in the midline, anterior and cranial to the bladder (*B*)

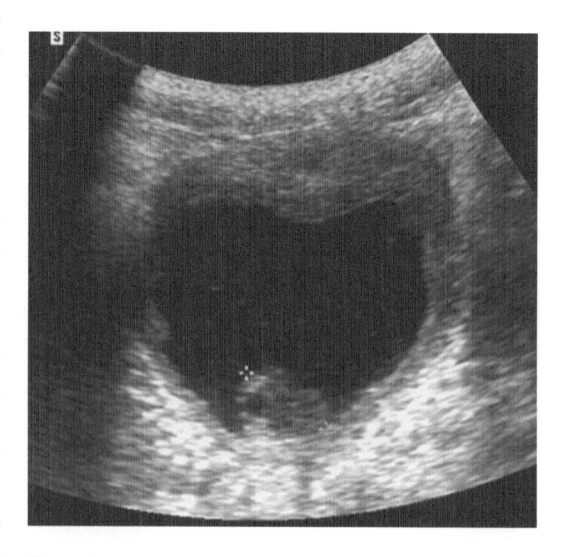

Fig. 36 Pseudotumoral cystitis. Ultrasound shows diffuse thickening of the bladder wall and a focal mass attached to the wall

2.2.5 Inflammation and Infection of the Prostate

Swelling due to inflammation of the prostate is rare in children. It is usually associated to a prostatic utricle cyst, and it can occur as a result to chronic voiding problems with high pressures (Hacker et al. 2009; Mong and Bellah 2006).

2.2.6 Scrotum

The paratesticular tissues consisting of the spermatic cord, epididymis, vestigial remnants, and tunica vaginalis may very rarely give rise to tumors other than RMS. In the prepubertal age group, benign tumors such as melanotic neuroectodermal tumor of infancy, leiomyoma, fibroma, lipoma, and hemangioma can be encountered (Ahmed et al. 2010). Adenomatoid tumor is a benign slow-growing tumor of the epididymis of the adult man, rarely occurring in adolescents (Guo et al. 2015). On US it is an oval-shaped tumor in the epididymis. The tumor is usually small, homogeneous, and encapsulated and cystic or solid and isoechoic or hypoechoic to normal epididymis (Akbar et al. 2003). CDS shows an isovascular or hypovascular tumor compared to the surrounding epididymis (Annam et al. 2015). Reported MRI findings are a slightly hypointense tumor relative to the testicular parenchyma on T2-weighted images and usually not enhancing more intensely than the testis (Patel and Silva 2004). Mimickers of paratesticular neoplasms are ectopic adrenal rests in the spermatic cord, often associated with synchronous intratesticular adrenal rests (Fig. 37), spermatic cord lipoma, splenogonadal fusion, accessory testicle, spermatocele, epidermoid cyst, inguinal hernia, inflammatory pseudotumor, cystic dysplasia of the epididymis, meconium peritonitis, and vascular malformations (Annam et al. 2015) (see also Chapter "Imaging in Male Genital Queries").

2.2.7 Vagina

There are two types of vaginal malignancies other than RMS occurring in children. In the younger age group, usually under 3 years, malignant germ cell tumors occur. Endodermal sinus or yolk sac tumors are the most frequent type with alpha-fetoprotein being a reliable marker. In prepuberal and puberal girls, vaginal clear cell adenocarcinoma occurs. All tumors present with vaginal bleeding or blood-stained discharge and/or a protrusion of a vaginal mass (Fernandez-Pineda et al. 2011; Goyal et al. 2014). Urothelial polyp of the anterior urethra has been described as a benign rare anomaly and mimicker of vaginal rhabdomyosarcoma by its presentation: an interlabial mass with bloody discharge (Akbarzadeh et al. 2014).

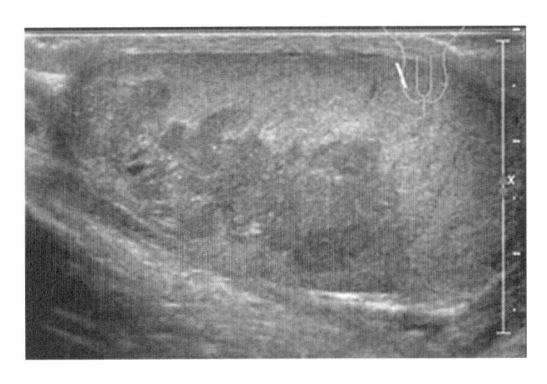

Fig. 37 Ectopic adrenal rest in boy with adrenogenital syndrome. Ultrasound shows a lobulated hypoechoic lesion within the testis

> **Take Away**
>
> Bladder lesions are usually benign tumors or of reactive, inflammatory, or infectious origin.
>
> Tumors other than RMS and inflammation and infection of the prostate are extremely rare in children.
>
> Paratesticular tumors other than RMS are rare in children.
>
> In young children, RMS and yolk sac tumor are the most frequent vaginal tumors.

References

Agrawal R, Jafri SZ, Gibson DP, Bis KG, Ali R (1995) Juxtaglomerular cell tumor: MR findings. J Comput Assist Tomogr 19(1):140–142

Agrons GA, Wagner BJ, Davidson AJ, Suarez ES (1995) Multilocular cystic renal tumor in children: radiologic-pathologic correlation. Radiographics Rev Publ Radiol Soc N Am Inc 15(3):653–669. doi:10.1148/radiographics.15.3.7624570

Ahmed HU, Arya M, Muneer A, Mushtaq I, Sebire NJ (2010) Testicular and paratesticular tumours in the prepubertal population. Lancet Oncol 11(5):476–483. doi:10.1016/s1470-2045(10)70012-7

Akbar SA, Sayyed TA, Jafri SZ, Hasteh F, Neill JS (2003) Multimodality imaging of paratesticular neoplasms and their rare mimics. Radiographics Rev Publ Radiol Soc N Am Inc 23(6):1461–1476. doi:10.1148/rg.236025174

Akbarzadeh A, Khorramirouz R, Saadat S, Hiradfar M, Kajbafzadeh AM (2014) Congenital urethral polyps in girls: as a differential diagnosis of interlabial masses. J Pediatr Adolesc Gynecol 27(6):330–334. doi:10.1016/j.jpag.2014.01.001

Alexander N, Lane S, Hitchcock R (2012) What is the evidence for radical surgery in the management of localized embryonal bladder/prostate rhabdomyosarcoma? Pediatr Blood Cancer 58(6):833–835. doi:10.1002/pbc.24087

Alvarez O, Rodriguez MM, Jordan L, Sarnaik S (2015) Renal medullary carcinoma and sickle cell trait: a systematic review. Pediatr Blood Cancer 62(10):1694–1699. doi:10.1002/pbc.25592

Amar AM, Tomlinson G, Green DM, Breslow NE, de Alarcon PA (2001) Clinical presentation of rhabdoid tumors of the kidney. J Pediatr Hematol Oncol 23(2):105–108

Annam A, Munden MM, Mehollin-Ray AR, Schady D, Browne LP (2015) Extratesticular masses in children: taking ultrasound beyond paratesticular rhabdomyosarcoma. Pediatr Radiol 45(9):1382–1391. doi:10.1007/s00247-015-3316-x

Argani P, Beckwith JB (2000) Metanephric stromal tumor: report of 31 cases of a distinctive pediatric renal neoplasm. Am J Surg Pathol 24(7):917–926

Argani P, Lae M, Ballard ET, Amin M, Manivel C, Hutchinson B, Reuter VE, Ladanyi M (2006) Translocation carcinomas of the kidney after chemotherapy in childhood. J Clin Oncol Off J Am Soc Clin Oncol 24(10):1529–1534. doi:10.1200/jco.2005.04.4693

Argani P, Perlman EJ, Breslow NE, Browning NG, Green DM, D'Angio GJ, Beckwith JB (2000) Clear cell sarcoma of the kidney: a review of 351 cases from the National Wilms Tumor Study Group Pathology Center. Am J Surg Pathol 24(1):4–18

Aronson DC, Slaar A, Heinen RC, de Kraker J, Heij HA (2011) Long-term outcome of bilateral Wilms tumors (BWT). Pediatr Blood Cancer 56(7):1110–1113. doi:10.1002/pbc.22881

Arroyo MR, Green DM, Perlman EJ, Beckwith JB, Argani P (2001) The spectrum of metanephric adenofibroma and related lesions: clinicopathologic study of 25 cases from the National Wilms Tumor Study Group Pathology Center. Am J Surg Pathol 25(4):433–444

Ashley RA, Figueroa TE (2010) Gross hematuria in a 3-year-old girl caused by a large isolated bladder hemangioma. Urology 76(4):952–954. doi:10.1016/j.urology.2010.03.062

Avni EF, Szliwowski H, Spehl M, Lelong B, Baudain P, Struyven J (1984) Renal involvement in tuberous sclerosis. Ann Radiol 27(2–3):207–214

Bahubeshi A, Bal N, Rio Frio T, Hamel N, Pouchet C, Yilmaz A, Bouron-Dal Soglio D, Williams GM, Tischkowitz M, Priest JR, Foulkes WD (2010) Germline DICER1 mutations and familial cystic nephroma. J Med Genet 47(12):863–866. doi:10.1136/jmg.2010.081216

Barese CN, Podestá M, Litvak E, Villa M, Rivas EM (2004) Recurrent eosinophilic cystitis in a child with chronic granulomatous disease. J Pediatr Hematol Oncol 26(3):2009–2012

Bayindir P, Guillerman RP, Hicks MJ, Chintagumpala MM (2009) Cellular mesoblastic nephroma (infantile renal fibrosarcoma): institutional review of the clinical, diagnostic imaging, and pathologic features of a distinctive neoplasm of infancy. Pediatr Radiol 39(10):1066–1074. doi:10.1007/s00247-009-1348-9

Beckwith JB (1993) Precursor lesions of Wilms tumor: clinical and biological implications. Med Pediatr Oncol 21(3):158–168

Beckwith JB (1998) Nephrogenic rests and the pathogenesis of Wilms tumor: developmental and clinical considerations. Am J Med Genet 79(4):268–273

Beckwith JB, Kiviat NB, Bonadio JF (1990) Nephrogenic rests, nephroblastomatosis, and the pathogenesis of Wilms' tumor. Pediatr Pathol Affiliated Int Paediatr Pathol Assoc 10(1–2):1–36

Beilan JA, Lawton A, Hajdenberg J, Rosser CJ (2013) Pheochromocytoma of the urinary bladder: a systematic review of the contemporary literature. BMC Urol 13:22. doi:10.1186/1471-2490-13-22

Bergeron C, Iliescu C, Thiesse P, Bouvier R, Dijoud F, Ranchere-Vince D, Basset T, Chappuis JP, Buclon M, Frappaz D, Brunat-Mentigny M, Philip T (2001) Does nephroblastomatosis influence the natural history and relapse rate in Wilms' tumour? A single centre experience over 11 years. Eur J Cancer (Oxford, England: 1990) 37(3):385–391

Bisogno G, Ferrari A (2012) Soft tissue sarcomas. In: Stevens MCGCH, Biondi A (eds) Cancer in children – clinical management. Oxford University Press, Oxford, pp 274–292

Bliek J, Gicquel C, Maas S, Gaston V, Le Bouc Y, Mannens M (2004) Epigenotyping as a tool for the prediction of tumor risk and tumor type in patients with Beckwith-Wiedemann syndrome (BWS). J Pediatr 145(6):796–799. doi:10.1016/j.jpeds.2004.08.007

Bolande RP, Brough AJ, Izant RJ Jr (1967) Congenital mesoblastic nephroma of infancy. A report of eight cases and the relationship to Wilms' tumor. Pediatrics 40(2):272–278

Breslow N, Olshan A, Beckwith JB, Green DM (1993) Epidemiology of Wilms tumor. Med Pediatr Oncol 21(3):172–181

Breslow N, Olshan A, Beckwith JB, Moksness J, Feigl P, Green D (1994) Ethnic variation in the incidence, diagnosis, prognosis, and follow-up of children with Wilms' tumor. J Natl Cancer Inst 86(1):49–51

Breslow NE, Olson J, Moksness J, Beckwith JB, Grundy P (1996) Familial Wilms' tumor: a descriptive study. Med Pediatr Oncol 27(5):398–403.

doi:10.1002/(sici)1096-911x(199611)27:5<398::aid-mpo2>3.0.co;2-h
Brisse H (2005) The radiologic contribution to surgical aspects of kidney tumors in children. JBR-BTR organe de la Societe royale belge de radiologie (SRBR) orgaan van de Koninklijke Belgische Vereniging voor Radiologie (KBVR) 88(5):250–253
Brisse HJ, Schleiermacher G, Sarnacki S, Helfre S, Philippe-Chomette P, Boccon-Gibod L, Peuchmaur M, Mosseri V, Aigrain Y, Neuenschwander S (2008a) Preoperative Wilms tumor rupture: a retrospective study of 57 patients. Cancer 113(1):202–213. doi:10.1002/cncr.23535
Brisse HJ, Smets AM, Kaste SC, Owens CM (2008b) Imaging in unilateral Wilms tumour. Pediatr Radiol 38(1):18–29. doi:10.1007/s00247-007-0677-9
Brucker BE, Ernst L, Meadows A, Zderic S (2006) A second leiomyosarcoma in the urinary bladder of a child with a history of retinoblastoma 12 years following partial cystectomy. Pediatr Blood Cancer 46(7):811–814. doi:10.1002/pbc.20506
Byerly D, Coley B, Ruymann F (2006) Perirenal hemorrhage as first presentation of Wilms tumor. Pediatr Radiol 36(7):714–717. doi:10.1007/s00247-006-0168-4
Casper KA, Donnelly LF, Chen B, Bissler JJ (2002) Tuberous sclerosis complex: renal imaging findings. Radiology 225(2):451–456. doi:10.1148/radiol.2252011584
Cesaro S, Spiller M, Sartori MT, Alaggio R, Peruzzo M, Saggiorato G, Bisogno G (2011) Veno-occlusive disease in pediatric patients affected by Wilms tumor. Pediatr Blood Cancer 57(2):258–261. doi:10.1002/pbc.22841
Chami R, Yin M, Marrano P, Teerapakpinyo C, Shuangshoti S, Thorner PS (2015) BRAF mutations in pediatric metanephric tumors. Hum Pathol 46(8):1153–1161. doi:10.1016/j.humpath.2015.03.019
Chan HS, Cheng MY, Mancer K, Payton D, Weitzman SS, Kotecha P, Daneman A (1987) Congenital mesoblastic nephroma: a clinicoradiologic study of 17 cases representing the pathologic spectrum of the disease. J Pediatr 111(1):64–70
Chang CY, Chiou TJ, Hsieh YL, Cheng SN (2003) Leukemic infiltration of the urinary bladder presenting as uncontrollable gross hematuria in a child with acute lymphoblastic leukemia. J Pediatr Hematol Oncol 25(9):735–739
Charlton J, Williams RD, Sebire NJ, Popov S, Vujanic G, Chagtai T, Alcaide-German M, Morris T, Butcher LM, Guilhamon P, Beck S, Pritchard-Jones K (2015) Comparative methylome analysis identifies new tumour subtypes and biomarkers for transformation of nephrogenic rests into Wilms tumour. Genome Medicine 7(1):11. doi:10.1186/s13073-015-0136-4
Chen H, Niu ZB, Yang Y (2012) Bladder leiomyoma in a 6-year-old boy. Urology 79(2):434–436. doi:10.1016/j.urology.2011.06.011
Chepuri NB, Strouse PJ, Yanik GA (2003) CT of renal lymphoma in children. AJR Am J Roentgenol 180(2):429–431. doi:10.2214/ajr.180.2.1800429

Choueiri TK, Cheville J, Palescandolo E, Fay AP, Kantoff PW, Atkins MB, McKenney JK, Brown V, Lampron ME, Zhou M, Hirsch MS, Signoretti S (2012) BRAF mutations in metanephric adenoma of the kidney. Eur Urol 62(5):917–922. doi:10.1016/j.eururo.2012.05.051
Christmann D, Becmeur F, Marcellin L, Dhaoui R, Roy E, Sauvage P, Walter JP (1990) Mesoblastic nephroma presenting as a haemorrhagic cyst. Pediatr Radiol 20(7):553
Chung CJ, Lorenzo R, Rayder S, Schemankewitz E, Guy CD, Cutting J, Munden M (1995) Rhabdoid tumors of the kidney in children: CT findings. AJR Am J Roentgenol 164(3):697–700. doi:10.2214/ajr.164.3.7863897
Cooper WN, Luharia A, Evans GA, Raza H, Haire AC, Grundy R, Bowdin SC, Riccio A, Sebastio G, Bliek J, Schofield PN, Reik W, Macdonald F, Maher ER (2005) Molecular subtypes and phenotypic expression of Beckwith-Wiedemann syndrome. Eur J Hum Genet EJHG 13(9):1025–1032. doi:10.1038/sj.ejhg.5201463
Coppes MJ, Arnold M, Beckwith JB, Ritchey ML, D'Angio GJ, Green DM, Breslow NE (1999) Factors affecting the risk of contralateral Wilms tumor development: a report from the National Wilms Tumor Study Group. Cancer 85(7):1616–1625
Cost NG, Cost CR, Geller JI, Cost NG, Cost CR, Geller JI, Defoor WR Jr (2014a) Adolescent urologic oncology: current issues and future directions. Urol Oncol 32(2):59–69. doi:10.1016/j.urolonc.2012.08.002
Cost NG, Sawicz-Birkowska K, Kajbafzadeh AM, Tourchi A, Parigi GB, Guillen G, DeFoor WR Jr, Apoznanski W (2014b) A comparison of renal function outcomes after nephron-sparing surgery and radical nephrectomy for nonsyndromic unilateral Wilms tumor. Urology 83(6):1388–1393. doi:10.1016/j.urology.2014.01.051
Cox SG, Kilborn T, Pillay K, Davidson A, Millar AJ (2014) Magnetic resonance imaging versus histopathology in Wilms tumor and nephroblastomatosis: 3 examples of noncorrelation. J Pediatr Hematol Oncol 36(2):e81–e84. doi:10.1097/MPH.0b013e318290c60d
Cozzi DA, Zani A (2006) Nephron-sparing surgery in children with primary renal tumor: indications and results. Semin Pediatr Surg 15(1):3–9. doi:10.1053/j.sempedsurg.2005.11.002
Daskas N, Argyropoulou M, Pavlou M, Andronikou S (2002) Congenital mesoblastic nephroma associated with polyhydramnios and hypercalcemia. Pediatr Nephrol (Berlin, Germany) 17(3):187–189. doi:10.1007/s00467-001-0779-9
Davidson AJ, Choyke PL, Hartman DS, Davis CJ Jr (1995) Renal medullary carcinoma associated with sickle cell trait: radiologic findings. Radiology 195(1):83–85. doi:10.1148/radiology.195.1.7892499
Davis CJ Jr, Barton JH, Sesterhenn IA, Mostofi FK (1995) Metanephric adenoma. Clinicopathological study of fifty patients. Am J Surg Pathol 19(10):1101–1114
Daw NC, Kauffman WM, Bodner SM, Pratt CB, Hoffer FA (2002) Patterns of abdominal relapse and role of sonography in Wilms tumor. Pediatr Hematol Oncol 19(2):107–115

de Kraker J, Graf N, Pritchard-Jones K, Pein F (2001) Nephroblastoma clinical trial and study SIOP 2001, Protocol. SIOP RTSG

de Kraker J, Jones KP (2005) Treatment of Wilms tumor: an international perspective. J Clin Oncol Off J Am Soc Clin Oncol 23(13):3156–3157. doi:10.1200/jco.2005.05.150; author reply 3157–3158

de Kraker J, Voute PA, Lemerle J, Tournade MF, Perry HJ (1982) Preoperative chemotherapy in Wilms' tumour. Results of clinical trials and studies on nephroblastomas conducted by the International Society of Paediatric Oncology (SIOP). Prog Clin Biol Res 100:131–144

De Waele L, Lagae L, Mekahli D (2015) Tuberous sclerosis complex: the past and the future. Pediatr Nephrol (Berlin, Germany) 30(10):1771–1780. doi:10.1007/s00467-014-3027-9

DeBaun MR, Tucker MA (1998) Risk of cancer during the first four years of life in children from The Beckwith-Wiedemann Syndrome Registry. J Pediatr 132(3 Pt 1):398–400

Defoor W, Minevich E, Sheldon C (2002) Unusual bladder masses in children. Urology 60(5):911

Dhall D, Al-Ahmadie HA, Dhall G, Shen-Schwarz S, Tickoo SK (2007) Pediatric renal cell carcinoma with oncocytoid features occurring in a child after chemotherapy for cardiac leiomyosarcoma. Urology 70(1):178.e113. doi:10.1016/j.urology.2007.03.055

Di Carlo D, Ferrari A, Perruccio K, D'Angelo P, Fagnani AM, Cecchetto G, Bisogno G (2014) Management and follow-up of urothelial neoplasms of the bladder in children: a report from the TREP project. Pediatr Blood Cancer 62:1000–1003. doi:10.1002/pbc.25380

Doerfler O, Reittner P, Groell R, Ratscheck M, Trummer H, Szolar D (2001) Peripheral primitive neuroectodermal tumour of the kidney: CT findings. Pediatr Radiol 31(2):117–119. doi:10.1007/s002470000392

Dome JS, Fernandez CV, Mullen EA, Kalapurakal JA, Geller JI, Huff V, Gratias EJ, Dix DB, Ehrlich PF, Khanna G, Malogolowkin MH, Anderson JR, Naranjo A, Perlman EJ (2013) Children's Oncology Group's 2013 blueprint for research: renal tumors. Pediatr Blood Cancer 60(6):994–1000. doi:10.1002/pbc.24419

Dome JS, Graf N, Geller JI, Fernandez CV, Mullen EA, Spreafico F, Van den Heuvel-Eibrink M, Pritchard-Jones K (2015) Advances in Wilms tumor treatment and biology: progress through International Collaboration. J Clin Oncol Off J Am Soc Clin Oncol 33(27):2999–3007. doi:10.1200/jco.2015.62.1888

Dome JS, Liu T, Krasin M, Lott L, Shearer P, Daw NC, Billups CA, Wilimas JA (2002) Improved survival for patients with recurrent Wilms tumor: the experience at St. Jude Children's Research Hospital. J Pediatr Hematol Oncol 24(3):192–198

Downey RT, Dillman JR, Ladino-Torres MF, McHugh JB, Ehrlich PF, Strouse PJ (2012) CT and MRI appearances and radiologic staging of pediatric renal cell carcinoma. Pediatr Radiol 42(4):410–417. doi:10.1007/s00247-011-2319-5; quiz 513–414

Dykes EH, Marwaha RK, Dicks-Mireaux C, Sams V, Risdon RA, Duffy PG, Ransley PG, Pritchard J (1991) Risks and benefits of percutaneous biopsy and primary chemotherapy in advanced Wilms' tumour. J Pediatr Surg 26(5):610–612

Ehrlich PF, Ferrer FA, Ritchey ML, Anderson JR, Green DM, Grundy PE, Dome JS, Kalapurakal JA, Perlman EJ, Shamberger RC (2009) Hepatic metastasis at diagnosis in patients with Wilms tumor is not an independent adverse prognostic factor for stage IV Wilms tumor: a report from the Children's Oncology Group/National Wilms Tumor Study Group. Ann Surg 250(4):642–648. doi:10.1097/SLA.0b013e3181b76f20

England RJ, Haider N, Vujanic GM, Kelsey A, Stiller CA, Pritchard-Jones K, Powis M (2011) Mesoblastic nephroma: a report the United Kingdom Children's Cancer and Leukaemia Group (CCLG). Pediatr Blood Cancer 56(5):744–748. doi:10.1002/pbc.22871

Esfahani SA, Montaser-Kouhsari L, Saeedi P, Sadeghi Z, Kajbafzadeh AM (2009) An antenatally diagnosed rhabdomyosarcoma of the bladder treated without extensive surgery. Nat Rev Urol 6(8):449–453. doi:10.1038/nrurol.2009.99

Farb JB, Lee EY (2006) Clinical image. Infiltrative renal lymphangioma in a pediatric patient. Pediatr Radiol 36(7):718. doi:10.1007/s00247-005-0108-8

Fernandes ET, Parham DM, Ribeiro RC, Douglass EC, Kumar AP, Wilimas J (1988) Teratoid Wilms' tumor: the St Jude experience. J Pediatr Surg 23(12):1131–1134

Fernandez-Pineda I, Spunt SL, Parida L, Krasin MJ, Davidoff AM, Rao BN (2011) Vaginal tumors in childhood: the experience of St. Jude Children's Research Hospital. J Pediatr Surg 46(11):2071–2075. doi:10.1016/j.jpedsurg.2011.05.003

Ferrari A, Bisogno G, Macaluso A, Casanova M, D'Angelo P, Pierani P, Zanetti I, Alaggio R, Cecchetto G, Carli M (2007) Soft-tissue sarcomas in children and adolescents with neurofibromatosis type 1. Cancer 109(7):1406–1412. doi:10.1002/cncr.22533

Ferraro EM, Klein SA, Fakhry J, Weingarten MJ, Rose JS (1986) Hypercalcemia in association with mesoblastic nephroma: report of a case and review of the literature. Pediatr Radiol 16(6):516–517

Filiatrault D, Hoyoux C, Benoit P, Garel L, Esseltine D (1987) Renal metastases from neuroblastoma. Report of two cases. Pediatr Radiol 17(2):137–138

Fleitz JM, Wootton-Gorges SL, Wyatt-Ashmead J, McGavran L, Koyle M, West DC, Kurzrock EA, Martin KW, Odom LF (2003) Renal cell carcinoma in long-term survivors of advanced stage neuroblastoma in early childhood. Pediatr Radiol 33(8):540–545. doi:10.1007/s00247-003-0913-x

Fuchs J, Szavay P, Seitz G, Handgretinger R, Schafer JF, Warmann SW (2011) Nephron sparing surgery for synchronous bilateral nephroblastoma involving the renal hilus. J Urol 186(4):1430–1436. doi:10.1016/j.juro.2011.05.068

Fuller TW, Dangle P, Reese JN, Ristau BT, Lyon TD, Jaffe R, Stephany HA (2015) Inflammatory myofibroblastic tumor of the bladder masquerading as eosinophilic cystitis: case report and review of the literature. Urology 85(4):921–923. doi:10.1016/j.urology.2015.01.005

Furtwaengler R, Reinhard H, Leuschner I, Schenk JP, Goebel U, Claviez A, Kulozik A, Zoubek A, von Schweinitz D, Graf N (2006) Mesoblastic nephroma – a report from the Gesellschaft fur Padiatrische Onkologie und Hamatologie (GPOH). Cancer 106(10):2275–2283. doi:10.1002/cncr.21836

Furtwangler R, Schmolze M, Graber S, Leuschner I, Amann G, Schenk JP, Niggli F, Kager L, von Schweinitz D, Graf N (2014) Pretreatment for bilateral nephroblastomatosis is an independent risk factor for progressive disease in patients with stage V nephroblastoma. Klin Padiatr 226(3):175–181. doi:10.1055/s-0034-1371840

Garel L, Robitaille P, Dubois J, Russo P (1993) Pediatric case of the day. Reninoma of the left kidney. Radiographics Rev Publ Radiol Soc N Am Inc 13(2):477–479. doi:10.1148/radiographics.13.2.8460232

Geller JI, Ehrlich PF, Cost NG, Khanna G, Mullen EA, Gratias EJ, Naranjo A, Dome JS, Perlman EJ (2015) Characterization of adolescent and pediatric renal cell carcinoma: A report from the Children's Oncology Group study AREN03B2. Cancer 121(14):2457–2464. doi:10.1002/cncr.29368

Godzinski J, Weirich A, Tournade MF, Gauthier F, Buerger D, Moorman-Voestermans CG, de Kraker J, Voute P, Ludwig R, Sawicz-Birkowska K, Vujanic G, Ducourtieux M (2001) Primary nephrectomy for emergency: a rare event in the International Society of Paediatric Oncology Nephroblastoma Trial and Study no. 9. Eur J Pediatr Surg Off J Aust Assoc Pediatr Surg [et al] Zeitschrift fur Kinderchirurgie 11(1):36–39

Gooskens SL, Furtwangler R, Vujanic GM, Dome JS, Graf N, van den Heuvel-Eibrink MM (2012) Clear cell sarcoma of the kidney: a review. Eur J Cancer (Oxford, England: 1990) 48(14):2219–2226. doi:10.1016/j.ejca.2012.04.009

Goske MJ, Mitchell C, Reslan WA (1999) Imaging of patients with Wilms' tumor. Semin Urol Oncol 17(1):11–20

Gow KW, Roberts IF, Jamieson DH, Bray H, Magee JF, Murphy JJ (2000) Local staging of Wilms' tumor – computerized tomography correlation with histological findings. J Pediatr Surg 35(5):677–679. doi:10.1053/jpsu.2000.5941

Goyal S, Puri A, Mishra K, Aggarwal SK, Kumar M, Sonaker P (2014) Endodermal sinus tumor of vagina posing a diagnostic challenge and managed by chemotherapy and novel posterior sagittal surgical approach: lessons learned. J Obstet Gynaecol Res 40(2):632–636. doi:10.1111/jog.12182

Graf N, van Tinteren H, Bergeron C, Pein F, van den Heuvel-Eibrink MM, Sandstedt B, Schenk JP, Godzinski J, Oldenburger F, Furtwangler R, de Kraker J (2012) Characteristics and outcome of stage II and III non-anaplastic Wilms' tumour treated according to the SIOP trial and study 93–01. Eur J Cancer (Oxford, England: 1990) 48(17):3240–3248. doi:10.1016/j.ejca.2012.06.007

Gratias EJ, Jennings LJ, Anderson JR, Dome JS, Grundy P, Perlman EJ (2013) Gain of 1q is associated with inferior event-free and overall survival in patients with favorable histology Wilms tumor: a report from the Children's Oncology Group. Cancer 119(21):3887–3894. doi:10.1002/cncr.28239

Green DM, Cotton CA, Malogolowkin M, Breslow NE, Perlman E, Miser J, Ritchey ML, Thomas PR, Grundy PE, D'Angio GJ, Beckwith JB, Shamberger RC, Haase GM, Donaldson M, Weetman R, Coppes MJ, Shearer P, Coccia P, Kletzel M, Macklis R, Tomlinson G, Huff V, Newbury R, Weeks D (2007) Treatment of Wilms tumor relapsing after initial treatment with vincristine and actinomycin D: a report from the National Wilms Tumor Study Group. Pediatr Blood Cancer 48(5):493–499. doi:10.1002/pbc.20822

Grundy P, Breslow N, Green DM, Sharples K, Evans A, D'Angio GJ (1989) Prognostic factors for children with recurrent Wilms' tumor: results from the Second and Third National Wilms' Tumor Study. J Clin Oncol Off J Am Soc Clin Oncol 7(5):638–647

Grundy PE, Breslow NE, Li S, Perlman E, Beckwith JB, Ritchey ML, Shamberger RC, Haase GM, D'Angio GJ, Donaldson M, Coppes MJ, Malogolowkin M, Shearer P, Thomas PR, Macklis R, Tomlinson G, Huff V, Green DM (2005) Loss of heterozygosity for chromosomes 1p and 16q is an adverse prognostic factor in favorable-histology Wilms tumor: a report from the National Wilms Tumor Study Group. J Clin Oncol Off J Am Soc Clin Oncol 23(29):7312–7321. doi:10.1200/jco.2005.01.2799

Grundy PE, Green DM, Coppes MJ (2002) Renal tumors. In: Pizzo PA (ed) Principles and practice of pediatric oncology. Lippincott Williams and Wilkins, Philadelphia, pp 865–893

Grundy PE, Green DM, Dirks AC, Berendt AE, Breslow NE, Anderson JR, Dome JS (2012) Clinical significance of pulmonary nodules detected by CT and Not CXR in patients treated for favorable histology Wilms tumor on national Wilms tumor studies-4 and −5: a report from the Children's Oncology Group. Pediatr Blood Cancer 59(4):631–635. doi:10.1002/pbc.24123

Guo K, Tian R, Liu L, Du C, Li F, Wang H (2015) Adenomatoid tumor of the tunica albuginea in a Boy: a case report and literature review. Case Rep Urol 2015:935193. doi:10.1155/2015/935193

Gururangan S, Wilimas JA, Fletcher BD (1994) Bone metastases in Wilms' tumor – report of three cases and review of literature. Pediatr Radiol 24(2):85–87

Gylys-Morin V, Hoffer FA, Kozakewich H, Shamberger RC (1993) Wilms tumor and nephroblastomatosis: imaging characteristics at gadolinium-enhanced MR imaging. Radiology 188(2):517–521. doi:10.1148/radiology.188.2.8392214

Hacker HW, Winiker H, Caduff J, Schwoebel MG (2009) Inflammatory tumour of the prostate in a 4-year-old boy. J Pediatr Urol 5(6):516–518. doi:10.1016/j.jpurol.2009.03.023

Haie-Meder C, Mazeron R, Martelli H, Oberlin O (2013) Brachytherapy role in pediatric rhabdomyosarcomas. Cancer radiotherapie Journal de la Societe francaise de radiotherapie oncologique 17(2):155–158. doi:10.1016/j.canrad.2012.12.011

Hales PW, Olsen OE, Sebire NJ, Pritchard-Jones K, Clark CA (2015) A multi-Gaussian model for apparent diffusion coefficient histogram analysis of Wilms' tumour subtype and response to chemotherapy. NMR Biomed 28(8):948–957. doi:10.1002/nbm.3337

Hamilton TE, Ritchey ML, Haase GM, Argani P, Peterson SM, Anderson JR, Green DM, Shamberger RC (2011) The management of synchronous bilateral Wilms tumor: a report from the National Wilms Tumor Study Group. Ann Surg 253(5):1004–1010. doi:10.1097/SLA.0b013e31821266a0

Han TI, Kim MJ, Yoon HK, Chung JY, Choeh K (2001) Rhabdoid tumour of the kidney: imaging findings. Pediatr Radiol 31(4):233–237. doi:10.1007/s002470000417

Harel M, Ferrer FA, Shapiro LH, Makari JH (2015) Future directions in risk stratification and therapy for advanced pediatric genitourinary rhabdomyosarcoma. Urol Oncol 34:103–115. doi:10.1016/j.urolonc.2015.09.013

Hartman DS, Lesar MS, Madewell JE, Lichtenstein JE, Davis CJ Jr (1981) Mesoblastic nephroma: radiologic-pathologic correlation of 20 cases. AJR Am J Roentgenol 136(1):69–74. doi:10.2214/ajr.136.1.69

Heidenreich A, Zirbes TK, Wolter S, Engelmann UH (1999) Nephrogenic adenoma: a rare bladder tumor in children. Eur Urol 36(4):348–353. https://doi.org/10.1159/000019998

Henno S, Loeuillet L, Henry C, D'Herve D, Azzis O, Ferrer J, Poulain P, Babut JM, Merlio JP, Jouan H, Dubus P (2003) Cellular mesoblastic nephroma: morphologic, cytogenetic and molecular links with congenital fibrosarcoma. Pathol Res Pract 199(1):35–40. doi:10.1078/0344-0338-00350

Herman TE, Shackelford GD, McAlister WH (1997) Pseudotumoral sarcoid granulomatous nephritis in a child: case presentation with sonographic and CT findings. Pediatr Radiol 27(9):752–754. doi:10.1007/s002470050218

Hugosson C, Mahr MA, Sabbah R (1997) Primary unilateral renal lymphoblastic lymphoma. Pediatr Radiol 27(1):23–25. doi:10.1007/s002470050056

Huppmann AR, Pawel BR (2011) Polyps and masses of the pediatric urinary bladder: a 21-year pathology review. Pediatr Dev Pathol Off J Soc Pediatr Pathol Paediatr Pathol Soc 14(6):438–444. doi:10.2350/11-01-0958-oa.1

Inoue M, Uchida K, Kohei O, Nashida Y, Deguchi T, Komada Y, Kusunoki M (2006) Teratoid Wilms' tumor: a case report with literature review. J Pediatr Surg 41(10):1759–1763. doi:10.1016/j.jpedsurg.2006.05.045

Irsutti M, Puget C, Baunin C, Duga I, Sarramon MF, Guitard J (2000) Mesoblastic nephroma: prenatal ultrasonographic and MRI features. Pediatr Radiol 30(3):147–150. doi:10.1007/s002470050033

Isaac J, Lowichik A, Cartwright P, Rohr R (2000) Inverted papilloma of the urinary bladder in children: case report and review of prognostic significance and biological potential behavior. J Pediatr Surg 35(10):1514–1516. doi:10.1053/jpsu.2000.16429

Isaacs H Jr (2008) Fetal and neonatal renal tumors. J Pediatr Surg 43(9):1587–1595. doi:10.1016/j.jpedsurg.2008.03.052

Ito J, Shinohara N, Koyanagi T, Hanioka K (1998) Ossifying renal tumor of infancy: the first Japanese case with long-term follow-up. Pathol Int 48(2):151–159

Jahn H, Nissen HM (1991) Haemangioma of the urinary tract: review of the literature. Br J Urol 68(2):113–117

Jeon A, Cramer BC, Walsh E, Pushpanathan C (1999) A spectrum of segmental multicystic renal dysplasia. Pediatr Radiol 29(5):309–315. doi:10.1007/s002470050595

Karaosmanoglu AD, Onur MR, Shirkhoda A, Ozmen M, Hahn PF (2015) Unusual benign solid neoplasms of the kidney: cross-sectional imaging findings. Diagn Interven Radiol (Ankara, Turkey) 21(5):376–381. doi:10.5152/dir.2015.14545

Kelner M, Droulle P, Didier F, Hoeffel JC (2003) The vascular "ring" sign in mesoblastic nephroma: report of two cases. Pediatr Radiol 33(2):123–128. doi:10.1007/s00247-002-0821-5

Khanna G, Naranjo A, Hoffer F, Mullen E, Geller J, Gratias EJ, Ehrlich PF, Perlman EJ, Rosen N, Grundy P, Dome JS (2013) Detection of preoperative wilms tumor rupture with CT: a report from the Children's Oncology Group. Radiology 266(2):610–617. doi:10.1148/radiol.12120670

Kieran K, Williams MA, McGregor LM, Dome JS, Krasin MJ, Davidoff AM (2014) Repeat nephron-sparing surgery for children with bilateral Wilms tumor. J Pediatr Surg 49(1):149–153. doi:10.1016/j.jpedsurg.2013.09.048

Knezevich SR, Garnett MJ, Pysher TJ, Beckwith JB, Grundy PE, Sorensen PH (1998) ETV6-NTRK3 gene fusions and trisomy 11 establish a histogenetic link between mesoblastic nephroma and congenital fibrosarcoma. Cancer Res 58(22):5046–5048

Kodet R, Fajstavr J, Kabelka Z, Koutecky J, Eckschlager T, Newton WA Jr (1991) Is fetal cellular rhabdomyoma an entity or a differentiated rhabdomyosarcoma? A study of patients with rhabdomyoma of the tongue and sarcoma of the tongue enrolled in the intergroup rhabdomyosarcoma studies I, II, and III. Cancer 67(11):2907–2913

Krasin MJ, Xiong X, Wu S, Merchant TE (2005) The effects of external beam irradiation on the growth of flat bones in children: modeling a dose-volume effect. Int J Radiat Oncol Biol Phys 62(5):1458–1463. doi:10.1016/j.ijrobp.2005.01.024

Kuo H, Cain MP (2004) Spontaneous bladder wall abscess in a child. Urology 63(4):778–779. doi:10.1016/j.urology.2003.12.013

Lalwani N, Prasad SR, Vikram R, Katabathina V, Shanbhogue A, Restrepo C (2011) Pediatric and adult primary sarcomas of the kidney: a cross-sectional imaging review. Acta Radiol (Stockholm, Sweden: 1987) 52(4):448–457. doi:10.1258/ar.2011.100376

Lam JS, Hensle TW, Debelenko L, Granowetter L, Tennenbaum SY (2003) Organ-confined primitive neuroectodermal tumor arising from the kidney. J Pediatr Surg 38(4):619–621. doi:10.1053/jpsu.2003.50135

Lee EY (2007) CT imaging of mass-like renal lesions in children. Pediatr Radiol 37(9):896–907. doi:10.1007/s00247-007-0548-4

Lee SH, Choi YH, Kim WS, Cheon JE, Moon KC (2014) Ossifying renal tumor of infancy: findings at ultrasound, CT and MRI. Pediatr Radiol 44(5):625–628. https://doi.org/10.1007/s00247-013-2855-2

Lobe TE, Wiener ES, Hays DM, Lawrence WH, Andrassy RJ, Johnston J, Wharam M, Webber B, Ragab A (1994) Neonatal rhabdomyosarcoma: the IRS experience. J Pediatr Surg 29(8):1167–1170

Lonergan GJ, Martinez-Leon MI, Agrons GA, Montemarano H, Suarez ES (1998) Nephrogenic rests, nephroblastomatosis, and associated lesions of the kidney. Radiographics Rev Publ Radiol Soc N Am Inc 18(4):947–968. doi:10.1148/radiographics.18.4.9672980

Lowe LH, Isuani BH, Heller RM, Stein SM, Johnson JE, Navarro OM, Hernanz-Schulman M (2000) Pediatric renal masses: Wilms tumor and beyond. Radiographics Rev Publ Radiol Soc N Am Inc 20(6):1585–1603. doi:10.1148/radiographics.20.6.g00nv051585

Luithle T, Szavay P, Furtwangler R, Graf N, Fuchs J (2007) Treatment of cystic nephroma and cystic partially differentiated nephroblastoma--a report from the SIOP/GPOH study group. J Urol 177(1):294–296. doi:10.1016/j.juro.2006.09.011

Maher ER, Neumann HP, Richard S (2011) von Hippel-Lindau disease: a clinical and scientific review. Eur J Hum Genet: EJHG 19(6):617–623. doi:10.1038/ejhg.2010.175

Malogolowkin M, Cotton CA, Green DM, Breslow NE, Perlman E, Miser J, Ritchey ML, Thomas PR, Grundy PE, D'Angio GJ, Beckwith JB, Shamberger RC, Haase GM, Donaldson M, Weetman R, Coppes MJ, Shearer P, Coccia P, Kletzel M, Macklis R, Tomlinson G, Huff V, Newbury R, Weeks D (2008) Treatment of Wilms tumor relapsing after initial treatment with vincristine, actinomycin D, and doxorubicin. A report from the National Wilms Tumor Study Group. Pediatr Blood Cancer 50(2):236–241. doi:10.1002/pbc.21267

Marietti S, Saenz N, Willert J, Holmes N (2013) Genitourinary rhabdomyosarcoma: unusual diagnosis presenting within hours of delivery. J Pediatr Urol 9(4):e139–e143. doi:10.1016/j.jpurol.2013.02.010

Marsden HB, Lawler W, Kumar PM (1978) Bone metastasizing renal tumor of childhood: morphological and clinical features, and differences from Wilms' tumor. Cancer 42(4):1922–1928

Marteinsson VT, Due J, Aagenaes I (1996) Focal xanthogranulomatous pyelonephritis presenting as renal tumour in children. Case report with a review of the literature. Scand J Urol Nephrol 30(3):235–239

Maschietto M, Williams RD, Chagtai T, Popov SD, Sebire NJ, Vujanic G, Perlman E, Anderson JR, Grundy P, Dome JS, Pritchard-Jones K (2014) TP53 mutational status is a potential marker for risk stratification in Wilms tumour with diffuse anaplasia. PLoS One 9(10):e109924. doi:10.1371/journal.pone.0109924

Matsunaga GS, Shanberg AM, Rajpoot D (2003) Prenatal ultrasonographic detection of bladder rhabdomyosarcoma. J Urol 169(4):1495–1496. doi:10.1097/01.ju.0000053462.98574.f7

McCarville MB, Hoffer FA, Howard SC, Goloubeva O, Kauffman WM (2001) Hepatic veno-occlusive disease in children undergoing bone-marrow transplantation: usefulness of sonographic findings. Pediatr Radiol 31(2):102–105. doi:10.1007/s002470000373

McCarville MB, Lederman HM, Santana VM, Daw NC, Shochat SJ, Li CS, Kaufman RA (2006) Distinguishing benign from malignant pulmonary nodules with helical chest CT in children with malignant solid tumors. Radiology 239(2):514–520. doi:10.1148/radiol.2392050631

Medeiros LJ, Palmedo G, Krigman HR, Kovacs G, Beckwith JB (1999) Oncocytoid renal cell carcinoma after neuroblastoma: a report of four cases of a distinct clinicopathologic entity. Am J Surg Pathol 23(7):772–780

Mong A, Bellah R (2006) Imaging the pediatric prostate. Radiol Clin North Am 44(5):749–756. doi:10.1016/j.rcl.2006.07.007, ix

Monsalve J, Kapur J, Malkin D, Babyn PS (2011) Imaging of cancer predisposition syndromes in children. Radiographics Rev Publ Radiol Soc N Am Inc 31(1):263–280. doi:10.1148/rg.311105099

Morgan E, Kidd JM (1978) Undifferentiated sarcoma of the kidney: a tumor of childhood with histopathologic and clinical characteristics distinct from Wilms' tumor. Cancer 42(4):1916–1921

Murthi GV, Carachi R, Howatson A (2003) Congenital cystic mesoblastic nephroma. Pediatr Surg Int 19(1–2):109–111. doi:10.1007/s00383-002-0833-0

Mynarek M, Hussein K, Kreipe HH, Maecker-Kolhoff B (2014) Malignancies after pediatric kidney transplantation: more than PTLD? Pediatr Nephrol (Berlin, Germany) 29(9):1517–1528. doi:10.1007/s00467-013-2622-5

Nagahara A, Kawagoe M, Matsumoto F, Tohda A, Shimada K, Yasui M, Inoue M, Kawa K, Hamana K, Nakayama M (2006) Botryoid Wilms' tumor of the renal pelvis extending into the bladder. Urology 67(4):845.e815. doi:10.1016/j.urology.2005.10.014

Navarro O, Conolly B, Taylor G, Bagli DJ (1999) Metanephric adenoma of the kidney: a case report. Pediatr Radiol 29(2):100–103. doi:10.1007/s002470050550

Navoy JF, Royal SA, Vaid YN, Mroczek-Musulman EC (1995) Wilms tumor: unusual manifestations. Pediatr Radiol 25(Suppl 1):S76–S86

Ng YY, Healy JC, Vincent JM, Kingston JE, Armstrong P, Reznek RH (1994) The radiology of non-Hodgkin's lymphoma in childhood: a review of 80 cases. Clin Radiol 49(9):594–600

Norman G, Fayter D, Lewis-Light K, Chisholm J, McHugh K, Levine D, Jenney M, Mandeville H, Gatz S, Phillips B (2015) An emerging evidence base for PET-CT in the management of childhood rhabdomyosarcoma: systematic review. BMJ Open 5(1):e006030. doi:10.1136/bmjopen-2014-006030

Oberlin O, Rey A, Lyden E, Bisogno G, Stevens MC, Meyer WH, Carli M, Anderson JR (2008) Prognostic factors in metastatic rhabdomyosarcomas: results of a pooled analysis from United States and European cooperative groups. J Clin Oncol Off J Am Soc Clin Oncol 26(14):2384–2389. doi:10.1200/jco.2007.14.7207

Ora I, van Tinteren H, Bergeron C, de Kraker J (2007) Progression of localised Wilms' tumour during preoperative chemotherapy is an independent prognostic factor: a report from the SIOP 93–01 nephroblastoma trial and study. Eur J Cancer (Oxford, England: 1990) 43(1):131–136. doi:10.1016/j.ejca.2006.08.033

Orbach D, Sarnacki S, Brisse HJ, Gauthier-Villars M, Jarreau PH, Tsatsaris V, Baruchel A, Zerah M, Seigneur E, Peuchmaur M, Doz F (2013) Neonatal cancer. Lancet Oncol 14(13):e609–e620. https://doi.org/10.1016/S1470-2045(13)70236-5

Owens CM, Brisse HJ, Olsen OE, Begent J, Smets AM (2008) Bilateral disease and new trends in Wilms tumour. Pediatr Radiol 38(1):30–39. doi:10.1007/s00247-007-0681-0

Panuel M, Bourliere-Najean B, Gentet JC, Scheiner C, Delarue A, Faure F, Devred P (1992) Aggressive neuroblastoma with initial pulmonary metastases and kidney involvement simulating Wilms' tumor. Eur J Radiol 14(3):201–203

Pappo AS, Anderson JR, Crist WM, Wharam MD, Breitfeld PP, Hawkins D, Raney RB, Womer RB, Parham DM, Qualman SJ, Grier HE (1999) Survival after relapse in children and adolescents with rhabdomyosarcoma: A report from the Intergroup Rhabdomyosarcoma Study Group. J Clin Oncol Off J Am Soc Clin Oncol 17(11):3487–3493

Parham DM, Barr FG (2013) Classification of rhabdomyosarcoma and its molecular basis. Adv Anat Pathol 20(6):387–397. doi:10.1097/PAP.0b013e3182a92d0d

Parham DM, Roloson GJ, Feely M, Green DM, Bridge JA, Beckwith JB (2001) Primary malignant neuroepithelial tumors of the kidney: a clinicopathologic analysis of 146 adult and pediatric cases from the National Wilms' Tumor Study Group Pathology Center. Am J Surg Pathol 25(2):133–146

Park CM, Kim WS, Cheon JE, Kim CJ, Kim WY, Kim IO, Shin HY, Yeon KM (2003) Teratoid Wilms tumor in childhood: CT and ultrasonographic appearances. Abdom Imaging 28(3):440–443. doi:10.1007/s00261-002-0044-0

Parvey LS, Warner RM, Callihan TR, Magill HL (1981) CT demonstration of fat tissue in malignant renal neoplasms: atypical Wilms' tumors. J Comput Assist Tomogr 5(6):851–854

Pastore G, Znaor A, Spreafico F, Graf N, Pritchard-Jones K, Steliarova-Foucher E (2006) Malignant renal tumours incidence and survival in European children (1978–1997): report from the Automated Childhood Cancer Information System project. Eur J Cancer (Oxford, England: 1990) 42(13):2103–2114. doi:10.1016/j.ejca.2006.05.010

Patel MD, Silva AC (2004) MRI of an adenomatoid tumor of the tunica albuginea. AJR Am J Roentgenol 182(2):415–417. doi:10.2214/ajr.182.2.1820415

Prasad SR, Humphrey PA, Menias CO, Middleton WD, Siegel MJ, Bae KT, Heiken JP (2005) Neoplasms of the renal medulla: radiologic-pathologic correlation. Radiographics Rev Publ Radiol Soc N Am Inc 25(2):369–380. doi:10.1148/rg.252045073

Priesemann M, Davies KM, Perry LA, Drake WM, Chew SL, Monson JP, Savage MO, Johnston LB (2006) Benefits of screening in von Hippel-Lindau disease-comparison of morbidity associated with initial tumours in affected parents and children. Horm Res 66(1):1–5. doi:10.1159/000093008

Raney B, Anderson J, Jenney M, Arndt C, Brecht I, Carli M, Bisogno G, Oberlin O, Rey A, Treuner J, Ullrich F, Stevens M (2006) Late effects in 164 patients with rhabdomyosarcoma of the bladder/prostate region: a report from the international workshop. J Urol 176(5):2190–2194. doi:10.1016/j.juro.2006.07.064; discussion 2194–2195

Raney RB Jr, Tefft M, Lawrence W Jr, Ragab AH, Soule EH, Beltangady M, Gehan EA (1987) Paratesticular sarcoma in childhood and adolescence. A report from the Intergroup Rhabdomyosarcoma Studies I and II, 1973–1983. Cancer 60(9):2337–2343

Rialon KL, Gulack BC, Englum BR, Routh JC, Rice HE (2015) Factors impacting survival in children with renal cell carcinoma. J Pediatr Surg 50(6):1014–1018. doi:10.1016/j.jpedsurg.2015.03.027

Riccabona M, Ring E, Hausler M, Ratschek M, Fotter R (1999) Neonatal segmental cystic nephroma. A case report. Z Geburtshilfe Neonatol 203(6):255–257

Rohrschneider WK, Weirich A, Rieden K, Darge K, Troger J, Graf N (1998) US, CT and MR imaging characteristics of nephroblastomatosis. Pediatr Radiol 28(6):435–443. doi:10.1007/s002470050378

Rossi E, Pavanello P, Marzola A, Franchella A (2011) Eosinophilic cystitis and nephrogenic adenoma of the bladder: a rare association of 2 unusual findings in childhood. J Pediatr Surg 46(4):31–34. doi:10.1016/j.jpedsurg.2010.12.027

Rump P, Zeegers MP, van Essen AJ (2005) Tumor risk in Beckwith-Wiedemann syndrome: a review and meta-analysis. Am J Med Genet A 136(1):95–104. doi:10.1002/ajmg.a.30729

Saarinen UM, Wikstrom S, Koskimies O, Sariola H (1991) Percutaneous needle biopsy preceding preoperative chemotherapy in the management of massive renal tumors in children. J Clin Oncol Off J Am Soc Clin Oncol 9(3):406–415

Sausville JE, Hernandez DJ, Argani P, Gearhart JP (2009) Pediatric renal cell carcinoma. J Pediatr Urol 5(4):308–314. doi:10.1016/j.jpurol.2009.04.007

Schafernak KT, Yang XJ, Hsueh W, Leestma JL, Stagl J, Goldman S (2007) Pediatric renal cell carcinoma as second malignancy: reports of two cases and a review of the literature. Can J Urol 14(6):3739–3744

Scheithauer BW, Santi M, Richter ER, Belman B, Rushing EJ (2008) Diffuse ganglioneuromatosis and plexiform neurofibroma of the urinary bladder: report of a pediatric example and literature review. Hum Pathol 39(11):1708–1712. doi:10.1016/j.humpath.2008.02.019

Schelling J, Schroder A, Stein R, Rosch WH (2007) Ossifying renal tumor of infancy. J Pediatr Urol 3(3):258–261. doi:10.1016/j.jpurol.2006.05.009

Schenk JP, Graf N, Gunther P, Ley S, Goppl M, Kulozik A, Rohrschneider WK, Troger J (2008) Role of MRI in the management of patients with nephroblastoma. Eur Radiol 18(4):683–691. doi:10.1007/s00330-007-0826-4

Schlesinger AE, Rosenfield NS, Castle VP, Jasty R (1995) Congenital mesoblastic nephroma metastatic to the brain: a report of two cases. Pediatr Radiol 25(Suppl 1):S73–S75

Schmidt D, Beckwith JB (1995) Histopathology of childhood renal tumors. Hematol Oncol Clin North Am 9(6):1179–1200

Scott RH, Stiller CA, Walker L, Rahman N (2006a) Syndromes and constitutional chromosomal abnormalities associated with Wilms tumour. J Med Genet 43(9):705–715. doi:10.1136/jmg.2006.041723

Scott RH, Walker L, Olsen OE, Levitt G, Kenney I, Maher E, Owens CM, Pritchard-Jones K, Craft A, Rahman N (2006b) Surveillance for Wilms tumour in at-risk children: pragmatic recommendations for best practice. Arch Dis Child 91(12):995–999. doi:10.1136/adc.2006.101295

Segers H, Kersseboom R, Alders M, Pieters R, Wagner A, van den Heuvel-Eibrink MM (2012) Frequency of WT1 and 11p15 constitutional aberrations and phenotypic correlation in childhood Wilms tumour patients. Eur J Cancer (Oxford, England: 1990) 48(17):3249–3256. doi:10.1016/j.ejca.2012.06.008

Selle B, Furtwangler R, Graf N, Kaatsch P, Bruder E, Leuschner I (2006) Population-based study of renal cell carcinoma in children in Germany, 1980–2005: more frequently localized tumors and underlying disorders compared with adult counterparts. Cancer 107(12):2906–2914. doi:10.1002/cncr.22346

Shamberger RC, Guthrie KA, Ritchey ML, Haase GM, Takashima J, Beckwith JB, D'Angio GJ, Green DM, Breslow NE (1999) Surgery-related factors and local recurrence of Wilms tumor in National Wilms Tumor Study 4. Ann Surg 229(2):292–297

Shimada H, Misugi K, Sasaki Y, Iizuka A, Nishihira H (1980) Carcinoma of the prostate in childhood and adolescence: report of a case and review of the literature. Cancer 46(11):2534–2542

Sinclair N, Babyn P, Kinloch M, Sinha R, Sinclair N, Babyn P, Kinloch M, Sinha R (2014) A rare and unusual case of Burkitt's lymphoma presenting with a prostate mass in a 12-year-Old Boy. Case Rep Radiol 42:233–238. doi:10.1155/2014/106176

Sköldenberg EG, Jakobson A, Elvin A, Sandstedt B, Läckgren G, Christofferson RH (1999) Pretreatment, ultrasound-guided cutting needle biopsies in childhood renal tumors. Med Pediatr Oncol 32(4):283–288

Slasky BS, Bar-Ziv J, Freeman AI, Peylan-Ramu N (1997) CT appearances of involvement of the peritoneum, mesentery and omentum in Wilms' tumor. Pediatr Radiol 27(1):14–17. doi:10.1007/s002470050053

Smets AM, de Kraker J (2010) Malignant tumours of the kidney: imaging strategy. Pediatr Radiol 40(6):1010–1018. doi:10.1007/s00247-010-1584-z

Smets AM, van Tinteren H, Bergeron C, De Camargo B, Graf N, Pritchard-Jones K, de Kraker J (2012) The contribution of chest CT-scan at diagnosis in children with unilateral Wilms' tumour. Results of the SIOP 2001 study. Eur J Cancer (Oxford, England: 1990) 48(7):1060–1065. doi:10.1016/j.ejca.2011.05.025

Sotelo-Avila C, Beckwith JB, Johnson JE (1995) Ossifying renal tumor of infancy: a clinicopathologic study of nine cases. Pediatr Pathol Lab Med J Socr Pediatr Pathol Affiliated Int Paediatr Pathol Assoc 15(5):745–762

Spreafico F, Pritchard-Jones K, Bergeron C, de Kraker J, Dallorso S, Graf N (2009) Value and difficulties of a common European strategy for recurrent Wilms' tumor. Expert Rev Anticancer Ther 9(6):693–696. doi:10.1586/era.09.45

Sredni ST, Tomita T (2015) Rhabdoid tumor predisposition syndrome. Pediatr Dev Pathol Off J Soc Pediatr Pathol Paediatr Pathol Soc 18(1):49–58. doi:10.2350/14-07-1531-misc.1

Strauss S, Libson E, Schwartz E, Peylan-Ramu N, Lebensart PD, Bloom RA, Itzchak Y (1986) Renal sonography in American Burkitt lymphoma. AJR Am J Roentgenol 146(3):549–552. doi:10.2214/ajr.146.3.549

Subhas N, Argani P, Gearhart JP, Siegelman SS (2004) Nephrogenic rests mimicking Wilms' tumor on CT. Pediatr Radiol 34(2):152–155. doi:10.1007/s00247-003-1008-4

Sudour H, Audry G, Schleimacher G, Patte C, Dussart S, Bergeron C (2012) Bilateral Wilms tumors (WT) treated with the SIOP 93 protocol in France: epidemiological survey and patient outcome. Pediatr Blood Cancer 59(1):57–61. doi:10.1002/pbc.24059

Sung L, Anderson JR, Arndt C, Raney RB, Meyer WH, Pappo AS (2004) Neurofibromatosis in children with Rhabdomyosarcoma: a report from the Intergroup Rhabdomyosarcoma study IV. J Pediatr 144(5):666–668. doi:10.1016/j.jpeds.2004.02.026

Swartz MA, Karth J, Schneider DT, Rodriguez R, Beckwith JB, Perlman EJ (2002) Renal medullary carcinoma: clinical, pathologic, immunohistochemical, and genetic analysis with pathogenetic implications. Urology 60(6):1083–1089

Szavay P, Luithle T, Graf N, Furtwangler R, Fuchs J (2006) Primary hepatic metastases in nephroblastoma – a report of the SIOP/GPOH Study. J Pediatr Surg 41(1):168–172. doi:10.1016/j.jpedsurg.2005.10.021; discussion 168–172

Thompson RH, Dicks D, Kramer SA, Thompson RH, Dicks D, Kramer SA (2005) Clinical manifestations and functional outcomes in children with eosinophilic cystitis. J Urol 174(6):2347–2349. doi:10.1097/01.ju.0000180423.06285.72

Tomlinson GE, Breslow NE, Dome J, Guthrie KA, Norkool P, Li S, Thomas PR, Perlman E, Beckwith JB, D'Angio GJ, Green DM (2005) Rhabdoid tumor of the kidney in the National Wilms' Tumor Study: age at diagnosis as a prognostic factor. J Clin Oncol Off J Am Soc Clin Oncol 23(30):7641–7645. doi:10.1200/jco.2004.00.8110

Trnka P, Orellana L, Walsh M, Pool L, Borzi P (2014) Reninoma: an uncommon cause of Renin-mediated hypertension. Front Pediatr 2:89. doi:10.3389/fped.2014.00089

van den Heuvel-Eibrink MM, Grundy P, Graf N, Pritchard-Jones K, Bergeron C, Patte C, van Tinteren H, Rey A, Langford C, Anderson JR, de Kraker J (2008) Characteristics and survival of 750 children diagnosed with a renal tumor in the first seven months of life: A collaborative study by the SIOP/GPOH/SFOP, NWTSG, and UKCCSG Wilms tumor study groups. Pediatr Blood Cancer 50(6):1130–1134. doi:10.1002/pbc.21389

van den Heuvel-Eibrink MM, van Tinteren H, Rehorst H, Coulombe A, Patte C, de Camargo B, de Kraker J, Leuschner I, Lugtenberg R, Pritchard-Jones K, Sandstedt B, Spreafico F, Graf N, Vujanic GM (2011) Malignant rhabdoid tumours of the kidney (MRTKs), registered on recent SIOP protocols from 1993 to 2005: a report of the SIOP renal tumour study group. Pediatr Blood Cancer 56(5):733–737. doi:10.1002/pbc.22922

van den Hoek J, de Krijger R, van de Ven K, Lequin M, van den Heuvel-Eibrink MM (2009) Cystic nephroma, cystic partially differentiated nephroblastoma and cystic Wilms' tumor in children: a spectrum with therapeutic dilemmas. Urol Int 82(1):65–70. doi:10.1159/000176028

Vazquez JL, Barnewolt CE, Shamberger RC, Chung T, Perez-Atayde AR (1998) Ossifying renal tumor of infancy presenting as a palpable abdominal mass. Pediatr Radiol 28(6):454–457. doi:10.1007/s002470050381

Vicha A, Stejskalova E, Sumerauer D, Kodet R, Malis J, Kucerova H, Bedrnicek J, Koutecky J, Eckschlager T (2002) Malignant peripheral primitive neuroectodermal tumor of the kidney. Cancer Genet Cytogenet 139(1):67–70

Vujanic GM, Harms D, Sandstedt B, Weirich A, de Kraker J, Delemarre JF (1999) New definitions of focal and diffuse anaplasia in Wilms tumor: the International Society of Paediatric Oncology (SIOP) experience. Med Pediatr Oncol 32(5):317–323

Vujanić GM, Kelsey A, Mitchell C, Shannon RS, Gornall P (2003) The role of biopsy in the diagnosis of renal tumors of childhood: results of the UKCCSG Wilms tumor study. Med Pediatr Oncol 40(1):18–22

Vujanic GM, Kelsey A, Perlman EJ, Sandstedt B, Beckwith JB (2007) Anaplastic sarcoma of the kidney: a clinicopathologic study of 20 cases of a new entity with polyphenotypic features. Am J Surg Pathol 31(10):1459–1468. doi:10.1097/PAS.0b013e31804d43a4

Vujanic GM, Sandstedt B, Dijoud F, Harms D, Delemarre JF (1995) Nephrogenic rest associated with a mesoblastic nephroma – what does it tell us? Pediatr Pathol Lab Med J Socr Pediatr Pathol Affiliated Int Paediatr Pathol Assoc 15(3):469–475

Vujanic GM, Sandstedt B, Harms D, Boccon-Gibod L, Delemarre JF (1996) Rhabdoid tumour of the kidney: a clinicopathological study of 22 patients from the International Society of Paediatric Oncology (SIOP) nephroblastoma file. Histopathology 28(4):333–340

Vujanic GM, Sandstedt B, Harms D, Kelsey A, Leuschner I, de Kraker J (2002) Revised International Society of Paediatric Oncology (SIOP) working classification of renal tumors of childhood. Med Pediatr Oncol 38(2):79–82

Waisman SS, Banko J, Cromie WJ (1990) Single polypoid cystitis cystica and glandularis presenting as benign bladder tumor. Urology 36(4):364–366

Wallace B, Organ M, Bagnell S, Rendon R, Merrimen J (2015) Renal cell carcinoma after neuroblastoma: A case study and review of the literature. Can Urol Assoc J Journal de l'Association des urologues du Canada 9(5–6):E316–E318. doi:10.5489/cuaj.2564

Wang ZP, Li K, Dong KR, Xiao XM, Zheng S (2014) Congenital mesoblastic nephroma: clinical analysis of eight cases and a review of the literature. Oncol Lett 8(5):2007–2011. doi:10.3892/ol.2014.2489

Warmann SW, Nourkami N, Fruhwald M, Leuschner I, Schenk JP, Fuchs J, Graf N (2012) Primary lung metastases in pediatric malignant non-Wilms renal tumors: data from SIOP 93-01/GPOH and SIOP 2001/GPOH. Klin Paediatr 224(3):148–152. doi:10.1055/s-0032-1304600

Weeks DA, Beckwith JB, Mierau GW, Luckey DW (1989) Rhabdoid tumor of kidney. A report of 111 cases from the National Wilms' Tumor Study Pathology Center. Am J Surg Pathol 13(6):439–458

Weinberger E, Rosenbaum DM, Pendergrass TW (1990) Renal involvement in children with lymphoma: comparison of CT with sonography. AJR Am J Roentgenol 155(2):347–349. doi:10.2214/ajr.155.2.2115266

Weiss AR, Lyden ER, Anderson JR, Hawkins DS, Spunt SL, Walterhouse DO, Wolden SL, Parham DM, Rodeberg DA, Kao SC, Womer RB (2013) Histologic and clinical characteristics can guide staging evaluations for children and adolescents with rhabdomyosarcoma: a report from the Children's Oncology Group Soft Tissue Sarcoma Committee. J Clin Oncol Off J Am Soc Clin Oncol 31(26):3226–3232. doi:10.1200/jco.2012.44.6476

Wilde JC, Aronson DC, Sznajder B, Van Tinteren H, Powis M, Okoye B, Cecchetto G, Audry G, Fuchs J, Schweinitz DV, Heij H, Graf N, Bergeron C, Pritchard-Jones K, Van Den Heuvel-Eibrink M, Carli M, Oldenburger F, Sandstedt B, De Kraker J, Godzinski J (2014) Nephron sparing surgery (NSS) for unilateral wilms tumor (UWT): the SIOP 2001 experience. Pediatr Blood Cancer 61(12):2175–2179. doi:10.1002/pbc.25185

Wilimas JA, Kaste SC, Kauffman WM, Winer-Muram H, Morris R, Luo X, Boyett JM (1997) Use of chest computed tomography in the staging of pediatric Wilms' tumor: interobserver variability and prognostic significance. J Clin Oncol Off J Am Soc Clin Oncol 15(7):2631–2635

Wootton-Gorges SL, Thomas KB, Harned RK, Wu SR, Stein-Wexler R, Strain JD (2005) Giant cystic abdominal masses in children. Pediatr Radiol 35(12):1277–1288. doi:10.1007/s00247-005-1559-7

Xu G, Hu J, Wu Y, Xiao Y, Xu M (2013) Botryoid Wilms' tumor: a case report and review of the literature. World J Surg Oncol 11:102. doi:10.1186/1477-7819-11-102

Zhuge Y, Cheung MC, Yang R, Perez EA, Koniaris LG, Sola JE (2010) Pediatric non-Wilms renal tumors: subtypes, survival, and prognostic indicators. J Surg Res 163(2):257–263. doi:10.1016/j.jss.2010.03.061

Zollner S, Dirksen U, Jurgens H, Ranft A (2013) Renal Ewing tumors. Ann Oncol Off J Eur Soc Med Oncol ESMO 24(9):2455–2461. doi:10.1093/annonc/mdt215

Zoubek A, Slavc I, Mann G, Trittenwein G, Gadner H (1999) Natural course of a Wilms' tumour. Lancet (London, England) 354(9175):344. doi:10.1016/s0140-6736(05)75257-0

Urinary Tract Trauma

Maria Luisa Lobo and Jean-Nicolas Dacher

Contents

1 Introduction: The Context 701
2 **Clinical Evaluation and Imaging Strategies** 703
2.1 Children with Severe Trauma and Multiple Injuries 703
2.2 Children with Minor and Moderate Trauma 704
2.3 Impact of Technical Environment on Imaging Strategy 705
2.4 Imaging Strategy 706
3 **Renal Injuries** 709
3.1 The AAST Classification 709
3.2 Ultrasound 711
3.3 Computed Tomography 712
3.4 Imaging Complications and Sequelae 713
4 **Bladder Injury** 714
5 **Urethral Injuries** 715
6 **Scrotal Injuries** 717
References 718

M.L. Lobo, MD (✉)
Department of Radiology, University Hospital of Santa Maria, HSM-CHLN, Avenida Professor Egas Moniz, 1649-035 Lisboa, Portugal

J.-N. Dacher, MD, PhD
Department of Radiology, University Hospital of Rouen 1, Rue de Germont, 76031 Rouen, France

1 Introduction: The Context

Evaluating a child who has sustained abdominal injury is daily practice in a department of pediatric radiology. In this chapter, emphasis will be put on pediatric particularities of urinary tract injuries, with special focus on renal trauma. Obviously, renal trauma cannot be separated from other associated traumatic lesions. This is especially true in organizing the imaging strategy.

The kidney is the most commonly injured organ of the urinary tract system and is affected in 10–20% of pediatric blunt abdominal trauma cases (Wessel et al. 2000; Grimsby et al. 2014); renal injuries, but also intraperitoneal bladder rupture, are more frequent in children than in adults.

Blunt abdominal trauma is much more frequent than penetrating injuries. Various mechanisms may be involved but discrepancy between the deceleration and severity of renal trauma can be encountered. Pre-existing renal abnormalities may lead to an increased susceptibility to injury, partially due to increased size or change in the position of the kidney. An underlying congenital renal anomaly may be found in about 8% of children who suffered a renal trauma, then most often related with low energy mechanism of trauma (McAleer et al. 2002). For example, a relatively minor trauma can induce a severe renal fracture in cases of

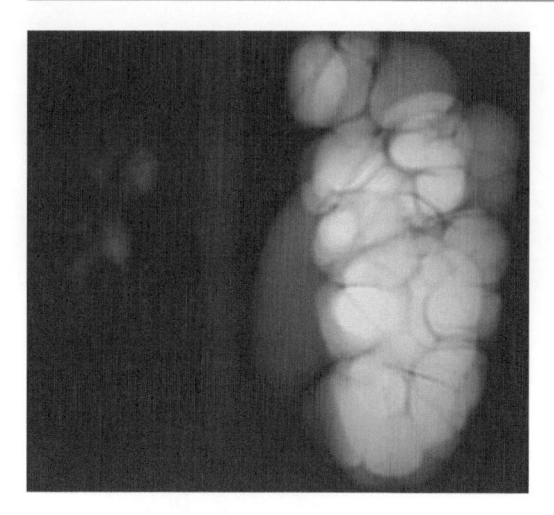

Fig. 1 A 12-year-old boy referred for evaluation of hematuria following minor trauma. US had revealed left hydronephrosis. MRI T2-weighted coronal image shows severe dilatation of multiple calyces contrasting with a slightly dilated pelvis. Megacalycosis was diagnosed

underlying kidney/urinary tract malformation (Fig. 1) or tumor. The most severe lesions are usually observed following high-energy trauma such as motor vehicle accident, pedestrian crash, or sport injury (biking, skiing, and horseback riding). On the other hand, minor trauma represents the most frequent situation: fall while playing for toddlers or bathroom accident for neonates and young children. Rarely, iatrogenic injury can also occur; inflicted injury should always be kept in mind as a potential cause.

Nowadays, in the vast majority of trauma patients, the management is nonoperative and noninterventional (Fig. 2). This principle was first applied in children; it is now becoming a rule in adult traumatology as well. A trend toward conservative management naturally impacts on imaging strategies.

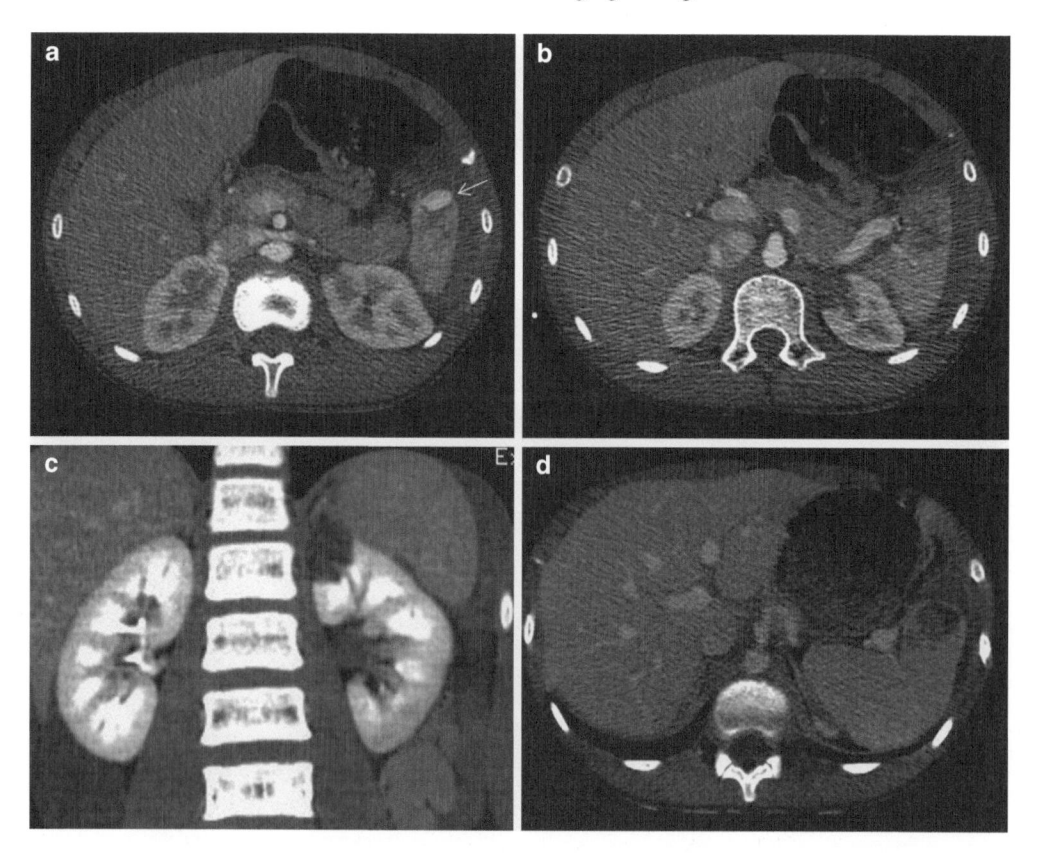

Fig. 2 Blunt abdominal trauma in a 12-year-old boy. On first evaluation (**a–c**), ce-CT showed a splenic fracture, hemoperitoneum, and contusion of the upper pole of the left kidney (**b**, **c**). A high-flow arteriovenous fistula (*arrow*) was disclosed in the spleen (note dilated splenic vein on **b**) and confirmed by aCDS (not shown). Intravascular closure of the fistula was discussed, but considering the absence of clinical symptoms and normal hemodynamics, it was not performed. One month later, clinical follow-up was unremarkable, splenic fistula was no longer permeable on ce-CT at portal time (**d**), and peritoneal free fluid had decreased

> **Take Away**
> Discrepancy between a relatively minor trauma and intense symptoms should raise suspicion of an underlying renal disease or malformation.

2 Clinical Evaluation and Imaging Strategies

2.1 Children with Severe Trauma and Multiple Injuries

Clinical findings are frequently limited, and even may be misleading. The mechanism of trauma and level of deceleration are essential elements of the diagnosis and imaging strategy. The presence of abdominal (the "seat belt sign") or lumbar ecchymosis correlates positively with severe intra-abdominal injuries. The gastrointestinal tract (duodenum) and the pancreas are more frequently involved (Sokolove et al. 2005), but it can also be associated with urinary bladder or even with a horseshoe kidney injury (Fig. 3). Skin lesions have to be considered in the imaging management, since they may represent a contraindication to ultrasound (US) examination. The localization of pain can point toward a specific organ lesion; for example, left upper quadrant pain points to the spleen and left kidney. Hemodynamic parameters (heart rate, blood pressure) are crucial in organizing the child's management and imaging workup. In this respect, one should remember that children have a higher physiologic circulatory reserve than adults; in children, the blood pressure is known to remain stable much longer than in adults in spite of a severe blood volume loss (Le Dosseur et al. 2005). The hematocrit can be a tricky marker as well.

In cases of unstable, non-transportable children, surgery is performed on an emergency basis. Then the role of imaging is extremely limited; a "focused assessment with sonography for trauma" (*FAST*) is able to identify the presence and rough location of peritoneal free fluid before proceeding to surgery (Walcher et al. 2006). Licensed emergency department physicians or professional sonographers can efficiently perform *FAST*.

In cases of severe and/or multiple trauma and a stable child, contrast-enhanced computed tomography (ce-CT) is unequivocally the modality of choice. If cranial trauma is present, a non-enhanced head CT is first performed in order to detect intracranial bleeding. Then a thoracic, abdominal and pelvic CT is carried out with contrast enhancement.

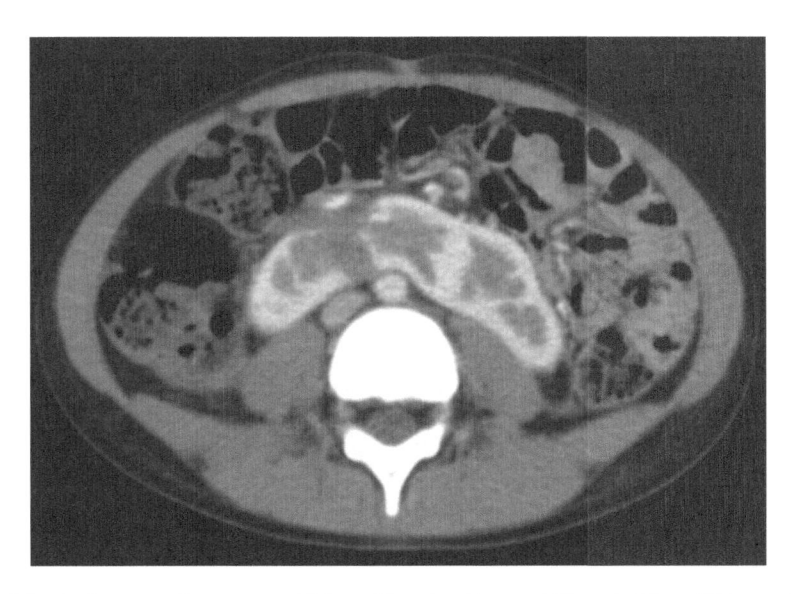

Fig. 3 Blunt abdominal trauma after motor vehicle accident in a 7-year-old boy. Axial ce-CT image depicting renal fracture in a previously unknown horseshoe kidney

Pediatric adapted CT protocols are mandatory, and multiphase scanning in every indiscriminate patient should be avoided (Riccabona et al. 2010; Damasio et al. 2013).

The priority of the radiologist is to detect the conditions that should lead to urgent treatment including resuscitation techniques, surgery, percutaneous drainage, or embolization. Among these conditions are hemopericardium, rupture of the thoracic aorta, compressive pneumothorax, post-traumatic diaphragmatic hernia, intraperitoneal rupture of the urinary bladder, pneumoperitoneum, potentially devascularized kidney, and an active intra-abdominal bleeding.

> **Take Away**
> In children, hypotension is a late sign of active bleeding.

2.2 Children with Minor and Moderate Trauma

In cases of blunt abdominal trauma, the kidneys seem to be more frequently injured in children than in adults (Brown et al. 1998). The reason could be the relative weight and mobility of kidneys in the pediatric abdomen as well as their only fair degree of protection (non-ossified thoracic cage covering less of the kidney, thin abdominal wall, and paucity of perirenal fat). Either gross or microscopic hematuria is frequent after urinary tract trauma. However, the severity of the renal lesion does not correlate with the degree of hematuria (Mayor et al. 1995). For example, the renal vascular pedicle lesion, one of the most severe renal injuries, rarely is revealed by gross hematuria. Moreover, gross hematuria is not always a sign of renal involvement; on the contrary, it is known to be an excellent marker of bladder injury (Stuhlfaut et al. 2007). Nevertheless, every child with haematuria after abdominal trauma should undergo renal and bladder imaging (Nguyen and Das 2002). It must be acknowledged that in those less severely injured children, the imaging strategy is not as straightforward as in severe and/or multiple trauma patients.

Enhanced CT remains the unquestionable reference technique, though it was shown to be non-cost effective when performed without prior selection of the patients; the rate of negative studies can be close to 80 % (Filiatriault and Garel 1995). Furthermore, the inevitable and significant radiation dose exposure is of special concern particularly in children (Brenner and Hall 2007). Other disadvantages of CT include those related with the need of intravenous iodine contrast medium administration and the availability of CT facilities. On the other hand, the limitations of US, the concurrent imaging modality, should be kept in mind. These limitations (diagnosis of free peritoneal gas, detection of spleen or liver injury during the first hours following trauma, difficult access due to skin lesion, and characterization of a solid organ injury) may decrease the sensitivity of the examination even in experienced hands (Richards et al. 2002).

The role of US in blunt abdominal trauma, both as initial screening and for follow-up, has been controversially debated (McKenney et al. 1998; Eeg et al 2009; Canon et al. 2014). US has been claimed and increasingly promoted as a valuable alternative initial imaging modality in pediatric renal trauma, particularly in cases of minor and moderate trauma (Fig. 4) or trauma restricted to the kidney area (Pietrera et al. 2001; Lougué-Sorgho et al. 2006; Riccabona et al. 2011; Amerstorfer et al. 2014). A complete US examination, including amplitude-coded color Doppler (aCDS) and sometimes spectral Doppler analysis, is often sufficient to reliably exclude major renal injuries, if performed under favorable conditions by a well-trained examiner. Furthermore, the use of intravenous US contrast agents seems to improve the potential of US in the detection and characterization of abdominal solid organ injuries (Valentino et al. 2006; Thorelius 2007). In the future, contrast-enhanced US (ce-US) may allow for further reduction of patient radiation exposure by decreasing the number of CT examinations needed (Riccabona et al. 2014) (Fig. 5).

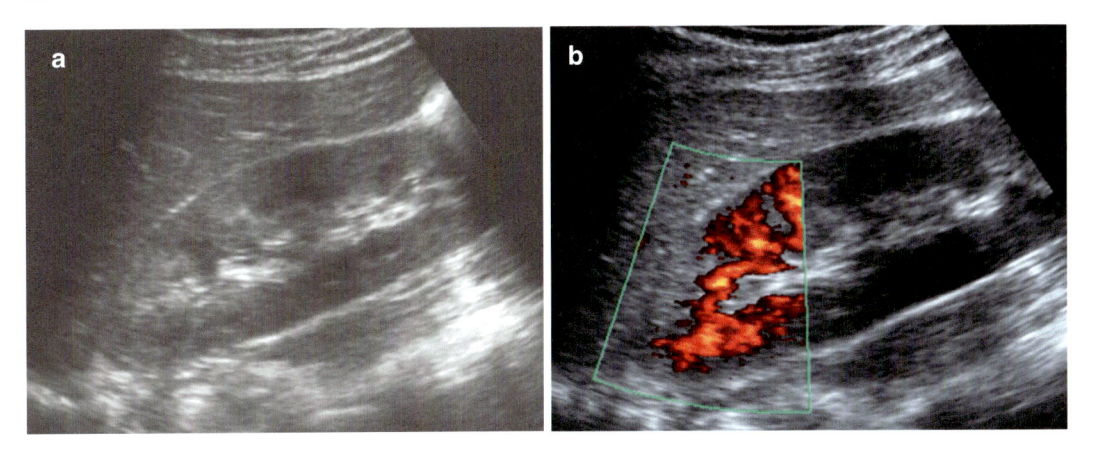

Fig. 4 Renal contusion following minor abdominal trauma in a 12-year-old boy with a single right kidney. US depicted a focal area of hyperechogenicity and loss of corticomedullary differentiation on grayscale US (**a**) and nonperfusion on aCDS (**b**). Note that the extent of the renal injury is clearly demonstrated on aCDS

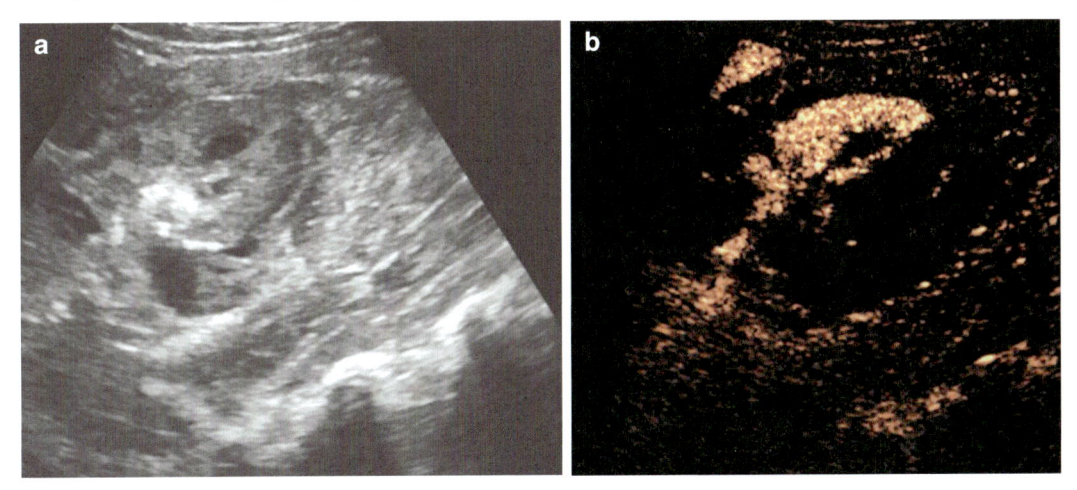

Fig. 5 Major renal trauma in a 16-year-old boy after motorcycle accident. US revealed an enlarged heterogeneous kidney (**a**) with clear demonstration of extensive parenchymal devascularization on ce-US (**b**) (Courtesy Dr. Schweintzger, Leoben, Austria)

> **Take Away**
> In children, hypotension is a late sign of active bleeding.

2.3 Impact of Technical Environment on Imaging Strategy

Non-medical aspects have to be considered in the imaging management of children with blunt abdominal trauma; the available imaging modalities and organization of the hospital obviously impact on the management of trauma children. For many years, the English literature has been reporting a poor sensitivity of US in the diagnosis of abdominal injuries (Benya et al. 2000). However, some conclusions were drawn from series of US examinations that had not been performed by expert pediatric radiologists. Results obtained by sonographers or emergency department physicians using portable equipment should not be compared with those from experts using last generation equipment, color Doppler and aCDS, high frequency transducers, and in some instances intravenous contrast agents. Due to differences in the practice of US, studies originating from different countries or institutions cannot be directly compared.

In many children's hospitals throughout the world, CT is not as easily available as in the United States, Japan, or Germany (Chirdan et al. 2007). For example, in the University Hospital of Rouen, short vehicle transportation to the adult hospital is required for every pediatric CT. This situation explains why many pediatric radiologists have had to develop expertise in emergency US. Any transportation outside the intensive care unit carries its own risk, particularly considering that cardiovascular shock occurs much more abruptly in children than in adults.

On the other hand, due to economic and financial reasons as well as local administration policies, there are an increasing number of radiology departments that do not hire enough medical staff to take over imaging examinations 24 hours a day throughout the year. This is particularly true for US, as more and more facilities keep CT available through teleradiology resources. Therefore, significant heterogeneities among different scenarios will influence imaging strategies in pediatric urinary tract trauma.

> **Take Away**
> US series should be interpreted with caution regarding the expertise of the operators, the employed equipment, and the local context.

2.4 Imaging Strategy

The aims of imaging are the early detection and accurate grading of significant urinary tract injuries (and other associated injuries), in order to timely provide the essential information needed for adequate therapeutic decision and optimal patient management.

Some algorithms have been suggested, for example, a group from Atlanta (Perez-Brayfield et al. 2002) proposed to limit the use of CT to traumatized children with >50 red blood cells/mm^3 on urinalysis, hypotension on presentation at the emergency room, or based on the severity and mechanism of injury. In Europe, the use of US with aCDS has been common practice for several years for the initial evaluation of a stable child with minor and moderate trauma and/or (microscopic) hematuria, with CT reserved only for selected cases (Pietrera et al. 2001; Lougué-Sorgho et al. 2006; Amerstorfer et al. 2014). The European Society of Paediatric Radiology abdominal (GI and GU) imaging task force and the European Society of Uroradiology paediatric working group have proposed a consensus-based imaging algorithm for pediatric urinary tract trauma (Riccabona et al. 2011). These consensus-based recommendations that have gained increasing acceptance throughout Europe (and even non-European countries) aim to standardize and improve imaging evaluation in pediatric urinary tract trauma by optimizing diagnostic imaging accuracy while reducing invasive imaging procedures.

CT is undoubtedly the primary imaging modality of choice in sufficiently stable patients who suffered from major trauma and polytrauma (Fig. 6). If an isolated direct flank injury has occurred and thus with less probability of other associated abdominal injuries, one should alternatively consider US as the first imaging choice provided a high-quality US examination is available. CT is recommended as the first step examination when US is not feasible either because of patient-related limitations (severe pain, obesity, or skin lesions) or local facility restrictions (unavailable minimal standard quality US), but CT can also be replaced by MRI if available and handling of a stable patient is feasible in the MR suite. A complete and comprehensive US examination of the entire abdominal and pelvic cavity, including aCDS of the kidney – and potentially supplemented with intravenous ce-US – is recommended as the initial choice pediatric renal imaging in cases of minor and moderate trauma (Fig. 7). Additional complementary ce-CT should be considered if US findings are abnormal (and further information is required for therapy decisions), inconclusive or discordant with more worrying clinical signs, or if there is (acute) clinical deterioration. US is certainly recommended as the method of choice

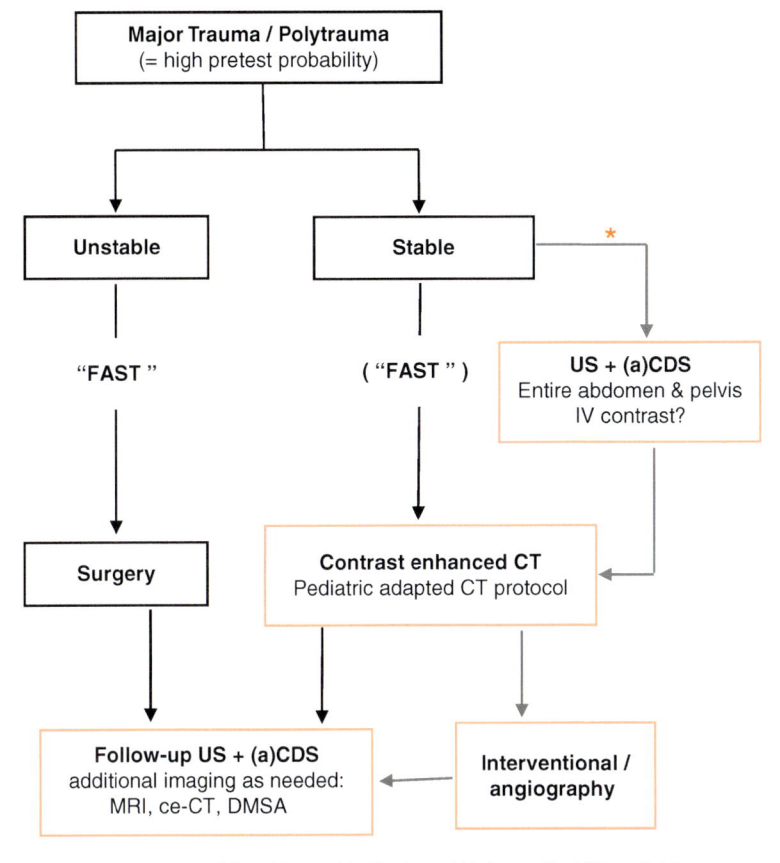

Fig. 6 Simplified flowchart on imaging strategy in suspected renal injury following major trauma and/or polytrauma in children, according to ESPR and ESUR recommendations (Riccabona et al. 2011)

for follow-up of children with traumatic renal lesions, even if the injuries were initially detected by CT. The systematic follow-up even of high-grade pediatric renal injuries with repeated CT as previously suggested (Buckley and McAninch 2004) does not seem justified (Amerstorfer et al. 2014).

MRI can be performed successfully instead of ce-CT, for example, in children with a known allergy to iodinated contrast media (Marcos et al. 1998). However, MRI is usually less available and more time consuming than CT, which is a crucial factor to consider in the acute trauma context. Otherwise, reliable monitoring of vital parameters inside the magnet requires sophisticated devices. On the contrary, MRI should be definitely considered whenever possible in non-emergent situations for suspected pediatric renal trauma with late presentation and for follow-up, particularly if US results are not conclusive (Riccabona et al. 2011). In the era of CT and MRI, intravenous urography (IVU) is no longer indicated, though in some rare instances an adapted focused IVU or simply an abdominal film taken approximately 15 min after injection of iodine contrast medium, the so-called one-shot IVU, may be helpful to assess renal function and urinary leakage and/or patency of the ureter in an unstable child that is taken directly into the operating room or to the intensive care after a trauma CT (without late excretion phase) (Riccabona et al. 2010).

No indication remains for angiography in the diagnostic evaluation of blunt abdominal trauma. On the one hand, the risk of the examination is relatively high. On the other hand, vascular injuries are extremely well depicted by aCDS and/or ce-CT. Angiography can be proposed in relatively rare instances when percutaneous treatment (embolization, angioplasty) appears to be the best option (Fig. 8). In the context of emergency, interventional radiology is an excellent tool to treat active bleeding. Later in the course, recurrent or persistent gross hematuria is an important indication; it is frequently due to a traumatic arteriovenous fistula (which can occur after blunt trauma). In cases

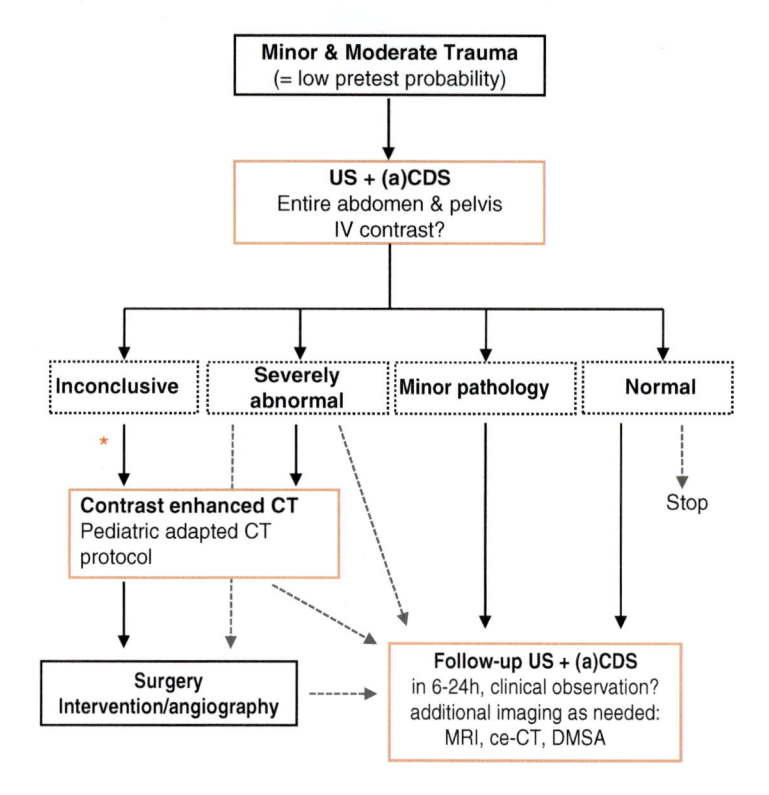

Fig. 7 Simplified flowchart on imaging strategy in suspected renal injury following minor and moderate trauma in children, according to ESPR and ESUR recommendations (Riccabona et al. 2011)

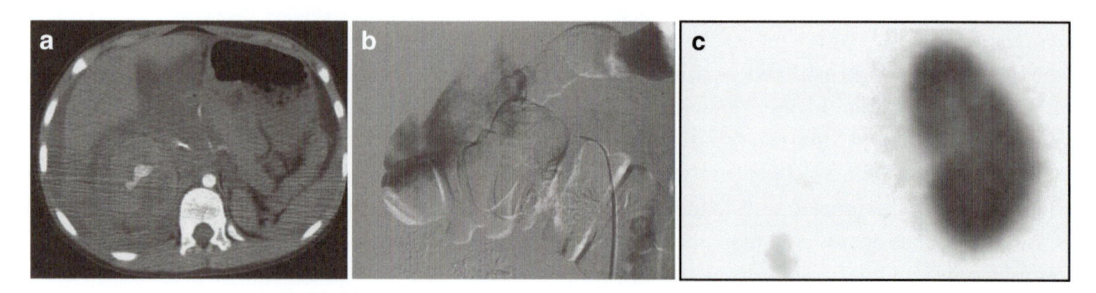

Fig. 8 Six-meter fall in a 10-year-old boy. Liver and right kidney injury. CT performed on admission showed intra- and retroperitoneal effusions (**a**). Active bleeding of the right renal artery was demonstrated by ce-CT and then confirmed by angiography (**b**). Selective embolization of the injured artery was carried out with immediate satisfactory result. Loss of renal function on the right side was detected 1 year later by DMSA scintigraphy (**c**)

of occlusion, dissection, or pseudoaneurysm of a renal artery, percutaneous treatment can be justified in order to recanalize or to occlude the involved arterial segment.

Imaging algorithms are a valuable support for daily practice at the emergency department but in children a challenge particularly for general radiologists not familiar with pediatric patients. Standardization of imaging strategies will facilitate future evidence-based studies.

> **Take Away**
> Imaging strategy aims to optimize diagnostic imaging accuracy while reducing (unnecessary) invasive imaging procedures.

3 Renal Injuries

3.1 The AAST Classification

The most commonly used classification was proposed by the American Association for the Surgery of Trauma (AAST) (Moore et al. 1989), which has been validated as predictive of clinical outcome and surgery (Santucci et al. 2001; Kuan et al. 2006; Shariat et al. 2007; Tasian et al. 2010). The ASST classification divides renal injuries in five grades, ranging from mild to severe lesion (Table 1). Minor injuries include grade I and II lesions (Figs. 9 and 10). Patients with minor injuries were shown to recover without sequelae; they represent 75 % of all blunt abdominal trauma cases (Wessel et al. 2000). Grade III lesions may be considered as intermediate injuries (Fig. 11), whereas major injuries include grades IV and V lesions (Figs. 12 and 13). It is noteworthy that treatment and prognosis of the two types of grade V injuries are completely different. Vascular pedicle lesion is considered as an extreme urgency; a revascularization procedure should be started within 6 (or even the first) hour following injury. In most cases, the functional prognosis of the kidney or involved segment is extremely poor (Fig. 8). On the contrary, renal fractures are usually managed nonoperatively, with a much better functional prognosis. Prognosis depends more or less on the volume of the devascularized kidney parenchyma. Similarly, significant differences in the management of grade IV injuries may also occur; for example, those patients with deep lacerations involving the collecting system have an increased risk to develop early urologic complication requiring intervention such as urinoma formation and even "auto-hemofiltration." They hence need close observation and sometimes more intense imaging surveillance (Bartley and Santucci 2012).

The ASST classification, though primarily based on surgical findings, has been shown to correlate with ce-CT findings. Improvement of CT technology – with resultant higher diagnostic capacities – and advances in interventional radiology approach, together with the increased knowledge of the natural history of renal trauma, have allowed for conservative treatment, either expectant or minimally invasive, to become the preferred management strategy for the majority of patients with renal injuries, even those with high-grade lesions (Rogers et al. 2004; Umbreit et al. 2009; Jacobs et al. 2012). Nowadays, indications for surgical treatment are getting rarer, with uncontrollable bleeding remaining the most important one, particularly if interventional angiography is unavailable or ineffective.

Table 1 Renal injury grading according to the ASST organ injury scale (Moore et al. 1989)

Renal injury	Description
Grade I	Contusion or non-enlarging subcapsular hematoma, no laceration
Grade II	Non-expanding perirenal hematoma Superficial laceration <1 cm depth, without urinary extravasation
Grade III	Laceration >1 cm depth Without extension into renal pelvis or collecting system No evidence of urine extravasation
Grade IV	Laceration extending to renal pelvis or urinary extravasation Renal artery or vein injury with contained hemorrhage (segmental infarct)
Grade V	Shattered kidney Avulsion of renal hilum with renal devascularization

Fig. 9 Renal injury ASST grade I (renal contusion) in a 13-year-old girl. US performed 24 h after the injury revealed swelling of the kidney with focal hyperechoic and loss of corticomedullary differentiation lesion with small amount of perirenal fluid (**a**), and hypoperfusion on aCDS (**b**)

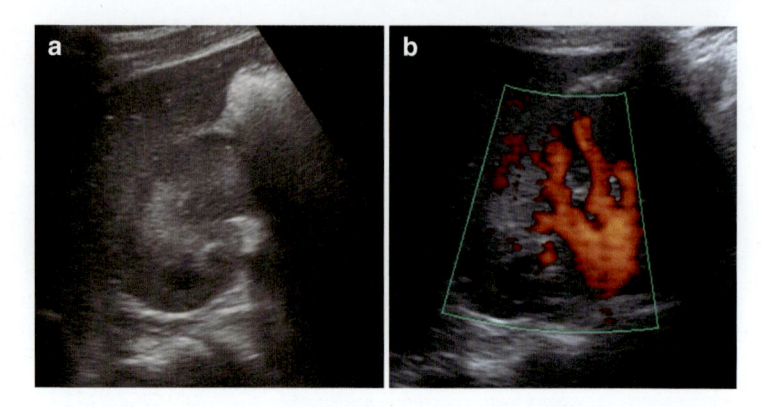

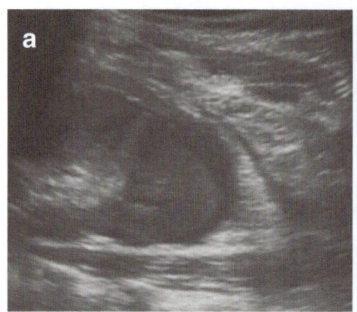

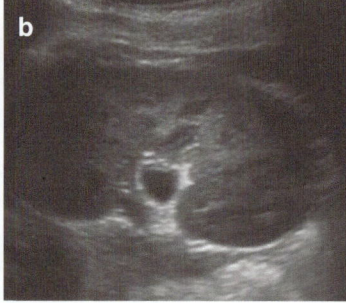

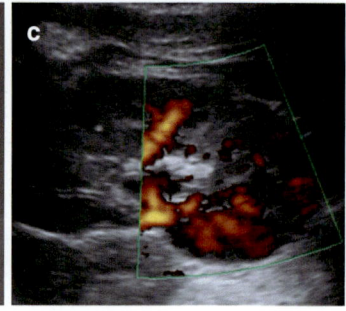

Fig. 10 Renal injury ASST grade II (renal laceration) in a 3-year-old boy after a fall with direct impact into the left flank. US on admission (**a**) with linear hypoechoic parenchymal disruption and irregular contour of the left kidney and perirenal fluid collection. Follow-up US showed persistent small perirenal fluid and heterogeneous hyperechoic parenchymal area at day 5 (**b**), with resolution of the perirenal hematoma and decreased size of the hypoperfused lesion on aCDS at day 12 (**c**)

Fig. 11 Renal injury ASST grade III in a 19-year-old woman after motor vehicle accident. Deep lacerations of the right kidney and perirenal hematoma seen on ce-CT at portal phase (**a**) with no evidence of urinary extravasation on excretory late phase (**b**)

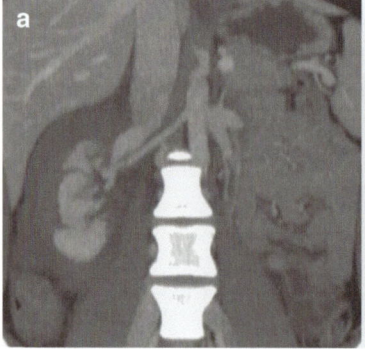

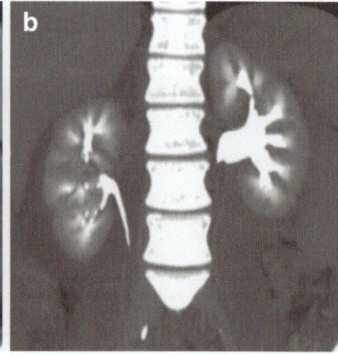

Other possible indications for surgery include urinary extravasation, high percentage of nonviable renal tissue and a large perirenal hematoma compressing the kidney (the so-called Page kidney).

However, this classification does not take the possible ureteric injuries into account that are known to be more frequent in children than in adults (Reda and Lebowitz 1986). Ureteropelvic junction disruption is the most common location in cases of blunt abdominal trauma; it predominates in children with ureteropelvic junction obstruction. Diagnosis is difficult due to the absence of hematuria. Other lesions do not belong

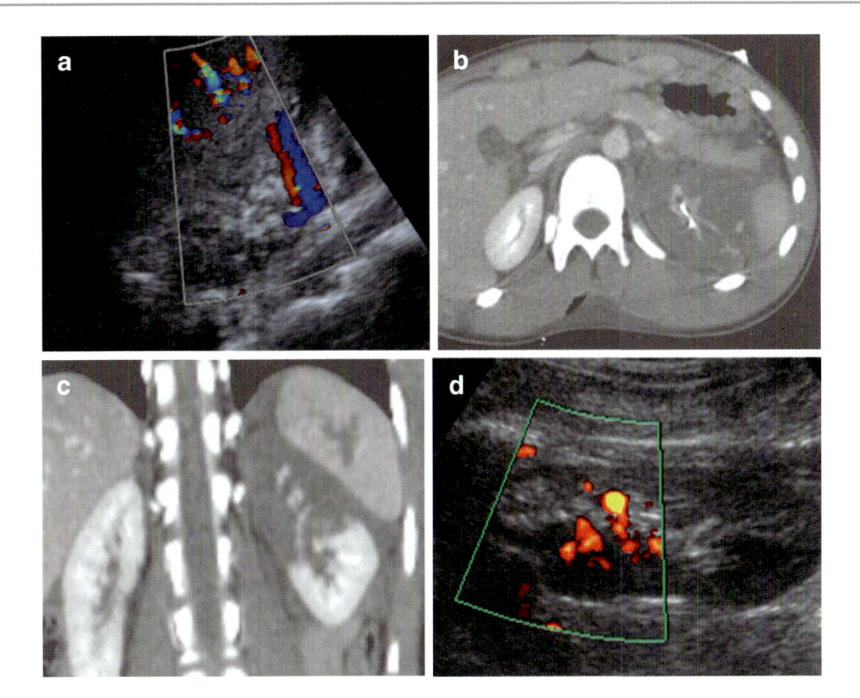

Fig. 12 Renal injury ASST grade IV (segmental infarction) in a 14-year-old boy after a fall from a horse. On admission, US showed slight parenchymal heterogeneity of the upper moiety of the left kidney with complete devascularization on aCDS (**a**). Immediate ce-CT confirmed segmental infarction of the left kidney (**b, c**). Spleen injury was also present (**c**). Follow-up US performed 4 months later revealed atrophy and nonperfusion of the upper third of the left kidney (**d**)

to this classification either. As stated above, intrarenal arteriovenous (or arteriocalyceal) fistulas or pseudoaneurysms can usually be treated successfully by super-selective angiography. Adrenal hematoma is frequently associated; the diagnosis by CT is straightforward, but feasible also on US. The endocrine prognosis is usually excellent, and calcification is frequent on follow-up.

Several authors have proposed modification of the ASST renal injury grading system in order to improve standardization as well as therapeutic guidance of high-grade renal injuries (Dugi et al. 2010; Buckley and McAninch 2011; Figler et al. 2013) – a formal revision has not yet taken place.

> **Take Away**
> Conservative, or minimally invasive, treatment has become the preferred therapeutic option for the majority of patients with renal injuries.

3.2 Ultrasound

US is efficient to show perirenal fluid collections (i.e., hematoma or a mixture of urine and blood), but it cannot assert the type of fluid. A focal impression on the kidney is identified in subcapsular hematoma, while a collection with a ruptured capsule tends to surround and displace the whole kidney. Subcapsular and perirenal hematoma may be difficult to detect on grayscale US, due to similar echogenicity with renal cortical parenchymal in early stages, a feature that can be overcome with the help of aCDS. Renal contusion can be identified as an initially isoechoic, then hyperechoic, and eventually even hypoechoic lesion with loss of corticomedullary differentiation and focally decreased signals on aCDS (Fig. 9) or on ce-US. Renal laceration can be difficult to detect, too – but usually an associated perirenal hematoma is present (Fig. 10). A careful search for central hilar structure abnormali-

Fig. 13 Renal injury ASST grade V in a 14-year-old boy after blunt abdominal trauma. Increased size and diffuse heterogeneity of the right kidney on US (**a**) with thrombus occlusion of the right renal vein on aCDS (**b**). Immediate ce-CT, portal (**c, e**), and late phases (**d, f**) showed renal fracture and perirenal hematoma (**c, e**), thrombosis of the right renal vein (*arrow*) (**d**), and contrast extravasation (*arrow*) with urinoma formation (**f**); note patency of the ureter. Nephrectomy was performed due to uncontrolled bleeding

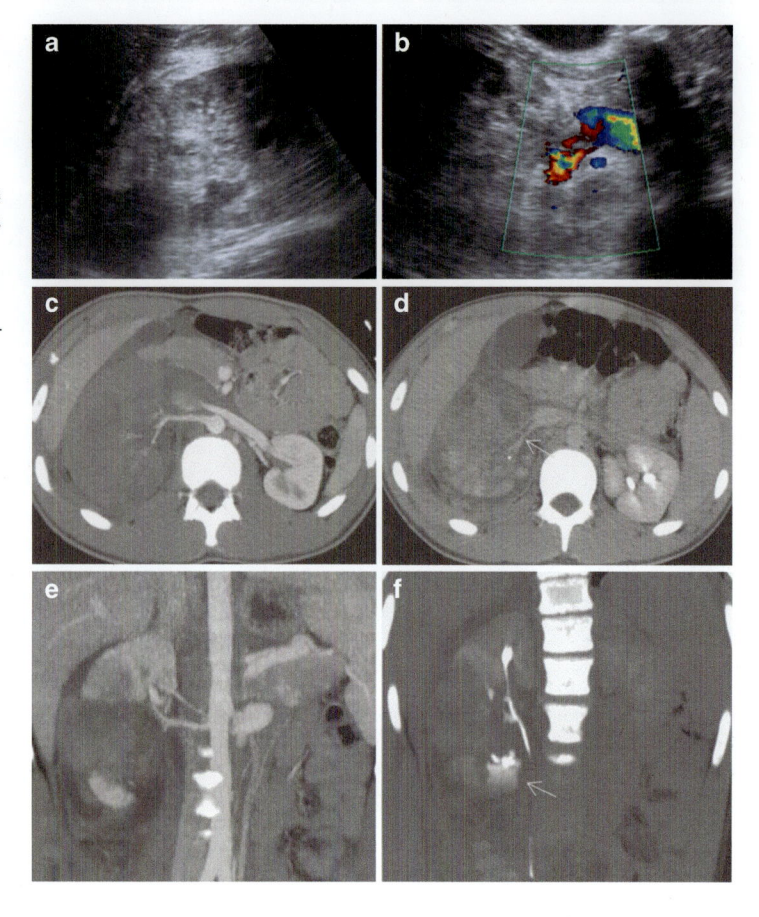

ties is necessary. A grayscale US examination can be completely normal in case of a vascular pedicle lesion; therefore, any examination should include aCDS which can detect complete or partial loss of vascularization (Fig. 12). If such an examination is not possible for any reason, CT should be performed. Ureteropelvic disruption is difficult to detect on US and only suspected by indirect signs with fluid collection formation (urinoma). Renal fracture is usually more difficult to characterize by grayscale US or aCDS (Pietrera et al. 2001); as for other vascular and parenchymal renal injuries, ce-US can help approach this diagnosis. Of course, the US examination should be completed by an entire survey of the whole abdominal cavity. For example, in cases of a right kidney lesion, it is common to find an associated liver lesion, whereas in left kidney lesions associated spleen injuries are likely.

> **Take Away**
> Always include aCDS in renal trauma US examination; particularly in early stages, grayscale US alone may miss significant renal injuries.

3.3 Computed Tomography

In case of severe trauma and/or polytrauma or if any abnormality is found by US that cannot be assessed accurately for therapy decision making, or in case of any discrepancy between clinical and biological findings and a normal US, ce-CT should be performed in an acute setting. The injection protocol and delay times can be tailored based on the previous results, and trauma CT protocols should be established in advance where pediatric CT adaptation needs should not be neglected (Damasio et al. 2013). In most cases, the child is scanned at the tubular phase (approximately 60 s after 1.5–2 ml/kg of contrast medium); this may be repeated after 10 min – if the first scan shows fracture and/or perirenal collection – in order to look for urinary contrast extravasation and/or ureter patency (Figs. 11 and 13). A preliminary non-enhanced acquisition is rarely useful; thus it should be avoided. An arterial phase scan can be performed when an arterial lesion is suspected, easily achieved by including the upper abdomen in the arterial chest phase range in a polytrauma CT protocol. Such a diagnosis is based on the following signs: decreased attenuation of the renal parenchyma at arterial phase, non- or delayed opacification of the excretory tract, and cortical rim sign as well as medullary enhancement (Malmed et al. 1992). Nowadays, ce-CT allows approaching the vascular lesion with good accuracy; it may show thrombosis, rupture, or dissection (Fig. 13). Multiplanar two- or three-dimensional reformatting is another advantage of multidetector CT.

On CT, the presence of intravascular contrast extravasation, medial laceration and perirenal hematoma with more than 3.5 cm thickness were recently identified as predictors of bleeding after renal injury (Dugi et al. 2010; Figler et al. 2013). On the other hand, medial urinary contrast extravasation and urinoma size were related with increasing need of urologic intervention (Bartley and Santucci 2012; Reese et al. 2014). The absence of contrast in the ipsilateral ureter in an excretion phase (if performed) or on a double/split bolus technique scan is always a worrying sign which may indicate ureteropelvic junction injury (Cannon et al. 2008; Bartley and Santucci 2012).

3.4 Imaging Complications and Sequelae

In the hours and days following the acute phase, intra- or extra-renal secondary bleeding is the main risk. It justifies hospitalizing traumatized children at the intensive care unit for a close clinical, biological, and imaging follow-up. US is the modality of choice for bedside follow-up when transportation to the radiology unit is considered difficult or even dangerous. The quality of equipment and experience of the examiner strongly impact the quality of information provided by bedside examinations. An increasing urinoma and/or perirenal hematoma size on US usually requires additional imaging with ce-CT or preferably MRI whenever possible. Otherwise, perirenal urinoma or hematoma can become infected and may justify percutaneous drainage under US or CT guidance, complemented by JJ drainage of the injured collecting system – which is the crucial point for healing. Later on, partial or complete lack of renal function is the most frequent complication in high-grade renal injuries (Fig. 8c). Arterial hypertension may develop in 7–10 % children with severe lesions (Delarue et al. 2002).

Nuclear medicine studies can be performed in the late stage of renal trauma to evaluate the residual renal function. Either DMSA-^{99m}Tc or MAG3-^{99m}Tc studies can be performed. MAG3-^{99m}Tc is preferred in patients in whom excretion should be assessed as well, and in kidneys with low function. Functional MR urography is a promising and emerging examination for this query (Fig. 14) (Grattan-Smith and Jones 2008).

> **Take Away**
> Pediatric adapted CT protocols are essential to optimize ce-CT diagnostic accuracy while reducing ionizing radiation exposure.

> **Take Away**
> MR and/or targeted isotopic examinations are the imaging techniques of choice for follow-up of high-grade injuries.

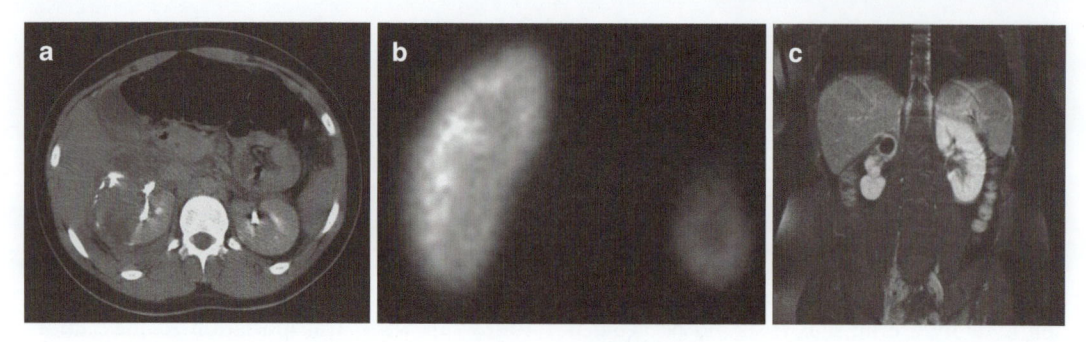

Fig. 14 Right renal fracture in a 15-year-old boy. Initial workup showed perirenal leak and two vascularized small fragments (**a**). Delayed DMSA scan showed severely decreased uptake of the right kidney (**b**). Delayed MRI provided the same functional results as DMSA scan, plus excellent depiction of renal morphology (**c**) (Courtesy of S. Hanquinet)

4 Bladder Injury

Bladder injury is relatively infrequent in children. It is usually the consequence of blunt abdominal trauma in a child with a full bladder. Motor vehicle accident is a common cause. Seat belt ecchymosis, hematuria, and pelvic fractures can be associated. Pelvic fractures are less common in children, and the incidence of significant lower genitourinary injury associated with pelvic fractures is also lower in children than in adults, being reported in only 0.5–3.7% (Tarman et al 2002; Gomez et al 2004). Bladder injuries are usually classified as intraperitoneal rupture, extraperitoneal rupture and combined lesions. Bladder contusion is a minor injury resulting from damage to the bladder mucosa or muscularis without full thickness loss of the bladder wall integrity; it may be revealed by a focal thickening of the bladder wall on US or an irregular contour on cystography without contrast extravasation (Fig. 15). Urinary leakage into the peritoneum is more frequent in children than in adults for anatomical reasons, due to the higher position of the child urinary bladder in the abdominal cavity (Sivit et al. 1995). Intraperitoneal bladder rupture is associated with high mortality and morbidity rates, requiring immediate surgical repair. On the contrary, extraperitoneal bladder rupture – causing prevesical hematoma or leakage into the prevesical space – is usually managed conservatively. US is not the modality of choice, although it may reveal secondary

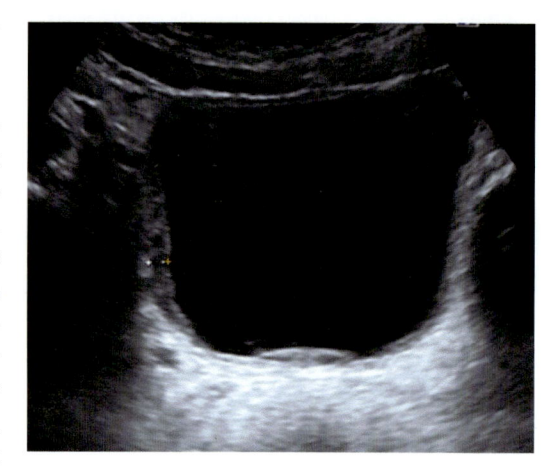

Fig. 15 Bladder contusion in a 7-year-old boy with hematuria after moderate abdominal blunt trauma. Focal thickening of the bladder wall (marked in the between x...x) and echogenic sediment in the bladder seen on US

signs; it can show hematoma and free fluid in the pelvic cavity that does not seem to be delineated by a normal bladder. Cystography, either conventional (VCUG) or by ce-CUS or CT cystography, is the preferred imaging tool to establish the diagnosis (Quagliano et al. 2006) (Fig. 16). Standard trauma CT with delayed images can also be used, although it should be recognized that it can miss significant bladder injuries if bladder distension is insufficient. When performing VCUG, it is recommended to start with careful opacification of the urethra to ensure there is no associated lesion and then complete the examination with bladder opacification (Bisset et al. 1991). Associated bone fractures should not be overlooked.

Take Away

Intraperitoneal bladder rupture, a surgical emergency, is more common in children than in adults.

5 Urethral Injuries

Urethral lesions occur much more frequently in male children for evident anatomical reasons. The adult-type lesion involving the membranous urethra complicates perineal injury and remains the most frequent one in adolescents. In adult men, the posterior urethra is relatively protected by the mature and firm prostate tissue. On the contrary, in children, urethral injuries may occur anywhere along the posterior urethra because the small soft prostate provides little stabilizing effect (Avanoglu et al. 1996). Hence, either partial tear or complete rupture of the posterior urethra can be observed. Management of partial tears is based on either prolonged catheter drainage of the urethra or suprapubic cystostomy (Glassberg et al. 1979).

In cases of complete disruption of the posterior urethra, the first step treatment is suprapubic drainage. The Mitrofanoff principle (interposition of the appendix between the urinary bladder and the abdominal wall) has been occasionally applied in severely crushed patients to divert the urine (Freitas Filho et al. 2003). Except in girls, in general immediate primary repair should be avoided, because of its associated high rates of complication (Pichler et al. 2012).

Anterior urethral injuries are usually straddle type. Unlike posterior urethral injuries, anterior urethra tears are rarely associated with pelvic fractures. Urethral injuries may be iatrogenic or inflicted. Bladder neck disruption seems to occur more frequently in children than in adults. It may be the consequence of blunt abdominal trauma and may be associated with pelvic fracture involving displacement of the pubic symphysis. It should be differentiated from urethral disruption because it may need primary repair rather than a cystostomy tube and secondary surgery. Anterior disruption at the bladder neck (vesicoprostatic junction) may occur in boys, while rupture through the vesicovaginal septum may occur in girls (Merchant et al. 1984).

The radiologist should avoid any urethral catheterization when urethral disruption is suspected. Secondary repair is the rule for urethral injuries, so that a minimal imaging evaluation should be performed in emergency situations

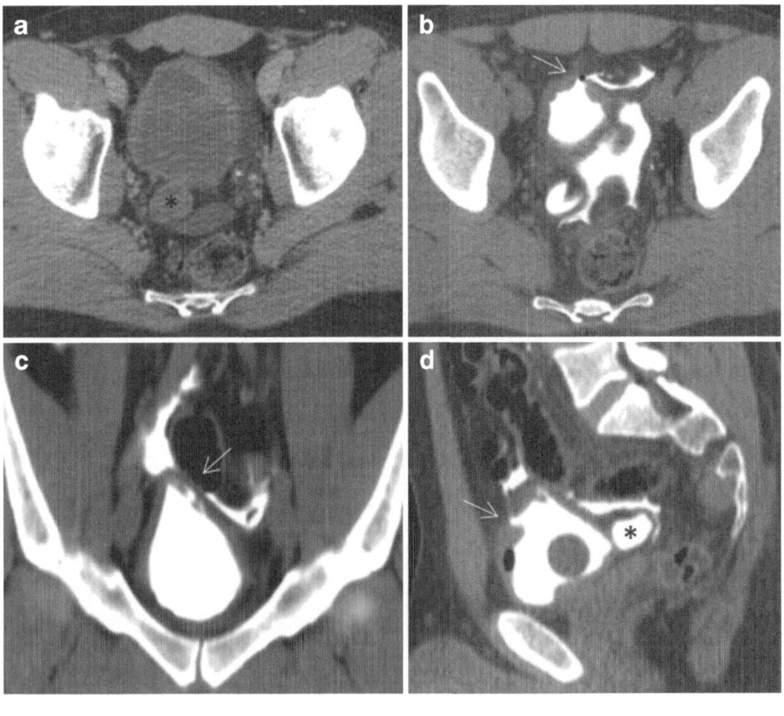

Fig. 16 Bladder intraperitoneal rupture. Initial ce-CT showed thickening of the anterior left sided wall of the bladder dome with some fluid in adjacent prevesical space (**a**); an incidental bladder diverticulum was also noted (*). CT cystography (**b–d**) confirmed the presence of a bladder leak (*arrow*) with contrast extravasation into the intraperitoneal cavity

(Baskin and McAninch 1993). Retrograde opacification of the urethra by water-soluble iodinated contrast medium is the reference examination (Riccabona et al. 2015) (Figs. 17 and 18b). A Foley catheter with a balloon inflated in the fossa navicularis is used. Combined retrograde urethrography with anterograde cystourethrography via a suprapubic catheter is helpful for full assessment of the site, severity, and length of the urethral injury (Fig. 18c). CT cystography can be considered in cases of bladder neck disruption and/or pelvic bones fractures for a comprehensive overview. Furthermore, signs of urethral injury such as obliteration of the fat plane around the urogenital diaphragm, ill-defined contour of the prostate gland, and obliteration of the internal obturator muscle should be recognized in any trauma CT (Fig. 18a).

The key questions to address by imaging are as follows: Is there any urethral leak (the absence of a leak cannot exclude hematoma or contusion) and is there any retrograde opacification of the bladder (allowing the differential diagnosis between complete and partial disruption of the urethra)? The follow-up of patients is of primary importance. The aim is to detect urethral stenosis or diverticulum (Fig. 18c). Again, prudent retrograde opacification is the optimal examination. Other imaging modalities, such as urethral US (or ce-US) and urethral MRI, may give additionally important information concerning the surrounding extraluminal soft tissue, which can be advantageous for surgical planning when delayed reconstruction is performed (Pichler et al. 2012).

Take Away

In urethral trauma, imaging studies should be scheduled and oriented accordingly with surgical management.

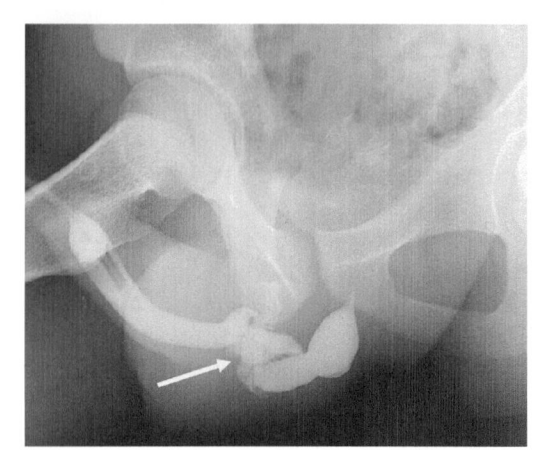

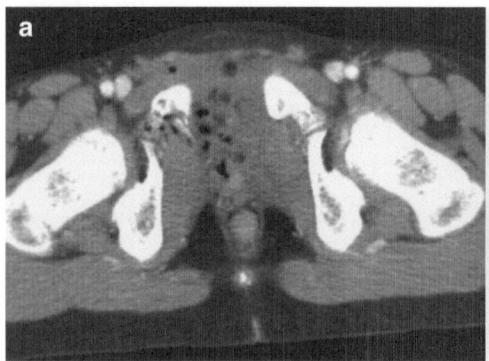

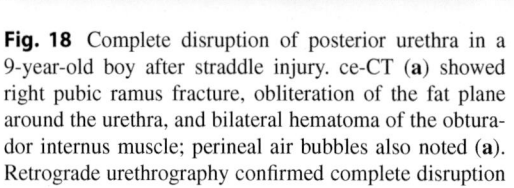

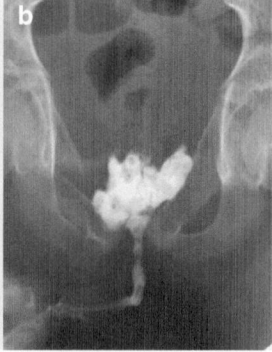

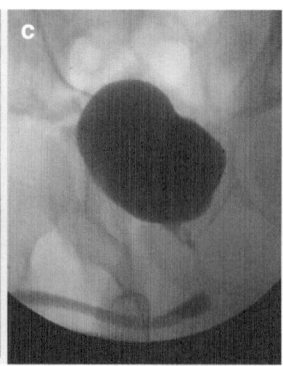

Fig. 17 Complete disruption of the membranous urethra in an adolescent boy shown by retrograde urethrography (*arrow*). Note the inflated balloon of the Foley catheter in the fossa navicularis

Fig. 18 Complete disruption of posterior urethra in a 9-year-old boy after straddle injury. ce-CT (**a**) showed right pubic ramus fracture, obliteration of the fat plane around the urethra, and bilateral hematoma of the obturador internus muscle; perineal air bubbles also noted (**a**). Retrograde urethrography confirmed complete disruption of the posterior urethra with contrast extravasation into the extraperitoneal pelvis; also note right pubic ramus fractures (**b**). Combined retrograde urethrography with anterograde cystography 9 months later showed a long segment stenosis of the posterior urethra; note contrast reflux into the prostatic ducts (**c**)

6 Scrotal Injuries

See also chapter "Imaging in Male genital Queries".

Scrotal trauma occurs more frequently in older boys and often results from blunt trauma during sport activities, motor vehicle accidents, falls, or straddle injuries. Sport accidents account for more than 50% of all cases of testicular injuries (Bhatt and Dogra 2008). The majority of scrotal injuries are managed conservatively. Testicular rupture is a surgical emergency, with a high rate of testicular salvage if surgical repair is performed within 72 hours of testicular injury. Disruption of tunica albuginea and compromised testicular blood flow are main indications for surgical exploration. Furthermore, high clinical suspicion of testicular rupture (despite equivocal US findings) and penetrating trauma should also prompt surgical exploration.

Clinical examination may be difficult. US with Doppler sonography is the imaging modality of choice to evaluate scrotal trauma. The primary goal of imaging is to assess the integrity of tunica albuginea and the vascularization of the testis. Scrotal US with aCDS has a high diagnostic accuracy for detection and characterization of scrotal injuries (Buckley and McAninch 2006). On US, intratesticular contusion or hematoma is seen as an avascular focal lesion, hyper-, iso-, or hypoechoic – depending on the time that has elapsed between the injury and US examination. In acute phases it might be difficult to differentiate it from the surrounding normal testis on grayscale US; thus aCDS is mandatory (Fig. 19). Testicular fracture refers to a break of the normal testicular parenchyma, whereas testicular rupture implies discontinuity of the tunica albuginea, with potential extrusion of the testicular components. US signs

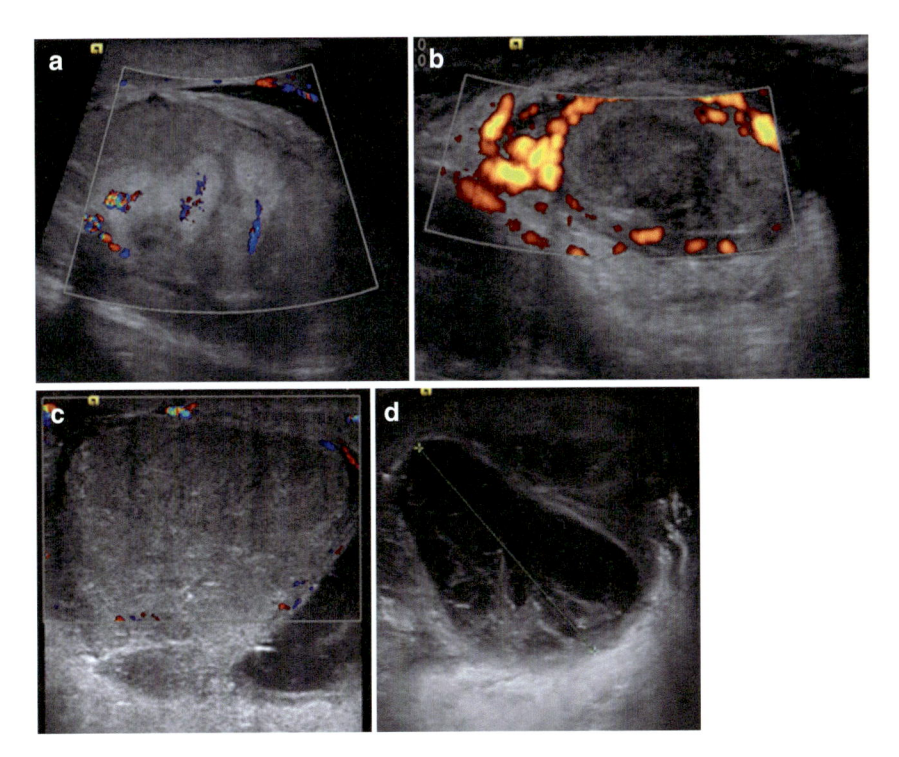

Fig. 19 Scrotal trauma on US and CDS. Testicular rupture in an 18-year-old boy (**a**) – testicular increased size, irregular contour, heterogeneous echotexture, and non-perfused parenchymal areas. Scrotal injury with extensive testicular devascularization in a 3-year-old boy (**b**). Testicular post-traumatic torsion in a 16-year-old boy (**c, d**) – testicular increased size and heterogeneous parenchyma with absent perfusion (**c**); associated extratesticular fluid collection (+…+) due to hematocele

of testicular rupture include disruption of the tunica albuginea, abnormal testicular contour, heterogeneous echogenicity, and loss of vascularization of the testis (Fig. 19a). The amount of nonviable testicular parenchyma on aCDS helps decide on the type of surgery (Bhatt and Dogra 2008) (Fig. 19b). Scrotal trauma may also result in testicular dislocation as well as in testicular torsion (Fig. 19c). Extratesticular hematoma (hematocele) and scrotal wall hematoma are common findings after scrotal blunt trauma (Fig. 19d). Post-traumatic epididymitis can also occur.

> **Take Away**
> US with CDS can accurately assess the integrity of tunica albuginea and the vascularization of the testis.

References

Amerstorfer EE, Haberlik A, Riccabona M (2015) Imaging assessment of renal injuries in children and adolescents: CT or ultrasound? J Ped Surg 50:448–455

Avanoglu A, Ulman I, Herek O, Ozok G, Gokdemir A (1996) Posterior urethral injuries in children. Br J Urol 77:597–600

Bartley JM, Santucci RA (2012) Computed tomography findings in patients with pediatric blunt renal trauma in whom expectant (nonoperative) management failed. Urology 80:1338–1343

Baskin LS, McAninch JW (1993) Childhood urethral injuries: perspectives on outcome and treatment. Br J Urol 72:241–246

Benya EC, Lim-Dunham JE, Landrum O, Statter M (2000) Abdominal sonography in examination of children with blunt abdominal trauma. Am J Roentgenol 174:1613–1616

Bhatt S, Dogra VS (2008) Role of US in testicular and scrotal trauma. Radiographics 28:1617–1629

Bisset GS, Strife JL, Kirks DR (1991) Genitourinary tract. In: Kirks D (ed) Practical pediatric imaging. Little, Brown, Boston, pp 905–1056

Brenner DJ, Hall EJ (2007) Computed tomography – an increasing source of radiation exposure. N Engl J Med 357:2277–2284

Brown SL, Elder JS, Spirnak JP (1998) Are pediatric patients more susceptible to major renal injury from blunt trauma? J Urol 160:138–140

Buckley JC, McAninch JW (2004) Pediatric renal injuries: management guidelines from a 25-year experience. J Urol 172:687–690

Buckley JC, McAninch JW (2006) Use of ultrasonography for the diagnosis of testicular injuries in blunt scrotal trauma. J Urol 175:175–178

Buckley JC, McAninch JW (2011) Revision of current American Association for the Surgery of Trauma Renal Injury grading system. J Trauma 70:35–37

Cannon GM Jr, Polsky EG, Smaldone MC et al (2008) Computerized tomography findings in pediatric renal trauma – indications for early intervention? J Urol 179:1529–1533

Canon S, Recicar J, Head B et al (2014) The utility of initial and follow-up ultrasound reevaluation for blunt renal trauma in children and adolescents. J of Pediatr Urol 10:815–818

Chirdan LB, Uba AF, Yiltok SJ, Ramyil VM (2007) Paediatric blunt abdominal trauma: challenges of management in a developing country. Eur J Pediatr Surg 17:90–95

Damasio MB, Darge K, Riccabona M (2013) Multidetector-CT in the paediatric urinary tract. Eur J Radiol 82:1118–1125

Delarue A, Merrot T, Fahkro A, Alessandrini P, Guys JM (2002) Major renal injuries in children: the real incidence of kidney loss. J Pediatr Surg 37:1446–1450

Dugi DD 3rd, Morey AF, Gupta A et al (2010) American Association for the Surgery of Trauma grade 4 renal injury substratification into grades 4a (low risk) and 4b (high risk). J Urol 183:592–597

Eeg KR, Khoury AE, Halachmi S et al (2009) Single center experience with application of the ALARA concept to serial imaging studies after blunt renal trauma in children – is ultrasound enough? J Urol 181:1834–1840

Figler BD, Malaeb BS, Voelzke B, Smith T, Wessells H (2013) External validation of a substratification of the American Association for the Surgery of Trauma renal injury scale for grade 4 injuries. J Am Coll Surg 217:924–928

Filiatriault D, Garel L (1995) Commentary: Pediatric blunt abdominal trauma: to sound or not to sound? Pediatr Radiol 25:329–331

Freitas Filho LG, Carnevale J, Melo Filho AR, Vicente NC, Heinisch AC, Martins JL (2003) Posterior urethral injuries and the Mitrofanoff principle in children. BJU Int 91:402–405

Glassberg KI, Tolete-Velcek F, Ashley R, Waterhouse K (1979) Partial tears of prostatomembranous urethra in children. Urology 13:500–504

Gomez RG, Ceballos L, Coburn M et al (2004) Consensus statement on bladder injuries. BJU Int 94:27–32

Grattan-Smith JD, Jones RA (2008) Magnetic resonance urography in children. Magn Reson Imaging Clin N Am 16:515–531

Grimsby GM, Voelzke B, Hotaling J, Sorensen MD, Koyle M, Jacobs MA (2014) Demographics of pediatric renal trauma. J Urol 192:1498–1502

Jacobs MA, Hotaling JM, Mueller BA et al (2012) Conservative management vs early surgery for high grade pediatric renal trauma – do nephrectomy rates differ? J Urol 187:1817–1822

Kuan JK, Wright JL, Nathens AB et al (2006) American Association for the Surgery of Trauma. AAST Organ Injury Scale for kidney injuries predicts nephrectomy, dialysis and death in patients with blunt injuries and nephrectomy for penetrating injuries. J Trauma 60:351–356

Le Dosseur P, Dacher JN, Pietrera P, Daudruy M, El Ferzli J (2005) Management of abdominal trauma in children. J Radiol 86:209–221

Lougué-Sorgho LC, Lambot K, Gorincour G et al (2006) Traumatisme du rein chez l'enfant: bonnes pratiques en imagerie médicale. J Radiol 87:275–283

Malmed AS, Love L, Jeffrey RB (1992) Medullary CT enhancement in acute renal artery occlusion. J Comput Assist Tomogr 16:107–109

Marcos HB, Noone TC, Semelka RC (1998) MRI evaluation of acute renal trauma. J Magn Reson 8:989–990

Mayor B, Gudinchet F, Wicky S, Reinberg O, Schnyder P (1995) Imaging evaluation of blunt renal trauma in children: diagnostic accuracy of intravenous pyelography and ultrasonography. Pediatr Radiol 25:214–218

McAleer IM, Kaplan GW, LoSasso BE (2002) Congenital urinary tract anomalies in pediatric renal trauma patients. J Urol 68:1808–1810

McKenney KL, Nunet DB Jr, McKenney MG (1998) Sonography as the primary screening technique for blunt abdominal trauma: experience with 899 patients. AJR Am J Roentgenol 170:979–985

Merchant WC 3rd, Gibbons MD, Gonzales ET Jr (1984) Trauma to the bladder neck, trigone and vagina in children. J Urol 131:747–750

Moore EE, Shackford SR, Pachter HL et al (1989) Organ injury scaling: spleen, liver, and kidney. J Trauma 29:1664–1666

Nguyen MM, Das S (2002) Pediatric renal trauma. Urology 59:762–766

Perez-Brayfield MR, Gatti JM, Smith EA et al (2002) Blunt traumatic hematuria in children: is a simplified algorithm justified? J Urol 167:2543–2546

Pichler R, Fritsch H, Skradski V et al (2012) Diagnosis and management of pediatric urethral injuries. Urol Int 89:136–142

Pietrera P, Badachi Y, Liard A, Dacher JN (2001) Les ultrasons dans l'évaluation initiale des lesions rénales post traumatiques chez l'enfant. J Radiol 82:833–838

Quagliano PV, Delair SM, Malhotra AK (2006) Diagnosis of blunt bladder injury: a prospective comparative study of computed tomography cystography and conventional retrograde cystography. J Trauma 61:410–421

Reda EF, Lebowitz RL (1986) Traumatic ureteropelvic junction disruption in the child. Pediatr Radiol 16:164–166

Reese JN, Fox JA, Cannon GM Jr, Ost MC (2014) Timing and predictors for urinary drainage in children with expectantly managed garde IV renal trauma. J Urol 192:512–517

Riccabona M, Avni F, Dacher JN et al (2010) ESPR uroradiology task force and ESUR paediatric working group: Imaging and procedural recommendations in paediatric uroradiology, Part III. Minutes of the ESPR uroradiology task force mini-symposium on intravenous urography, uro-CT and MR-urography in childhood. Pediatr Radiol 40:1315–1320

Riccabona M, Avni F, Dacher JN et al (2011) ESPR uroradiology task force and ESUR paediatric working group: imaging recommendations in paediatric uroradiology, part IV Minutes of the ESPR uroradiology task force mini-symposium on imaging in childhood renal hypertension and imaging of renal trauma in children. Pediatr Radiol 41:939–944

Riccabona M, Vivier PH, Ntoulia A et al (2014) ESPR uroradiology task force imaging recommendations in paediatric uroradiology, part VII: standardised terminology, impact of existing recommendations, and update on contrast-enhanced ultrasound of the paediatric urogenital tract. Pediatr Radiol 44:1478–1484

Ricabbona M, Darge K, Lobo ML et al (2015) ESPR uroradiology taskforce – imaging recommendations in paediatric uroradiology, part VIII: retrograde urethrography, imaging disorder of sexual development and imaging childhood testicular torsion. Pediatr Radiol 45:2023–2028

Richards JR, Knopf NA, Wang L, McGahan JP (2002) Blunt abdominal trauma in children: evaluation with emergency US. Radiology 222:749–754

Rogers CG, Knight V, MacUra KJ et al (2004) High-grade renal injuries in children – is conservative management possible? Urology 64:574–579

Santucci RA, McAninch JW, Safir M et al (2001) Validation of the American Association for the Surgery of Trauma organ injury severity scale for the kidney. J Trauma 50:195–200

Shariat SF, Roehrborn CG, Karakiewicz PI et al (2007) Evidence-based validation of the predictive value of the American Association for the Surgery of Trauma kidney injury scale. J Trauma 62:933–939

Sivit CJ, Cutting JP, Eichelberger MR (1995) CT diagnosis and localization of rupture of the bladder in children with blunt abdominal trauma: significance of contrast material extravasation in the pelvis. AJR Am J Roentgenol 164:1243–1246

Sokolove PE, Kuppermann N, Holmes JF (2005) Association between the seat belt sign and intraabdominal injury in children with blunt torso trauma. Acad Emerg Med 12:808–813

Stuhlfaut JW, Anderson SW, Soto JA (2007) Blunt abdominal trauma: current imaging techniques and CT findings in patients with solid organ, bowel and mesenteric injury. Semin Ultrasound CT MRI 28:115–129

Tasian GE, Aaronson DS, McAninch JW (2010) Evaluation of renal function after major renal injury: correlation with the American Association for the Surgery of Trauma injury scale. J Urol 183:196–200

Tarman GJ, Kaplan GW, Lerman SL, McAleer IM, Losasso BE (2002) Lower genitourinary injury and pelvic fractures in pediatric patients. Urology 59:123–126

Thorelius L (2007) Emergency real-time contrast-enhanced sonography for detection of solid organ injuries. Eur Radiol 17:F107–F111

Umbreit EC, Routh JC, Husmann DA (2009) Nonoperative management of nonvascular grade IV blunt renal trauma in children: meta-analysis and systematic review. Urology 74:579–582

Valentino M, Serra C, Zironi G et al (2006) Blunt abdominal trauma: emergency contrast-enhanced sonography for detection of solid organ injuries. AJR Am J Roentgenol 186:1361–1367

Walcher F, Weinlich M, Conrad G et al (2006) Prehospital ultrasound imaging improves management of abdominal trauma. Br J Surg 93:238–242

Wessel LM, Scholz S, Jester I et al (2000) Management of kidney injuries in children with blunt abdominal trauma. J Pediatr Surg 35:1326–1330

Pediatric Genitourinary Intervention

Richard Towbin, David Aria, Trevor Davis, Robin Kaye, and Carrie Schaefer

Contents

1 Introduction 721
2 **Nonvascular Interventions** 722
2.1 Whitaker (Pressure-Flow) Perfusion Test 722
2.2 Percutaneous Nephrostomy 723
2.3 Nephrostomy Track Dilatation 728
2.4 Endourologic Techniques 728
2.5 Percutaneous Renal Biopsy 737
2.6 Percutaneous Cystostomy 739
3 **Vascular Interventions** 740
3.1 Percutaneous Renal Angioplasty 740
3.2 Embolotherapy of the Genitourinary System 744
4 **Summary** 748
References 748

R. Towbin, MD (✉) • D. Aria, MD • R. Kaye, MD
C. Schaefer, MD
Department of Medical Imaging, Phoenix Children's Hospital, 1919 East Thomas Road, Phoenix, AZ 85016, USA
e-mail: rtowbin@phoenixchildrens.com

T. Davis, DO
Pediatric Interventional Radiology, Phoenix Children's Hospital, 1919 East Thomas Road, Phoenix, AZ 85016, USA

1 Introduction

Percutaneous techniques offer several advantages over open surgery in the treatment of many pediatric genitourinary diseases. The pediatric interventionalist routinely performs minimally invasive procedures on patients, frequently as outpatients utilizing procedural sedation, which would otherwise require general anesthesia and lengthy hospital admissions if treated surgically. The minimally invasive nature of percutaneous therapy also results in cost reduction. The outcomes of percutaneous techniques have now been established as equal to or better than the corresponding surgical techniques in many instances. In spite of this, pediatric genitourinary intervention has grown relatively slowly over the past decade. Limited growth in this area is likely due to a variety of factors, especially the preference of urologists to perform combined percutaneous and surgical procedures in the operating room. Most referrals to pediatric interventional radiologists are cases that are difficult to treat operatively or with endoscopic techniques. Consequently, a relatively small number of children are referred to pediatric interventionalists for routine percutaneous urologic procedures. This trend continues today.

Percutaneous treatment of diseases affecting the urinary tract most often begins with accessing the collecting system and placing a nephrostomy tube. Thus, nephrostomy insertion is the basic technique upon which percutaneous surgical procedures are built. This chapter discusses diagnostic and therapeutic interventional procedures of the genitourinary (GU) tract, including percutaneous nephrostomy tube and ureteral stent insertion, ureteral stricture dilatation, nephrostomy tract dilatation, percutaneous removal of calculi, endopyelotomy techniques used in the treatment of ureteropelvic junction (UPJ) strictures, percutaneous renal angioplasty for treatment of renovascular hypertension, and embolotherapy of the GU system.

2 Nonvascular Interventions

2.1 Whitaker (Pressure-Flow) Perfusion Test

In 1973, Dr. Whitaker described the pressure-flow stress test to help understand the physiologic aspects of a dilated urinary tract. Dr. Whitaker determined that urine flow at the time of maximum diuresis was 10 ml/min, reasoning that a normal ureter should be able to tolerate this rate without a significant increase in intrapelvic pressure. The initial approach to testing was to infuse saline into the renal pelvis at a rate of 10 ml/min while simultaneously measuring the intrarenal and bladder pressure and determining the difference between the two pressure measurements. Normal pressure gradient was considered below 15 cm of water and abnormal above 22 cm of water, with a zone of uncertainty for pressures between the two. In practice, we prefer to consider pressure gradients less than 22 cm of water as normal or insignificantly elevated and pressure gradients of greater than 22 cm of water as abnormal, with increasing grades of obstruction based on opening pressures closest to 35 cm of water. At levels >35 cm of water, high-grade obstruction with possible pyelotubular reflux may occur if an infusion is performed. In our hands, the routine Whitaker test is a combination of a pressure-volume test using one (Fig. 1) or two needles or catheters and an antegrade pyelogram using contrast to define the urinary anatomy and peristaltic function.

With opening pressures below 25 cm of water, our initial rate of contrast infusion is 6 ml/min over 5 min followed by an infusion rate of 10 ml/min if there is no significant elevation in pressure. When the opening pressure is higher, a more conservative approach is taken with infusion rates beginning at 2–4 ml/min with a slow increase in rate based on the response to 5 min infusion increments. When the opening pressure is near 35 cm of water, a 1:1 exchange of urine for contrast is performed to opacify the urinary tract in order to identify the site of obstruction without further pressure

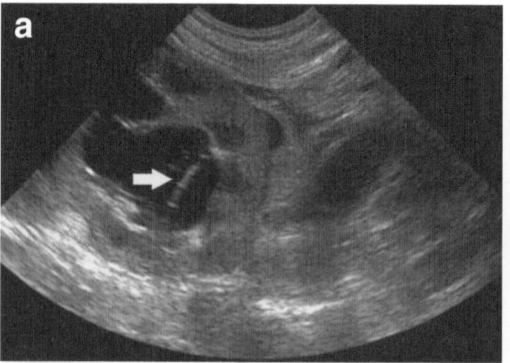

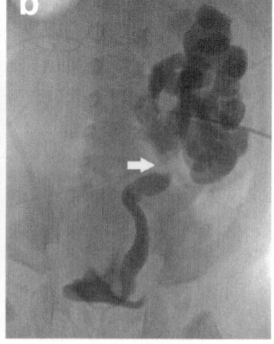

Fig. 1 6-month-old male with congenital right UPJ obstruction status post-dismembered pyeloplasty presents with persistent dilatation of the right renal collecting system. (**a**) Ultrasound-guided access of the distended right renal pelvis with a 5-French Yueh catheter (*arrow*). (**b**) Whitaker test via the Yueh sheath (single-needle technique) demonstrates calyceal dilatation and blunting with a focal, nonocclusive stenosis at the pyeloplasty site (*arrow*). Pressure measurements were mildly elevated post-pyeloplasty with associated pelvicaliectasis

elevation. In our view, these small incremental volume increases help to define the degree of obstruction, with slower pressure rises associated with less severe obstruction.

Procedural Details and Technique

The technical approach to the Whitaker test may vary slightly depending upon operator preferences, the presence of a nephrostomy tube, and test goals. Our preferred approach is to use a two-needle technique, although a single-needle approach also works well but can be cumbersome due to the frequent need to switch from infusion to pressure measurement (Fig. 2). Although a variety of needles or small catheters can be used, we prefer to use the 5-French Yueh Centesis Disposable Catheter Needle (Cook Medical, Bloomington, IN, USA) since they deliver a sheath that works well for both infusion and pressure measurement functions. When two needles or catheters are used, the infusion and pressure measurements are done continuously. The pressure monitoring can be accomplished with a manometer or electronic pressure-measuring device. If a single needle is used, a three-way stopcock is required, and pressure is measured immediately after a volume infusion has been completed. The infusate is a nonionic contrast to allow for simultaneous infusion and to visualize the urinary tract anatomy and peristalsis under fluoroscopy.

We have found this test to be useful in confidently identifying whether there is an element of obstruction to the dilated urinary tract when there is an equivocal nuclear renogram or when there are symptoms of uncertain significance or etiology.

> **Take Away**
> The Whitaker test is used infrequently; however, in cases that are indeterminate by nuclear imaging, it is a valuable tool to demonstrate the presence of partial or complete obstruction. Also, it may help decide whether or not to insert a drainage catheter.

2.2 Percutaneous Nephrostomy

Nephrostomy insertion is the building block for most urinary tract interventions. The percutaneous nephrostomy technique was first described for the treatment of hydronephrosis (Goodwin et al. 1955). About 20 years later, the first percutaneous stone removal was performed (Fernstrom and Johanasson 1976). Endourologic technology was further extended when electrosurgical instruments were safely used. These developments, combined with new interventional and endoscopic equipment, have led to the development of complex endourologic techniques. These advances have led to better patient care and a closer working relationship among the nephrologist, urologist, pediatric surgeon, transplant surgeon, and pediatric interventionalist. In many instances, these collaborations have led to a reduced need for open surgical procedures.

Percutaneous nephrostomy has been successful in over 97 % of pediatric patients ranging in age from 1 day to 18 years (Irving et al. 1987; Winfield et al. 1984; Lipuma et al. 1984). These results compare favorably with surgical management (Gonzalez-Serva et al. 1977).

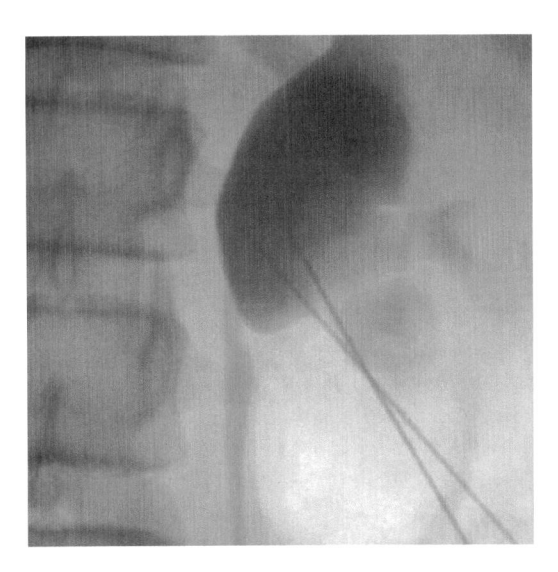

Fig. 2 Teenage girl with a dilated right renal pelvis and equivocal Lasix renogram after a dismembered pyeloplasty. Whitaker test performed using a two-needle technique demonstrating an enlarged renal pelvis due to persistent UPJ obstruction

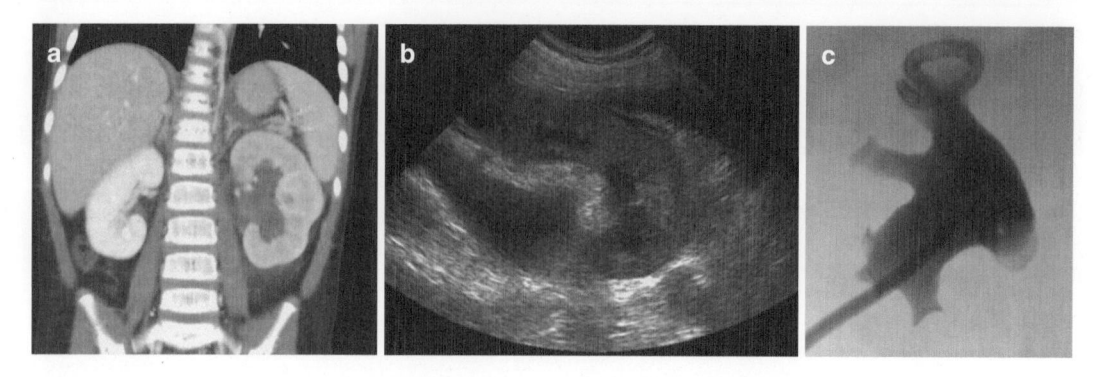

Fig. 3 4-year-old male with fever and abdominal pain. (**a**) Coronal contrast-enhanced CT demonstrates left pyelonephritis with a delayed left nephrogram and a dilated renal pelvis secondary to a proximal ureteral calculus (not shown). The Hounsfield units suggest complex fluid. (**b**) Gray-scale ultrasound demonstrates increased echogenicity of the renal pelvis, consistent with proteinaceous fluid. (**c**) Nephrostomy tube placement with decompression of the renal pelvis and mild residual blunting of calyces. Aspiration yielded cloudy, debris-containing urine. Cultures came back positive for Klebsiella pneumonia

The most common indications for percutaneous nephrostomy are for relief of symptomatic urinary tract obstruction (Fig. 3) and pyonephrosis (Man et al. 1983; Pode et al. 1982). In a series of 50 percutaneous nephrostomies in the pediatric population reported by Stanley and colleagues (1983), the most frequent causes of obstruction were ureteropelvic junction (UPJ) narrowing and obstruction after ureteral reimplantation.

The benefits of percutaneous nephrostomy are related to the ease of placement under sedation and to the rapid relief of obstruction and improved renal function. Infected and obstructed systems can be drained, and fever management becomes possible (Gonzalez-Serva et al. 1977). Other indications for percutaneous nephrostomy include assessment of renal function, demonstration of pathologic anatomy, and differentiation between obstructed and nonobstructed dilated systems using a Whitaker perfusion test (Whitaker 1981).

Percutaneous nephrostomy can be utilized as a temporizing measure prior to definitive therapy of underlying obstruction (Fig. 4). Percutaneous decompression of the obstruction allows time for improvement in renal function, treatment of urinary sepsis, and for a more accurate assessment of the urinary collecting system. Children with postoperative ureteral edema, leakage, or obstruction from extrinsic compression may benefit from percutaneous nephrostomy.

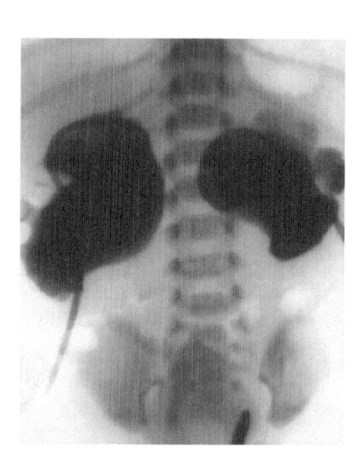

Fig. 4 Neonate with bilateral UPJ obstructions. Fluoroscopic image demonstrates marked dilatation of both pelvises with 5-French nephrostomy tubes placed

In rare instances, obstruction caused by a fungus ball may be treated with a combination of percutaneous nephrostomy and infusion of amphotericin (Fig. 5) (Matsumoto et al. 1990). In asymptomatic children with hydronephrosis, antegrade pyelography and pressure measurement (Whitaker test) may be performed prior to surgical or endourologic correction to document the level and nature of the obstruction. Finally, percutaneous nephrostomy may be the initial procedure required to gain access prior to other endourologic procedures. Examples of these include percutaneous stone removal and percutaneous endopyelotomy.

Fig. 5 (**a**) Neonate with complicated course developed UPJ obstruction secondary to a fungus ball (*arrow*). (**b**) Nephrostomy drainage (5-French system) and amphotericin infusion showed partial resolution in 2 weeks. Eventually the obstruction resolved (not shown)

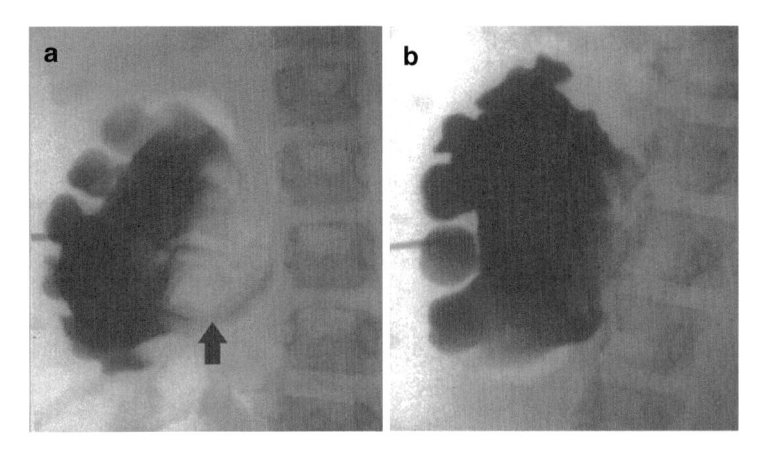

Contraindications to percutaneous nephrostomy are uncommon and include an uncorrectable coagulopathy and an unfavorable anatomy, making percutaneous access impossible or dangerous.

Procedural Details and Technique/Technical Remarks

Properly sized equipment is essential to safely perform percutaneous nephrostomy in children. Equipment routinely used in adults may be ineffective or dangerous, especially in the perinate and young infant. For example, the Cope introducer system (Cook Inc., Bloomington, IN), which facilitates exchanging a 0.035-in. or 0.038-in. guidewire for a 0.018-in. guidewire after puncture of the renal pelvis with a 22-gauge Chiba needle, is problematic in small infants. While this system works well in older children, its side port design (through which the 0.035-in. or 0.038-in. guidewire will exit) will often lie outside the renal pelvis making guidewire exchange difficult or impossible. Also, if the sheath is advanced, it likely will kink at the side port, again making a guidewire exchange problematic. Thus, it is preferable to use an end-hole coaxial dilator, such as the coaxial dilator system, the Micropuncture set (Cook Inc.), or a sheathed needle to insert a 0.035-in. or 0.038-in. guidewire into a small renal pelvis.

It is important to carefully consider the guidewire selection. Standard and stiff guidewires are of value in both older children and adults. In perinates and small infants, a standard 0.035-in. or 0.038-in. guidewire may injure or lacerate the thin renal parenchyma. In the perinate, the thin skin, minimal paraspinal musculature, and short distance from the flank to the renal pelvis offer little resistance to track dilation. The only barrier to catheter insertion is the renal capsule, which may be surprisingly tough. Thus, a guidewire that does not kink, such as a 0.018-in. angled nitinol glidewire, is useful. If a 0.018-in. mandril guidewire is used, one must be careful that the floppy tip does not kink, making wire withdrawal difficult. If one attempts to pull the guidewire back into the Chiba needle, the floppy tip may shear off. If a kink occurs, it might be necessary to remove the entire system and repuncture the renal pelvis. Because of these issues, the mandril guidewire is now rarely used. Regardless of the guidewire selected, it is important to maintain a straight catheter-guidewire course during tube placement to avoid buckling in the retroperitoneal soft tissues.

For insertion of standard drains (≥8 French), a variety of guidewires perform well, including the Newton, angled glidewire, Rosen, and Amplatz guidewires. In patients who are muscular, obese, or those in whom catheter insertion is difficult, a stiff guidewire such as a stiff glidewire, Amplatz, and Rosen provides greater stability and facilitates passage of the nephrostomy catheter.

Selection of the nephrostomy catheter depends upon the age and size of the patient, as well as the anticipated contents of the collecting system. The choice of catheter is usually determined by physician preference. In perinates and small children, smaller catheters are used, specifically a 5- or

6-French pigtail catheter with a small distal loop (1 cm). The drain side ports are positioned along the inner curve of the pigtail catheter, which prevents catheter occlusion resulting from contact with the wall of the renal pelvis. The operator can be confident that all drainage holes are satisfactorily positioned within the renal pelvis once the catheter reforms (Fig. 6).

Image guidance for percutaneous nephrostomy usually consists of a combination of fluoroscopy and ultrasound, although either modality can be used alone. The use of ultrasound obviates the need for opacification of the collecting system in most instances and is especially useful in patients with impaired renal function or contrast allergy. In the pediatric population, CT is rarely necessary for guidance and is only considered for children with unusual renal anatomy or when other guidance methods have failed. Patients with severe hydronephrosis may not require imaging guidance for puncture of the renal pelvis.

Local anesthetic and intravenous sedation or anesthesia are used in almost all cases for placement of a nephrostomy catheter. The patient is placed either in a prone or prone-oblique position. An entry site is selected on the flank using anatomic landmarks alone or with imaging. With ultrasound, an entry site is selected beneath the costal margin approximately along the midscapular line. The puncture site selected should allow for puncture into a posterior middle or lower pole calyx. If a percutaneous surgical procedure is planned, it is usually best to enter the renal pelvis via a middle pole calyx. However, the best entry site depends on the procedure to be performed.

The skin is prepared and draped in sterile fashion, and local anesthesia is injected into the skin and deep soft tissues along the planned needle course, using a 30-gauge needle when procedural sedation is being utilized. One percent buffered 1 % lidocaine minimizes discomfort. Inadequate local anesthesia may result in pain that will awaken the sedated child and make the procedure more difficult and time-consuming. A skin incision is then made with a no. 11 scalpel blade and enlarged with blunt dissection.

Puncture of the renal parenchyma and into the calyx is made with a Chiba needle or a 19-gauge sheathed needle. A posterolateral approach angling the needle toward the costovertebral junction is used. Direct puncture of the renal pelvis is avoided to minimize the chance of injury to the posterior branch of the renal artery. In addition, the renal pelvis lacks supporting parenchyma to provide tamponade against bleeding or urine leakage or premature catheter loss. After the kidney is punctured and a guidewire coiled within the renal

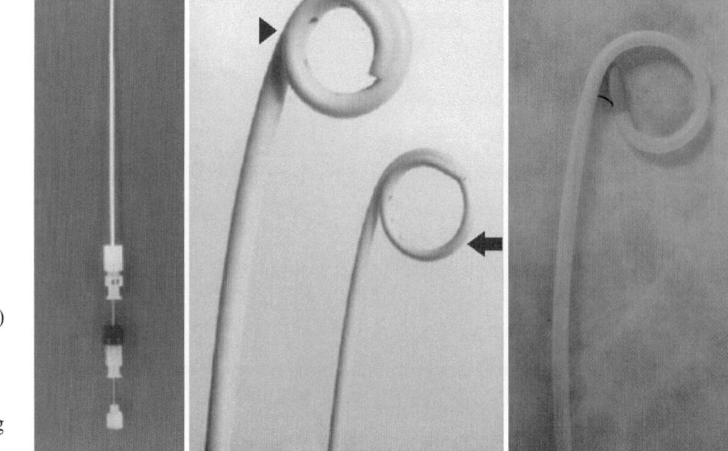

Fig. 6 (**a**) Modified 5-French neonatal nephrostomy drain. (**b**) Comparison of a 5-French (*arrow*) and standard 8-French (*arrowhead*) nephrostomy drains. Note side holes positioned along the inner curvature of the pigtails. (**c**) 6.3-French Dawson-Muller locking pigtail drainage catheter

pelvis, the track may be dilated up to 2 French larger than the nephrostomy catheter to ease insertion of the drain. Overdilation is especially helpful in some perinates because of the resistant renal capsule and relative mobility of the kidney.

In patients with renal transplants, the approach to percutaneous nephrostomy depends upon the surgical anatomy. Renal transplants may be placed intraperitoneal or extraperitoneal, typically in the iliac fossa. An intraperitoneal approach is more common in smaller children; however, approaches vary by institution. Given the location of the renal allograft, the renal pelvis usually faces medially or posteromedially. As a result, an anterolateral approach is usually best for nephrostomy tube placement. Real-time ultrasound is used to guide needle puncture to avoid inadvertent injury to the bowel. CT guidance is rarely utilized for nephrostomy tube placement in transplants.

Major complications resulting from insertion of a percutaneous nephrostomy are unusual in children. Initially, percutaneous nephrostomy was considered less applicable to the pediatric population because of the need for general anesthesia. However, improvements in sedation techniques, monitoring equipment, catheters, and the widespread use of ultrasound for needle puncture guidance have helped percutaneous nephrostomy become a safe and effective procedure in the pediatric population (Ball et al. 1986; Pfister et al. 1981).

The two most serious complications of percutaneous nephrostomy are sepsis and bleeding. Overdistension of the collecting system at the time of catheter placement is likely the most significant factor leading to bacteremia. Decompressing the renal pelvis prior to performing an antegrade nephrostogram, especially in patients with pyonephrosis, is important to minimize this problem. For this reason, it is preferable to delay a diagnostic antegrade nephrostogram for 24–72 h to allow for decompression of the obstructed system and sterilization of urine. Patients with suspected or documented pyonephrosis require antibiotic coverage before and after the procedure.

Transient mild hematuria is common after percutaneous nephrostomy and usually clears within 48 h. This can be expected and should not be considered a complication. Severe bleeding at the time of catheter insertion or later is unusual and may indicate vascular injury, a clotting disorder, or an unsuspected vascular malformation. Occasionally blood clots will cause catheter obstruction. If significant bleeding occurs, arteriography may be required to establish the site and etiology of bleeding, e.g., vessel laceration, pseudoaneurysm, or arteriovenous fistula (Pode et al. 1982; Stanley and Diament 1986; Cope and Zeit 1982; Boddy et al. 1987). If a vascular injury is identified, it can be treated by selective embolization. The risk of vascular injury is reduced by using a posterolateral approach for renal pelvic access. Also, arterial injury and severe bleeding are minimized by parenchymal tamponade.

Nephrostomy-related urinoma formation has been reported in the pediatric population. This complication is more likely when the renal parenchyma is thin, as in children with severe vesicoureteral reflux, or when the free wall of the renal pelvis is punctured. If the urinoma is large or becomes infected, percutaneous drainage may be required (Gonzalez-Serva et al. 1977). While a small amount of urine leakage around the nephrostomy catheter can be considered normal, excessive leakage is usually due to catheter obstruction, especially in patients with pyonephrosis or excessive bleeding.

With the use of ultrasound for guidance, misadventures due to needle malposition are unusual. Pneumothorax is now rarely reported as puncture above the 12th rib is usually avoided.

Take Away

Nephrostomy tube insertion is the building block for a variety of interventions involving the urinary tract. Nephrostomy tube insertion is highly successful for treating urinary tract obstruction and pyonephrosis. Properly sized equipment is necessary for safe and effective treatment of urinary tract abnormalities.

2.3 Nephrostomy Track Dilatation

This simple technique enlarges a nephrostomy track so that larger equipment can be safety inserted into the renal pelvis or distal urinary tract for the purpose of an endourological procedure.

Dilatation of a nephrostomy track facilitates insertion of a stent or angioplasty balloon catheter and provides a bridging technique for endourological procedures that require larger diameter devices. In the latter case, large diameter sheaths (12–24 French) or balloon dilatation is needed for track enlargement. The contraindications for track dilatation are the same as those discussed for nephrostomy insertion. It is important to keep the child's size in mind when choosing the diameter of the sheath to be left in place. In general, the recommended sheath size is 2 French larger than the diameter of the largest instrument to be used. Overdilatation of a track can lead to renal injury.

Once access to the renal pelvis is achieved, either by direct puncture or via an indwelling nephrostomy catheter, a non-kinkable guidewire is inserted and coiled within the renal pelvis or directed into the ureter or bladder. The track is then serially dilated to the predetermined diameter by upsizing the dilators at 2–4-French increments. Alternatively, an angioplasty balloon can be used for track dilatation. After track dilatation, a sheath is positioned in the renal pelvis. If endoscopy is to be used, a Rutner adapter (Cook Inc.) is fitted into the sheath to make a watertight connection. In many cases, the sheath needs to be shortened by cutting it with scissors. The shorter sheath is easier to work with and better adapted for the pediatric endoscope.

> **Take Away**
> Nephrostomy tract dilatation is a procedure that translates a simple drainage entry procedure into percutaneous surgery and/or allows the introduction of stents or other devices.

2.4 Endourologic Techniques

Endourology is defined as minimally invasive surgical therapy involving the urinary tract. Percutaneous access to the renal collecting system is frequently required for these procedures and is via a puncture identical to that used in placement of percutaneous nephrostomy tubes. Sequential dilatation of the track allows for placement of an introducer sheath, which then allows for the endourologic treatment of a variety of conditions. Endourologic procedures include ureteral dilatation, ureteral stenting, calculus removal (percutaneous nephrolithotomy), and endopyelotomy (percutaneous pyeloplasty). Preprocedure discussion between the interventionalist and urologist should include which calyx to traverse for access (upper, mid, or lower pole) and goals of the interventional component of the procedure.

2.4.1 Ureteral Dilatation and Stenting

Dilation of the ureter was initially reported by Dourmashkin in 1926. It was not until the development of the percutaneous angioplasty balloon catheter that equipment effective for percutaneous dilatation became readily available. Subsequent research with animal models confirmed that ureteral strictures could be treated using a percutaneous approach (Barbaric et al. 1977). Percutaneous endourologic treatment of calculi and ureteropelvic junction strictures was initially described in adults and subsequently in children (Gedroyc et al. 1989; Kadir et al. 1982; Lee et al. 1988; Towbin et al. 1987). Since its introduction, ureteral stenting has become a well-established procedure for the management of ureteral obstruction of varying etiologies. As a result of continual improvements in technique and equipment, the percutaneous approach is currently utilized both as a primary therapy and as an adjunct to open and endourologic surgery.

Although permanent metallic stents are widely utilized in adults for treatment of malignant obstruction, they are not routinely used in the pediatric urinary tract. In almost all cases, temporary internal (double J) (Fig. 7) ureteral or internal-external nephroureterostomy stents (universal stent) (Fig. 8) are preferred to treat strictures in children.

Stents may be placed either antegrade via a nephrostomy track or retrograde through the bladder using cystoscopy. Advantages of the antegrade approach include the ability to perform other antegrade diagnostic procedures of the urinary tract, including antegrade pyelography and Whitaker perfusion testing, to identify the genitourinary tract anatomy and to assess for obstruction. A combined approach involving both the interventionalist and urologist may be valuable in children with an ileal loop who have an ileoureteral anasto-

Fig. 7 13-month-old male with history of bilateral vesicoureteral reflux status post-ureteral implantation now presents with hydronephrosis suspicious for bilateral UVJ obstruction. (**a**) Nephrostomy tube placed on postoperative day no. 4 for immediate decompression. (**b**) Double J ureteral stents placed on postoperative day no. 6

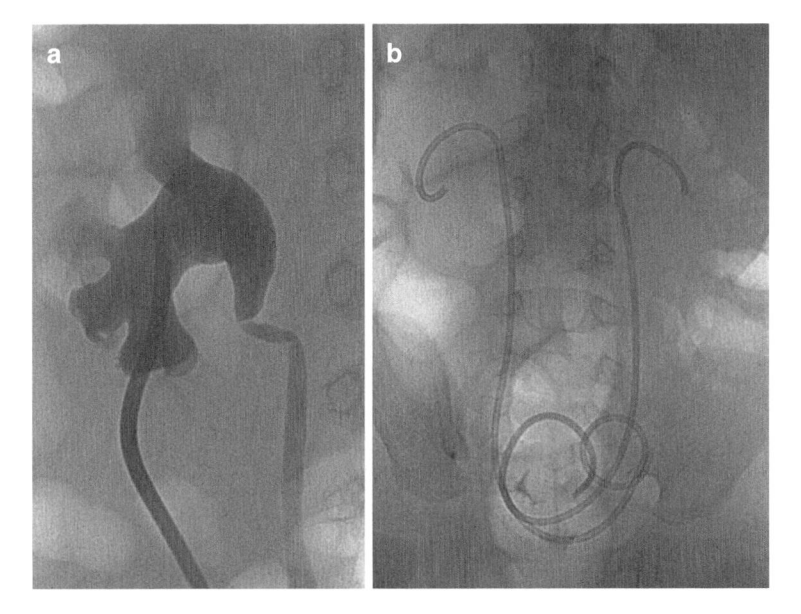

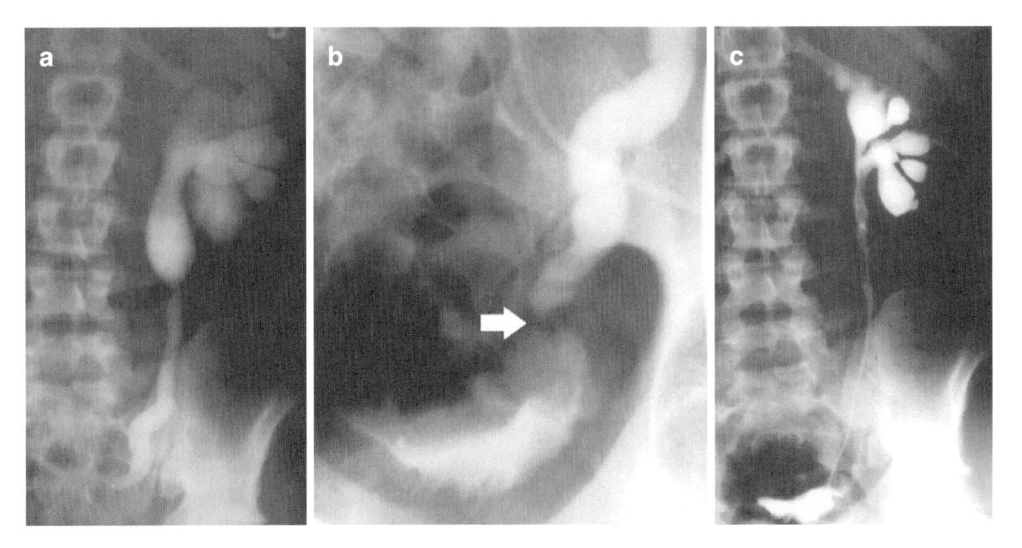

Fig. 8 (**a**) A 19-year-old patient with a UVJ obstruction and secondary hydronephrosis and hydroureter. (**b**) A coned-down view of the UVJ confirms the site of obstruction (*arrow*). (**c**) Treatment with a universal drain was effective

motic stricture or those with a pelvi-ureteric junction (PUJ) obstruction (PUJO) needing an endopyelotomy or to treat stone disease.

Percutaneous management of an isolated ureteral stricture is often effective. Ureteral narrowing may result from intraluminal or extrinsic obstruction, including following ureteral reimplantation or urinary diversion. The likelihood of successful dilatation of a stricture will depend upon the cause, length, and duration of the stricture. In the presence of impaired blood supply to the ureter, a successful result is uncertain, but strictures present for less than 3 months and postoperative strictures generally respond well to balloon dilatation. The location of a ureteral stricture does not appear to be of prognostic importance in predicting its response to balloon dilatation. However, for successful percutaneous therapy, one must be able to cross the stricture with a guidewire and catheter or other instruments.

Indications for ureteral stenting include relief of a ureteral obstruction from any cause, providing drainage while a ureteral injury heals, maintaining ureteral caliber until edema or mass effect subsides, stone removal, or surgery. Antegrade ureteral stent placement may be performed as the initial treatment or after failure of the endoscopic approach due to unfavorable anatomy.

Stent insertion should be avoided or delayed in the presence of significant hemorrhage or urinary tract infection. An indwelling ureteral stent can become the nidus for infection and may be obstructed by purulent material or blood clot. In patients with a ureteral fistula and a nondilated upper collecting system, retrograde stent insertion is the preferred route because of the ease of insertion.

Procedural Details and Technique

Many interventionalists prefer to perform ureteral dilatation and stent insertion under general anesthesia. However, a successful outcome can also be achieved with procedural sedation. A Foley catheter is inserted into the bladder once the child is asleep. The child is usually in the prone or prone-oblique position to allow optimal access to the collecting system and is secured to the tabletop with Velcro straps. The skin entry site is selected so that the puncture is cephalad to the PUJ, frequently the mid pole calyx, which allows for more direct access to the PUJ and facilitates stent insertion. The intercostal approach is avoided to make track dilatation and catheter insertion easier and to minimize the chance of hydrothorax and other thoracic complications.

After access to the renal pelvis is achieved, a guidewire is coiled within the renal pelvis or maneuvered into the ureter. The track is then progressively dilated to accommodate a peel-away or hemostasis sheath that is 2 French larger than the stent. Ultimately, a stiff guidewire (stiff-angled glidewire, Rosen, Roadrunner, Amplatz, etc.) is helpful to avoid buckling and/or telescoping of the stent as it is positioned across the stricture. A directional catheter (JB-1) and guidewire system are used to catheterize the ureter. Once the guidewire and catheter are within the proximal ureter, contrast is injected, and the location and extent of the stricture are identified. The length and diameter of the stricture are measured and the appropriate balloon is selected. The directional catheter and guidewire are then maneuvered through the ureter, and the guidewire is looped in the bladder.

Strictures that are difficult to pass often require patience and various technical manipulations to cross. Opacification of the ureter can simplify the task of crossing a tight stricture. After the stricture is identified, a radiopaque marker or hemostat is attached to the drape at the level of the stricture to aid in crossing and dilatation of the stricture. Contrast is injected into the ureter and the pathologic anatomy is documented with a road map or digital image. The guidewire and directional catheter are manipulated until the guidewire and catheter are across the stricture. If necessary, a 0.018-in. guidewire can be substituted for the larger guidewire to initially cross the stricture. Once the catheter is within the bladder, the guidewire is exchanged for a stiff or superstiff guidewire.

Treatment of strictures may be carried out with a variety of balloons. Initially, the diameter and length of the stricture are measured. The percutaneous transluminal angioplasty (PTA) balloon selected is at least 1 cm longer than the stricture and equal to or slightly wider (1–2 mm) than the expected normal ureteral diameter as measured distal to the stricture. In all cases, the balloon with the highest burst pressure is selected. Under fluoroscopic visualization, the balloon is centered across the stricture and inflated with dilute contrast while balloon pressure is monitored with a gauge. Balloon inflation progresses until the stricture waist disappears, visualized fluoroscopically. If the stricture persists, the process may be repeated with a cutting angioplasty balloon or Acucise device (Applied Medical Inc., Rancho Santa Margarita, CA). If the post-dilatation ureterogram still shows obstruction without significant change in the stricture diameter, surgery may be required.

After dilatation of a stricture has been completed, placement of a stent is needed to maintain the enlarged lumen. Stent selection depends upon a number of factors, including personal preference, available equipment, and the duration of the stenting. Each stent type has its advantages and disadvantages. Internal double J stents have a higher patient satisfaction rate because they are not visible, are less apt to be inadvertently pulled out, require no maintenance, and have a lower infection rate. They also have a number of disadvantages in that they are more difficult to insert, are only available in specific sizes that must be stocked, are more difficult to remove, and gross hematuria and infection limit their use. The internal-external (universal) stent is more flexible, easier to tailor to length, and easier to remove. Removal of the drain is performed on an outpatient basis without sedation or anesthesia in most instances. In spite of its disadvantages, the internal double J stent is usually preferred since it has greater stability and easier postprocedural care.

Placement of an internal stent is performed under fluoroscopic guidance. Prior to beginning ureteral stent placement, a second (safety) guidewire is inserted through the sheath and coiled in the renal pelvis. This guidewire is then secured to the drape with a hemostat and covered with a sterile towel. After a stiff guidewire has been maneuvered into the bladder, a 5-French catheter is positioned over the guidewire with the tip just distal to the ureterovesical junction (UVJ). The length of the ureter is measured so that the proper stent length can be selected. A catheter or guidewire (bent guidewire technique) can be used as a measurement tool to obtain the ureteral length. Ureteral length is determined by positioning the tip of the catheter or guidewire at a point just distal to the UVJ, under fluoroscopic guidance. The catheter is marked with a Steri-Strip or marker, or the guidewire is then bent at the sheath hub. Alternatively, a hemostat may be clipped to the guidewire at this point and left in position. Next, the catheter or guidewire is pulled back so that the tip is at the PUJ, and again the catheter is marked or the wire bent or clipped with a hemostat at the level of the sheath hub. The distance between the catheter marks or the wire bends or hemostats is the length of the ureter, which determines the internal stent length. Depending on the age and height of the child, stent length usually varies between 8 and 24 cm. Alternatively, the proper double J ureteral stent length in children can be determined by adding ten to the patient's age in years (Palmer and Palmer 2007).

If there is not a string attached to the ureteral stent when manufactured, a suture is inserted through the proximal end-hole and used as a safety to pull the stent back into the renal pelvis if inadvertently advanced beyond the renal pelvis. The stent is then fed over the guidewire and pushed through the peel-away sheath into the renal pelvis and ureter. To maneuver the stent, a stent positioner is advanced over the guidewire and used to push the stent into its final position, with the distal loop in the bladder and proximal loop in the renal pelvis. Stent positioning is intermittently monitored under fluoroscopy. In order to complete the procedure, the guidewire must be removed. This step is crucial to the success of the procedure and although technically easy, often leads to problems. Once the stent is in satisfactory position, the positioner is kept abutted to the stent and counterpressure applied while the wire is slowly withdrawn to form the distal bladder loop. The stent can be repositioned at this point by readvancing the wire or pulling back on the string, as needed. Again, the stent is maintained in a satisfactory position by applying counterpressure with the positioner as the guidewire is slowly removed to form the proximal loop in the renal pelvis. If the proximal loop of the stent is too distal, it may be pulled back into the pelvis with retraction on the tether, under fluoroscopy, prior to removal of the string. If a safety guidewire is in position, the guidewire traversing the stent can be completely removed. If not, the guidewire is withdrawn until it exits the stent, but is still within the renal pelvis. At this point the guidewire is advanced and coiled in the renal pelvis to assist placement of the nephrostomy catheter. If this maneuver fails, the renal pelvis can be re-catheterized via the peel-away sheath.

Next, a nephrostomy catheter is inserted and secured to the skin. The nephrostomy catheter should be equal to the diameter of the track to prevent leakage of urine. The nephrostomy tube may be left in place as long as clinically indicated and may be capped. If another procedure is necessary, the nephrostomy is left in place for access. If no procedure is planned and no problem has occurred, the nephrostomy tube is removed after 24–72 h. Prior to removal, a nephrostogram may be performed to confirm satisfactory position and function of the stent. If the ureter drains well, the nephrostomy is removed and covered with a dry, sterile dressing. The child is usually followed clinically, and when the ureteral stent is no longer needed, it is removed cystoscopically from the bladder. In rare cases, the stent may be removed from above after a nephrostomy track has been reestablished.

Regardless of the stent used, duration of stent placement will vary according to the underlying etiology of the stricture. Short-term placement (3–5 days) is required for treatment of ureteral edema, while 10–21 days is usually needed after ureteral surgery. Longer time periods (6–8 weeks) are usually needed to maintain ureteral caliber after endopyelotomy, even longer sometimes after dilatation of a stenosis.

In the immediate postprocedural period, care centers around recovery of the child from sedation or general anesthesia, and treatment of complications. Children awakening from sedation have their vital signs monitored and recorded per institutional guidelines. In addition to monitoring the vital signs, the nephrostomy site and drainage are checked for bleeding. If no hematuria is identified, the Foley catheter is removed before the child awakens. Any complication identified is immediately treated, and the appropriate clinical service and referring physician are notified.

When the child is discharged home, verbal and written instructions are provided, including a list of the more common delayed complications and contact numbers for questions. If necessary, a prescription is given for antibiotics or analgesics. In general, mild analgesics such as acetaminophen, ibuprofen, or acetaminophen with codeine are recommended. Occasionally, oral Toradol will be prescribed if significant flank pain is encountered. If there is severe pain, it is recommended that the child return to the hospital to be reexamined by the interventionalist or referring service, since this level of discomfort is unexpected.

Any reported complication resulting from nephrostomy insertion such as bleeding, sepsis, or urine extravasation secondary to a leak or laceration, may also be noted after a percutaneous surgical procedure. Complications specific to percutaneous stricture dilatation include ureteral perforation or rupture and intraluminal or submucosal hematoma. Surprisingly, these problems have rarely been reported in adults or children. Untoward effects related to stent placement are more common, but still unusual in the pediatric population (Woodside et al. 1985). Stent occlusion is probably the most common and occurs secondary to encrustation, bleeding, or rarely, infection. An encrusted stent is prone to secondary infection, which may lead to sepsis. Therefore, it is important to keep the urine dilute and infection-free. Stent occlusion can be detected by cystography, antegrade pyelography, excretory urography, or if present, nephrostomy injection. In most instances, cystography is performed: stent patency is inferred if vesicoureteral reflux occurs. The ideal timing for stent removal or replacement remains controversial. Twelve weeks is the preferable limit of time that the stent is left in situ. With high-risk children, such as those with a renal transplant on immune suppression, shorter intervals are recommended.

Stent migration occurs if the stent is not adequately positioned or if it is not the correct length. This problem is avoided by careful technique and accurate measurement of ureteral length and selection of a stent of appropriate diameter and length.

When stents are too long, bladder irritation may occur. If unavoidable, bladder spasms can be treated with urinary anesthetics such as Pyridium.

> **Take Away**
> Ureteral dilatation with stenting is an effective method for treating ureteral strictures. Either internal or external drainage may be effective for treating strictures. Ureteral dilatation and stenting can be safely performed under sedation or general anesthesia.

2.4.2 Percutaneous Nephrolithotomy

The fundamental techniques of nephrostomy insertion, track dilatation, and stent insertion have led to the development of more sophisticated endourologic procedures. The initial percutaneous technique developed was for removal of renal calculi. Within a short time, techniques for treatment of ureteropelvic junction and ureteral strictures were developed. Today percutaneous nephrolithotomy has been replaced in many situations by extracorporeal shock wave lithotripsy (ESWL) and ureteroscopic techniques. However, minimally invasive management of staghorn calculi, infected lower pole calculi, and cystine stones via percutaneous nephrolithotomy and lithotripsy is still indicated.

In industrialized countries, urinary calculi are less common in the pediatric population. When stones occur, they are often metabolic or infectious in origin. Prior to the advent of percutaneous nephrostomy and ESWL, surgical procedures were required for treatment of recurrent stone disease. Current management of renal calculi in both adults and children may require a combination of techniques. Either alone or in combination with ESWL, percutaneous nephrolithotomy and ureteroscopy may be helpful for management of calculi without surgery. Chemical dissolution of calculi is an alternative to surgery in adults, but has not been used in the treatment of calculi in children. Both ESWL and endoscopic techniques have had a profound impact on the management of renal calculi and now limit the use of percutaneous techniques. Prior to the availability of ESWL, percutaneous techniques were considered superior to open surgery because of reduced cost, decreased morbidity, and shortened convalescence and hospital stay. In addition, the presence of a nephrostomy track enabled subsequent removal of any residual stone fragments. Although its role has changed, the need for percutaneous stone removal persists.

Indications for calculus removal include pain, urinary tract infection, and obstruction. Percutaneous nephrolithotomy is preferable for patients with large stone volumes such as staghorn or branched calculi, which if fragmented, are likely to cause obstruction (Shepard et al. 1988). Percutaneous evacuation of the stone material, combined with fragmentation using ESWL, laser energy, or percutaneous ultrasonic lithotripsy offers a safe alternative. Renal calculi associated with obstruction either at the PUJ or in the ureter may be better managed percutaneously. ESWL is also precluded when spinal stabilization hardware is present, as in children with myelodysplasias, a group making up a significant proportion of the pediatric renal calculi population.

Contraindications to percutaneous nephrolithotomy are infrequent, but include a child with an uncorrectable coagulopathy. Children with a small renal pelvis cause technical problems. Renal access may be difficult, and there may be insufficient room to maneuver instruments if the collecting system is not large enough. Also, in small children, the size of the kidneys may make dilatation to greater than 10–12 French dangerous for fear of a renal fracture.

Procedural Details and Technique
Percutaneous nephrolithotomy is performed under fluoroscopic guidance. In most cases, single-plane C-arm fluoroscopy is adequate. However, in some instances, biplane fluoroscopy is useful.

Nephrolithotomy requires the establishment of a nephrostomy track from 10.5 to 24 French, depending on the size of nephroscope used. A pediatric nephroscope (approximately 10.5 French) is used whenever possible to minimize potential complications. Stone removal can be performed in one or two stages. The two-stage approach is establishment of a track on day one, followed by track enlargement and stone removal at a later date. The two-stage approach allows for greater flexibility, especially if nephrostomy track creation is difficult. A single-stage procedure involves establishment of a track and nephrolithotomy procedure under the same general anesthesia. This typically requires the patient to be transferred from the interventional suite to the surgical suite under anesthesia.

The location and size of the renal calculi are initially determined by ultrasound or unenhanced low-dose CT (see also Chaps. 1 and 33). The most important factor for successful percutaneous nephrolithotomy is appropriate placement of the nephrostomy track. A posterolateral puncture of a middle calyx is preferred so that a direct route to the ureter is obtained and an effective tamponade achieved to limit bleeding. However, the target calyx depends on the location of the calculus.

After access to the renal pelvis has been achieved, a 0.035-in. or 0.038-in. guidewire is advanced into the ureter or preferably to the bladder. The presence of a long, stiff guidewire makes later manipulations easier. If the guidewire cannot be passed through the PUJ into the ureter, it is initially coiled in the renal pelvis or upper pole calyx. A directional catheter (JB-1) is used if traversing the PUJ proves difficult. In some cases, retrograde insertion of a guidewire via the bladder may be helpful. Prior to track dilatation, a generous skin incision is made. Track enlargement is accomplished with either progressive dilators or an angioplasty balloon of appropriate size. Final track size is predetermined by the diameter of the endoscope selected. The sheath acts to tamponade the fresh track to prevent bleeding, reduce renal injury, and maintain access to the renal pelvis for insertion of instruments and catheters.

There are multiple techniques that can be used alone or in combination to remove renal calculi. Small stones may be removed under direct vision or fluoroscopic guidance with a stone basket or forceps (Fig. 9). Irrigation and aspiration with saline may be successful in removing stones or fragments smaller than the diameter of the sheath. Occlusion balloon catheters inflated in the ureter distal to the stone may be helpful in preventing dislodgment and passage of fragments into the ureter. Stones larger than 1.5 cm usually require fragmentation prior to removal. Calculi can be crushed mechanically or fragmented by using a laser fiber ≥ 200 micra or with an ultrasonic lithotriptor.

At the conclusion of the procedure, a plain radiograph or CT scan may be obtained to look for residual fragments not visible fluoroscopically. With a guidewire in place, the sheath is removed, and a council catheter (end-hole Foley) or pigtail catheter, measuring the same diameter as the track, is inserted to provide access to the renal pelvis if needed and to provide continued tamponade. At 48 h, a repeat abdominal radiograph, supplemented by a CT scan if necessary, is obtained to look for residual stones or fragments. If no residual is found, a nephrostogram is performed to confirm patency of the ureter. If the ureter is normal, the nephrostomy tube is clamped for 24–48 h, and if no problems occur, the tube is removed.

The excellent results with nephrolithotomy in adults (Ball et al. 1986; Boddy et al. 1987; Hulbert et al. 1985) led to its application in children. Although most children were over 5 years of age in the reported pediatric series, percutaneous stone removal in younger children has been successful (Ball et al. 1986). The percutaneous approach has been especially useful in managing recurrent renal calculi in children who have had multiple open surgical procedures.

Bleeding and sepsis are the most frequent complications of percutaneous nephrolithotomy (Lee et al. 1985; LeRoy and Segura 1986). Some degree of hematuria occurs in most patients, and although it is usually not of clinical significance, occasionally a transfusion is needed. Delayed bleeding due to a leaking pseudoaneurysm or arteriovenous fistula has been reported in adult series, but not in children. Infection resulting from accessing an infected urinary tract or infected calculus may also occur. Using antibiotics before the procedure, avoiding overdistension of the renal pelvis and collecting system, and adequately draining the collecting system minimize this risk.

Perforation of the renal pelvis or ureter may occur. These tears usually seal spontaneously within 72 h if adequate drainage is provided. Renal pelvic and ureteral edema requiring prolonged nephrostomy drainage is uncommon, and delayed ureteral or ureteropelvic stricture has not

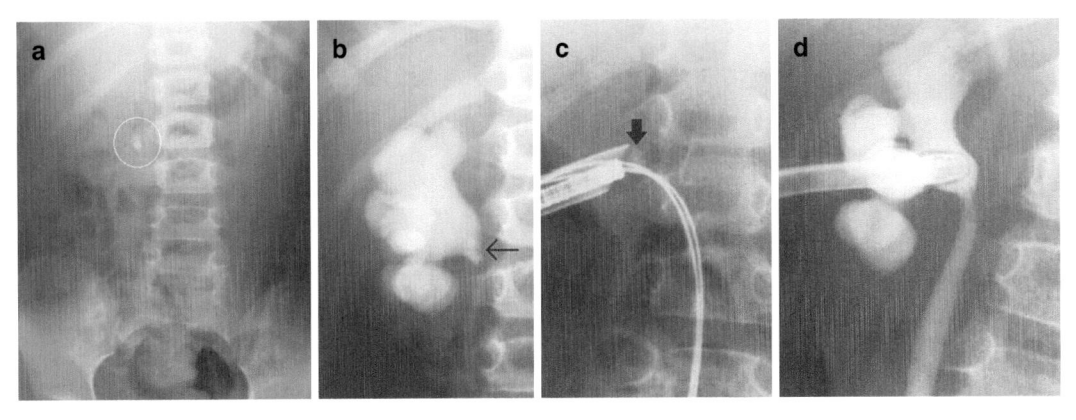

Fig. 9 (**a**) An 8-year-old boy presenting with renal colic secondary to a stone obstruction at the right UPJ (*white circle*). (**b**) Excretory nephroureterogram confirms stone position (*arrow*) and demonstrates moderate hydronephrosis. (**c**) After puncture of the middle pole calyx, tract dilation, and insertion of guidewires and a sheath, the stone (*arrow*) was removed endoscopically. (**d**) A Council tube was inserted at the completion of the procedure for drainage and to maintain renal access

been reported in children. A potential complication is extravasation of irrigation fluid from the percutaneous track producing fluid overload, pleural effusion, and retroperitoneal collections. A postprocedural chest radiograph is routinely obtained when an intercostal approach has been used to exclude hydrothorax or even pneumothorax; increasingly US is used for this purpose.

> **Take Away**
> Renal stones can be safely and effectively removed using percutaneous surgical techniques. An interventionalist working with urologists makes a good team for treatment of renal stones. Procedures are usually performed under general anesthesia.

2.4.3 Percutaneous Endopyelotomy (Percutaneous Pyeloplasty)

In 1943, Davis described the intubated ureterostomy for treatment of ureteral and PUJ strictures (David 1943). In this procedure the ureter was incised from the outside and stented. He showed that the ureter would heal and maintain a larger diameter, thereby resolving the obstruction. Forty years later, the endoscopic counterpart to the Davis intubated ureterostomy was described (Wickham and Kellett 1983; Whitfield et al. 1983). Using a nephroscope, PUJ obstruction was treated by incising the stricture under direct vision using a cold knife. The work of these pioneers and others provided the foundation for developing percutaneous surgical treatment of ureteral strictures in children. Badlani and Smith (1986) later popularized the endopyelotomy technique. Their results and those of other investigators compared favorably to those achieved by open pyeloplasty. In 1987, Towbin and colleagues proved that the percutaneous approach could be successfully performed in children with congenital PUJ obstruction. Dismembered pyeloplasty remains the mainstay for treating children with strictures of the PUJ. However, with the development of percutaneous surgical techniques, percutaneous endopyelotomy (PE) has become an acceptable alternative. PE can be performed as a one- or two-step procedure, as is the case for nephrolithotomy; the one-step approach is preferable.

The indications for an endopyelotomy are similar to those for an open surgical procedure. Children with congenital or acquired strictures of the ureteropelvic junction or ureteral strictures elsewhere are candidates for endopyelotomy (Fig. 10). Although there are few absolute contraindications to either the percutaneous (antegrade) or endoscopic (retrograde) approach, children with long (>2 cm) strictures respond poorly to PE and should likely go directly to an open procedure. Very small children may also benefit from open surgery. As is true for other genitourinary interventions, children with an uncorrectable coagulopathy, those who are medically unstable, and those with inaccessible anatomy are not candidates for percutaneous endopyelotomy.

Procedural Details and Technique

An endopyelotomy is begun with a guidewire inserted into the renal pelvis in retrograde fashion. Retrograde guidewire placement is often easier, especially in patients with an eccentric stenosis of the PUJ. If difficulty passing the guidewire is encountered, the antegrade approach may be utilized. With the antegrade approach, a directional catheter and guidewire are used to probe until the guidewire is directed past the stricture into the bladder.

The child is positioned prone or prone-oblique, and a percutaneous nephrostomy is performed. Once renal access has been obtained, the track is dilated to the predetermined size. A sheath 2 French larger than the diameter of the largest instrument to be used is left in place. After the stenosis has been crossed with a guidewire, it is retrieved and pulled out of the urethra or renal pelvis, depending on the site of insertion. A hemostat is fastened to the distal end (urethral side) so that the guidewire cannot be inadvertently removed during the procedure. In this circumstance, a second guidewire (safety wire) is not necessary. A Rutner valve (Cook Inc.) is connected to the sheath so that an endoscope can be used without using large volumes of water while maintaining a dry field. Using a combination of direct vision and fluoroscopy, the endoscope is maneuvered to the PUJ, and an incision is made with electrocautery (Fig. 10), knife blade, laser, or an Acucise cutting balloon (Applied Medical Resource Company, Laguna Hills, CA), through the posterolateral wall of the PUJ. The posterolateral wall is selected for the site of incision since this is an unlikely area for vessels to course. Regardless of the instrument used, the incision is made through the full thickness of the PUJ until periureteric fat is identified. The procedure is completed by insertion of a 5- or 6-French internal stent and nephrostomy tube (Fig. 10).

The best results with percutaneous endopyelotomy have been achieved in children with a stricture occurring within a few months of an injury or surgery. In addition to postoperative strictures, congenital PUJ narrowing, strictures associated with stones, and those secondary to tumors have all been successfully managed with percutaneous treatment. Variable results have been seen with long segment ureteral strictures. Results with balloon dilatation of congenital and acquired PUJ strictures have been mixed. Percutaneous pyeloplasty has been an effective method of treatment in children with congenital PUJ strictures and is a good alternative for children who have contraindications to surgery or whose family prefers the percutaneous approach.

Following PE, the child is typically admitted overnight to monitor vital signs and assess for and

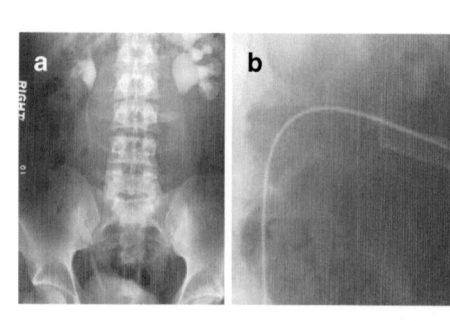

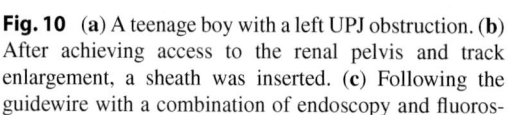

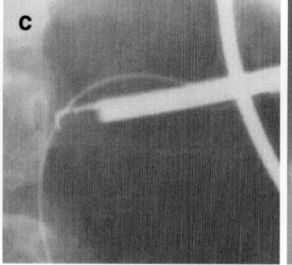

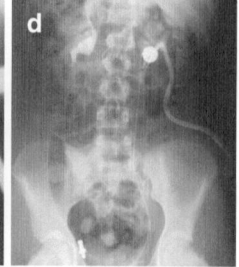

Fig. 10 (a) A teenage boy with a left UPJ obstruction. (b) After achieving access to the renal pelvis and track enlargement, a sheath was inserted. (c) Following the guidewire with a combination of endoscopy and fluoroscopy, the posterolateral UPJ stricture was inserted using electrocautery. (d) The UPJ was stented with an internal (double J) stent and a nephrostomy inserted

treat untoward effects. Most children require analgesia for mild to moderate discomfort. After discharge, the child is instructed to resume normal activity as tolerated. Two weeks after the percutaneous endopyelotomy, a nephrostogram is performed in interventional radiology. If there is prompt antegrade flow of contrast and there is no extravasation or other complication, the nephrostomy tube is removed. The internal stent is kept in place for 6–8 weeks to allow the PUJ incision to heal. The stent is subsequently removed cystoscopically.

The success rate of an endopyelotomy for treatment of strictures at the PUJ is about 85 % with a range of 57–100 % (Towbin et al. 1987; Badlani et al. 1986; Capulicchio et al. 1997; Khan et al. 1997; Kavoussi et al. 1993; Motola et al. 1993). It appears that a failed endopyelotomy does not jeopardize the success of a subsequently performed open surgical procedure. The success rates achieved for endoscopic and percutaneous endopyelotomy are similar (Kavoussi et al. 1993; Brooks et al. 1995).

The complication rate is low with endopyelotomy. The exact rate and type of complications depend somewhat upon the technical approach selected and the indication for therapy. Major complications have been reported and include hemorrhage requiring transfusion or occasionally embolization, ureteral necrosis, and ureteral avulsion. However, minor problems occur more frequently (10–23 %) and include stent or nephrostomy-related problems. Minor complications include stent repositioning, retroperitoneal hematoma, dysuria, flank pain, and stenoses in the ureter, UVJ, or urethra. The incidence and type of complications occurring using the Acucise device appear to be similar to the other methods. It is important to acknowledge that it is possible to lacerate adjacent blood vessels and cause major hemorrhage. Fortunately, vascular injury is uncommon and occurs in less than 1 % of cases (Gerber and Lyon 1994; Bogaert et al. 1996; Figenshau et al. 1996). Other possible untoward effects include congestive heart failure, oliguria, hematuria, intrarenal clots, recurrent strictures, and hydrothorax or pneumothorax. The latter two problems can occur when the pleural space is transgressed at the time of renal access. Therefore, it is imperative that the operator be aware of the position of the posterior costophrenic sulcus.

Percutaneous endopyelotomy appears to be a safe and effective method for the treatment of both primary and secondary strictures of the ureter and PUJ. Each approach appears to result in a successful outcome with a low complication rate and good long-term patency. Open surgery still remains the gold standard for the treatment of either primary or secondary PUJ obstruction in most institutions. Proponents of endopyelotomy suggest that the reduced overall morbidity, decreased postoperative analgesic requirements, shortened hospital stay, and diminished time to return to normal activity favor the endourologic approach.

Minimally invasive diagnostic and therapeutic procedures are well suited for the pediatric urinary tract. It seems that the advantages of the percutaneous approach may be ideal for treating children and are especially cost-effective. Thus, one can expect that the interventional approach will continue to grow with a broadening of indications.

> **Take Away**
> Percutaneous surgery is best performed under general anesthesia. Incision of the PUJ can be achieved using a variety of methods including a cold knife, electrocautery, or a laser. Percutaneous endopyelotomy is an acceptable alternative for treating congenital PUJ stenosis. Other ureteric strictures/stenoses may be approached in a similar way.

2.5 Percutaneous Renal Biopsy

Prior to 1951, renal biopsies were performed by open surgical procedures. The change to a percutaneous biopsy occurred after the publication by Iverson and Brun. In the beginning, percutaneous biopsies were guided by excretory urography or anatomic landmarks (Uppot et al. 2010). Imaging-guided renal biopsy began in the early 1960s, and the imaging guidance component has become more sophisticated and the standard for renal biopsy over time and has led to increased safety and accuracy.

Percutaneous renal biopsy using ultrasound (US) guidance can be expected to be successful in almost all cases. In our practice, renal biopsy to diagnose medical renal diseases or for transplant surveillance is the most common indication. Technical success in obtaining diagnostic specimens has occurred in about 99 % of cases. Today, the percutaneous approach is the procedure of choice for both routine and targeted renal biopsies. Open surgical biopsies are now rarely performed and are considered when percutaneous biopsy fails to provide a diagnosis or if surgical resection can be carried out at the time of biopsy.

The most common indications for renal biopsy in the pediatric population include:

1. Medical renal disease: hematuria, proteinuria, renal failure or impending renal failure, and renal transplant surveillance (possible rejection, BK nephropathy, drug toxicity, and possible recurrent disease) (see Chaps. 12, 32, and 34)
2. Mass lesions (see also Chap. 36)

Although uncommon, absolute and relative contraindications to percutaneous renal biopsy are present. The absolute contraindications include uncorrectable coagulopathy, uncontrolled severe hypertension, and, in some cases, a solitary kidney. Relative contraindications may include azotemia, unfavorable anatomy, acute urinary tract infection and pyonephrosis, and morbid obesity making US guidance challenging. In this latter situation, CT guidance may be a solution.

Procedural Details and Technique
(See Also Chap. 32)
To maximize patient safety and technical success when performing percutaneous renal biopsy, one must take patient preparation seriously. It is our preference to obtain a complete blood count, coagulation profile, INR and pre-procedural US prior to the biopsy. The purpose of the pre-procedural imaging is to identify an anatomic abnormality such as a pelvic kidney, renal cystic disease, or any condition that can alter the technical approach. If the hemoglobin is too low (<8 g/dL), platelets are less than 50,000/uL, or the PT/aPTT is abnormal, the abnormality is corrected by giving the appropriate blood product and correction verified with the appropriate follow-up laboratory study. In addition, in these situations or when there is concern for a higher risk of bleeding, e.g., systemic lupus erythematosus, a coaxial biopsy technique with track embolization using Gelfoam slurry through the introducer needle may be utilized.

All renal biopsies are performed using real-time US guidance if possible. In the rare instance when real-time US is not helpful, CT guidance is substituted. When the goal of the procedure is obtaining tissue for medical renal disease in native kidneys, an 18-gauge end-cutting biopsy needle is utilized, and two to three specimens are obtained from the lower pole of typically the left kidney (Fig. 11). However, when a renal mass is present, a 16-gauge needle is preferred and a coaxial technique is always used. Also, if the mass is large, we obtain samples from many quadrants of the lesion and try to avoid sampling the center of the lesion because this area most often has areas of necrosis. The goal of a mass lesion biopsy is to obtain five to ten cores, more if the pathologist requires more material.

Our standard procedure is to perform the biopsy under sedation or general anesthesia, although the latter is currently more common. Prior to sterile preparation, a survey US is performed to examine the renal anatomy or the location and size of the mass. The preferred needle size and type and transport materials are selected depending on the preference of the pathology department. The preferred US transducer is selected and draped in sterile fashion. The biopsy is carried out using real-time US guidance and the specimens are obtained as described above. In our practice, the specimens are reviewed by the pathologist to ensure that diagnostic tissue is obtained before the procedure is considered complete. If needed, additional specimens are obtained. If, after pathologic review, the specimens are adequate, postprocedural US with Doppler is performed to exclude a

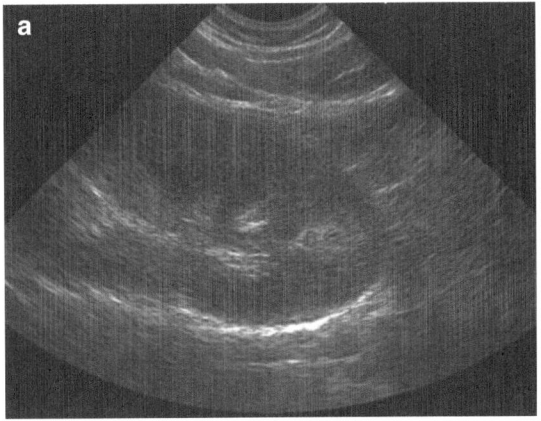

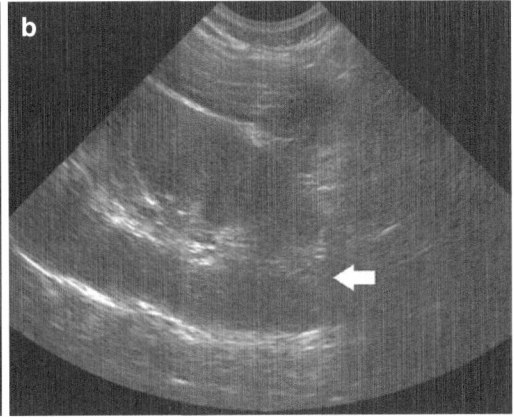

Fig. 11 13-year-old female with Henoch-Schonlein purpura and new onset hematuria. (**a**) Sagittal grayscale ultrasound along the long axis of the kidney to identify lower pole cortex for biopsy. (**b**) 18-gauge biopsy needle traversing the lower pole calyx (*arrow*). Core specimens revealed IgA nephropathy

bleeding complication. If stable, the child is discharged to the recovery room for observation. While in the recovery room, the child's vital signs are continuously monitored, urine output is observed, and if there is gross hematuria, a urine rack is set up and urine samples (<5 ml) collected in a test tube so that the color can be compared to prior specimens. This approach makes it easy to follow the evolution of the blood loss. If the child has gross hematuria and/or pain, a follow-up US is performed, and if there is a significant hematoma, the child is admitted to the hospital for 24 h observation. If bleeding is severe, persists, or is associated with a pseudoaneurysm or an arteriovenous fistula, renal angiography with potential therapeutic embolization is considered. In the past the child was observed for 23 h or overnight. Today, children are discharged after 4 h of observation if no complication has occurred.

Since 2010, we have performed an increasing number of renal biopsies on an outpatient basis. A postprocedure CBC is obtained at 4 h. We anticipate the hematocrit will fall by three to six points while the hemoglobin will drop by less than 2 gm/dL. If these criteria are present and the child is asymptomatic, the child is discharged to home. If symptoms are present and/or there is a fall in hematocrit or hemoglobin beyond this range, the child will be assessed. The decision to discharge the child is always made in the most conservative manner. We also tend to observe patients for a longer period of time if they live significant distances from the hospital; other places have other routines, often a standard follow-up US is performed after 4–6 h or before discharge.

Take Away
Renal biopsies are performed for a wide range of indications. Currently, whenever possible, we perform ultrasound-guided biopsies on an outpatient basis. If after 4 h of observation no complications are identified, the child may be discharged to home.

2.6 Percutaneous Cystostomy

The creation of suprapubic access to the urinary bladder has historically been performed surgically. When surgery is performed, a stoma is created between the skin and urinary bladder, and a collection bag is usually attached directly to the skin with adhesive, and urine exits the cystostomy and collects in the bag. Although the surgical approach is still an option, percutaneous puncture of the bladder with insertion of an indwelling catheter is now the preferred approach in most cases (Irby and Stoller 1993). This approach creates a track between the urinary bladder and skin, and urine is drained via the catheter into a collection bag.

The indications for insertion of a percutaneous suprapubic cystostomy vary and include any child that needs a urinary catheter but cannot be catheterized via the urethra. The most common indications are bladder outlet obstruction and perineal/pelvic trauma, e.g., a straddle injury.

Procedural Details and Technique

Technically, the insertion of a suprapubic cystostomy is usually straightforward and can be placed using local anesthesia, sedation, or general anesthesia, depending on the situation. Today, US guidance is utilized to guide needle puncture in most cases also to assure a sufficient bladder filling. While a midline approach via the linea alba inferior to the umbilicus is the classic skin entry site, US guidance allows for bladder entry at almost any location and helps avoid injury to blood vessels and adjacent structures. We prefer to use a 5-French Yueh sheathed needle to traverse the bladder using US guidance, followed by placement of an angled guidewire through the sheath, which is then looped in the bladder, visualized under fluoroscopy. Subsequently, the track is serially dilated, and an 8.5-French locking pigtail drainage catheter is placed in the bladder over the guidewire. In most cases, gravity drainage is all that is needed.

> **Take Away**
> Percutaneous cystostomy is a simple procedure that may have an important role in the management of children with poorly functioning bladders. Although a midline puncture is preferred, ultrasound-guided paramedian punctures are also safe and effective when needed.

3 Vascular Interventions

3.1 Percutaneous Renal Angioplasty

Renovascular hypertension continues to be a diagnostic and therapeutic challenge in the pediatric population (see Chap. 35). Up to 2 % of children suffer from systemic hypertension, and in as many as 20 % of these individuals, the underlying pathology involves the renal arteries (Haas et al. 2002). Treatment of this subgroup of children depends largely on the location and underlying pathology of the renal artery stenosis (RAS). Fortunately, the most common etiology of main or branch renal artery stenosis in children is fibromuscular dysplasia (FMD), which is amenable to percutaneous transluminal renal angioplasty (PTRA). PTRA has a high technical and clinical success rate. Also, PTRA is currently considered the treatment of choice for RAS due to FMD (Levy et al. 2000). Renal artery ostial and aorto-renal narrowing is often associated with syndromes such as neurofibromatosis or Williams syndrome or is due to arteritis or mid-aortic syndrome (Courtel et al. 1998; Lund et al. 1984; Booth et al. 2002; Robinson et al. 1991; Kurien et al. 1997; Haas et al. 2002; Shroff et al. 2006; Panayiotopoulos et al. 1996; Daniels et al. 1987; Mali et al. 1987; Ellis et al. 1995; Arora et al. 1997; Fostera et al. 2000; Cura et al. 2002; Hughes et al. 2004). These lesions are often resistant to percutaneous transluminal angioplasty (PTA) and in the past have required surgical revascularization when medical therapy failed.

In a prospective study of 35 children with renovascular hypertension, Tyagi and colleagues (1997) found PTRA to have a beneficial effect on blood pressure in 93.1 % of children. Unfortunately, restenosis occurred in 25.8 % of lesions treated percutaneously. In adults, renal artery stenting is commonplace for lesions not responding to PTRA. However, renal artery stenting (Ing et al. 1995) has been avoided in children whenever possible due to technical issues (McLaren and Roebuck 2003) related to the size of the vessels and concerns that stents may limit arterial growth, make subsequent surgical revascularization more complicated, and predispose to renal artery thrombosis.

The equipment necessary to perform a PTRA in a child is generally available today and should be tailored to the size and weight of the child. The first step in a child with hypertension, suspected of having main or branch renal artery narrowing, is to do cross-sectional imaging.

Although noninvasive imaging cannot definitively rule out renal artery stenosis, it is important to evaluate the child for nonrenal causes of hypertension as well as renal arterial disease. Cross-sectional imaging is also valuable for planning of an interventional procedure. In our practice, renal vein and inferior vena cava renin levels are collected to help localize a lesion. Renal vein renin sampling is performed just prior to the renal angiogram, under the same sedation or anesthetic. Next, diagnostic abdominal aortography and selective renal angiography are performed to define the pathologic anatomy. In most children, AP and oblique projections are performed to best evaluate the renal vasculature. The most common site for stenosis is the main renal artery. However, the most challenging area for diagnosis is the branch renal arteries. Often the angiographer needs to look carefully and have a high level of suspicion to find these subtle lesions. If necessary, selective injections in a variety of obliquities may be required to confirm the diagnosis.

Procedural Details and Technique

Our approach to the angiographic examination of these children is to begin with an abdominal aortogram in frontal projection to evaluate the aortorenal junction and main renal arteries. The examination begins with puncture of the right common femoral artery. In all children >10 kg, a hemostasis sheath is inserted into the artery. The sheath must be large enough to accept an angioplasty catheter. Initially, a 3–5-French pigtail catheter is inserted and positioned in the aorta just cephalad to the origin of the renal arteries, and approximately 1.0–1.5 ml/kg of contrast agent (maximum 40 mL) is power injected over two seconds, and the aortogram images are obtained at three frames/s. In selected instances (rapid heart rates, high-flow lesions) faster film rates (up to six frames/s) are utilized. Next, a selective catheter (RIM, C-1, JB-1) is positioned in the proximal renal artery. In the anterior oblique projection [usually 30°], a selective renal angiogram is performed with a contrast injection over 2 s using a volume of 0.25–0.5 ml/kg (maximum 10 mL). Again images are obtained at a minimum of 3 frames/s. When possible, pressure measurements are obtained across the area of stenosis.

If an area of stenosis >50% is identified, the child is considered for PTRA after consultation with the nephrologist. In preparation for PTRA, the narrowest diameter and length of the stenosis are measured as is the diameter of the adjacent normal caliber renal artery. We prefer to select the angioplasty balloon that most closely approximates the normal arterial size and will not dilate the stenotic artery to greater than 10% more than the predicted normal diameter. In addition, the balloon selected will generally be the one with the highest inflation pressure. Our goal is to dilate the artery to the measured level on the initial attempt. Before PTRA, the child is heparinized to reduce the incidence of renal artery thrombosis and renal loss. A successful PTRA is often signaled by elimination of the "waist" as the balloon inflates to size and improvement in the pressure measurement across the lesion (Fig. 12). At the completion of the angioplasty, a follow-up angiogram is performed to assess outcome and to identify complications if present. If there is significant improvement in the stenosis post PTRA, no further treatment is performed. If there is significant residual stenosis, repeat angioplasty with a larger balloon or stenting may be considered. Since there may be clinical improvement even in children with disappointing visual results, a conservative approach is preferred. The procedure is concluded if the visual result suggests less than 50% narrowing, if there is a reduction in the measured gradient across the stenosis, if the collateral vessels are no longer seen, or if the operator is uncomfortable with additional treatment (Fig. 13). At the conclusion of the procedure, the child is taken to the intensive care unit for observation and continuous monitoring of blood pressure and vital signs. Heparin is continued until discharge or converted to oral medications, which are continued for several months.

If, upon clinical follow-up, there is improvement in blood pressure, no additional intervention may be needed. However, if hypertension persists, repeat US, CTA, or MRA can be performed to evaluate renal artery anatomy and flow. If further vascular intervention is considered, repeat angiography is performed. If re-treatment is needed, repeat PTRA or cutting balloon angioplasty (CBA) may be considered. Stenting is less desirable in younger children.

In 1991, Barath and colleagues (1991) introduced the cutting balloon, a device consisting of three or four metal blades mounted on the surface of the balloon catheter parallel to the long axis of the catheter (Fig. 14). Upon inflation of the balloon, the blades are exposed and create radially distributed longitudinal atherotome incisions into the intimal and medial lay-

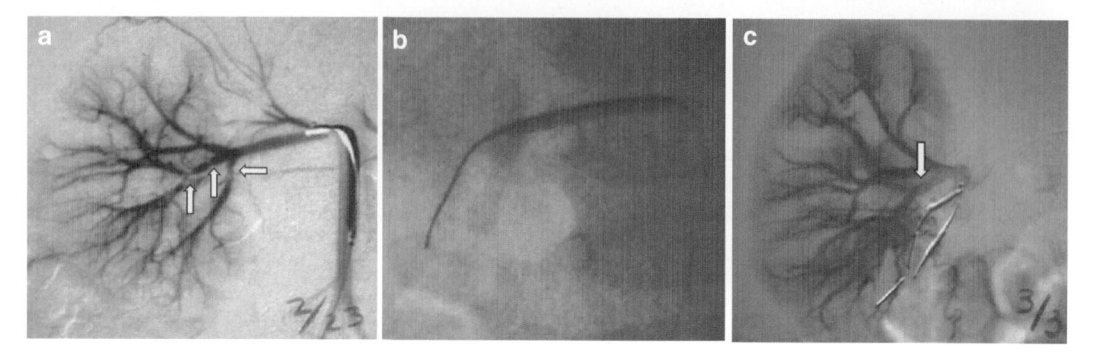

Fig. 12 4-year-old girl with severe hypertension that failed medical therapy. (**a**) Selective right renal arteriography demonstrates branch renal artery stenosis (*arrows*) with the presumed diagnosis of fibromuscular dysplasia. (**b**) Using a microangioplasty balloon, the middle pole segmental renal artery branch was dilated. However, the stenotic lower pole segmental artery could not be accessed with an angioplasty balloon. Therefore, segmental embolization was performed. (**c**) Postangioplasty resolution of middle branch stenosis (*arrow*) and microcoil embolization of the lower pole branches. Postprocedure, the hypertension was treated with fewer drugs but not cured

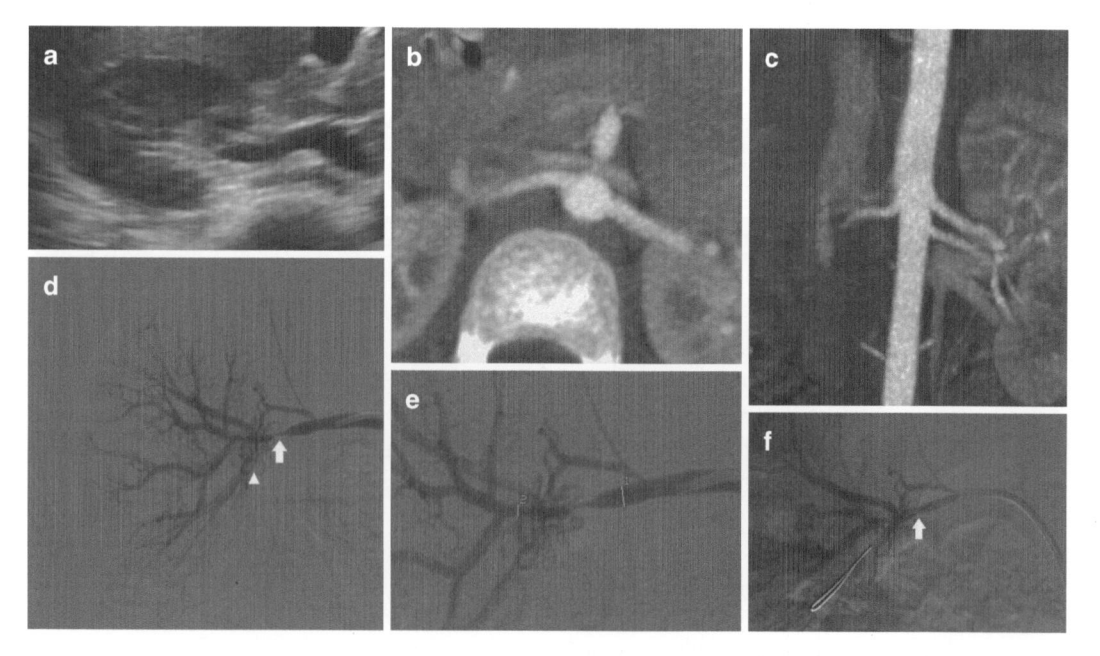

Fig. 13 7-year-old male with hypertension refractory to medical therapy. (**a**) Ultrasound evaluation of the renal arteries was normal. (**b, c**) CTA of the renal arteries was unable to provide definitive diagnosis. (**d**) Digital subtraction angiography of the main right renal artery demonstrates focal, high-grade stenosis (*arrow*) with intrarenal collaterals (*arrowhead*). (**e**) Pre- and post-stenotic vessel measurements for selection of appropriate balloon catheter. (**f**) Postangioplasty image demonstrating almost complete resolution of the stenosis with only a minimal residual waist (*arrow*)

ers of the artery. Unterberg et al. (1993) reported the first clinical use of the cutting balloon for the treatment of a coronary artery stenosis. Since then, the use of the cutting balloon in children has been reported for the treatment of peripheral pulmonary artery stenosis (Rhodes et al. 2002) and in a small number of adolescents and young adults (Haas et al. 2002; Lupatteli et al. 2005; Oguzkurt et al. 2005; Tanemoto et al. 2005) and in children (Caramella et al. 2005; Towbin et al. 2007) with resistant RAS. This new technology may allow for treatment of resistant stenosis, especially in children with syndromes and arteritides that result in renal artery stenoses. In the past, these lesions responded poorly to PTRA and usually required open surgery. In these conditions there is typically aorto-renal or proximal renal artery involvement. This pattern of involvement makes treatment with PTRA less effective with a high rate of failure (Booth et al. 2002; Ing et al. 1995). In patients with syndromic causes, renal artery lesions are more often bilateral and are usually localized to the ostia of the renal arteries (Ing et al. 1995). In these children cutting balloon angioplasty is the most effective choice for treatment of hypertension due to resistant RAS (Haas et al. 2002) (Fig. 15). Cutting balloons are now available in a wider variety of diameters and lengths, with a range suitable for treatment of pediatric lesions.

The complications associated with the use of cutting balloons for the treatment of hypertension related to resistant RAS are similar to those described for PTRA, including dissection, rupture, delayed pseudoaneurysm, and renal artery thrombosis. The possibility of arterial injury should be communicated during the informed consent process, and specific surveillance should be employed to exclude this complication at the conclusion of the CBA procedure.

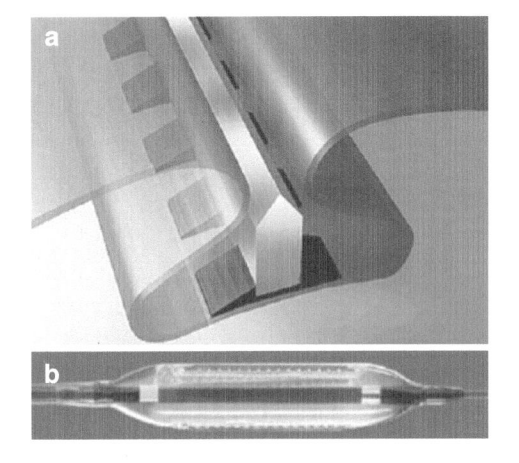

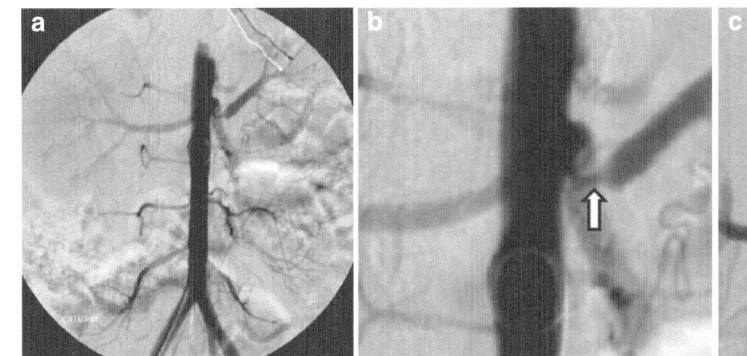

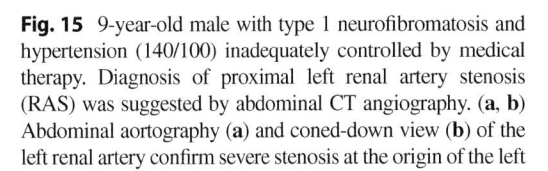

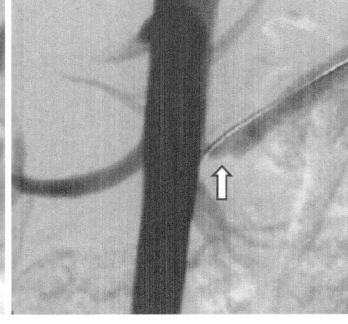

Fig. 14 Cutting balloon angioplasty. (**a**) An artistic drawing of a cutting balloon blade. (**b**) Picture of a cutting balloon catheter

Fig. 15 9-year-old male with type 1 neurofibromatosis and hypertension (140/100) inadequately controlled by medical therapy. Diagnosis of proximal left renal artery stenosis (RAS) was suggested by abdominal CT angiography. (**a, b**) Abdominal aortography (**a**) and coned-down view (**b**) of the left renal artery confirm severe stenosis at the origin of the left renal artery (*arrow*) with associated post-stenotic dilatation. (**c**) Balloon angioplasty was performed without success with a residual pressure gradient of 45 mmHg. A cutting balloon (Interventional Technologies, San Diego, CA) was utilized with follow-up angiography (*arrow*) showing mild residual stenosis with a pressure gradient less than 15 mmHg

In the rare instance of arterial rupture with associated hemorrhage, balloon tamponade of arterial extravasation (Towbin et al. 2007) offers at least one salvage strategy that may preserve a successful final outcome. Additional recommendations that may increase safety include pre-procedure imaging of the arterial wall, such as with intravascular ultrasound (Lupatteli et al. 2005), to place the cutting balloon in the safest position. We agree with Tanemoto and colleagues (2005) that it may be a safer strategy to limit the cutting balloon diameter to no more than the normal vessel diameter in the incisional phase. Then, if necessary, the lumen can be further enlarged with PTRA.

> **Take Away**
> PTRA has long been an option for the minimally invasive treatment of children with renovascular hypertension. Angioplasty is especially effective in children with fibromuscular dysplasia. With the advent of the cutting balloon, children with lesions resistant to traditional angioplasty, such as those with syndromes and arteritis, can now be considered for interventional therapy, though long-term follow-up is still pending.

3.2 Embolotherapy of the Genitourinary System

3.2.1 Renal Arterial Embolization

Since the development of renal artery embolization in the 1970s, it has become a versatile therapeutic and supportive technique for the treatment of a variety of conditions affecting the kidney in the pediatric population. Prior to the development of renal endovascular techniques, open surgery was the only option to improve normal renal parenchymal perfusion due to renal arterial anomalies or to decrease perfusion to renal masses. Although the open surgical approach was effective, it was associated with high morbidity and mortality. Today, selective renal angiography with embolization is the treatment of choice for children with renovascular trauma associated with major blood loss and hemodynamic instability, congenital or acquired (iatrogenic) arteriovenous fistulas, and arteriovenous malformations and for treatment of complications of angiomyolipomas (Fig. 16) and complications following renal transplantation. Although rare, embolization may be an option for small-branch stenosis not amenable to angioplasty and as presurgical treatment for vascular neoplasms to reduce blood loss during surgery.

Procedural Details and Technique

Technically the same approach is used for embolization of the renal artery as would be used for any vessel in a child. The choice of sheath with hemostasis valve, directional catheter, and guidewire depends upon the patient's weight and common femoral artery and target vessel size. In general, we try to use a 4-French hemostasis sheath for children weighing between 11 and 30 kg and a 5-French sheath for children over 30 kg. The most difficult decision is what to choose for children <10 kg since in this group, a 3-French hemostasis sheath is preferred but, for the most part, is not available. Therefore, it is important to realize that the outer diameter of a 3-French sheath is about 4.5 French and requires a vessel with an inner diameter of at least two mm. It is also important to remember that in these small children, it is essential to maintain temperature control and carefully monitor contrast administered and total fluid volume to avoid fluid overload. Additionally, heparin should be administered in children <10 kg after accessing the common femoral artery.

After selective catheterization of the target vessel with a directional catheter or microcatheter, embolization can be accomplished using a variety of materials, depending on the lesion type. For example, particles would not be appropriate for the treatment of an AV fistula because it would result in distant embolization. In this situation, coils, Amplatzer plugs, and/or tissue adhesives would be a good choice. Particles, however, are a good choice for the treatment of traumatic bleeds and angiomyolipomas. In general, the choice of embolic material often depends on the preference of the interventionalist.

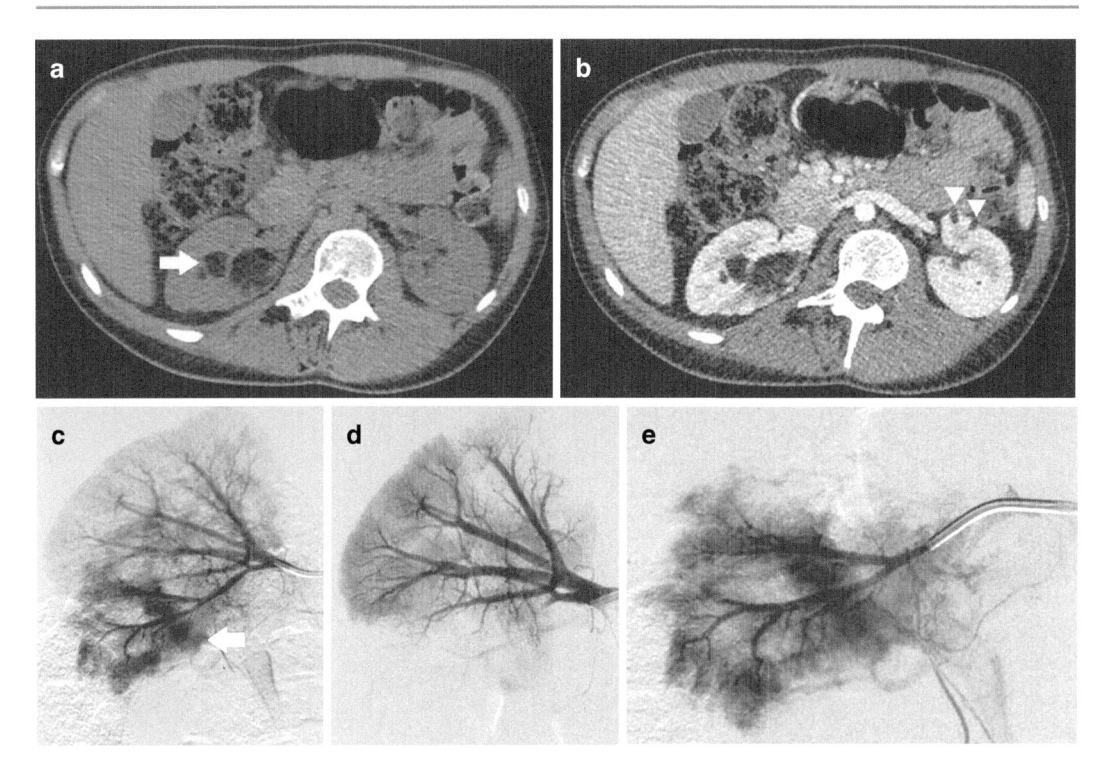

Fig. 16 21-year-old female with tuberous sclerosis and right flank pain. (**a, b**) Pre- and post-contrast abdominal CT demonstrates a large, multi-lobulated right renal angiomyolipoma (*arrow*) with several subcentimeter similar left renal masses (*arrowheads*). (**c**) Distal right renal digital subtraction angiography demonstrates abnormal patchy enhancement of the right lower pole angiomyolipoma (*arrow*). (**d**) Super-selective angiography of the right lower pole arterial branch just prior to embolization with 300–500 micron embospheres. (**e**) Post-embolization angiography demonstrates no residual arterial supply to the mass

> **Take Away**
> Embolization of renal lesions is uncommon in the pediatric population but when necessary is quite effective. In experienced hands, renal embolization can be utilized in children of all ages. However, in children less than 10 kg, special precautions should be taken.

3.2.2 Priapism

Priapism can occur at any age and is defined as a prolonged involuntary penile erection not caused by sexual arousal. The condition may be classified as either high flow or low flow depending upon the underlying cause. Low-flow priapism is more common in childhood and results from obstructed outflow from the corpora cavernosa with secondary venous stasis, acidosis, and in some cases ischemia. When there is ischemia, pain is usually present. The most common etiologies include sickle cell anemia, hypercoagulable states, leukemia, and medications. Low-flow priapism should be treated immediately, because delayed therapy may result in corporal smooth muscle injury with subsequent fibrosis and cavernosal artery thrombosis and occlusion, with potential irreversible impotence.

In contrast, high-flow priapism is usually non-painful and results from excessive arterial inflow that is secondary to arterial injury with a fistula between the artery and corpus cavernosum. The typical clinical presentation is an erection without involvement of the corpus spongiosum (glans). There is often a delay in the onset of symptoms, typically about 3 days post-injury. In childhood, the most common cause of high-flow priapism is a straddle injury.

It is important to differentiate between high- and low-flow priapism because the approach to therapy is different. The history and physical examination is helpful, but not always accurate. However, the presence of pain is an important marker since it strongly supports the diagnosis of low-flow priapism. It is helpful to obtain a penile US including Doppler and a cavernosal blood gas to clarify the diagnosis. In children with high-flow priapism, the cavernosal blood gas is arterial and bright red, and the blood gas levels are as expected for any arterial sample. US will reveal hypoechoic cavernosal bodies in the acute phase; Doppler evaluation demonstrates normal to high blood flow and may identify the fistulous connection. In the chronic phase, there may be a pseudoaneurysm with a hyperechoic rim in a cavernous body. A common site for a fistula is in the region of the distal internal pudendal artery, common penile artery, and the cavernosal, dorsal penile, and bulbourethral arteries. In low-flow conditions, (amplitude coded) color Doppler sonography demonstrates minimal to absent flow in the cavernosal arteries. Additionally, blood aspirated from the corpus cavernosum is darker in color and usually acidotic. Also, it may be difficult aspirate blood from the corpus cavernosum because it may be clotted.

Today, the treatment of choice for high-flow priapism is selective embolization of the internal pudendal artery or a branch feeding the arteriovenous fistula. As per the American Urological Association Guideline on the Management of Priapism (2003), embolization utilizing absorbable material has a lower rate of erectile dysfunction than when compared to embolization with permanent materials. Additionally, the rate of resolution of nonischemic priapism following embolization with absorbable and nonabsorbable material is similar. In a small percentage of cases, bilateral internal pudendal artery occlusion may be necessary. If successful, detumescence can be expected over the next several days.

Procedural Details and Technique
The technique used begins with ultrasound-guided puncture of the common femoral artery and insertion of a 4–5-French sheath with hemostasis valve. Next, a unilateral or bilateral common or internal iliac angiogram is performed via a directional catheter, to identify the site of the AVF. Next, in most cases, the internal pudendal artery is selectively catheterized and an angiogram is performed. Once the vascular pathology is demonstrated, a catheter, usually a microcatheter, is superselectively positioned in the feeding artery, and the vessel is occluded. In our practice, we have successfully utilized both Gelfoam and microcoils for embolization.

The treatment of children with low-flow priapism should be undertaken as quickly as possible and, whenever possible, a urologist should be consulted. Treatment is usually stepwise (see the American Urological Association Guideline on the Management of Priapism; 2003) and begins with aspiration of the corpus cavernosum, with or without irrigation, and intracavernous injection of a sympathomimetic agent. If detumescence cannot be achieved, a surgical shunt may be needed. Unfortunately, impotence may result in at least 50 % of patients.

Take Away
Embolotherapy should be considered in young males with priapism resistant to medical therapy.

3.2.3 Internal Spermatic Vein Embolization for Varicocele

The most common intervention involving the renal venous system is for the treatment of a varicocele. Embolization as primary therapy was first promoted in the 1970s and over the years has increased in popularity. Today it is widely accepted as the first line of therapy in most practices. A varicocele is an abnormal enlargement of the pampiniform plexus secondary to gonadal vein insufficiency or uncommonly left renal vein compression. In almost all instances, the left testis is involved. The incidence ranges between 8 and 23 % in boys with the primary reason for treatment being testicular pain or atrophy since fertility is usually unknown at this age (Urbano et al. 2014).

The technique used for embolization is based on selective catheterization of the spermatic vein followed by a gonadal venogram to determine the pathologic anatomy. Historically, a wide variety of materials have been utilized for vein occlusion including boiling contrast, particles, detachable balloons, and absolute alcohol. These agents are rarely used today and have been replaced by coils with or without a sclerosant (sodium tetradecyl or polidocanol foam), tissue adhesive, or Amplatzer plugs. It is currently our preference to use the "sandwich technique" with Gianturco coils (Cook Inc., Bloomington, IN) and sodium tetradecyl (Fig. 17). We place the initial coil at the level of the inferior sacroiliac (SI) joint followed by sclerosant foam. The next coil is deployed at the top of the SI joint followed by foam, with the final coil placed safely below the renal vein or above the highest parallel channel. If needed, sclerosant can be injected into a high parallel channel after selective catheterization with a microcatheter if possible.

The reported recurrence rate post-varicocele embolization is about 12 %, although in our experience, recurrence has occurred in less than 5 % of cases. The risks of embolotherapy include a groin hematoma, pain, gonadal vein perforation, renal vein thrombosis, and distant embolization. Complication rates have been reported to be as high as 11 %; however, in our experience, it is less than 2 %.

> **Take Away**
> Spermatic vein embolization has become the procedure of choice for the treatment of symptomatic varicoceles in young males. It is a safe and effective technique with a technical success rate of nearly 100 %.

3.2.4 Renal Vein Stenting for Nutcracker Phenomenon/Syndrome

The nutcracker syndrome (NCS) is a clinical presentation resulting from renal vein compression between the abdominal aorta and superior mesenteric artery. The condition was first reported in 1950 (El-Sadr and Mina 1950). The condition usually presents with hematuria with or without abdominal or left flank pain. Imaging may demonstrate the presence of collateral veins. In the pediatric age range, this syndrome most often presents in otherwise healthy adolescents (Kurklinsky and Rooke 2010). As a result of the somewhat vague symptoms, diagnosis is often late and indirect. Radiologic evaluation using cross-sectional imaging may be used and is the primary tool for diagnosis. Ultrasound with Doppler is helpful, and, if NCS is considered, should be the first modality utilized (see Chap. 32). When asymmetric enlargement of the left renal vein is noted and

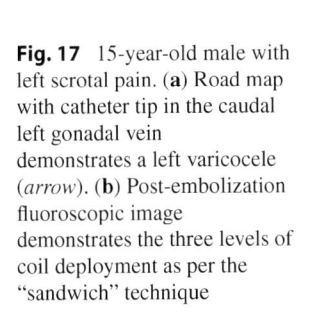

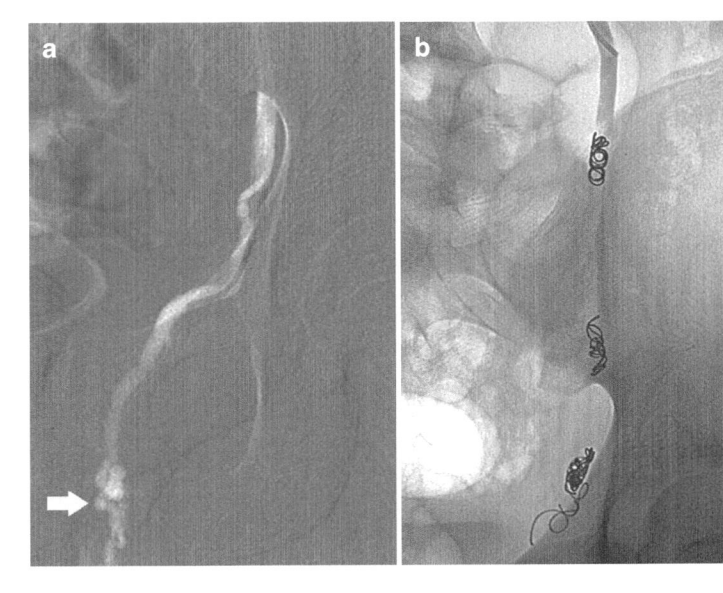

Fig. 17 15-year-old male with left scrotal pain. (**a**) Road map with catheter tip in the caudal left gonadal vein demonstrates a left varicocele (*arrow*). (**b**) Post-embolization fluoroscopic image demonstrates the three levels of coil deployment as per the "sandwich" technique

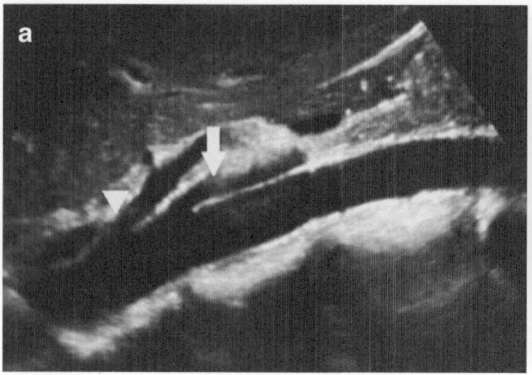

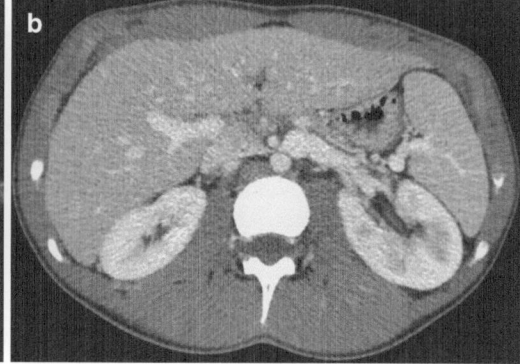

Fig. 18 17-year-old male with chronic abdominal pain secondary to Nutcracker syndrome. (**a**) Sagittal grayscale ultrasound demonstrates a steep course at the origin of the superior mesenteric artery (*arrow*) just below the celiac axis (*arrowhead*). (**b**) Contrast-enhanced CT demonstrates the SMA immediately anterior to the abdominal aorta with abnormal dilatation of the proximal, draining left renal vein

there is a large discrepancy in size between the distended and non-distended segments with collateral vessels, the diagnosis should be considered. When CT or MR is performed, in addition to asymmetric renal vein distention and perirenal collaterals, a 3-D reconstruction may demonstrate the area of extrinsic compression and demonstrate the crossing vessel (Fig. 18), though this can usually be demonstrated with a meticulous US and Doppler study.

Treatment of NCS was first reported in 1974 (Pastershank 1974). In children, the best option may be a conservative approach since the long-term outcomes of many interventional and surgical therapies have not been fully assessed. Also, spontaneous remission has been seen in children during growth. When more aggressive therapy is needed, placement of a stent within the renal vein is a consideration since angioplasty alone will not be successful in most cases. If a stent is placed, anticoagulation is recommended for 2–3 months until stent endothelialization occurs. Alternatively, some patients have been successfully managed with antiplatelet drugs alone. Another therapeutic approach for treatment of NCS has been gonadal vein embolization to treat the symptoms of pelvic congestion or varicocele. This approach may successfully treat the symptoms; however, embolotherapy may be complicated by worsening of left renal vein outflow and increased renal vein pressure, recurrence of pelvic congestion or varicocele, and onset of new renal symptoms.

> **Take Away**
> Children, usually teenagers, with NCS are effectively treated with minimally invasive techniques. It is likely that image-guided stent placement is the first-line procedure for most of these individuals.

4 Summary

Minimally invasive techniques are extremely well suited for the GU system of children. In order to maximize the therapeutic success in this patient group, it is important to work closely and collaboratively with urologists, nephrologists, hospitalists, and pediatricians. Minimally invasive approaches should be the procedures of choice whenever possible since they provide the best outcomes at the lowest risk and cost in most situations. Over the past decade, a greater number of treatment options have become available and proven to be safe even when performed in an outpatient setting.

References

Arora P, Kher V, Singhal MK et al (1997) Renal artery stenosis in aortoarteritis: spectrum of disease in children and adults. Kidney Blood Press Res 20:285–289

Badlani G, Eshghi M, Smith A (1986) Percutaneous surgery for ureteropelvic junction obstruction (endopyelotomy): technique and early results. J Urol 135:26–28

Ball WS, Towbin R, Strife JL, Spencer R (1986) Interventional genitourinary radiology in children: a review of GI procedures. AJR Am J Roentgenol 147:791–797

Barath P, Fishbein MC, Vari S, Forrester JS (1991) Cutting balloon: a novel approach to percutaneous angioplasty. Am J Cardiol 68:1249–1252

Barbaric ZL, Göthlin JH, Davies RS (1977) Transluminal dilatation and stent placement in obstructed ureters in dogs through the use of percutaneous nephropyelostomy. Invest Radiol 12:534–536

Boddy SAM, Kellett MJ, Fletcher MS et al (1987) Extracorporeal shock wave lithotripsy and percutaneous nephrolithotomy in children. J Pediatr Surg 22:223–227

Bogaert GA, Kogan BA, Mevorach RA et al (1996) Efficacy of retrograde endopyelotomy in children. J Urol 156:734–737

Booth C, Preston R, Clark G, Reidy J (2002) Management of renal vascular disease in neurofibromatosis type 1 and the role of percutaneous transluminal angioplasty. Nephrol Dial Transplant 17:1235–1240

Brooks JD, Kavoussi LR, Preminger GM et al (1995) Comparison of open and endourologic approaches to the obstructed ureteropelvic junction. Urology 46:791–795

Capulicchio G, Homsy YL, Houle AM et al (1997) Long-term results of percutaneous endopyelotomy in the treatment of children with failed open pyeloplasty. J Urol 158:1534–1537

Caramella T, Lahoche A, Negaiwi Z et al (2005) False aneurysm formation following cutting balloon angioplasty in the renal artery of a child. J Endovasc Ther 12:746–749

Cope C, Zeit RM (1982) Pseudoaneurysms after nephrostomy. AJR Am J Roentgenol 139:255–261

Courtel V, Soto B, Niauet P et al (1998) Percutaneous transluminal angioplasty of renal artery stenosis in children. Pediatr Radiol 28:58–63

Cura MA, Bugnone A, Becker GJ (2002) Midaortic syndrome associated with fetal alcohol syndrome. J Vasc Interv Radiol 13:1167–1170

Daniels SR, Loggie JM, McEnery PT, Towbin RB (1987) Clinical spectrum of intrinsic renovascular hypertension in children. Pediatrics 80:698–704

David SM (1943) Intubated ureterotomy, new operations for ureteral and ureteropelvic stricture. Surg Gynecol Obstet 76:513–523

Ellis D, Shapiro R, Scantlebury VP, Simmons R, Towbin R (1995) Evaluation and management of bilateral renal artery stenosis in children: a case series and review. Pediatr Nephrol 9:259–267

El-Sadr AR, Mina E (1950) Anatomical and surgical aspects in the operative management of varicocele. Urol Cutaneous Rev 54(5):257–262

Fernstrom I, Johanasson B (1976) Percutaneous pyelolithotomy. A new extraction technique. Scand J Urol Nephrol 10:257–259

Figenshau RS, Clayman RV, Colberg JW et al (1996) Pediatric endopyelotomy: the Washington University experience. J Urol 156:2025–2030

Fostera BJ, Bernardb C, Drummond KN (2000) Kawasaki disease complicated by renal artery stenosis. Arch Dis Child 83:253–255

Gedroyc WM, MacIver D, Joyce MR et al (1989) Percutaneous stone and stent removal from renal transplants. Radiology 40:174–177

Gerber GS, Lyon ES (1994) Endopyelotomy: patient selection, results and complications. Urology 43:2–10

Gonzalez-Serva L, Weinerth JL, Glenn JF (1977) Minimal mortality of renal surgery. Urology 9:253–255

Goodwin WE, Casey WC, Woolf W (1955) Percutaneous trocar (needle) in hydronephrosis. JAMA 157:891–894

Haas NA, Ocker V, Knirsch W et al (2002) Successful management of a resistant renal artery stenosis in a child using a 4-mm cutting balloon catheter. Catheter Cardiovasc Interv 56:227–231

Hughes RJ, Scoble JE, Reidy JF (2004) Renal angioplasty in non-atheromatous renal artery stenosis: technical results and clinical outcome in 43 patients. Cardiovasc Intervent Radiol 27:435–440

Hulbert JC, Reddy PK, Gonzales R et al (1985) Percutaneous nephrolithotomy: an alternative approach to the management of pediatric calculus disease. Pediatrics 76:610–612

Ing FF, Goldberg B, Siegel DH, Trachtman H, Bierman FZ (1995) Arterial stents in the management of neurofibromatosis and renovascular hypertension in a pediatric patient: case report of a new treatment modality. Cardiovasc Intervent Radiol 18:414–418

Irby PB, Stoller ML (1993) Percutaneous suprapubic cystostomy. J Endourol 7(2):125–130

Irving HC, Arthur RJ, Thomas DF (1987) Percutaneous nephrostomy in pediatrics. Clin Radiol 38:245–248

Kadir S, White RI, Engel R (1982) Balloon dilatation of a ureteropelvic junction obstruction. Radiology 143:263–264

Kavoussi LR, Albala DM, Clayman R (1993) Outcome of secondary open surgical procedure in patients who fail primary endopyelotomy. Br J Urol 72:157–160

Khan AM, Holman E, Pasztor I et al (1997) Endopyelotomy: experience with 320 cases. J Endourol 11:243–246

Kurien A, John PR, Milford DV (1997) Hypertension secondary to progressive vascular neurofibromatosis. Arch Dis Child 76:454–455

Kurklinsky AK, Rooke TW (2010) Nutcracker phenomenon and nutcracker syndrome. Mayo Clin Proc 85(6):552–559

Lee WJ, Loh G, Smith AD et al (1985) Percutaneous extraction of renal stones: experience in 100 patients. AJR Am J Roentgenol 144:457–462

Lee WJ, Badlani GH, Karlin GS et al (1988) Treatment of ureteropelvic strictures with percutaneous pyeloplasty: experience in 62 patients. AJR Am J Roentgenol 151:515–518

LeRoy AJ, Segura JW (1986) Percutaneous removal of renal calculi. Radiol Clin North Am 24:615–622

Levy JM, Duszak RL Jr, Akins EW et al (2000) Percutaneous transluminal renal angioplasty. American College of Radiology. ACR appropriateness criteria. Radiology 215(Suppl):1015–1028

LiPuma JP, Hoaga JR, Bryan PJ et al (1984) Percutaneous nephrostomy in neonates and infants. J Urol 132:722–724

Lund G, Sinaiko A, Castaneda-Zuniga W, Cragg A, Salomonowitz E, Amplatz K (1984) Percutaneous transluminal angioplasty for treatment of renal artery stenosis in children. Eur J Radiol 4:254–257

Lupattelli T, Nano G, Inglese L (2005) Regarding "cutting balloon angioplasty of renal fibromuscular dysplasia: a word of caution.". J Vasc Surg 42:1038–1039, author reply 1039–1040

Mali WP, Puijlaert CB, Kouwenberg HJ et al (1987) Percutaneous transluminal renal angioplasty in children and adolescents. Radiology 165:391–394

Man DWK, Hendry GMA, Hamdy MH (1983) Percutaneous nephrostomy in pelviureteric junction obstruction in children. Br J Urol 55:356–360

Matsumoto AH, Dejter SW Jr, Barth KH et al (1990) Percutaneous nephrostomy drainage in the management of neonatal anuria secondary to renal candidiasis. J Pediatr Surg 25:1295–1297

McLaren CA, Roebuck DJ (2003) Interventional radiology for renovascular hypertension in children. Tech Vasc Interv Radiol 6:150–157

Motola JA, Badlani GH, Smith AD (1993) Results of 212 consecutive endopyelotomies: an 8-year follow-up. J Urol 149:453–456

Oguzkurt L, Tercan F, Gulcan O, Turkoz R (2005) Rupture of the renal artery after cutting balloon angioplasty in a young woman with fibromuscular dysplasia. Cardiovasc Intervent Radiol 28:360–363

Palmer JS, Palmer LS (2007) Determining the proper stent length to use in children: age plus 10. J Urol 178(4 Pt 2):1566–1569

Panayiotopoulos YP, Tyrrell MR, Koffman G et al (1996) Mid-aortic syndrome presenting in childhood. Br J Surg 83:235–240

Pastershank SP (1974) Left renal vein obstruction by a superior mesenteric artery. J Can Assoc Radiol 25(1):52–54

Pfister RC, Yoder IC, Newhouse JH (1981) Percutaneous uroradiologic procedures. Semin Roentgenol 16:135–151

Pode D, Shapiro A, Gordon R, Lebensart P (1982) Percutaneous nephrostomy for assessment of functional recovery of obstructed kidneys. Urology 19:482–485

Rhodes JF, Lane GK, Mesia CI et al (2002) Cutting balloon angioplasty for children with small-vessel pulmonary artery stenoses. Catheter Cardiovasc Interv 55:73–77

Robinson L, Gedroyc W, Reidy J, Saxton HM (1991) Renal artery stenosis in children. Clin Radiol 44:376–382

Shepard P, Thomas R, Harmon EP (1988) Urolithiasis in children: innovations in management. J Urol 140:790–792

Shroff R, Roebuck DJ, Gordon I et al (2006) Angioplasty for renovascular hypertension in children: 20-year experience. Pediatrics 118:268–275

Stanley P, Bear JW, Reid BS (1983) Percutaneous nephrostomy in infants and children. AJR Am J Roentgenol 141:473–477

Stanley P, Diament MJ (1986) Pediatric percutaneous nephrostomy: experience with 50 patients. J Urol 135:1223–1226

Tanemoto M, Abe T, Chaki T et al (2005) Cutting balloon angioplasty of resistant renal artery stenosis caused by fibromuscular dysplasia. J Vasc Surg 41:898–901

Towbin RB, Wacksman J, Ball WS et al (1987) Percutaneous pyeloplasty in children: experience in three patients. Radiology 163:381–384

Towbin RB, Pelchovitz DJ, Baskin KM et al (2007) Cutting balloon angioplasty in children with resistant renal artery stenosis. J Vasc Interv Radiol 18:663–669

Tyagi S, Kaul UA, Satsangi DK, Arora R (1997) Percutaneous transluminal angioplasty for renovascular hypertension in children: initial and long-term results. Pediatrics 99:44–49

Unterberg C, Buchwald AB, Barath P et al (1993) Cutting balloon coronary angioplasty-initial clinical experience. Clin Cardiol 16:660–666

Uppot R, Harisinghani M, Gervais D (2010) Imaging-guided percutaneous renal biopsy: rationale and approach. Am J Roentgenol 194:1443–1449

Urbano J, Cabrera M, Alonso-Burgos A (2014) Sclerosis and varicocele embolization with N-butyl cyanoacrylate: experience in 41 patients. Acta Radiol 55(2):179–185

Whitaker RH (1981) Percutaneous upper urinary tract dynamics in equivocal obstruction. Urol Radiol 2:187–189

Whitfield HN, Mills V, Miller RA et al (1983) Percutaneous pyelolysis: an alternative to pyeloplasty. Br J Urol 53(Suppl):93–96

Wickham JEA, Kellett MJ (1983) Percutaneous pyelolysis. Eur Urol 9:122–124

Winfield AC, Kirchner SG, Brun ME et al (1984) Percutaneous nephrostomy in neonates, infants and children. Radiology 151:617–619

Woodside JR, Stevens GF, Stark GL et al (1985) Percutaneous stone removal in children. J Urol 134:1166–1167

Part VIII

Management, Guidelines, Recommendations and Beyond Including Normal Values

Clinical Management of Common Nephrourologic Disorders (Guidelines and Beyond)

Michael Riccabona, Ekkehard Ring, and Hans-Joachim Mentzel

Contents

1	Introduction...	753
2	**What Clinicians Should Know**.........................	754
3	**What Clinicians Expect from Imaging**.........	754
4	**What Pediatric Radiologists Should Know About Treatment**..	755
4.1	Urinary Tract Infection...	755
4.2	Vesicoureteral Reflux..	756
4.3	Fetal and Neonatal Urinary Tract Dilatation.....	759
4.4	Other Common Conditions.................................	761
5	**Guidelines and Beyond**..................................	762
5.1	General Considerations.......................................	762
5.2	Urinary Tract Infection and Vesicoureteric Reflux..	763
5.3	Fetal Urinary Tract Dilatation (UTD).................	764
5.4	Other Common and Important Conditions........	764
6	**Imaging Algorithms and Procedural Recommendations**...	766
	Conclusion..	768
	References...	768

M. Riccabona, MD (✉)
Department of Radiology, Division of Pediatric Radiology, University Hospital Graz,
Auenbruggerplatz 34, 8036 Graz, Austria
e-mail: michael.riccabona@medunigraz.at

E. Ring, MD (Retired)
Department of Pediatrics, Division of General Pediatrics, University Hospital Graz,
Auenbruggerplatz 30, 8036 Graz, Austria

H.-J. Mentzel, MD
Section of Paediatric Radiology, Institute of Diagnostic and Interventional Radiology, University Hospital Jena, Erlanger Allee 101,
D – 0774 Jena, Germany

1 Introduction

It is not the aim and is beyond the scope of this chapter to show and to discuss all issues concerning treating nephrourological disorders. In many aspects, we can refer to other chapters of this book. Basically, pediatric radiologists are responsible for imaging, clinicians (pediatric nephrologists, pediatric urologists, general pediatricians, etc.) for treatment. This strict separation is valid, but somewhat questionable for optimal diagnosis and treatment. The task of preserving renal parenchyma, to the best of our knowledge, can be achieved only by cooperation and an interdisciplinary approach in many situations. The partners need to know about each other's thinking, intentions, and expectations. Interdisciplinary discussions with an exchange of knowledge are of value. This chapter is dedicated to discussing the cooperation between subspecialties and to showing aspects of the treatment of disorders. The discussion will include the dilemma of guidelines in general and in the daily routine of single centers. Disorders with minimal or no contribution of imaging to clinical decisions (e.g., dosage or duration of steroid treatment in glomerular disorders) are excluded. Quite a few aspects of this clinical management are shown in other respective chapters – the overlap with other parts of this book is desired as this chapter tries to provide a more clinically oriented practical approach.

2 What Clinicians Should Know

Basically, one could recommend clinicians to read this book entirely. Yet this is not realistic as, conversely, radiologists will not read a textbook of pediatric nephrology as well. Clinicians referring a child to imaging procedures – especially when working in a center for pediatric nephrology/urology – must have a basic knowledge about the imaging procedures, radiation burden, the respective potential of specific studies as well as their limitations, and the impact of the different investigations. Aside from reviewing the literature, personal communication is of importance for quick information about trends in imaging, changes in the performance of established investigations, and indications for new imaging procedures. And it is essential for defining a personalized imaging and treatment increasingly more important in these days. Urinary tract ultrasound (US) is the basic and often single investigation and frequently guides further imaging. However, the level of available US expertise is essential and thus the value of US often has to be seen with respect to local practice. And in some situations high level dedicated pediatric urinary tract US is not available 24/7, which also impacts on imaging algorithms and their practical usability. Nevertheless it must be stressed that it is also our task to make this dedicated high level and noninvasive imaging modality available for all children at all times when they need it.

But it is wrong to rely exclusively upon US for answering all questions; this would be giving too much credit to US. No other imaging technique is more investigator-dependent and prone to errors and pitfalls if not performed correctly. This should be kept in mind as the use of US has partially shifted to other specialists such as general pediatricians, pediatric urologists, and pediatric nephrologists, or to obstetricians in the case of fetal imaging. Particularly fetal US is part of the daily obstetrical routine. It may be that some special issues of imaging can be discussed with the pediatric radiologist. After birth, pediatric radiologists should know the results of previous imaging in order to plan and perform further radiological imaging properly.

3 What Clinicians Expect from Imaging

Clinicians expect the investigations to give clear answers to their questions. It would be optimal to perform just one or two investigations – as minimally invasively as possible – to know all about the patient's disorder (Ring et al. 2002). The daily routine is as follows: the families get a sheet of paper with hopefully sufficient information about the disease and the questions for the current investigation. They come back to the clinician with at least a preliminary report about the result of the investigation to clarify and discuss the results and to plan the treatment including further investigations and the next outpatient visit. This situation requires several basic conditions to function. The clinical information must be sufficient, the ordered investigation must be capable of answering the questions, and the setting must be appropriate. This way probably is appropriate for most routine situations, but requires modifications in special and emergency situations. Important initial results or major changes during follow-up need a rapid personal communication for properly planning the immediate treatment or urgent additional investigations. If many investigations are performed (e.g., US, VCUG, and DMSA-scan), a summarized radiological diagnosis may be of value for clinicians. Basically, a few images are superior to a thousand words. Thus, radiological documentation programs must include rapid access to images for clinicians. If requested, pediatric radiologists should find enough time to participate in interdisciplinary conferences on special patients to demonstrate the results of imaging and discuss further imaging options if necessary. However, these discussions are time consuming and seem to be unnecessary in most routine situations as often clinicians are capable of interpreting imaging to a certain extent. But local interdisciplinary meetings, additionally focusing on the current knowledge and future aspects of imaging in urinary tract disorders, seem to be also of educational value. Here pediatric radiologists can clarify why, e.g., IVU nowadays is no longer the routine investigation in urinary obstruction if new investigations such as MRI are available or why echo-enhanced voiding urosonography (ce-VUS), if locally available, should replace conventional voiding cystourethrography (VCUG) in certain clinical settings (Riccabona et al. 2010, 2012). All this should lead to an improvement of imaging settings, to prevention of invalid performances, and to a better understanding of each other, consecutively enabling an optimal management of our children.

4 What Pediatric Radiologists Should Know About Treatment

4.1 Urinary Tract Infection (See Also Chapters "UTI and VUR" and "Imaging in Urinary Tract Infections")

Urinary tract infection (UTI) is the second most frequent bacterial infection during childhood defined by the presence of bacteria within the bladder, the kidneys and/or the urinary tract. Demographic data on UTI have remained unchanged during the last decades with an overall female predominance, an equal gender distribution during infancy, and with infant boys having UTI earlier than girls (Ring and Zobel 1988; Hansson et al. 1999). UTI in boys aged more than 2 years is exceptional and mostly related to some underlying condition. Many factors are involved in the pathogenesis of UTI. We are on the way to a better understanding of the innate and adaptive immunity of the urinary tract and the impact of Toll-like receptors or cytokines on host defense mechanisms. Detection of immunologic disturbances or of genetic polymorphisms could contribute to the identification of children susceptible to recurrent UTI and to renal scarring (Saemann et al. 2005; Mak and Kuo 2006). So far, no single clinical or laboratory factor can identify children at risk. Nevertheless, it is no longer accepted nowadays that renal damage following UTI is predominantly the consequence of VUR as there seems to be an equal distribution of renal scarring in refluxing and nonrefluxing renal units (Hellerstein 2006; Moorthy et al. 2005). Sometimes VUR is found contralateral to a severely compromised kidney (Fig. 1). In general, children with UTI but without renal and urinary tract malformations have no risk for chronic renal failure. Aside from looking for UT malformations, functional disturbances of the bladder must be addressed especially in children with recurrent UTI. Nevertheless – there is a general trend of questioning the number of investigations and strategise them according to age and risks (Marks et al. 2008, Tsai et al. 2012, Tse et al. 2009, Riccabona 2016). Appropriate treatment of non-neurogenic bladder-sphincter dysfunction with drugs such as anticholinergics and/or behavioral therapy and treatment of constipation are of importance in reducing the number of recurrent UTIs (see chapter "Non-Neurogenic Bladder-Sphincter Dysfunction ("Voiding Dysfunction")"). Selected cases need imaging to exclude neurological deficits such as occult dysraphia, lipoma, or a tethered cord. It is well recognized that circumcision is associated with a significantly reduced risk of UTI in infant boys (Schoen 2005). This could be of value in boys with severe UT malformations. From a European view, there is no benefit of circumcision to prevent UTI in the general male population (Malone 2005).

Symptomatic UTI needs immediate antibiotic treatment, and a delay of diagnosis and treatment may be associated with renal scarring (Jodal 1987, Bouissou et al. 2008). Therapy needs to be appropriate for the severity of infection shown by clinical symptoms such as vomiting, fever, or shock. Treatment for lower UTI can be shorter than treatment of febrile upper UTI where an

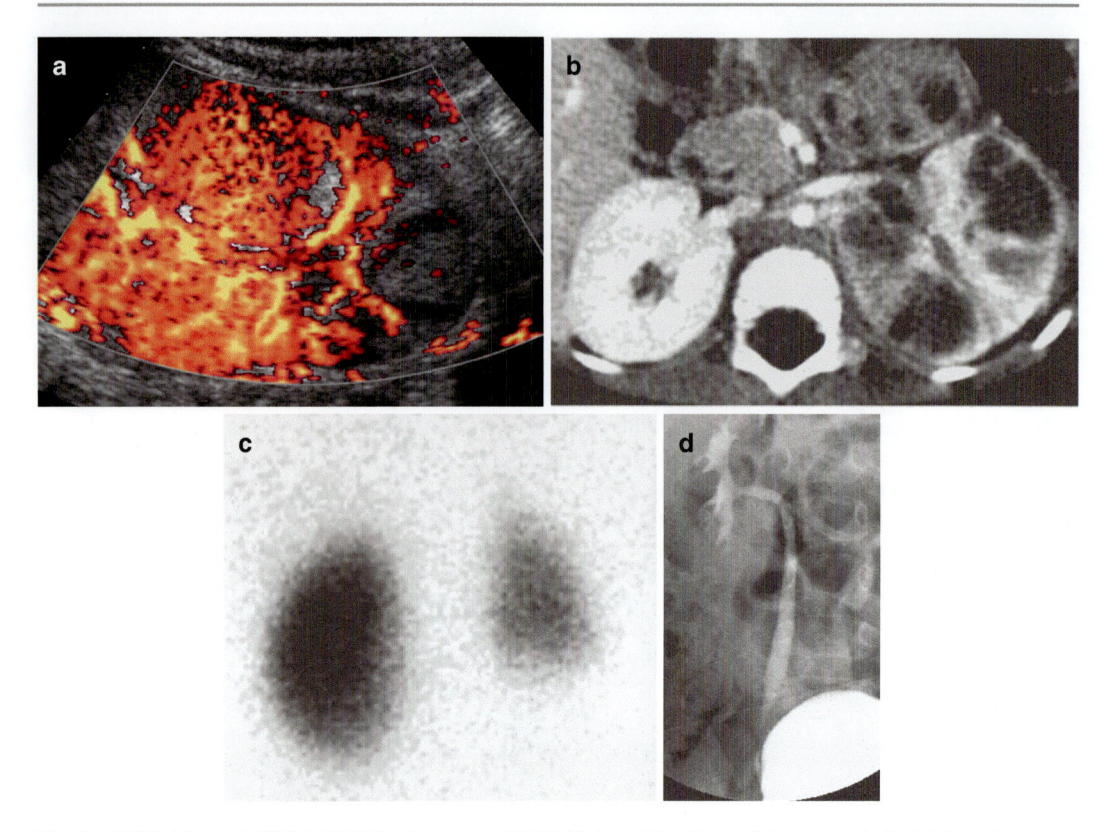

Fig. 1 ACDS (**a**), renal CT (**b**), DMSA (**c**) scan, and VCU (**d**) in a girl with renal abscesses. Left-sided renal scarring is the outcome (split-function 23 %), but VUR is on the right side into a normal kidney

antibiotic course of 10 days is adequate. Bacteria can persist within the bladder tissue in a quiescent state and may serve as a reservoir for recurrent infections (Mulvey et al. 2000). Antibiotic prophylaxis for a few weeks, especially after severe infections, could be the consequence. But what about long-term prophylaxis? For decades, long-term prophylaxis – even for many years – was an accepted treatment for children with recurrent UTI in preventing renal scarring, but this effect is questioned nowadays (Pennesi et al. 2008; Williams et al. 2001; Beetz 2006; Montini et al. 2008, Conway et al. 2007, Marcus et al. 2005). Nevertheless, prophylaxis can be recommended in children with a normal urinary tract and problems such as recurrent pyelonephritis, infection stones, or functional bladder disorders as adjunct to bladder therapy. The most frequently used substances are trimethoprim, co-trimoxazole, and nitrofurantoin. Cephalosporins are a reasonable alternative as the number of bacterial strains resistant to trimethoprim is increasing (Kaneko et al. 2003). Each center or region separately must decide on the best drug according to the local bacteriological findings and resistance. Fianlly one needs to refer to the various national and international guidelines and recommendations that additionally change over time making the individual imaging strategy and mangement decisions sometimes difficult (De Palma and Manzoni 2013, National Institute for Health and Clinical Excellence 2007, Royal College of Physicians 1992, Saadeh and Mattoo 2011, Roberts 2011, Tse et al. 2009).

4.2 Vesicoureteral Reflux

No other clinical entity of pediatric nephrology and urology causes more interdisciplinary discussions than VUR, and the most frequent clinical situations associated with VUR are shown in Table 1. A reorientation concerning diagnosis, treatment, and outcome of VUR

Table 1 Clinical situations with an increased probability of VUR

Urinary tract infection
Fetal hydroureteronephrosis (= distention of the collecting system and the ureter)
Family member with VUR (sibling, parents)
Unilateral multicystic dysplasia or renal agenesis
Neurogenic and nonneurogenic bladder dysfunction

Table 2 Treatment options for children with primary VUR

1. Observation without continuous medication
(a) Frequent urinanalysis (partially at home)
(b) Immediate treatment of UTI
2. Antibiotic prophylaxis
(a) Prophylaxis until VUR resolves
(b) Stopping prophylaxis despite VUR persistence and observation as in option 1
(c) Prophylaxis for a defined period without reevaluation. Observation as in option 1
3. Primary surgical treatment (with or without postoperative prophylaxis)
(a) Subureteral injection
(b) Open surgery
4. Combined conservative and surgical approach
(a) Elective primary surgery (e.g., paraostial diverticulum)
(b) Surgery following conservative treatment
Recurrent UTI with options 1 or 2
New scarring
Preservation of bladder function (e.g., megacystis-megaureter syndrome)
(c) Failure of surgery – with second surgery and/or options 1 or 2
Invalid technique
Not recognized nonneurogenic bladder-sphincter dysfunction or neurogenic bladder
5. Proceeding based on parental preferences and compliance to treatment

Supportive measures such as awareness of UTI, treatment of nonneurogenic bladder-sphincter dysfunction, constipation, vulvitis, and phimosis are mandatory in all.
RTx renal transplantation, *CRF* chronic renal failure

took place during the past years and is going on still, particularly as one realised that VUR may spontaneously disappear without any sequalae or clinical symptoms (Schwab et al. 2002). The International Reflux Study in Children gave the final report after 10 years of follow-up. There were no differences in the outcome (scarring, renal growth, UTI recurrence rate) under medical or surgical management except that medically treated children more often had febrile UTIs. The importance of continuous surveillance of VUR patients was emphasized (Jodal et al. 2006). Children with VUR do not necessarily suffer from recurrent UTI. Consequently, the need and the duration of antibiotic prophylaxis have to be questioned (Pennesi et al. 2008). There is evidence that VUR grade 3–5 (international classification) is a risk factor for UTI, but VUR grade 1–2 not so (Nuutinen and Uhari 2001; Hellerstein and Nickell 2002). Stopping long-term prophylaxis in children with persisting VUR was found to be safe without an increased risk for UTI or renal scarring, mostly in school-aged children with nondilating low grade VUR (Cooper et al. 2000; Thompson et al. 2001; Al-Sayyad et al. 2005; Garin et al. 2006). The above-mentioned gender differences in UTI could influence the decision to stop prophylaxis, being earlier in boys than in girls. Discontinuing or not even starting prophylaxis in cases with VUR (no prophylaxis in VUR grade 1–2; stopping prophylaxis in persisting VUR grade 3–4 after 1 year, at least in boys) is more often accepted in Europe and was proposed as an alternative much earlier than in North America (Jodal and Lindberg 1999). The data of the RIVUR study were published recently; they confirmed prophylaxis to be better than placebo in children with high-grade VUR (The RIVUR Trial Investigators 2014).

The American Urological Association recommended continuous antibiotic prophylaxis as initial treatment for most children with VUR (Peters et al. 2010). Surgery (mostly open surgery) was recommended in children with persistent dilating VUR (Elder et al. 1997). Nowadays, surgically oriented institutions mostly emphasize endoscopic treatment (subureteral injection) not only as an alternative to prophylaxis and to open surgery, but sometimes also as the first-line treatment for most children with high-grade or intrarenal VUR (Puri et al. 2006; Capozza and Caione 2007).

What is our ultimate goal? Is it prevention of renal damage or is it cure of VUR? Treatment options for children with VUR are shown in

Table 2. Physicians are obliged to inform families about all treatment options. Parental preferences have to be respected and need to be incorporated into ultimate decisions, as well as the compliance. A recent questionnaire study showed that the majority of parents favored antibiotic prophylaxis over surgery as initial treatment. If a long-term treatment course was predicted, surgery and especially endoscopic treatment were preferred (Ogan et al. 2001). Information given to parents for decisions should be objective, but certainly are biased by center preferences. This has to be considered in interpreting a questionnaire study of a surgical center showing an 80% parental preference of endoscopic treatment (Capozza et al. 2003). Whatever the individual situation, spontaneous resolution or surgical repair of VUR is not the endpoint of treatment and observation. Long-term studies showed that UTI is independent from VUR, and it was found in up to 74% of patients 20 years even after successful antireflux surgery (Beetz et al. 2002; Mor et al. 2003). Women with or without renal scarring (RNP) are prone to UTI during pregnancy, abortion may occur in 37% of pregnancies, and chronic renal failure will deteriorate in approximately 20% of cases (Jungers et al. 1996). Arterial hypertension is found in 10–20% of all patients with scars or reflux nephropathy (RNP). Patients with chronic renal failure (CRF) due to bilateral RNP or RNP in a single kidney are especially prone to these long-term sequelae (Smellie et al. 2001).

It is well recognized that particularly boys with bilateral high-grade VUR present with renal hypodysplasia, also called congenital RN (Ring et al. 1993; Yeung et al. 1997; Wennerström et al. 2000; Marra et al. 2004). Hypodysplasia with VUR is the most frequent single cause of CRF during childhood, accounting for 26% of cases (Ardissino et al. 2003). Future end-stage renal failure cannot be prevented in these children, but the progression of CRF can be delayed. Proper nephrological treatment is essential to avoid complications such as hypertension, renal anemia, or renal osteodystrophy and must start early in CRF.

Statements such as "… it is not clear whether any intervention for children with primary VUR does more good than harm …" or "… it is uncertain whether the identification and treatment of children with VUR confers clinically important benefit …" are questionable (Wheeler et al. 2003). The presence of renal hypodysplasia cannot be changed by any treatment. However, early identification of children with congenital renal compromise, particularly those with CRF, is essential for adequate nephrological treatment. The rationale for treatment of VUR can only be the prevention of acquired renal scarring. Scars may cause renal morbidity in patients born with normal kidneys or can accelerate the progression of CRF in patients with renal hypodysplasia. Therefore, we need identification, observation, and probably treatment of VUR patients at risk for renal scarring. As a negative example, a study of 115 adults (99 females) – all born before 1968 – with VUR detected in adulthood and without diagnosis of VUR during childhood showed that 88% of patients had RNP, 34% were hypertensive, and 19% suffered from CRF. Females more often had UTI, while CRF was predominant in males (Köhler et al. 1997). These data of a special group of adults indicate that we should not leave our children without long-term care and surveillance. Gender differences of VUR and of RNP have to be considered as they may influence management significantly (Fanos and Cataldi 2004). And in addition, developing countries strongly await our decisions and proposals, and also need our support (Xhepa et al. 2004).

Decisions about treatment are influenced by guidelines – commonly accepted or not – which are discussed below. Clinically oriented decisions, individually influenced by our knowledge about the family situation, the estimated compliance with medical treatment, and the adherence to follow-up investigations, seem to be of equal importance. Aside from patients being involved in multicenter studies with strict protocols, treatment of many children with VUR is based on individual experience, local attitudes, parent's preference, and the specialization of the center. Our current knowledge seems to raise more questions than solutions concerning evidence-based treatment of children with VUR.

4.3 Fetal and Neonatal Urinary Tract Dilatation

Formerly, the term "hydronephrosis" (HN) indicated obstructive uropathy with compromise of the renal parenchyma; therefore it has been recently suggested to introduce a new classification system using the term "urinary tract or pelvicaliceal dilatation/distension" (UTD/PCD) (Nguyen et al. 2014; Riccabona et al. 2014a; Riccabona et al. 2017 in press; Vivier 2015). Nowadays, this term usually refers to different grades of renal pelvic dilatation on US investigation (prenatally and after birth) as a sonographic grading scale mostly classified as proposed by the Society for Fetal Urology, based on the Hofman US classification, and adapted by the ESPR uroradiology task force (Fernbach et al. 1993; Riccabona et al. 2008); however, different grading systems exist. A major point of discussion is what extent of fetal UTD at which gestational age reliably predicts significant postpartum renal and urinary tract disease (Toiviainen-Salo et al. 2004). Recent publications could show that severe degrees of UTD (HN-SFU grades 3–4) and an anterior-posterior renal pelvic diameter of >12 mm on a third trimester US are highly predictive for significant postpartum pathology (Lee et al. 2006a, b; Sidhu et al. 2006). Some reports even suggest to repeated prenatal US scans and then perform a detailed postnatal evaluation in patients with much smaller distention – increasing detection rate, but also causing a higher number of negative studies (John et al. 2004). UTD per se does not necessarily indicate a special disease, and a correct final diagnosis is warranted. US devices applicable to small fetuses enabling diagnosis of urinary tract disease in early pregnancy have become standard. Yet the actual diagnostic potential during fetal life is limited, and the correct postpartum diagnosis cannot be obtained in many cases.

The diagnosis of fetal renal failure is based on US findings of the kidneys (no kidneys present, a single dysplastic kidney, renal cysts, hyperechogenic renal parenchyma), the calculation of the amount of amniotic fluid as oligohydramnios indicating renal failure, and the measurement of electrolytes in fetal urine (see also chapter "Anomalies of Kidney Rotation, Position and Fusion"). Sometimes repeated US and analyses of fetal urine indicate an adverse outcome justifying elective termination of pregnancy. MRI of the fetal kidneys and urinary tract sometimes may clarify inconclusive findings on US and may serve as a valuable future tool (see chapter "Anomalies of Kidney Rotation, Position and Fusion") (Hörmann et al. 2006; Cassart et al. 2004). Fetal interventions nowadays are mostly restricted to boys with oligohydramnios and bilateral urinary tract obstruction caused by posterior urethral valves. Fetal rupture within the urinary tract may cause concern on postpartum renal and pulmonary function (Fig. 2). Fetal interventions must be discussed interdisciplinarily in these rare but important situations. If not indicated or performed, early imaging and emergency treatment immediately after birth are mandatory, and the long-term renal outcome may be poor.

Most fetuses with isolated UTD survive and are asymptomatic neonates after birth. Further imaging is needed frequently to clarify the fetal findings. Sometimes the parents may not know enough about the significance of prenatal findings and their postpartum diagnostic and therapeutic management. Such a situation leads to a long period of uncertainty and anxiety for the parents who have been worried about their

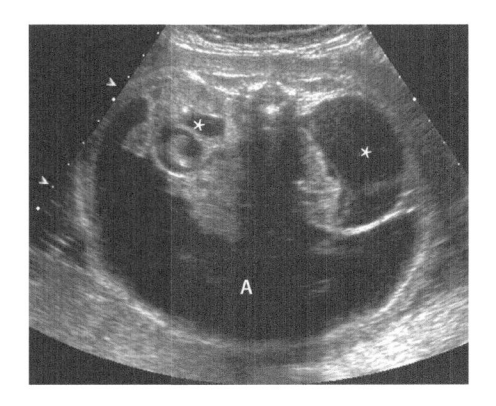

Fig. 2 Oligohydramnios, fetal urinary ascites (*A*), and bilateral urinoma (*asterisks*) in a boy with posterior urethral valve recognized in the 32nd week of gestation

child's renal outcome since the first recognition of fetal UTD. Correct information for the parents from the obstetricians is therefore mandatory, with pediatric radiologists eventually being helpful in interpreting US. Especially in severe findings on fetal US, the direct contact to neonatologists, pediatricians, or preferably to pediatric nephrologists already during pregnancy is of utmost importance. They should inform the parents what will happen after birth and which investigations (mostly imaging) should be performed at which postpartum age. Appropriate information about prognosis and therapeutic options (antibiotic prophylaxis, indications for surgery, etc.) should be provided in time. In strictly unilateral renal compromise with a normal contralateral kidney showing compensatory hypertrophy, the global renal outcome will be favorable.

Fetal UTD is found in up to 5% of pregnancies. It is transient or physiological without renal compromise in approximately 60% of cases. Nearly half of the neonates with significant pathology suffer from pelvi-ureteric junction obstruction (PUJO) and one third from VUR. In the early years of US, most of us were deeply impressed by the magnitude of neonatal UTD, and probably too many children had early operations. A recent retrospective survey carried out for 19 years showed that prenatal diagnosis led to earlier detection of PUJO and to earlier surgical repair. The total number of operations remained unchanged (Capello et al. 2005). The "wait and see" strategy, nowadays successfully applied in many centers, may reduce the number of surgically treated neonates and infants significantly. Dilatation is not necessarily equal to obstruction. Obstruction basically means development of renal damage if left untreated and is a retrospective assessment. However, acquired irreversible renal damage should not be the rationale for therapeutic decisions. In this dilemma of operating only on children with proven obstruction and not losing renal parenchyma, we must accept investigations felt to be somewhat invalid (e.g., MAG3 isotope washout curves) or rely on repeated US and split renal function on isotope investigation with deterioration being an indication for surgery. Permanent loss of renal parenchyma may occur within few months (Dejter and Gibbons 1989), is accepted to occur in some studies (Dhillon 1998), and a close follow-up can prevent this irreversible renal damage (Thorup et al. 2000, 2003; Onen et al. 2002). A survey of French-speaking European pediatric nephrologists and urologists showed that about 61% rely on 99m Tc-MAG3 curves to recommend surgery or not (Ismaïli et al. 2004). In recent years, functional MRU providing also information on regional and split glomerular filtration rate as well as renal transit times (not only on anatomic information, split size, and drainage pattern) is partially advocated for more accurately determining which kidneys may benefit from surgery (see chapter "MR of the Urogenital Tract in Children").

The long-term outcome of children with prenatally recognized PUJO is favorable in general. Deterioration on long-term surveillance seems to be rare, and the outcome of the affected kidney mostly is determined at birth. Children with a moderate reduction of neonatal split renal function may benefit from pyeloplasty, while poorly functioning kidneys mostly will not recover despite surgery (Ylinen et al. 2004). In the latter cases, pelvic dilatation on US may be moderate due to the decreased urine output. Increased parenchymal echogenicity, cortical cysts, and a reduced perfusion indicate a congenital lesion already in neonates

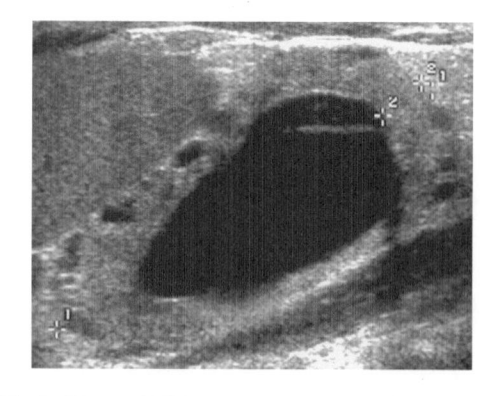

Fig. 3 Neonatal US in pelvi-ureteric junction obstruction with moderate renal pelvic dilatation. Increased parenchymal echogenicity and cortical cysts indicate severe obstructive dysplasia and poor renal function

(Fig. 3) (see also chapters "Congenital Urinary Tract Dilatation and Obstructive Uropathy" and "Upper Urinary Tract Dilatation in Newborns and Infants and the Postnatal Work up of Congenital Uro-nephropathies").

Although performed frequently, it is unclear whether all neonates with fetal UTD should receive an antibiotic prophylaxis starting at birth. Infants with urinary tract obstruction had an increased incidence of UTI in an early study (Ring and Zobel 1988). A 36 % incidence of UTI – predominantly during the first 6 months of life – in infants with severe obstructive UTD and left without antibiotic prophylaxis was reported recently. UTI was more frequent in infants with ureterovesical junction obstruction than with PUJO (Song et al. 2007). Prophylaxis given to all neonates with all grades of fetal UTD and starting with birth may be a prerequisite for large prospective multicenter trials, but otherwise is not timely. Just 23 % of pediatric nephrologists and 31 % of pediatric urologists would recommend prophylaxis immediately after birth, more often in VUR than in urinary tract obstruction (Ismaïli et al. 2004). Table 3 shows possible indications for antibiotic prophylaxis in neonates depending on the severity of fetal and neonatal findings. If prophylaxis is questioned in cases with low grade VUR, indications for VCUG or ce-VUS in asymptomatic neonates with mild to moderate fetal and neonatal UTD but a normal appearance of renal parenchyma should be modified (Ismaïli et al. 2006; Lidefelt et al. 2006). VCUG (or ce-VUS) should be selectively used accepting that some neonates with predominantly mild VUR may be missed (which however might well be without any consequence). Renal parenchymal lesions on US, known to be associated with severe VUR, and indirect signs of dilating VUR, such as ureteral distension, urothelial thickening, or a changing ureteral or renal pelvic width, are in favor of an immediate or at least delayed VUR evaluation test.

4.4 Other Common Conditions

There are a few other common pediatric urinary tract conditions that have specific implications on imaging and where understanding of treatment is essential for pediatric radiologists. In renal cystic disease, new treatment options may be available in the near future – the indication for treating probably will be based on the patients age, on the number of cysts, and the speed of disease evolution; thus a more detailed description of number and size of cysts has become essential (see also chapter "Renal Agenesis, Dysplasia, Hypoplasia and Cystic Diseases of the Kidney" and "Imaging in Renal Agenesis, Dysplasia, Hypoplasia and Cystic Diseases of the Kidney"). In urinary tract trauma, most conditions can be managed conservatively – only severe renal trauma, bladder, or caliceal or urethra/ureter rupture need prompt intervention. Thus the initial assessment is crucial, sometimes necessitating a ce-CT or ce-MRU, whereas in most other cases particularly with blunt or moderate trauma can be managed based on US findings (Amerstorfer et al. 2015) (see also chapter "Urinary Tract Trauma"). For urethral trauma retro- and/or antegrade urethrography is necessary. In childhood urolithiasis, the clinical and therapeutic consequences should govern imaging, too – as children are more susceptible to radiation, and patients with stone disease will have to undergo repeated studies during their life potentially accumulating a very high overall dose, radiation sparing imaging is of even higher importance (see also chapters "Urolithiasis and

Table 3 Indications where antibiotic prophylaxis in neonates with fetal UTD should be considered

Neonates after fetal interventions
Severe fetal findings leading to immediate neonatal investigations
Suspicion of posterior urethral valves
Complex obstructive uropathy (e.g., duplication with ureterocele)
Uni- or bilateral severe supravesical UTD
Dilating VUR (grades 3–5, international classification)
Single functioning kidney with severe UTD

Abbreviations: *UTD* urinary tract distension, *VUR* vesicoureteric reflux

Nephrocalcinosis" and "Imaging of Urolithiasis and Nephrocalcinosis"). Therefore US should always be the first imaging step, as most stones are located at the renal pelvis and the pelvi-ureteric or the ureterovesical junction, all areas ideally accessible by US. And small stones <5 mm usually pass spontaneously if they have reached the ureter, at least to the distal prevesical part – thus depiction of those sitting in the mid ureter portion is of no consequence, and therefore CT is rarely needed and indicated. Additionally, childhood urolithiasis should also prompt a search for underlying conditions such as metabolic disturbances (hypercalciuria, hyperoxaluria, etc.). Finally (glomerulo)nephritis needs to be considered; the most important clinical aspects are diagnosing and managing these conditions trying to avoid permanent renal damage and renal failure. The contribution of imaging is limited to US and US-guided renal biopsy as shown in chapters "Renal Parenchymal Disease" and "Imaging in Renal Parenchymal Disease".

> **Take Away**
> Knowledge about clinical aspects is essential for performing imaging in a way that aids diagnosis and treatment. Imaging results should be quickly transferred to clinicians. US is the basic and sometimes single investigation and should guide the need for additional studies like VCUG or DMSA-scan. VCUG is needed just in a part of the children with UTI, and isotope studies frequently are decisive for treatment of children with urinary tract obstruction. Special attention is necessary in renal cystic disease, renal trauma, and urolithiasis.

5 Guidelines and Beyond

5.1 General Considerations

Guidelines permanently accompany our work in the daily routine. Young colleagues eagerly follow the proposals of the local specialists, making the daily work much easier. Specialists themselves are involved in the interdisciplinary approach to special disorders within their own countries or in the setting of international cooperation or societies. Consequently, clinical and basic research continuously modifies our approach to disorders (Marks 2007; Ulman et al. 2000). The resulting guidelines influence the clinical management and represent a continuum to better care for our children. But are our guidelines always followed? A recent study showed that less than half of infants with UTI received the recommended care including diagnostic imaging. Hospitalized infants were more likely to get imaging (Cohen et al. 2005). Another point of concern is the practicability of a given guideline. Adequacy for a tertiary center may be a challenge for primary or secondary care or for countries with limited resources. We have to accept that not all can follow new concepts. Modifications according to local circumstances or adherence to previous proposals are the consequence.

It is the current attitude to question approved approaches to diagnosis and therapy and to ask for evidence-based medicine. If the treatment of special disorders is not evidence based, prospective, multicenter, randomized trials are proposed and "… further decisions strongly will depend on these findings …". Meanwhile and for the years up to the first results of ongoing or planned studies, we are in a vacuum, not knowing what should be done – lacking evidence in many such situations, in particular concerning imaging. But our patients and their disorders cannot wait years for such suggestions as treatment has to be done immediately.

Meta-analyses showing that current approaches are not evidence based and proposing studies to clarify these issues are of importance. Yet there is no proof that omitting all current imaging and treatment protocols is better and does not harm our children; actually some recent papers suggest that strategies that have been proposed based on the lack of evidence of benefit of a certain test risk missing a relevant number of patients who suffer from treatable conditions thus increasing morbidity for the benefit of being more "economic" (McDonald and Kenney 2014).

Timely individual management, partially influenced by personal experience and local preferences, and sometimes being different from proposed guidelines, must parallel clinical research. Guidelines are as good as they allow modifications for the individual patient. It is not our intention to give new proposals or algorithms with the presumption of being superior to previous recommendations. The impact of investigations in disease entities must be discussed from a clinically oriented view. This hopefully will contribute to the best decision on imaging in children with UTI, VUR, and fetal UTD where doctors from several subspecialties are involved.

5.2 Urinary Tract Infection and Vesicoureteric Reflux

It is almost universally accepted that all infants and children with (febrile, upper) UTI should undergo imaging starting with US. Yet one prospective study found US to be of limited value if performed at the time of acute UTI as the impact on treatment is low (Hoberman et al. 2003). No other imaging procedure is more investigator-dependent than US. But high-quality modern US including (amplitude-coded) color Doppler sonography (CDS) has the potential to influence and to guide further imaging, thereby reducing the total radiation burden. This is to some extent a local decision. If local clinicians rely on the results of US, recommended subsequent imaging eventually can be delayed, performed just in selective cases, or be omitted. Inconsistencies and failures need reevaluation of such an approach mostly going back to an imaging protocol following generally recommended guidelines.

Discussion on imaging following UTI is based on the correlation of UTI with renal scarring, VUR, other malformations of the kidneys and the urinary tract, and nonneurogenic bladder-sphincter dysfunction. VCUG is still the central point of discussion and is an invasive investigation with radiation burden, discomfort, and a small risk of causing a UTI. The American Academy of Pediatrics and a Swedish state-of-the-art conference recommended US and VCUG in all infants and young children up to 2 years of age with UTI to detect VUR (American Academy of Pediatrics. Committee on Quality Improvement. Subcommittee on Urinary Tract Infection 1999; Jodal and Lindberg 1999). This imaging policy is no more accepted nowadays and the American Academy of Pediatrics basically changed their attitude (American Academy of Pediatrics 2011). The number of investigations can be reduced and VCUG not necessarily has to be performed in all children with UTI, only those with indirect signs on US or complicating clinical circumstances. In infants with febrile UTI, an US of the bladder and the kidney should be performed during the first 2 days of treatment to identify serious complications such as pyonephrosis or abscesses formation – when the clinical situation is severe or if there is no clinical improvement. Nuclear scanning with DMSA is not recommended as part of routine evaluation in the first febrile UTI. Radionuclide cystography (RNC) with low-dose radiation or ce-VUS without radiation are alternatives to conventional fluoroscopic VCUG, but both also require catheterization of the bladder. As stated above, it is the ultimate goal to recognize and to prevent renal damage. Renal scarring without VUR is frequent. Conversely, detecting VUR is not a good predictor of renal damage after UTI and cannot serve as a screening investigation for renal damage (Gordon et al. 2003).

Siblings of an index patient more often have VUR, mostly low-grade VUR, and the mean incidence is 32 % (Hollowell 2002). Scarring is infrequent in this special, mostly asymptomatic population, and no increased risk for UTI has been reported. Performing a VCUG seems to be advisable just in siblings with UTI or with proven renal damage. Elective screening with RNC was recommended (Lee et al. 2006b), but close surveillance including repeated US and immediate urinalysis in febrile states could be an alternative.

VCUG in children older than 2 years is a matter of debate. A DMSA scan – if available – was recommended 6–12 months after an upper UTI and VCUG was performed only if a renal lesion was recognized (Jodal and Lindberg 1999). In contrast, others recommended VCUG in all prepubertal children (Lee et al. 2006b).

There is increasing evidence that an imaging policy using US and DMSA (or today also MRI) could be a reasonable alternative to strict adherence to VCUG in all cases (Riccabona and Fotter 2004a, b). Two recent studies with this approach could reduce the number of VCUGs by 49 % and 30 %, respectively (Hansson et al. 2004; Tseng et al. 2007). It is important to note that – taking these two studies with 445 patients together – a small number of children with VUR grade 1–2 and just one child with a renal lesion were missed. This is acceptable, especially if one feels that some children with VUR can be left without prophylaxis.

Another point of concern is the timing of repeated VCUG (or ce-VUS/RNC) once VUR is detected. Most centers probably would accept a follow-up VUR test in yearly intervals while children are on prophylaxis. A recent study analyzed a schedule of delaying VCUG, thereby taking into account the resolution rates of different VUR grades. A delay of 2 years in clinically uneventful children with mild VUR and of 3 years with severe VUR would have reduced the number of VCUGs by 19 % with a moderate prolongation of giving prophylactic antibiotics (Thompson et al. 2005). In cases in which prophylaxis is stopped despite persisting VUR, the need for a repeated VUR test basically has to be questioned in an uneventful course without UTI.

There is a significant change in the approach to children with VUR concerning treatment and imaging. The central point of concern is the renal parenchyma and not VUR itself. If we can accept that all children with renal compromise but not all children with VUR have to be detected, a significant reduction of radiation and invasiveness seems to be possible. Nevertheless, even nowadays there is no ideal universally accepted protocol for imaging following UTI and looking for VUR (La Scola et al. 2013).

5.3 Fetal Urinary Tract Dilatation (UTD)

Imaging protocols following fetal UTD should be dedicated to identifying neonates with renal dysplasia, complex uropathies, obstructive uropathy, single functioning kidneys, or severe VUR with or without congenital RNP. Fetal findings do not necessarily equal postpartum findings. High-quality fetal US is not performed in all pregnancies, and some renal or urinary tract malformations can be missed including VUR. Consequently, a recently reported approach not to perform renal US in children with UTI and a reportedly normal fetal US has to be questioned (Hoberman et al. 2003).

Severe fetal findings suggesting important diagnoses such as posterior urethral valves are a neonatal emergency, and US (as well as a VCUG) is needed immediately after birth. Otherwise, neonatal US can (and should) be delayed up to the end of the first week of life. Timely imaging algorithms basically including VCUG or ce-VUS were shown (Riccabona and Fotter 2004a, b; Lee et al. 2006a, b; Riccabona et al. 2008). Neonatal US is the first investigation, but VCUG or ce-VUS in all neonates even with unilateral severe fetal UTD but without dilated ureter has to be questioned nowadays. Antibiotic prophylaxis is prescribed in most of these neonates, obviating the need for immediate VCUG or ce-VUS that can be performed later and electively. Modern high resolution US can guide further imaging in a more individually based fashion and should be performed by an experienced investigator. Preservation of renal parenchyma is the ultimate task in cases with fetal UTD, but the radiation burden can be lowered with modified imaging protocols.

5.4 Other Common and Important Conditions

In renal cystic disease not only a more detailed description of number and size of cysts has become essential (see also chapter "Renal Agenesis, Dysplasia, Hypoplasia and Cystic Diseases of the Kidney" and "Imaging in Renal Agenesis, Dysplasia, Hypoplasia and Cystic Diseases of the Kidney"); it has also become possible by using modern high resolution US and MRI. This is important for early recognition, even in neonates relatively small cysts that have not been detectable a decade ago can now be depicted and thus earlier diagnosis has become possible, with all its implications on possible future treatment and prognosis (see Figs. 7d and 8). But one has to consider that therefore treatment concepts that are based on the "old" imaging potential may need to be revisited – also the constantly increasing importance of genetics and the new insight into the disease pathophysiology (the concept of ciliopathies and uromodulin) that indicates to extend imaging to other organs such as major vessels (e.g., for aneurysm) and other organs (e.g., liver fibrosis, cysts in other parenchymal organ).

In urinary tract trauma, US with its modern options such as (amplitude-coded) CDS and contrast-enhanced US has become an accepted alternative to ce-CT (Fig. 4); new imaging algorithms for mild to moderate blunt renal trauma tribute to this development (Amerstorfer et al. 2015; Riccabona et al. 2011) (see also chapter "Urinary Tract Trauma"). For severe (or multiple) and penetrating renal/urinary tract trauma, a ce-CT (in the acute setting) or ce-MRU (in the delayed setting or for follow-up) still remain the gold standard – better devices, modern detectors, and reconstruction algorithms and improved intelligent contrast application techniques as well as dedicated pediatric CT protocols have, however, helped to reduce the burden on the patient without sacrificing diagnostic accuracy (see also chapters "Diagnostic Procedures: Excluding MRI, Nuclear Medicine and Video-Urodynamics", "MR of the Urogenital Tract in Children", "Contrast Agents in Childhood: Application and Safety Considerations", and "Urinary Tract Trauma").

In childhood urolithiasis, the shift towards US as the main and initial imaging modality has implications on the details of the procedure (see also chapter "Imaging of Urolithiasis and Nephrocalcinosis"). Adequate scanning condi-

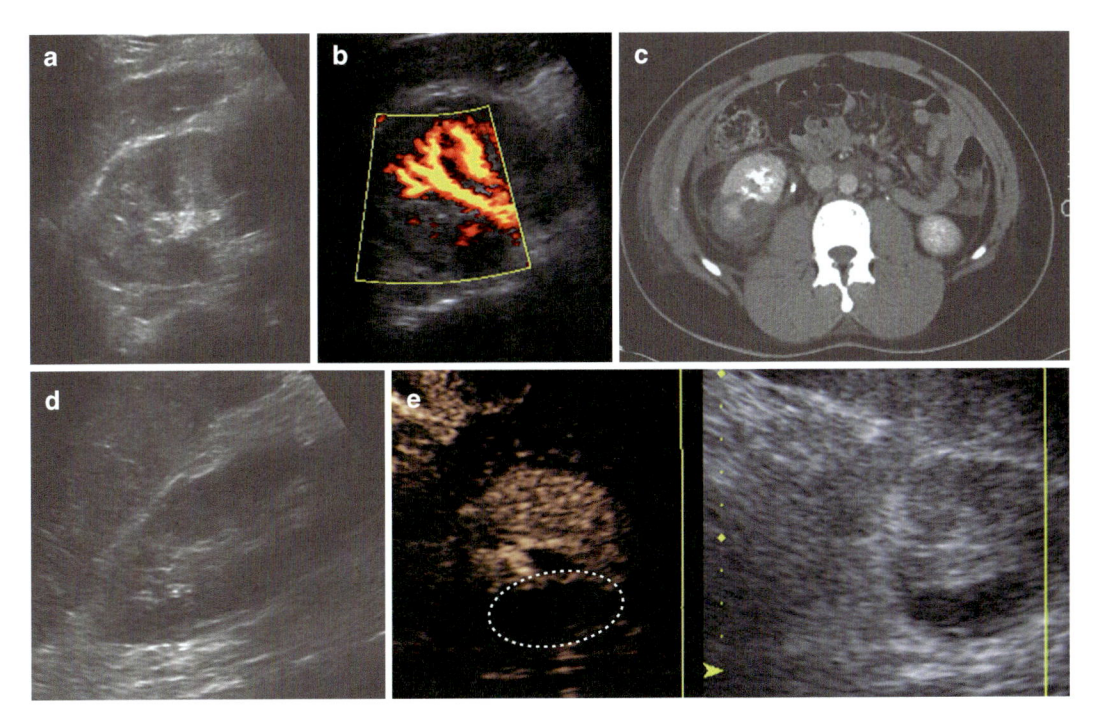

Fig. 4 Potential of aCDS and ce-US in renal trauma: excellent early depiction of renal injury after moderate abdominal trauma by aCDS (**b**), not really convincingly depictable on gray scale imaging (**a**) in the early phase after the accident. Corresponding ce-CT image (**c**). The renal injury in another patient with splenic laceration is hardly seen on the gray scale image (**d**), whereas ce-US (dual/split image display, left side is the contrast image) nicely delineates the nonperfused (= noncontrasted, *dotted circle*) area (**e**)

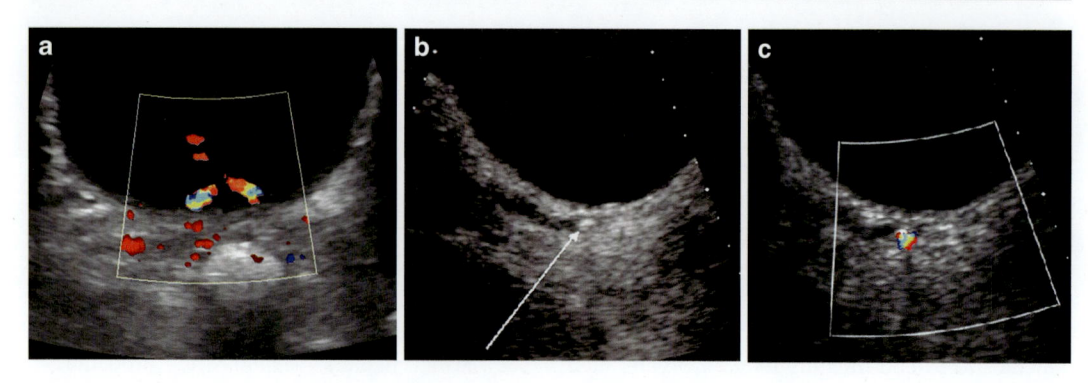

Fig. 5 Potential of modern CDS in urolithiasis: (**a**) CDS depicts the symmetric ureteral inflow jet proving patency of the ureter; (**b**) a small calculus in the distal ureter is depicted (*arrow*) – becoming much more obvious by the "twinkling sign" using CDS (**c**) than on pure gray scale imaging

tions have become more important, such as a full bladder as a requirement for being able to visualize the distal ureter; new CDS applications such as the ureteral jet and the twinkling sign have further increased US potential – therefore US is recommended as the first imaging step, and low-dose "stone-CT" only rarely becomes necessary (Riccabona et al. 2009) (Fig. 5).

In childhood (glomerulo-) nephritis imaging usually does not play such an essential role as in other nephrourological conditions. It often cannot offer a definite diagnosis. But there are some specific findings which can be important and need to be known and looked for; furthermore additional information on the intravascular fluid load, potential effusions, other potentially related manifestations (e.g., bowel involvement in hemolytic-uremic syndrome), or renal perfusion (reflecting the disease severity, sometimes with high prognostic value) must be offered and are valuable details for patient management.

> **Take Away**
> Guidelines and recommendations on imaging procedures and algorithms exist and are helpful for standardizing imaging. They have changed over time and are constantly evolving, too. However, not for all queries these are ideal and universally accepted; furthermore there is some local and individual variation.

6 Imaging Algorithms and Procedural Recommendations

There are numerous guidelines and recommendations from different national and international groups (mostly scientific associations and societies) and issued by the different specialties involved; sometimes, every institution has its own rules. The most commonly used are from clinical fields and issued by national groups or institutions such as those from the American Academy/Association and the British National Institute for Health and Clinical Excellence (NICE) (McDonald and Kenney 2014); In pediatric uroradiology there are by far less, on supranational level these are the joint recommendations of the ESPR abdominal (GI and GU) imaging task force and the ESUR pediatric working group. How did this pile of partially contradicting numerous guidelines arise? It happened in the last two decades, driven partially by economic reasons, partially by legal and regulatory intentions, and only in part based on the real interest of our patients. Evidence and evidence based has become the magic word – or better the spell – during the last decade, with all its restrictions and limitations. Nobody dares to question this Holy Grail of ultimate proof; however, there are restrictions in many regards: are these available for pediatric (imaging) queries? Has the right question been posed? Which is the evidence level – have they been questioned in the light of long-term consequences and impact on the entire socioeconomical life time balance? Are the proposed guidelines applicable throughout the world, and are the respective tests available 24/7 for the entire pediatric population? Still at present there are no better tools for evaluating the correctness of our measures, and thus we have to use them to the best of our knowledge, but baring in mind those restrictions.

Why still try to create such recommendations? Why to adhere to them? There are a number of reasons: They have the potential to increase patient safety and reduce unnecessary burden – e.g., by invasive tests that can be replaced by other methods or are not useful in terms of "diagnostic thinking efficacy". They definitely can provide guidance for less specialized colleagues and centers, define a quality standard, and also may help to reduce costs – where achievable without endangering patient care and well-being, particularly in children who are the future of our society and who will possibly suffer life-long morbidity from mistakes that happened during their childhood, impacting not only the individual and their life quality. And eventually a standardized imaging will enable future meta-analysis and more knowledge and "evidence" for deepening our knowledge and improving imaging as well as selection of the individual method.

For pediatric uroradiology, nearly all relevant procedures and conditions have been addressed by the ESPR and ESUR procedural recommendations and imaging algorithms in a way that they respect local needs and options, integrate existing other guidelines and clinical needs, and are adaptable towards the local and individual needs and options. These procedural recommendations are all available as free/open access articles and cover US, ce-VUS, ce-US, VCUG, IVU, CT, and MRI, but also less frequently performed examinations such as retrograde urethrography or colonography and (fluoroscopic or sonographic) genitography, or interventional procedures such as renal biopsy (Riccabona et al. 2008, 2009, 2012, 2014a, b, 2015, 2016). The imaging algorithms include suggestions for a work-up in childhood UTI, fetal/neonatal moderate or gross (hydronephrosis) UTD, suspected obstructive uropathy, childhood urolithiasis, childhood hypertension, genital and anorectal malformations, disorders of sex development, hematuria, renal trauma, testicular and ovarian torsion, childhood cystic kidney disease, and renal transplantation (Riccabona et al. 2008, 2009, 2014a, b, 2015, 2016). But also with these – as with many pediatric (radiologic) recommendations – evidence is scarce and most of the proposals are consensus statements from expert groups ("eminence based") trying to integrate the available literature. We also have to be aware that there may be some differences to algorithms and suggestions offered by pediatric nephrology and pediatric urology.

Guidelines and recommendations are helpful but shall not completely govern our professional practice. It is and hopefully will remain the individual patient and their wellbeing that should define our proceedings and procedures, indications, and performance. This is reflected by the increasing importance and acceptance of "personalized" medicine, a trend also supported by research and newest treatment developments. And it is of utmost importance that – before following a certain guideline – one has to make oneself knowledgeable about the topic and select the proper recommendation, abandon the idea of having to reinvent the wheel all the time over and over again, find out if it is applicable in the respective local circumstances and patient population, and then be consistent in the daily routine. Only if these are used prudently, they have the chance to improve patient care and reduce invasiveness (and potentially costs).

Take Away

Various guidelines and suggestion exist with sometimes differing implications and recommendation – partially depending on which group has issued them for which purpose. They often are more experience- and eminence-based, as evidence is scarce for many pediatric queries. And above all, the individual patient care is the most important aspect governing imaging – trying to be as little burdening and invasive as possible without missing a possibly treatable condition that might impact morbidity.

Conclusion

Interdisciplinary communication and cooperation are necessary for optimal treatment of children with renal disorders where imaging significantly contributes to management.

Infants and children with UTI need appropriate treatment. Antibiotic prophylaxis is recommended in selected cases, but imaging is required in all. Renal scarring following UTI is equally found in patients with and without VUR. Prospective studies eventually modifying the current treatment of infants and children with VUR are welcome. Long-term renal morbidity is significant, and prevention of renal damage is the ultimate goal. It is not an option to reduce all imaging to detect VUR nearly to zero. Not to identify children with dilating VUR and a high risk for renal compromise may increase long-term renal morbidity.

Fetal UTD frequently is a transient feature, but postpartum renal US is needed in all with a significant distention. The majority of infants with significant postpartum findings have PUJO. Follow-up studies with renal US and isotope investigations (or fMRU) decide between the more frequently applied "wait and see strategy" and surgery.

Guidelines and recommendations are important for the daily routine and are permanently influenced by the results of new research, thus they need revisiting and updates. They should be appropriate for most countries and centers, and evidence based – if available (which is only rarely the case in pediatric radiology). Modifications according to preferences of single centers and necessities of the individual patient ("personalized medicine") are acceptable unless the timely treatment and long-term prognosis of the neonates, infants, and children are not challenged.

References

Al-Sayyad AJ, Pike JG, Leonard MP (2005) Can prophylactic antibiotics safely be discontinued in children with vesicoureteral reflux? J Urol 174:1587–1589
American Academy of Pediatrics. Committee on Quality Improvement. Subcommittee on Urinary Tract Infection (1999) Practice parameter: the diagnosis, treatment, and evaluation of the initial urinary tract infection in febrile infants and young children. Pediatrics 103:843–852
American Academy of Pediatrics (2011) Urinary tract infection: clinical practice guideline for the diagnosis and management of the initial UTI in febrile infants and children 2 to 24 months. Pediatrics 128:595–610
Amerstorfer EE, Haberlik A, Riccabona M (2015) Imaging assessment of renal injuries in children and adolescents: CT or ultrasound? Eur J Pediatr Surg 50:448–455
Ardissino G, Dacco V, Testa S et al (2003) Epidemiology of chronic renal failure in children: data from the ItalKid project. Pediatrics 111:382–387
Beetz R (2006) May we go on with antibacterial prophylaxis for urinary tract infections? Pediatr Nephrol 21:5–13
Beetz R, Mannhardt W, Fisch M et al (2002) Long-term follow-up of 158 young adults surgically treated for vesicoureteral reflux in childhood: the ongoing risk of urinary tract infections. J Urol 168:704–707
Bouissou F, Munzer C, Decramer S et al (2008) Prospective, randomized trial comparing short and long intravenous antibiotic treatment of acute pyelonephritis in children: dimercaptosuccinic acid scintigraphic evaluation at 9 months. Pediatrics 121(3):e553–e560
Capello SA, Kogan BA, Giorgi LJ Jr et al (2005) Prenatal ultrasound has led to earlier detection and repair of ureteropelvic junction obstruction. J Urol 174:1425–1428
Capozza N, Lais A, Matarazzo E et al (2003) Treatment of vesico-ureteric reflux: a new algorithm based on parental preference. BJU Int 92:285–288
Capozza N, Caione P (2007) Vesicoureteral reflux: surgical and endoscopic treatment. Pediatr Nephrol 22:1261–1265
Cassart M, Massez A, Metens T et al (2004) Complementary role of MRI after sonography in assessing bilateral urinary tract anomalies in the fetus. Am J Roentgenol 182:689–695
Cohen AL, Rivara FP, Davis R et al (2005) Compliance with guidelines for the medical care of first urinary tract infections in infants: a population-based study. Pediatrics 115:1474–1478
Conway PH, Cnaan A, Zaoutis T, Henry BV, Grundmeier RW, Keren R (2007) Recurrent urinary tract infections in children: risk factors and association with prophylactic antimicrobials. JAMA 298:179–186
Cooper CS, Chung BI, Kirsch AJ et al (2000) The outcome of stopping prophylactic antibiotics in older children with vesicoureteral reflux. J Urol 163:269–272
De Palma D, Manzoni G (2013) Different imaging strategies in febrile urinary tract infection in childhood. What, when, why? Pediatr Radiol 43:436–443
Dejter SW Jr, Gibbons MD (1989) The fate of infant kidneys with fetal hydronephrosis but initially normal postnatal sonography. J Urol 142:661–662
Dhillon HK (1998) Prenatally diagnosed hydronephrosis: the great ormond street experience. BJU Int 81(Suppl 2):39–44
Elder JS, Peters CA, Arant BS Jr et al (1997) Pediatric vesicoureteral reflux guidelines panel summary report

on the management of primary vesicoureteral reflux in children. J Urol 157:1846–1851

Fanos V, Cataldi L (2004) Antibiotics or surgery for vesicoureteric reflux in children. Lancet 364:1720–1722

Fernbach SK, Maizels M, Conway JJ (1993) Ultrasound grading of hydronephrosis: introduction to the system used by the society for fetal urology. Pediatr Radiol 23:478–480

Garin EH, Olavarria F, Nieto VC et al (2006) Clinical significance of primary vesicoureteral reflux and urinary antibiotic prophylaxis after acute pyelonephritis: a multicenter, randomized, controlled study. Pediatrics 117:626–632

Gordon I, Barkovics M, Pindoria S et al (2003) Primary vesicoureteric reflux as a predictor of renal damage in children hospitalized with urinary tract infection: a systematic review and meta-analysis. J Am Soc Nephrol 14:739–744

Hansson S, Bollgren I, Esbjorner E et al (1999) Urinary infections in children below two years of age: a quality assurance project in Sweden. The swedish pediatric nephrology association. Acta Paediatr 88:270–274

Hansson S, Dhamey M, Sigström O et al (2004) Dimercaptosuccinic acid scintigraphy instead of voiding cystourethrography for infants with urinary tract infection. J Urol 172:1071–1074

Hellerstein S (2006) Acute urinary tract infection–evaluation and treatment. Curr Opin Pediatr 18:134–138

Hellerstein S, Nickell E (2002) Prophylactic antibiotics in children at risk for urinary tract infection. Pediatr Nephrol 17:506–510

Hoberman A, Charron M, Hickey RW et al (2003) Imaging studies after first febrile urinary tract infection in young children. N Engl J Med 348:195–202

Hollowell JG (2002) Screening siblings for vesivoureteral reflux. J Urol 168:2138–2141

Hörmann M, Brugger PC, Balassy C et al (2006) Fetal MRI of the urinary system. Eur J Radiol 57:303–311

Ismaïli K, Avni FE, Piepsz A et al (2004) Current management of infants with fetal renal pelvis dilatation: a survey by French-speaking pediatric nephrologists and urologists. Pediatr Nephrol 19:966–971

Ismaïli K, Hall M, Piepsz A et al (2006) Primary vesicoureteral reflux detected in neonates with a history of fetal renal pelvis dilatation: a prospective clinical and imagig study. J Pediatr 148:222–227

Jodal U (1987) The natural history of bacteriuria in childhood. Infect Dis North Am 1:713–729

Jodal U, Lindberg U (1999) Guidelines for management of children with urinary tract infection and vesicoureteric reflux. Recommendations from a Swedish state-of-the-art conference. Acta Paediatr 88(Suppl 431):87–89

Jodal U, Smellie JM, Lax H et al (2006) Ten-year results of randomized treatment of children with severe vesicoureteral reflux. Final report of the international reflux study in children. Pediatr Nephrol 21:785–792

John U et al (2004) The impact of fetal renal pelvic diameter on postnatal outcome. Prenat Diagn 24:591–595

Jungers P, Houillier P, Chauveau D et al (1996) Pregnancy in women with reflux nephropathy. Kidney Int 50:593–599

Kaneko K, Ohtomo Y, Shimizu T et al (2003) Antibiotic prophylaxis by low-dose cefaclor in children with vesicoureteral reflux. Pediatr Nephrol 18:468–470

Köhler J, Tencer J, Thysell H et al (1997) Vesicoureteral reflux diagnosed in adulthood. Incidence of urinary tract infections, hypertension, proteinuria, back pain and renal calculi. Nephrol Dial Transplant 12:2580–2587

La Scola C, De Mutiis C, Hewitt IK et al (2013) Different guidelines for imaging after first UTI in febrile infants: yield, cost, and radiation. Pediatrics 131:e665–e671

Lee RS, Cendron M, Kinnamon DD et al (2006a) Antenatal hydronephrosis as a predictor of postnatal outcome: a meta-analysis. Pediatrics 118:586–593

Lee RS, Diamond DA, Chow JS (2006b) Applying the ALARA concept to the evaluation of vesicoureteral reflux. Pediatr Radiol 36(Suppl 2):185–191

Lidefelt KJ, Ek S, Mihocsa L (2006) Is screening for vesicoureteral reflux mandatory in infants with antenatal renal pelvis dilatation? Acta Paediatr 95:1653–1656

Mak RH, Kuo HJ (2006) Pathogenesis of urinary tract infection: an update. Curr Opin Pediatr 18:148–152

Malone PSJ (2005) Circumcision for preventing urinary tract infection in boys: European view. Arch Dis Child 90:774–774

Marcus N, Ashkenazi S, Yaari A, Samra Z, Livni G (2005) Non-Escherichia coli versus Escherichia coli community-acquired urinary tract infections in children hospitalized in a tertiary centre: relative frequency, risk factors, anti-microbial resistance and outcome. Pediatr Infect Dis J 24:581–585

Marks SD, Gordon I, Tullus K (2008) Imaging in childhood urinary tract infections: time to reduce investigations. Pediatr Nephrol 23:9–17

Marks SD (2007) How have the past 5 years of research changed clinical practice in paediatric nephrology? Arch Dis Child 92:357–361

Marra G, Oppezzo C, Ardissino G et al (2004) Severe vesicoureteral reflux and chronic renal failure: a condition peculiar to male gender? data from the ItalKid project. J Pediatr 144:677–681

McDonald K, Kenney I (2014) Being NICE to Paediatric UTIs: a retrospective application of the NICE guidelines to a large general practitioner referred historical cohort. Pediatr Radiol 44:1085–1092

Montini G, Rigon L, Zucchetta P et al (2008) Prophylaxis after the first febrile urinary tract infection in children? a multicenter, randomized, controlled, noninferiority trial. Pediatrics 122:1064–1071

Moorthy I, Easty M, McHugh K et al (2005) The presence of vesicoureteric reflux does not identify a population at risk for renal scarring following a first urinary tract infection. Arch Dis Child 90:733–736

Mor Y, Leibovitch I, Zalts R et al (2003) Analysis of the longterm outcome of surgically corrected vesicoureteric reflux. BJU Int 92:97–100

Mulvey MA, Schilling JD, Martinez JJ et al (2000) Bad bugs and beleaguered bladders: interplay between uropathogenic escherichia coli and innate host defenses. Proc Natl Acad Sci U S A 97:8829–8835

National Institute for Health and Clinical Excellence (2007) Urinary tract infection in children: diagnosis, treatment and long-term management. 2007. http://www.nice.org.uk/nicemedia/pdf/CG54fullguideline.pdf

Nguyen HT, Benson CB, Bromley B, Campbell JB, Chow J, Coleman B, Cooper C, Crino J, Darge K, Herndon CDA, Odibo AO, Somers MJG, Stein DR (2014) Multidisciplinary consensus on the classification of prenatal and postnatal urinary tract dilation (UTD classification system). J Pediatr Urol 10(6):982–998

Nuutinen M, Uhari M (2001) Recurrence and follow-up after urinary tract infection under the age of 1 year. Pediatr Nephrol 16:69–72

Ogan K, Pohl HG, Carlson D et al (2001) Parental preferences in the management of vesicoureteral reflux. J Urol 166:240–243

Onen A, Jayanthi VR, Koff SA (2002) Long-term follow-up of prenatally detected severe bilateral newborn hydronephrosis initially managed nonoperatively. J Urol 168:1118–1120

Pennesi M, Travan L, Peratoner L et al (2008) Is antibiotic prophylaxis in children with vesicoureteral reflux effective in preventing pyelonephritis and renal scars? a randomized, controlled trial. Pediatrics 121:e1489–e1494

Peters CA, Skoog SJ, Arant BS Jr et al (2010) Summary of the AUA guideline on management of primary vesicoureteral reflux in children. J Urol 184:1134–1144

Puri P, Pirker M, Mohanan N et al (2006) Subureteral dextranomer/hyaluronic acid injection as first line treatment in the management of high grade vesicoureteral reflux. J Urol 176:1856–1859

Riccabona M (2016) Imaging in childhood urinary tract infection. Radiol Medica 121(3):238–239. doi: 10.1007/s11547-015-0594-1

Riccabona M, Fotter R (2004a) Reorientation and future trends in paediatric uroradiology. Pediatr Radiol 34:295–301

Riccabona M, Fotter R (2004b) Urinary tract infection in infants and children: an update with special regard to the changing role of reflux. Eur Radiol 14(Suppl 4):L78–L88

Riccabona M, Avni FE, Blickman JG, Darge K, Dacher JN, Lobo LM, Willi U (2008) Imaging recommendations in paediatric uroradiology: minutes of the ESPR workgroup session on urinary tract infection, fetal hydronephrosis, urinary tract ultrasonography and voiding cysto-urethrography. ESPR-Meeting, Barcelona/Spain, June 2007. ESUR Paediatric guideline subcommittee and ESPR paediatric uroradiology work group. Pediatr Radiol 38:138–145

Riccabona M, Avni FE, Blickman JG, Dacher JN, Darge K, Lobo ML, Willi U (2009) (Members of the ESUR paediatric paediatric recommendation work group and ESPR paediatric uroradiology work group). Imaging recommendations in paediatric uroradiology, part II: urolithiasis and haematuria in children, paediatric obstructive uropathy, and postnatal work-up of foetally diagnosed high grade hydronephrosis. Minutes of a mini-symposium at the ESPR annual meeting, Edinburg, June. Pediatr Radiol 39 (8):891–898

Riccabona M, Avni FE, Dacher JN, Damasio B, Darge K, Lobo ML, Ording-Müller LS, Papado-polos F, Willi U (2010) ESPR uroradiology task force and ESUR paediatric working group: Imaging and procedural recommendations in paediatric uroradiology, Part III. Minutes of the ESPR uroradiology task force mini-symposium on intravenous urography, uro-CT and MR-urography in childhood. Pediatr Radiol 40(7):1315–1320

Riccabona M, Avni F, Dacher JN, Damasio B, Darge K, Lobo ML, Ording-Müller LS, Papado-poulou F, Vivier P, Willi U (2011) ESPR uroradiology task force and ESUR paediatric working group: imaging recommendations in paediatric uroradiology, part IV minutes of the ESPR urora-diology task force mini-symposium on imaging in childhood renal hypertension and imaging of renal trauma in children. Pediatr Radiol 41(7):939–944

Riccabona M, Avni F, Damasio B, Ordning-Mueller LS, Lobo ML, Darge K, Papadopoulou F, Willi U, Blickmann J, Vivier PH (2012) ESPR uroradiology task force and ESUR paediatric working group - imaging recommendations in paediatric uroradiology, part V: childhood cystic kidney disease, childhood renal transplantation, and contrast-enhanced ultrasound in children. Pediatr Radiol 42:1275–1283

Riccabona M, Lobo ML, Willi U, Avni F, Blickmann J, Damasio B, Ordning-Mueller LS, Darge K, Papadopoulou F, Vivier PH (2014a) ESPR uroradiology task force and ESUR paediatric working group - imaging recommendations in paediatric uroradiology, part VI: childhood renal biopsy and imaging of neonatal and infant genital tract. Pediatr Radiol 44:496–502

Riccabona M, Vivier HP, Ntoulj A, Darge K, Avni F, Papadopoulou F, Damasio B, Ordning-Mueller LS, Blickmann J, Lobo ML, Willi U (2014b) ESPR uroradiology task force – imaging recommendations in paediatric uroradiology - part VII: standardized terminology, impact of existing recommendations, and update on contrast-enhanced ultrasound of the paediatric urogenital tract. Pediatr Radiol 44:1478–1484

Riccabona M, Darge K, Lobo ML, Orling-Muller LS, Augdal TA, Avni FE, Blickman J, Damasio BM, Ntoulia A, Papadopoulou F, Vivier PH, Willi U (2015) ESPR Uroradiology Task Force – imaging recommendations in paediatric uroradiology – part VIII: rethrograde urethrography, imaging in disorders of sexual development, and imaging in childhood testicular torsion. Report on the mini-symposium at the ESPR meeting in Amsterdam, June 2014. Pediatr Radiol 45:2023–2028

Riccabona M, Lobo ML, Ording-Mueller LS et al (2017) ESPR Abdominal (GU and GI) Imaging Task Force – Imaging Recommendations in Paediatric Uroradiology, Part IX: imaging in anorectal and cloacal malformation, imaging in childhood ovarian torsion, and efforts in standardising pediatric uroradiology terminology. Report on the mini-symposium at the ESPR meeting in Graz, June 2015, Pediatr Radiol 47; in press

Ring E, Mache CJ, Vilits P (2002) Future expectations - what paediatric nephrologists and urologists await from paediatric uroradiology. Eur J Radiol 43:94–99

Ring E, Petritsch P, Riccabona M et al (1993) Primary VUR in infants with a dilated fetal urinary tract. Eur J Pediatr 152:523–525

Ring E, Zobel G (1988) Urinary infection and malformations of urinary tract in infancy. Arch Dis Child 63:818–820

Royal College of Physicians (1992) Guidelines for the management of acute urinary tract infection in childhood. Report of a working group of the research unit, royal college of physicians. J R Coll Physicians Lond 25:36–42

Saadeh SA, Mattoo TK (2011) Managing urinary tract infections. Pediatr Nephrol 26:1967–1976

Saemann MC, Weichhart T, Horl WH et al (2005) Tamm- Horsfall protein: a multilayered defence molecule against urinary tract infection. Eur J Clin Invest 35:227–235

Schwab CW Jr, Wu HY, Selman H, Smith GH, Snyder HM III, Canning DA (2002) Spontaneous resolution of vesico-ureteric reflux: a 15 year perspective. J Urol 168:2594–2599

Schoen EJ (2005) Circumcision for preventing urinary tract infection in boys: north American view. Arch Dis Child 90:772–773

Sidhu G, Beyene J, Rosenblum ND (2006) Outcome of isolated antenatal hydronephrosis: a systematic review and meta-analysis. Pediatr Nephrol 21:218–224

Smellie JM, Barratt TM, Chantler C et al (2001) Medical versus surgical treatment in children with severe bilateral vesicoureteric reflux and bilateral nephropathy: a randomised trial. Lancet 357:1329–1333

Song SH, Lee SB, Park YS et al (2007) Is antibiotic prophylaxis necessary in infants with obstructive hydronephrosis? J Urol 177:1098–1101

Roberts KB, Subcommittee on Urinary Tract Infection, Steering Committee on Quality Improvement and Management (2011) Urinary tract infection: clinical practice guideline for the diagnosis and management of the initial UTI in febrile infants and children 2 to 24 months. Pediatrics 128:595–610

The RIVUR Trial Investigators (2014) Antimicrobial prophylaxis for children with vesicoureteral reflux. N Engl J Med 370:2367–2376

Thompson M, Simon SD, Sharma V et al (2005) Timing of follow-up voiding cystourethrogram in children with primary vesicoureteral reflux: development and application of a clinical algorithm. Pediatrics 115:426–434

Thompson RH, Chen JJ, Pugach J et al (2001) Cessation of prophylactic antibiotics for managing persistent vesicoureteral reflux. J Urol 166:1465–1469

Thorup J, Jokela R, Cortes D et al (2003) The results of 15 years of consistent strategy in treating antenatally suspected pelvi-ureteric junction obstruction. BJU Int 91:850–852

Toiviainen-Salo S, Garel L, Grignon A et al (2004) Fetal hydronephrosis: is there hope for consensus? Pediatr Radiol 34:519–529

Tsai JD, Huang CT, Lin PY et al (2012) Screening high grade vesicoureteral reflux in young infants with a febrile urinary tract infection. Pediatr Nephrol 27:955–963

Tse NK, Yuen SL, Chiu MC, Lai WM, Tong PC (2009) Imaging studies for first urinary tract infection in infants less than 6 months old: can they be more selective? Pediatr Nephrol 24:1699–1703

Tseng MH, Lin WJ, Lo WT et al (2007) Does a normal DMSA obviate the performance of voiding cystourethrography in evaluation of young children after their first urinary tract infection? J Pediatr 150:96–99

Ulman I, Venkata R, Jayanthi R et al (2000) The long-term follow-up of newborns with severe unilateral hydronephrosis initially treated nonoperatively. J Urol 164:1101–1105

Vivier PH (2015) How to report using standardised terminology. Pediatr Radiol 45(S2):S 269–S 270

Wennerström M, Hansson S, Jodal U et al (2000) Primary and acquired renal scarring in boys and girls with urinary tract infection. J Pediatr 136:30–34

Wheeler D, Vimalachandra D, Hodson EM, Roy LP, Smith G, Craig JC (2003) Antibiotics and surgery for vesicoureteric reflux: a meta-analysis of randomised controlled trials. Arch Dis Child 88:688–694

Williams G, Lee A, Craig J (2001) Antibiotics for the prevention of urinary tract infection in children: a systematic review of randomized controlled trials. J Pediatr 138:868–874

Xhepa R, Bosio M, Manzoni G (2004) Voiding cystourethrosonography for the diagnosis of vesicoureteral reflux in a developing country. Pediatr Nephrol 19:638–643

Yeung CK, Godley ML, Dhillon HK et al (1997) The characteristics of primary vesico-ureteric reflux in male and female infants with pre-natal hydronephrosis. BJU Int 80:319–327

Ylinen E, Ala-Houhala M, Wikstrom S (2004) Outcome of patients with antenatally detected pelviureteric junction obstruction. Pediatr Nephrol 19:880–887

Normal Values

Ekkehard Ring, Hans-Joachim Mentzel, and Michael Riccabona

Contents

1	**Introduction**	773
2	**Physiologic Data**	773
3	**Laboratory Values**	774
3.1	Serum Creatinine and Cystatin C	774
3.2	Combined Serum and Urinary Values	774
3.3	Clearance (C), Glomerular Filtration Rate (GFR)	775
3.4	Fractional Excretion	777
4	**Radiological Data**	778
4.1	Ultrasonography	778
4.2	Voiding Cystourethrography	780
4.3	Other Methods	780
References		782

E. Ring, MD (Retired)
Department of Pediatrics, Division of General Pediatrics, University Hospital Graz, Auenbruggerplatz 30, A-8036 Graz, Austria
e-mail: ekkehard.ring@medunigraz.at

H.-J. Mentzel, MD
Section of Paediatric Radiology, Institute of Diagnostic and Interventional Radiology, University Hospital Jena, Erlanger Allee 101, D-07740 Jena, Germany
e-mail: Hans-Joachim.Mentzel@med.uni-jena.de

M. Riccabona, MD (✉)
Department of Radiology, Division of Pediatric Radiology, University Hospital Graz, Auenbruggerplatz 34, A-8036 Graz, Austria
e-mail: michael.riccabona@medunigraz.at

1 Introduction

Correct interpretation of different data in disease states requires comparison with data obtained in a normal situation. This is valid especially during childhood as, for example, a given value may be normal for an adolescent but is pathologic for an infant. Selected data important for daily routine are discussed in this chapter. For some data, the reader is referred to other chapters of this book. Comments are added where appropriate. However, as intrinsically with all measurements, they always have to be seen in the individual context taking variability and assessment restrictions into consideration; calculating mean values from several measurements will help to reduce errors. A properly standardized initial technique however is mandatory, though even this approach may reveal some variance of measurements taken from the same object during the same investigation (e.g., sonographically measured kidney length, particularly if taken from different access or positions).

2 Physiologic Data

Percentiles for body length and body weight, as well as normograms to calculate body surface area (BSA), are found in most pediatric textbooks or as charts in every pediatric department.

Table 1 Normal heart rate in children: variations according to age

Age	Mean heart rate (bpm)	Range
Neonates	123	(88–168)
1–3 weeks	148	(96–188)
1–12 months	137	(100–176)
1–2 years	119	(68–165)
3–4 years	108	(68–145)
5–7 years	100	(60–139)
8–11 years	91	(51–145)
12–15 years	85	(51–133)

Table 2 Mean systolic blood pressure during the first week of life

Gestational age	Mean systolic blood pressure
<29 weeks	45–57 mmHg
29–32 weeks	50–62 mmHg
33–36 weeks	58–69 mmHg
>37 weeks	66–77 mmHg

A simple estimation of BSA is possible with an empirically derived formula.

$$\mathrm{BSA}(m^2) = \text{square root of} \left[\frac{\text{body weight}(kg) \times \text{body length}(cm)}{3600} \right]$$

Heart rate in children (Table 1) depends on age and factors like sleep, excitement, intravascular volume, or cardiac function. This, as well as many other systemic factors such as intravascular volume or vaso-active drugs need to be considered for correct interpretation of values obtained by Doppler sonography such as resistive index (RI).

Blood pressure in neonates depends on the gestational age (Table 2). Later, blood pressure is influenced by age, gender, and height adjusted to the height percentile at a given age. Figure 1a, b show the upper limit of normal blood pressure related to gender, age, and 5th, 50th, and 95th height percentile.

3 Laboratory Values

Two different units are used worldwide for reporting laboratory values, conventional units, and SI units. Table 3 shows some frequently needed data and the conversion factors between the units. Conventional units have to be multiplied to get SI units. SI units divided by the conversion factor lead to conventional units.

3.1 Serum Creatinine and Cystatin C

Determining serum creatinine is of utmost importance in calculating renal function. Normal values vary strongly with age and this is shown in Table 4 and in Fig. 2. Note that creatinine derives from the metabolism of muscle cells thereby reflecting the muscle mass of the body. Children with muscle deficit like neuromuscular disorders (cerebral palsy, muscle dystrophy, and atrophy), dystrophy, anorexia, or oncologic disorders have lower normal values of creatinine. Yet no standardized values for these subgroups of children exist.

Cystatin C (CysC) is a small protein produced by all nucleated cells in a constant rate, excreted exclusively by glomerular filtration, and totally reabsorbed and degraded in the tubular cells. Normally, there is no excretion into the urine. Not all laboratories measure CysC and determination is more expensive than measuring creatinine. Yet CysC seems to reflect renal function and minor variations better than creatinine. It is a reasonable alternative in selected situations (such as borderline renal function or malnourished children with malignancies). Beyond infancy, CysC values are mostly independent from age, gender, body length, and of muscle mass. The normal value measured by a nephelometric assay is 0.62–1.11 mg/L, but different laboratory kits have to be considered.

Additional important blood and urine values are shown in Tables 5, 6, 7, 8, and 9.

3.2 Combined Serum and Urinary Values

Combined determination of serum and urinary values of markers allow for refinement in determination of different renal functions.

Normal Values

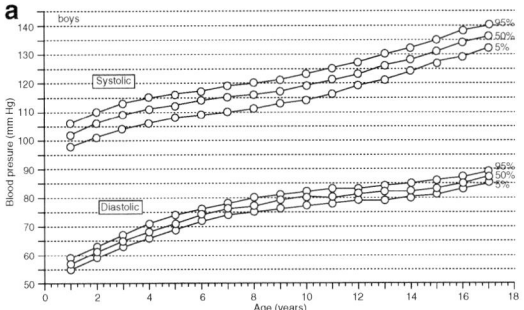

Fig. 1 Normograms for systolic and diastolic blood pressure in boys (**a**) and girls (**b**). The upper limit of normal blood pressure (95th percentile) is shown according to age and percentile for body length (5th, 50th, and 95th percentiles are shown) (Adapted from: The Fourth Report on the Diagnosis, Evaluation, and Treatment of High Blood Pressure in Children and Adolescents (2004))

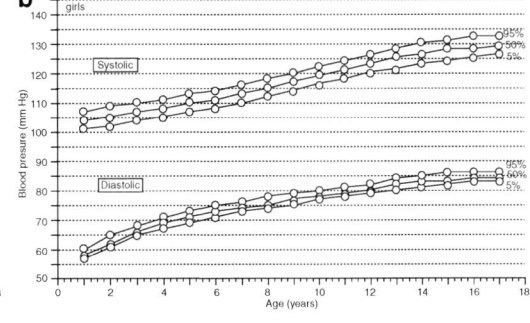

Table 3 Conversion table to standard international (SI) units for commonly used parameters

Component	Present unit	Conversion factor	SI unit
Erythrocytes	per mm^3	1	10^6/l
Leucocytes	per mm^3	1	10^6/l
Platelet count	10^3/mm^3	1	10^9/l
Calcium	mg/dl	0.2495	mmol/l
Phosphorus	mg/dl	0.3229	mmol/l
Creatinine	mg/dl	88.4	µmol/l
Urea nitrogen	mg/dl	0.357	mmol/l
Uric acid	mg/dl	59.48	mmol/l

Table 4 Serum creatinine values in preterm and term neonates during the first 3 weeks of life

Weight	Age 1–2 days	1 week	2 weeks	3 weeks
Preterm 1,000–1,500 g	1.10	0.72	0.55	0.40
Preterm 1,500–2,000 g	1.00	0.65	0.56	0.34
Preterm 2,000–2,500 g	0.94	0.53	0.43	0.34
Full term	0.75	0.45	0.34	0.31

Adapted from Bueva and Guignard (1994)
Mean values, mg/dl

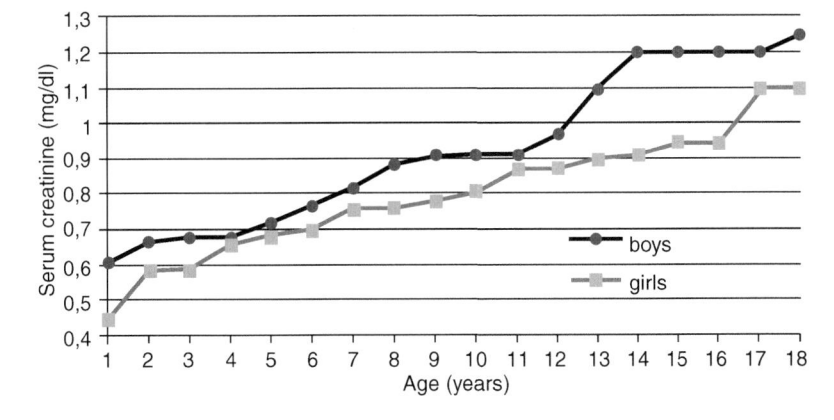

Fig. 2 Serum creatinine values (upper limit of normal) during childhood and adolescence (Adapted from Schwartz et al. (1976))

Calculating clearance and excretion values is possible. These calculations are extremely dependent on urine collection, which may be inappropriate. Formulas without the need for urine collection are derived to overcome this problem.

3.3 Clearance (C), Glomerular Filtration Rate (GFR)

Clearance is defined as the blood volume being cleared of a substance during a certain time. The general clearance formula is $U/P \times V$, where U

Table 5 Selected blood values at different ages

	Neonates	Infants	Age 1–6 years	Age 6–16 years
Leukocytes/mm^3	9,000–30,000	6,000–17,500	5,000–15,000	4,500–13,000
Erythrocytes_10^6/mm^3	4.2–5.8	3.1–4.6	3.7–5.1	3.9–5.3
Hemoglobin (g/dl)	14.00–20.0	11.0–13.5	11.5–13.5	11.5–15.5
Platelet count_10^3/mm^3	150–350	–	140–440	–

Table 6 Selected serum values at different ages

	Neonates	Infants	Age 1–6 years	Age 6–16 years
Sodium (mmol/l)	130–143	–	135–145	–
Potassium (mmol/l)	3.7–5.9	3.9–5.5	3.5–5.0	–
Calcium (mmol/l)	1.9–2.9	–	2.2–2.7	–
Phosphorus (mmol/l)	1.3–2.3	1.25–2.0	1.1–1.75	1.0–1.7
Urea (mg/dl)	10–30	–	10–40	–
Uric acid (mg/dl)	3.6–6.0	–	3.0–6.4	–
Total protein (g/dl)	5.6–8.0	5.6–7.4	5.8–8.0	6.4–8.2

Table 7 Urine values – commonly used parameters

	Normal	*Questionable*	*Pathologic*
Leucocytes/mm^3	<10		>10
Erythrocytes/mm^3	<5	5–10	>10
Bacteriuria (bacterial count/ml urine)			
	Normal		*Pathologic*
Bag urine specimen	≤105		≥106
Mid-stream collection	≤104		≥105
Bladder catheterization	≤103		≥104
Suprapubic aspiration	No bacteria		Each count

Table 8 Proteinuria – normal values and findings for typical conditions

Level of proteinuria	Values
24-h collection	
Normal	<4 mg/m^2 per h
Significant proteinuria	4–40 mg/m^2 per h
Nephrotic range proteinuria	>40 mg/m^2 per h
Spot urine (urine protein/creatinine ratio)	
Normal	<0.2 mg/mg
Minimal proteinuria	0.2–0.5 mg/mg
Moderate proteinuria	0.5–2.0 mg/mg
Nephrotic range proteinuria	>2.0 mg/mg

Table 9 Urinary excretion of electrolytes – normal values

Electrolytes	Values
Sodium	2–4 mmol/kg per day
Potassium	1–2 mmol/kg per day
Calcium	<0.1 mmol/kg per day
Calcium in spot urine	
<1 year	<1.0 mmol/mmol creatinine
>1 year	<0.6 mmol/mmol creatinine

and *P* indicate urinary and plasma (serum) concentrations of a substance, and *V* is urinary volume mostly in 24 h. Correction for time (minute) and BSA are easy to calculate. If a substance with a stable plasma concentration is exclusively excreted by glomerular filtration and not modified or metabolized by the tubular system, the amount found in urine is equal to the filtered amount meaning the glomerular filtration rate (GFR). Inulin is such an ideal substance and inulin clearance is the gold standard for measuring GFR. Iohexol or nuclear medicine substances like ^{51}Cr-EDTA could be an alternative. All these methods are time consuming, invasive, may cause radiation exposure, etc., and are not feasible for daily routine. Creatinine and creatinine clearance are the most widely used markers to measure GFR. CysC is no alternative as it is not found in urine.

$$C_{crea}\left(ml/min/1.73m^2\right) = \frac{U_{crea} \times V(ml\,in\,24h) \times 1.73}{P_{crea} \times 24 \times 60 \times BSA(m^2)}$$

The creatinine clearance roughly equals the GFR. The tubular secretion of creatinine leads to an overestimation of GFR in chronic renal failure where GFR is used to define the five stages of chronic kidney disease shown in Table 10 (K/DOQI 2002; KDIGO 2013). Children <2 years of age do not apply to the five stages and should be categorized as having normal, moderately reduced, or severely reduced GFR. Age dependent normal values of creatinine clearance are shown in Table 11.

GFR estimation models (eGFR) obviating urine sampling were developed to improve correct GFR determination. Some formulae use creatinine, some CysC, and some complex formula both markers (Filler et al. 2012). The Schwartz formula is most frequently used in pediatric nephrology and is shown in Table 12 (Schwartz et al. 1976).

If the local laboratory uses the enzymatic method for determination of serum creatinine instead of the kinetic Jaffe method, the new adapted Schwartz formula should be used: eGFR = 0.413 × height/crea (mg/dl) (Schwartz et al. 2009).

CysC based formulae or complex formulae may offer advantages over the Schwartz formula and two simple CysC formulae are shown:

Formula of Le Bricon: eGFR = (78/CysC) + 4. (Le Bricon et al. 2005)
Formula of Bökenkamp: eGFR = 137/CysC − 20.4. (Bökenkamp et al. 1998)
For additional formulae, the reader is referred to three recent publications (Bacchetta et al. 2011; Filler et al. 2012; Andersen et al. 2013).

Table 10 Stages of chronic kidney disease (CKD) according to GFR

CKD/GFR category	GFR (ml/min/1.73 m²)	Terms
G1	≥90	Normal or high
G2	60–89	Mildly decreased
G3a	45–59	Mildly to moderately decreased
G3b	30–44	Moderately to severely decreased
G4	15–29	Severely decreased
G5	<15	Kidney failure

Table 11 Normal values of creatinine clearance

Age group	Values
Neonates	10–20 ml/min per 1.73 m²
Infants	20–40–60 ml/min per 1.73 m²
1–18 years	80–140 ml/min per 1.73 m²

Table 12 The adapted Schwartz formula applicable for calculating pediatric GFR values $GFR\left(ml/min/1.73m^2\right) = \frac{Body\,length(cm) \times k}{Serum\,creatinine(mg/dl\,or\,mol/L)}$

Table of k	Crea (mg/dl)	Crea (µmol/L)
Low birth weight infants <1 year	0.33	29.2
Term infants <1 year	0.45	39.8
Children 2–12 years	0.55	48.6
Girls 13–18 years	0.55	48.6
Boys 13–18 years	0.70	61.9

3.4 Fractional Excretion

Calculation of fractional excretion (FE) makes it possible to study certain tubular functions. "Fractional" means relative to creatinine. Most frequently, the FE of sodium (FE$_{Na}$) is calculated. For calculation, simultaneous determination of creatinine and of sodium in the serum and in spot urine is needed. FE$_{Na}$ is helpful to distinguish prerenal failure from intrinsic renal failure.

$$FE_{Na}(\%) = \frac{U_{Na} \times P_{Crea} \times 100}{P_{Na} \times U_{Crea}}$$

4 Radiological Data

4.1 Ultrasonography

Body height and body weight influence renal size and volume. In addition, as characteristics of a population may be of value, the data depicted here are valid in most situations, but some populations may require special growth charts (Kasiske and Umen 1986). For estimating kidney volume prone position is recommended because the variance in repeated measurements is smaller than in supine position; at least the same position should be used for follow-up. The kidney volume is calculated using the formula:

$$\text{Kidney volume (ml)} = L \times W \times \left[(D_1 + D_2) : 2\right] \times 0.523$$

where L is bipolar length in the longitudinal plane, W is width, D_1 is longitudinal depth, and D_2 is transverse depth in the axial plane. In the daily routine it is sufficient to sample only D_2 (anteroposterior diameter) in the transverse plane. Thus the formula can be varied to:

$$\text{Kidney volume (ml)} = L \times \left[W \times D_2\right] : 2 \times 0.523$$

Tables 13 and 14 as well as Figs. 3, 4, 5, and 6 show important age adapted normal pediatric sonographic values and how measurements are done Figs. 7 and 8.

Table 7 demonstrates a grading system most commonly used for grading pelvi-caliceal distension (PCD – former term "hydronephrosis").

Bladder volume calculation as well as bladder wall measurements are addressed in Table 8.

Table 13 Urinary bladder measurements

Bladder volume (ml) $= L \times W \times \left[(D_1 + D_2) : 2\right] \times K$ (normal volumes see Fig. 9)	
Bladder wall thickness (upper limit of normal)	
Almost empty bladder	5.0 mm (some use 7 mm as threshold for definite pathology)
Full bladder	3.0 mm (some use 2 mm as additional measure in oversized and overextended bladders)

The factor K ranges from 0.5 to 1.1 depending on the shape of the bladder (Knorr et al. 1990). The other numbers adapted from Jequier and Rousseau (1987)

Comment: Bladder volume measured by ultrasonography reflects the current filling of the bladder which does not necessarily equal the maximal or functional bladder capacity. Measurement of residual urine after voiding seems to be appropriate and 3DUS can significantly improve the accuracy of the results (Riccabona et al. 1996). Bladder wall thickness should be measured at a significant filling of the bladder, best measured on an axial median section of the ventral bladder wall – with the bladder wall in a 90° angle to the US beam direction, and sufficiently away from the bladder trigone and the urachal insertion, using a linear transducer. There is a linear relationship between bladder filling and bladder wall thickness. However, the orienting cut-off point of 3–5 mm seems to be independent of age and gender and is also valid in adults (Jequier and Rousseau 1987; Manieri et al. 1998)

Abbreviations: L length, W width, D_1 longitudinal depth, D_2 transversal depth, K correction factor

Table 14 Normal values for typical common renal Doppler US measurements

	RA	SA	ILA
Neonates	25.3 ± 10.3	a	a
Infants	51.5 ± 13.4	33.0 ± 8.0	19.5 ± 5.0
Toddlers	71.3 ± 13.5	43.6 ± 8.0	28.3 ± 6.8
School age children	80.0 ± 18.0	45.5 ± 9.1	27.9 ± 5.3
Adolescents	80.7 ± 13.7	46.8 ± 11.8	28.0 ± 6.1
Resistive indices (RI)[a]			
	RA	SA	ILA
Neonates	0.79 ± 0.1	a	a
Infants	0.82 ± 0.1	0.81 ± 0.1	0.73 ± 0.2
Toddlers	0.71 ± 0.1	0.67 ± 0.1	0.65 ± 0.1
School age children	0.71 ± 0.1	0.66 ± 0.1	0.58 ± 0.1

Table 14 (continued)

	RA	SA	ILA
Adolescents	0.69 ± 0.1	0.63 ± 0.1	0.60 ± 0.1
Renal blood flow:	4.1 ± 1.2 ml/min/g kidney		

Systolic peak flow velocity in renal arteries, V_{systmax} (cm/s)
Values derived from recent literature (Deeg et al. 1994 and Deeg et al. 2014; Yildirim et al. 2005; Grunert et al. 1990)
Comment: Determination of RI is the most common measure giving information on renal perfusion and on vascular resistance. Several renal arteries must be checked for correct interpretation. RI is angle-independent but influenced by many other (systemic) factors such as heart rate, cardiac output, blood viscosity, circulating blood volume, and medications such as vasopressor support. Thus, pathologic values should be compared to values of other low resistive arteries to exclude systemic changes. A side difference of RI may indicate unilateral renal disease
Defined measurements points:
    Main renal artery close to the origin from abdominal aorta and/or close to entering the kidney at the renal hilus
    Segmental arteries intrarenal in central echo complex
    Interlobar arteries at the level of the mid-medullar pyramid
    Arcuate arteries at transition from medulla to cortex
Abbreviations: *RA* renal artery, *SA* segmental artery, *ILA* interlobular artery, * not available, *RI* resistive index
[a]RI is calculated by the formula $\text{RI} = (V_s - V_d)/V_s$, [$V_s$ is the maximum peak-systolic flow velocity and V_d is the end-diastolic flow velocity]

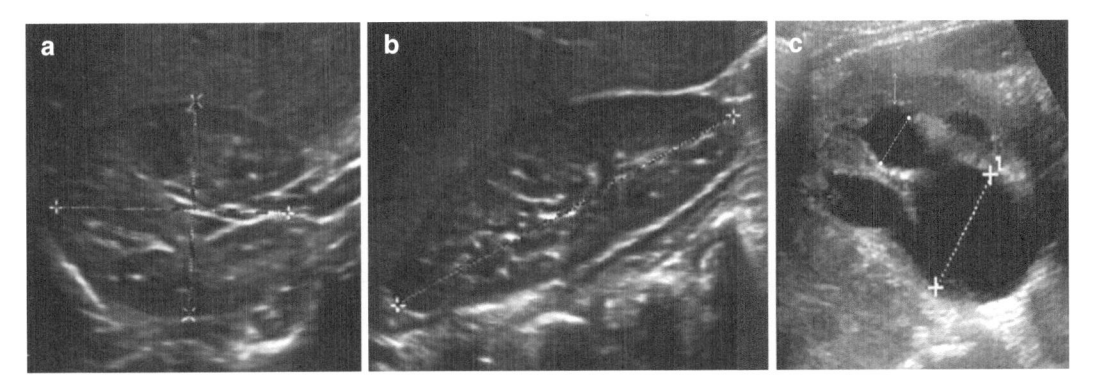

Fig. 3 US images demonstrating the correct planes for measurement of renal size. *Comment*: Exact measurement of real maximal length and diameters of the kidneys is of utmost importance. Most inaccuracies derive from measurements taken in a slightly oblique or displaced section

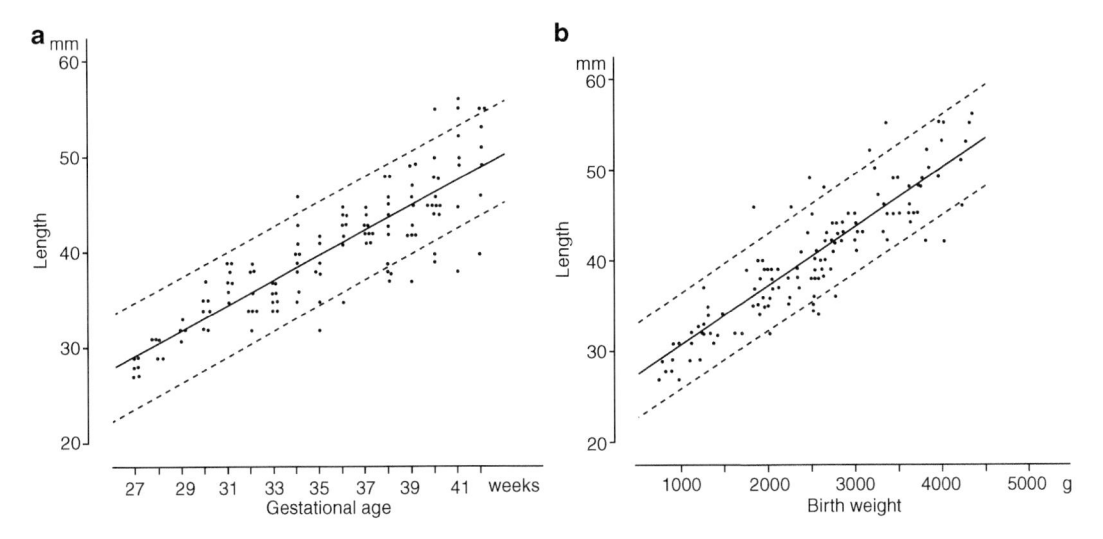

Fig. 4 Kidney length related to (**a**) gestational age and (**b**) birth weight in term and preterm neonates (Data derived from ultrasonography. From Chiara et al. (1989))

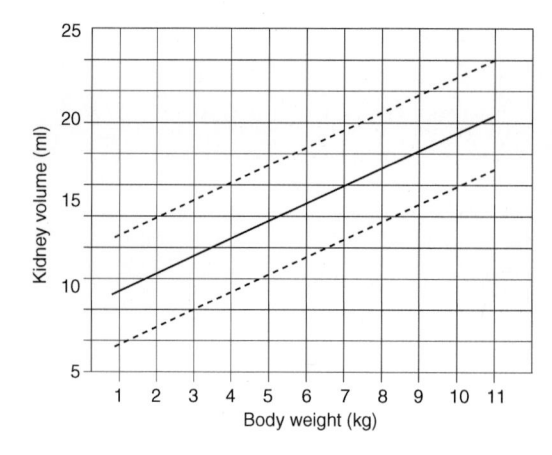

Fig. 5 Kidney volume of neonates and infants related to body weight. Mean ±2 SD are shown. Data derived from ultrasonography (Modified from Peters et al. (1986))

4.2 Voiding Cystourethrography

A formula-derived estimation of bladder capacity (BC) is shown in Table 15. Data of BC obtained during VCUG are compared with formula-derived BC in Fig. 9.

4.3 Other Methods

Data for IVU are not addressed as hardly used any longer; the relevant data and information (not really typical "normal values") for CT, MRI, as well as nuclear medicine are outlined in the various chapters when presenting the dedicated indications, conditions, and protocols.

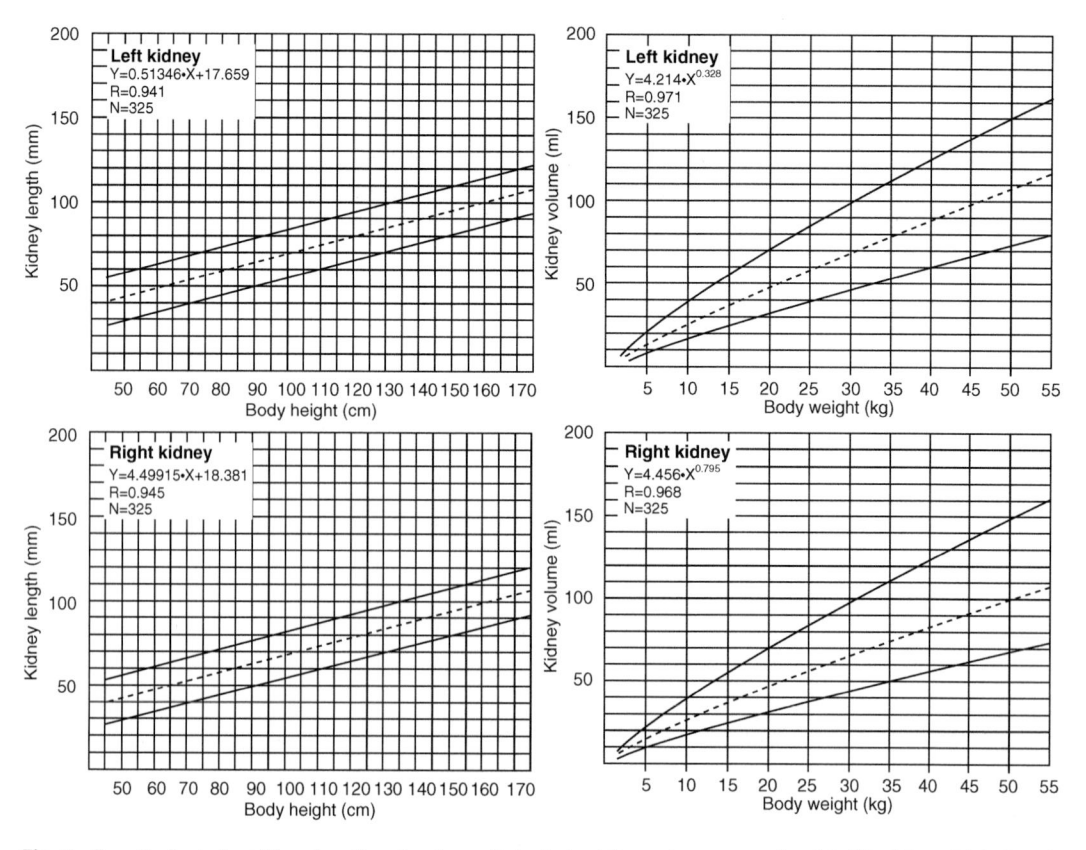

Fig. 6 Growth charts for kidney length and volume. Data derived from ultrasonography (Modified from Dinkel et al. (1985))

US grading of pelvi-caliceal distention / dilatation / width (PCD) in neonates and infants

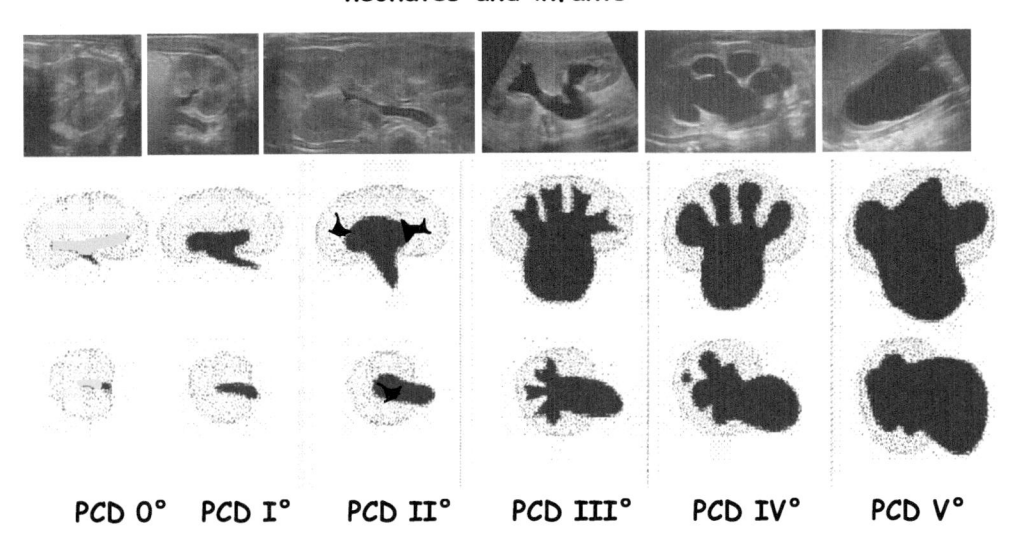

PCD 0°   PCD I°   PCD II°   PCD III°   PCD IV°   PCD V°

PCD 0   =   collecting system not or hardy visible, normal
PCD I   =   just renal pelvis clearly visible, calices not depictable
            axial plevic diameter less than 7 mm, considered normal
PCD II =   axial renal pelvis diameter less than 10 mm , (some) calices visible, but with
            normal forniceal and papillar shape / configuration (often normal variation)
PCD III =   marked dilatation of calices and pelvis, the pelvic axial width usually >10 mm
            with flattened papilla and rounded fornices, but without parenchymal narrowing
PCD IV =   gross dilatation of entire collecting system + narrowing of renal parenchyma
(PCD V =   additionally used in some places, to describe an extreme PCD IV°
            with only a thin, membrane-like residual renal parenchymal rim)

Fig. 7 Grading of pelvi-caliceal distension (PCD) on US – old "hydronephrosis (HN) grading" grade 0: closely apposed central renal echo complex; grade 1: slight separation of the central renal echo complex; grade 2: further dilatation of the renal pelvis, a single or a few calices are visible; grade 3: dilated renal pelvis, all calices are fluid filled, normal thickness of renal parenchyma; grade 4: as in grade 3, but thinning of the renal parenchyma over the calices (Adapted from the ESPR grading proposal (Riccabona et al. 2008, updated 2016) based on Hofmann's pediatric ultrasonographic (Hofmann 1981) and the Society of fetal urology's grading system (Fernbach et al. 1993).

Grading system for dilated ureter: grade 1: ureter dilated less than 7 mm; grade 2: ureter 7–10 mm; grade 3: ureter greater than 10 mm (Adapted from Fernbach et al. (1993)).

Comment: The grading system was first introduced for pediatric ultrasonography by Hofmann, then introduced to standardize the degree of hydronephrosis primarily in fetuses with prenatally recognized hydronephrosis and to allow comparison between institutions. Finally, the ESPR recommendation for renal pelvo-caliceal distension, based from Hofmann's ultrasonographic pediatric grading proposal and the fetal classification described by Fernbach et al. was introduced to allow comparison between prenatal and postnatal findings, for descriptive postnatal use in sonographic studies – this is the grading system listed and illustrated above (Riccabona et al. 2008, updated 2016). As calyceal distension depends on urine production, standardized and optimized hydration is crucial. In addition to the grading, accurate measurement of pelvic, calyceal, and ureteral diameters are helpful and must be read with considering calyceal and forniceal morphology. Note that these grades are different from those commonly used in adult urology, and that this system does not address renal parenchymal pathology except for parenchymal narrowing. Furthermore, the degree ("grade") of pelvic and calyceal distension does not define the entity, and even high degree dilatation does not necessarily equal obstruction. Also note that PCD 0–II may often represent normal findings

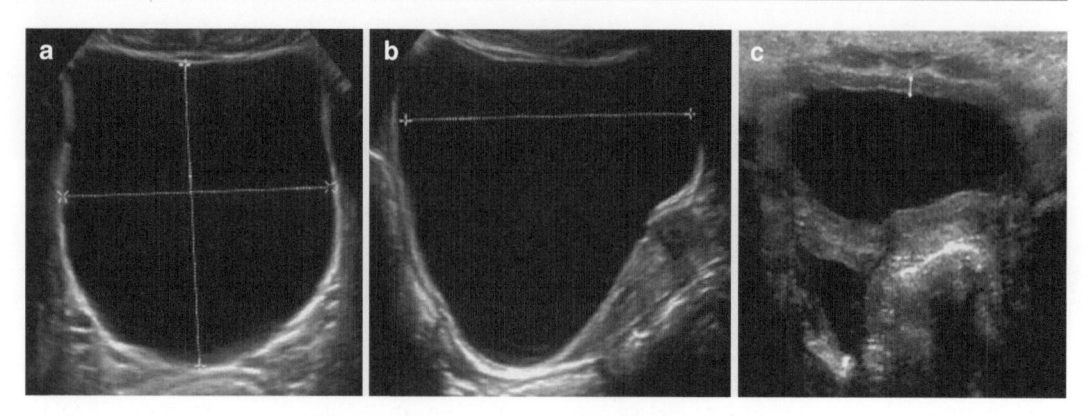

Fig. 8 (**a–c**) Urinary bladder measurements on ultrasonography. Axial (**a**) and sagittal (**b**) diameters (+.... +) as used for bladder volume calculation. Note that these measurements should represent the geometrical axes of the geometric model used as the base for the calculation. Note that in (**b**) there is a typical mistake – the upper border cross is placed inside the bladder (not realized on the small US screen, only afterwards when reviewing it), and the lower cross is just placed at an estimate of the bladder wall, as it was not depictable on the US screen. (**c**) Measurement of bladder wall thickness (◆———◆) in the near field using a linear transducer and a section with the US-beam orthogonal to the bladder wall. Note some ascites behind the bladder in this cross-section view with a thick-walled bladder which is only insufficiently filled – not reliably useful for proper wall thickness assessment

Table 15 Bladder capacity (BC): age dependent bladder capacity (both formulas are identical)

$BC(ml) = (Age\ in\ years + 2) \times 30$
$BC(ml) = (30 \times age\ in\ years) + 60$
Bladder capacity in children with myelodysplasia
$BC(ml) = (24.5 \times age\ in\ years) + 62$

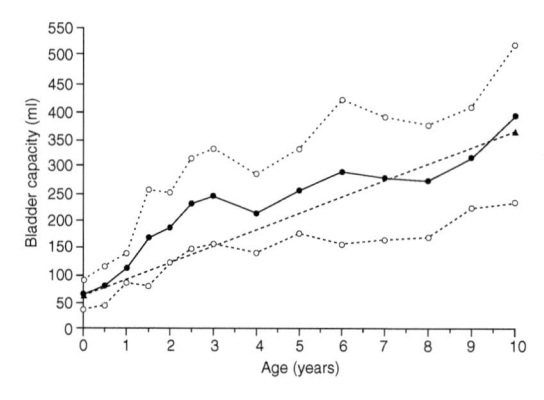

Fig. 9 Bladder capacity (BC) (mean ± 1 SD) during childhood. The *dotted line* represents the formula-derived estimation of BC (Data obtained from Zerin et al. (1993)). *Comment*: The above-mentioned formula seems to underestimate mean BC during the first few years of life. This may reflect the normal development of BC but could be influenced by bladder training to reach continence. Children with myelodysplasia seem to have a BC approximately 20–25 % lower than neurologically intact children (Palmer et al. 1997)

References

Andersen TB, Jodal L, Erlandsen EJ et al (2013) Detecting reduced renal function in children: comparison of GFR-models and serum markers. Pediatr Nephrol 28:83–92

Bacchetta J, Cochat P, Rognant N et al (2011) Which creatinine and cystatin c equations can be reliably used in children? Clin J Am Soc Nephrol 6:552–560

Bueva A, Guignard JP (1994) Renal function in preterm neonates. Pediatr Res 36:572–577

Bökenkamp A, Domanetzki M, Zinck R et al (1998) Cystatin C – a new marker of glomerular filtration rate in childfrren independent of age and height. Pediatrics 101:875–881

Chiara A, Chirico G, Barbarini M et al (1989) Ultrasonic evaluation of kidney length in term and preterm infants. Eur J Pediatr 149:94–95

Deeg KH, Wörle K, Wolf A (1994) Doppler sonographic estimation of normal values for flow velocity and resistance indices in renal arteries of healthy infant. Ultraschall Med 24:312–322

Deeg KH, Hofmann V, Hoyer PF (2014) Ultraschalldiagnostik in Pädiatrie und Kinderchrirurgie. Georg Thieme Verlag

Dinkel E, Ertel M, Dittrich M et al (1985) Kidney size in childhood: sonographical growth charts for kidney length and volume. Pediatr Radiol 15:38–43

Fernbach SK, Maizels M, Conway JJ (1993) Ultrasound grading of hydronephrosis: introduction to the system used by the society for Fetal Urology. Pediatr Radiol 23:478–480

Filler G, Huang SS, Yasin A (2012) The usefulness of cystatin C and related formulae in pediatrics. Clin Chem Lab Med 50:2081–2091

Grunert D, Schöning M, Rosendahl W (1990) Renal blood flow and flow velocity in children and adolescents: duplex Doppler evaluation. Eur J Pediatr 149:287–292

Hofmann V (1981) Ultraschalldiagnostik (B-Scan) im Kindesalter. VEB Georg Thieme Verlag, Leipzig

Jequier S, Rousseau O (1987) Sonographic measurements of the normal bladder wall in children. Am J Roentgenol 149:563–566

Kasiske BL, Umen AJ (1986) The influence of age, sex, race, and body habitus on kidney weight in humans. Arch Pathol Lab Med 110:55–60

KDIGO Clinical practice guideline for the evaluation and management of chronic kidney disease (2013) Kidney Int Suppl 3:19–62

K/DOQI National Kidney Foundation (2002) Clinical practice guidelines for chronic kidney disease: evaluation, definition, and stratification. Am J Kidney Dis 39:S46–S75

Knorr H, Strauss I, Seichert N (1990) Ultrasound cystometry with reference to urinary bladder form and filling. Ultraschall Med 11:150–154

Le Bricon T, Leblanc I, Benlakehal M et al (2005) Evaluation of renal function in intensive care: plasma cystatin C vs. creatinine and derived glomerular filtration rate estimates. Clin Chem Lab Med 43:953–957

Manieri C, Carter SS, Romano G et al (1998) The diagnosis of bladder outlet obstruction in men by ultrasound measurement of bladder wall thickness. J Urol 159:761–765

Palmer LS, Richards I, Kaplan WE (1997) Age-related bladder capacity and bladder capacity growth in children with myelomeningocele. J Urol 158:1261–1264

Peters H, Weitzel D, Humburg C et al (1986) Sonographische Bestimmung des normalen Nierenvolumens bei Neugeborenen und Säuglingen. Ultraschall Med 7:25–29

Riccabona M, Nelson TR, Pretorius DH et al (1996) In vivo three-dimensional sonographic measurement of organ volume: validation in the urinary bladder. J Ultrasound Med 15:627–632

Riccabona M, Avni FE, Blickman JG et al (2008) Imaging recommendations in paediatric uroradiology: minutes of the ESPR workgroup session on urinary tract infection, fetal hydronephrosis, urinary tract ultrasonography and voiding cysto-urethrography. ESPR-Meeting, Barcelona/Spain, June 2007. ESUR Paediatric guideline subcommittee and ESPR paediatric uroradiology work group. Pediatr Radiol 38:138–145

Riccabona M; Lobo ML, Ording-Muller LS, Augdal TA, Avni FE, Blickman J, Bruno C, Damasio BM, Darge K, Ntoulia A, Papadopoulou F, Vivier PH (2017) ESPR abdominal (GU and GI) imaging task force – imaging recommendations in paediatric uroradiology, part IX: imaging in anorectal and cloacal malformation, imaging in childhood ovarian torsion, and efforts in standardising pediatric uroradiology terminology. Report on the mini-symposium at the ESPR meeting in Graz, June 2015. Pediatr Radiol (in press)

Schwartz GJ, Haycock GB, Spitzer A (1976) Plasma creatinine and urea concentration in children. Normal values for age and sex J Pediatr 88:928–830

Schwartz GJ, Munoz A, Schneider MF et al (2009) New equations to estimate GFR in children with CKD. J Am Soc Nephrol 20:629–637

The fourth report on the diagnosis, evaluation, and treatment of high blood pressure in children and adolescents (2004) Pediatrics 114:555–576

Yildirim H, Gungor S, Cihangiroglu MM et al (2005) Doppler studies in normal kidneys of preterm and term neonates: changes in relation to gestational age and birth weight. J Ultrasound Med 24:623–627

Zerin JM, Chen E, Ritchey ML et al (1993) Bladder capacity as measured at voiding cystourethrography in children: relationship to toilet training and frequency of micturition. Radiology 187:803–806

Index

A

Abdominal muscular deficiency syndrome. *See* Prune-belly syndrome
Abscesses, 238, 643
ABU. *See* Asymptomatic bacteriuria (ABU)
aCDS. *See* Amplitude-coded color Doppler sonography (aCDS)
ACEI. *See* Angiotensin-converting enzyme inhibitors (ACEI)
Acquired pyelonephritic renal damage, 243
Acquired renal cyst, 580–582, 632
Acucise device, 743, 749
Acute bacterial nephritis, 556–557
Acute catheter dysfunction, 302, 631
Acute focal bacterial nephritis, 237–238
Acute kidney injury (AKI), 219
    causes of, 296–297
    childhood renal failure, 628
    classification, 296
    definition, 296
    diagnosis, 297
    imaging, 634
    prognosis, 297
    RPD and, 592–593
    treatment, 297
    US, 629
Acute postinfectious glomerulonephritis, 220
Acute renal failure (ARF). *See* Acute kidney injury (AKI)
Acute scrotum, male genital tract
    acute epididymitis, 370
    acute idiopathic scrotal oedema, 373
    causes, 370
    clinical history, 370
    epididymitis, 373, 374
    epididymoorchitis, 373
    Henoch-Schönlein purpura, 373–374
    hydroceles, 369–370
    imaging algorithms, 370–371
    immediate surgical treatment, 370
    intrascrotal appendage torsion, 372–373
    perinatal testicular torsion, 372
    symptoms and signs, 370
    testicular appendages, 370
    testicular torsion
        history and clinical findings, 371
        and tumours, 370
Acute tubular necrosis (ATN), 113, 296, 303, 594, 642
Adenine phosphoribosyltransferase (APRT), 288, 289
Adenomatoid tumour, 378
ADPKD. *See* Autosomal dominant polycystic kidney disease (ADPKD)
AKI. *See* Acute kidney injury (AKI)
Allograft transplants, 638
Allopurinol, 290
Alport syndrome (AS), 196, 203–204, 219–220, 630
Alveolar type rhabdomyosarcoma (A-RMS), 695, 699
American Association for the Surgery of Trauma (AAST), renal injuries
    grade I, 720
    grade II, 720, 721
    grade III, 720, 721
    grade IV, 720, 721
    grade V, 720, 722
    ureteropelvic junction disruption, 722
American College of Radiology (ACR), 43
American Urological Association (AUA), 245
Aminoglycoside, 237
Ammonia, 289
Ampillicin, 237
Amplitude-coded color Doppler sonography (aCDS)
    children with minor and moderate trauma, 716–717
    neonatal oligoanuria and RF, 635–636
    nephrourologic disorders, 777, 778
    PTLD, 646, 647
    renal dysplasia, 569–570
    renal injuries, 720, 721
    renal scarring, 558–559
    scrotal injuries, 728
    urinary tract trauma, 718, 719, 722
    UTI, 767, 768
Amyloidosis, 227, 604
Anaplastic sarcoma, 683–684
Androgen insensitivity syndrome (AIS)
    CAIS, 348
    diagnostic imaging, 349
    PAIS, 348

Angiography
  abdominal CT, 355, 757
  CE-MRA, 42–43, 93
  conventional, 640
  CTA, 635, 657–658
  DSA, 385, 659
  MRA, 93, 452, 454, 594, 609, 659
  post-embolization, 757
  super-selective, 757
  urinary tract injuries, 719
Angiomyolipoma, 11, 690, 691, 756
Angioplasty, 659, 660, 754–756
Angiotensin-converting enzyme inhibitors (ACEI), 290, 298, 300
Anorectal malformations (ARMs), imperforate anus
  anal incontinence, 392
  associated malformations, 387–389
  associated vertebral anomalies, 388, 389
  atresia level, 388
  embryology, 386–387
  high-intermediate-low classification, 386
  Krickenbeck classification, 386
  partial/complete sacral agenesis, 388
  stool evacuation, 392
Antegrade pyelography, 643
Antibacterial therapy, 236–238
Antibiotic prophylaxis, 262, 768, 769, 773, 776
Antiphospholipid syndrome (APS), 226
Antireflux surgery techniques, 418–419
ARPKD. *See* Autosomal recessive polycystic kidney disease (ARPKD)
Arterial spin labeling (ASL), 41–42
Arteriovenous fistula (AVF)
  hemodialysis, 302, 632
  renal biopsy, 608, 609
ASL. *See* Arterial spin labeling (ASL)
Asphyxia, 6
Asymptomatic bacteriuria (ABU), 238
ATN. *See* Acute tubular necrosis (ATN)
Attention-deficit/hyperactivity disorder, 421
AUA. *See* American Urological Association (AUA)
Autosomal dominant polycystic kidney disease (ADPKD)
  autosomal dominant, 210, 211
  fetal nephropathies, 169–170
  genetic basis, 194, 201, 202
  polycystic kidney disease, 574
  uro-nephropathies, 487–
Autosomal recessive cystinuria, 204
Autosomal recessive polycystic kidney disease (ARPKD), 5
  cystic kidney disease, 209–213
  fetal nephropathies, 170
  genetic basis, 201
  polycystic kidney disease, 573–577

B

Bartter's syndrome, 204, 225, 284, 286, 602
BBD. *See* Bladder and bowel dysfunction (BBD)
BC. *See* Bladder capacity (BC)

Beckwith-Wiedemann syndrome (BWS), 10, 203, 333, 666
Benign cysts, 378
Benign familial hematuria, 203
Benign tumors
  angiomyolipoma, 690
  bladder tumors, 699–700
  CMN, 686–687
  juxtaglomerular cell tumor, 690–691
  multilocular cystic nephroma, 688
  ossifying renal tumor of infancy, 689–690
  stromal tumors
    metanephric adenofibroma, 689
    metanephric adenoma, 688, 689
    metanephric stromal tumor, 688–689
Bifid collecting systems, 447–463
Bifid ureter, 128
Bilateral disease, 208, 655, 670–672, 676, 677
Bilateral herniation, 156
Bilateral hydronephrosis, 68, 69, 485
Bilateral ovarian cysts, 357–358
Bilateral Wilms' tumor, 666, 676
Bilharziasis, 562
BK virus (BKV), 304, 646–647
Bladder and bowel dysfunction (BBD), 233
Bladder capacity (BC), 792, 794
Bladder contusion, 725–726
Bladder diverticulum, 323, 519, 540
Bladder dysfunction
  cystitis, 560–561
  IRC, 117
  in neonates and infants, 424
  postoperative imaging and findings, 537
  treatment for, 241
  UTIs, 233
  VUR, 245–246
Bladder exstrophy
  anatomical description, 400
  bladder function, 404
  continence, 404–405
  fetal bladder anomalies, 172–173
  musculoskeletal features, 401
  with normal infraumbilical wall, 402
  with normal umbilicus, 402
  OEIS complex, 402
  prenatal diagnosis, 398
  psychosexual function and fertility, 405
  repair of, 538
  urogenital features, 400–401
  vesicoureteral reflux, 404
Bladder injury, 725–726
Bladder outlet obstruction
  Cobb's collar, 320–321
  Cowper's gland cysts, 320–321
  tumor
    reference imaging modality, 322
    rhabdomyosarcoma, 321
  ureterocele prolapse, 320
  urethral diverticula, 320–321
  urethral polyp, 320
Blastemal Wilms' tumor, 668

Blunt abdominal trauma, 11, 90, 713–716, 719–722, 727
Body surface area (BSA), 785–786
Branchio-oto-renal syndrome, 209
Breast milk feeding, 241
Brödel effect, 259
Bud theory, 242
Burkitt's lymphoma, 684, 685

C

CAKUT. *See* Congenital abnormalities of kidney and urinary tract (CAKUT)
Calcineurin inhibitors, 303, 645
Calcium oxalate stones, 283, 285
Calcium phosphate stones, 283, 285, 286
Calyceal cyst, 566, 581, 582, 617
Calyceal diverticulum, 74, 78, 447, 567, 618
CAN. *See* Chronic allograft nephropathy (CAN)
Carbohydrate-deficient glycoprotein (CDG) syndromes, 596–598, 605
Cardiovascular disease, 304
Catecholamines, 298
CCSK. *See* Clear cell sarcoma of the kidney (CCSK)
CDG syndromes. *See* Carbohydrate-deficient glycoprotein (CDG) syndromes
CDS. *See* Color Doppler sonography (CDS)
ce-CT. *See* Contrast-enhanced computed tomography (ce-CT)
Cefaclor, 245
Cephalosporin, 237
Cerebral atrophy, 605
ce-VUS. *See* Contrast-enhanced voiding urosonography (ce-VUS)
CFU. *See* Colony-forming units (CFU)
Chemoprophylaxis, 241
Chest X-ray (CXR)
 CRF, 633
 nephroblastoma, 674–679
Chiba needle, 737, 738
Childhood renal failure, 628
Chronic allograft injury, 642
Chronic allograft nephropathy (CAN), 304
Chronic obstruction, 130
Chronic renal failure (CRF), 295, 595, 627, 789
 children with, 297, 634
 CT, 634
 definitions, 299–301
 diagnosis, 300–301
 epidemiology, 299–300
 GFR, 789
 MRI, 634
 pathophysiology, 300
 planning dialysis, 301
 transplantation, 301
 treatment, 300–301
 US, 634
Circumcision, 241, 767
Clearance (C), 787–789
Clear cell sarcoma of the kidney (CCSK), 678–679
Cloacal dysgenesis, 173

Cloacal exstrophy, 312, 350, 397, 402–403, 406, 407, 537
Cloacal malformation
 diagnostic imaging
  balloon catheter, 355
  fetal MRI, 352
  fluid-debris level, 343
  fluoroscopic studies, 354
  genital secretion, 352
  granular abdominal calcifications, 354
  intrapelvic structures, 352
  prenatal US, 352
  rotational fluoroscopy, 355
  spinal cord anomalies, 354
  3D reconstruction, 355
  urethral sphincter, 355
  US evaluation, newborn, 352
  uterus malformations, 352
  vaginal and bladder duplication, 352
  voiding cystourethrogram, 355
 and genital anomalies, 351, 352
 immediate colostomy, 351
 incomplete, 351
 pelvic osseous structures, 351
 perineal anatomy, 350
 posterior, 351
 with uterus didelphys, 350, 353
 vaginal anomalies, 350
Cohen procedure, 270
Colony-forming units (CFU), 235
Color Doppler sonography (CDS)
 ADPKD, 571
 drug toxicity, 645, 646
 epispadias-exstrophy complex, 406
 graft dysfunction, 642
 HUS, 628
 left renal vein, 153
 locoregional tumor extent, 672, 691, 695
 MCDK, 577–579
 neonatal oligoanuria and RF, 635–636
 neoplasms, 691
 nephrocalcinosis, 623
 nephrourologic disorders, 777, 779
 ovarian torsion, 359
 peritoneal dialysis, 632
 priapism, 757–758
 renal allograft, 640
 renal arteries, 153
 renal biopsy, 608
 renal transplantation, 645
 renal tumors, 583
 RMS, 694
 RPD, 594, 606
 rTX, 633, 635, 636, 639–640, 644
 scrotal injuries, 728–729
 scrotum, 701
 sickle cell disease, 604, 607
 spermatic cord, torsion of, 371
 urinary tract infection and vesicoureteric reflux, 775
 urolithiasis, 616, 618–620
 UTI, 236, 775

Color Doppler sonography (CDS) (cont.)
   vasculitis, 600
   VUR, 508–510, 542
Computed tomographic angiography (CTA)
   CA, 136
   hypertension, 753–756
   planning transplantation, 633
   rTX, 633
   RVH, 657–658
   urogenital tract, 43
Computed tomography (CT)
   abdomen, 149, 154
   CA, 136
   calyceal diverticulum, 447
   CCSK, 678, 679
   children with minor and moderate trauma, 716
   children with severe trauma and multiple injuries, 715
   CMN, 687
   complicated cyst, 582
   CPDN, 671
   CRF, 634
   diffuse nephroblastomatosis, 671, 672
   intraperitoneal WT rupture, 672, 675
   metanephric adenoma, 688
   moderate trauma, 10, 11
   NC, 282
   nephroblastoma, 671–675
   nephrocalcinosis, 623–624
   oncological surgery, 542, 543
   ossifying renal tumor of infancy, 689–690
   ovarian torsion, 360
   pelvis and ureter, 446–447
   percutaneous nephrostomy, 738
   planning transplantation, 633
   PTLD, 119
   renal failure, 636
   renal fibrosarcoma, 687
   renal injuries, 723–724
   renal tumors, 583
   retrocaval ureter, 460
   surgery, surgical procedures and indications, 278
   technical environment, 717–718
   urinary tract injuries, 718–720
   urolithiasis, 283, 620–622
   UTI, 555
Computed tomography of the urinary tract (uro-CT)
   abdominal distention, 28
   acquisition technique, 27–29
   indications, 26
   of left kidney, 27
   preparation, 27
   of right kidney, 28
Congenital abnormalities of kidney and urinary tract (CAKUT), 161, 238, 242, 243
   bilateral renal dysplasia, 72
   calyceal diverticulum, 74, 78
   cystic kidney disease
      ADPKD, 210
      ARPKD, 209–210
      complicated cyst, 213, 582–584
      GCKD, 211
      MCDK, 212
      MCKD, 211
      MSK, 212
      NPHP, 211
      simple renal cyst, 212–213
   ectopic kidney, 72, 76
   horseshoe kidney, 75
   hydrocalyx, 74, 79
   hypoplasia, 213
   hypoplastic ectopic right kidney, 73, 77
   management, 208
   pathology of, 70
   prognosis, 208
   prune belly syndrome, 74
   renal agenesis, 208–209
   renal dysplasia, 209
   renal hypodysplasia, 71
   structural and functional malformations, 500
   unilateral renal dysplasia, 72, 73
Congenital adrenal hyperplasia
   adrenal steroidogenesis, 347
   diagnostic imaging, 349–350
   severe and mild forms, 347
   3β-hydroxysteroid dehydrogenase deficiency, 347
   21-hydroxylase deficiency, 347
Congenital anomalies, urinary bladder
   appendicovesicostomy, 538
   bladder exstrophy, 537
   cloacal exstrophy, 537
   epispadias, 537
   posterior urethral valve
      abnormal detrusor function, 539–540
      renal functional imaging, 541
      severe renal disease, 538
      urine drainage, 539
   urinary tract diversion, 537, 538
   VUR, 541–542
Congenital cystic disease, 323
Congenital hydronephrosis. See also Hydronephrosis
   calyceal transit time, 54
   compensated, 55, 57
   decompensated, 56, 57
   delayed cortical transit time, 54
   delayed parenchymal transit time, 53–54
   diuretic renal scintigraphy, 50
   fluid levels, 52, 54
   MR urography, 50
   Patlak number, 54
   pyeloplasty, 57–59
   renal damage, 52, 53
   renal parenchyma, 52
   RTT, 52
   uropathy, 52, 53, 57
Congenital mesoblastic nephroma (CMN), 686–687
Congenital nephrotic syndrome
   Finnish type of, 576
   syndromal cystic renal disease, 577

Congenital obstructive posterior urethral membrane (COPUM), 314, 426
Congenital reflux nephropathy, 242–243, 512, 629
Congenital renal disorders, 299
Congenital ureter disorders
  bilateral ureterocele repair, 537
  bladder dysfunction, 537
  documented persistent symptomatic VUR, 536
  primary endoscopic incision, ectopic ureterocele, 537
  secondary surgical procedure, 537
  sheath reimplantation technique, 536
  ureteric duplication, 535–537
  UVJO, 551–552
Contrast agents (CA), 636–637
  ASL, 41–42
  CE-MRA, 42–43
  dose, 136, 137
  gadolinium-based, 43
  Gd-based MR, 137–139
  in pregnancy, 134
  radiopaque iodine-based, 135–137
  US, 134–137
Contrast-enhanced computed tomography (ce-CT), 715
  abscesses, 643
  blunt abdominal trauma, 714
  complicated cyst, 582
  cystic renal disease, 571
  PTLD, 647
  renal injuries, 720–726
  trauma and multiple injuries, 715
  urinary tract trauma, 718, 719, 777
Contrast-enhanced MR angiography (ce-MRA), 42–43, 93
Contrast-enhanced ultrasonography (ce-US), 15–16, 18–19, 543, 639
  children with trauma, 717
  with intravenous UCA administration procedure, 19
  renal stone disease, 543
  rTX, 639, 640
  urinary tract trauma, 723, 777, 779
  VUR, 542
Contrast-enhanced voiding urosonography (ce-VUS), 269
  contrast agents, 135
  cystic renal disease, 571
  definition, 16
  nephrourologic disorders, 773, 777, 779
  procedure, 16–18
  renal agenesis, 566–568
  renal failure, 637
  UTD, 776
  UTI, 775
  vesicoureteric reflux, 510–512
Contrast-induced nephropathy (CIN), 136, 636
Conventional angiography, 640
Cope introducer system, 737
Coronary angioplasty systems, 660
Cortex, 149
  blood supply, 151–154
  dysplasia, 570

echogenicity, 14, 170
initial enhancement, 54
internal anatomy, 150–151
MR urography, 45, 52
periphery of, 669
renal parenchyma, 591
Cortical scars, 77, 82, 129
Corticomedullary differentiation, 129, 173
Covered exstrophy, bladder, 402
CPDN. See Cystic partially differentiated nephroblastoma (CPDN)
CRF. See Chronic renal failure (CRF)
Crossed renal ectopia
  IVU, 188
  MRI, 187
  types, 186–188
  VCUG, 187
  VUR, 188
Cryptorchidism, 370
CT. See Computed tomography (CT)
CTA. See Computed tomographic angiography (CTA)
Cushing syndrome, 357
Cutting balloon angioplasty (CBA), 754, 755
CXR. See Chest X-ray (CXR)
Cyst
  acquired renal, 580–582, 632
  benign, 378
  calyceal, 581
  complicated, 213
  multiloculated, 213, 582–584
  neonatal ovarian, 356–358
  renal parenchymal morphology, 130
  simple renal, 215, 580–582
Cystatin C (CysC), 786, 789
Cystic dysplasia, rete testis, 378
Cystic kidney diseases, 208, 571–574
  acquired renal cyst, 580–582
  ADPKD, 201, 210, 574–576
  ARPKD, 201, 209–210, 573–574
  complicated cyst, 213, 582–584
  GCKD, 201, 211, 576–577
  juvenile nephronophthisis, 201–202
  MCDC, 576
  MCDK, 212, 577–579
  MCKD, 211
  MSK, 202, 212, 579–580
  multiloculated cyst, 582–584
  NPHP, 213, 576
  renal tumor, 582–584
  simple renal cyst, 212–213, 580–582
Cystic partially differentiated nephroblastoma (CPDN), 668, 671, 688, 693
Cystic renal tumor, 213, 582–584
Cystine stones, 283, 290
Cystinosis
  encephalopathy, 605
  genetic basis, 205
  nephropathic, 227, 605
Cystinuria, 288, 602

Cystitis, 560–561. *See also* Urinary tract infections (UTIs)
   glandularis, 700
   pseudotumoral, 700
   therapy for, 238
   urinary tract infection, 324, 560–561
   vs. pyelonephritis, 236
Cystostomy, percutaneous, 751–752
Cystourethritis, 238

D

Davis intubated ureterostomy, 747
Defensins, 233
Deflux®, 246
Delayed dense nephrogram, 49, 56, 66, 67
Dense deposit disease (DDD), 222
DES. *See* Dysfunctional elimination syndrome (DES)
Detrusor pressure, 125
Diabetic nephropathy, 605
Dialysis, 630–631
   HD, 302, 632
   PD, 301–302, 631–632
   planning and transplantation, 301
Differential renal function (DRF), 262, 451, 485
   contrast agent, 46, 47
   DMSA, 108
   DRS, 44
   dynamic renography, 104
   GFR, 45, 46
   Rutland-Patlak technique, 46
   signal intensity *vs.* time curves, 45
   volumetric differential function, 44, 45
Diffuse nephroblastomatosis, 671, 672
Diffusion-weighted imaging (DWI), 40–41
   adrenal neuroblastoma, 692, 693
   Burkitt's lymphoma, 684
   malignant rhabdoid tumor of the kidney, 680
   non-Hodgkin lymphoma, 684
   pyelonephritis, 75–77
   renal transplantation, 92
   rhabdomyosarcoma, 696
   vaginal rhabdomyosarcoma, 698
   Wilms' tumor, 670
Digital subtraction angiography (DSA), 42
   hypertension, 754
   percutaneous renal angioplasty, 753, 754
   renal arterial embolization, 756–757
   RVH, 659
   tuberous sclerosis, 757
Dilative uremic cardiomyopathy, 633
Dimercaptosuccinic acid (DMSA), 498–499, 550, 554
   DRF, 111
   immobilisation, 105, 106
   precautions, 105
   PUV, 106
   radiopharmaceutical, 106–107
   SPECT CT, 107, 119
   static renal scan, 498–499
   Tc-99m DMSA scan, 107, 108
   Tc-99m MAG3, 108
   transplant kidney, views of, 106

UTI, 104, 236, 240, 550
VUR, 243
Direct radioisotope cystography (DIC)
   advantages, 116
   uses, 116
   with VUR, 116
Direct radionuclide cystography (DRNC), 244, 505–506
Disorders of sexual development (DSD), 83
   classification, 346
   46,XX disorders
      androgenic drugs administration, pregnant women, 348
      congenital adrenal hyperplasia, 347
      placental aromatase deficiency, 347–348
      virilizing maternal tumors, 348
   46,XY disorders
      AIS, 348
      5-alpha reductase deficiency, 348
      mixed gonadal dysgenesis, 348
Distal renal tubular acidosis (dRTA), 286
Distant metastases, 675, 696, 697, 699
Diuretic renography, 109, 261, 263, 498
DMSA. *See* Dimercaptosuccinic acid (DMSA)
Doppler sonography
   CDS (*see* Color Doppler sonography (CDS))
   hemodialysis, 632
   power, 9, 10, 12, 14
   renal failure, 594, 634
   RPD, 605–607
   RVH, 654
DRF. *See* Differential renal function (DRF)
dRTA. *See* Distal renal tubular acidosis (dRTA)
DSA. *See* Digital subtraction angiography (DSA)
Duplex collecting systems
   abnormal kidneys, 464
   complications, 463
   diagnosis, 463–464
   duplication and VUR
      lower-pole VUR, 464, 466
      reflux nephropathy, 465
      upper pole VUR, 465
   dysplasia, upper pole, 470–472
   etiology and epidemiology, 463
   MR urography, 464, 467
   PUJ obstruction, 472
   ureteral ectopia, 466–469
   ureterocele, 470
   ureterohydronephrosis, 464
   UVJ obstruction, 472
   VCUG, 464
Duplex Doppler sonography
   lupus nephritis, 603
   renal dysplasia, 569–570
   renal parenchymal disease, 592, 606
   RPD, 592
Duplex kidney, 128
   complicated, 489
   cystic dysplasia, 471
   evaluation, 45
   obstruction, 472
   upper pole, 66, 470–471

ureteral ectopia, 461
uretero-pelvic duplication, 166, 167
VUR and, 518
work-up of, 464, 465
Duplex systems with ectopic ureter
  imaging, 275
  postoperative imaging, 275
  surgical approaches, 275
  Weigert-Meyer rule, 275
Duplicated ureter, 128, 535
Duplicate exstrophy, 402
Dynamic renography, 109, 498
Dysfunctional elimination syndrome (DES), 233, 409, 414, 416–418

E

Eagle-Barrett syndrome. *See* Prune-belly syndrome
Echo-planar imaging (EPI), 41–42
Ectopic kidney, 72, 76, 128, 180–181
Ectopic ureter, 65–69
  Duplex systems with
    imaging, 275
    postoperative imaging, 275
    surgical approaches, 275
    Weigert-Meyer rule, 275
  renal pelvis and ureter
    duplex collecting systems, 466–469
    in single and bifid collecting systems, 461–463
EEC syndrome, 333
Electrolytes, 219, 788
Ellipsoid formula, 129, 150
Embolotherapy
  NCS, renal vein stenting, 759–760
  priapism, 757–758
  renal arterial embolization, 756–757
  varicocele, internal spermatic vein embolization, 758–759
Embryology
  of epispadias-exstrophy complex, 398–399
  female genitalia
    cloacal development, 331
    gonad development, 330
    mesonephric ducts, 330, 331
    Müllerian-inhibiting substance, 330
    partitioning process, 331, 332
    primary sex reversal, 330
    sex determination, chromosome level, 330
    sinovaginal bulbs, 331
    urinary and anorectal system, 330
    uterovaginal canal, 331
    Wolffian ducts, 330, 331
  imperforate anus, 386–387
  of male genital tract, 367–368
Embryonal type rhabdomyosarcoma (E-RMS), 695
Endogenous toxins, 296
Endopyelotomy, percutaneous
  Davis intubated ureterostomy, 747
  indications, endopyelotomy, 747–748
  PE, 750
  procedural details and technique, 748–749

Endourologic techniques, 740
  percutaneous cystostomy, 751–752
  percutaneous endopyelotomy
    Davis intubated ureterostomy, 747
    indications, endopyelotomy, 747–748
    PE, 750
    procedural details and technique, 748–749
  percutaneous nephrolithotomy
    contraindications, 745
    ESWL and ureteroscopic techniques, 745
    indications, 745
    procedural details and technique, 745–747
  percutaneous renal biopsy, 749–751
  ureteral dilatation and stenting
    antegrade approach, 741
    indications, 742
    internal-external nephroureterostomy stents, 741
    metallic stents, 740
    percutaneous approach, 740
    percutaneous management, 742
    procedural details and technique, 742–745
End-stage renal disease (ESRD), 72, 295, 299–302, 304, 628, 632–634
Epididymitis, 373, 374
Epididymoorchitis, 373
Epispadias, 322
  balanitic, 399
  cross-sectional anatomy, 399
  females, 400
  males, 399–400
  musculoskeletal deformities, 399–400
  penile, 399
  penopubic, 399
  repair, 404
  types, 399
Epispadias-exstrophy complex
  anatomy
    classical bladder exstrophy, 400–401
    cloacal exstrophy, 402
    covered exstrophy, bladder, 402
    duplicate exstrophy, 402
    epispadias, 399–400
    inferior vesical fissure, 402
    with normal infraumbilical wall, 402
    with normal umbilicus, 402
    OEIS complex, 402
    pseudoexstrophy, bladder, 401–402
    superior vesical fissure, 402
  embryology, 398–399
  imaging, 405–406
  incidence, 398
  multistage surgical repair, 397
  prenatal diagnosis, 398
  risk of occurrence, 398
  surgical repair
    bladder neck reconstruction, 404
    epispadias repair, 404
    initial bladder closure, 403–404
    staged, 402–403, 406
    urinary diversion, bowel segments, 403
  types and frequencies, 397, 398

ESPR. *See* European Society of Pediatric Radiology (ESPR)
ESRD. *See* End-stage renal disease (ESRD)
ESWL. *See* Extracorporeal shock wave lithotripsy (ESWL)
Ethanol, 660
European Medicines Agency (EMA), 43
European Society of Pediatric Radiology (ESPR), 127, 261
Ewing's sarcoma family of tumors, 682–683
Exogenous toxins, 296
Extracorporeal shock wave lithotripsy (ESWL), 283, 290, 745
Extraosseous Ewing sarcoma, 682–683
Extraperitoneal bladder rupture, 725
Extravesical reimplantation, 270
Extrinsic stenosis, 258–259

F

Familial Mediterranean fever (FMF), 227, 604
Fanconi syndrome, 225, 227
FAST. *See* Focused assessment with sonography for trauma (FAST)
Female genital anomalies
  embryology, 330–332
  Müllerian duct (*see* Müllerian duct anomalies)
  ovarian conditions, 355–361
  ovarian cysts, 329–330
  radiological and biochemical examinations, 329
  urogenital sinus (*see* Urogenital sinus malformations)
Female hypospadias, 345
Femoral artery, 659
Fetal bladder anomalies
  bladder exstrophy, 172–173
  megabladder, 171–172
Fetal homeostasis, 298
Fetal magnetic resonance imaging
  of cloacal malformation, 175
  normal fetal kidney, 163
  normal fetal pelvic, 164
  normal fetal urinary tract, 164
  of urogenital sinus malformation, 173–174
Fetal nephropathies
  MCDK, 168–169
  polycystic kidneys, 169–170
  renal dysplasia, 170, 171
  renal vein thrombosis, 170–171
Fetal urinary tract dilatation (UTD), 771–773, 776
Fetal uropathies
  antenatal diagnosis and postnatal follow-up, 450
  neonatal work-up of, 479, 480
  obstruction, 164–166
  postnatal workup of, 512–513
  uretero-pelvic duplication, 166–168
  VUR, 167–168
Fibroepithelial polyps, 63, 64
Fibromuscular dysplasia (FMD), 655, 752, 754
5-French neonatal nephrostomy drain, 738
Fluorodeoxyglucose positron emission tomography/computerised tomography (FDG PET-CT), 104, 119

FMD. *See* Fibromuscular dysplasia (FMD)
Focal dysplasia, 570
Focal renal infarction, 607
Focused assessment with sonography for trauma (FAST), 276, 715
Foley catheter, 24, 274, 354, 727, 742, 744
Fractional excretion (FE), 789
Fractional excretion of sodium (FENa), 297, 298
Fraley's syndrome, 74, 448
Fraser syndrome, 199, 333
Functional diuretic MR urography (fMRU), 263, 489, 533, 573
Furosemide, 36, 38, 39, 110, 451, 483, 486

G

Gadolinium-based contrast agents (GBCAs), 42–43, 137–139, 637
GCKD. *See* Glomerulocystic kidney disease (GCKD)
Genetic counseling, 196–198
Genetic heterogeneity, 195, 196
Genetics
  databases, 205
  formal, 194, 195
  molecular
    genetic complexity, of genes, 195
    genetic counseling, 196–198
    genetic heterogeneity, 195, 196
    genotype-phenotype correlation, 195
    inherited disorders, 196
  nephropathies
    AS, 203–204
    Bartter syndrome, 204
    cystinosis, 205
    nephrogenic diabetes insipidus, 204
    nephrolithiasis, 204
    nephrotic syndromes, 204–205
    nocturnal enuresis, 204
  urogenital system
    ciliopathies, 200–202
    duplication malformations, 198, 199
    hydronephrosis, 198, 199
    hypospadias, 200
    kidney, hereditary tumors, 200
    renal agenesis, 198, 199
    VUR, 200
Genital anomalies
  female
    embryology, 330–332
    Müllerian duct (*see* Müllerian duct anomalies)
    ovarian conditions, 355–361
    ovarian cysts, 329–330
    radiological and biochemical examinations, 329
    urogenital sinus (*see* Urogenital sinus malformations)
  urethra
    appendicovesicostomy, 538
    bladder exstrophy, 537
    cloacal exstrophy, 537
    epispadias, 537
    posterior urethral valve, 538–540
    urinary tract diversion, 538

VUR, 541–542
Genitourinary system
  benign tumors
    angiomyolipoma, 690
    benign stromal tumors, 688–689
    CMN, 686–687
    juxtaglomerular cell tumor, 690–691
    multilocular cystic nephroma, 688
    ossifying renal tumor of infancy, 689–690
  diagnostic strategy, 691–694
  differential diagnosis
    benign bladder tumors, 699–700
    inflammation and infection, prostate, 701
    reactive, inflammatory and infectious lesions of bladder, 700
    scrotum, 701
    tumors, prostate, 700
    urothelial neoplasms, 699
    vagina, 701
  embolotherapy
    NCS, renal vein stenting, 759–760
    priapism, 757–758
    renal arterial embolization, 756–757
    varicocele, internal spermatic vein embolization, 758–759
  infectious diseases, 691, 692
  malformations, 691
  malignant hematologic diseases
    Burkitt's lymphoma, 684, 685
    with non-Hodgkin lymphoma, 684, 685
    primary unilateral renal lymphoma, 684
    T-ALL, 684, 686
  miscellaneous, 691
  non-Wilms' malignant tumors
    anaplastic sarcoma, 683–684
    CCSK, 678–679
    Ewing's sarcoma family of tumors, 682–683
    malignant hematologic diseases, 684–686
    MRTK, 680–681
    RCC, 681, 682
    renal medullary carcinoma, 681–682
    renal metastases, 686
  RMS
    clinical features, 695
    epidemiology, 694–695
    follow-up, 699
    histopathology and genetics, 695
    imaging, 695–698
    treatment principles and prognosis, 698–699
Genotype-phenotype correlation, 195
Germ cell tumours, 376, 377
GFR. See Glomerular filtration rate (GFR)
Giant multicystic dysplastic kidney, 454, 456, 487, 489, 577–578
Giggle incontinence, 421
Gitelman syndrome, 204, 225
Glomerular basement membrane (GBM), 220, 221, 600
Glomerular disease
  AS, 219–220
  acute postinfectious glomerulonephritis, 220
  congenital and inherited, 599

HSP, 221, 600
IgAN, 221, 600
INS, 222–223, 600–601
membranoproliferative and membranous glomerulopathy, 221–222, 601
MN, 222
post-/parainfectious, 600
rapidly progressive, 600
RPGN, 220–221
Glomerular filtration rate (GFR), 136–137, 297–299, 787–789
Glomeruli, 146, 151, 155, 602, 635
Glomerulocystic kidney disease (GCKD), 201, 211, 576–577
Glomerulonephritis
  acute postinfectious, 220
  membranoproliferative, 221–222
  RPGN, 220–221
  ultrasound findings in, 593
Glomerulosclerosis, 300
Glycogen storage diseases (GSD), 227, 605
Gonadoblastoma, 376
Goodpasture's syndrome, 221, 600
Graft dysfunction, 92, 642
Graft thrombosis, 303
Granulomatosis with polyangiitis (GPA), 224
Grayscale ultrasound
  IVC thrombosis, 672
  minor and moderate trauma, 716–717
  nutcracker syndrome, 759–760
  percutaneous renal biopsy, 749–750
  renal injury, 720
  testicular rupture, 728
  urolithiasis, 616–618

H
Haemolytic-uraemic syndrome (HUS), 224–225, 594, 601, 602, 607
Hand-foot-genital syndrome, 333
HD. See Hemodialysis (HD)
Hematomas
  PUJ, 269
  UVJ, 280
  VUR, 271
Hematuria, 218, 297, 680, 682, 695
  ADPKD, 210
  benign familial, 203
  bleeding and sepsis, 746
  clear cell sarcoma, 666
  familial benign, 220
  Henoch-Schonlein purpura and, 751
  medical renal disease, 750
  microscopic, 221, 716
  MSK, 212
  and nephritic syndrome, 218
  ossifying renal tumor of infancy, 690
  and proteinuria, 297
  RCC, 681
  SCN, 226
  sporadic Wilms' tumor, 669
  transient mild, 739

Hemodialysis (HD), 301, 302, 630, 632
Hemostat, 742, 743, 753
Henoch-Schönlein purpura (HSP)
    acute scrotum, male genital tract, 373–374
    glomerular disease, 220–221, 600
    and hematuria, 751
    RPGN, 220–221
Heparin, 753, 756
Hereditary amyloidosis, 604
Hereditary tyrosinaemia, 605
Herlyn-Werner-Wunderlich syndrome, 85–86, 337
Heterozygosity testing, 197–198
High-turnover disease, 633–634
Hinman syndrome, 410, 421
HN. See Hydronephrosis (HN)
Horseshoe kidney, 75
    definition, 182
    diagnosis, 182–185
    hydronephrosis, 184
    trisomy 18, 183
    Turner's syndrome, 184
    Wilms' tumor, 185
HTN. See Hypertension (HTN)
HUS. See Haemolytic-uraemic syndrome (HUS)
Hydatid disease, 562
Hydrocalyx, 73, 79, 448
Hydrocolpos, 84, 342, 351
Hydronephrosis (HN), 198, 256, 688
    congenital, 50–60
    follow-up of, 456
    genetic basis, 198, 200
    obstruction diagnosis, 48–50
    PUJ obstruction, 60–63
    renal parenchymal morphology, 129–130
    ureteric anomalies, 63–64
    ureteroceles, 69–70
    UVJ obstruction, 64–69
Hydroureter, 457
    IRC, 117
    secondary
        crural hernia, 460
        extrinsic causes, 460
        intrinsic causes, 459–460
        midureteral stenosis, 459
        retrocaval ureter, 460
        retroperitoneal malignant fibrosis, 460, 461
        ureterohydronephrosis, fecaloma, 460, 461
Hypercalcaemia, 6, 286
Hypercalciuria, 78, 212, 285–286, 604
Hyperfiltration, 300, 523
Hyperoxaluria
    primary
        type I, 286–287
        type II, 287
    secondary/enteric, 287–288
Hyperperfusion, 300
Hypertension (HTN), 219
    ADPKD, 574
    blunt abdominal trauma, 11
    children born, 72
    complications, 755
    definition, 653–654
    DSA, 659
    focal renal infarction, 607
    renal hypoplasia, 568–569
    renovascular (see Renovascular hypertension)
    in RPD, 219
    secondary, 561, 654–655
    US, 10
    VUR, 521
Hyperuricosuria, 288–289
Hypervitaminosis D, 286
Hypocitraturia, 278, 289
Hypodysplasia, 71, 300, 630, 770
Hypospadias
    female, 345–346
    genetic basis, 200
    male genital tract, congenital anomalies, 368
Hypoxanthine phosphoribosyltransferase (HPRT), 288

I
Idiopathic hypercalciuria, 285–286
Idiopathic nephrotic syndrome (INS), 222–223, 600–601
Idiopathic scrotal oedema, 373
IgA glomerular disease, 600
IgA nephropathy (IgAN), 221, 600, 751
Imaging
    acute scrotum, male genital tract, 370–371
    AKI, 634
    cloacal malformation, balloon catheter, 355
    congenital anomalies of urinary bladder, 541
    cystic kidney diseases (see Cystic kidney diseases)
    duplex systems with ectopic ureter, 275
    dysplasia (see Renal dysplasia)
    episadias-exstrophy complex, 405–406
    hypoplasia (see Renal hypoplasia)
    imperforate anus, 392–394
    intravenous urography, 272
    male genital tract
        corpus spongiosum, 367
        low-resistance spectral Doppler tracing, 366–367
        magnetic resonance imaging, 367
        normal prepubertal testicle, 366
        penile shaft, 367
        spermatic cord, 366
        tunica albuginea, 366
        ultrasonography, 366
    Müllerian duct anomalies
        distal vaginal atresia, hematocolpos, 338, 339
        hydro-/hematocolpos and hydrometro-/
            hematometrocolpos, 342, 343
        pelvic sonography, 339
        renal US and voiding cystourethrography, 339
        ultrasound, 338
        of vaginal anomalies, 344
    neonatal oligoanuria
        ARF, 634
        CA, 636–637
        CDS and aCDS, 635–636

Index 795

childhood, CRF in, 634
CT and intravenous pyelography, 636
isotope investigations, 636
MRI, 638
plain films, 636, 637
support therapeutic measures, 634
ultrasound, 635
VCUG, 637–638
nephroblastoma
atypical patterns, 670, 671
bilateral disease, 670–672
common WT radiological pattern, 669–670
distant metastases, 675
locoregional tumor extent, 672–675
preoperative imaging, 675–676
nephrocalcinosis (*see* Nephrocalcinosis)
neurogenic bladders
drip infusion dropping speed, 456
modified VCUG technique
modified VCUG technique: bladder compliance, 439
modified VCUG technique: detrusor function, 440
modified VCUG technique: filling phase, 437
modified VCUG technique: leak point pressure estimation, 440
modified VCUG technique: safe storage volume, 439–440
modified VCUG technique: sphincter detrusor dyssynergia, 440
modified VCUG technique: unstable detrusor contraction, 439
video urodynamics, 437
renal agenesis (*see* Renal agenesis)
renal failure (*see* Renal failure)
renal parenchymal disease (*see* Renal parenchymal disease)
renal pelvis and ureter, 446–447
rhabdomyosarcoma,
distant metastases, 696, 697
locoregional tumor extent, 695–696
staging, 697–698
tissue harmonic, 11
transplantation (*see* Renal transplantation (RTx))
UPJO, 578
upper urinary tract dilatation, 482
urinary tract infections (*see* Urinary tract infections (UTIs))
urolithiasis (*see* Urolithiasis)
US (*see* Ultrasound (US))
Immobilisation, 26, 105, 106, 286, 288, 608
Immunosuppressive therapy, 303, 639, 647
Imperforate anus, 385, 402
ARMs, 386–389
anal incontinence, 392
associated malformations, 387–389
associated vertebral anomalies, 388, 389
atresia level, 388
embryology, 386–387
high-intermediate-low classification, 386
Krickenbeck classification, 386
partial/complete sacral agenesis, 388
stool evacuation, 392
cloacal malformation, 312, 350
functional disorders of the urinary system, 385
imaging, 392–394
maldevelopment, 385
therapy, 394
types, 385
urinary tract anomalies, 385, 389–390
VUD, 124, 125
Incisura, 157
Indirect radioisotope cystography (IRC)
method, 118
recurrent urinary tract infection, 117
strength, 117
VUR detection, 117–118
weakness, 117
Indirect radionuclide cystography (IRC), 104, 115, 116, 506–507
Indomethacin, 298
Infectious diseases, 691
Infectious stones, 284, 285, 289
Inflammatory renal parenchymal disease, 606–607
Infundibular stenosis, pelvic urolithiasis, 448, 449
Inheritance modes, 194, 195
Inherited glomerular disease, 599–600
Interlobar arteries, 150, 152
Interlobular veins, 152
Internal spermatic vein embolization, 749–750
International Reflux Study (IRS), 245, 504, 769
Interstitium, 146, 225, 591, 633
Intracavitarily applied radiopaque iodine-based contrast agents, 135–136
Intraperitoneal bladder rupture, 713, 725
Intrarenal pelvis, 130, 156
Intrarenal reflux, 23, 151, 152, 506, 510, 541
Intravascularly applied iodine-based contrast agents, 136–137
Intravenous pyelography, 636
Intravenous urography (IVU)
acute obstruction, 48
in adult, 272, 283
diagnostic procedures, 4, 26
inferior ectopia, 186, 188
MSK, 212
nephrocalcinosis, 624
obstruction diagnosis, 48
one-shot, 719
postnatal diagnostic approach, 499
and radiography, 622, 624
tuberculous, 562
upper urinary tract, 406
ureteral quadruplication, 473
urinary tract diversion, 537
urolithiasis, 622
uro-nephropathies, work-up of, 446
use of, 533
Intravesical reimplantation, 270
Intrinsic stenosis, 258
Inulin, 45, 788

IRC. *See* Indirect radioisotope cystography (IRC)
IRS. *See* International Reflux Study (IRS)
Ischemia, 275, 276, 296, 403, 404, 541
Isotope cystography
    DIC, 116
    IRC, 116–118
IVU. *See* Intravenous urography (IVU)

J

Jarcho-Levin syndrome, 333
JB-1 catheter, 742, 746, 753
Junctional parenchymal defect (JPD), 130, 148
Juvenile granulosa cell tumours, 376
Juvenile nephronophthisis, 201–202, 576, 630
Juxtaglomerular cell tumor, 690–691

K

Kawasaki disease (KD), 223
Kidney
    anatomy and variants
        blood supply, 151–154
        internal, 150–152
        measurements, 149
        position, 148
        shape, 148–150
        size, 148–150
        US, 155
    Bertin, 149, 150
    development, 145–147
    fusion anomalies
        crossed renal ectopia, 185–188
        horseshoe kidney, 182–185
    grooves, 148
    hereditary tumors of, 202–203
    in infants, 149
    JPD, 148
    left, 150
    lobar architecture in, 150
    in newborn, 148
    position anomalies
        renal ectopy, 180–181
        supernumerary kidney, 181–182
        thoracic kidney, 181, 182
    right, 149, 151
    rotation anomalies, 181–182
    structural organization of, 152
    transplantation, 92–93
    vascular supply of, 152
    VCUG, 151
    volume, 129
Kidney stones, 278, 283, 284, 287
Kidneys-ureter-bladder (KUB) radiograph, 25
    acquisition technique, 6–7
    asphyxia, 6
    definition, 4
    equipment, 5–6
    hypercalcaemia, 6
    indications, 4–7
    in neonate, 5
    palpable abdominal mass, 5, 7
    systemic lupus erythematosus, 6
    urolithiasis diasgnosis, 622
Koff formula, 16, 22
KUB radiograph. *See* Kidneys-ureter-bladder (KUB) radiograph

L

Lazy bladder syndrome, 415, 417–418, 428
Leak point pressure, 125, 436, 440
Left ventricular hypertrophy, 633, 654
Leydig cell tumour, 376
Lich-Gregoir procedure, 270
Lipomas, 378
Lobar nephronia. *See* Pseudotumoral acute pyelonephritis
Locoregional tumor extent, 695–697
Lower genitourinary tract, neoplasms
Lower urinary tract, 414, 415, 418, 421, 426, 550, 552
    assessment of, 426
    bladder outlet obstruction, 321–322
    differential diagnosis, neoplasms
        benign bladder tumors, 699–700
        inflammation and infection, prostate, 701
        reactive, inflammatory and infectious lesions of bladder, 700
        scrotum, 701
        tumors, prostate, 700
        urothelial neoplasms, 699
        vagina, 701
    endemic bladder stones, 324
    infection (*see* Urinary tract infections (UTIs))
    malformations, 390
        cloacal dysgenesis, 175
        fetal MRI, 173
        urogenital sinus anomalies, 173–174
    prenatal diagnosis, 311–314
        assessment, 314
        karyotyping, 314
        management, 313–314
        maternal-fetal sonography, 314
        of megacystis, 313
        plain film post delivery, 312
        visible bladder absence, 312–313
    PUV (*see* Posterior urethral valves (PUV))
    RMS
        clinical features, 695
        epidemiology, 694–695
        follow-up, 699
        histopathology and genetics, 695
        imaging, 695–698
        treatment principles and prognosis, 698–699
    scanning technique, 13–15
    symptoms, in young children, 234
    and urachus, 325–326
    urogenital sinus malformations
        chromosomal and hormonal abnormalities, 345
        female hypospadias, 345

Index

neonates with, 345
physical examination, newborn, 344
Low-turnover disease, 634
Lupus nephritis, 226, 603
Lymphoceles, 303, 643, 644

M

Magnetic resonance angiography (MRA), 43, 93
  renal arteries, 153
  rTX, 644
  RVH, 655, 659
Magnetic resonance genitography, 83–86
  cloacal malformations, 84
  DSD, 83
  genitogram, 83, 84
  Herlyn-Werner-Wunderlich syndrome, 85–86
  hydrocolpos, 84
  Mayer-Rokitansky-Kuster-Hauser syndrome, 85
  Mullerian duct anomalies, 84
  urogenital sinus, 84
  US, 83
Magnetic resonance imaging (MRI), 312, 322, 367, 406, 537, 566, 569, 643, 771
  ADPKD, 574
  ARPKD, 575
  bilateral disease, 670
  Burkitt's lymphoma, 684, 685
  CCSK, 678, 679
  children, urogenital tract in, 44, 45
  CMN, 686
  complicated cyst, 582
  coronal T2, 187
  cortical scarring, 129
  corticomedullary differentiation, 129, 151
  CPDN, 669, 670
  CRF, 634
  CT, 581
  cyst detection, 573, 580–581
  epispadias-exstrophy complex, 406
  Ewing's sarcoma family of tumors, 682–684
  fat suppression, T2-weighted sequence with, 156
  female genital anomalies, 350, 360
  genitourinary system, neoplasms of, 675, 701
  heterogeneous lesion, 670
  HUS, 601, 602
  juxtaglomerular cell tumor, 691
  locoregional tumor extent, 697
  MA, 688
  macrocyclic gadolinium-based agents, 134
  male genital queries, 367–370, 375, 378
  malignant hematologic diseases, 684–686
  MCDC, 576
  MRTK, 680
  MSK, 580
  multicystic nephroma and multiloculated cysts, 583
  nephrogenic rests, 673
  NPHP, 576
  nuclear medicine, 104, 120
  pelvic cavity, 312

renal agenesis, 566–567
renal dysplasia, 569–570
renal failure, 634, 638
renal hypoplasia, 568–569
renal neoplasms, 694
renal parenchymal disease, 601, 610
renal scarring, 558–559
renal tumors, 583
rhabdomyosarcoma, 695
RMS, 695, 699
scrotum, 701
simple renal cyst and acquired renal cyst, 580–582
testes, 277
thinned pelvic floor muscles, 392
upper urinary tract dilatation, in children, 499
urinary problems associated with imperforate anus, 392
urinary tract
  infections, 554–555
  injuries, 718–720
  trauma, 718, 724, 728
urogenital fetal imaging, 162–164, 167, 168, 172–175
WT, 670–673, 677–681
Magnetic resonance urography (MRU), 4, 447, 499, 570, 578
  antenatal hydronephrosis, 37
  CAKUT, 70–80
  contrast agents, 43–44
  core protocol, 36–40
  dilatation detection, 538
  genitography, 83–86
  hydronephrosis evaluation
    congenital, 50–59
    obstruction diagnosis, 48–50
    PUJ obstruction, 60–62
    ureteric anomalies, 63–64
    ureteroceles, 69–70
    UVJ obstruction, 64–69
  MCDK, 577–579
  nephrocalcinosis, 624
  optional sequences
    ASL, 41–42
    CE-MRA, 42–43
    DWI, 41
  postoperative imaging and findings, 538
  post-processing, 44–47
  pyelonephritis and renal scarring, 75–77, 81
  in renal transplantation, 92–93
  in renal trauma, 90–92
  of renal tumors, 87–90
  RN, 522
  3D sequences *vs.* 2D sequences, 36
  urolithiasis, 622
  vesicoureteric reflux, 519, 520, 522, 523
  volume-rendered T2-weighted images, 39
  VUR, 511, 520
  for VUR assessment, 83
Major genetic syndromes, 667

le genital tract
acute epididymitis, 371
acute idiopathic scrotal oedema, 373
acute scrotal pain, 370–371
    causes, 370
    clinical history, 370
    congenital and acquired conditions, 365
    congenital anomalies
        hypospadias, 368
        penile anomalies, 368–369
        scrotal anomalies, 369
    cryptorchidism, 370
    embryology, 367–368
    epididymitis, 373, 374
    epididymoorchitis, 373
    haemorrhage and trauma, 374–375
    Henoch-Schönlein purpura, 373–374
    hydroceles, 370
    hydroceles and hernias, 369–370
    imaging
        algorithms, 370–371
        technique, 366–367
    immediate surgical treatment, 370
    inguinal canal, 369–370
    intrascrotal appendage torsion, 372–373
    perinatal testicular torsion, 372
    priapism, 379
    pseudotumours, 375
    superficial lesions, 380
    symptoms and signs, 370
    testicular and paratesticular tumours, 375–378
    testicular appendages, 370
    testicular torsion
        history and clinical findings, 371
        and tumours, 370
    varicocele, 380
    vascular lesions, genitalia, 379
Malformations
    ARM, simperforate anus
        anal incontinence, 392
        associated malformations, 387, 388
        associated vertebral anomalies, 388, 389
        atresia level, 388
        embryology, 386–387
        high-intermediate-low classification, 386
        Krickenbeck classification, 386
        partial/complete sacral agenesis, 388
        stool evacuation, 392
    associated, 387–389, 391
    CAKUT, 209, 500
    duplication, 200
    genitourinary system, neoplasms, 692
    lower urinary tract
        cloacal dysgenesis, 175
        fetal MRI, 173
        urogenital fetal imaging, 173–175
    MR genitography, 83
    MSK, 212
    Müllerian duct anomalies, uterovaginal, 332
    renal tumors, 691
    upper urinary tract, 333
    ureteroceles, 69
    urinary tract, 300, 500–501, 637
    urogenital sinus, 173–174
        adrenogenital syndrome, 345
        chromosomal and hormonal abnormalities, 345
        clitoric hypertrophy, 350
        cloacal (*see* Cloacal malformation)
        diagnostic imaging, 349–350
        in DSD, 346–350
        female hypospadias, 344–345
        fluoroscopic genitography, 349
        genitourinary tract malformations, 350
        neonates with, 345
        physical examination, newborn, 344
        sex determination, 345
        US, 162–163
    vascular, 379
Malignant hematologic diseases
    Burkitt's lymphoma, 684, 685
    with non-Hodgkin lymphoma, 684–685
    primary unilateral renal lymphoma, 684
    T-ALL, 684, 686
Malignant paratesticular tumours, 378
Malignant rhabdoid tumors of the kidney (MRTK), 680–681
Malrotation, 179–181, 318
Maternal-fetal sonography, 311
Maximum intensity projection (MIP), 154, 460, 620
    arterial, 61
    coronal, 55, 58, 59, 61, 62, 64, 66–68, 73, 74, 76, 77, 79, 80
    delayed coronal, 63, 67–69, 71–74, 76–78, 80, 82, 91
    sagittal, 462
    T2-weighted, 51
Mayer-Rokitansky-Küster-Hauser syndrome, 85
    developmental defects, 332, 333
    genital anomalies, 333, 334
    primary amenorrhea, 333
    Turner syndrome, 335
    type A (typical form), 333
    type B (atypical form), 333
    upper urinary tract malformations, 333
McCune-Albright syndrome, 357–358
MCDC. *See* Medullary cystic disease complex (MCDC)
MCDK. *See* Multicystic dysplastic kidney (MCDK)
Meconium periorchitis, 378
Mediterranean fever, 227, 604
Medulla, 41, 45, 49, 67, 150, 152, 574, 576, 591
    ARPKD, 170
    echogenicity, 14–15
    hyperechogenicity, 623
    hyperechoic patches, 579
    hypertonic, 226
    hypoechoic, 151
    in neonate, 155
    renal medullary carcinoma, 681–682
    renal parenchymal involvement, 605
    zones, 151
Medullary cystic disease complex (MCDC), 576

Medullary sponge kidney (MSK), 202, 212, 579–580, 598
Megabladder, 22, 171–172, 484
Megacalycosis, 74, 80, 449, 450
Megacystis, 313, 316, 318–320, 498
Megacystis-microcolon hypoperistalsis (MMH) syndrome, 172
Megaureter (MU), 64–67, 75, 131, 165, 259. *See also* Uretero-vesical junction obstruction (UVJO)
  antibiotic prophylaxis, 262
  antireflux reimplantation, 459
  crural hernia, 460
  development of, 423
  and megacalycosis, 449
  on MR urography, 458
  natural history, 460
  non-refluxing primary, 534–535
  primary, 269–270, 450, 457–459
  reflux, 459
  ureteral modeling, 459
  urinary tract dilatation, 457
  on US, 457, 458
Membranoproliferative glomerulonephritis (MPGN), 221–222, 601
Membranous glomerulopathy, 601
Membranous nephropathy (MN), 219, 222–223
Mesonephros, 145, 146, 330
Metanephric adenofibroma, 689
Metanephric adenoma (MA), 688
Metanephric blastema, 146, 180, 330, 669
Metanephric stromal tumor, 688–690
Metanephros, 72, 145, 146
Microscopic polyangiitis (MPA), 224, 601
Middle aortic syndrome, 656–658
Midstream urine (MSU), 235
Mitrofanoff principle, 726
Mixed gonadal dysgenesis, 348
Modified VCUG (mVCUG) technique
  neurogenic bladder, diagnostic imaging, 437
  non-neurogenic bladder-sphincter dysfunction
    bladder filling, 425
    COPUM, 426
    cystographic signs, 425
    electromyographic assessment, pelvic floor muscles, 425
    lower urinary tract assessment, 426
    unstable detrusor contractions, 425
    urethral morphology, 426
    WBNA, 426
MRA. *See* Magnetic resonance angiography (MRA)
MRTK. *See* Malignant rhabdoid tumors of the kidney (MRTK)
MRU. *See* Magnetic resonance urography (MRU)
MSK. *See* Medullary sponge kidney (MSK)
MSU. *See* Midstream urine (MSU)
99mTc-mertiatide, 640
MU. *See* Megaureter (MU)
Müllerian duct anomalies, 84
  bicornuate uterus, 332, 333, 336
  diagnostic imaging
    distal vaginal atresia, hematocolpos, 338, 340
    hydro-/hematocolpos and hydrometro-/hematometrocolpos, 342, 343
    pelvic sonography, 339–340
    renal US and voiding cystourethrography, 339
    ultrasound, 338
    of vaginal anomalies, 344
  imperforate hymen
    with excessive hydrocolpos, 342, 343
    with hydrometrocolpos and ascites, 343
    with moderate hydrocolpos, 342, 343
  lateral fusion disorders, 332, 336, 338
  morphologic features
    neonatal uterus, 338–341
    postpubertal uterus, 341–342, 344
    prepubertal uterus, 341
    pubertal uterus, estrogen stimulation, 340
  Müllerian agenesis/hypoplasia, 332–335
  septate uterus, 333
  unicornuate uterus, 332
  uterovaginal malformations, 332
  uterus didelphys
    with double vagina, 336, 337
    with left-sided vaginal atresia, 340
  uterus duplex unicollis, 336
  vaginal anomalies with/without obstruction, 333, 337–338
  vertical fusion disorders, 332, 335–336
Mullerian structures, 175
Multicystic dysplastic kidney (MCDK), 168–169, 212
  cystic renal lesion, 577–578
  PUJO, differential diagnosis, 456
  renal hypodysplasia contralateral to, 71
  spontaneous involution of, 487
  ureteric obstruction, 337
  uro-nephropathies, 487–488
  VUR, 519
Multicystic nephroma, 583
Multilocular cystic nephroma, 688
Multiloculated cyst, 213, 583
mVCUG. *See* Modified VCUG (mVCUG) technique

N

nAKI. *See* Neonatal acute kidney injury (nAKI)
NC. *See* Nephrocalcinosis (NC)
NCS. *See* Nutcracker syndrome (NCS)
Neonatal acute kidney injury (nAKI), 295
  ACEI/ATII-RB, 298
  characterization, 298
  congenital renal disorders, 299
  diagnosis, 298–299
  fetal and neonatal renal function, 297–298
  indomethacin, 298
  oliguria, 298
  sepsis-associated, 298
  stages, 298
  treatment, 298–299
Neonatal intensive care unit (NICU), 298, 628, 637

Neonatal oligoanuria, 628
    diagnostic workup and imaging, 630, 631
    imaging methods and findings
        ARF, 634
        CA, 636–637
        CDS and aCDS, 635–636
        childhood, CRF in, 634
        CT and intravenous pyelography, 636
        isotope investigations, 636
        MRI, 638
        plain films, 636, 637
        support therapeutic measures, 634
        ultrasound, 635
        VCUG, 637–638
    planning transplantation, imaging for, 633
Neonatal ovarian cysts, 356–358
Neonatal renal failure. *See* Neonatal acute kidney injury (nAKI)
Neonatal urinary tract dilatation, 771–773
Neoplasms, genitourinary system
    benign tumors
        angiomyolipoma, 690
        benign stromal tumors, 688–689
        CMN, 686–687
        juxtaglomerular cell tumor, 690–691
        multilocular cystic nephroma, 688
        ossifying renal tumor of infancy, 689–690
    diagnostic strategy, 691–694
    differential diagnosis
        benign bladder tumors, 699–700
        inflammation and infection, prostate, 701
        reactive, inflammatory and infectious lesions of bladder, 700
        scrotum, 701
        tumors, prostate, 700
        urothelial neoplasms, 699
        vagina, 701
    infectious diseases, 691
    malformations, 691
    malignant hematologic diseases
        Burkitt's lymphoma, 684, 685
        with non-Hodgkin lymphoma, 684, 686
        primary unilateral renal lymphoma, 684
        T-ALL, 686
    miscellaneous, 691
    nephroblastoma (*see* Nephroblastoma)
    non-Wilms' malignant tumors
        anaplastic sarcoma, 683–684
        CCSK, 678–679
        Ewing's sarcoma family of tumors, 682–683
        malignant hematologic diseases, 684–686
        MRTK, 680–681
        RCC, 681
        renal medullary carcinoma, 681–682
        renal metastases, 686
    RCC
        clinical findings, 681
        complication, 681
        with hematuria, 681
        majority of, 681
        survival, 681
        von Hippel-Lindau syndrome, 681
    RMS
        clinical features, 695
        epidemiology, 694–695
        follow-up, 699
        histopathology and genetics, 695
        imaging, 695–698
        treatment principles and prognosis, 698–699
Nephrectomy, 212, 534, 537, 676, 677, 687
    CMN, 686
    compensatory hypertrophy, 149
    Giant PUJO, 455
    MCKD, 212
    PUJ obstruction, 60
    SIOP protocol, 676
    urolithiasis, 615
    VUR, 423
Nephritic syndrome (NS), 217–223
Nephroblastoma, 184, 666
    clinical features
        patients with predisposing syndromes, 669
        sporadic Wilms' tumor, 669
    epidemiology, 666
    FDG PET-CT in, 119–120
    genetic basis, 203
    imaging
        atypical patterns, 670, 671
        bilateral disease, 670–672
        common WT radiological pattern, 669–671
        distant metastases, 675
        locoregional tumor extent, 672–675
        preoperative imaging, 675–676
    management, 87
    MR imaging, 87–90
    nephroblastomatosis, 87–89
    nephrogenic rests, 87
    pathology
        focal anaplasia, 668–669
        high-risk tumors, 668
        intermediate-risk tumors, 668
        NRs and nephroblastomatosis, 669
        SIOP working classification, 668
        triphasic tumor, 666
    prognosis and follow-up
        imaging during follow-up, 677–678
        prognostic factors, 677
        relapses, 677
        survival, 677
    treatment principles
        bilateral Wilms' tumor, 676
        unilateral Wilms' tumor, 676
Nephroblastomatosis, 87, 89, 119, 669, 671, 672, 676, 688
Nephrocalcinosis (NC), 603, 605, 615, 637
    classification of, 616
    clinical findings, 281–282
    CT, 623–624
    definition, 281
    diagnostic imaging, 282–283

diagnostic procedure, 285, 288
etiology of, 616
extra-urinary calcifications, 5
incidence, 284, 616
infectious stones, 289
inhibitors
   hypocitraturia, 289
   THP kidneys, 289
medication, 290
MRU, 624
MSK, 579–580
promotors
   cystinuria, 288
   hypercalciuria, 285–286
   hyperoxaluria, 286–288
   hyperuricosuria, 288–289
radiographs and IVU, 624
and renal stones, 225
surgery, 290
ultrasound, 623
Nephrogenic diabetes insipidus, 204, 225, 602
Nephrogenic rests (NRs), 87, 666, 669, 671, 673, 677, 694
Nephrogenic systemic fibrosis (NSF), 40, 42, 44, 138–139, 638
Nephrolithiasis, 204, 579, 623
Nephrolithotomy, percutaneous
contraindications, 745
ESWL and ureteroscopic techniques, 745
indications, 745
procedural details and technique, 745–747
Nephron, 46, 48–50, 54, 72, 151, 295
acute pyelonephritis, 556–557
consists of, 151
CRF, 595
DMSA static renography, 554
fetal and neonatal renal function, 146
formation, 146
glomerular hypertrophy, 300
hypoplasia, 170, 208
renal development, 146
renal hypoplasia, 568–569
Nephronophthisis (NPHP), 201, 211, 576, 630
Nephron-sparing surgery (NSS), 105, 119, 669, 675
Nephropathic cystinosis, 227, 605
Nephropathies, 489–490
AS, 203–204
Bartter syndrome, 204, 225
cystinosis, 205
nephrogenic diabetes insipidus, 204
nephrolithiasis, 204
nephrotic syndromes, 204–205
nocturnal enuresis, 204
postnatal work-up, 486–487
Nephrostomy, percutaneous
benefits of, 736
contraindications, 737
endourologic technology, 735–736
indications, 736
insertion, 735
neonate with bilateral UPJ obstructions, 736
procedural details and technique/technical remarks
   complications, 739
   equipment, 737
   image guidance, 738
   local anesthetic and intravenous sedation/anesthesia, 738
   nephrostomy catheter, selection of, 737
   nephrostomy-related urinoma formation, 739
   posterolateral approach, 739
   standard and stiff guidewires, 737
   standard drains, insertion of, 737
   transient mild hematuria, 739
   ultrasound, 739
Nephrostomy track dilatation, 740
Nephrotic syndromes (NS)
Finnish type, 576
genetic basis, 205
and proteinuria, 218–219
Wilms tumors, 203
Nephrourologic disorders
clinicians, 766
guidelines and beyond
   conditions, 776–778
   considerations, 774–775
   fetal UTD, 776
   urinary tract infection and vesicoureteric reflux, 775–776
imaging
   algorithms and procedural recommendations, 778–779
   clinicians expectation, 766–767
treatment, pediatric radiologists
   conditions, 773–774
   fetal and neonatal urinary tract dilatation, 771–773
   UTI, 767–768
   vesicoureteral reflux, 768–771
Neurofibromatosis type 1, 655, 656, 694
Neurogenic bladders, 323, 391
anatomy and physiology, 435–436
classification, 436–437
continence, 436
diagnostic imaging, 437–440
dysfunction, 125, 390, 394
etiology, 436
imperforate anus, 391
secondary VUR, 514
voiding, 436
Next-generation sequencing (NGS), 194, 195
NICU. *See* Neonatal intensive care unit (NICU)
Nitrofurantoin, 245, 768
Nocturnal enuresis
causal mechanisms, 419
genetic basis, 203
incidence of, 419
monosymptomatic, 419, 421
pathogenesis of, 419
primary, 415, 419, 420, 429
secondary, 419

Non-neurogenic bladder-sphincter dysfunction
  categorizations
    bladder and striated urethral muscle, overactivity, 410
    diagnosis, 410
    dysfunctional voiding, 410–412
    "functional" urinary symptoms, 410
    Hinman syndrome, 410, 411
    non-neurogenic neurogenic bladder, 418
    non-neuropathic/non-neurogenic bladder-sphincter dysfunction, 410, 411
    non-neuropathic vesicourethral dysfunction, 410
    pathophysiology, 410
    unstable bladder, 410–412
    urodynamic classifications, 411
  clinical presentations
    daytime and/or nighttime wetting, 409
    recurrent urinary tract infections, 409
    vesicoureteral reflux, 409
  constipation, 416–417
  definitions, 410
  detrusor-sphincter dysfunction
    during bladder filling, 415
    during micturition, 415
  enuresis
    causal mechanisms, 419, 420
    clinical symptoms, 421
    definition, 419
    monosymptomatic bedwetting, 419, 421
    pathological factors, 420
    primary nocturnal, 419
    secondary nocturnal, 419
    stool retention, 420
    and urinary incontinence, 419–421
  evaluation process
    clinical symptoms, 428
    dysfunctional voiding and unstable bladder, 428
    enuretic children, 428
    incontinence symptoms, 427
    indications, VCUG, 428
    primary monosymptomatic enuresis nocturna, 429
    radiological assessment, children, 427
    scoring system, 427
    upper urinary tract dilatation, 428
    urodynamic abnormalities, 428
    videourodynamic studies, 428
  incidence, 412–413
  modified VCUG technique, 425–426
  in neonates and infants
    bilateral abnormal kidneys, high-grade VUR, 422
    bilateral high-grade fetal dilatation, 422, 424
    detrusor hypercontractility, 422
    detrusor pressure with micturition, 422
    external urinary sphincter after birth, 422
    functional bladder capacity, 423
    hypercontractile detrusor, 424
    moderate bilateral fetal hydronephrosis, 422, 423
    sex-linked developmental anatomy, 422
    transient fetal urethral obstruction, 424
    unstable detrusor contractions, 422
    upper tract pathology, 423
    ureteral bud and bladder trigone differentiation, 423
  pathophysiology
    fractionated voiding, 415
    staccato voiding, 415
    therapeutic efficacy, 414
    types, 414–415
    unstable/overactive bladder, 415
    upper tract dilatation, 416
    wetting, fractionated voiding, 416
  patient management, 430
  physiology, 413
  reimplantation surgery failure, 410
  with renal transplantation, 417
  toilet training (bladder control), 414
  UTI, 417–419
  VUR, 417–419
Nonobstructive vaginal anomalies, 336
Nonvascular interventions
  endourologic techniques (see Endourologic techniques)
  nephrostomy track dilatation, 740
  percutaneous cystostomy, 751
  percutaneous nephrostomy (see Percutaneous nephrostomy)
  percutaneous renal biopsy
    imaging-guided renal biopsy, 749–750
    indications, 749
    procedural details and technique, 750–751
    US guidance, 750
  Whitaker perfusion test, 734–735
Non-Wilms' malignant tumors
  anaplastic sarcoma, 683
  CCSK, 679
  Ewing's sarcoma family of tumors, 683–686
  malignant hematologic diseases, 684–686
  MRTK, 680–681
  RCC, 681
  renal medullary carcinoma, 681–682
  renal metastases, 686
NS. See Nephrotic syndromes (NS)
NSF. See Nephrogenic systemic fibrosis (NSF)
NSS. See Nephron-sparing surgery (NSS)
Nuclear medicine, studies and
  differential renal function, 485, 486
  drainage stimulation, 486
  functional deterioration, 486
  radionuclide renogram, 485
  renal trauma, 724
  tubular tracers, 485
Nutcracker syndrome (NCS), 154, 606, 760

O
Obstipation, treatment for, 241
Obstruction of an unilateral rudimentary horn, 338
Obstructive uropathies, 48, 256, 299, 562, 594, 771
  CRF, 299
  MR urography, 59, 454
  pelvi-ureteric junction, 164, 165
  secondary hypertension, causes of, 654

ureterovesical junction, 165
urethral, 165–166
VCUG, 21
Occlusion balloon catheters, 746
Ochoa syndrome, 421
Oligohydramnios, 165, 166, 170, 208, 210, 272, 298, 299, 493–496, 517, 568, 573, 771
Omphalocele-exstrophy-imperforate anus-spinal defects (OEIS) complex, 398, 402
Oncological surgery, 542–543
One-shot intravenous urography, 719
Ossifying renal tumor of infancy, 689
Ovarian disorders
  characteristics
    neonatal ovary-containing indirect inguinal hernia, 356
    normal ovarian appearance, neonate, 356, 357
  neonatal cysts, 356–358
  torsion
    adnexectomy, 360
    circulatory impairment, 359
    Color and spectral Doppler sonography, 359
    diagnosis, 359
    diffusion-weighted sequences, 360
    features, 359
    hemorrhagic necrosis, 359, 360
    multiple cortical follicles, 359
    pelvic pain, 359
    risk of torsion, 359
    sonography, 359
    stages, 359
    symptoms, 359
    twisted ischemic ovary, 360
    twisted vascular pedicle and the whirlpool sign, 359–360
Ovotesticular disorder, chimeric, 348–349

P
Paediatric renal radionuclide imaging
  DMSA
    indications, 109–115
    SPECT, 119
  dynamic renography, 109
  FDG PET-CT, 119
  isotope cystography
    DIC, 116
    IRC, 116–118
  MAG3 Tc99m renography, 109–115
  PTLD, 119–120
  static renal scan, 104–105
Page kidney, 276, 643, 721
Pallister-Hall syndrome (vaginal atresia), 333
Patlak-Rutland plot method, 111, 113
PCD. *See* Pelvicalyceal dilatation/distension (PCD)
PD. *See* Peritoneal dialysis (PD)
PE. *See* Percutaneous endopyelotomy (PE)
Pediatric genitourinary intervention
  nonvascular
    endourologic techniques (*see* Endourologic techniques)

nephrostomy track dilatation, 740
percutaneous cystostomy, 751–752
percutaneous nephrostomy (*see* Percutaneous nephrostomy)
percutaneous renal biopsy, 749–751
Whitaker perfusion test, 736
percutaneous techniques, 733
percutaneous treatment, 733–734
vascular (*see* Vascular interventions)
Pediatric intensive care unit (PICU), 297
Pediatric-modified RIFLE criteria (pRIFLE), 296
Pelvicalyceal dilatation/distension (PCD), 129–131, 155, 256–261, 263, 793
Pelvi-calyceal system, 155–156, 515, 516, 521–523
Pelvic excretion efficiency (PEE), 109, 111, 114
Pelvic fractures, 725, 727
Pelvi-ureteric junction obstruction (PUJO), 164, 165, 257, 260, 772
  active intervention, 530
  anatomic anomalies, 454
  clinical symptoms, 530
  complications, 268, 530
  crossing vessels, 60
  differential diagnosis, 456
  extrinsic stenosis, 258–259
  failed pyeloplasty, 60, 62
  forms of
    Dietl's crisis, 456
    giant PUJO, 454
    and horseshoe kidney, 456, 458
    intermittent obstruction, 456
    and ureterovesical junction obstruction, 456
    and urinoma, 456
    and urolithiasis, 456, 457
  functional diuretic MR urography, 533, 534
  impaired renal function, 530
  interventional treatments, 263
  intrinsic stenosis, 258
  natural history and treatment, 456
  nephrostogram, nephrostomy catheter, 530, 532
  open pyeloplasty, 530, 532
  postoperative drainage system, 532, 533
  postoperative image, 268
  progression of obstruction, 457
  surgery
    findings and indication for, 268
    management, 530
    procedure, 268
  symptoms, 454
  ureteric anomalies, 63–64
  uro-nephropathies, 487
Penile anomalies, 368–369
Pepper-salt kidney, 574
Percutaneous cystostomy, 751–752
Percutaneous endopyelotomy (PE), 747
  Davis intubated ureterostomy, 747
  indications, endopyelotomy, 747, 748
  PE, 747
  procedural details and technique, 748–749

Percutaneous nephrolithotomy
  contraindications, 745
  ESWL and ureteroscopic techniques, 745
  indications, 745
  procedural details and technique, 745–747
Percutaneous nephrostomy, 748
  benefits of, 736
  contraindications, 737
  endourologic technology, 735–736
  indications, 736, 737
  insertion, 735
  neonate with bilateral UPJ obstructions, 736
  procedural details and technique/technical remarks
    complications, 739
    equipment, 737
    image guidance, 738
    local anesthetic and intravenous sedation/
      anesthesia, 738
    nephrostomy catheter, selection of, 738
    nephrostomy-related urinoma formation, 739
    posterolateral approach, 739
    standard and stiff guidewires, 736, 737
    standard drains, insertion of, 737
    transient mild hematuria, 739
    ultrasound, 739
  PUJO, 530, 534
Percutaneous pyeloplasty. *See* Percutaneous
  endopyelotomy
Percutaneous renal angioplasty
  cross-sectional imaging, 752–753
  procedural details and technique, 753–756
    angiographic examination, 753
    CBA, 754, 755
    complications, 753
    follow-up angiogram, 753–754
    selective catheter, 753
  PTRA, 752
  renal vein renin sampling, 753
  renovascular hypertension, 752–753
Percutaneous renal biopsy
  imaging-guided renal biopsy, 750
  indications, 750
  procedural details and technique, 750–751
  US guidance, 750
Percutaneous transluminal renal angioplasty (PTRA),
  752–756
Perinephric hematoma, 90, 643
Peripheral primitive neuroectodermal tumor (pPNET),
  682–683
Peritoneal dialysis (PD), 301, 302, 630–632, 638
Peritoneal equilibration test (PET), 119, 302
Periureteral edema, 621, 622
Persistence fetal lobulation, 148
Persistent hypocomplementemia, 221
Persistent urinary tract infection, 5
PET. *See* Peritoneal equilibration test (PET)
Physiologic data, 785–786
PICU. *See* Pediatric intensive care unit (PICU)
Placental aromatase deficiency, 347–348
Plain films

abdomen, 392–393, 457, 482, 517
associated malformations, 388, 389
bladder stones, 324
KUB, 4
lumbar spine, 405
MSK, 579–580
normal bladder, absence of, 312–313
PUJ obstruction and lithiasis, 456, 457
reflux and lithiasis, 515, 517
renal failure, 636, 637
renal parenchymal disease, 609, 610
Politano-Leadbetter reimplantation, 270
Polycystic kidney disease
  ADPKD, 574
  ARPKD, 573–574
  GCKD, 576–577
  MCDC and NPHP, 576
  recessive-type, 480
Polycystic ovarian disease, 357
Positron emission tomography (PET)-CT
  rTX, 647
  staging, 698
Posterior reversible encephalopathy syndrome (PRES),
  219, 645, 646
Posterior urethral valves (PUV), 8, 16, 17, 23, 106, 269,
  480, 481, 496, 538–541, 771
  abnormal mucosal folds, 314
  complications, 273
  live-related donor transplant, 106
  lower urinary tract obstruction, in male fetuses, 165
  megacystis–megaureter association, 517
  membranous obstruction, 314
  mesoderm formation, primary defect in, 495
  in neonates
    bilateral dilatation fo teh ureters, 315
    cystic dysplastic appearance, kidneys, 315, 316
    differential diagnosis, 316
    pelvicaliceal system, 315
    iodinated contrast medium, 318
    management, 313–314
    neuropathic causes, dysfunctional voiding, 318,
      319
    perirenal urinoma, 315
    radiological evaluation, 315
    renal dysplasia, 315
    retrograde catheterization, 316
    suprapubic micturating cystourethrography, 316,
      317
    voiding cystourethrogram, 315
  obstructive forms, 314
  in older boys, diagnosis, 319
  postoperative image, 273
  PUJO, 455
  renal consequences, 314
  surgery, findings and indication for, 271–273
  surgical procedure, 273
  types, 314
  UTD, 259–260
  VCUG, 637
Post-/parainfectious glomerular disease, 600

Posttransplant lymphoproliferative disorder (PTLD), 119–120, 304, 647–648
Potter's syndrome, 567, 573
Predictive testing, 197
Preimplantation genetic diagnosis (PGD), 197
Prenatal diagnosis (PD), 161
    ARPKD, 201
    bladder exstrophy, 398
    female fetuses, 316
    fetal intervention, 314
    genetic counseling, 196
    hydronephrosis, 8
    lower urinary tract obstruction, 13
    megacystis, 313
    normal bladder, absence of, 312–313
    PUV, 314
    unilateral hydronephrosis, 114, 116
Pressure-flow perfusion test, 734–735
Priapism, 757, 758
    ischaemic, 379
    neonatal, 379
    non-ischaemic, 379
pRIFLE. *See* Pediatric-modified RIFLE criteria (pRIFLE)
Primary bladder stones, 284
Primary hypercalciuria, 285–286
Primary hyperparathyroidism, 286
Pronephros, 145–146
Prostate
    inflammation and infection, 701
    RMS, 695, 696
    tumors, 700
Proteinuria, 218–219, 221, 227, 247, 286, 297, 576, 600, 788
Prune-belly syndrome, 322, 326
    clinical presentation, 494
    with dysplastic calyces, 74
    fetal US, 165, 166
    incidence, 494
    management, 499–500
    megacystis, 313
    obstetric ultrasound and antenatal diagnosis, 496–497
    pathogenesis
        bladder histology, fetuses, 495
        primary defect, mesoderm formation, 495
        urethral obstruction, 496
    pathogenetic mechanism, 493
    pathology, 494
    postnatal diagnostic approach
        computed tomography, 499
        dynamic renography, 498
        intravenous urography, 499
        magnetic resonance imaging, 499
        megacystis, 498
        renal and urinary tract ultrasonography, 497
        static renal scan, 498–499
        VCUG, 315, 317, 498
    prognosis, 499
    treatment of, 499–500
    urethral aplasia, oligohydramnios syndrome, 493

Pseudoexstrophy, bladder, 401–402
Pseudo-nutcracker syndrome, 593, 606
Pseudo-prune belly syndrome. *See* Prune-belly syndrome
Pseudotumoral acute pyelonephritis, 691
Pseudotumoral cystitis, 324, 325, 700
Pseudoureterocele, 70, 274
Psoas-hitch technique, 246, 271, 272
PTLD. *See* Posttransplant lymphoproliferative disorder (PTLD)
PTRA. *See* Percutaneous transluminal renal angioplasty (PTRA)
PUJO. *See* Pelvi-ureteric junction obstruction (PUJO)
Pulse repetition frequency (PRF), 619
PUV. *See* Posterior urethral valves (PUV)
Pyelonephritis, 231, 489, 499, 554, 556, 646, 736
    ABU, 238
    acute bacterial nephritis, 556–557
    characterization, 231
    complicated, 237
    CT, 555
    and cystitis, 236
    DMSA scan, 238–239
    late infancy and childhood, 237
    MRI, 554–555
    newborns and early infancy, 236–237
    pseudotumoral acute, 691
    renal abscess, 557–558
    and renal scarring, 75, 77, 82, 92, 93, 404, 550, 558–559
    sonographic signs, 552–554
    in transplanted kidney, 93
    US, 552–554
    VUR, 241–247
    XPN, 559–560, 691
Pyeloplasty, 52, 53, 57, 60–62, 258, 261, 735
    open, 530
    percutaneous, 747–749
    PUJ obstruction, 60–62, 532, 533
    ureteral reimplantation, 262–263

R
Radiography
    after ureteric reimplantation, 552
    high-end digital systems, 5
    kidney-ureter-bladder (KUB) film, 622
    nephrocalcinosis, 622
    surgical complications, 541
    urolithiasis, 622
Radiopaque iodine-based contrast agents, 135–137
Rapidly progressive glomerulonephritis (RPGN), 220–221, 594
RBF. *See* Renal blood flow (RBF)
RCC. *See* Renal cell carcinoma (RCC)
RD. *See* Renal dysplasia (RD)
Reflux nephropathy (RNP), 234, 242–243, 247, 392, 522, 770
Renal abscess, 237, 557–558, 692

Renal agenesis, 128
  bilateral, 209
  CAKUT, 209
  contralateral kidney, 488
  cystoscopy, 568
  genetic basis, 203–204
  MRI, 566
  postnatal imaging, 566
  unilateral, 208
  US, 566, 567
Renal allograft
  rTX, 640–641
  US evaluation, 640, 641
  VUR, 418
Renal arterial embolization, 756, 760
Renal artery stenosis (RAS), 42, 569, 654, 656, 755
Renal biopsy
  complications, 607–610
  extra-renal complications, 609–610
  histological classification, 607
  imaging findings, 609
  plain film, 609
  US-guided, 608
Renal blood flow (RBF), 298, 594, 601
Renal cell carcinoma (RCC)
  clinical findings, 681
  complication, 680
  with hematuria, 682
  majority of, 681
  survival, 681
  von Hippel-Lindau syndrome, 681
Renal coloboma syndrome, 198, 500
Renal corticomedullary abscesses, 238
Renal dysplasia (RD), 170, 172, 209, 244, 577
Renal ectopy, 180–181
Renal failure, 219
  CRF, extrarenal imaging in, 633–634
  definitions, 628
  imaging methods and findings
    ARF, 634
    CA, 636–637
    CDS and aCDS, 635–636
    childhood, CRF in, 634
    CT and intravenous pyelography, 636
    isotope investigations, 636
    MRI, 638
    plain films, 636, 637
    support therapeutic measures, 634
    ultrasound, 635
    VCUG, 637–638
  planning transplantation, imaging for, 633
  renal imaging, 628–630
  RPD and
    acute presentation, 592–593
    causes, 592, 593
    clinical aspects, 592–594
    initial imaging, 592
    manifestation, 594
    mechanisms, 594
Renal fibrosarcoma, 687

Renal-genital-ear anomalies, 333
Renal hypodysplasia, 71, 300, 770
Renal hypoplasia
  aCDS, 569, 570
  catheter angiography, 569
  definition, 209, 568
  with massive hydroureteronephrosis, 66
  mixed renal hypoplasia, 568
  simple renal hypoplasia, 568
  standardized volume calculations, 568
Renal injuries
  AAST classification
    grade I, 720
    grade II, 720, 721
    grade III, 720, 721
    grade IV, 720, 722
    grade V, 720, 723
    ureteropelvic junction disruption, 722
  CT, 723–724
  imaging complications and sequelae, 724–725
  ultrasound, 722–723
Renal medullary carcinoma, 604, 681–682
Renal osteodystrophy (ROD), 300, 633
Renal parenchymal disease (RPD)
  advanced imaging
    biopsy, 607–609
    ultrasonography and Doppler sonography, 605–607
  causes, 592
  classic entities, 592
  compartments, renal parenchyma, 591
  definition, 591
  glomerular disease, 219–223
  hematuria, 218
  hypertension, 219
  imaging findings
    glomerular disease, 599–601
    HUS, 601, 602
    systemic disease, 603–605
    tubular disorders, 602
    tubulointerstitial nephritis, 602
    vasculitis, 601
  nephritic syndrome, 218
  presentation, 218
  primary imaging management
    clinical symptoms and laboratory findings, 695
    differential diagnosis, sonographic renal changes, 596–597
    hydration and diuresis, 599
    initial assessment, 599
    initial study, 595, 598
    intravascular volume and potential effusions, 598
    urinary system, dilatation and differentiation, 598
  proteinuria, 218–219
  and renal failure, 219
    acute presentation, 592–593
    causes, 592, 593
    clinical aspects, 592–594
    initial imaging, 692
    manifestation, 594

Index

mechanisms, 594
systemic disease, 225–227
tubular dysfunction, 219
vascular and tubulointerstitial disease, 223–225
Renal pelvis and ureter, 771
 causes, 446
 congenital anomalies, 446
 duplex collecting systems (*see* Duplex collecting systems)
 imaging, 446–447
 in single and bifid collecting systems
  bifid collecting systems, 462, 463
  calyceal diverticulum, 447
  ectopic ureter, 461–462
  Fraley's syndrome, 448
  hydrocalyx, 448, 449
  hydroureter, 457, 458
  infundibular stenosis, 448, 449
  megacalycosis, 446, 448, 450
  megaureter, 457–458
  polycalicosis, 449, 450
  ureteral wall lesions, 460
  ureterocele and single collecting system, 462
  ureteropelvic obstruction (*see* Ureteropelvic junction obstruction (UPJO))
 triplication and quadruplication, 473
Renal ptosis, 180–181
Renal scarring, 234, 558–559
Renal stone disease, 287, 543–544
Renal transit time (RTT), 52, 62
Renal transplantation (RTx), 289
 acute problems, 303
 acute rejection, 303
 considerations, 638–639
 infections, 303–304
 living-related donor, 303
 MR imaging in, 92–93
 postoperative and surveillance imaging, 639–640
 posttransplant complications, 641, 642
  drug toxicity, 645–646
  graft dysfunction, 642
  infections, 645–647
  surgical complications, 643–645
 prognosis, 304
 PTLD, 304, 647–648
 regular follow-up, 303
 renal allograft, 640–641
 surgical technique, 639
 tacrolimus, 303
Renal trauma. *See also* Urinary tract trauma
 clinical management, 276
 complications, 276
 imaging, 276
 MR imaging in, 90–92
 postoperative/follow-up imaging, 276
 surgical procedures, 276
Renal tubular dysgenesis (RTD), 298
Renal tumors, 202, 583–584
 benign tumors
  angiomyolipoma, 690

  benign stromal tumors, 688–689
  CMN, 686–687
  juxtaglomerular cell tumor, 690–691
  multilocular cystic nephroma, 688
  ossifying renal tumor of infancy, 689–690
 cystic, 213, 566, 583
 diagnostic strategy, 694–697
 infectious diseases, 691
 malformations, 691
 malignant hematologic diseases
  Burkitt's lymphoma, 684, 685
  with non-Hodgkin lymphoma, 684–685
  primary unilateral renal lymphoma, 684
  T-ALL, 684, 686
 miscellaneous, 691
 MRI, 87–89
  multicentric Wilms' tumor, 87, 88
  nephroblastomatosis, 87, 89
 non-Wilms' malignant tumors
  anaplastic sarcoma, 683–684
  CCSK, 678–680
  Ewing's sarcoma family of tumors, 682–683
  malignant hematologic diseases, 684–686
  MRTK, 680–682
  RCC, 681–686
  renal medullary carcinoma, 681–682
  renal metastases, 686
Renal vasculature, 14, 153
Renal vein, 152, 154, 593, 606, 759–760
Renal venous thrombosis, 10, 168, 297, 596, 616
Reninoma. *See* Juxtaglomerular cell tumor
Renovascular disease (RVD). *See* Renovascular hypertension (RVH)
Renovascular hypertension (RVH), 654
 causes, 654–655
 clinical presentation, 654
 endovascular treatment, 659–660
 imaging
  CTA, 657–658
  DSA, 659
  MRA, 659
  post-captopril renal scintigraphy, 657
  US with Doppler, 655–657
Retrograde urethrography (RUG), 24–25, 368
Rhabdomyosarcoma (RMS)
 clinical features, 695
 epidemiology, 695
 follow-up, 699
 histopathology and genetics, 695
 imaging
  distant metastases, 697, 698
  locoregional tumor extent, 695–697
  staging, 697–698
 treatment principles and prognosis, 698–699
Risk, Injury, Failure, Loss, and End-stage renal disease (RIFLE), 296
RMS. *See* Rhabdomyosarcoma (RMS)
RNP. *See* Reflux nephropathy (RNP)
Roberts syndrome, 333
RPD. *See* Renal parenchymal disease (RPD)

RTD. *See* Renal tubular dysgenesis (RTD)
RTx. *See* Renal transplantation (RTx)
Rutland-Patlak technique, 46
Rutner valve, 748
RVH. *See* Renovascular hypertension (RVH)

S
Sandwich technique, 759
Schinzel-Giedion syndrome, 333
Scintigraphy
 cortical, 236
 cystic renal disease, 571
 DMSA (*see* Dimercaptosuccinic acid (DMSA))
 DRF, 57
 impaired drainage, 50
 MAG3, 54
 renal hypoplasia, 568–569
SCr. *See* Serum creatinine (SCr)
Scrotal anomalies, 369
Scrotal haematoma, 375
Scrotal injuries, 728–729
Scrotum
 acute testicular torsion, 371
 causes, 370
 clinical history, 370
 imaging algorithms, 370–371
 perinatal testicular torsion, 372
 right-sided testicular torsion, 371
 signs, 370
 symptoms, 370
Secondary/enteric hyperoxaluria, 287–288
Secondary hypertension, 561, 654–655
Secondary testicular malignancy, 376
Sertoli cell tumour, 376
Serum creatinine (SCr), 297, 298, 786
Serum procalcitonin, 236, 240
Sex chromosome disorders, sexual development, 248–249
Sex cord-stromal tumours, 376
SFU grading system. *See* Society for Fetal Urology (SFU) grading system
Sickle cell disease, 226, 603–604
Sickle cell nephropathy (SCN), 226
Simple renal cysts, 212–213, 580–582, 584
Society for Fetal Urology (SFU) grading system, 261, 262
Sono-elastography, 20
Sonography. *See also* Doppler sonography
 fetal, 311
 in haemolytic-uraemic syndrome, 601, 602
 in HUS, 601, 602
 M-mode, 12
 ovarian torsion, 359
 pelvic, 339
 renal and vascular injury, 276
 ureteral jets, 13
Spectral Doppler analysis, 640, 641
Spermatoceles, 378
Split-bolus technique, 27, 137

Sporadic Wilms' tumor, 669
Steroid-resistant nephrotic syndrome (SRNS), 222
Steroid-sparing therapy, 222
Strain elastography, 20
Strict ROD therapy, 301
Struvite stones, 283, 289
Supernumerary kidneys, 128, 181–182
Suprapubic micturating cystourethrography, 317
Systemic lupus erythematosus (SLE), 225–226, 603

T
Tacrolimus, 303, 645
Tamm–Horsfall protein (THP), 129, 155, 289, 565
Tc-99m MAG3 renography
 adequate hydration, 112
 advantages, 112
 disadvantages, 113
 diuretic administration, 110
 dose, 110
 DRF, 111
 limitations, 110
 Patlak-Rutland plot method, 111
 PEE, 111, 114
 post-micturition images, 110, 112, 115
 renal cadaveric transplant, after, 111, 113
 ROI, 111
Technetium-99m di-mercapto-succinic acid (Tc-99m DMSA)
 advantages, 108
 disadvantages, 108
 DRF, 108
 SPECT, 107
 UTI, 104, 105
Testes
 complications, 277
 imaging, 277
 postoperative/follow-up imaging, 277
 surgery, 277
 UDT, 277
Testicular fracture, 374, 728
Testicular microlithiasis, 377–378
Testicular trauma, 374–375
Thoracic kidney, 181, 182
Three-dimensional US (3DUS), 567
Thrombocytopenic purpura (TTP), 224
Thrombotic microangiopathy (TMA), 224–226, 296
Tissue rim sign, 621, 622
Toilet training, 414
Transient mild hematuria, 739
Transplant renal artery stenosis (TRAS), 92–93
Triad syndrome. *See* Prune-belly syndrome
Trimethoprim, 245, 768
Triphasic tumor, 666
Tuberculous, 562
Tubular dysfunction, 219, 225
Tubulointerstitial fibrosis, 300
Tubulointerstitial nephritis (TIN), 225, 602–603
Twinkling sign, 618–620, 623, 778
Tyrosinemia, 286

Index

U

UDT. *See* Undescended testes (UDT)
Ultrasound (US), 566, 567, 790, 792–794
  acute pyelonephritis, 9
  ADPKD, 169–170, 574
  applications, 7
  ARF, 628
  ARPKD, 170, 573–574
  botryoid type of Wilms' tumor, 670, 671
  CA, 134–135
  colour Doppler sonography, 13, 14
  complicated cyst, 582–584
  corticomedullary differentiation, 9
  CRF, 630
  equipment, 11–12
  fetal malformations, 162–163
  in glomerulonephritis, 593
  greyscale, 12
  HUS, 601, 602
  hydronephrosis, 8
  indications, 8–11
  inferior vena cava thrombosis, 672, 673
  lymphoceles, 643, 644
  malignant hematologic diseases, 684, 697
  MCDC and NPHP, 576
  in MCDK, 168–169
  in megaureter, 165
  M-mode sonography, 12
  MR angiography, 601
  multicystic nephroma and multiloculated cysts, 583
  NCS, 759
  neonatal kidney by, 154–156
  neonatal oligoanuria, 630
  nephrocalcinosis, 623
  nephrogenic rests and Wilms' tumors, 671, 673
  nephrourologic disorders, 765
  normal fetal bladder, 163
  normal fetal renal, 162
  ossifying renal tumor of infancy, 689–690
  in pelvi-ureteric junction obstruction, 164
  percutaneous nephrostomy, 740
  percutaneous renal biopsy, 749
  preparation, 12–13
  priapism, 757
  of proximal urethra, 166
  in prune belly syndrome, 165, 166
  in pseudo-nutcracker syndrome, 593
  pseudotumoral cystitis, 700
  RCC, 681
  renal
    abscess, 691
    biopsy, 608
    dysplasia, 569, 570
    failure, 594, 629, 635
    hypoplasia, 567
    injuries, 720–722
    scarring, 558–559
    vein thrombosis, 10
  of renal cystic dysplasia, 170, 171
  in renal duplication, 166–168
  in renal vein thrombosis, 171
  right kidney, 11
  right renal vein tumor thrombosis, 673
  RMS, 694, 695
  RPD, 605–607
  RVH, 655–656
  scanning technique
    lower urinary tract, 13, 14
    upper urinary tract, 13–15
  scrotal injuries, 728–729
  scrotum, 701
  sickle cell disease, 604
  simple renal cyst and acquired renal cyst, 582
  SLE, 603
  in tissue harmonic imaging, 12, 14
  ureterocele, 13, 167
  urinary tract infection and vesicoureteric reflux, 775, 776
  urolithiasis, 616
    color Doppler, 618–620
    grayscale, 616–618
  UTI, 552–554
  vasculitis, 601
Undescended testes (UDT), 277
Unilateral obstructive vaginal septum, 337–338
Unilateral renal dysplasia, 74, 76
Unilateral Wilms' tumor (UWT), 673
Upper urinary tract dilatation
  antenatal detection, 477
  postnatal work-up
    antenatal diagnosis, 480
    bilateral lung hypoplasia, 480
    clinical situations, 480
    ectopic ureterocele, 480
    functional assessment (*see* Nuclear medicine, studies and)
    giant PUJO, 480, 482
    imaging algorithm, 478, 479
    morphological assessment, 484
    MR imaging, complicated duplex kidney, 485
    neonatal MR urography, left megaureter, 483, 484
    neonatal puncture of ureterocele, 480, 481
    of nephropathies, 486–487
    posterior urethral valves, 480, 481
    right pneumothorax, 480
    sonographic classification, 478, 479
    ureterocele prolapse, 480, 481
    of uropathies, 480–483
    VCUG, 480, 482
    VUR, 482
Urachus, 325–326
Ureteral dilatation and stenting
  antegrade approach, 741–742
  indications, 742
  internal-external nephroureterostomy stents, 741
  metallic stents, 740
  percutaneous approach, 740
  percutaneous management, 742
  procedural details and technique, 742–745

Ureteral necrosis, 645
Ureteral peristalsis, 12, 269, 541
Ureteral reimplantation, 262
Ureteral stone, 283, 284, 290
Ureteric bud, 146, 242
Ureteric stricture, 63
Ureterocele (U-cele) system
　complications, 274
　definition, 69
　duplex collecting systems
　　cecoureterocele, 469, 470
　　small obstructive U-cele, 469, 472
　　ureterocele eversion, 471, 472
　ectopic, 69
　management, 69
　orthotopic, 69, 70
　postoperative imaging, 574
　and single collecting system, 462
　surgery, findings and indication for, 273–274
　surgical procedure, 274
　VCUG, 22–24
Uretero-pelvic duplication, 166–167
Ureteropelvic junction obstruction (UPJO)
　diagnosis
　　differential renal function, 451
　　diuretic renogram, 451, 452
　　Doppler analysis, renal arteries, 450
　　fetal uropathies, 450
　　functional deterioration, risk factors, 452
　　grading systems, 450
　　imaging techniques, 450
　　MR urography, 452
　　normalized residual activity, 451
　　output efficiency, 451–452
　　pressure measurements, 452
　　radioisotope study, furosemide injection, 451
　　renal drainage interpretation, 451
　　urinary tract dilatation, 446, 450
　　Whitaker test, 452
　PUJO (*see* Pelvi-ureteric junction obstruction (PUJO))
Uretero-vesical junction obstruction (UVJO), 164–165, 489, 534–535
　bilateral hydronephrosis, 67, 68
　bilateral ureteral dilatation, 269
　complications, 270
　dilated tortuous ureter, 269
　ectopic upper pole insertion, 65, 68
　follow-up, 269
　megaureters, 64, 65, 67
　MR urography, 65, 66
　renal hypoplasia, 66
　surgery, findings and indication for, 269
　surgical procedure, 269
　UTD, 61, 260, 261
　VUR, 65
Urethra
　congenital anomalies
　　appendicovesicostomy, 538
　　bladder exstrophy, 537
　　cloacal exstrophy, 537
　　epispadias, 537
　　posterior urethral valve, 538–539, 541
　　urinary tract diversion, 537
　　VUR, 541–542
　development, 147
　female, 158, 159
　incisura, 157
　male, 157–158
　micturition, 158
　VCUG, 156, 158
Urethral congenital abnormalities
　bulbous urethra duplication, 322, 323
　cystourethroscopy, 322
　epispadias, 322
　exstrophy-epispadias complex, 322
　hypospadias, 322
　megalourethra, 322
Urethral injuries, 726–728
Urethral obstruction, 165–166, 496, 504
Urge syndrome, 410–412
Uric acid stones, 284, 285, 288
Urinary bladder, 131
　anatomy and variants, 156–157
　bilateral herniation, 156
　congenital anomalies
　　appendicovesicostomy, 538
　　bladder exstrophy, 537
　　cloacal exstrophy, 537
　　epispadias, 537
　　posterior urethral valve, 538–539, 541
　　urinary tract diversion, 537
　　VUR, 541–542
　development, 147
　measurements, 790, 794
　VCUGs, 156
Urinary tract dilatation (UTD)
　antenatal detection, 477
　epidemiology, 255–257
　etiology, 257
　examinations, 261
　grading systems, 261, 262
　obstruction, definition of, 256–257
　PCD, 257, 260
　postnatal work-up
　　antenatal diagnosis, 480
　　bilateral lung hypoplasia, 480
　　clinical situations, 480
　　ectopic ureterocele, 480
　　functional assessment (*see* Nuclear medicine, studies and)
　　giant PUJO, 480, 482
　　imaging algorithm, 478, 479
　　morphological assessment, 484
　　MR imaging, complicated duplex kidney, 485
　　neonatal MR urography, left megaureter, 483, 484
　　neonatal puncture of ureterocele, 480, 481
　　of nephropathies, 486–487
　　posterior urethral valves, 480, 481
　　right pneumothorax, 480
　　sonographic classification, 478, 479
　　ureterocele prolapse, 480, 481

Index

of uropathies, 480–483
VCUG, 480, 482
VUR, 482
PUJ, 260
    extrinsic stenosis, 258–259
    intrinsic stenosis, 258
subvesical obstruction, 259–260
treatment
    antibiotic prophylaxis, 262
    interventional treatment, 263
    postoperative imaging, 263
    pyeloplasty, 262
    ureteral reimplantation, 262
UVJ, obstruction at, 259
VUR, 260
Urinary tract infections (UTIs), 9, 104, 549–550, 767–768, 775–776
acute focal bacterial nephritis, 237–238
antibacterial therapy, 236
antibiotics, 236
asymptomatic bacteriuria, 238
classification, 231–232
colour/power Doppler sonography techniques, 9
complications
    acute bacterial nephritis, 556–557
    cystitis, 560–561
    renal abscess, 557–558
    renal scarring, 558–559
    XPN, 559–560
cystitis, 238, 324
cystourethritis, therapy for, 238
definition, 231
diagnosis
    dipstick test and microscopy, 235
    pyelonephritis *vs.* cystitis, 38
    urine culture, 235–236
    urine sampling, 235
diagnostic work-up
    bladder function diagnostics, 240
    imaging, 238–241
    serum and urine markers, 240
epidemiology, 232
etiology, 232–233
infravesical obstruction, bilateral hydronephrosis, 227
nodular echogenic lesion, 226
parasitic infection, 226
pathogenesis, 232–233
and patient selection, imaging, 550–551
progression of, 555
prophylaxis, 240–241
pyelonephritis, 234
    complicated, 237
    late infancy and childhood, 237
    newborns and early infancy, 236–237
radiological examinations
    DMSA, 555
    IVU, 555
    MRI, 554–555
    US, 552–554
    VCUG, 555
renal cortical abscesses, 237–238
renal corticomedullary abscesses, 238
renal scarring, 234
schistosomiasis, 325
symptoms, 234
therapeutic success, control of, 238
unusual infections
    bilharziasis, 562
    hydatid disease, 562
    renal candidiasis, 561
    tuberculous, 562
voiding dysfunction
    risk factors, 417
    toilet training, 417
Urinary tract malformations
cloacal malformation, 175
gene defect, syndromes associated with, 500
prune belly syndrome, 497
urogenital sinus malformation, 173–175
voiding cystourethrography, 637–638
Urinary tract trauma
bladder injury, 725
blunt abdominal trauma, 713–715
clinical evaluation
    children with minor and moderate trauma, 716–717
    children with severe trauma and multiple injuries, 715
    imaging strategy, 718–720
    technical environment, impact, 717–718
renal injuries, 720–723
scrotal injuries, 728–729
urethral injuries, 726–728
Urinary values, 786
Urine extravasation
PUJ, 269
renal trauma, 276
UVJ, 270
VUR, 271
Urine markers, 240
Urine production, 628
Urine values, 788
Urinoma. *See* Urine extravasation
Urogenital fetal imaging
complex lower urinary tract malformations, 173–175
fetal bladder anomalies, 171–173
fetal nephropathies, 168–171
fetal uropathies, 164–168
MRI, 163–167
US, 162–163
Urogenital sinus malformation, 84, 149, 173–175
adrenogenital syndrome, 345
chromosomal and hormonal abnormalities, 345
clitoric hypertrophy, 350
cloacal (*see* Cloacal malformation)
diagnostic imaging, 349–350
in DSD, 346–350
female hypospadias, 345
fluoroscopic genitography, 349
genitourinary tract malformations, 350
neonates with, 344–345
physical examination, newborn, 344
sex determination, 345

Urogenital system
  ciliopathies, 200–202
  duplication malformations, 200
  hydronephrosis, 198, 199
  hypospadias, 200
  kidney, hereditary tumors, 202–203
  renal agenesis, 198
  VUR, 200
Urolithiasis, 615–616
  clinical findings, 281–282
  complications, 277
  CT, 620–622
  definition, 281
  diagnostic imaging, 282–283
  diagnostic procedure, 285, 288
  extrinsic factors, 289
  imaging, 277
  incidence, 284
  infectious stones, 289
  inhibitors
    hypocitraturia, 289
    THP kidneys, 289
  kidney stones, 278
  medication, 290
  MRU, 622
  promotors
    cystinuria, 288
    hypercalciuria, 285–287
    hyperoxaluria, 286–288
    hyperuricosuria, 288–289
  radiography and intravenous urography, 622
  surgery, 290
  treatment, indications for, 278
  ultrasound, 616
    color Doppler, 618–620
    grayscale, 616–618
Urologic anomalies
  complications, 389–390
  functional anomalies, 391–392
  incidence, 390
  occult spinal dysraphism, 391
  radiological/urologic evaluation, 389–390
  rectourethral fistula, 394
  structural anomalies, 390–391
Uromodulin (UMOD), 565
Uro-nephropathies
  ADPKD evolution, 490
  complicated duplex collecting systems, 489
  management, 489, 490
  MCDK, 489
  multicystic dysplastic kidney, 487
  prophylactic treatment, 487
  PUJ obstruction, 488–489
  renal ectopia, 487
  renal functional impairment, 486
  small cysts, diagnosis, 486, 487
  unilateral agenesis, 487
  UVJ obstruction, 489
  VURs, 487, 488
Uropathy(ies)
  ante-and postnatal diagnosis, PUJ obstruction, 482, 483
  high-grade VUR, 21
  neonatal VUR, 480–482, 487
  obstructive (see Obstructive uropathies)
  preoperative diagnosis, 52
  US examination, 483
Uroradiology
  ESPR, 346, 793
  pediatric application, 135, 268
  reports in
    kidneys, 128
    pelvicaliceal dilatation, 130–131
    renal parenchymal morphology, 129–130
    renal size, 128–129
    urethra, 131
    urinary bladder, 131
    urogenital tract, anatomy of, 128
Urosepsis, 232, 233, 236–237
Urothelial neoplasms, 699
US. See Ultrasound (US)
US contrast agent (UCA), 15
  ce-VUS, 17, 18
  in paediatric applications, 16
  techniques, 17
US Food and Drug Administration (FDA), 43
UTD. See Urinary tract dilatation (UTD)
UTIs. See Urinary tract infections (UTIs)

V
Vaginal malignancies, 701
Varicocele, 380, 669, 758–759
Vascular access, 301, 302, 631, 632
Vascular interventions
  embolotherapy, genitourinary system
    NCS, renal vein stenting, 759–760
    priapism, 757–758
    renal arterial embolization, 756–757
    varicocele, internal spermatic vein embolization, 758–759
  percutaneous renal angioplasty
    cross-sectional imaging, 752, 753
    procedural and technique, 753–756
    PTRA, 752–756
    renal vein renin sampling, 753
    renovascular hypertension, 752–753
Vascular supply, 151, 152, 639
Vasculitis, 223–224, 601
Vasoactive factors, 48, 49
VCUG. See Voiding cystourethrography (VCUG)
Veno-occlusive disease (VOD), 676
Vesicoureteral reflux (VUR), 9, 16, 270, 274, 767–769, 775–776
  and bladder diverticulum, 519
  chemoprophylaxis, 241
  classification, 241–242
  complications, 271, 521
  conservative treatment, 520
  contrast-enhanced voiding urosonography, 510–511

continuing susceptibility, patients with, 247
cystoscopic injection, 516
definition, 241–242
de novo VUR, 274
detection of
    familial occurrence, 514, 515
    fetal anomalies, antenatal diagnosis, 512–513
    nonneurogenic bladder-sphincter dysfunction, 513
    urinary tract infection, 513–514
diagnosis, 243–244
DMSA scanning, 522
DRNC, 505–506
and duplex kidneys, 518
ectopic kidney, 163, 518
endoscopic treatment, 521
epidemiology, 243
etiology, 242
fetal reflux nephropathy, 512, 521–522
genetic basis, 200
grading of, 504, 505
iatrogenic, 518–519
intrarenal dilatation, 541
intravenous urography, 511
IRC, 506–507
management, 541
megacystis-megaureter association, 517, 518
multicystic dysplastic kidney, 519, 520
natural history, 520
pathogenesis, 242
postoperative imaging, 270–271
primary fetal reflux, 520
progressive renal damage, 503
and PUJO, 515, 516
reflux and lithiasis, 515, 517
reflux nephropathy, 242–243, 247
renal damage, 234
renal disease progression
    antireflux bulcking material injection, 521, 522
    reflux nephropathy, 522, 523
    UTI nephropathy, 522
renal scarring, 242–243
secondary, 513
submucosal agent injection, 541
suprainfection, 516
surgery
    findings and indication for, 270
    procedures, 270
    treatment, 520–521
symptoms, 243
therapy
    long-term antibacterial prophylaxis, 245–246
    surgical correction, 246
US, 167–168
    anomalies, 508, 509
    Color Doppler sonography, 508
    direct cystography, 509
    non-irradiating technique, 504
    patient screening, 507
    signs, 508

uro-nephropathies, 487, 488
UTD, 260, 262
and UVJ obstruction, 515, 516
VCUG, 239, 504–505
voiding dysfunction
    anticholinergics, 417, 418
    antirefluxive surgery techniques, 418–419
    clinical implication, 417
    daytime urinary incontinence, 418
    dysfunctional elimination syndromes, 418
    non-neurogenic neurogenic bladder, 417
    reflux nephropathy, 417, 418
    unstable bladder, 417, 418
    upper urinary tract abnormalities, 418
yo-yo reflux, 516
Video urodynamics (VUD)
    applications, 125
    EMG tracings, 124
    findings, 125
    indications, 125
    neurogenic bladder dysfunction, 125
    procedure, 124
Virtual contrast technique, 621
VOD. See Veno-occlusive disease (VOD)
Voiding cystourethrography (VCUG), 792, 794
    boy with dysuria, 319
    cyclic, 504, 507
    cystic renal disease, 573
    ectopic kidney, 181
    equipment, 21
    indications, 21
    kidney malrotation, 179, 180
    limitations, 504, 507
    micturition phase, 504–505
    MR, 83
    in neonates
        prune-belly syndrome, 317, 318
        suprapubic catheter, 316, 317
        and ultrasound, 317, 318
    preparation, 21–22
    procedure, 22–24
    prune belly syndrome, 497–498
    pulsed fluoroscopy cystographic technique, 504
    PUV, 272–273
    renal failure, 657–658
    retrograde filling, vagina, 507
    urethral obstruction, 504, 507
    urinary tract infection and vesicoureteric reflux, 775–776
    UTD, 260, 261
    UTI, 239, 550
    UVJ, 269
    VUR, 244, 246, 270
        left grade I, 504, 505
        bilateral grade II, 504, 505
        bilateral grade III, 504, 506
        bilateral grade IV, 504, 506
        bilateral grade V, 504, 506
Voiding dysfunction. See Non-neurogenic bladder-sphincter dysfunction

Volumetric differential function, 44, 45
Von Hippel-Lindau (VHL) syndrome, 202–203, 681
VUD. *See* Video urodynamics (VUD)
VUR. *See* Vesicoureteral reflux (VUR)

W
Wegener's granulomatosis, 600, 601
Whitaker perfusion test, 734–736, 741
Wide bladder neck anomaly (WBNA), 426
William's syndrome, 286, 421, 655
Wilms' tumor (WT). *See* Nephroblastoma

X
Xanthinuria, 289
Xanthogranulomatous pyelonephritis (XPN), 559–560, 691
X-linked hypophosphatemic rickets, 225, 602
X-linked Lesch–Nyhan syndrome, 288

Y
Yolk sac tumour, 376, 377

Printed by Printforce, the Netherlands